CONQUER MEDICAL CODING

A Critical Thinking Approach
with Coding Simulations

2018

CONQUER MEDICAL CODING

2018

A Critical Thinking Approach with Coding Simulations

Jean H. Jurek, MS, RHIA
President
Jean Jurek Associates Inc., Medical Coding Solutions Company
Clarence, NY

Stacey Mosay, RHIA, CCS-P, COC
Policy Solutions Manager
Cotiviti Healthcare, Atlanta, GA
Consultant
Private Practice Solutions, Charleston, SC

Daphne Neris, CPC, CCS-P, CPC-I
Consultant
Branford, CT

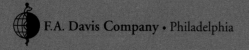
F.A. Davis Company • Philadelphia

F.A. Davis Company
1915 Arch Street
Philadelphia, PA 19103
www.fadavis.com

Printed in the United States of America

Last digit indicates print number: 10 9 8 7 6 5 4 3 2 1

Publisher, Health Professions: Quincy McDonald
Director of Content Development: George W. Lang
Senior Developmental Editor: Dean W. DeChambeau
Developmental Editor, Digital Products: Amelia Blevins
Content Project Manager: Julie Chase
Art and Design Manager: Carolyn O'Brien

As new scientific information becomes available through basic and clinical research, recommended treatments and drug therapies undergo changes. The author(s) and publisher have done everything possible to make this book accurate, up to date, and in accord with accepted standards at the time of publication. The author(s), editors, and publisher are not responsible for errors or omissions or for consequences from application of the book, and make no warranty, expressed or implied, in regard to the contents of the book. Any practice described in this book should be applied by the reader in accordance with professional standards of care used in regard to the unique circumstances that may apply in each situation. The reader is advised always to check product information (package inserts) for changes and new information regarding dose and contraindications before administering any drug. Caution is especially urged when using new or infrequently ordered drugs.

Library of Congress Cataloging-in-Publication Data

Names: Jurek, Jean H., author. | Mosay, Stacey, author. | Neris, Daphne,
    author.
Title: Conquer medical coding : a critical thinking approach with coding
    simulations 2018 / Jean H. Jurek, Stacey Mosay, Daphne Neris.
Description: Third edition. | Philadelphia : F.A. Davis Company, [2017] |
    Includes index.
Identifiers: LCCN 2017052974| ISBN 9780803669390 | ISBN 0803669399
Subjects: | MESH: International statistical classification of diseases and
    related health problems. 10th revision. | Clinical Coding--methods |
    International Classification of Diseases
Classification: LCC RB115 | NLM W 80 | DDC 616.001/2--dc23
LC record available at https://lccn.loc.gov/2017052974

I would like to dedicate this book to the late Myrna Breskin, without whose foresight, professionalism, and patience, this project would have not been possible.

—J. J.

To my children Zachary, Jeremy, and Abbey. I hope this book makes you proud of me and shows you that with a vision, a great deal of grit and grime, a dash of perseverance, and a lot of faith, you can reach your goal, despite obstacles that may appear as mountains.

To my mother, my best friend, who taught me to believe in myself, trust my instincts, and leave my mark on this earth, teaching others what I know.

To my husband Ted, who picked me up when I fell, who searched for lost files, brought dinner to my desk, and endured many years of stops and starts and meltdowns, but never stopped believing in me. I love you.

—S. M.

To my family and friends, who suffered through the sturm und drang of my becoming a textbook author, and to Myrna Breskin, who believed in this book and its authors.

—D. N.

Welcome to *Conquer Medical Coding: A Critical Thinking Approach with Coding Simulations 2018*, a textbook for students learning the ins and outs of medical coding. Medical coding is one of the fastest-growing health occupations worldwide, a result in part of the increased medical needs of an aging population, advances in technology, and the growing number of health-care providers and facilities that require the services that only trained coders can provide. Medical coders play an important role in gathering and analyzing data for quality health care and help ensure the financial well-being of health-care organizations in every delivery setting.

Medical coding is a challenging, fascinating, and rewarding career in which coders are compensated according to the level of their skills and how effectively they put them to use. Individuals with the right combination of skills and abilities have the opportunity to advance to management positions, such as coding supervision, or to higher-paid specialty coding positions, such as anesthesiology or radiology coding.

Education, coupled with national certification, brings more employment options and advancement opportunities. Individuals who have a firm understanding of the medical coding process will find themselves well prepared to enter this ever-changing field. And because coding is the basis for billing in health care, medical coders also become familiar with the rules and guidelines of each health-care plan, so the facility they work in can receive the maximum allowable reimbursement for the services it provides.

How You'll Conquer Coding

Whether your course of study is medical coding, medical assisting, medical insurance and billing, or health information technology or management, this text will give you a strong foundation in medical coding. The textbook and its accompanying print and digital assets focus on four key aspects of the medical coding process:

1. Knowledge of HIPAA-mandated medical code sets, which include the ICD-10-CM diagnosis code set, ICD-10-PCS procedure code set, CPT procedure code set, and the HCPCS code set.
2. Skill in applying HIPAA-compliant guidelines for the correct use of medical code sets, such as the *Official Guidelines for Coding and Reporting* that define correct diagnosis coding.
3. Understanding of the correct procedures for code assignments, explained in carefully sequenced presentations of coding principles and in flowcharts that reinforce the correct steps to follow.
4. Ability to use the Internet and other resources to stay current in the field.

Navigating the Textbook

The instructional parts of the text and accompanying workbook follow a logical, purposeful sequence. Part One, "Medical Coding and the World of Health Care," introduces you to medical coding as a health-care field. It talks about the importance of medical coding, a medical coder's working environment, what skills it takes to be a medical coder, and how to move ahead in your chosen career. This section also covers a number of important regulations that all coders need to understand and abide by, including the requirements of the Health Information Portability and Accountability Act (HIPAA), the rules of meaningful use, regulations regarding fraud and abuse, and an overview of compliance plans.

Part Two, "ICD-10-CM Coding," provides fundamental information about diagnosis coding. Chapters 3 and 4 discuss the history of the current diagnosis code set, ICD-10-CM, the coding process used, and various ICD-10 Indexes, conventions, and resources. Before covering specific ICD-10 codes, these chapters provides general inpatient and outpatient coding guidelines, how to identify a principal diagnosis, and admission guidelines.

The remaining chapters in this section, Chapters 5 through 11, focus on common code assignment decisions and complex coding scenarios for diseases and disorders for each body system, from the nervous system through factors influencing health status and contact with health services. The organization of those chapters follows exactly the organization of the official ICD-10-CM codebook, contained in the *International Classification of Diseases, Tenth Revision, Clinical Modification* (ICD-10-CM). Part Two also covers outpatient ICD-10-CM coding (Chapter 10) and an overview of ICD-10-PCS (Chapter 11), a type of coding used only in hospitals.

Part Three, "CPT and HCPCS Coding," provides in-depth information on procedural coding, including the history of Current Procedural Terminology (CPT) coding and CPT organization, modifiers, updates, and resources. It also compares ICD-10-CM and CPT and explains how to assign CPT codes. Part Three goes on to cover evaluation and management (E&M) codes and procedural coding for various body systems, organized precisely the way the CPT codebook, *CPT® 2018 Professional Edition*, published by the American Medical Association, is organized. Starting with anesthesia codes and ending with medicine codes, Chapters 15 through 29 cover terminology, modifiers, an anatomy overview, descriptions of a wide variety of diseases and disorders commonly seen in medical offices and other outpatient facilities, and a large number of procedures designed to treat those conditions. New to the 2018 edition is a significant expansion of the Breast Procedures section in Chapter 17, Integumentary System, to include additional mastectomy procedures and breast reconstruction. Chapter 18, Musculoskeletal System, has new sections on the spine and its common problems and procedures.

Finally, Chapter 30 covers the Healthcare Common Procedure Coding System (HCPCS) Level II codes. This code set describes items and services used in a health-care environment in addition to CPT codes and sometimes in place of CPT codes. For example, HCPCS codes are used to bill for prosthetic limbs and ambulance transfers.

Features

You will find a number of features designed to help you understand the information, remember it, and then apply your knowledge to realistic coding scenarios:

- **The latest ICD-10-CM, CPT, and HCPCS code changes** for 2018 are incorporated into the text to help you learn the most current information available.
- **Learning outcomes** show you exactly what information you need to master in each chapter.
- **Pinpoint the Code.** These unique flowcharts show essential steps for accurate coding. Each key step is shown in a clear, concise manner.
- **Case scenarios.** Brief case studies throughout the book provide examples of the kinds of coding cases you'll see in actual medical offices and outpatient facilities.
- **Coding alerts, caution, and tip boxes** alert you to common coding stumbling blocks and offer hints for successful coding.
- **Simulated medical documentation** provides a realistic coding experience.
- **Checkpoints** provide quick checks on your knowledge of material just presented and give you a chance to test your comprehension on your own.
- **Big green boxes.** We've designed several sidebars, each with a green background, that provide quick-review information on topics you might have learned in other courses but that remain relevant for proper coding. Those sidebars include:
  - Anatomy Review
  - Pathophysiology Connection
  - Pharmacology Connection
  - Reimbursement Review
- **Chapter Summary.** This section recaps key information within the chapter.
- **Review questions** provide an extra opportunity to check your knowledge of the coding process.

Medical Coding Lab

Medical Coding Lab is an online activity center where you can practice applying your coding knowledge in a completely safe environment, and it comes free when you purchase the book. Here you'll find a variety of exercises, including:

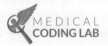

- Case studies, realistic coding scenarios that test your coding knowledge
- Flash cards
- Don't Tip the Scale, a hangman-like game for fun and learning
- Short-answer exercises
- Build Medical Codes exercises
- Analyze Medical Codes exercises

In addition, a special set of complex cases, called Capstone Cases, is provided that will really test your decision-making skills. Each case study presents a patient with a complex medical history and, often, multiple procedures. You're asked to assign the proper ICD, CPT, or HCPCS codes for the case. Your instructor may choose to use the Capstone Cases as a final exam or assign them as a review for a final exam. Either way, your successful completion of these cases will help prepare you for actual coding situations in the workforce.

Workbook to Accompany *Conquer Medical Coding 2018*

Written by the authors of *Conquer Medical Coding 2018*, this workbook helps you to develop into a skilled and proficient coder and to prepare for your AAPC or AHIMA certification exam. Each chapter in the workbook corresponds to a chapter in *Conquer Medical Coding 2018* and contains practice exam questions and coding exercises.

Tips for Using *Conquer Medical Coding*

We want every student to succeed, so we've put together some tips for getting the most out of the *Conquer Medical Coding* textbook, workbook, and the accompanying Medical Coding Lab.

- Before reading a chapter, review the Learning Outcomes, so you'll know what you're expected to learn.
- Read the summary at the end of the chapter. It will give you the highlights of that chapter and a clear sense of what's to come.
- Take notes of key points as you go along. Then study the notes whenever you need to review the content.
- Pay attention to the headings. They give you a clear idea of overall organization and allow you to find particular pieces of information easily.
- Give yourself enough time to read thoroughly. Cornell College tells its students to "multiply the number of pages you have to read by five minutes. That is the amount of time the average college student needs to spend on their reading assignment." Sound advice.
- Complete the exercises at the end of each chapter even if your instructor doesn't assign them. Doing so will help you retain the information you've learned even longer.
- Visit Medical Coding Lab after every chapter and do the exercises there. You're likely to find that the time you spend there is the most fun and effective of all!

One Last Note

We hope you consider *Conquer Medical Coding 2018* your guide into the world of medical coding. The foundational knowledge you'll gain through its pages, activities, and case studies will give you the confidence you need to succeed as a professional coder. Use the book and its assets wisely, and there is no telling how far you can go in this wonderful career.

Good luck!

Jean H. Jurek
Stacey Mosay
Daphne Neris

Cindy A. Akkerman, MBA, MBA-HCA, CPC, CPPM
Brown Mackie
Tulsa, OK

Rhona Alboucq, BAS, CPC
Lewis-Clark State College
Lewiston, ID

Eleonora Alvarado RN, MHA, CPC
Nashville State Community College
Nashville, TN

Beverly Bartholomew, M.Ed., CPC
Wake Tech Community College
Raleigh, NC

Christine M. Christensen, CCA
Williston State College
Williston, ND

Susan E. Coon, RMA, AHI, MAOL
Brown Mackie College
Tucson, AZ

Denise Cross, CMA (AAMA)
Jackson Community College
Jackson, MI

Cathy Davis, MHCL, CPC, CMBS
Wichita Technical Institute
Wichita, KS

Brian Dickens, MBA, CHI
Southeastern College
Greenacres, FL

Judith A. Dietz, CPC
Mercyhurst Northeast University
Erie, PA

Barbara J. Diveley-Wiedenmann, MLT/MT (ASCP), CMA (AAMA), MSED
Black Hawk College
Moline, IL

Linda H. Donahue, RHIT, CCS, CCS-P, CPC
Delgado Community College
New Orleans, LA

Evelun Fazel, RMA
Central Florida Institute
Palm Harbor, FL

William C. Fiala, MA, CCS-P, CPC
University of Akron
Akron, OH

Thomas F. Finnegan, IV, DC, MBA, FABDA, DAAIM, DAAETS
Minnesota School of Business
Blaine, MN

Lillian J. Galindo-Bryson, CPC
Martinez Adult Education
Martinez, CA

Donna L. Gilbert, CPC, CPC-I
Greenville Health System
Greenville, SC

Sharon Haas, CPC, CPC-I, CCS
Lorain County Community College
Elyria, OH

Melissa D. Hibbard, MSEd, CEHRS, CMRS, CPC, CPhT
Miami-Jacobs Career College
Dayton, OH

Annette Hoffman, MSM, CMT, CPC-A
Globe University/Minnesota School of Business
Woodbury, MN

Deborah J. Honstad, MA, RHIA
San Juan College
Farmington, NM

Linda Howrey, EJD
PMG Consulting
Warwick, RI

Carolyn M. Hutt, CPC, CPC-I
McKesson Specialty Health
The Woodlands, TX

Margo Imel, RHIT, MBA/TM
Arapahoe Community College
Littleton, CO

Carolyn B. Jackson, MHA, CPC, MA, MBS
Medical Program Coordinator
BIR Training Center
Chicago, IL

Acknowledgments

In preparing this textbook, we received assistance directly or indirectly from many people. Speaking for myself, initial inspiration was provided by Cynthia Newby, CPC, CPC-P, who persuaded me that writing a coding text was indeed possible.

The support, encouragement, and love provided by my husband Mike and children, Amy and Michael, were essential for the completion of this project. The acknowledgment of their priceless contributions toward my professional goals can hardly be overstated. The current text would be impossible without the knowledge and patience from the F.A. Davis staff.

—J. J.

With thanks to Cynthia Newby, who started us down this yellow brick road, and to the staff at F.A. Davis Publishing, the wizards behind the curtain who made it all happen.

—S. M., D. N.

Contents in Brief

Contents

Chapter 15   CPT: Anesthesia Codes   505

Chapter 16   CPT: Surgery Codes   525

painting a picture of a data set

PART I

Medical Coding and the World of Health Care

CHAPTER 1

Your Career as a Medical Coder

CHAPTER OUTLINE

The Importance of Medical Coding

A Medical Coder's Working Environment

Medical Coding: Accurate and Compliant

Coding Skills, Personal Attributes, and Ethics

Moving Ahead in Your Career

LEARNING OUTCOMES

After studying this chapter, you should be able to:

1. Describe the purposes of medical coding.
2. Define medical necessity, and discuss the way that medical coding links diagnoses and procedures to establish it.
3. Discuss the types of health-care organizations that employ medical coders, comparing facility (inpatient and outpatient) and physician practice coding environments.
4. Describe the relationship between documentation, coding, and billing.
5. List the basic steps in the medical coding process.
6. Identify the skills, attributes, and ethical behaviors that successful medical coders exemplify.
7. Define the opportunities for professional certification as a medical coder.

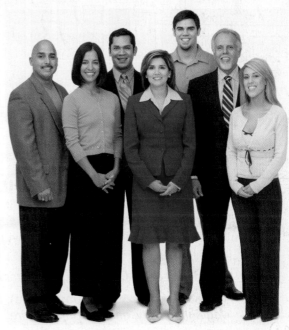

Jack Hollingsworth/Photodisc/Thinkstock

When health-care providers examine or treat patients, they use clinical terms to document the patients' medical diagnoses and procedures in medical records. To be able to analyze and track how these conditions are treated and to bill for the medical services, medical codes must be assigned to the narrative clinical text. The role of the medical coder is to determine the correct codes for diagnoses and procedures. Coders are health information practitioners who are skilled in classifying medical information from patient records. Job titles for coders include health information coders, medical record coders, coder/abstractors, and medical coding specialists. Knowledgeable medical coders who can accurately report the medical services provided are in demand because they help ensure the correct appropriate payment for medical services and facilitate payment for the billed services. Rising medical costs affect patients and providers alike (Fig. 1.1). Patients need to understand the health-care charges they are incurring in order to plan for payment. Health-care providers, such as doctors and hospitals, must carefully manage their business functions so they can continue to serve their patients' needs. Successful completion of this program is your first step on the path to a rewarding career as a medical coder.

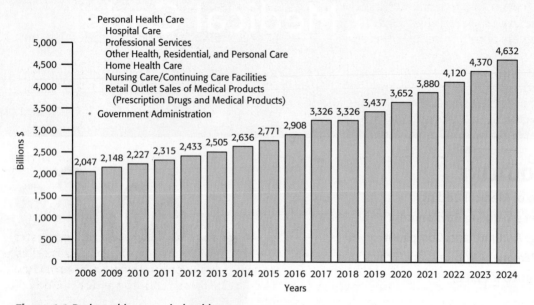

Figure 1.1 Projected increase in health-care expenses.

THE IMPORTANCE OF MEDICAL CODING

Can a code, like a picture, be worth a thousand words? It is clear from the following example that numbers can be very effective in portraying complex meanings.

EXAMPLES

Diagnosis codes: O80, Z37.0, *Encounter for full-term uncomplicated delivery, single live birth.*

Procedure code: 59400 (Obstetrician), *Routine obstetrical care including antepartum care, vaginal delivery, and postpartum care.*

ICD-10-PCS Procedure code: 10E0XZZ (Hospital), *Normal vaginal delivery.*

A code set is any group of codes used for encoding data elements, such as tables of terms, medical concepts, and diseases. The patient's primary illness or symptoms and other treated conditions are assigned diagnosis codes selected from the code set contained in the *International Classification of Diseases, Tenth Revision, Clinical Modification* (ICD-10-CM). Similarly, procedures that are performed are assigned procedure codes that stand for particular services, treatments, or tests. Most procedure codes are selected from the Current Procedural Terminology (CPT). A large group of CPT codes covers the physician's evaluation and management of a patient's condition at particular places of service, such as an office, a hospital, or a nursing home. Other codes cover specific procedures, such as surgery, pathology, and radiology. Another group of codes called the *Healthcare Common Procedure Coding System* (HCPCS) covers supplies and other services. Facilities use a separate set of codes called ICD-10 Procedure Coding System (ICD-10-PCS) to code for and bill the costs of procedures that occur in the hospital setting.

Medical Data

The coded data that the medical coding process produces are easier to study and [...] numbers are efficient, translating long descriptions so they can be universally u[...] exchanged, regardless of the different medical terms physicians might use. The cl[...] medical coders provide may be used to help plan for needed health-care services, [...] tient care, to control costs, in legal actions, and for research studies. Examples are[...]

- Pay-for-performance measurements that financially reward physicians for fol[...] medical practices to ensure patients' health, such as prescribing a beta blocker after a p[...] has had a myocardial infarction (MI, or heart attack)
- Cancer (tumor) registries that collect information about cancer—the types diagnosed, their locations in the body, the extent of the cancers when diagnosed, the treatments provided, and the outcomes—to improve care
- Alerts that advise providers about preventive immunizations, such as flu shots
- Reports of patients' mortality, of births, and of cases of abuse that must be released to state health or social services departments under state law
- Reports of communicable diseases such as Ebola, tuberculosis, hepatitis, and rabies that must be reported to authorities to monitor public health and risks
- A special category of communicable disease control for patients with diagnoses of HIV infection and AIDS: Every state requires AIDS cases to be reported, and most states also require reporting of the HIV infection that causes the syndrome
- Data that identify fraudulent activities
- Data that help consumers compare costs and outcomes of treatment options

Study the coding tips in the margin. Throughout your text, these notes in the margin advise you on correct coding.

Medical Necessity for Payment

Medical coding creates a bridge between the clinical data and the billing process that generates payment for medical services to physicians and facilities (Fig. 1.2). The billing process is called the revenue cycle, because the business side of medicine is a continual process of providing clinical services, billing, collecting payments, and then using these funds to pay for the cost of operations, such as salaries and medical equipment.

The costs for most medical services that patients receive are covered, in part or in full, by medical insurance. Nearly 272 million people in the United States have some form of insurance through either their employers, government programs, or individual insurance. To be paid for by insurance payers (see the Reimbursement Review), treatments and procedures must be medically necessary. Medical necessity means that the services are reasonable and are required for the diagnosis or treatment of a condition, illness, or injury or to improve the functioning of a malformed body part. Services also may not be elective, experimental, or performed for the convenience of the patient or the patient's family.

> Successful coders research the meaning of unfamiliar medical and anatomical terms to improve their coding skills.

EXAMPLES

Medically necessary:

  Diagnosis: Nasal obstruction

  Procedure: Nasal surgery

Not medically necessary:

  Diagnosis: Overly large nose

  Procedure: Cosmetic nasal surgery performed to improve a patient's appearance

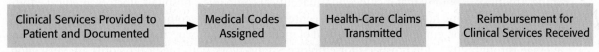

| Clinical Services Provided to Patient and Documented | → | Medical Codes Assigned | → | Health-Care Claims Transmitted | → | Reimbursement for Clinical Services Received |

Figure 1.2 Medical coding links clinical services to reimbursement.

Medical Insurance

Medical insurance (or health insurance) is a written policy between an individual, called the *policyholder*, and a health plan—an insurance company or government program that is the *payer*. The policyholder pays a specified amount of money called a *premium*. In exchange, the payer provides benefits—defined by the America's Health Insurance Plans (AHIP) association as payments for covered medical services—for a specific period of time.

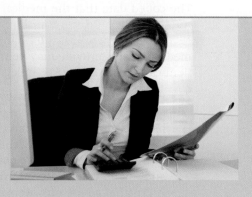

The major types of payers are:

- *Private plans:* Large insurance companies that dominate the national market and offer all types of health plans, such as Anthem, UnitedHealth Group, Aetna, Kaiser Permanente, and the members of the Blue Cross and Blue Shield Association
- *Self-funded health plans:* Health plans set up by employers that assume the risk of paying directly for medical services
- *Government-sponsored health-care programs:* Four major government-sponsored health-care programs offer benefits for which various groups in the population are eligible:
  — Medicare is a 100% federally funded health plan that covers people ages 65 and older and those who are disabled or have permanent kidney failure (end-stage renal disease [ESRD]).
  — Medicaid, a federal program that is jointly funded by federal and state governments, covers low-income people who cannot afford medical care. Each state administers its own Medicaid program, determining the program's qualifications and benefits under broad federal guidelines.
  — TRICARE, a Department of Defense program, covers medical expenses for active-duty members of the uniformed services and their spouses, children, and other dependents; retired military personnel and their dependents; and family members of deceased active-duty personnel.

The provider of the service must also meet the payer's professional standards. Providers include all types of licensed health-care professionals, such as physicians, nurse practitioners, physician's assistants, and therapists, as well as facilities (e.g., hospitals and their departments for therapy and radiology) and suppliers (e.g., pharmacies and medical supply companies). Providers must have the payer's required medical credentials and follow the payer's other *conditions of participation* relating to patient care.

Study the Reimbursement Reviews. At appropriate points in your text, these overviews provide you with background information on the key components of the revenue cycle and explain how they are related to medical coding.

A MEDICAL CODER'S WORKING ENVIRONMENT

Medical coders are part of the trillion-dollar health-care industry, a fast-growing and dynamic sector of the American economy that includes pharmaceutical companies, hospitals, doctors, medical equipment makers, nursing homes, assisted-living centers, and insurance companies. According to the U.S. Department of Labor, employment in the field of medical coding is expected to grow much faster than average through 2022. Job prospects for employees who work with medical records are very good, and people with strong backgrounds in medical coding will be in particularly high demand (Fig. 1.3).

— CHAMPVA, the Civilian Health and Medical Program of the Department of Veterans Affairs, covers veterans with permanent service-related disabilities and their dependents. It also covers surviving spouses and dependent children of veterans who died from service-related disabilities.

Note that under the federal *Emergency Medical Treatment and Active Labor Act (EMTALA)*, hospital emergency departments must provide care for all patients in need of medical services, regardless of their ability to pay. More than $100 billion in unpaid health care is provided annually for uninsured and underinsured patients.

Covered services are listed on the schedule of benefits. These services may include primary care, emergency care, medical specialists' services, and surgery. Coverage of some services is mandated by state or federal law; coverage of others is optional. Some policies provide benefits only for loss resulting from illnesses or diseases, while others also cover accidents or injuries. Many health plans cover *preventive medical services*, such as annual physical examinations, pediatric and adolescent immunizations, prenatal care, and routine screening procedures such as mammograms.

The medical insurance policy also describes noncovered services (excluded)—those for which it does not pay—which may include some or all of the following:

- Most medical policies do not cover dental services, eye examinations or eyeglasses, employment-related injuries, cosmetic procedures, or experimental procedures.
- Policies may exclude specific items, such as vocational rehabilitation or surgical treatment of obesity.
- Many policies do not have prescription drug benefits.

Providers send a health-care claim—a formal insurance claim, in either electronic or hardcopy format, that reports data about the patient and the services provided—to the payer on behalf of the patient. Payers scrutinize the need for medical procedures, examining each bill to make sure it meets their medical necessity guidelines.

CHECKPOINT 1.1

In your opinion, is each of the following diagnoses and procedures correctly linked to show medical necessity? Why or why not?

1. Diagnosis: deviated septum

   Procedure: nasal surgery _____

2. Diagnosis: mole on a female patient's cheek, questionable nature

   Procedure: surgical removal and biopsy _____

3. Diagnosis: male syndrome hair loss

   Procedure: implant hair plugs on scalp _____

4. Diagnosis: probable broken wrist

   Procedure: comprehensive full-body examination, with complete set of lab tests, chest x-ray, and

   ECG _____

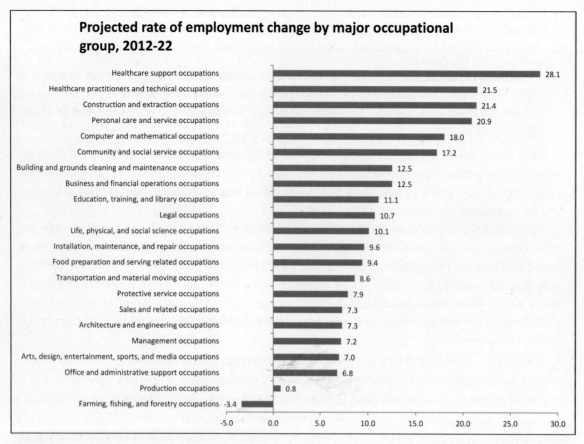

Figure 1.3 U.S. Department of Labor employment projections.

Medical coders may work in traditional health-care delivery environments or in nontraditional jobs. Traditional employers include both facilities and physician practices:

- Acute care hospitals
- Various hospital departments, such as same-day surgery, radiology, laboratory departments, and emergency departments
- Skilled nursing facilities (SNFs)
- Long-term acute care (LTAC) facilities
- Rehabilitation facilities
- Home health agencies (HHAs)
- Hospices
- Military treatment facilities
- Special care facilities, such as ESRD and cancer facilities
- Durable medical equipment (DME) suppliers and ambulance service providers
- Physician practices (solo, single specialty, multispecialty)
- Ambulatory surgery centers (ASCs)
- Clinics

Facility-Based Employment

Facilities were the first employers of medical coders, and currently two out of five coders work in hospital settings. Because facilities are very large institutions with many employees and complex functions, they are organized into departments:

- Administrative departments perform general business support functions, such as human resources (the hiring of personnel), public relations, purchasing, and legal services.
- Financial departments perform accounting functions, including registration (collecting patient information relating to payment at admissions); patient financial services, such as explaining anticipated bills; and payment plans, billing, and collections.

- Clinical departments provide medical, surgical, rehabilitation, and psychiatric servic[e] patients. Clinical tasks include ancillary services, such as departments for nursing; r[a] laboratory; physical, occupational, speech, and respiratory therapy; social services; a[n] management functions.

- Operational departments help run the facility and include the health information ma[nage]ment (HIM) department—sometimes called the *medical records department*—which is re[spon]sible for collecting, organizing, maintaining, storing, and disseminating the medical rec[ords] of patients, both internally and externally. Several areas make up the HIM department, including coding, tumor registry, transcription, and release of information (staff members who handle proper release of patients' data).

Inpatient Versus Outpatient Services

Facilities have two categories of services that are based on the status of the patient. Inpatient (IP) services are provided when the patient is admitted to the facility for care with the expectation of at least an overnight stay. Outpatient (OP) services, in contrast, are for patients who are not expected to stay overnight in the hospital. Hospital-based OP services may be performed in the hospital or in an outside facility that the hospital owns and runs. Hospital outpatient care is also called *ambulatory service*, because the patient is not bedridden.

The major hospital-based OP services are:

- Emergency department visits, during which the patient is assessed and treated or admitted as an IP, if required
- Diagnostic testing
- Ambulatory surgery unit visits, such as for a colonoscopy
- Observation encounters in which patients with symptoms, such as shortness of breath and chest pain, are assessed and either admitted or discharged from the hospital

Outpatient Care Not Provided in Facilities

Driven by advances in medical technology and anesthesia monitoring, many procedures that used to be done during a hospital stay are now provided on an outpatient basis. Examples include same-day surgical procedures and screening examinations, such as colonoscopies. OP services are cheaper and take less time than services in a traditional hospital operating room, so there has been explosive growth of the demand for these ambulatory procedures. Hospitals compete for OP business with physicians who set up OP clinics and ASCs. Care provided in these places of service is outpatient care but not *facility-based outpatient care*. Likewise, care in the physician office is outpatient care. A physician who sends a patient to a hospital on an ambulatory basis for a laboratory test is not transferring care to the hospital; the hospital provides the technical service the physician orders, and the physician continues to be responsible for the patient's care.

Physician Practice Employment

Many millions of visits to physicians each year are for ambulatory services. Physician practices range from solo practices to large groups of thousands of doctors. Some practices are made up of physicians of one specialty, such as family medicine, cardiology, pediatrics, or urology; others are multispecialty organizations. Specialties that require a lot of technology, such as radiology, tend to have large single-specialty medical groups.

Typically, *front office* staff members handle duties such as reception (registration) and scheduling. *Back office* staff duties are related to coding, billing, insurance, and collections. In small offices, the same person may handle both coding and billing of insurance payers and patients. In large groups, coders may handle just coding tasks and may be assigned a coding specialty, such as Medicare coding.

Nontraditional Employers

Medical coders are also employed in many different nontraditional settings. These include working for health plans to review coded data that are sent for payment; working as a consultant to physician practices, hospitals, law firms, or other health-care settings; working in educational and research institutions, public health and government agencies, and correctional facilities; and jobs with health information system computer vendors. Some coders also work for traditional

...mployers but are home based. Called *remote coders*, they are either employed by or have contracts with a hospital or physician practice. Coding service companies also employ qualified coders who travel to assignments in other locations.

MEDICAL CODING: ACCURATE AND COMPLIANT

The work that medical coders do is based on the medical records (charts) that providers create in physician practices and facilities. These records contain facts, findings, and observations about patients' health histories that are shared among health-care professionals and nonclinicians to provide continuity of care. The records help in making accurate diagnoses of patients' conditions and in tracing the course of treatment.

EXAMPLE

A primary care physician (PCP) creates a patient's medical record that contains the results of all tests ordered during a comprehensive physical examination. To follow up on a problem, the PCP refers the patient to a cardiologist, also sending the pertinent data for that specialist's review. By studying the medical record, the cardiologist treating the referred patient learns the outcome of previous tests and avoids repeating them unnecessarily. Instead, the cardiologist orders a needed test to be done on an outpatient basis at the hospital's radiology department, which also documents its results for interpretation by the cardiologist.

Medical liability cases can result in lawsuits. Physicians and facilities purchase professional liability insurance to cover such legal expenses. Although they are covered under these policies, other medical professionals often purchase their own liability insurance. Medical coders are advised to have professional liability insurance called error and omission (E&O) insurance, which protects against financial loss due to intentional or unintentional failure to perform work correctly (but not against fraud and abuse cases).

Documentation

The process of creating medical records is called *documentation*. It involves organizing a patient's health record in chronological order using a systematic, logical, and consistent method. A patient's health history, examinations, tests, and results of treatments are all documented. Providers need complete and comprehensive documentation to show that they have followed the medical standards of care that apply in their state. Medical standards of care are state-specified performance measures for the delivery of health care by medical professionals. Health-care providers are liable (that is, legally responsible) for providing this level of care to their patients. The term *medical professional liability* describes this responsibility of licensed health-care professionals.

The connection between documentation and coding is essential. A service that is not documented cannot be coded—and, hence, cannot be billed.

Patient medical records are legal documents. Good medical records are part of the provider's defense against accusations that patients were not treated correctly. They clearly state who performed what service and describe why, where, when, and how it was done. Providers document the rationale behind their treatment decisions. This rationale is the basis for medical necessity—the clinically logical link between a patient's condition and a treatment or procedure.

Accurate and compliant medical coding follows a basic process that begins when the patient is given care in a physician's office, hospital, or other setting, and the provider documents the service. The medical coder works with this documentation, in full or in summary form, to follow the coding steps summarized in Figure 1.4.

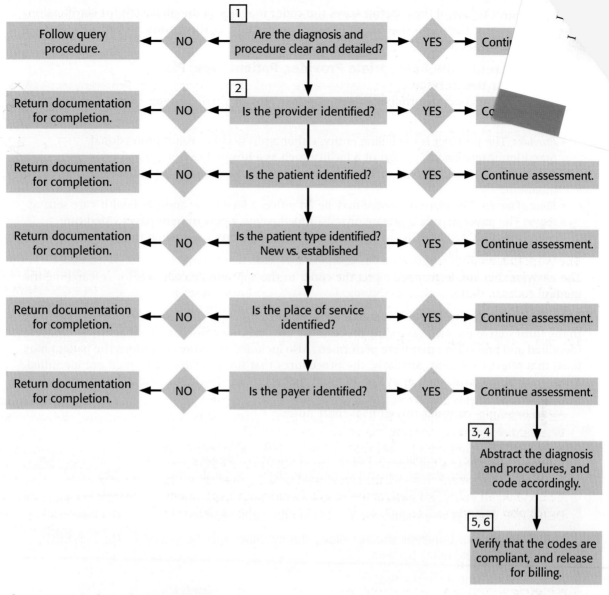

Figure 1.4 Basic document assessment.

1. Assess the documentation for completeness and clarity.
2. Determine the appropriate provider, patient type, place, and payer for the service.
3. Abstract the diagnoses that were identified and procedures that were performed.
4. Assign accurate, complete diagnosis and procedure codes.
5. Verify that the assigned codes are compliant.
6. Release the assigned codes for billing.

Step 1: Assess the Diagnosis and Procedure Documentation for Completeness and Clarity

The medical coder first assesses the available diagnosis and procedure documentation. Is the documentation complete, containing all the expected elements for the type of medical situation? Is the record legible, if written? Are diagnoses clearly stated, with sufficient detail about related conditions that affect the main condition?

the answer to any of these points is *no*, the coder may query the physician for clarification. ._ most situations, the medical coder follows the practice or facility query procedure to secure the needed information.

Step 2: Determine the Appropriate Provider, Patient Type, Place, and Payer for the Service

Next, the medical coder determines the appropriate provider, patient type, place, and payer for the service:

- *Provider:* The provider is the billing entity, either a physician or other professional practitioner (*professional billing*) or a facility such as a hospital (*facility billing*).
- *Patient type:* The patient type is determined by status as an outpatient (ambulatory) or inpatient.
- *Place of service:* The place of service may be an office, a facility, or another health-care setting.
- *Payer:* The payer may be a private or self-funded payer, a government payer (Medicare, Medicaid, TRICARE, or CHAMPVA), or a *self-payer,* the term used when the patient is responsible for the bills.

The answers that are determined direct the coder to the appropriate code sets for researching the medical codes.

Step 3: Abstract the Diagnoses and Procedures

In the third step of the medical coding process, the medical coder abstracts the diagnoses that were identified and procedures that were performed. Also included are other conditions the patient may have that affect treatment. Similarly, the procedures that the provider performed are identified. These may be medical, such as evaluation and management, diagnostic, therapeutic, or surgical in nature.

As an example, consider this clinical chart note:

> SUBJECTIVE: Patient complains of frequency of urination, urgency, and burning sensation for about 3–5 days. She denies hematuria. She has slight suprapubic discomfort. She has been treated for bladder infection in the past. Her last menstrual period was 4 days ago.
>
> OBJECTIVE: She has very vague tenderness over the suprapubic area. Flanks are clear.
>
> LAB: WBC 11,200. Urinalysis shows yellow, cloudy urine; specific gravity 1.015; 3–5 RBCs; 80–100 WBCs; and many bacteria.
>
> ASSESSMENT: Urinary tract infection.
>
> PLAN: Septra DS 1 bid × 10 days. Repeat urinalysis after that.

In this case, the patient's diagnosis can be isolated as urinary tract infection (UTI), and the procedure performed by the physician is an evaluation and management of her condition, as well as a urinalysis and blood work. The doctor has prescribed medication as a result of the evaluation and orders a follow-up test postmedication.

Step 4: Assign Accurate and Complete Diagnosis and Procedure Codes

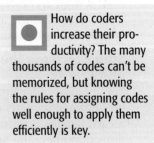

How do coders increase their productivity? The many thousands of codes can't be memorized, but knowing the rules for assigning codes well enough to apply them efficiently is key.

In the fourth step of the medical coding process, the coder researches the code sets and selects the correct medical codes to assign. The diagnosis and the procedures that are documented in the patient's medical record should be logically connected (linked) to demonstrate the medical necessity of the charges. Codes cannot be based on what a coder assumed took place, only on what the documentation supports.

Step 5: Verify That the Assigned Codes Are Compliant

Compliance means that actions have been performed that satisfy requirements. In the area of coding, compliance involves following the guidelines for correct code assignment and then following

all other regulations to verify the code choice. Chapter 2 of your text explains the m
that cover medical coding and how to comply with them.

Step 6: Release the Assigned Codes for Billing

The final step in the medical coding process is to release the verified codes for billing fu
ers then develop the health-care claims, transmit them to payers, and receive payment
received are posted in the financial record, and patients are billed as appropriate for th
that insurance did not cover.

CHECKPOINT 1.3

The following chart note contains typical documentation abbreviations and shortened forms for words.

> 65-yo female; hx of right breast ca seen in SurgiCenter for bx of breast mass. Frozen section reported as benign tumor. Bleeding followed the biopsy. Reopened the breast along site of previous incision with coagulation of bleeders. Wound sutured. Pt adm. for observation of post-op bleeding. Discharged with no bleeding recurrence.
>
> Final Dx: Benign neoplasm, left breast.

Research each abbreviation using an online resource and record their meanings on the lines provided.

1. yo _Years old_
2. hx _History_
3. ca _Cancer_
4. bx _Biopsy_
5. Pt _prothrombin_
6. adm _Addmission_
7. op _Out patient_
8. Dx _Diagnosis_

CODING SKILLS, PERSONAL ATTRIBUTES, AND ETHICS

Along with the importance of medical coding to physician practices and hospitals come the professional responsibilities of medical coders. Preparing for, securing, and advancing in medical coding positions require skills, particular attributes, and ethical behavior that demonstrate competence in the field.

Coding Skills

Medical coders need three types of skills for success in their work:

1. Coding skill
2. Communications skill
3. Information technology (IT) skill

Coding Skill

Coding skill is developed through study, followed by application, practice, and experience during employment. This skill is built on a strong foundation of medical terminology, anatomy, and physiology. Medical coders are knowledgeable about *pathophysiology*—identifying the clinical signs,

Charge Capture: Physician and Facility

The medical billing process followed in physician practices and hospitals is aimed at effective charge capture to ensure payment for all the medical services and procedures that patients receive. The basic steps of charge capture are similar for offices and facilities:

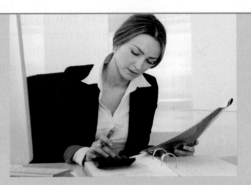

1. Preregister patients.
2. Establish financial responsibility for visits.
3. Check patients in.
4. Check patients out.
5. Review coding compliance.
6. Check billing compliance.
7. Prepare and transmit claims.
8. Monitor payer adjudication.
9. Generate patient statements.
10. Follow up on patient payments and handle collections.

Two tools are used in these environments to help capture the work done: the encounter form and the charge description master.

Encounter Form

In the professional setting, an encounter form (also called a *superbill*) may be completed by the provider after a patient's visit. The encounter form contains a summary of the provider's major or frequent services. The provider uses the form to check off procedures done, and the medical coder examines the documentation to verify the code selection. The encounter form is also used by billing staff to update the diagnosis and procedure information for the patient in the practice management program (PMP) (the software used to run day-to-day operations). The updated data are used to create health-care claims and patients' bills.

Charge Description Master

Likewise, facilities have tools for charge capture. But because the number of possible services is vastly greater, hospitals use a computerized list of all billable services, procedures, devices, medications, and supplies that can be provided to inpatients and outpatients. This list is called the charge description master (CDM). The typical hospital CDM encompasses thousands of service line items ranging from drugs, medical supplies, and equipment to ancillary department tests and procedures. For example, the following departments are included:

- Ambulatory surgery
- Anesthesia
- Cardiac catheterization
- Cardiology/cardiopulmonary
- Chemotherapy

- Clinics (pain, wound)
- Coronary care
- Emergency department
- Intensive care
- Laboratory
- Medical imaging/interventional procedures
- Nursery
- Observation room
- Operating room
- Pharmacy
- Radiology
- Recovery room
- Rehabilitation (physical, speech, occupational, cardiac, and pulmonary therapies)
- Room and board
- Sleep studies/neurology
- Surgery supplies
- Tissue pathology and cytology

The CDM contains the hospital's billing structure for creating claims and bills. Typically, for each item, there is the hospital's own master charge code (digits that stand for the department and the item), a description (the name of the procedure or service), a HCPCS/CPT code if the item is an outpatient procedure, a three-digit revenue code for billing purposes, a quantity or dose indicator, and a price. The facility's finance department has the main responsibility for assigning the numbers and keeping the CDM current, but other departments help as well.

In each hospital department, electronic forms in the computerized departmental charge entry system, called *charge slips* (or *charge tickets*), are used to input the services the patient has received. For example, in the ancillary service departments, to capture charges, the physician or the technician enters data from a requisition form, physician order, or other order into the hospital's charge description master, and those data are translated into CPT/HCPCS codes. Therefore, coders typically do not directly assign the radiology, pathology, and laboratory codes. The HIM department assigns codes for diagnoses and major inpatient procedures.

CHARGE CODE	DESCRIPTION	REVENUE CODE	CPT CODE	UNITS	CHARGE
55438867	Doxycycline tablet, 200 mg	250		1	$4.52
56637740	Established pt, Level 4	510	99214	1	$235.00
75436610	Wrist, complete	320	73110	1	$112.00
77749348	ICU, per diem	202		1	$1,897.00

Current Procedural Terminology © 2010 American Medical Association. All Rights Reserved.

symptoms, disease processes, and treatments of patients' conditions—and know how to relate these descriptions to diagnosis and procedure codes. They learn through training and experience to translate the clinical terms used in documentation into terms that relate directly to medical codes.

Communications Skill

Communications skill—both written and verbal—is as important as knowing about specific code sets and regulations. Using a pleasant tone, a friendly attitude, and a helpful manner when gathering information increases patient satisfaction. Having interpersonal skills enhances the coding process by establishing professional, courteous relationships with people of different backgrounds and communication styles, both fellow workers and other people. Effective communicators have the skill of empathy; their actions convey that they understand the feelings of others.

Equally important are effective communications with physicians and other professional medical staff members. The correct terminology, used in the correct context, demonstrates knowledge of the clinical topic. Written requests for information should be brief and clear and should follow the query process and procedures. Conversations must be brief and to the point, showing that the speaker values the provider's time. People are more likely to listen when the speaker is smiling and has an interested expression, so speakers should be aware of their facial expressions and should maintain moderate eye contact.

IT Skill

Medical coders use IT—computer hardware and software information systems—in almost all of the health-care environments in which they work. Computers not only improve business functions, such as billing and collecting payments, but also aid the coding process in many ways.

Because IT is used daily by most medical coders, the basic skills of file management with Microsoft Windows and document/spreadsheet management using Microsoft Office are generally considered essential. Also essential is skill in Internet research. Using the Internet effectively and gaining the ability to judge the quality of information received are valuable skills. In addition, social media networks are used in some situations for communications with patients and between providers, so the medical coder should be familiar with how to use these effectively.

Building on this foundation, depending on the work setting, medical coders may receive training in the use of the following major types of computer programs that relate to coding and billing work:

> Although IT increases efficiency and reduces errors, it is no more accurate than the individual who is entering the data. If people make mistakes while entering data, the information the program produces will be incorrect. Computer applications can be very precise and also very unforgiving. While the human brain knows that flu is short for influenza, some programs might regard them as two distinct conditions. If a computer user accidentally enters a name as ORourke instead of O'Rourke, a human might know what is meant, but the program might not. It would probably respond with a message such as "No such patient exists in the database."

- *Billing-related (charge capture) programs* such as PMPs that are used for billing in physician practices and CDM programs in facilities that maintain a database of all medical services provided with their billing codes
- *Electronic health record (EHR)* programs that allow providers to create digital files of patients' care
- *Encoder* products that store digital versions of code sets, guidelines, and payer requirements; some of these programs electronically examine documentation and suggest codes for the medical coder to validate
- *Grouper* programs that are licensed by many facilities to analyze coded data and then produce reimbursement-related information; for example, a grouper can collect the diagnosis codes for all of a hospitalized patient's conditions and calculate the expected Medicare payment for that stay

These various programs may be supplied in one of two ways in practices and facilities:

1. *Turnkey systems*, which are hardware and software owned by the practice or facility on which various programs are set up. These systems may be loaded on individual personal computers or on a multiuser network.
2. *Cloud-computing service*, in which a vendor's software and data are accessed by users over the Internet. Billed on a monthly subscription basis, Active Server Pages (ASP) installations—which are also called *host based*—have many advantages. Data are often updated, as are code sets, with annual or more frequent code updates.

Personal Attributes

A number of personal attributes are also very important contributors to success in medical coding. Most have to do with the quality of professionalism, which is key to getting and keeping employment:

- *Appearance:* A neat, clean, professional appearance increases other people's confidence in your skills and abilities. When you are well groomed, with clean hair, nails, and clothing, patients and other staff members see your demeanor as businesslike.
- *Attendance:* Being on time for work demonstrates that you are reliable and dependable.
- *Initiative:* Being able to start a course of action and stay on task is an important quality to demonstrate.
- *Courtesy:* Treating patients and fellow workers with dignity and respect helps build solid professional relationships at work.
- *Attention to detail:* Most aspects of the job involve paying close attention to detail, so this characteristic is essential for success.
- *Flexibility:* Working in an environment in which codes, regulations, and technology constantly change requires the ability to adapt to new procedures and to handle varying kinds of problems and interactions during a busy day.
- *Ability to work as a team member:* Patient service is a team effort. To do their part, medical coders must be cooperative and must focus on the best interests of the patients and the practice or facility.

ETHICS

Medical Ethics

Medical ethics are standards of behavior requiring truthfulness, honesty, and integrity. Ethics guide the behavior of physicians, who have the training, the primary responsibility, and the legal right to diagnose and treat human illness and injury. All individuals working in health-related professions share responsibility for observing the ethical code.

Each professional organization has a code of ethics that is to be followed by its members. In general, this code states that information about patients and other employees and confidential business matters should not be discussed with anyone not directly concerned with them. Behavior should be consistent with the values of the profession. For example, it is unethical for an employee to take money or gifts from a company in exchange for giving the company business.

CHECKPOINT 1.4

Consider medical ethics, and answer the questions that follow.

1. Sallie Smith, who works for the Clark Clinic, ordered medical office supplies from her cousin, David Hand. When the supplies arrived, David came to the office to check on them and to take Sallie out to lunch.

   Is Sallie's purchase of supplies from her cousin ethical? Why or why not? _____

   _____

2. Davon Singh is a medical coder in the practice of Dr. Karen Kline. During the past few weeks, Dr. Kline has consistently written down codes that stand for 1-hour appointments, but Davon knows that these visits were all very short, no longer than 15 minutes each.

   Is it ethical for Davon to code these visits as hour-long appointments? _____

   _____

Formal Education

Completion of a medical coding or HIM program at a postsecondary institution provides an excellent background for a coding position. Another possibility is to earn an associate degree or a certificate in a related curriculum area, such as health-care business services, and learn on the job.

Job Experience

Securing the first position can be challenging. Many jobs in hospitals and physician practices require both actual coding experience and coding certification. Simulated or actual experience starts with internships and/or externships. One type of internship is a capstone course in the curriculum in which students in class code de-identified patient charts, starting with simple cases and moving to more complex assignments; in another type, students are placed in physician offices and hospital coding departments for hands-on experience. Employers evaluate student work. Externships place students as unpaid assistants and provide mentoring, giving prospective employers a way to evaluate coding students.

> **INTERNET RESOURCE:**
> The Internet is a valuable source of information about many topics of interest to medical coders. For example, to explore career opportunities, study the job statistics gathered by the *Occupational Outlook Handbook* of the U.S. Department of Labor Bureau of Labor Statistics. Using the search tool, enter a job title of interest, such as health information technician. In particular, review the job outlook information.
> http://stats.bls.gov/oco

Membership in Professional Organizations

Moving ahead in a coding career is often aided by membership in and credentials from professional organizations. Student memberships are often available at a reduced cost. Recent graduates benefit from becoming full members by joining the local chapter of one of the national professional associations and volunteering to help with the chapter's activities. Some chapters of professional organizations may offer mentoring programs in which a recently certified coder is employed in an entry-level job under the tutelage of an established coding manager to "learn the ropes."

Certification as a Medical Coder

Becoming a credentialed coder is also an important step, because it shows prospective employers that the applicant has demonstrated a superior level of skill in medical coding. Certification is achieved by passing a written proficiency test given by a nationally recognized professional organization. Many job descriptions list certification as one of the hiring criteria for coding positions. Certification has a positive effect on the salaries of coders.

American Health Information Management Association

Two major organizations offer credentialing tests in the professional area of medical coding. AHIMA is the oldest association of HIM professionals. AHIMA's 50,000 members are dedicated to the effective management of personal health information needed to deliver quality health care to the public. Founded in 1928 to improve the quality of medical records, AHIMA is committed to advancing the HIM profession in an increasingly electronic and global environment through leadership in advocacy, education, certification, and lifelong learning.

AHIMA offers three coding certifications: the Certified Coding Associate (CCA), intended as a starting point for entering a new career as a coder; the Certified Coding Specialist (CCS); and the Certified Coding Specialist–Physician-based (CCS-P).

American Health Information Management Association (AHIMA)
233 North Michigan Avenue, 21st Floor
Chicago, IL 60601-5809
800-335-5535

INTERNET RESOURCE: AHIMA
www.ahima.org

American Academy of Professional Coders

AAPC's mission incorporates the establishment and maintenance of professional, ethical, and educational standards for all parties concerned with medical coding. The AAPC also offers training and credentials in documentation and coding audits, inpatient hospital/facility coding, regulatory compliance, and physician practice management. Currently, the AAPC has a membership base of more than 141,000 worldwide, of which nearly 98,000 are certified.

By becoming a member of the AAPC, a coder not only obtains a greater understanding of the coding field through education and networking but also receives much deserved recognition as a coding professional.

The AAPC grants the Certified Professional Coder (CPC), Certified Outpatient Coder (COC), Certified Inpatient Coder (CIC), Certified Risk Adjustment Coder (CRC), and Certified Professional Coder-Payer (CPC-P) certifications. It also offers more than 20 advanced specialty coding certifications, including

- Certified Evaluation and Management Coder (CEMC)
- Certified General Surgery Coder (CGSC)
- Certified Obstetrics Gynecology Coder (COBGC)
- Certified Orthopaedics Surgery Coder (COSC)
- Certified Emergency Medicine Coder (CEDC)

American Academy of Professional Coders
2480 South 3850 West, Suite B
Salt Lake City, UT 84120
800-626-2633

INTERNET RESOURCE: AAPC
www.aapc.com

Health Information Management Education and Certification

Students who are interested in the professional area of HIM (also known as medical records) may complete an associate degree from an AHIMA-accredited college program and pass a credentialing test to be certified as a Registered Health Information Technician, or RHIT. An RHIT examines medical records for accuracy, reports patient data for reimbursement, and also helps with information for medical research and statistical data.

Students can also receive credentialing as a Registered Health Information Administrator (RHIA), which requires a baccalaureate (four-year) degree and national certification. RHIAs are skilled in the collection, interpretation, and analysis of patient data. Additionally, they receive the training necessary to manage these functions. RHIAs manage patient health information and medical records and administer computer information systems that collect and analyze patient data.

The RHIA is knowledgeable about medical, administrative, ethical, and legal requirements and the standards of health-care delivery and the privacy of protected patient information. They manage people and operational units, participate in administrative committees, and prepare budgets and participate with all levels of an organization—clinical, financial, administrative, and information systems—that employ patient data in decision making and everyday operations. Both the RHIA and the RHIT national certification examinations have a coding component aimed at demonstrating the knowledge needed to supervise or manage the coding function.

Two other advanced certifications are available from AHIMA. With the National Cancer Registrars Association (NCRA), AHIMA provides certification in the cancer registry profession through the Certified Tumor Registrar (CTR) examination. To show proficiency in the Health Insurance Portability and Accountability Act (HIPAA), AHIMA has a Certified in Healthcare Privacy and Security (CHPS) certification.

Continuing Your Education Throughout Your Career

Most professional organizations require credentialed members to keep up to date by taking annual training courses to refresh or extend their knowledge. Continuing education sessions are assigned course credits by the credentialing organizations, and satisfactory completion of a test on the material is often required for credit.

Under their compliance plans, employers often approve attendance at coding seminars that apply to the practice or facility's medical setting and ask the person who attends to update other staff members.

Further baccalaureate and graduate study can enable advancement to managerial positions in physician practices and HIM departments. As shown in Table 1.1, there are many opportunities for coding and HIM personnel at all levels.

Professional certification, additional study, and work experience contribute to advancement to positions such as medical coding manager. Coders may also advance through specialization in a field, such as radiology coding.

Table 1.1 Selected Job Titles and Descriptions

JOB TITLE	DESCRIPTION
Entry-level coder	Coding basics/CCA or CPC-A
Coding specialist	On-the-job training/CCS, CCS-P, or CPC/CPC-H
Coding manager	Supervisory position: bachelor of science degree, RHIT or RHIA certification, and 5+ years of experience
Coding consultant/auditor	Consulting position: 4-year degree with management experience and business experience

A Look to the Future

Many experts think that technology will continue to change the work of medical coders. Coders' skills will remain in demand but in a different form. It is likely that initial code assignment will increasingly be done using computer-assisted coding, but the final coding will be validated by coders who act as editors, using their critical thinking and communication skills to ensure accurate coding that reflects documentation, whether in printed or electronic form. In any event, the demand for and rewards of a medical coding career appear to have a very strong future.

CHECKPOINT 1.5

1. Visit AHIMA's website for information about certification (www.ahima.org/certification), and review the criteria for applying for the CCS versus the CCA examinations. Report on the major differences in their requirements.
2. Visit the AAPC website to learn more about certification (www.aapc.com/certification), and report on three of the certifications that are offered.

Chapter Summary

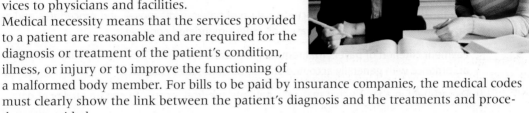

1. Medical coding creates coded data based on the documentation of patients' medical diagnoses and services. The data are used both to continually improve the delivery of health care and to provide a bridge between the clinical data and the billing process that generates payment for medical services to physicians and facilities.

2. Medical necessity means that the services provided to a patient are reasonable and are required for the diagnosis or treatment of the patient's condition, illness, or injury or to improve the functioning of a malformed body member. For bills to be paid by insurance companies, the medical codes must clearly show the link between the patient's diagnosis and the treatments and procedures provided.

3. Medical coders may be employed by facilities such as hospitals in the inpatient coding setting or by hospital ambulatory departments or physician practices for outpatient coding. Nontraditional employment includes positions at insurance companies and consulting, teaching, and auditing positions.

4. The connection between documentation and coding is essential. A service that is not documented cannot be coded—and, hence, cannot be billed.

5. The basic steps in the medical coding process are to (1) assess the documentation for completeness and clarity; (2) determine the appropriate provider, patient type, place, and payer for the service; (3) abstract the diagnoses that were made and procedures that were performed; (4) assign accurate, complete diagnosis and procedure codes; (5) verify that the assigned codes are compliant; and (6) release the assigned codes for billing.

6. Medical coders must exhibit three kinds of skills for career success: clinical coding, IT, and communication. Important attributes are professional appearance, punctual attendance, initiative, courtesy, attention to detail, flexibility, and ability to work as a team member. Medical ethics are standards of behavior requiring truthfulness, honesty, and integrity.

7. Certification as a medical coder is achieved by passing a written proficiency test given by one of two nationally recognized professional organizations, AHIMA and the AAPC. AHIMA has three coding certifications: the Certified Coding Associate (CCA), the Certified Coding Specialist (CCS), and the Certified Coding Specialist–Physician-based (CCS-P). The AAPC grants the Certified Professional Coder (CPC) and the Certified Professional Coder-Hospital (Outpatient) (CPC-H) certifications. The AAPC also offers the CPC-P, a payer certification; the CPC-A, an apprentice level for those who do not yet have medical coding work experience; and advanced specialty coding certifications.

Review Questions

Matching

Match the key terms with their definitions.

A. health information management (HIM)
B. ethics
C. provider
D. medical necessity
E. code set

F. compliance
G. diagnosis code
H. certification
I. documentation
J. medical coding

1. ___B___ Standards of conduct based on moral principles

2. _____ The systematic, logical, and consistent recording of a patient's health status—history, examinations, tests, results of treatments, and observations—in chronological order in a patient's medical record

3. _____ A coding system used to encode elements of data

4. _____ The completion of actions that follow and satisfy official guidelines and requirements

5. _____ Number assigned to a patient's documented illness or condition

6. _____ Process of earning a credential through a combination of education and experience followed by successful performance on a national examination

7. _____ Person or entity that supplies medical or health services and bills for or is paid for the services in the normal course of business; may be a professional member of the health-care team such as a physician, or a facility such as a hospital or skilled nursing home

8. _____ The process of analyzing the documentation of patients' diagnoses and procedures and assigning accurate, compliant codes based on HIPAA-mandated code sets

9. _____ Payment criterion of payers that requires medical treatments to be appropriate and provided in accordance with generally accepted standards of medical practice

10. _____ Department in a facility that manages patients' medical records to ensure quality of data

True or False

Decide whether each statement is true or false.

1. _____ The terms *outpatient* and *ambulatory* have the same meaning.

2. _____ The particular tests, services, and treatments a patient receives are assigned procedure codes based on the medical record.

3. _____ The medical billing process is called the *resource cycle*.

4. __F__ An inpatient is usually released from a facility within 15 to 18 hours.

5. __F__ Providers work only in the hospital setting.

6. __F__ Medical coders work only for hospitals.

7. __T__ Information technology, communications, and coding skills are needed for success as a medical coder.

8. _____ Compliance can involve actions that ignore regulations.

9. _____ The fourth step in the medical coding process is to assign accurate, complete diagnosis and procedure codes.

10. __F__ Most successful coders need professional certification to advance in their careers.

Multiple Choice

Select the letter that best completes the statement or answers the question.

1. The correct link between a patient's condition and the services a provider performed demonstrates the
   A. Minimum necessary standard
   B. HIPAA Security Rule
   C. Medical necessity of the services for payment
   D. Release of information

2. Coding credentials that can be earned include
   A. CCP-A, CPC, CCS, and CCS-P
   B. RHIT, RHIA, and MBA
   C. CHS, ROI, and MRN
   D. None of the above

3. Skills required for medical coding include knowledge of
   A. Anatomy and physiology
   B. Disease processes
   C. Medical terminology
   D. All of the above

4. Medical necessity means the patient's treatments/services are
   A. Reasonable
   B. Required for the diagnosis
   C. Not experimental
   D. All of the above

5. The major types of payers are
   A. Private, self-funded, and government sponsored
   B. Medicare, Medicaid, and TRICARE
   C. TRICARE and CHAMPVA
   D. None of the above

6. The health information management department may also be known as
   A. The clinical area
   B. The medical records department
   C. Human resources
   D. Registration

7. The medical *billing* process is aimed at
   A. Effective charge capture
   B. Efficient use of facility resources
   C. Documentation improvement
   D. Increasing information technology use

8. In the second step of the medical coding process, the coder determines the appropriate
   A. Diagnosis and procedure
   B. Supply use and place of service
   C. Prognosis, provider, and payer
   D. Provider, patient type, place of service, and payer

9. Which of the following is an example of using information technology?
   A. Using encoder products
   B. Using empathy
   C. Gaining certification
   D. Ethical actions

10. Earning certification as a medical coder requires
    A. Education
    B. Experience
    C. Successful completion of an examination
    D. All of the above

CHAPTER 2

The Regulatory Environment of Coding

CHAPTER OUTLINE

Documenting Encounters

HIPAA

Governmental Regulations/Fraud and Abuse

Compliance Plans

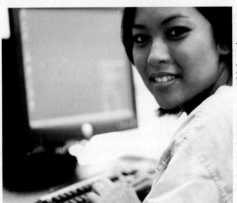

Jupiterimages/PHOTOS.com/Thinkstock

LEARNING OUTCOMES

After studying this chapter, you should be able to:

1. Describe the importance of the documentation in medical records in the medical coding process.
2. Understand the requirements and procedures for guarding the confidentiality of patients' protected health information under the HIPAA Privacy Rule.
3. Briefly describe the purpose of the HIPAA Security Rule and the breach notification rule.
4. State the required disease, procedure, and supply code sets under the HIPAA Electronic Health Care Transactions and Code Sets standards.
5. Define fraud and abuse in health care.
6. Describe the use of compliance plans to ensure accurate and compliant medical coding.

This chapter on the laws and regulations that apply to coding begins by explaining the types of documentation with which coders work, followed by the regulations that guide the coder's interaction with these medical records. It concludes with a description of the compliance plans that help ensure that coders are well trained in the use of current code sets.

DOCUMENTING ENCOUNTERS

Patients' medical records contain the complete, chronological, and comprehensive documentation of their health history and status. The records are used by providers to communicate and coordinate health care and as the basis for medical coding. An encounter (also called a *visit*) is a direct personal contact between a patient and a provider in any place of service (medical office, clinic, hospital, or other location) for the diagnosis and treatment of an illness or injury. At a minimum, each encounter should be documented with the following information:

- Patient's name
- Encounter date and reason
- Appropriate history and physical examination
- Review of all tests and drugs that were ordered
- Diagnosis
- Plan of care, or notes on procedures or treatments that were given
- Instructions or recommendations that were given to the patient
- Signature of the physician or other licensed health-care professional who saw the patient

In physician practices, the medical record for a patient usually contains the following data:

- Biographical and personal information, including the patient's full name, date of birth, gender, race/ethnicity, residence address, marital status, identification numbers, home and work telephone numbers, and employer information as applicable
- Copies of all communications with the patient, including letters, telephone calls, faxes, and e-mail messages; the patient's responses; and a note of the time, date, topic, and physician's response to each communication
- Copies of prescriptions and instructions given to the patient, including refills
- Original documents that the patient has signed, such as an advance directive
- Medical allergies and reactions, or their absence
- Up-to-date immunization record and history, if appropriate, such as for a child
- Previous and current diagnoses, test results, health risks, and progress, including hospitalizations
- Copies of referral or consultation letters
- Records of any missed or cancelled appointments
- Requests for information about the patient (from a health plan or an attorney, for example) and release data

For each hospital encounter, additional information is recorded:

- Type of encounter
- Date of encounter, including admission and discharge dates for inpatient admissions
- Physicians involved with the patient's care
- Patient's diagnoses and procedures
- Medications prescribed
- Disposition of the patient (i.e., the arrangements for the next steps in the patient's care, such as transfer to a skilled nursing facility or to home)

Hospitals need complete patient information to support high-quality medical care, with the typical goal of creating a unit record that brings together all documented treatment information, both inpatient and outpatient, for a patient in a single facility. The flow of information into and out of the patient record is typically funneled through a master person index (MPI)—a master list of patients—that has a unique medical record

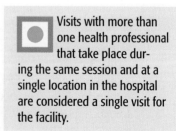 Visits with more than one health professional that take place during the same session and at a single location in the hospital are considered a single visit for the facility.

number (MRN) for each patient. This same number is used whenever the patient has [...] counter with the facility.

Evaluation and Management Services Documentation

When providers diagnose a patient's condition and decide on a course of treatment, the [...] called *evaluation and management (E/M)*. There are many types of E/M encounters, such [...] patient visit, an encounter about a patient's current complaint, a visit to decide whether surgery is needed, and a hospital postoperative visit.

Evaluation and management services often include an interview (history) and physical (an examination). A history and physical (H&P) is documented with four types of information: (1) the chief complaint, (2) the history and physical examination, (3) the diagnosis/assessment, and (4) the treatment plan (Box 2.1).

BOX 2.1 Example of History and Physical Examination Documentation

Samson, Arthur   Date of Birth: 7/23/1960

Date of Service: 2/24/20--

CHIEF COMPLAINT: Left leg muscle pain

History of present illness: Patient with left leg muscle pain for 2 weeks. The pain became worse 2 days ago and he feels weak and tired all the time. Patient states he is not short of breath, and has no stomach pain. He does have environmental allergies. There is nothing relevant in his family history, he is married and has two children, and works as a car dealer. He does not take any medication other than Claritin, an over-the-counter allergy medication. He has not had any past surgeries. He has taken ibuprofen on occasion for the leg pain but it has not helped.

Examination: Blood pressure 130/80, weight 155, afebrile, the lungs are clear to auscultation, no evidence of hepatosplenomegaly, neck is supple, cardiovascular exam shows a regular rhythm without murmur, both legs appear normal, gait is normal but legs are painful when manipulated. The general muscle tone is normal and there is no skin rash, the skin texture and color are normal.

An EKG done here today is normal.

DIAGNOSIS: Mr. Samson may have an underlying infection/virus, or possible chronic fatigue syndrome.

TREATMENT: I am sending him for x-rays, blood count, and metabolic panel. I have prescribed Celebrex to help with the pain. The patient is to return in 1 week.

● Medicare requires a medical history and physical examination (H&P) within 30 days before, or 24 hours after, a patient's inpatient admission.

The physician documents the patient's reason for the visit, called the *chief complaint (CC)*, often using the patient's own words to describe the symptom, problem, condition, diagnosis, or other factor. For clarity, the physician may restate the reason as a "presenting problem," using clinical terminology. The physician also documents the patient's relevant medical history. The extent of the history is based on what the physician considers appropriate. It may include the history of the present illness (HPI), past medical history (PMH), and family and social history. There is usually also a review of systems (ROS) in which the doctor asks questions about the function of each body system considered appropriate to the problem.

The physician performs a physical examination and documents the diagnosis—the interpretation of the information that has been gathered—or the suspected problem if more tests or procedures are needed for a diagnosis, and describes the treatment plan, or plan of care.

Physician Orders

Physician orders are another important type of documentation. Orders in the physician practice include documentation of requested laboratory, pathology, and radiology tests; consultations or referrals to other physicians; and prescriptions. In the hospital inpatient setting, orders from the physician who admits the patient (the *admitting physician*) and from the physician who is primarily responsible for taking care of the patient during the stay (the *attending physician*) include all instructions for the patient's treatment. The admitting physician and attending physician are often the same physician.

Procedural Services Documentation

If the plan of care involves significant risk (e.g., surgery), state laws require the physician to have the patient's informed consent in advance. The physician discusses the assessment, risks, and recommendations with the patient and documents this conversation in the patient's record. Usually, the patient signs either a chart entry or a consent form to indicate agreement.

Other common types of documentation are for specific procedures done in a physician office, ambulatory surgery center, hospital surgical suite, or elsewhere:

- Procedure or operative reports for simple or complex surgery (Box 2.2)
- Laboratory reports for laboratory tests
- Radiology reports on the results of x-rays, computed tomography (CT) scans, magnetic resonance imaging (MRI), and similar services
- Forms for a specific purpose, such as immunization records, preemployment physicals, and disability reports

---

BOX 2.2 Example of an Operative Report

Patient Name: Torres, Felix
Hospital No.: 567A
Room No.: 590
Date of Surgery: 10/20/20--
Admitting Physician: Gloria Bevilacque, MD
Surgeon: Francis Lee, MD

PREOPERATIVE DIAGNOSIS: Intermittent atrial flutter/fibrillation with severe ventricular bradycardia.

POSTOPERATIVE DIAGNOSIS: Intermittent atrial flutter/fibrillation with severe ventricular bradycardia.

PROCEDURE: Implantation of permanent transvenous cardiac pacemaker.

ANESTHESIA: Local, 1% Xylocaine.

FINDINGS (including the condition of all organs examined): The patient was admitted with episodes of atrial flutter/fibrillation with very slow ventricular response in the low 40s. The patient was entirely uncooperative and combative during the course of operation. It took five people to hold him on the catheterization table. Also, his heart rate was between 140 and 180. He had very small veins in the region of the deltopectoral groove. All these problems led to great difficulty putting this pacemaker in. However, the electrode was finally positioned in the apex of the right ventricle, and I assumed that this threshold was satisfactory; but we could not be entirely sure of this because of his very fast ventricular rate of 140 to 160. It appeared that the threshold was an MA of 0.8, voltage 0.5, with resistance of 610 ohms. R-wave sensitivity was 7.3.

PROCEDURE IN DETAIL: With the patient in the supine position, the right pectoral region was prepped and draped in the usual fashion. As mentioned above, the patient was entirely combative and uncooperative so that five people had to hold him down. After satisfactory local anesthesia and regional anesthesia were induced, a transverse incision was made and the deltopectoral groove was dissected. One vein appeared to be slightly larger than the rest of the very small venules in this area; and it was cannulated with a cardiac electrode, which with some difficulty was placed into the apex of the right ventricle under fluoroscopic control. As mentioned above, the patient's threshold appeared to be satisfactory, though this was not entirely certain. Electrode was ligated in place with heavy silk, after which it was attached to the Medtronic pacemaker model 5985. The unit was implanted into the subcutaneous pocket. It should be noted that the patient had practically no subcutaneous fat, so that only a very, very thin layer of subcutaneous tissue and skin overlies the pacemaker. The wound was closed in two layers. Dressings were applied, and the patient was taken back to his room.

Francis Lee, MD

FL:BJ
D: 10/20/20--
T: 10/21/20--

Other Chart Notes

Many other types of chart notes appear in patients' medical records. Progress notes, a[s in] Box 2.3, document a patient's progress and response to a treatment plan. They expl[ain] the plan should be continued or changed. Progress notes include

- Comparisons of objective data with the patient's statements
- Goals and progress toward the goals
- The patient's current condition and prognosis
- Type of treatment still needed and for how long

BOX 2.3 Example of a Progress Note

Davidson, Christine   Date of Birth: 4/17/2001

Date of Service: 8/31/20--

SUBJECTIVE: Patient has had a history of occasional redness in the left eye but no trauma or foreign body irritation. She now complains of itching and a purulent discharge in the left eye. She has had no visual changes.

OBJECTIVE: Her blood pressure is 110/60, her weight is 105, and her respiration is normal. Both eyes are examined today and the right eye is normal. The left eye is again red but with a purulent exudate. Her extraocular muscles are intact bilaterally. A fundoscopic exam was benign and there is no evidence of corneal abrasion.

ASSESSMENT: Acute bacterial conjunctivitis left eye.

PLAN: Patient is to apply sodium sulamyd ophthalmic solution three times a day into the left eye for 1 week and to apply warm, moist compresses as needed.

Discharge summaries, as shown in Box 2.4, are prepared during a patient's final visit for a particular treatment plan or hospitalization. Discharge summaries include

- Final diagnosis
- Comparisons of objective data with the patient's statements
- Whether goals were achieved
- Reason for and date of discharge
- Patient's current condition, status, and final prognosis
- Instructions given to the patient, noting any special needs such as restrictions in activities and medications

Electronic Health and Medical Records

In the course of a lifetime, a patient may receive care from many different providers in physician offices, hospitals, emergency departments, and home health settings. The patient's medical records are created and stored electronically, on paper, or in some combination called a *hybrid record*. Because of their advantages and because of government mandates, many hospitals and provider practices now use electronic health records (EHRs). An EHR is a digital health record. It holds a person's health data as documented by all the providers who have cared for the individual. Once information is updated in a patient record, it is available to all who need access, whether across the hall or across town.

EHRs offer improved communications across the continuum of care—from the primary care physician to the hospital and to other locations of patient care. The advantages of EHRs are summarized in Table 2.1.

For example, one hospital's EHR system is set up so both the hospital staff and physicians who visit patients at the hospital can use it. In the hospital, an EHR contains nursing and ancillary department documentation, laboratory and radiology results, reports from the health

BOX 2.4 Example of a Discharge Summary

Patient Name: Donaldson, Gerald
Hospital No.: 4903982
Admitted: 06/08/20--
Discharged: 06/11/20--

DIAGNOSIS:
1. Atrophic gastritis.
2. Irritable bowel syndrome.

OPERATION: Esophagogastroduodenoscopy 6/11/20--

This 78-year-old white male was admitted for evaluation of abdominal pain, nausea, and vomiting and reports of coffee-ground emesis. Several weeks ago, he was evaluated at Rangely Hospital for similar symptoms and was told he had several ulcers in his distal esophagus, and that he might require surgery. He was subsequently started on medications. He did fairly well after the initiation of medication, but over 3 days prior to admission, he had increasing left upper quadrant discomfort along with nausea, vomiting, and hematemesis. He also gives history of 35-pound weight loss over the last 18 months. In October 2015, he underwent evaluation at Rangely Hospital and was found to have erosive gastritis with duodenitis as well as reflux esophagitis. He also had some left upper quadrant pain at that time that was attributed to some post-herpes zoster neuritis. The patient has previously had cholecystectomy and appendectomy.

Physical exam on admission showed multiple well-healed abdominal scars. No masses were palpable. There was some mild discomfort in the left upper quadrant on palpation and bowel sounds were normal.

LABORATORY DATA ON ADMISSION: Hemoglobin 13.8. WBC 8000. Urinalysis showed 3+ protein with 1 to 3 RBCs/HPF. SMAC was normal except for slight elevation of BUN at 38.

HOSPITAL COURSE: The patient underwent EGD by Dr. Arun Ramanathan on June 11, with findings of some mild erythema in the prepyloric area, but otherwise was unremarkable. CT scan of the abdomen was normal. Serum gastrin was slightly elevated at 256, and gastric analysis was done, which showed basal of 0.3 mEq/hr, which was quite low; maximal acid output 7.1, which is also low; and peak acid output of 10 mEq/hr. The Zantac had been discontinued about 24 hours prior to gastric analysis. Lactose tolerance test was done and this showed normal curve. Barium enema was done, which was grossly normal.

My impression is that the patient has elements of atrophic gastritis. He was started on Reglan while in the hospital and has shown marked improvement with regard to his nausea and abdominal discomfort. I suspect that he has some element of irritable bowel syndrome, and we are instituting a high-fiber diet and continuing Reglan and Zantac. He has been instructed to continue a bland diet and to add additional foods one at a time. He is to return to my office in 3 weeks for follow-up.

DISCHARGE MEDICATIONS:
1. Zantac 150 mg po bid
2. Reglan 10 mg po ac and hs
3. Restoril 30 mg hs prn sleep
4. Darvocet-N 100 1 q4h prn pain

Davida Hammett, MD

DH:BJ

D: 6/14/20--
T: 6/14/20--

Table 2.1 Advantages of Electronic Health Records

Immediate access to health information	The EHR is simultaneously accessible to all qualified user[s]... [com]pared to sorting through papers in a paper folder, an EH[R] can save time when vital patient information is needed.
Computerized physician order management	Physicians can enter orders for prescriptions, tests, and o[ther ser]vices at any time, along with the patient's diagnosis.
Clinical decision support	An EHR system can provide access to the latest medical research on approved medical websites to help in medical decision making.
Automated alerts and reminders	The system can provide medical alerts and reminders for staff to ensure that patients are scheduled for regular screenings and other preventive practices. Alerts can also be created to identify patient safety issues, such as possible drug interactions.
Electronic communication and connectivity	An EHR system can provide a means of secure and easily accessible communication between physicians and staff and, in some offices, between physicians and patients.
Patient support	Some EHR programs allow patients to access their medical records and request appointments. These programs also offer patient education on health topics and instructions on preparing for common medical tests, such as cholesterol tests.
Administration and reporting	The EHR may provide administrative tools, including reporting systems that enable facilities and medical practices to comply with federal and state reporting requirements.
Error reduction	An EHR can decrease medical errors that result from illegible chart notes, because notes are entered electronically on a computer or a handheld device. Nevertheless, the accuracy of the information in the EHR is only as good as the accuracy of the person entering the data; it is still possible to click the wrong button or enter the wrong letter.

information management (HIM) department, and electronic dates/signatures. A physician who comes to the hospital opens an electronic "storage box" that contains documentation for him or her to read, correct, and sign. The documentation may have questions from coders in the HIM department for the doctor to resolve.

Individual physicians have digitized records of their encounters with patients, called *electronic medical records*, which are maintained and stored to provide documentation of the physician's treatment. Individual patients have their own version of digital records, called *personal health records*, that they use to create and store their own health information.

The American Recovery and Reinvestment Act (ARRA) of 2009, also known as the "stimulus package," contains additional provisions concerning the standards for electronic transmission of health-care data. The most important rules are in the *Health Information Technology for Economic and Clinical Health (HITECH) Act*, which is Title XIII of ARRA. This law guides the use of federal stimulus money to promote the adoption and use of EHRs.

The HITECH Act and subsequent financial incentive programs encourage and motivate health-care providers into meaningful use of technology to improve patient care. Meaningful use is the application of certified EHR technology to improve quality, efficiency, and patient safety in the health-care system. Providers must meet the objectives required to demonstrate that they are meeting the thresholds for a certain quantity of objectives through utilization of their EHR. If the levels of meaningful use are on target, providers are eligible for financial incentives. If not, payments are reduced. Over the reporting years, incentives and penalties gradually increase.

Read the following cases and answer the questions.

A. The following chart note is on file for a female patient:

Rayelle Smith-Jones   2/14/20--

SUBJECTIVE: The mother brought in this 1-month-old female. The patient is doing very well. They have been using the phototherapy blanket. She is thirsty, has good yellow stooling, and continues on formula. Her alertness is normal. Other pertinent ROS is noncontributory.

OBJECTIVE: Afebrile. Comfortable. Jaundice is only minimal at this time. No scleral icterus. Good activity level. Normal fontanel. TMs, nose, mouth, pharynx, neck, heart, lungs, abdomen, liver, spleen, and groin are normal. Good extremities.

ASSESSMENT: Resolving physiological jaundice on phototherapy.

PLAN: Will stop phototherapy and do a bilirubin level for a couple of days to make sure there is no rebound. The patient is to be seen in 1 week. Push fluids. Routine care was discussed.

MD/xx

1. Identify the patient: _____

2. What abnormal condition does the patient have? _____

3. Is the abnormal condition getting better or worse? _____

4. What test is ordered? _____

B. This letter is in the patient medical record of John W. Wu:

Nicholas J. Kramer, MD
2200 Carriage Lane
Currituck, CT 07886

Consultation Report
on John W. Wu
(Birth date 12/06/1942)

Dear Dr. Kramer:

At your request, I saw Mr. Wu today. This is a 65-year-old male who stopped smoking cigarettes 20 years ago but continues to be a heavy pipe smoker. He has had several episodes of hemoptysis; a small amount of blood was produced along with some white phlegm. He denies any upper respiratory tract infection or symptoms on those occasions. He does not present with chronic cough, chest pain, or shortness of breath. I reviewed the chest x-ray done by you, which exhibits no acute process. His examination was normal.

A bronchoscopy was performed, which produced some evidence of laryngitis, tracheitis, and bronchitis, but no tumor was noted. Bronchial washings were negative.

I find that his bleeding is caused by chronic inflammation of his hypopharynx and bronchial tree, which is related to pipe smoking. There is no present evidence of malignancy.

Thank you for requesting this consultation.

Sincerely,

Mary Lakeland Georges, MD

1. What is the purpose of the letter? _____

2. How does it demonstrate the use of a patient medical record for continuity of care?

   _____

HIPAA

Medical coders work intensively with patients' medical documentation, so they must u[nderstand] the laws that govern the use of medical records. The foundational legislation is called [Health] Insurance Portability and Accountability Act (HIPAA) of 1996. This law is designed to [do] the following:

- Protect people's private health information.
- Ensure health insurance coverage for workers and their families when they change or lose their jobs.
- Uncover fraud and abuse.
- Create standards for electronic transmission of health-care transactions.

Medical coders are required by this law to protect the information in patients' records. At times, they need to know what information can be released about patients' conditions and treatments. What information can be legally shared among providers and payers? What information must patients specifically authorize to be released? The answers to these questions are based on the three Administrative Simplification provisions of HIPAA:

1. *HIPAA Privacy Rule:* The privacy requirements cover patients' health information.
2. *HIPAA Security Rule:* The security requirements state the administrative, technical, and physical safeguards that are required to protect patients' health information.
3. *HIPAA Electronic Transaction and Code Sets standards:* The standards require every provider who does business electronically to use the same health-care transactions and code sets.

The Administrative Simplification provisions encourage the use of electronic data interchange (EDI). EDI is the computer-to-computer exchange of routine business information using publicly available standards. Practice staff members use EDI to exchange health information about their practice's patients with other providers and with payers.

Health-care organizations that are required by law to obey the HIPAA regulations are called _covered entities_. A covered entity is an organization that electronically transmits any information that is protected under HIPAA. Three types of covered entities must follow the regulations:

> HIPAA laws go through a lengthy review process before being released as final rules. Future changes are expected. Stay current with the changes that affect medical coders' areas of responsibility.

1. Health plans: the individual or group health plan that provides or pays for medical care
2. Health-care clearinghouses: companies that help providers handle such electronic transactions as submitting claims and that manage electronic medical record systems
3. Health-care providers: people or organizations that furnish, bill, or are paid for health care in the normal course of business

Other organizations that work for the covered entities, called _business associates_, must also agree to follow the HIPAA rules.

HIPAA Privacy Rule

The HIPAA *Standards for Privacy of Individually Identifiable Health Information* section is known as the HIPAA Privacy Rule. The HIPAA Privacy Rule is also often referred to by its number in the Federal Register, which is 45 CFR Parts 160 and 164. It represents the first comprehensive federal protection for the privacy of health information. Its national standards protect individuals' medical records and other personal health information.

Patients' medical records are legal documents that belong to the provider who created them. But the provider cannot withhold the information in the records from patients unless providing it would be detrimental to the person's health. This information belongs to the patient. Patients control the amount and type of information that is released, except for the use of the data to treat them or to conduct normal business transactions. Under HIPAA, only patients or

...eir legally appointed representatives have the authority to authorize the release of information to anyone not directly involved in their care.

Before the HIPAA Privacy Rule became law, the personal information stored in hospitals, physician practices, and health plans was governed by a patchwork of federal and state laws. Some state laws were strict, but others were not.

The Privacy Rule says that a covered entity must do the following:

- Have privacy practices in place that are appropriate for its health-care services.
- Notify patients about their privacy rights and how their information can be used or disclosed; have patients review and sign a form stating that they have received and reviewed this notification.
- Train employees so that they understand the privacy practices.
- Appoint a privacy official who is responsible for seeing that the privacy practices are adopted and followed.
- Safeguard patients' records.

Protected Health Information

The HIPAA Privacy Rule covers the use and disclosure of patients' protected health information (PHI). PHI is defined as individually identifiable health information that is transmitted or maintained by electronic media, such as over the Internet, by computer modem, or on magnetic tape or compact disks. This information includes a person's

- Name
- Address (including street address, city, county, zip code)
- Relatives' and employers' names
- Birth date
- Telephone numbers
- Fax number
- E-mail address
- Social Security number
- Medical record number (MRN)
- Health plan beneficiary number
- Account number
- Certificate or license number
- Serial number of vehicle or other device
- Website address
- Fingerprints or voiceprints
- Photographic images

Disclosure for Treatment, Payment, and Health-Care Operations. Both using and disclosing patients' PHI under HIPAA are permitted under certain circumstances. Use of PHI involves sharing and analyzing data within the entity that holds the information during routine daily operations. Disclosure of PHI means the release, transfer, provision of access to, or divulging of PHI outside the entity holding the information.

Both use and disclosure of PHI are necessary and permitted for patients' treatment, payment, and health-care operations (TPO). *Treatment* means providing and coordinating the patient's medical care; *payment* refers to the exchange of information with health plans; and *health-care operations* are the general business management functions.

A covered entity must try to limit the use or disclosure of protected health informat[ion] minimum amount of PHI necessary for the intended purpose. This minimum necessary refers to taking reasonable safeguards to protect PHI from incidental disclosure.

EXAMPLES

These examples comply with HIPAA:

- A medical coder does not disclose a patient's history of cance[r] workers' compensation claim for a sprained ankle. Only the info[rma]tion the recipient needs to know is given.
- A physician's assistant faxes appropriate patient cardiology test results before scheduled surgery at the hospital.
- A physician sends an e-mail message to another physician requesting a consultation on a patient's case.
- A patient's authorized family member picks up medical supplies and a prescription.

> The minimum necessary standard does not apply to any type of disclosure—oral, written, phone, fax, e-mail, or other—among healthcare providers for treatment purposes.

Designated Record Set. A covered entity must disclose individuals' PHI to them (or to their personal representatives) when they request access to, or an accounting of disclosures of, their PHI. Patients' rights apply only to a designated record set (DRS) that does not include all items. For example, in a physician office, the DRS denotes the medical and billing records the provider maintains. It does not include appointment and surgery schedules, requests for lab tests, and birth and death records. It also does not include mental health information, psychotherapy notes, and genetic information.

Within this DRS, patients have the right to

- Access, copy, and inspect their PHI.
- Request amendments to their health information.
- Obtain accounting of most disclosures of their health information.
- Receive communications as needed from providers via means such as in braille or a foreign language.
- Complain about alleged violations of the regulations and the provider's own information policies.

> Take care not to discuss patients' cases with anyone not directly involved with their care, including family and friends. Avoid talking about cases, too, in areas where other patients might hear. Close charts on desks when they are not being worked on. Position computer screens so that only the person working with a file can view it.

INTERNET RESOURCE: Questions and Answers on Privacy of Health Information (HIPAA)
http://answers.hhs.gov

Authorizations. A patient release of information document is not needed when PHI is shared for TPO under HIPAA. However, state law may require authorization to release data, and under HIPAA, the strictest rule is enforced, so many practices and facilities ask patients to sign releases. For use of PHI or disclosure other than for TPO, the covered entity must have the patient sign an authorization to release the information (Box 2.5). Processing a request for information involves careful checking and following applicable release of information (ROI) procedures.

BOX 2.5 Example of an Authorization to Use or Disclose Information

Patient Name: _____

Health Record Number: _____

Date of Birth: _____

1. I authorize the use or disclosure of the above-named individual's health information as described below.

2. The following individual(s) or organization(s) is/are authorized to make the disclosure:
_____

3. The type of information to be used or disclosed is as follows (check the appropriate boxes and include other information where indicated):
   □ Problem list
   □ Medication list
   □ List of allergies
   □ Immunization records
   □ Most recent history
   □ Most recent discharge summary
   □ Lab results (please describe the dates or types of lab tests you would like disclosed):
   _____
   □ X-ray and imaging reports (please describe the dates or types of x-rays or images you would like disclosed): _____
   □ Consultation reports from (please supply doctors' names): _____
   □ Entire record
   □ Other (please describe): _____

4. I understand that the information in my health record may include information relating to sexually transmitted disease, acquired immunodeficiency syndrome (AIDS), or human immunodeficiency virus (HIV). It may also include information about behavioral or mental health services, and treatment for alcohol and drug abuse.

5. The information identified above may be used by or disclosed to the following individuals or organization(s):
   Name: _____
   Address: _____
   Name: _____
   Address: _____

6. This information for which I'm authorizing disclosure will be used for the following purpose:
   □ My personal records
   □ Sharing with other health-care providers as needed/other (please describe):
   _____

7. I understand that I have a right to revoke this authorization at any time. I understand that if I revoke this authorization, I must do so in writing and present my written revocation to the health information management department. I understand that the revocation will not apply to information that has already been released in response to this authorization. I understand that the revocation will not apply to my insurance company when the law provides my insurer with the right to contest a claim under my policy.

8. This authorization will expire (insert date or event) on: _____
   If I fail to specify an expiration date or event, this authorization will expire six months from the date on which it was signed.

9. I understand that once the above information is disclosed, it may be redisclosed by the recipient, and the information may not be protected by federal privacy laws or regulations.

10. I understand authorizing the use or disclosure of the information identified above is voluntary. I need not sign this form to ensure health-care treatment.

Signature of patient or legal representative: _____Date: _____

If signed by legal representative, relationship to patient: _____

Signature of witness: _____ Date: _____

Distribution of copies: Original to provider; copy to patient; copy to accompany use or disclosure
Note: This sample form was developed by the American Health Information Management Association for discussion purposes. It should not be used without review by the issuing organization's legal counsel to ensure compliance with other federal and state laws and regulations.

To legally release PHI for purposes other than treatment, payment, or health-care operations, a signed authorization document is required.

The American Association for Medical Transcription (AAMT) advises against using a patient's name in the body of a medical report. Instead, place any data related to the patient's identification in the demographic section of the report only, where it can be easily deleted when the data are needed for research.

Information about substance (alcohol and drug) abuse, transmitted diseases (STDs), HIV, and behavioral/mental health may not be released without a specific authorization from the The authorization document must be in plain language and clude the following:

- A description of the information to be used or disclosed
- The name or other specific identification of the person(s) a rized to use or disclose the information
- The name of the person(s) or group of people to whom the covered entity may make the use or disclosure
- A description of each purpose of the requested use or disclosure
- An expiration date
- The signature of the individual (or authorized representative) and the date

In addition, the rule states that a valid authorization must include a statement about the following:

- The individual's right to revoke the authorization in writing
- Whether the covered entity is able to base treatment, payment, enrollment, or eligibility for benefits on the authorization
- The fact that information used or disclosed after the authorization may be disclosed again by the recipient and may no longer be protected by the rule

Uses or disclosures for which the covered entity has received specific authorization from the patient do not have to follow the minimum necessary standard. Incidental use and disclosure are also allowed.

Exceptions. There are a number of exceptions to the usual rules for release:

- Court orders
- Workers' compensation cases
- Statutory reports
- Research

All these types of disclosures must be logged, and the released information must be available to the patient who requests it.

De-Identified Health Information. There are no restrictions on disclosing de-identified health information that neither identifies nor provides a reasonable basis to identify an individual. To prepare this type of document, all identifiers must be removed, such as names, medical record numbers, health plan beneficiary numbers, device identifiers (such as pacemakers), and biometric identifiers, such as fingerprints and voiceprints. Such de-identified records are also called *blinded* or *redacted* documents.

Enforcement of HIPAA Privacy Rules

HIPAA privacy regulations are enforced by the Office for Civil Rights (OCR). When the OCR investigates a complaint, the covered entity must cooperate and provide access to its facilities, books, records, and systems, including relevant PHI. People who do not comply with HIPAA may be fined. Providers can also lose their contracts with payers and can be excluded from participation in all government health-care programs.

INTERNET RESOURCE: OCR Privacy Fact Sheets
www.hhs.gov/ocr/hipaa

In each of the following cases of release of PHI, was the HIPAA Privacy Rule followed?

1. A laboratory communicates a patient's medical test results to a physician by phone. _____

2. A physician mails a copy of a patient's medical record to a specialist who intends to treat the patient. _____

3. A hospital faxes a patient's health-care instructions to a nursing home to which the patient is being transferred. _____

4. A doctor discusses a patient's condition over the phone with an emergency department physician who is providing the patient with emergency care. _____

5. Bedside, a doctor orally discusses a patient's treatment regimen with a nurse who will be involved in the patient's care. _____

6. A physician consults with another physician by e-mail about a patient's condition. _____

7. A hospital shares an organ donor's medical information with another hospital that is treating the organ recipient. _____

8. A medical assistant answers a health plan's questions about a patient's dates of service on a submitted health claim over the phone. _____

HIPAA Security Rule and Breach Notification Rule

The HIPAA Security Rule requires covered entities to establish safeguards to protect PHI. This rule focuses specifically on electronic health information—that is, PHI that is created, received, maintained, or transmitted in electronic form. The Security Rule provides guidelines on how to secure such PHI on computer networks, the Internet, and electronic storage media. Security measures rely on *encryption*, the process of encoding information in such a way that only the person (or computer) with the key can decode it.

The security standards contain requirements for three types of safeguards to prevent security breaches: administrative, physical, and technical.

Administrative, Physical, and Technical Safeguards

Administrative safeguards are the administrative actions that a covered entity must perform, or train staff to do, to carry out security requirements. These actions include implementing office policies and procedures to prevent, detect, contain, and correct security violations. Examples include a disaster recovery plan and an emergency mode operation plan. Security training is provided to educate staff members on the policies and to raise awareness of security and privacy issues.

Physical safeguards are ways to protect electronic systems, equipment, and data from threats, environmental hazards, and unauthorized intrusion. Physical security also includes maintaining appropriate controls of files that are retained, stored, or scheduled for destruction.

Technical safeguards are the technology and related policies and procedures used to protect electronic data and control access to it. They include the use of the following:

- Firewalls that check data entering and leaving a computer network, using defined rules to determine whether to allow it to continue toward its destination
- Intrusion detection systems that provide constant surveillance of the network
- User authentication procedures and passwords to confirm the claimed identity of all users who access the data

Breach Notification Rule

A breach is an impermissible use or disclosure under the Privacy Rule that compromises the security or privacy of PHI in a way that could pose a significant risk of financial, reputational, or other harm to the affected person. Covered entities and their business associates are responsible for determining whether a breach has occurred under the Privacy Rule. If they determine a breach has occurred, they must follow required breach notification procedures.

Following the discovery of a breach of unsecured PHI, a covered entity must notify each individual whose unsecured PHI has been, or is reasonably believed to have been, inappropriately accessed, acquired, or disclosed. The document notifying an individual of a breach, called the *breach notification*, must include (1) a brief description of what happened; (2) a description of the types of unsecured PHI that were involved in the breach (e.g., full name, Social Security number, date of birth, home address, account number, or disability code); (3) the steps individuals should take to protect themselves from potential harm resulting from the breach; (4) a brief description of what the covered entity is doing to investigate the breach, to mitigate losses, and to protect against further breaches; and (5) contact procedures for individuals who have questions or want additional information, including a toll-free telephone number, an e-mail address, a website, or a postal address.

CHECKPOINT 2.3

Read the following case and answer the questions.

Gloria Traylor, an employee of National Bank, called Marilyn Rennagel, a medical coder who works for Dr. Judy Fisk. The bank is considering hiring one of Dr. Fisk's patients, Juan Ramirez, and Ms. Traylor would like to know whether he has any known medical problems. Marilyn, in a hurry to complete the call and get back to work on this week's charts, quickly explains that she remembers that Mr. Ramirez was treated for depression some years ago, but that he has been fine since that time. She adds that she thinks he would make an excellent employee.

1. In your opinion, did Marilyn handle this call correctly? _____

2. What problems might result from her answers? _____

INTERNET RESOURCE: Breach Notification Rule
www.hhs.gov/ocr/privacy/hipaa/administrative/breachnotificationrule

HIPAA Electronic Health-Care Transactions and Code Sets

The HIPAA Electronic Health-Care Transactions and Code Sets (TCS) standards require providers and payers to exchange electronic data using a standard format and standard code sets.

Standard Transactions

The HIPAA TCS standards apply to the electronic data that are regularly sent back and forth between providers, health plans, and employers. Each standard is labeled with both a number and a name. Either the number (such as "the 837") or the name (such as the "HIPAA claim") may be used to refer to the particular electronic document format.

Standard Code Sets

Throughout this text, the correct use of HIPAA code sets will be explained and demonstrated so that you can increase your coding skills.

Of great importance to medical coders are the code sets HIPAA requires for diseases, medical procedures, and supplies. The codes assigned by coders must be accurate in terms of HIPAA. For example, HIPAA requires the use of codes that are current as of the date of service. Because codes are updated and changed every year (and sometimes more often), medical coders research the codes that are in use at that point. Medical coders also must assign codes based on the rules found in the published guidelines for the HIPAA code sets. As shown in Table 2.2, both the diagnosis and procedure codes have particular guidelines to be observed.

Table 2.2 HIPAA Standard Code Sets as of October 1, 2016

PURPOSE	STANDARD	GUIDELINE
Codes for diseases, injuries, impairments, and other health-related problems	*International Classification of Diseases, Tenth Revision, Clinical Modification* (ICD-10-CM)	*ICD-10-CM Official Guidelines for Coding and Reporting; Coding Clinic* (American Hospital Association)
Codes for procedures or other actions taken to prevent, diagnose, treat, or manage diseases, injuries, and impairments	Physicians' services: Current Procedural Terminology (CPT) Inpatient hospital services: *International Classification of Diseases, Tenth Revision, Clinical Modification, Procedure Classification System*	Guidelines within the code set and in the *CPT Assistant* (American Medical Association) *ICD-10-CM Official Guidelines for Coding and Reporting; Coding Clinic* (American Hospital Association)
Codes for supplies, durable medical equipment, and other medical services	Healthcare Common Procedures Coding System (HCPCS)	Guidelines from the Centers for Medicare and Medicaid Services (CMS) and private payers

CHECKPOINT 2.4

Use the letter from Dr. Georges to Dr. Kramer provided in Checkpoint 2.1 to answer the following questions.

1. Identify and define the patient's symptom using clinical terms: _____

2. What procedure did Dr. Georges perform? _____

GOVERNMENTAL REGULATIONS/FRAUD AND ABUSE

Regulations

Regulations are issued by the federal and state governments, as well as by other organizations that guard the interest of consumers receiving health care. The main federal government agency responsible for health-care regulation is the Centers for Medicare and Medicaid Services (CMS), formerly the Health Care Financing Administration, or HCFA. An agency of the U.S. Department of Health and Human Services (HHS), CMS administers the Medicare and Medicaid programs to more than 100 million Americans. Every provider that receives payment from CMS, whether a professional or a facility, must comply with the *conditions of participation* that are issued by CMS. Individual states help CMS conduct surveys to certify Medicare and Medicaid providers and also regulate health care by licensing physicians and other clinical professionals to provide care.

INTERNET RESOURCE: CMS Home Page
www.cms.gov

A number of other nongovernmental organizations also regulate providers and health plans:

- *The Joint Commission*: Formerly named the Joint Commission on Accreditation of Health-care Organizations (JCAHO), The Joint Commission evaluates and accredits more than 20,500 health-care organizations and programs in the United States. For accreditation, an organization must undergo an on-site survey by a Joint Commission survey team at least every 3 years. (Laboratories must be surveyed every 2 years.) Joint Commission standards address the organization's level of performance in key functional areas, such as patient rights, patient treatment, and infection control. The Joint Commission also awards Disease-Specific Care Certification to health plans, disease management service companies, hospitals, and other care-delivery settings that provide disease management and chronic care services for asthma, diabetes, congestive heart failure, coronary artery disease, chronic obstructive pulmonary disease, chronic kidney disease, skin and wound management, and primary stroke care.

INTERNET RESOURCE: The Joint Commission
www.jointcommission.org

- *Agency for Healthcare Research and Quality (AHRQ)*: A division of the HHS, AHRQ measures the various quality aspects of health care. It has established a scale of measurements called *quality indicators* that assess the results of patients' health-care encounters, such as surgical complications.

INTERNET RESOURCE: AHRQ
www.ahrq.gov

- *URAC*: Formerly known as the Utilization Review Accreditation Commission, URAC is an independent nonprofit organization that promotes health-care quality through its accreditation and certification programs. URAC offers a wide range of quality benchmarking programs and ensures that all stakeholders are represented in establishing meaningful quality measures for the entire health-care industry.

INTERNET RESOURCE: URAC
www.urac.org

- *National Committee for Quality Assurance (NCQA)*: A private, not-for-profit organization dedicated to improving health-care quality. The NCQA seal is a widely recognized symbol of quality. Organizations incorporating the seal into advertising and marketing materials must first pass a rigorous, comprehensive review and must annually report on their performance. For consumers and employers, the seal is a reliable indicator that an organization is well managed and delivers high-quality care and service.
- *The Healthcare Effectiveness Data and Information Set (HEDIS)*: HEDIS is a rating tool created by the NCQA that is used by more than 90% of America's health plans to measure performance on important dimensions of care and service. Altogether, HEDIS consists of 81 measures across five domains of care. Because so many plans collect HEDIS data and the measures are so specifically defined, HEDIS makes it possible to compare the performance of health plans on an "apples-to-apples" basis.

INTERNET RESOURCE: NCQA
www.ncqa.org

Payer Policies

Although a separate fee is associated with each code, each code is not necessarily payable. Whether a code will be reimbursed depends on whether it has been correctly coded. Some payers include particular codes in the payment for another code, which may or may not be a correct inclusion. Medical coders learn coding rules and will work with payers' guidelines while verifying if the payers have appropriately reimbursed the physician's service.

Through the policies they issue, payers also regulate the medical services that are covered as well as the coding and billing process used to submit health-care claims. For example, some payers do not pay for certain procedure codes that are reported together for the same patient on the same day. Some policies do not cover preexisting conditions—those the patient had before signing an insurance contract—so if such a condition is the cause of the medical service, it is not paid by the insurance company.

ent Protection and Affordable Care Act (ACA)

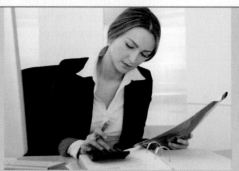

th system reform legislation signed into law in 2010, called Affordable Care Act, introduced a number of significant benefits for patients. Some benefits took effect immediately, and others are being phased in gradually. The following is an overview of the improvements that are now in effect for patients with private health insurance:

- A payer can no longer drop a beneficiary from a plan because of a preexisting illness or a new condition, a practice known as *rescission*.
- Children, ages 18 and younger, cannot be denied private insurance coverage if they have a preexisting medical condition.
- Young adults up to age 26 can remain as dependents on their parents' private health insurance plan.
- Payers cannot impose lifetime financial limits on benefits.
- Insurance plan beneficiaries have expanded rights to appeal denials or cancellation of coverage.
- Insurance companies must spend at least 80 cents of every dollar they collect from customers on providing health care, limiting salaries and profits. If this is not the case, health plan subscribers will get a tax-free rebate.
- Preventive services for women, such as mammograms, and immunizations for children must be covered by insurers with no copayments or deductibles required.
- Preventive services for all patients in new health plans, such as annual physicals and dozens of screening tests, must be completely covered by payers as long as in-network providers are used.

Fraud and Abuse

Another aspect of coding compliance is the potential for fraud and abuse. Although almost everyone involved in the delivery of health care is trustworthy and is devoted to patients' welfare, some are not. Health-care fraud and abuse laws help control cheating in the health-care system. Is this really necessary? The evidence says that it is. Health care is a tempting target for thieves. Total health spending in America is $2.9 trillion, and while no one knows for sure how much of that is embezzled, CMS has estimated that fraud (and the extra rules and inspections required to fight it) has added as much as $98 billion, or roughly 10%, to annual Medicare and Medicaid spending—and up to $272 billion across the entire health system.

> To bill when the task was not done is fraud; to bill when it was not necessary is an example of abuse. Remember the rule: If a service was not documented, in the view of the payer, it was not done and cannot be coded and billed. To bill for undocumented services is fraudulent.

Fraud and Abuse Defined

Fraud is an act of deception used to take advantage of another person. For example, misrepresenting professional credentials and forging another person's signature on a check are fraudulent. Pretending to be a physician and treating patients without a valid medical license is also fraudulent. Fraudulent acts are intentional; the individual expects an illegal or unauthorized benefit to result.

Claims fraud occurs when health-care providers or others falsely report charges to payers. A provider may bill for services that were not performed, overcharge for services, or fail to provide complete services under a contract. A patient may exaggerate an injury to get a settlement from an insurance company.

- U.S. citizens and legal residents cannot be denied private health insurance coverage for any reason, and they must obtain health insurance coverage or pay a minor tax penalty (although there are some exemptions).
- State-based health insurance exchanges are in place to enable people who do not have access to employer-based insurance to compare the benefits and costs of private health insurance plans. These exchanges have created insurance pools that allow people to choose among affordable coverage options. All insurance companies in the exchange must provide at least a minimum benefit package, as well as additional coverage options beyond a basic plan.
- Federal subsidies through tax credits or vouchers are being provided to people who cannot afford the full cost to help them purchase coverage through the exchanges.

For patients enrolled in Medicare or Medicaid:

- Preventive services recommended by the U.S. Preventive Services Task Force (USPSTF), which uses a letter grading system to determine when a service is appropriate, are now provided without deductible or coinsurance requirements. Examples include bone mass measurement, colorectal cancer screening, influenza and pneumococcal vaccines, and ultrasound abdominal aortic aneurysm screening.
- The cost of Medicare drug coverage is reduced.
- A series of pilot programs will be implemented to help find new ways to improve quality and lower the cost of care.
- Medicaid coverage is being expanded to all eligible children, pregnant women, and parents and childless adults under age 65 who have incomes at or below 138% of the federal poverty level.

In federal law, abuse means an action that misuses money that the government has allocated, such as Medicare funds. Abuse is illegal because it results in taxpayers' dollars being misspent. An example of abuse is an ambulance service that billed Medicare for transporting a patient to the hospital when the patient did not need ambulance service. This abuse—billing for services that were not medically necessary—resulted in improper payment to the ambulance company. Abuse is not necessarily intentional. It may be the result of ignorance of a billing rule or of inaccurate coding.

Fraud and Abuse Laws

The major laws that address fraud and abuse include the following:

- The *Health Care Fraud and Abuse Control Program* was created under HIPAA and is enforced by the U.S. Department of Health and Human Services Office of the Inspector General (OIG). This program has the task of detecting health-care fraud and abuse and enforcing all laws relating to them. The OIG works with the U.S. Department of Justice (DOJ), which includes the Federal Bureau of Investigation (FBI), under the direction of the U.S. Attorney General, to prosecute those suspected of medical fraud and abuse.
- The federal *False Claims Act (FCA)*, a related law, prohibits submitting a fraudulent claim or making a false statement or representation in connection with a claim. It also encourages reporting suspected fraud and abuse against the government by protecting and rewarding people involved in *qui tam*, or whistle-blower, cases. People who blow the whistle are current or former employees of insurance companies or of medical facilities, program beneficiaries, and independent contractors.

e *Deficit Reduction Act (DRA) of 2005* gives states financial incentives for setting up their own
se claims acts to prevent false claims under the Medicaid program. This act also requires
ining of hospital staff and outside vendors to make sure they investigate and report fraud.

INET RESOURCE: OIG Home Page
/oig.hhs.gov

OIG Enforcement

The OIG enforces rules relating to fraud and abuse. The intent to commit fraud does not have to be proved by the accuser for the provider to be found guilty. Actions that might be viewed as errors or occasional slips might also be seen as establishing a pattern of violations, which constitutes the knowledge meant by "providers knew or should have known."

OIG has the authority to investigate suspected fraud cases and to *audit* the records of providers and payers. In an audit (which is a methodical examination), investigators review selected medical records to see whether the documentation supports the coding. The accounting records are often reviewed as well. When problems are found, the investigation proceeds and may result in charges of fraud or abuse against the provider.

Investigators look for patterns like these:

• Intentionally coding services that were not performed or documented

EXAMPLES

A lab bills Medicare for two tests when only one was done.

A physician asks a coder to report a physical examination that was just a telephone conversation.

• Coding services at a higher level than was carried out

EXAMPLE

After a visit for a flu shot, the provider bills the encounter as a comprehensive physical examination plus a vaccination.

• Performing and billing for procedures that are not related to the patient's condition and, therefore, are not medically necessary

EXAMPLE

After reading an article about Lyme disease, a patient is worried about having worked in her garden over the summer, and she requests a Lyme disease diagnostic test. Although no symptoms or signs have been reported, the physician orders and bills for the *Borrelia burgdorferi* (Lyme disease) confirmatory immunoblot test using the diagnosis of Lyme disease.

CHECKPOINT 2.5

Read the following case and answer the questions.

Mary Kelley, a patient of the Good Health Clinic, asked Kathleen Culpepper, the employee who handles medical coding and billing, to help her out of a tough financial spot. Her medical insurance authorized her to receive four radiation treatments for her condition, one every 35 days. Because she was out of town, she did not schedule her appointment for the last treatment until today, which is 1 week beyond the approved period. The insurance company will not reimburse Mary for this procedure. She asks Kathleen to change the date on the record to last Wednesday so that it will be covered, explaining that no one will be hurt by this change and, anyway, she pays the insurance company plenty.

1. What type of action is Mary asking Kathleen to do? _____

2. How should Kathleen handle Mary's request? _____

COMPLIANCE PLANS

Because of the risk of fraud and abuse liability, and to ensure full compliance with HIPAA/HITECH, providers must be sure that rules and regulations are followed by all staff members. For this reason, physician practices and hospitals are required to have compliance plans to uncover and correct compliance problems to avoid risking liability.

A compliance plan is a written document that describes a process for finding, correcting, and preventing illegal activities. It is prepared by a *compliance officer* and committee that sets up the steps needed to (1) monitor compliance with government regulations, especially in the area of coding and billing; (2) ensure that policies and procedures are consistent; (3) provide for ongoing staff training and communication; and (4) respond to and correct errors. Having a compliance plan demonstrates to outside investigators like the OIG that honest, ongoing attempts have been made to find and fix weak areas. A wise slogan is that "the best defense is a good offense."

Compliance plans cover more than coding and billing. They also cover other areas of government regulation, such as Equal Employment Opportunity (EEO) regulations (e.g., hiring and promotion policies) and Occupational Safety and Health Administration (OSHA) regulations (e.g., fire safety and handling of hazardous materials, such as blood-borne pathogens).

Two parts of compliance plans are especially important to coders: physician training and staff training.

Physician Training

Part of the compliance plan is a commitment to keep physicians trained in pertinent coding and regulatory matters. A medical coder may be assigned the task of briefing physicians on changed codes or medical necessity regulations. The following guidelines are helpful in conducting physician training classes:

> OIG has developed a series of compliance program guidelines (CPGs) for a wide variety of specific health-care providers and suppliers. CPGs are intended to encourage the development and use of internal controls to monitor adherence to applicable statutes, regulations, and program requirements.

- Keep the presentation as brief and straightforward as possible.
- In a multispecialty practice, issues should be discussed by specialty; all physicians do not need to know changed rules on dermatology, for example.
- Use actual examples, and stick to the facts when presenting material.
- Explain the benefits of coding compliance to the physicians, and listen to their feedback to improve job performance.
- Set up a way to address additional changes during the year, such as a newsletter or compliance meetings.

Staff Training

> Do not code or bill services that are not supported by documentation, even if instructed to so do by a physician. Instead, report this kind of situation, ideally to a compliance officer, if the situation warrants doing so.

The other key part of the compliance plan is a commitment to train staff members who are involved with coding and billing. Ongoing training also requires providing annual updates, reading health plan bulletins and periodicals, and researching changed regulations. Compliance officers often conduct refresher classes in proper coding and billing techniques. Review the compliance plan elements for providers shown in Box 2.6.

INTERNET RESOURCE: Model Compliance Programs
http://oig.hhs.gov/compliance/compliance-guidance

BOX 2.6 Provider Compliance Program Core Elements Checklist

1. Written Policies, Procedures, and Standards of Conduct
- ☐ Clearly write and describe expectations in detail.
- ☐ Include detailed "code of conduct" and reporting mechanisms.
- ☐ Policies include compliance staff roles and responsibilities.
- ☐ Procedures show training plans and operational details of the program, including interactions with other departments.
- ☐ Readily available to all employees.
- ☐ Reviewed by employees within 90 days of hire and annually.
- ☐ Regularly reviewed and updated.

2. Compliance Program Oversight

Compliance Officer/Committee Duties:
- ☐ Develop and/or review policies and procedures that implement the compliance program.
- ☐ Attend operations staff meetings.
- ☐ Monitor compliance performance by operational areas.
- ☐ Enforce disciplinary standards, ensuring consistency.
- ☐ Implement system for assessment of risk.
- ☐ Develop auditing work plan.
- ☐ Review auditing and monitoring reports.
- ☐ Coordinate with Human Resources.
- ☐ Monitor effectiveness of corrective actions.

Compliance Officer/Committee Authority:
- ☐ Interview employees.
- ☐ Review collected data.
- ☐ Seek advice from legal counsel.
- ☐ Report potential fraud, waste, and abuse within the organization.

3. Training and Education
- ☐ Conduct general compliance training for all employees, managers, and supervisors who effectively communicate compliance program requirements, including the company's code of conduct.
- ☐ Conduct initial training for new employees at or near the date of hire.
- ☐ Conduct annual refresher compliance training that re-emphasizes the code of conduct and highlights compliance program changes.
- ☐ Include compliance scenarios and/or investigations of noncompliance.
- ☐ Communicate compliance messages using training methods such as posters, newsletters, and intranet communications.

4. Opening the Lines of Communication
- ☐ Establish an "Open Door" policy with compliance officer/committee.
- ☐ Compliance staff answers routine questions regarding compliance or ethics issues.
- ☐ Make several methods available for employees to report compliance issues (e.g., in person, electronically, or by anonymous drop box or toll-free hotline).

5. Auditing and Monitoring

Auditing and Monitoring System:
- ☐ Include internal monitoring and audits and external audits, as appropriate.
- ☐ Monitoring occurs on a regular basis during normal operations and is performed by staff.
- ☐ Auditing is performed at least annually, or more frequently, as appropriate.
- ☐ Auditing includes written reports containing findings, recommendations, and proposed corrective actions.
- ☐ High-risk areas are audited regularly.

Risk Assessment:
- ☐ Includes areas of concern.
- ☐ Identifies risk levels (e.g., high, medium, or low).
- ☐ Results are included in monitoring and auditing work plans.

Monitoring and Auditing Work Plans:
- ☐ Outline monitoring/auditing specifics.
- ☐ Base on results of risk assessment.
- ☐ Include a process for responding to results.
- ☐ Include corrective actions (e.g., repayment of overpayments or disciplinary action against responsible employees).

Written Policies and Procedures Regarding Response to Detected Offenses:
- ☐ Outline a plan of how internal investigations should be conducted.
- ☐ Identify a time limit for closing an investigation.
- ☐ Include options for corrective action.
- ☐ Include when to have an investigation performed by an outside, independent contractor.
- ☐ State how and when to refer an act of noncompliance to CMS or law enforcement authorities.

6. Consistent Discipline
- ☐ Write clearly.
- ☐ Describe expectations as well as consequences for noncompliant, unethical, and illegal behaviors.
- ☐ Include sanctions for noncompliance, failure to detect noncompliance when routine observation should have provided adequate clues, and failure to report actual or suspected noncompliance.
- ☐ Review with staff regularly (at least annually).
- ☐ Deal with in a timely manner and enforce consistently.

7. Corrective Actions
- ☐ Conduct in response to potential violations (e.g., repayment of overpayments or disciplinary action against responsible employees).

CHECKPOINT 2.6

As a medical coder, do you think that ongoing training will be important to you? _____

Chapter Summary

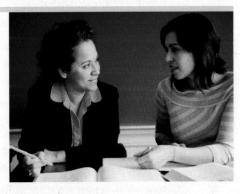

1. Documentation of an examination includes the chief complaint (CC), the history, the examination, the diagnosis/assessment, and the treatment plan. The process leading to the patient's informed consent for procedures is also documented. A progress report documents a patient's response to a treatment plan and provides justification for continued treatment. At the end of a treatment plan, a discharge summary documents the patient's final status and prognosis. The importance of the documentation in medical records in the medical coding process cannot be overstated: If a diagnosis or procedure is not documented, it cannot be coded, and therefore it cannot be billed.

2. The HIPAA Privacy Rule regulates the use and disclosure of patients' protected health information (PHI). Under HIPAA, covered entities are required to safeguard PHI, defined as individually identifiable health information that is transmitted or maintained by electronic media, including data such as a patient's name, Social Security number, address, and phone number. For use or disclosure for treatment, payment, or health-care operations (TPO), no release is required from the patient. To release PHI for other than TPO, a covered entity must have an authorization signed by the patient. The authorization document must be in plain language and have a description of the information to be used, who can disclose it and for what purpose, who will receive it, an expiration date, and the patient's signature.

3. The HIPAA Security Rule requires covered entities to establish administrative, physical, and technical safeguards to protect the confidentiality, integrity, and availability of health

information. The breach notification rule of the HITECH Act is aimed at preventing unauthorized disclosure of unsecured PHI.

4. The HIPAA Electronic Health Care Transactions and Code Sets establish standards for the exchange of financial and administrative data among covered entities. HIPAA requires accurate coding using current code sets and following published coding guidelines. Federal and state regulations, voluntary accreditation organizations, and payers' policies dictate the terms of compliant medical coding. As of October 1, 2016, the current code sets are ICD-10-CM/PCS, CPT, and HCPCS.

5 Fraud is an intentional act of deception for the purpose of taking financial advantage of another person; abuse is an action that misuses the government's resources.

6. A medical practice compliance plan covers the ongoing training of coders so that they can comply with the requirement to correctly use current code sets.

Review Questions

Matching

Match the key terms with their definitions.

A. Joint Commission
B. HIPAA Privacy Rule
C. HIPAA Security Rule
D. informed consent
E. minimum necessary standard
F. Affordable Care Act
G. protected health information (PHI)
H. treatment, payment, and health-care operations (TPO)
I. meaningful use
J. covered entity

1. _____ HIPAA law regulating the use and disclosure of patients' protected health information—individually identifiable health information that is transmitted or maintained by electronic media

2. _____ Using certified EHR technology to improve quality, efficiency, and patient safety in the health-care system

3. _____ Principle that individually identifiable health information should be disclosed only to the extent needed to support the purpose of the disclosure

4. _____ Under HIPAA, a health plan, clearinghouse, or provider who transmits any health information electronically

5. _____ Under HIPAA, the purposes for which patients' protected health information may be shared without authorization

6. _____ Individually identifiable health information that is transmitted or maintained by electronic media

7. _____ Organization that accredits and certifies hospitals and other health-care organizations/programs

8. _____ HIPAA law that requires covered entities to establish administrative, physical, and technical safeguards to protect health information

9. _____ Process by which a patient authorizes a planned treatment following discussion concerning its nature and risks

10. _____ Common name for the 2010 health system reform legislation that provides significant patient benefits

True or False

Decide whether each statement is true or false.

1. _F___ When a state law and the federal HIPAA provision both cover a particular situation, the state law is followed.

2. _F___ Fraud is not intentional.

3. _T___ The chief complaint is usually documented using clinical terminology.

4. __T__ Electronic health records have advantages over paper records.

5. __T__ A compliance plan includes measures to ensure that coders are trained in current code sets.

6. __T__ Business associates of providers must follow the same privacy rules as the providers for whom they work.

7. __T__ Protected health information includes the various numbers assigned to patients, such as their medical record numbers.

8. __T__ The minimum necessary standard does not refer to the patient's health history.

9. __F__ Patients do not have the right to access, copy, inspect, and request amendment of their medical records.

10. __T__ A patient's authorization is needed to disclose protected information for payment purposes.

Multiple Choice

Select the letter that best completes the statement or answers the question.

1. Health information that does not identify an individual is referred to as
   A. Protected health information
   B. Authorized health release
   C. Statutory data
   D. De-identified health information

2. An encounter is
   A. An operation
   B. An office visit
   C. A chemotherapy infusion
   D. All of the above

3. A patient's PHI may be released without authorization to
   A. Local newspapers
   B. An anesthesiologist who will anesthetize the patient during a scheduled surgery
   C. Friends who visit the patient during a hospital stay
   D. A lawyer who calls for information

4. Which government group has the authority to enforce the HIPAA Privacy Rule?
   A. FBI
   B. OIG
   C. OCR
   D. Medicaid

5. When PHI is correctly requested, what is the only information the HIM department releases?
   A. De-identified information
   B. Code set data
   C. Minimum necessary data
   D. A copy of the entire file

6. The authorization to release information of an unsecured breach of PHI must specify the
   A. Number of pages to be released
   B. Social Security number of the patient
   C. Entity to whom the information is to be released
   D. Name of the treating physician

7. The main purpose of the HIPAA Security Rule is to
   A. Regulate bank transactions
   B. Protect research data
   C. Control access to protected health information
   D. Protect medical facilities from break-ins and robbery

8. The _____ codes used in the United States are based on the International Classification of Diseases (ICD).
   A. Diagnosis
   B. Treatment
   C. Procedure
   D. Transaction

9. Medical coders assign codes based on the requirements of the
   A. HIPAA Privacy Rule
   B. HIPAA Security Rule
   C. HIPAA Electronic Health-Care Transactions and Code Sets standards
   D. Health Care Fraud and Abuse Control Program

10. Patients' protected health information may be released for
    A. Treatment
    B. Payment
    C. Operations
    D. All of the above

PART II

ICD-10-CM Coding

CHAPTER 3

ICD-10-CM Basics

CHAPTER OUTLINE

History of ICD-10-CM

Purpose of ICD-10-CM

Organizational and Structural Changes in ICD-10-CM

ICD-10-CM Basic Coding Process

ICD-10-CM Alphabetic Index

ICD-10-CM Tabular List of Diseases and Injuries

ICD-10-CM Coding Conventions

ICD-10-CM Coding Resources

Jack Hollingsworth/Photodisc/Thinkstock

LEARNING OUTCOMES

After studying this chapter, you should be able to:

1. Briefly discuss the background and history of ICD-10-CM.
2. Discuss the roles of the NCHS, CMS, AHIMA, and AHA in maintaining and updating ICD-10-CM codes.
3. Explain how to locate the periodic updates to ICD-10-CM codes using the Internet.
4. Identify five uses of ICD-10-CM.
5. Discuss the importance of the *ICD-10-CM Official Guidelines for Coding and Reporting.*
6. Describe the organization and content of Volumes 1 and 2 of ICD-10-CM.
7. Interpret the formats, conventions, and symbols used in ICD-10-CM.
8. List the basic process of assigning ICD-10-CM diagnosis codes.
9. Describe the meaning of coding to the highest level of specificity.
10. Identify common medical resources used to assist in the assignment of accurate ICD-10-CM codes.

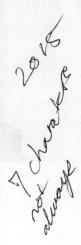

...gnosis codes represent diseases, injuries, and conditions that affect health. Because ...s reflect the reasons for services rendered and the medical complexity of the pa-...ns, accurately reporting them is important for health-care reimbursement, research, ...rement, and management decisions. Reporting a diagnosis code communicates the ...edical visit, such as chest pain, and demonstrates the medical necessity of the ser-...al diagnosis codes are reported for coexisting conditions or complications of medical ...ge of medical terminology, anatomy and physiology, and current coding guidelines ...ccurately assign all diagnosis codes and sequence those codes in the correct order. ...vailable for coders to use, such as printed codebooks with useful enhancements, medical dictionaries, drug references, and national guidelines.

HISTORY OF ICD-10-CM

The current classification system to record all diagnoses for medical visits in the United States is the *International Classification of Diseases, Tenth Revision, Clinical Modification*, often just called ICD-10-CM. This coding system is maintained by the National Center for Health Statistics (NCHS) and the Centers for Medicare and Medicaid Services (CMS), both of which are departments of the U.S. Department of Health and Human Services (HHS). ICD-10-CM replaced ICD-9-CM. It is organized into two sections that are used to classify diagnoses: the Index to Diseases and Injuries and the Tabular List of Diseases and Injuries.

Procedures (covered in Chapter 11 of this text) are classified using a new coding system named the *International Classification of Diseases, Tenth Revision, Procedure Coding System* (ICD-10-PCS). This coding system is used to classify inpatient procedures reported by hospitals and replaces Volume III of ICD-9-CM. An inpatient is an individual who has been formally admitted to a hospital and is receiving services from that hospital.

Prior to implementation of ICD-10-CM on October 1, 2015, the three-volume ICD-9-CM code set was used. The ICD-9-CM code set was modeled after the International Classification of Diseases, which is used throughout the world and maintained by the World Health Organization (WHO). In 1959, the U.S. Public Health Service (USPHS) published the *International Classification of Diseases, Adapted for Indexing of Hospital Records and Operation Classification* (ICDA). This system was revised over the years to accommodate the need to classify morbidity, the rate of incidences of diseases, and mortality (death) in the United States. In 1978, WHO published a ninth revision of ICD called ICD-9. The next year, in order to meet statistical data needs in the United States, the USPHS published its modified code set, ICD-9-CM. ICD-9-CM included more than 13,000 codes and used more digits in those codes than ICD-9, making it possible to specifically describe more diseases.

ICD-10 Versus ICD-9

A tenth edition of the ICD code set was published by WHO in 1990. The changes from ICD-9 to ICD-10 are summarized here:

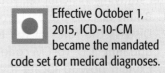

Effective October 1, 2015, ICD-10-CM became the mandated code set for medical diagnoses.

- The ICD-10 contains more than 2,000 categories of disease, many more than the ICD-9. These expanded categories permit more specific reporting of diseases and newly recognized conditions.
- Codes are alphanumeric, starting with a letter followed by up to six numbers.
- A sixth digit is added to capture clinical details. For example, all codes that relate to pregnancy, labor, and childbirth include a digit that indicates the patient's trimester.
- The second and third character are alphanumeric and combined with the first character to create a category.
- The fourth, fifth, and sixth digit is added to capture clinical details.

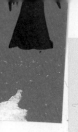

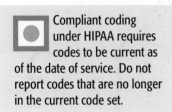

Use ICD-10-PCS for coding *inpatient* procedures reported by the facility (overview in Chapter 11), and use CPT/HCPCS (covered in Chapters 12–30) for coding *outpatient* procedures for the facility and physician and inpatient procedures reported by the physician.

- A seventh character provides information regarding the episode of care. For example, the seventh character of "A" in code S36.299A means "initial encounter" for that injury.
- More than one code may be required to show which side of the body is affected for a disease or condition that can be involved with the right side, the left side, or bilaterally. For example, separate codes are listed for a malignant neoplasm of the right upper-inner quadrant of the female breast and for a malignant neoplasm of the left upper-inner quadrant of the female breast.

Again, the USPHS published a modified code set—ICD-10-CM—in response. The Health Insurance Portability and Accountability Act of 1996 (HIPAA) considers ICD-10-CM to be the required code set for diseases, injuries, impairments, other health problems and their manifestations, and other causes of injury, disease, and impairment.

ICD-10-CM Today: Maintenance and Updates

To keep current with medical trends in disease management, the new ICD-10-CM system will be updated every year. The responsibility for maintaining ICD-10-CM is divided between the NCHS, a part of the Centers for Disease Control and Prevention (CDC), and 3M, which maintains ICD-10-PCS, the facility procedure coding system.

Compliant coding under HIPAA requires codes to be current as of the date of service. Do not report codes that are no longer in the current code set.

The federal ICD-10-CM Coordination and Maintenance Committee (CMS) considers coding modifications that have been proposed to ICD-10-CM. This committee is cochaired by representatives from CMS and NCHS. Interested parties from the public and private sectors can propose changes to ICD-10-CM. The committee's role is advisory, and the final determination of code changes is made by the administrator of CMS and the director of NCHS. The updates to these systems and associated publications are noted here.

INTERNET RESOURCES: ICD-10-CM Coordination and Maintenance Committee
http://www.cdc.gov/nchs/icd/icd10cm_maintenance.htm

ICD-10-CM Code Updates
www.cms.hhs.gov/ICD9ProviderDiagnosticCodes

The Addenda

NCHS and CMS release ICD-10-CM updates called *addenda* that take effect on October 1 and April 1 of every year. The October 1 changes are the major updates; the April 1 changes catch up on codes that were not included in the major changes. The major new, invalid, and revised codes are posted on the CMS website by the beginning of July for HIPAA-mandated use as of October 1 of the current year. New codes must be used as of the date they go into effect, and invalid (deleted or changed) codes must not be used.

Codebooks

The U.S. Government Printing Office (GPO) publishes the official ICD-10-CM code set on the Internet and in CD-ROM format every year. Various commercial publishers include the updated codes in annual coding books that are printed soon after the major updates are released. Many different features are available in these codebooks, ranging from straightforward code listings to enhanced manuals with many notes, illustrations, and helpful tips for coders. No matter which codebook is chosen, medical coders must have the current reference in order to select HIPAA-compliant codes.

The *Federal Register*

The *Federal Register* is the daily journal of the U.S. government and the government resource for official coding requirements and guidelines. These medical coding regulations are published in the *Federal Register* and are listed under CMS. Annual ICD-10-CM and ICD-10-PCS code changes are published in the *Federal Register* every year. The Office of the Federal Register is responsible for publishing the official text of federal laws, regulatory material, and presidential documents. The *Federal Register* and many other government documents can be found at www.ofr.gov. The HIPAA Final Rule mandating the ICD-10-CM code set was published in the January 16, 2009 issue of the *Federal Register*.

ICD-10-CM Official Guidelines

The HIPAA Final Rule requires the use of the *ICD-10-CM Official Guidelines for Coding and Reporting* when codes are selected. The guidelines assist in standardizing the assignment of ICD-10-CM codes for all users. For example, they include the rules for selecting the principal diagnosis when a patient has more than a single condition, assist the coder in understanding the basic rules of code selection using ICD-10-CM, and explain certain coding rules for specific medical conditions. The *Official Guidelines* are covered in detail in Chapter 4 of this text.

The *Official Guidelines* are the basis of consistent and accurate ICD-10-CM reporting. They are written by NCHS and CMS and approved by the cooperating parties, made up of the American Hospital Association (AHA), the American Health Information Management Association (AHIMA), CMS, and NCHS.

> Always base assignment of ICD-10-CM codes on the *Official Guidelines*.

PURPOSE OF ICD-10-CM

ICD-10-CM is a statistical tool used to convert medical diagnoses into alphanumeric codes, and ICD-10-PCS converts inpatient hospital procedures into alphanumeric codes. The code set has five primary applications.

Reporting and Research

ICD-10-CM/PCS statistical data are used in the United States to track morbidity, mortality, and other health-care information with a consistent, defined way of reporting. For example, to report that patients have the condition of chest pain, medical coders assign an ICD-10-CM code that always classifies chest pain the same way. Imagine trying to gather data on diseases if the conditions were listed alphabetically; chest pain could be reported in different ways, such as "pain in the chest" and "pain: chest." Having diagnoses and procedures reported in a consistent manner is essential for accurate tracking. At the national and state levels, the code set is used to track cases of prevalent conditions such as HIV, influenza, pneumonia, and other communicable diseases.

ICD-10-CM codes are also very important in medical and health-care research. For example, if a pharmaceutical company wants to research the effects of a new drug on patients with lung cancer, ICD-10-CM codes can be used to identify a patient population with that disease and to include those patients in the study. Researchers can also use ICD-10-CM to look at trends in health care among different patient groups. Federal agencies such as the CDC conduct research and report health-care data using ICD-10-CM codes (Fig. 3.1). The CDC's annual report of the number of patients discharged from hospitals by disease and by age is based on ICD-10-CM codes.

> **INTERNET RESOURCE: ICD-10-CM Home Page**
> www.cdc.gov/nchs/icd/icd10cm.htm

Monitoring the Quality of Patient Care

The quality of the care provided to patients can be measured in many ways, and ICD-10-CM often plays an important role. For example, all of a hospital's patients with hip replacements may be asked to complete questionnaires about their pain control after surgery. To perform this survey, researchers identify the patients who underwent hip replacements by the ICD-10-PCS code reported

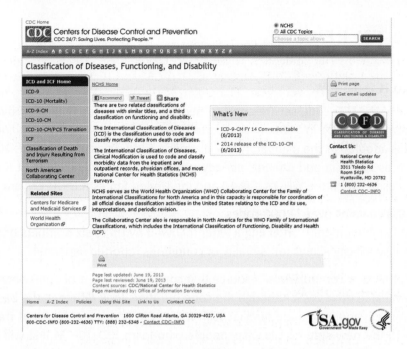

Figure 3.1 CDC/NCHS ICD-10-CM home page (the page changes as new information is included).

for their inpatient visit. Other examples include monitoring quality of care by collecting statistics on treatment for heart attacks and death rates of patients with particular diseases. ICD-10-CM can also be used in evaluating quality of care for people with certain diagnoses or procedures, which allows health-care providers to improve services.

Communications and Transactions

Because ICD-10-CM is a nationally used classification system, the code meanings provide a method of consistent communication. Providers can communicate with payers about the reason for services (the diagnosis in ICD-10-CM) and the services provided (the procedures in ICD-10-CM or CPT/ HCPCS). Payer policies often use code numbers in communications to providers. For example, a Medicare coverage policy is often explained by listing the diagnosis codes that are appropriate for a set of procedure codes. The searchable index and a specific example of a Medicare coverage policy can be found at www.cms.gov/medicare-coverage-database/indexes/national-and-local-indexes.aspx.

Reimbursement

Much of the focus of ICD-10-CM is insurance reimbursement. Payment for services rendered to hospital inpatients is based on their diseases and conditions. If the health-care visit is not coded correctly, payment to the hospital could be incorrect. All hospital inpatients must have their visits coded using ICD-10-CM and ICD-10-PCS. For Medicare patients, these codes are then used to calculate a Medicare Severity Diagnosis-Related Group (MS-DRG) payment. Consideration of the diagnoses and procedures and the patient's gender, disposition, and age all contribute to the MS-DRG calculation and thus to a payment. Other payers (e.g., Medicaid) have developed their own payment systems such as All Patient Refined Diagnosis-Related Groups (APR-DRGs) for hospital inpatient services.

ICD-10-CM diagnosis codes assigned to outpatients also affect payment. ICD-10-CM is used to indicate the medical necessity of (i.e., reason for) patients' health-care visits to physician offices, clinics, and outpatient hospital departments. For example, a diagnosis of chest pain is the reason for a chest x-ray. The diagnosis code explains why the procedure was performed.

Administrative Uses

Because ICD-10-CM is a standardized data set used throughout the country, it is easy to use coded data to study the types of patients seen and the services provided. For example, staffing

Why Move to ICD-10-CM?

A 10th edition of the ICD code set (referred to here as ICD-10) was published by the World Health Organization (WHO) in 1990. In the United States, the new *Clinical Modification,* the ICD-10-CM, was adopted as the mandatory U.S. diagnosis code set as of October 1, 2015. (Other countries, such as Australia and Canada, already use their own modifications of ICD-10.) The major differences between the WHO's ICD-10 and the United States ICD-10-CM are as follows:

- ICD-10-CM contains over 71,000 codes.
- Codes are alphanumeric, containing a letter followed by up to six numbers or letters.
- Additional specificity allows for laterality of conditions reported separately.

A crosswalk (a printed or computerized resource that connects two sets of data) between ICD-9 and ICD-10 is available from CMS. Although the code numbers look different, the basic systems are very much alike. People who are familiar with ICD-9-CM codes will find that their training quickly applies to the new system. Likewise, people who learn ICD-10-CM first will be able to use the crosswalk to find equivalent older codes if needed for previous years' claim questions.

decisions can be made based on the number of patients with a certain diagnosis. Using ICD-10-CM data, a hospital director knows that the hospital treats a certain number of patients each month, and can schedule the appropriate amount of specialized nursing care for those patients. Administrative budgeting, staffing, and marketing tasks that require the evaluation of patient types and services can be supported by review of the ICD-10-CM/PCS or CPT codes reported for each patient.

ORGANIZATIONAL AND STRUCTURAL CHANGES IN ICD-10-CM

ICD-10-CM represents an improvement over ICD-9-CM in regard to specificity and comprehensiveness. ICD-10-CM has the same hierarchical structure as ICD-9-CM in that the first three characters are the category of the code and all codes within the same category have similar traits. In addition, a comparison of the two coding systems highlights the organizational and structural changes. The hierarchical structure is the same, yet the following differences can be noted:

- ICD-10-CM consists of 21 chapters compared with 17 chapters in ICD-9-CM.
- ICD-9-CM's V and E code supplemental classifications are incorporated into the main classification in ICD-10-CM.
- ICD-10-CM codes are alphanumeric and can be up to seven characters in length; ICD-9-CM codes are only three to five characters in length.
- ICD-10-CM includes the addition of a placeholder character (x).
- ICD-9-CM had fewer codes (approximately 14,000 in ICD-9) than ICD-10-CM, which makes approximately 71,000 codes available.
- Postoperative complications have been moved to procedure-specific body system chapters.

- ICD-10-CM includes full code titles for all codes (no reference back to common fourth and fifth digits).
- ICD-9-CM lacks laterality, which is now incorporated into ICD-10-CM.

Transitioning From ICD-9-CM to ICD-10-CM

The CMS coordinated the transition from ICD-9-CM. A partial freeze on new codes was implemented to help in this transition and can be summarized as follows:

- October 1, 2011, was the last major update of ICD-9-CM.
- After October 1, 2011, there were no further releases of ICD-9-CM on CD-ROM.
- October 1, 2011, was the last major update of ICD-10-CM/PCS until October 1, 2015.
- Between October 1, 2011, and October 1, 2015, revisions to ICD-10-CM/PCS were made only for new diseases/new technology procedures and for any minor revisions to correct reported errors in these classifications.
- Regular (at least annual) updates to ICD-10-CM/PCS resumed on October 1, 2016.
- ICD-10-CM/PCS, on CD-ROM, was released 1 year prior to implementation.

Effective October 1, 2015, all codes had to be reported using ICD-10-CM. To make an effective transition, tools called *general equivalence mappings (GEMs)* were created. The GEMs tool converts ICD-9-CM diagnosis codes to ICD-10-CM, but it is only a tool. In some instances there is a "one-to-one" match—meaning that the ICD-9-CM code translates to one code in ICD-10-CM. In other instances there is a "one-to-many" mapping. In other words, there is no perfect match per se—one code in ICD-9-CM may equate to three codes in ICD-10-CM, and one code in ICD-10-CM may require two codes in ICD-9-CM. The GEMs point the coder in the right direction or to a starting point but a codebook is required to finalize the exact ICD-10-CM code. CMS has also developed a GEMs tool to convert ICD-10-CM back to ICD-9-CM, and this is termed *backward mapping*. In electronic data transmission, Medicare uses a flag to denote the matching between a specific ICD-9-CM code and an ICD-10-CM code. A flag has five characters that relate to a specific code pair. For example:

ICD-10-CM source code: T15.00xA
ICD-9-CM target code: 930.0
Flag: 10111

The flag identifies how well the codes match in meaning. The first character in the flag code is a "1," which denotes that the codes mapped are "approximate" (a "0" would mean the translation is an identical match). The second and third characters of the flag also have meaning regarding the source code and the translation of the code. See Table 3.1 for examples of bidirectional conversions. An overview of the GEMs tool and flag system can be found at www.cms.gov/medicare/coding/icd10/downloads/gems-crosswalksbasicfaq.pdf.

Table 3.1 Transition Table

ICD-9-CM CODE	=	ICD-10-CM CODE
824.4 Bimalleolar fracture, left ankle	=	S82.842A Displaced bimalleolar fracture of the left lower leg, initial encounter S82.845A Nondisplaced bimalleolar fracture of the left lower leg, initial encounter
995.92 Severe sepsis AND 785.52 Septic shock	=	R65.21 Severe sepsis with septic shock
None	=	Z72.3 Lack of physical exercise

A. Identify the purpose of ICD-10-CM coding in the following case scenarios as research (R), quality (Q), communication (C), payment (P), or administrative (A).

1. A hospital board would like to develop a chemotherapy marketing campaign because the hospital has had a reduction in services to patients during the past year.

_____

2. A physician reported the wrong ICD-10-CM codes to Medicare and was reimbursed incorrectly; the codes had to be resubmitted on a new health-care claim.

_____

3. A hospital wants to send a patient survey to all patients to determine whether the services they received were satisfactory. _____

4. A trend showed an increase in hospital postoperative complications, and a hospital wanted to investigate this trend. _____

5. A company wants to determine whether its new drug for the treatment of diabetes is effective. _____

B. Identify which coding system (ICD-9-CM and/or ICD-10-CM) is referenced in the following statements.

6. Classifies laterality. _____

7. Contains a separate classification for external causes of injury (E codes).

_____

8. Contains 21 chapters. _____

9. The code 410.11 is a sample from this system. _____

10. GEMs helps transition which coding system(s)? _____

ICD-10-CM BASIC CODING PROCESS

Diagnostic coding requires knowledge of the format of each ICD-10-CM section and of the conventions and rules each uses to assist the coder in finding different types of codes, such as those describing external causes of injuries rather than codes describing the injuries themselves. A codebook is the source of the codes; the *ICD-10-CM Official Guidelines for Coding and Reporting* is the source of the conventions and rules.

The two sections of ICD-10-CM are:

1. The Alphabetic Index contains four sections: the Index to Diseases and Injuries, the Neoplasm Table, Table of Drugs and Chemicals, and Index to External Causes of Injuries.
2. *Tabular List of Diseases and Injuries:* The Tabular List is made up of 21 chapters and is organized by code numbers and their descriptions.

> The first part of Section I of the *Official Guidelines* is "A. Conventions for the ICD-10-CM."

> The correct coding process is to locate a main term and its code in the Index and to verify the code selection in the Tabular List.

ICD-10-CM is used for diagnostic coding, and the coding process starts with looking up words. Thus, the ICD-10-CM Alphabetic Index, which contains medical terms, is used first. After a code has been located in the Alphabetic Index based on the diagnostic statement and the main term identified, it is verified in the ICD-10-CM Tabular List of Diseases and Injuries (Tabular List). See

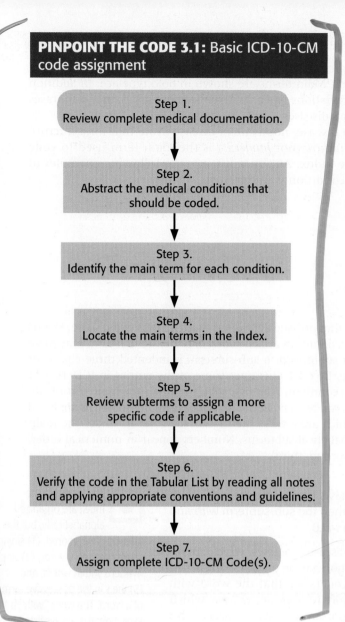

PINPOINT THE CODE 3.1: Basic ICD-10-CM code assignment

Step 1.
Review complete medical documentation.

↓

Step 2.
Abstract the medical conditions that should be coded.

↓

Step 3.
Identify the main term for each condition.

↓

Step 4.
Locate the main terms in the Index.

↓

Step 5.
Review subterms to assign a more specific code if applicable.

↓

Step 6.
Verify the code in the Tabular List by reading all notes and applying appropriate conventions and guidelines.

↓

Step 7.
Assign complete ICD-10-CM Code(s).

Pinpoint the Code 3.1, which de[...] all the steps in the coding process[...] focus on the use of the Disease In[...] Tabular List in this chapter. This t[...] process must be followed in order [...] correctly. This chapter follows th[...] order of use, with the Disease Ind[...] cussed first, followed by discussion of the Tabular List.

ICD-10-CM ALPHABETIC INDEX

The ICD-10-CM Alphabetic Index has four main sections:

a. Index of Diseases and Injuries (Disease Index)
b. Table of Neoplasms (Neoplasm Table)
c. Table of Drugs and Chemicals
d. External Cause of Injuries Index (Index of External Causes of Injury or External Cause Index)

The Disease Index lists words that describe diseases or injuries, such as *pneumonia, bronchitis, infection*, and *fracture*. The Table of Drugs and Chemicals is an alphabetical listing of drugs and chemicals such as aspirin, alcohol, gasoline, and penicillin. The Table of Neoplasms identifies the site of a neoplasm and its behavior. In coding external causes of diseases, coders start with words such as *fall, accident, burn*, and *cut* that can be found in the External Cause of Injuries Index. Examples of entries in the four sections of the Index are listed in Table 3.2.

Table 3.2 Organization of the ICD-10-CM Index to Diseases and Injuries

SECTION DESCRIPTION	SAMPLE ENTRIES
Index to Diseases and Injuries (A–Z)	Angina Fracture Pneumonia
The Table of Neoplasms	Lung
Table of Drugs and Chemicals (A–Z)	Aspirin Coumadin Petroleum
External Cause of Injuries Index (A–Z)	Fire Hit Sting

Main Terms

The Disease Index lists main terms that represent diseases, injuries, problems, complaints, drugs, and external causes of diseases or conditions. Main terms are shown in bold typeface. In addition to common nouns, main terms can be abbreviations (such as AAT) or eponyms, names or phrases based on people's names, such as Gamstorp's disease.

Usually the main term in the Index is a disease, not a site of disease. Note that for a fracture of the humerus, for example, the term *fracture* (not *humerus*) is the main term used to code the condition and the starting point in the Index. As you can see in the following examples of diseases, the main term used to code the condition is underlined.

- Urinary tract <u>infection</u>
- Benign prostatic <u>hypertrophy</u>
- Aspiration <u>pneumonia</u>
- <u>Fractured</u> humerus
- Chronic obstructive pulmonary <u>disease</u>

Subterms

Main terms are followed by indented words that provide additional specifications of a disease. Words that are indented under a main term are called *subterms*. Each subterm under a main term may have additional indented terms (*sub-subterms*). A subterm or a sub-subterm is indented three character spaces from the term above it. For example, Box 3.1 illustrates some of the entries in ICD-10-CM relating to bronchitis, a common respiratory condition. The first subterm under the main term *bronchitis* is *with*. The second subterm under the main term *bronchitis* is *acute or subacute*. Subterms are listed alphabetically except for *with* or *without*, which are always the first listed subterms under the main term. Numeric subterms appear before alphabetical subterms. Numbers appear in numerical order, even if they are spelled out as words (first, second, third).

EXAMPLE

To code acute bronchitis with bronchiectasis, first locate the main term *bronchitis*, then the subterm *acute*, and then the sub-subterm *with* and then *bronchiectasis.* This results in code J47.0.

Coders will need to be familiar with the disease processes, which are reviewed in the basic Pathophysiology Connection box on the following pages.

The use of the indented format helps coders see that the word with bronchiectasis (in Box 3.1) refers specifically to *acute or subacute,* which refers to the main term *bronchitis*. It is important to always observe this pattern of indention.

> The entries in the Index are organized alphabetically, but the following are ignored: (1) single spaces between words, (2) single hyphens within words, and (3) the *s* in the possessive form of a word. The word "with" is the exception; it is always listed first.

BOX 3.1 Format of the ICD-10-CM Index of Diseases and Injuries (Disease Index)

Bronchitis (diffuse, fibrinous, hypostatic, infective, membranous) J40	Carryover line
with	Subterm
influenza, flu, or grippe—*see* Influenza, with,	Sub-subterm
respiratory manifestations	Carryover line
obstruction (airway)(lung) J44.9	Sub-subterm
tracheitis (15 years and above) J40	Sub-subterm
acute or subacute J20.9	Sub-sub-subterm
chronic J42	Sub-sub-subterm
under 15 years of age J20.9	Sub-sub-subterm
Acute or subacute (with bronchospasm or	Subterm
obstruction) J20.9	Carryover line
with	Subterm
bronchiectasis J47.0	Sub-sub-subterm
chronic obstructive pulmonary disease J44.0	Sub-sub-subterm

There are other types of indentions. Indentions that are six characters in length represent carryover lines. These lines are used when an entry will not fit on a single line. For example, the terms in parentheses after the main term *bronchitis* (*diffuse, fibrinous, hypostatic, infective, membranous, with tracheitis*) are related to bronchitis, but because they all do not fit on one line, they are carried over to the next line and indented 6 spaces.

CHECKPOINT 3.2

Using the entire ICD-10-CM Alphabetic Index, identify which specific section in the Index—Disease index (A), Neoplasm table (B), Table of Drugs and Chemicals (T) or the External cause of injury index (E)—the coder would reference for the following examples:

1. Carbon monoxide _____
2. Chronic obstructive pulmonary disease _____
3. Parachuting _____
4. Tylenol _____
5. Infection _____

Underline the main term in the following examples that the coder would use to begin the coding process.

6. Burn of the hand
7. Fall from tree
8. Poisoning from cocaine
9. Chronic cystitis
10. Automobile accident
11. Acute appendicitis
12. Malignant neoplasm of the colon
13. Allergic reaction to shellfish
14. Closed fracture of the lateral condyle of the left humerus
15. Struck by lightning

Answer the following using the Disease Index.

16. What is the first subterm under the main term edema? _____
17. What is the first subterm under the main term drowning? (*Hint*: See the External Cause of Injuries Index.) _____
18. What is the first subterm under the main term pain? _____
19. Is there a carryover line at the main term pneumonia? _____
20. What is the first sub-subterm under the main term accident, subterm transport? _____

Using the Index only, code the following.

21. Urinary tract infection _____
22. Progressive atrophic paralysis _____
23. Insomnia due to alcohol abuse _____
24. Ski lift accident _____
25. Regional enteritis with complication of intestinal obstruction _____

PATHOPHYSIOLOGY CONNECTION

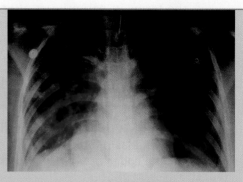

Overview

Pathophysiology combines the study of *pathology*—the origins, causes, and course of disease—with *physiology,* the study of how living things function. Pathophysiology is the study of how diseases arise and how they affect the normal functioning of the body.

Origins and Causes of Diseases and Disorders

Diseases and disorders occur in one of two ways. They may be part of a person's genetic makeup, or they may be acquired. Some individuals have complex genetic makeups that predispose them to a particular disease, but they may never actually get the disease. For example, type 2 diabetes mellitus may tend to occur in a family, but some family members do not develop it. Other people have a genetic tendency for a particular disease but may be able to avoid it through careful lifestyle management. While people with the inherited gene for breast cancer have a greater likelihood of getting breast cancer, it is not absolutely certain that they will.

Acquired diseases or disorders are caused by coming into contact with a *pathogen* (a disease-causing agent) or an *allergen,* or they may result from a number of factors or situations. The state of a person's immune system can determine resistance to disease. Bacteria, fungi, and viruses are some of the pathogens that cause disease. Accidents and traumas cause injuries and possible psychological disorders. Environmental causes of disease can include exposure to hazardous substances, overexposure to the ultraviolet rays of the sun, and poor diet and lack

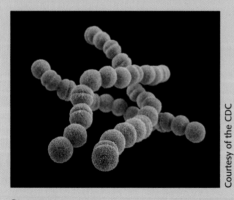

Streptococcus.

Courtesy of the CDC

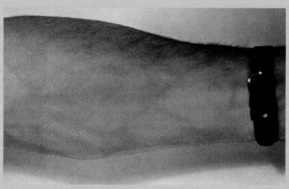

Skin test for a fungal infection.

Courtesy of the CDC

of exercise. Factors such as age, gender, genetic makeup, lifestyle, access to health care, and environment are called *predisposing* factors.

SOAP and the Understanding of Disease

When medical professionals examine patients, they often use the SOAP method of observation and treatment. Sometimes the signs and symptoms of disease are reported by a patient as the chief complaint. In such cases, the physician diagnoses the disease using a standard examination process. Other times, a screening service, such as a mammogram or a blood pressure test, uncovers signs of a disease for which there is no external evidence, such as a breast tumor or hypertension. *SOAP* stands for *subjective, objective, assessment, plan:*

S: The *subjective* information is what the patient relates as the problems or complaints.

O: The *objective* information is what the physician finds during the examination of the patient. It may include the results of laboratory tests or other procedures.

A: The *assessment,* also called the "conclusion," is the physician's diagnosis.

P: The *plan,* also called "advice" or "recommendations," is the course of treatment for the patient, such as surgery, medications, other tests, further patient monitoring, follow-up, and instructions to the patient.

The Vocabulary of Pathophysiology

Many terms used with diseases and disorders are general terms that cover a number of diseases with certain common characteristics. For example, *cancer* is a term for any disease that involves malignant growths. A specific cancer, such as leukemia, may also include a number of different variations of the disorder. In addition, individual diseases are characterized by certain terms that indicate the type, severity, or some other aspect of the disease. Many diseases are either *acute* (brief and severe) or *chronic* (of long duration). Some symptoms may be *integral* (part of the disease process) or *nonintegral* (not directly connected with the disease). A tumor may be *benign* (located in one area and not spreading) or *malignant* (spreading in an uncontrolled manner). *Necrotic* or *necrotizing* indicates that tissue is dying; for example, *acute necrotizing pancreatitis* is a severe attack of pancreatitis accompanied by the death of some tissue. *Suppurative* indicates the discharge of pus. *Exfoliative* indicates scaling or flaking. *Infantile* indicates very young; *senile* indicates very old. Treatments may be *invasive* (requiring incision or puncture) or *noninvasive* (not requiring incision or puncture). These and other characteristics are used to classify diseases.

...CD-10-CM Tabular List contains 21 chapters representing body systems or conditions by
...gy or nature of disease. For example, Chapter 6 represents diseases of the nervous system
...-G99) and Chapter 1 represents infectious and parasitic diseases (A00–B99). The chapters of
...osis codes are used to verify codes first looked up in the index. For example, to verify the
...J81.1, the coder looks in the Diseases of the Respiratory System chapter in the Tabular List,
which describes chronic pulmonary edema. ICD-10-CM incorporates External Causes of Injuries
and Poisonings and the Factors Influencing Health Status and Contact with Human Services into
the core classification. ICD-10-CM codes begin with a letter and range from A00 to Z99.89, but
the letter U is not used.

The structure of the ICD-10-CM Tabular List of Diseases and Injuries (Tabular List) is shown in
Table 3.3.

ICD-10-CM Tabular List of Diseases and Injuries Format

ICD-10-CM diagnosis codes range from an alpha character plus two digits to an alpha character plus
six digits. The first three digits identify the broad category of the disease, and the additional digits are
used to more specifically identify the details of the disease. The format of the Tabular List reflects this
method of identifying diagnoses:

Chapter	Range of codes
Block	Range of codes within a chapter
Category	Three-digit code within a block
Subcategory	Four-, five-, six-, or seven-digit code within a category

Table 3.3 Organization of the ICD-10-CM Tabular List of Diseases and Injuries

CHAPTER	DESCRIPTION	CODE RANGE
Classification of Diseases and Injuries		
1	Certain infectious and parasitic diseases	A00–B99
2	Neoplasms	C00–D49
3	Diseases of the blood and blood-forming organs and certain disorders involving the immune mechanism	D50–D89
4	Endocrine, nutritional, and metabolic diseases	E00–E89
5	Mental, behavioral, and neurodevelopmental disorders	F01–F99
6	Diseases of the nervous system	G00–G99
7	Diseases of the eye and adnexa	H00–H59
8	Diseases of the ear and mastoid process	H60–H95
9	Diseases of the circulatory system	I00–I99
10	Diseases of the respiratory system	J00–J99
11	Diseases of the digestive system	K00–K95
12	Diseases of the skin and subcutaneous tissue	L00–L99
13	Diseases of the musculoskeletal system and connective tissue	M00–M99
14	Diseases of the genitourinary system	N00–N99
15	Pregnancy, childbirth, and the puerperium	O00–O9A
16	Certain conditions originating in the perinatal period	P00–P96
17	Congenital malformations, deformations, and chromosomal abnormalities	Q00–Q99
18	Symptoms, signs, and abnormal clinical laboratory findings, not elsewhere classified	R00–R99
19	Injury, poisoning, and certain other consequences of external causes	S00–T88
20	External causes of morbidity	V00–Y99
21	Factors influencing health status and contact with health services	Z00–Z99

Find the following codes in the ICD-10-CM Tabular List of Diseases and Injuries (Tabular List) and state their meaning.

1. M26.02 _Maxillary hypoplasia_
2. H92.02 _Otalgia, left ear_
3. W59.02xA _Struck by nonvenomous lizard, inital encounter_
4. Z62.891 _____
5. R71.0 _____
6. D23.71 _____
7. K56.1 _____
8. B35.3 _____
9. S09.21xA _____
10. O40.2xx2 _____

_3-7_
+ placeholder

Chapters and Blocks

Each of the 21 chapters in the Tabular List contains a series of three-digit codes that represent a body system or group of diseases. Chapters are divided into *blocks*. A block contains a group of codes related to a more specific disease group within a chapter. For example, Chapter 1 covers infectious and parasitic diseases (A00–B99). The first block in the chapter is titled Intestinal Infectious Diseases (A00–A09), and the second block in this chapter is titled Tuberculosis (A15–A19). The blocks are located at the beginning of each chapter, but are also located at the beginning of the noted code range. Take the time to find the block titled Tuberculosis; it is found between codes A09 and A15. The blocks are not quite as easy to find, but they are important in understanding the format of the tabular list. Box 3.2 shows a chapter and the first block in that chapter.

Categories and Subcategories

Two terms are used to identify the types of specific codes within a chapter and block: category and subcategory. Category codes are three digits in length; subcategories classify etiology, anatomical site, and/or severity of the disease or injury. The subcategories can extend the code using a fourth, fifth, sixth, and seventh alphanumerical character. Not all codes are seven digits in length; rather, a valid code can be three, four, five, six, or seven digits in length. To interpret each code, the medical coder reads the description at the complete code level. It is important to note that notes at the chapter or block level apply to the entire chapter or block. The following is a list of valid codes representing different character lengths:

- I10—Hypertension
- M54.9—Back pain
- G81.11—Spastic hemiplegia affecting right dominant side
- G90.511—Complex regional pain syndrome 1 of right upper limb
- S72.041A—Displaced fracture of base of neck, right femur, initial encounter for closed fracture

When reading the Tabular List the coder can find the entire description of the code, but be careful that the code is reported with the most number of digits available. To see how this works, the following example shows the relationship between the category (three-digit code) and the subcategory characters that provide additional meaning.

EXAMPLE

To find the correct code for transient arthropathy of the right shoulder, which is M12.811, notice that the description at the category level (Other specified arthropathy) is carried over to the code description. Notice that at the subcategory level (code M12.8), these classify Other specific arthropathies, not elsewhere classified, which includes transient arthropathy. This is further refined to identify the Other specific arthropathies, not elsewhere classified, shoulder, right shoulder. Therefore, the code M12.811 classifies a very specific disease and its location.

An important coding rule is that *a disease must be classified to its highest level of specificity*. This means that all digits assignable for a specific disease must be used. For example, code S43.014A, "anterior subluxation and anterior dislocation of the right humerus, initial encounter," requires the use of seven digits. It would be incorrect to use only the first three digits—category code S43—which reports only that the patient has dislocation and sprain of joints and ligaments of the shoulder girdle. Correct diagnosis coding using ICD-10-CM requires adding a fourth and a fifth digit to explain the type and specific site of the dislocation, a sixth digit to identify laterality, and a seventh digit to identify the type of encounter.

Seventh-digit character values can be found in the Tabular List at the category level (i.e., after the three-digit code). The subcategory codes are found indented under the category codes. See Box 3.3.

BOX 3.2 Example of Tabular List Entries in ICD-10-CM

CHAPTER 1
Certain Infectious and Parasitic Diseases (A00–B99)
Includes: diseases generally recognized as communicable or transmissible
Use Additional code to identify resistance to antimicrobial drugs (Z16.-)
Excludes1: certain localized infections—see body system-related chapters
Excludes2: carrier or suspected carrier of infectious disease (Z22.-)
　　　　　　 infectious and parasitic diseases complicating pregnancy, childbirth and the puerperium (O98.-)
　　　　　　 infectious and parasitic diseases specific to the perinatal period (P35–P39)
　　　　　　 influenza and other acute respiratory infections (J00–J22)

This chapter contains the following blocks:

A00–A09	Intestinal infectious diseases
A15–A19	Tuberculosis
A20–A28	Certain zoonotic bacterial diseases
A30–A49	Other bacterial diseases
A50–A64	Infections with a predominantly sexual mode of transmission
A65–A69	Other spirochetal diseases
A70–A74	Other diseases caused by chlamydiae
A75–A79	Rickettsioses
A80–A89	Viral and prion infections of the central nervous system
A90–A99	Arthropod-borne viral fevers and viral hemorrhagic fevers
B00–B09	Viral infections characterized by skin and mucous membrane lesions
B10	Other human herpesviruses
B15–B19	Viral hepatitis
B20	Human immunodeficiency virus [HIV] disease
B25–B34	Other viral diseases
B35–B49	Mycoses
B50–B64	Protozoal diseases
B65–B83	Helminthiases
B85–B89	Pediculosis, acariasis, and other infestations
B90–B94	Sequelae of infectious and parasitic diseases
B95–B97	Bacterial and viral infectious agents
B99	Other infectious diseases

Intestinal Infectious Diseases (A00–A09)

A00 Cholera

Intestinal Infectious Diseases (A00–A09)
A00 Cholera
　　　 A00.0　　Cholera due to Vibrio cholerae 01, biovar cholerae
　　　　　　　 Classical cholera

A00.1   Cholera due to Vibrio cholerae 01, biovar eltor
         Cholera eltor
A00.9   Cholera, unspecified
A01 Typhoid and Paratyphoid Fevers
A01.0   Typhoid fever
         Infection due to Salmonella typhi
A01.00 Typhoid fever, unspecified
A01.01 Typhoid meningitis
A01.02 Typhoid fever with heart involvement
         Typhoid endocarditis
         Typhoid myocarditis

BOX 3.3 Seventh-Digit Values

The appropriate seventh character is to be added to each code from category S30:
A = initial encounter
D = subsequent encounter
S = sequelae

When a five-digit code is not available, a four-digit code is correct. For example, if a patient has a malignant neoplasm of the stomach (category 151), a fourth digit is required to reflect the exact location of the neoplasm in the stomach, such as 151.4 for a malignant neoplasm of the body of the stomach.

Placeholder characters are used to maintain the format of ICD-10-CM and its seven digits when a seventh character is required. Remember that the "x" is used as the placeholder. A capital X at the beginning of a code is NOT a placeholder.

Always code to the highest level of specificity—the most number of digits available.

BOX 3.4 Example of Tabular List Requiring Seventh Character

Y21 Drowning and submersion, undetermined intent

The appropriate seventh character is to be added to each code from category Y21

   A - initial encounter
   D - subsequent encounter
   S - sequela

Y21.0   Drowning and submersion while in the bathtub, undetermined intent

Y21.1   Drowning and submersion after fall into bathtub, undetermined intent

Y21.2   Drowning and submersion while in swimming pool, undetermined intent

Y21.3   Drowning and submersion after fall into swimming pool, undetermined intent

Y21.4   Drowning and submersion in natural water, undetermined intent

Y21.8   Other drowning and submersion, undetermined intent

Y21.9   Unspecified drowning and submersion, undetermined intent

The placeholder character "x" is used to maintain the format of a ICD-10-CM seven-digit code when required. The placeholder character holds a place in the event a fifth or sixth subcategory is not present but a seventh character is required. The ICD-10-CM code might look like this: Y21.3xxA. See Box 3.4, which shows the Tabular List entries for code Y21.3. Note that a seventh character is required to classify the type of encounter, yet category Y21 extends only to a fourth character. A placeholder character (x) fills the fifth- and sixth-digit spaces so that the seventh-digit character stays in its place. The code Y21.3xxA is the correct code for drowning and submersion after fall into swimming pool, undetermined intent, initial encounter.

Basic Anatomy and Physiology for ICD-10-CM

ICD-10-CM requires a clear understanding of basic anatomy and physiology. Codes in ICD-10-CM denote location and specificity. In previous code sets, this was not generally indicated by the code itself. For example, the ICD-9-CM code for an ankle fracture is 824.8. In ICD-10-CM, the code S82.63xA now indicates laterality, either right or left side, as well as the specific site of the fracture (as in the lateral malleolus).

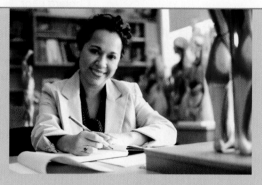

Anatomy and physiology are the sciences that describe the normal functioning of the body. Generally, the body is divided into body systems as listed in the table below.

BODY SYSTEM(S)	MAJOR STRUCTURE(S)	ESSENTIAL FUNCTION(S)
Integumentary	Skin, hair, nails, sweat glands, oil glands	Protection of organs, temperature regulation
Musculoskeletal	Muscles, bones, cartilage	Supports body, protects organs, provides movement
Cardiovascular	Heart, blood vessels	Transports blood throughout body, carries nutrients, and removes wastes
Respiratory	Lungs, airways	Performs respiration
Nervous	Brain, spinal cord, peripheral nerves	Regulates body activities and sends and receives sensory messages
Urinary	Kidney, bladder, ureters, urethra	Eliminates metabolic waste, regulates acid–base and water–salt balances, helps regulate blood pressure
Reproductive	Male and female reproductive organs	Controls reproduction and heredity
Hemic	Blood	Transports nutrients and removes waste from all body tissue
Lymphatic and Immune	Lymph, lymphatic vessels and glands, nonspecific defenses of the immune system	Lymphatic: Transports lymph, a clear, colorless fluid containing white blood cells that helps rid the body of toxins, waste, and other unwanted materials. Immune system identifies abnormal or foreign antigens and pathogens
Endocrine	Glands that secrete hormones	Hormones regulate various bodily functions
Digestive	All structures involved in digestion and excretion of waste	Digestion and excretion
Sensory	Eyes and ears and other structures involved in the five senses	Reaction to the five senses

Pathophysiology and Medical Terminology

The coder is usually involved with diagnoses and procedures that address abnormal body functioning. As such, it is invaluable for the coder to understand normal functions as well as pathophysiology, the diseases and disorders of the body. All these subjects use medical terminology to describe structures, functions, and malfunctions of the body. If you are studying for a career in health care, you will most likely take courses that cover these subjects. That knowledge will be invaluable to you in your work life.

ICD-10-CM Coding Examples

The examples listed here for each organ system include location and specificity within the code itself:

Integumentary system: Pressure ulcer of the left upper back, stage 1 (L89.121)
Musculoskeletal system: Felty's syndrome, right elbow (M05.021)
Circulatory system: Cerebral infarction due to thrombosis of the right cerebral artery (I63.341)
Respiratory system: Chronic maxillary sinusitis (J32.0)
Nervous system: Quadriplegia, C1–C4 complete (G82.51)
Genitourinary system: Small kidney, bilateral (N27.1)
Digestive system: Diverticulitis of the small intestine with bleeding (K57.11)
Hemic system: Drug-induced aplastic anemia (D61.1)
Endocrine system: Type I diabetic with polyneuropathy (E10.42)
Sensory system: Hypotony of the left eye due to ocular fistula (H44.422)

following questions using the ICD-10-CM Tabular List of Diseases and Injuries.

1. ...e block associated with code N36.41? _____

2. ...the sixth digit classify in code H10.423? _____

3. ...the fourth digit classify in code N70.11? _____

4. ...is code S00.252 reported at the highest level of specificity? _____

5. What chapter is represented by code O9A.312? _____

Match the following terms.

6. Chapter	A. a three-digit code
7. Block	B. a character that maintains the seven digits
8. Category	C. the last digit in an ICD-10-CM code
9. Subcategory	D. a fourth, fifth, or sixth digit is assigned
10. Placeholder character	E. a range of codes representing a body system or disease state
11. Seventh character	F. a group of codes within a chapter

ICD-10-CM CODING CONVENTIONS

Just as the basic rules of the road help people drive safely, so do coding conventions guide the use of ICD-10-CM. Conventions, or notations, appear throughout ICD-10-CM. The cardinal rule is that codes are never selected from one section alone; always start with the Index and finish by verifying the code in the Tabular List. Specific details and examples of coding conventions follow and are summarized in Table 3.4. Coders should always follow the *Official Guidelines* for conventions and rules.

Acronyms

Acronyms are used in all sections of ICD-10-CM.

Not Elsewhere Classified (NEC)

Not elsewhere classified (NEC) means that ICD-10-CM does not have a code for the documented condition. The acronym appears in the Index, and the code must be verified in the Tabular List. Often the Tabular List uses a grouping of such conditions. When NEC is used, additional information will not alter the code assignment; often, there is a precise statement but no correlated code. The acronym often directs the coder to an "other specified" code in the Tabular List. This application of NEC refers to the fact that a more specific category is not provided and that additional information will not alter code assignment. The entries in the Tabular List for codes S01.81 and S01.91 are noted in the example that follows. Notice that the subcategory (fourth digit) value of 8 reflects other specified (aka NEC).

> **EXAMPLE**
> **Laceration**
> Head (S01.91-)
> Specified site NEC S01.81

In this example from the Index, NEC is used to classify a specified site of a laceration to the head (S01.81). When verified in the ICD-10-CM Tabular List of Diseases and Injuries, code S01.81 classifies "laceration without foreign body of other parts of head" and a seventh character value is required.

Table 3.4 Summary List of Conventions Used in ICD-10-CM

CONVENTION	CONVENTION LOCATION	MEANING
Acronyms		
NEC	Index, Tabular	Not elsewhere classified or otherwise specified, or a more specific category is not provided.
NOS	Tabular	Not otherwise specified, or unspecified.
Punctuation		
Brackets [ ]	Index	Enclose manifestation codes, or codes that should be listed second.
Parentheses ( )	Index, Tabular	Enclose supplemental words or nonessential modifiers.
Colon :	Tabular	Placed after an incomplete term that needs one or more of the modifying terms to assign that code.
Terms		
Includes	Tabular	Further defines or gives examples of terms included in that code or code section.
Excludes1	Tabular	A pure excludes note meaning NOT CODED here. Refers to the situation where two conditions cannot occur together. The note lists terms that are excluded from or are to be coded elsewhere.
Excludes2	Tabular	Means "not included here." The condition listed after an "excludes note 2" is not included in that code, but the excluded condition may also be coded when appropriate (i.e., when both conditions exist).
Inclusion terms	Tabular	These are terms included in the code. These may be various conditions or synonyms. These are not exhaustive; thus, the code may classify other conditions as well.
Cross-References		
See	Index	Follows a main term and provides a new main term that should be referenced.
See also	Index	Follows a main term to instruct the coder to see additional entries that may apply.
And	Index	Should be interpreted as meaning "and" or "or."
With	Index	The word *with* is sequenced first following a main term and is not in alphabetical order. The word *with* also means "associated with" or "due to" and these terms presume a causal relationship between the two conditions linked by the terms in the Alphabetic Index or Tabular List.
Typeface		
Bold	Tabular	Font of all codes and titles.
	Index	Font of all main terms.
Instructions		
Use additional code	Tabular	Instructs the coder to assign an additional code to give more information if known. This instruction is located at the etiology code and instructs the coder to use an additional code for the manifestation.
Code first	Tabular	Instructs the coder to code an underlying condition first, then the other code second (the code containing the instruction). This instruction is often a manifestation code.

Continued

TION	CONVENTION LOCATION	MEANING
s classified	Tabular	Found in the title of a code and means "this code is a component code and this code is a manifestation."
	Tabular	Also means "other specified," and relates to index entries of NEC. Detail is available, yet the specific code does not exist.
Unspecified	Tabular	Reflects codes that often have a fourth digit of 9 or fifth digit of 0, and the title states unspecified. Often, documentation in the medical record lacks the detail to assign a more specific code (NOS).
Code also	Tabular	Instructs the coder that two codes may be required to classify a condition with no sequencing direction.
Default codes	Index	Default codes are listed next to a main term.
Syndromes	Index	Guidance in the Index should be followed for syndromes because codes for documented manifestations of the syndrome should be reported.

Not Otherwise Specified (NOS)

Not otherwise specified (NOS) is used in the Tabular List to indicate a code that should be used when the documentation does not supply a more specific condition for code assignment. In other words, typically the coder does not have information to code a specific disease and would need such information to assign a different code. The acronym NOS is the same as "unspecified."

EXAMPLE
S01.91xA   Laceration without foreign body of unspecified part of head, initial encounter.

This code has a subcategory value of 9 (unspecified). Often, codes that end in 9 classify conditions that are unspecified.

> Essentially, NEC indicates a classification failure of the ICD-10-CM, and NOS indicates a documentation failure.

EXAMPLES
A22.9   Anthrax, unspecified.
Z80.9   Family history of malignant neoplasm, unspecified.
M85.069   Fibrous dysplasia, unspecified, lower leg.

CHECKPOINT 3.5

Code the following medical conditions in ICD-10-CM and identify the convention that applies: NEC or NOS.

	Code	Convention
1. Specified contraception management	_____	_____
2. Lipoma of unspecified site	_____	_____
3. Viral gastroenteritis	_____	_____
4. Accidental food poisoning, initial encounter	_____	_____
5. Specified malformation of the heart	_____	_____

Terms

Certain notes, words, or terms provide instruction to the coder regarding the meaning of codes, identify which conditions might be included or excluded, or provide additional information. Notes can also provide further clarification or definitions of disease. For example, see Notes at the beginning of Chapter 2 Neoplasms (C00–D49) that describe the functional activity and morphology of neoplasms.

Includes

The term *includes* refers to a list of terms that are included in that code. These additi[...] can provide further definition or give additional examples of conditions classified using [...] These terms can be found at the chapter level (i.e., the terms included apply to the entir[...] or they can be found at the other code levels (block, category, subcategory, etc.). Ther[...] includes note at the block level, such as for the block of tuberculosis codes, instructs the c[...] infection by *Mycobacterium tuberculosis* and *Mycobacterium bovis* are included for any code[...] from A15 to A19.

EXAMPLE
TUBERCULOSIS (A15–A19)

> **Includes:** Infections due to *Mycobacterium tuberculosis* and *Mycobacterium bovis.*

An includes note at the category level can provide definitions or examples for that category.

EXAMPLE
I65 OCCLUSION AND STENOSIS OF PRECEREBRAL ARTERIES, Not resulting in cerebral infarction

> **Includes:** Embolism of precerebral artery.
> Narrowing of precerebral artery.
> Obstruction (complete) (partial) of precerebral artery.
> Thrombosis of precerebral artery.

In this example, category I65 includes the conditions of embolism of precerebral artery.

EXAMPLE
M87 OSTEONECROSIS

> **Includes:** Avascular necrosis of bone.

Looking at the includes note at category M87 helps the coder know that osteonecrosis is classified the same as avascular necrosis of bone.

Excludes

There are two types of excludes notes in the Tabular List of Diseases and Injuries. These are denoted as "Excludes1" and "Excludes2."

"EXCLUDES1: An exception to the Excludes1 definition is the circumstance when the two conditions are unrelated to each other." An Excludes1 note refers to conditions that should be coded elsewhere. In other words, these conditions are not included in the code and should not be coded here, but coded elsewhere.

EXAMPLE
G43.0 MIGRAINE WITHOUT AURA

> Common migraine
> **Excludes1:** *chronic migraine without aura (G43.7-).*

In this example, the excludes note is at the subcategory level. This means that if documentation states that a migraine without an aura is specified as "chronic," then code G43.0 should not be assigned; rather, the code G43.7 should be assigned. These two conditions would not occur together.

EXCLUDES2: An Excludes2 note refers to conditions that are not included here and that condition should be classified elsewhere. The Excludes2 note also means that the condition excluded is not included in the condition represented, yet the patient may have both conditions. If documentation supports both conditions, then both codes can be assigned. Thus, the condition and the Excludes2 condition can both be reported.

EXAMPLE
F14 COCAINE-RELATED DISORDERS

> **Excludes2:** *other stimulant-related disorders (F15.-).*

The excludes note here is at the category level and states that other stimulant-related disorders are not included in cocaine-related disorders. Yet, if the patient has both types of disorders, codes from both categories F14 and F15 can be assigned.

[handwritten margin note: Never never]

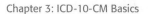

When documentation states the patient has one condition "with" another, this is interpreted to mean "associated with" or "due to" when it appears in a code title, Disease Index, or as an instructional note in the Tabular List. There is a presumption that a causal relationship exists between the two conditions when the two conditions or terms are linked in the Index or Tabular List. If the provider documentation states the conditions are not related, the code which combines the conditions cannot be assigned.

When two conditions are not specifically linked by the relational terms in the Index or Tabular, the documentation must state the association or link. If documentation supports that link, the coder assigns the code that relates the conditions. If not, the conditions are reported separately or the physician is queried to clarify the absence or presence of a relationship.

EXAMPLES
- Head injury and loss of consciousness, the coder would assign the combination code head injury with loss of consciousness (S06.9-).

- Gastrointestinal bleeding and sigmoid diverticulitis. Documentation by the provider must state linkage between these conditions in order to assign diverticulitis with bleeding (K57.33). If no linkage is documented, then the two conditions are reported separately: Gastrointestinal bleeding (K92.2) and sigmoid diverticulitis (K57.32).

Cross-References

In the ICD-10-CM Index, the terms *see* and *see also* indicate cross-references, meaning that the coder must look elsewhere to code a particular condition.

See
The cross-reference *see* refers the coder to another main term under which the information about a specific disease or injury will be found.

> When the cross-reference *see* appears, look at the new main term and all subterms listed. Subterms are separated by commas.

EXAMPLES
Parkinson's disease, syndrome, or tremor—*see Parkinsonism.*
Myringitis with otitis media—*see Otitis Media.*
Deformity, Dandy-Walker with spina bifida—*see Spina Bifida.*

Notice that the comma separates a main term from a subterm when the cross-reference refers to a more specific disease. In the example of deformity above, the coder would follow the cross-reference to the main term *Spina Bifida.*

See Also
The cross-reference term *see also* directs the coder to check another main term that may have additional information if the first main term the coder looks up does not provide a correct match for the diagnostic statement.

EXAMPLES
Paresthesia—*see also Disturbance, sensation.*
Dilatation, cardiac (acute) (chronic)—*see also Hypertrophy, cardiac.*
Neuroma—*see also Neoplasm, nerve, benign.*

In the first example, to code paresthesia of smell and taste, the cross-reference *Disturbance, sensation* tells the coder to go to the main term *Disturbance.* By following this cross-reference, the specific code for disturbance of smell and taste can be located (R43.8).

Punctuation

ICD-10-CM uses various punctuation marks that direct the coder to follow certain rules, provide additional meaning, or explain terms.

Answer the following questions using the Index and tabular List of ICD-10-CM.

1. What does the note at Chapter 13 instruct the coder to do? _____

2. What is the cross-reference used to code Crohn's disease? _____

3. What does the note refer to at category G43? _____

4. Which cross-reference should the coder follow when coding *depressive psychosis*?

   _____

5. What does the note specify at code S45? _____

6. Is the diagnosis of fainting classified as code R55? _____

7. Does code R68.11 include excessive crying of a child? _____

8. Which conditions are excluded (NOT CODED HERE) when reporting the code false labor (O47)?

   _____

9. Can codes N40.0 (enlarged prostate without lower urinary tract symptoms (LUTS)) and C61 (malignant neoplasm of the prostate) both be reported when documented for the same visit of the same patient? _____

10. Can Baker's cyst of the right knee, without rupture be classified using code M66.0?

    _____

Brackets [ ]

Brackets enclose manifestation codes and are located in the Index. Some conditions may require two codes, one for the etiology, the cause or origin of the condition, and a second for the manifestation, a disease resulting from a different underlying disease or disorder. For example, Parkinson's disease (underlying cause) can manifest to dementia. When brackets appear, both codes must be reported; the etiology code should be listed first and the manifestation code in brackets reported second.

EXAMPLE
Parkinsonism . . .
Dementia G31.83 [F02.80]

The Index entry above indicates that the diagnostic statement "Parkinson's dementia" requires two codes, one for the etiology (Parkinson's disease) and one for the manifestation (dementia).

EXAMPLE
Aphasia   R47.01

   Progressive isolated G31.01 [F02.80]

   In this example from the Index, both codes G31.01 and F02.80 should be reported. When these codes are verified in the Tabular List, code G31.01 represents Pick's disease (etiology) with the manifestation of dementia.

Parentheses ( )

Parentheses are used in both the Index and the Tabular List to enclose terms that are supplementary, that may or may not be present in the disease statement, and that do not affect code assignment. Parentheses are always used to enclose these nonessential terms.

Influenza (bronchial, epidemic, respiratory (upper)).
(unidentified influenza virus) J11.1.

Colon

The colon is used in the Tabular List after an incomplete term that needs one or more of the terms or modifiers that follow it in order to assign a code. These are used sparingly and may depend on the codebook's publisher.

Comma

Words in the Index following a comma are *essential* modifiers. These words must be present in the documentation in order to assign that code. Commas separate descriptive terms as shown in the following example.

EXAMPLE

Obstruction, lacteal, with steatorrhea K90.2

The example above, which depicts the Index at the main term "obstruction" and subterm "lacteal," shows that in order to assign the code K90.2 documentation must include the presence of steatorrhea.

Typeface

Boldface and *italic* type are special typeface settings that provide coding instructions.

Bold: Boldface print is used to identify main terms and titles in the Alphabetic Index. Bold type in the Tabular List depicts each code and code title.

Italics: In the Tabular List of Diseases and Injuries, *italics* may indicate an excludes note, as discussed earlier.

NOTE: Sequencing of multiple codes is covered in Chapter 4 of this text.

CHECKPOINT 3.7

Apply the ICD-10-CM punctuation and typeface conventions to answer the following questions.

1. Would the diagnosis of tropical sprue be classified to code K90.1? _____

2. Which two codes should be reported when coding Lewy body dementia? (*Hint*: Report in the correct sequence.) _____

3. When reporting the external cause of injury as "cutting," does the specific body part cut impact the code assignment? (*Hint*: See the Index to External Causes.) _____
   _____

4. When looking up the main term *Stenosis*, subterm *colon*, in the Index, does the documentation need to support that this is a congenital disorder when assigning code Q42.9?
   _____

5. Would the diagnosis of acute coronary embolism without myocardial infarction be classified to code I24.0? _____

6. Does code L97.101 include a chronic topical ulcer of unspecified thigh limited to breakdown of skin? _____

7. Can alcoholic cirrhosis of the liver be reported using code K74.3? _____

8. Code poorly controlled diabetes mellitus, type 2. _____

9. What is the significance of the terms in parentheses located at the main term *bronchitis*?
   _____

10. Code anterior dislocation of the lens, left eye. _____

Instructional Notations

ICD-10-CM also includes terms that are instructional in nature. These notations tell the coder to do something (e.g., use an additional code); these notations are found in the Tabular List.

Use Additional Code

The instruction *use additional code* tells the coder to also code further information if it is documented. For example, in the Tabular List, this instruction means to use an additional code for a condition if in fact that condition is documented.

> ### EXAMPLE
> **H44.0 Purulent endophthalmitis.**
> **Use additional code** to identify organism.

This notation instructs the coder that the organism causing panophthalmitis should be coded if it is identified in the documentation. The following example shows the notation instructing the coder to identify report of any associated fever with sickle-cell disorders.

> ### EXAMPLE
> **D57 SICKLE-CELL DISORDERS.**
> **Use additional code** for any associated fever (R50.81).
> **D57.0 Hb-SS disease with crisis, unspecified.**
> **D57.01 Hb-SS disease with acute chest pain syndrome.**

Code First

The instruction *code first* is located only in the Tabular List with codes that are not intended to be selected as a primary diagnosis because they are manifestations of other underlying diseases. Sometimes, these codes are in italics. The underlying disease or disorder or drug should be coded first, when applicable, followed by the code with the notation *Code First*.

> ### EXAMPLE
> F06 Other mental disorders due to known physiological condition.
>   Code first the underlying physiological condition.

Code F06.1 should be coded second, and the underlying physiological condition code (e.g., endocrine disorder) should be coded and sequenced first.

Code Also

The instructional notation *Code also* is found only in the Tabular List. This note instructs that two codes may be required to fully describe a condition, but there is no sequencing direction as noted in "Code first" or "Use additional code." It is located at any code level and instructs the coder to code another diagnosis, yet either code can be listed first.

> ### EXAMPLE
> S51 Open wound of elbow and forearm
>   Code also any associated wound infection.

In the above example, a patient may have an open wound of the elbow and an infection of that wound. In this case, two codes would be reported: one for the wound and another code for the infection (S51.002A and L08.9)—*see* infection, skin.

Code Assignment and Clinical Criteria

A new instructional notation was added to the *Official Coding Guidelines* in 2017 which advises the coder to report conditions based on provider documentation rather than clinical criteria. The provider's statement that the patient has a condition, is sufficient to report that condition, keeping in mind all other coding conventions and guidelines. Code assignment is not based on clinical criteria used by the provider to establish the diagnosis.

For example: The diagnosis of urinary tract infection documented by the provider is sufficient to report the code N39.0 even in the absence of clinical signs or symptoms or positive urine culture.

CHECKPOINT 3.8

Using all sections of ICD-10-CM, indicate whether each of the following statements is *true* or *false*.

1. The sequencing of the following codes is correct: L24.0, T49.0x5A. _____

2. Solar urticaria due to ultraviolet radiation is reported using code L56.3. _____

3. Moderate persistent asthma with acute exacerbation due to exposure to secondhand tobacco smoke is reported using codes J45.41 and Z77.22. _____

4. Code F04 should always be listed first. _____

5. The instruction "code also" dictates sequencing of codes. _____

Code the following medical conditions in ICD-10-CM.

6. Acute cystitis due to *Escherichia coli* (*E. coli*) _____

7. Benign prostatic hypertrophy with lower urinary tract symptom of urinary retention.

   _____

8. Alcohol abuse with uncomplicated intoxication, blood alcohol level is 65 mg/100 mL.

   _____

9. Bilateral Kearns-Sayre syndrome with heart block. _____

10. Encounter for adequacy testing for hemodialysis in a patient with end-stage renal disease.

    _____

Tables

Two tables in ICD-10-CM are used to provide an organized structure for the coding of neoplasms, drugs and chemicals. The format of each table is based on the need to classify different types of conditions, sites, or circumstances.

Table of Neoplasms

Neoplasm codes can be located two different ways in the Index. The first way may be by morphology, meaning the histological type such as carcinoma, sarcoma, adenoma, or histiocytoma and the code is identified in the Index. The second listing is found in the Table of Neoplasms. The coder must always be directed to the neoplasms table when coding first by morphology. The table is organized alphabetically by body or anatomical site. The first column lists the anatomical location, and the next six columns relate to the behavior of the neoplasm, described as a malignant tumor, a benign tumor, a tumor of uncertain behavior, or a tumor of unspecified nature.

There are three types of malignant tumors. Each is progressive, rapid growing, life threatening, and made of cancerous cells:

1. *Primary*: The neoplasm is the site of origin.
2. *Secondary*: The neoplasm has metastasized (spread) to an additional body site from the site of origin.
3. *Carcinoma in situ*: The neoplasm is restricted to one site (a noninvasive type); this may also be referred to as *preinvasive cancer*.

A benign tumor is slow growing, not life threatening, and is made of normal or near-normal cells. A tumor of uncertain behavior was not classifiable when the cells were examined, and one of unspecified nature is one for which there is no documentation of the nature of the neoplasm. Coders will need familiarity with these diseases, which are reviewed in the Pathophysiology Connection on cancer.

The following entries from the neoplasms table are for a neoplasm of the lower lobe of the lung:

	MALIGNANT PRIMARY	MALIGNANT SECONDARY	CANCER *IN SITU*	BENIGN	UNCERTAIN	UNSPECIFIED BEHAVIOR
Lung, lower lobe	C34.3-	C78.0-	D02.2-	D14.3-	D38.1	D49.1

Table of Drugs and Chemicals

The Table of Drugs and Chemicals is used to classify poisoning, adverse effects, or underdosing, which are conditions caused by the use or underuse of a drug or chemical. The table is organized alphabetically by drug or chemical name. Columns across the table provide codes to identify that a poisoning, adverse effect, or underdosing has occurred.

CHECKPOINT 3.9

Using the ICD-10-CM, answer the following questions.

1. Which type of term is used as a subterm in the neoplasm table: *site, etiology,* or *manifestation*?

   _____

2. What is the code for benign neoplasm of the left lower female breast? _____

3. What is the accidental poisoning code for aspirin seen for the initial encounter? _____

4. Starting with the main term *Sarcoma*, report the code for sarcoma of the left arm. _____

5. How would an underdose of digoxin be reported (subsequent encounter)? _____

ICD-10-CM CODING RESOURCES

To assign ICD-10-CM codes correctly, the coder must use the current code set and follow the *Official Guidelines*. Correct coding also requires a variety of resources for understanding the medical terms, diseases, and procedures to assign accurate ICD-10-CM codes.

AHA Coding Clinic® for ICD-10-CM

AHA Coding Clinic® for ICD-10-CM is published by the AHA. The AHA Central Office handles all ICD-10-CM coding-related issues and works with NCHS and CMS to maintain integrity of the coding system. *AHA Coding Clinic* provides advice on coding certain diseases.

The *AHA Coding Clinic* is published quarterly or as needed and can be purchased from the AHA. The coding advice is approved by CMS for Medicare reimbursement and is also accepted by many other payers.

> INTERNET RESOURCE: AHA *Coding Clinic*® *for ICD-10-CM*
> www.aha.org/aha/issues/Medicare/IPPS/coding.html

NCHS Website

A list of all ICD-10-CM diagnosis code changes can be found at the NCHS website. Also available is an ICD-10-CM conversion table that shows new and replaced codes used to classify the same conditions. This ICD-10-CM conversion table includes code changes made between 1986 and the current year. Coders use this resource to update old codes reported in earlier years. For example, dehydration was coded differently before 2005 than it is today (it is currently coded as E86.0).

> INTERNET RESOURCE: ICD-10-CM Code Conversion Table
> www.cdc.gov/nchs/icd/icd9cm_addenda_guidelines.htm

PATHOPHYSIOLOGY CONNECTION

Cancer

Cancer is a general term for any of a number of diseases with malignant growths. *Tumors* or *neoplasms* are growths. *Benign* growths are generally located within a limited area and do not spread. *Malignant* growths sometimes spread within the organ or part in which they originate. If they spread to other organs or parts, they are said to *metastasize*.

Neoplasms are grouped according to whether they are *primary* (located in a specific originating site, except for lymphatic tissue), *primary of lymphatic tissue*, *secondary* (originating from another site), *unspecified* (as to location), *benign*, *carcinoma in situ* (meaning a localized cluster of malignant cells), or of *uncertain behavior*. In addition, neoplasms are categorized by where they occur, such as *abdominopelvic, brain,* and *breast.* Subcategories within the sites indicate more specific locations (e.g., brain cancer is sub-categorized as *basal ganglia, cerebrum, cerebellum, midbrain,* and so on).

Neoplasms are also *staged* (graded) by the TNM system. *T* stands for tumor; *N* stands for spread to the lymph nodes; and *M* stands for metastasis (spreading to other sites). The TNM system rates tumors from 1 to 4 depending on the severity of the malignancy.

Cancer is the second leading cause of death in the United States, following heart disease, the number one killer. The most deadly form of cancer is lung cancer.

Common Cancers

Cancer can occur anywhere in the body. For women, breast, cervical, and ovarian cancers occur frequently. *Breast cancer* is classified by *glandular tissue* or *soft tissue,* and it is categorized by location (such as the quadrant or the nipple). *Cervical cancer* is categorized by location (*endocervix* or *external os,* for example). *Ovarian cancer* may be categorized according to the parts involved, such as *fallopian tube* or *parametrium.*

For men, *prostate cancer* may be aggressive and require treatment, or it may be slow growing and just need watching. *Testicular cancer* is more common in men who have had an undescended testicle or abnormal testicular development.

Lung cancer is widespread, especially among smokers. It is categorized by location (e.g., *middle lobe* or *main bronchus*). *Colon cancer* is also categorized by location (e.g., *sigmoid* or *ascending*).

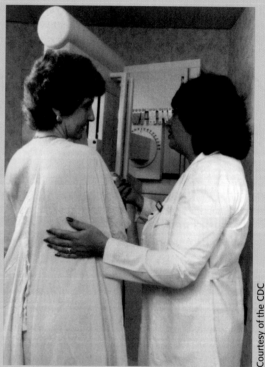

A mammogram.

Courtesy of the CDC

Some glandular cancers can be fairly contained and easily treated; for example, *thyroid cancer* usually requires surgical removal and limited treatment, followed by hormone replacement. However, other cancers such as *pancreatic cancer,* are difficult to treat and are usually fatal.

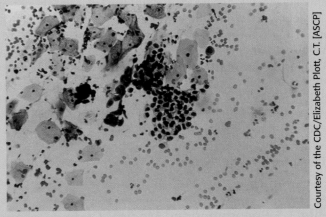

A cancer cell.

Skin cancer is categorized by location, such as *hand* or *thigh.* Moles on the skin are either benign or malignant (the latter are usually dark and irregular). Skin cancer is on the rise as a result of increasing exposure to ultraviolet rays from the sun.

Leukemia is a general term for blood or bone marrow cancer. Leukemias are classified either *without mention of remission* or *with remission.* They are either *acute* (having an overgrowth of immature blood cells) or *chronic* (having an overgrowth of mature blood cells). There is also an early stage of leukemia called *myelodysplastic syndrome (MDS)* in which bone marrow does not produce enough blood cells.

Cancer Prevention and Treatment

Cancer is not always preventable; however, avoidance of *carcinogens* (things that are known to cause cancer) is the best way to prevent it. Some known carcinogens are tobacco smoke, asbestos, ultraviolet rays of the sun, and certain chemicals. The next best thing to total avoidance is early detection. Some symptoms clearly indicate possible cancer: rectal bleeding; dark, irregular skin moles; breast lumps; and persistent coughing of unknown cause. Other symptoms are more subtle, but can be detected by cancer screenings, now common procedures. Mammograms (breast cancer screening) are recommended at certain intervals for women depending on age and family history. Prostate-specific antigen (PSA) tests (prostate cancer screening) are routine for males at certain ages and with certain histories. A colonoscopy provides a clear picture of any suspicious polyps. Chest x-rays can detect lung cancer, and MRIs and CAT scans can see tumors in various locations.

Cancer treatment has advanced greatly in the early 21st century. Radical surgeries are still sometimes necessary, but radiation and chemotherapy have replaced some surgical procedures. New targeted therapies, such as hormone receptor treatments, show promise for limiting tumor growth in certain cases.

Medical References

A basic understanding of medical terms, the disease process, and current medical procedures is required in medical coding, but no one can possibly remember all the medical terms and anatomy, physiology, disease, and procedural information. It is important for coders to have references available to help when a documented health issue needs further investigation. For example, if a medical record includes terms a coder has never seen before, a medical dictionary would be helpful. If a physician documents a blockage of a specific artery, the coder may need to consult an anatomy book to locate that artery in the vascular system.

Documented medications can be investigated in a drug manual to determine the category of drug. Internet research is helpful in understanding new technology in the treatment of disease. Researching and understanding a new medical technique can help a coder assign the correct ICD-10-CM diagnosis code. Pathophysiology books discuss the disease process and treatment, including the signs and symptoms of disease. Table 3.5 is a basic listing of medical references used by coders.

Table 3.5 Recommended Medical Coding Resources

CODING RESOURCE	INFORMATION
CD-10-CM Official Guidelines for Coding and Reporting	Contains the most current rules for ICD-10-CM coding.
AHA Coding Clinic® for ICD-10-CM	Provides advice on ICD-10 coding issues.
AMA CPT Assistant	Provides advice on CPT coding issues.
Centers for Medicare and Medicaid website at www.cms.gov	Lists most current ICD-10-PCS procedure codes.
National Center for Health Statistics website at www.cdc.gov/nchs	Lists most current ICD-10-CM diagnosis codes (Volumes 1 and 2).
Medical dictionaries	Define medical terms.
Anatomy and physiology books	Identify location of body organs and explain different body systems.
Pathophysiology books	Explain the disease process.
Drug references	List medications and their actions, indications, and side effects.
Abbreviation books	List abbreviations and their meanings.
Internet medical sites	Provide resources for new technology and endless health-care information.
Medical terminology books	Define medical terms.

Computer-Aided Coding

Today many larger health-care facilities use computer programs to assign ICD-10-CM codes. This computer-aided coding software called an "encoder" can be based on the logic behind selecting codes or on a computerized version of the actual ICD-10-CM code set.

Logic-based encoders contain a system of questions and answers that help the coder assign the correct ICD-10-CM code. Book-based encoders provide computerized versions of the actual ICD-10-CM codebook, allowing the coder to access the Tabular List and Index on screen. Built into these software encoding systems are alerts, edits, and references. For example, if the coder enters an invalid ICD-10-CM code, the software alerts the coder to make a correction. If the coder selects a code for a male when the patient is female, the encoder system alerts the coder about that error. Other edits alert the coder that two codes cannot be reported together in combination, or that an additional digit is required. References to *Coding Clinic* and *CPT Assistant* can also be linked to codes in the Tabular List, allowing the coder to access specific guidelines immediately. CPT codes for procedures are covered in Part III of this text.

The use of encoders does not replace the need for knowledge of the ICD-10-CM coding guidelines. These computer-aided systems provide a tool for coders that can be useful to improve consistency, efficiency, and accuracy by putting alerts, edits, and references at the coder's fingertips. A list of diagnosis codes and their descriptions in a billing software package or file is not the same as using an encoder. The list in billing software primarily includes the diagnoses most commonly used in a physician's practice. It does not contain specific coding edits, alerts, or references.

Computer-Assisted Coding Systems (CACS)

A computer-assisted coding system (CACS) is a computer software application that analyzes health-care documents and produces appropriate medical codes for specific phrases and terms within the electronic document. For example, the CACS could code hypertension (I10) from an electronic history and physical by recognizing the medical term. This software uses natural language processing (NLP) to highlight key phrases in the electronic health-care document. The CACS also analyze the context to determine whether an instance requires coding. For example, the software can determine that the term "hypertension" requires a diagnosis code, yet text stating "family history of hypertension" would not be coded. A CACS is especially efficient to assist in straightforward coding, allowing the coders to perform coding for more complex scenarios. With the expansion of electronic health records, computer-assisted coding systems can be implemented and aid in the transition to ICD-10-CM.

CHECKPOINT 3.10

Using the coding resources listed in Table 3.5, identify a resource that could be used to find the medical information below.

1. The meaning of *CHF* _____
2. Coding advice regarding a patient who has uncontrolled diabetes _____
3. The medical indications for the drug Zantac _____
4. The ICD-10-CM code changes effective October 1, 2015 _____
5. The signs and symptoms of gastric ulcer _____
6. In which part of the body the talus is located _____
7. The code for sleep apnea effective October 1, 2005 _____
8. The latest technology for heart transplants _____
9. The rules for sequencing ICD-10-CM diagnosis codes _____
10. Medical term for gallbladder removal _____

Chapter Summary

1. ICD-10-CM is the *International Classification of Diseases, Tenth Revision, Clinical Modification*. This coding system is modeled after the *International Classification of Disease, Ninth Revision*, which is maintained by the World Health Organization. ICD-10-CM can be traced to 1959, when the U.S. Public Health Service published the *International Classification of Diseases, Adapted for Indexing of Hospital Records and Operation Classification* (ICDA). Over the years, the ICDA was revised, updated, and adapted for the United States as ICD-10-CM. This code set contains more than 71,000 codes and is updated annually.

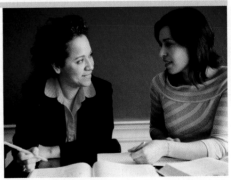

2. The responsibility for maintaining ICD-10-CM is divided between the National Center for Health Statistics (NCHS) and the Centers for Disease Control and Prevention (CDC). The ICD-10-CM Coordination and Maintenance Committee considers proposed coding modifications to ICD-10-CM. In order to maintain the coding system, the cooperating parties, which represent NCHS, CMS, AHIMA, and AHA, meet regularly. Interested parties from either the public or private sectors can propose a change in ICD-10-CM. Changes to ICD-10-CM are published annually on October 1 and April 1.

3. The best way to keep up to date on ICD-10-CM code changes is to use the Internet. The website for ICD-10-CM updates from the National Center for Health Care Statistics (www.cdc.gov/nchs/icd/icd10cm.htm) contains the latest information on ICD-10-CM codes. This website includes a crosswalk tool from old codes to new codes called GEMs. The website also includes the addenda and updated guidelines.

4. ICD-10-CM is the medical coding system used throughout the United States for reporting medical conditions and factors influencing health status. The code set is used to transform medical words into code numbers for data reporting. The ICD-10-CM codes are used by a variety of health-care providers, payers, and agencies for data reporting. The actual coded data are used for health-care payment, health-care communication, measurement of health-care quality, research and education, and administrative decision making.

5. For all health-care providers to use ICD-10-CM accurately and consistently, national guidelines for its use must be followed. ICD-10-CM guidelines are published in the *ICD-10-CM Official Guidelines for Coding and Reporting*, and HIPAA legislation mandates their use effective October 1, 2015. The guidelines address basic coding steps, conventions, sequencing, and chapter-specific guidelines. National guidelines provide coders with consistent, comprehensive instructions on the use of ICD-10-CM.

6. The structure and content of ICD-10-CM differs depending on which part of ICD-10-CM is being used. For example, the Alphabetic Index is formatted in four main sections: The Index to Diseases and Injuries, Table of Neoplasms, Table of Drugs and Chemicals, External Causes of Injuries Index. The Tabular List of Diseases and Injuries contains 21 chapters organized by code.

7. The format of an ICD-10-CM code consists of three to seven characters with a decimal point after the third character. All codes begin with a letter (except U) and may contain letters or numbers for the additional characters. The use of placeholder characters allows for this new format. Conventions, or rules of coding, are specific to the use of ICD-10-CM. For example, punctuation such as parentheses, brackets, and colons instruct the coder. Other conventions such as notes, includes, and excludes instruct the coder regarding certain conditions and how those conditions should be coded. Cross-references and terms such as *see* and *see also* provide instructions. It is imperative to understand and apply these conventions in order to assign codes accurately.

8. The basic coding process begins with review of complete medical documentation and abstraction of conditions. Each condition is coded by identifying the main term representing it. The main term is one word in the diagnostic statement that the coder uses to find the code. Indented subterms are used to provide specificity in coding a condition. Once a code has been located in the Index, that code is verified in the Tabular List. All conventions and instructions must be followed for accuracy in coding.

9. The requirement to code to the highest level of specificity means that the most digits available for a particular category must be assigned. The use of a fourth-, fifth-, sixth- or seventh-digit extension is prominent throughout ICD-10-CM. The fourth, fifth, or sixth digits assigned to a particular category may have an indented format, and instructions to use a seventh digit can be located in notes. Remember to always code to the highest level of specificity.

10. Having the resources to assign ICD-10-CM codes accurately is essential. Access to national coding guidelines, published coding advice, medical dictionaries, and medical Internet sites and use of encoders are some of the resources coders use to keep current with medical practice, understand medical documentation, and assign accurate codes.

Matching

Match the key terms with their definitions.

A. WHO
B. cooperating parties
C. *ICD-10-CM Official Guidelines for Coding and Reporting*
D. External Cause of Injuries Index
E. brackets

F. block
G. includes note
H. subcategory
I. colon
J. letter "x"

1. _____ Coding convention that encloses codes that should be reported second; these codes rep___ manifestation of a disease

2. _____ Organization responsible for maintaining ICD-9 and ICD-10

3. _____ Character used as a placeholder

4. _____ An ICD-10-CM code with five digits

5. _____ Publication that contains rules on ICD-10-CM coding and sequencing

6. _____ A range of codes within a chapter

7. _____ A coding convention that combines a term on the left with a term on the right

8. _____ A coding convention that instructs the coder that these conditions are not excluded

9. _____ The group of organizations that includes representatives from the NCHS, CMS, AHIMA, and AHA

10. _____ A portion of ICD-10-CM, the Index of Diseases and Injuries

True or False

Decide whether each statement is true or false.

1. __F__ A coder is finished coding once a code is found in the Index.

2. __F__ ICD-10-CM codes are never used for health-care reimbursement.

3. __T__ HIPAA legislation mandates the use of ICD-10-CM.

4. __F__ ICD-10-CM codes are updated annually on January 1.

5. __T__ A Z code can never be used as a principal diagnosis.

6. __T__ The first step in assigning an ICD-10-CM code is reviewing complete documentation.

7. __T__ When coding to the highest level of specificity, the coder must assign a code using the most digits available.

8. __F__ The comma is a convention used in ICD-10-CM to list nonessential modifiers.

9. __F__ An encoder can replace a knowledgeable coder.

10. __F__ The Tabular List of ICD-10-CM has 20 chapters.

Multiple Choice

Select the letter that best completes the statement or answers the question.

1. Which code(s) would be used to classify an individual with insulin-dependent type 2 diabetes with diabetic polyneuropathy?
   A. E11.42
   B. E11.610, Z79.4
   C. E11.42, Z79.4
   D. E11.40, Z79.4

2. Which convention instructs the coder to go to a different word in the Alphabetic Index?
    A. Bold typeface
    B. Parentheses
    C. See
    D. Code first

3. Which of the following codes are invalid (may be more than one)?
    A. I22.9
    B. I11.9
    C. S84.111A
    D. S89.019

4. Which codes represent initial encounter for open fracture of the distal tibia due to fall from a ladder at home?
    A. S82.90xB, W11.xxxA, Y92.9
    B. S82.309, W19.xxxA, Y92.9
    C. S82.899A, W19.xxxA, Y92.009
    D. S82.309B, W11.xxxA, Y92.009

5. Which codes represent acute pyelonephritis due to pseudomonas in a patient with a history of urinary tract infections?
    A. N10, B96.5, Z87.410
    B. N11, B95.0, Z80.59
    C. N10, B95.0, Z80.59
    D. N10, B96.5, Z87.440

6. Code A54.00 describes which disease?
    A. Gonorrhea not otherwise specified
    B. Acute gonococcal infection of the lower genitourinary tract
    C. Gonococcal urethritis
    D. All of the above

7. Which code or codes represent acute and chronic cholecystitis with choledocholithiasis?
    A. K81.2, K80.66
    B. K80.44
    C. K80.46
    D. K80.50, K81.2

8. Which codes represent hypertension with stage V chronic kidney disease?
    A. I13.11, N18.5
    B. I12.0, N18.5
    C. I12.9, N18.5
    D. I13.0, N18.5

9. Which E code would be assigned when coding an initial encounter for suicide attempt by morphine?
    A. T40.2x1A
    B. T40.2x5A
    C. T40.2x2A
    D. T40.2x3A

10. Which of the following represents pyrophosphate crystal–induced arthritis of the left knee?
    A. M11.879
    B. M11.859
    C. M11.862
    D. M11.869

CHAPTER 4

ICD-10-CM Coding Guidelines

CHAPTER OUTLINE

Official Guidelines Content

General Coding Guidelines: Inpatient and Outpatient

Selection of Principal Diagnosis/Additional Diagnoses for the Inpatient Setting

Present on Admission (POA) Guidelines

LEARNING OUTCOMES

After studying the general coding guidelines in this chapter, you should be able to:

1. Understand the content and source of the ICD-10-CM General Coding Guidelines. Describe how the correct coding process uses both the Index and the Tabular List to assign codes.
2. Understand the concept of level of detail.
3. Explain the coding of conditions that are an integral part of the disease process.
4. Explain the coding of conditions that are not an integral part of the disease process.
5. Differentiate coding guidelines for multiple codes and combination codes.
6. Understand the guidelines for coding acute and chronic conditions.
7. Explain the rules governing the coding of the sequelae (late effects) of previous diseases and conditions.
8. Understand the coding implications of diagnostic terms stated as *impending* or *threatened*.

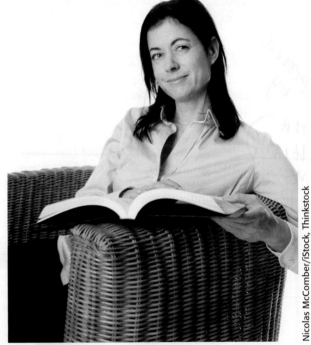

Nicolas McComber/iStock, Thinkstock

studying the inpatient coding sections in this chapter, you should be able to:

scuss the importance of the UHDDS and its relationship to diagnostic coding.

escribe the patient care flow and associated documentation in the inpatient setting.

fine the term *principal diagnosis* as it relates to the inpatient setting.

scribe the specific sequencing rule that is followed when multiple diagnoses are documented.

5. Apply diagnostic coding sequencing rules to these coding situations:
   (a) two or more principal diagnoses
   (b) treatment plan not carried out
   (c) complications
   (d) uncertain diagnoses
6. Describe the guidelines for selecting the principal diagnosis following admission from an observation unit or from an outpatient surgery.
7. Discuss the criteria for reporting additional diagnoses.
8. Define *POA* and describe how it is assigned.
9. Based on diagnostic statements, correctly assign diagnosis codes for the inpatient setting.

The Health Insurance Portability and Accountability Act (HIPAA) mandates the use of ICD-10-CM to report codes for diseases, injuries, impairments, and other health-related problems. As every beginning coder has learned, knowing the basics of how to select codes from the ICD-10-CM Alphabetic Index and Tabular List is only the first step toward coding competency. Moving ahead requires familiarity with the *ICD-10-CM Official Guidelines for Coding and Reporting*.

This chapter covers the basic coding guidelines found in Sections IB, II, III, and IV of the *ICD-10-CM Official Guidelines for Coding and Reporting*. The major benefit of the national standard for reporting is data consistency. Adherence to these guidelines when assigning ICD-10-CM diagnosis codes is required under HIPAA.

OFFICIAL GUIDELINES CONTENT

The *ICD-10-CM Official Guidelines for Coding and Reporting* (called the *Official Guidelines* for short) have these sections:

I   Conventions, General Coding Guidelines, and Chapter-Specific Guidelines
II   Selection of Principal Diagnosis
III   Reporting Additional Diagnoses
IV   Diagnostic Coding and Reporting Guidelines for Outpatient Services
Appendix I   Present on Admission Reporting Guidelines

As stated in the preface to the *Official Guidelines*:

> These guidelines have been approved by the four organizations that make up the Cooperating Parties for the ICD-10-CM: the American Hospital Association (AHA), the American Health Information Management Association (AHIMA), CMS [the Centers for Medicare and Medicaid Services], and NCHS [the National Center for Health Statistics].

The *Official Guidelines* are updated as necessitated by newly released ICD-10-CM codes. Coders should be sure they are using the current version. The version used in your text is available at www.cdc.gov/nchs/data/icd/icd10cm_guidelines_2018.pdf

These guidelines are a set of rules that have been developed to accompany and complement the official conventions and instructions provided within the ICD-10-CM itself. The instructions and conventions of the classification take precedence over the guidelines. These guidelines are based on the coding and sequencing instructions in the Tabular List and Alphabetic Index of ICD-10-CM, but provide additional instruction. Because code assignment is based on provider documentation, a joint effort is required between the provider and coder to achieve accurate and complete coded diagnostic data. The guidelines have been developed to support consistent, accurate, and complete diagnosis code reporting after review of the entire medical record.

Understanding these guidelines is essential in assigning accurate ICD-10-CM codes and sequencing them correctly. These guidelines also assist the coder with decisions regarding reporting additional conditions that may coexist or a history of a condition or medical status that should be reported. The basic guidelines clarify the use of both the Alphabetic Index and Tabular List and the need to code to the highest level of specificity. Guidelines also address the coding of conditions that may or may not be integral to a disease process. The coder learns when to assign multiple codes for a single condition and when to assign combination codes to reflect multiple conditions. The rules on coding both acute and chronic conditions are covered, as are the definition of sequelae (late effects) and the way to code conditions that are impending or threatened. When assigning codes in the inpatient setting, additional information regarding the presence on admission for each diagnosis code is collected. The additional inpatient coding qualifier "Present on Admission" is reviewed in this chapter because different values may impact the Medicare payment system.

GENERAL CODING GUIDELINES: INPATIENT AND OUTPATIENT

Section I.B of the *Official Guidelines*, as shown in Box 4.1, includes general coding guidelines, which apply to all settings and all providers of health care. For example, physicians, hospitals, and nursing homes would all utilize these guidelines for diagnosis reporting. The guidelines apply whether coding in the outpatient or the inpatient setting.

Use of Both the Index and the Tabular List

> The Index drives code assignment; verification of codes is completed using the Tabular List.

Points 1 and 2 of the General Coding Guidelines (see Box 4.1), explain the basic correct coding process. The coder must use both the Alphabetic Index and the Tabular List when locating and assigning codes and must not rely solely on only one or the other, because errors will occur in code assignment if only one section of the codebook is used. For example, by

---

BOX 4.1 Section I.B, General Coding Guidelines

1. Locating a Code in the ICD-10-CM
To select a code in the classification that corresponds to a diagnosis or reason for visit documented in a medical record, first locate the term in the Index, and then verify the code in the Tabular List. Read and be guided by instructional notations that appear in both the Index and the Tabular List.

It is essential to use both the Index and Tabular List when locating and assigning a code. The Index does not always provide the full code. Selection of the full code, including laterality and any applicable seventh character can only be done in the Tabular List. A dash (-) at the end of an Index entry indicates that additional characters are required. Even if a dash is not included at the Index entry, it is necessary to refer to the Tabular List to verify that no seventh character is required.

2. Level of Detail in Coding
Diagnosis codes are to be used and reported at their highest number of characters available.

ICD-10-CM diagnosis codes are composed of codes with 3, 4, 5, 6, or 7 characters. Codes with three characters are included in ICD-10-CM as the heading of a category of codes that may be further subdivided by the use of fourth and/or fifth characters and/or sixth characters, which provide greater detail.

A three-character code is to be used only if it is not further subdivided. A code is invalid if it has not been coded to the full number of characters required for that code, including the seventh character, if applicable.

3. Code or Codes From A00.0 Through T88.9, Z00–Z99.8
The appropriate code or codes from A00.0 through T88.9, Z00–Z99.8 must be used to identify diagnoses, symptoms, conditions, problems, complaints, or other reason(s) for the encounter/visit.

4. Signs and Symptoms
Codes that describe symptoms and signs, as opposed to diagnoses, are acceptable for reporting purposes when a related definitive diagnosis has not been established (confirmed) by the provider. Chapter 18 of ICD-10-CM, Symptoms, Signs, and Abnormal Clinical and Laboratory Findings, Not Elsewhere Classified (codes R00.0–R99) contains many, but not all codes for symptoms.
See Section I.B.18 Use of Signs/Symptom/Unspecified Codes

5. Conditions That Are an Integral Part of a Disease Process
Signs and symptoms that are associated routinely with a disease process should not be assigned as additional codes, unless otherwise instructed by the classification.

Continued

BOX 4.1 *Continued*

6. Conditions That Are Not an Integral Part of a Disease Process

Additional signs and symptoms that may not be associated routinely with a disease process should be coded when present.

7. Multiple Coding for a Single Condition

In addition to the etiology/manifestation convention that requires two codes to fully describe a single condition that affects multiple body systems, there are other single conditions that also require more than one code. "Use additional code" notes are found in the Tabular List at codes that are not part of an etiology/manifestation pair where a secondary code is useful to fully describe a condition. The sequencing rule is the same as the etiology/manifestation pair, "use additional code" indicates that a secondary code should be added, if known.

For example, for bacterial infections that are not included in Chapter 1, a secondary code from category B95, Streptococcus, Staphylococcus, and Enterococcus, as the cause of diseases classified elsewhere, or B96, Other bacterial agents as the cause of diseases classified elsewhere, may be required to identify the bacterial organism causing the infection. A "use additional code" note will normally be found at the infectious disease code, indicating a need for the organism code to be added as a secondary code.

"Code first" notes are also under certain codes that are not specifically manifestation codes but may be due to an underlying cause. When there is a "code first" note and an underlying condition is present, the underlying condition should be sequenced first, if known.

"Code, if applicable, any causal condition first" notes indicate that this code may be assigned as a principal diagnosis when the causal condition is unknown or not applicable. If a causal condition is known, then the code for that condition should be sequenced as the principal or first-listed diagnosis.

Multiple codes may be needed for sequela, complication codes and obstetric codes to more fully describe a condition. See the specific guidelines for these conditions for further instruction.

8. Acute and Chronic Conditions

If the same condition is described as both acute (subacute) and chronic, and separate subentries exist in the Index at the same indentation level, code both and sequence the acute (subacute) code first.

9. Combination Code

A combination code is a single code used to classify

Two diagnoses, or

A diagnosis with an associated secondary process (manifestation)

A diagnosis with an associated complication

Combination codes are identified by referring to subterm entries in the Index and by reading the inclusion and exclusion notes in the Tabular List.

Assign only the combination code when that code fully identifies the diagnostic conditions involved or when the Index so directs. Multiple coding should not be used when the classification provides a combination code that clearly identifies all of the elements documented in the diagnosis. When the combination code lacks necessary specificity in describing the manifestation or complication, an additional code should be used as a secondary code.

10. Sequelae (Late Effects)

A sequela is the residual effect (condition produced) after the acute phase of an illness or injury has terminated. There is no time limit on when a sequela code can be used. The residual may be apparent early, such as in cerebral infarction, or it may occur months or years later, such as that due to a previous injury. Coding of a sequela generally requires two codes sequenced in the following order: The condition or nature of the sequela is sequenced first. The sequela code is sequenced second.

An exception to the above guidelines are those instances where the code for the sequela is followed by a manifestation code identified in the Tabular List and title, or the sequela code has been expanded (at the fourth, fifth, or sixth character levels) to include the manifestation(s). The code for the acute phase of an illness or injury that led to the sequela is never used with a code for the late effect.

See Section I.C.9. Sequelae of cerebrovascular disease

See Section I.C.15. Sequelae of complication of pregnancy, childbirth and the puerperium

See Section I.C.19. Application of 7th characters for Chapter 19

11. Impending or Threatened Condition

Code any condition described at the time of discharge as "impending" or "threatened" as follows:

If it did occur, code as confirmed diagnosis.

If it did not occur, reference the Index to determine if the condition has a subentry term for "impending" or "threatened" and also reference main term entries for "Impending" and for "Threatened."

If the subterms are listed, assign the given code.

If the subterms are not listed, code the existing underlying condition(s) and not the condition described as impending or threatened.

12. Reporting Same Diagnosis Code More Than Once

Each unique ICD-10-CM diagnosis code may be reported only once for an encounter. This applies to bilateral conditions when there are no distinct codes identifying laterality or two different conditions classified to the same ICD-10-CM diagnosis code.

13. Laterality

Some ICD-10-CM codes indicate laterality, specifying whether the condition occurs on the left, right or is bilateral. If no bilateral code is provided and the condition is bilateral, assign separate codes for both the left and right side. If the side is not identified in the medical record, assign the code for the unspecified side.

When a patient has a bilateral condition and each side is treated during separate encounters, assign the "bilateral" code (as the condition still exists on both sides), including for the encounter to treat the first side. For the second encounter for treatment after one side has previously been treated and the condition no longer exists on that side, assign the appropriate unilateral code for the side where the condition still exists (e.g., cataract surgery performed on each eye in separate encounters). The bilateral code would not be assigned for the subsequent encounter, as the patient no longer has the condition in the previously-treated site. If the treatment on the first side did not completely resolve the condition, then the bilateral code would still be appropriate.

14. Documentation for BMI, *Depth of* Non-Pressure Ulcers, Pressure Ulcer Stages, Coma Scale, *and NIH Stroke Scale*

For the Body Mass Index (BMI), depth of non-pressure chronic ulcers, pressure ulcer stage, coma scale, and NIH stroke scale (NIHSS) codes, code assignment may be based on medical record documentation from clinicians who are not the patient's provider (i.e., physician or other qualified healthcare practitioner legally accountable for establishing the patient's diagnosis), since this information is typically documented by other clinicians involved in the care of the patient (e.g., a dietitian often documents the BMI, a nurse often documents the pressure ulcer stages, and an emergency medical technician often documents the coma scale). However, the associated diagnosis (such as overweight, obesity, acute stroke, or pressure ulcer) must be documented by the patient's provider. If there is conflicting medical record documentation, either from the same clinician or different clinicians, the patient's attending provider should be queried for clarification.

The BMI, coma scale, and NIHSS codes should only be reported as secondary diagnoses.

15. Syndromes

Follow the Index guidance when coding Syndromes. In the absence of Index guidance, assign codes for the documented manifestations of the Syndrome.

16. Documentation of Complications of Care

Code assignment is based on the provider's documentation of the relationship between the condition and the care or procedure, unless otherwise instructed by the classification. The guideline extends to any complications of care, regardless of the chapter the code is located in. It is important to note that not all conditions that occur during or following medical care or surgery are classified as complications. There must be a cause-and-effect relationship between the care provided and the condition, and an indication in the documentation that it is a complication. Query the provider for clarification, if the complication is not clearly documented.

17. Borderline Diagnosis

If the provider documents a "borderline" diagnosis at the time of discharge, the diagnosis is coded as confirmed, unless the classification provides a specific entry (e.g., borderline diabetes). If a borderline condition has a specific index entry in ICD-10-CM, it should be coded as such. Because borderline conditions are not uncertain diagnoses, no distinction is made between the care setting (inpatient versus outpatient). Whenever the documentation is unclear regarding a borderline condition, coders are encouraged to query for clarification.

18. Use of Sign/Symptom/Unspecified Codes

Sign/symptom and "unspecified" codes have acceptable, even necessary, uses. While specific diagnosis codes should be reported when they are supported by the available medical record documentation and clinical knowledge of the patient's health condition, there are instances when signs/symptoms or unspecified codes are the best choices for accurately reflecting the health-care encounter. Each health-care encounter should be coded to the level of certainty known for that encounter.

If a definitive diagnosis has not been established by the end of the encounter, it is appropriate to report codes for sign(s) and/or symptom(s) in lieu of a definitive diagnosis. When sufficient clinical information isn't known or available about a particular health condition to assign a more specific code, it is acceptable to report the appropriate "unspecified" code (e.g., a diagnosis of pneumonia

Continued

using the Index only to code the condition of right ankle pain, the code M25.57- would be assigned. This code is incorrect; the Tabular List indicates that a sixth digit is required to identify the laterality (right) of the ankle pain. Code M25.571 correctly reports the diagnosis of right ankle pain. It is also important for the coder to read and follow any notes that appear in either section.

Level of Detail in Coding

Points 2 and 3 of the General Coding Guidelines (see Box 4.1) explain how to assign the most specific code. The primary rule states that both diagnosis and procedure codes are to include the highest number of digits available for the highest level of specificity. This does not mean, however, that every code will be seven digits in length.

ICD-10-CM Diagnosis Codes

ICD-10-CM diagnosis codes are composed of either three, four, five, six, or seven characters, with three characters always before the decimal point. Codes with three characters are categories, and a category may be subdivided by a fourth, fifth, sixth, or seventh subcategory. The seventh character must always be the last character. Typically the fourth, fifth, and sixth characters provide additional specificity regarding the type of disease, the cause of disease, or the site of disease.

In other words, a three-character code is to be used only if it is not further subdivided. If a particular category includes fourth-, fifth-, sixth-, or seventh-digit subcategories, then they must be assigned. A code is incorrect or invalid if it has not been coded to the full number of digits available (also known as to the highest level of specificity).

EXAMPLES
J20 Acute bronchitis

    Includes: acute and subacute bronchitis (with) bronchospasm.
              acute and subacute bronchitis (with) tracheitis.
              acute and subacute bronchitis (with) tracheobronchitis, acute.
              acute and subacute fibrinous bronchitis.
              acute and subacute membranous bronchitis.
              acute and subacute purulent bronchitis.
              acute and subacute septic bronchitis.

    Excludes2: acute bronchitis with bronchiectasis (J47.0).
              acute bronchitis with chronic obstructive asthma (J44.0).
              acute bronchitis with chronic obstructive pulmonary disease (J44.0).
              allergic bronchitis NOS (J45.909-).
              bronchitis due to chemicals, fumes and vapors (J68.0).
              bronchitis NOS (J40).
              chronic bronchitis NOS (J42).
              chronic mucopurulent bronchitis (J41.1).
              chronic obstructive bronchitis (J44.-).
              chronic obstructive tracheobronchitis (J44.-).
              chronic simple bronchitis (J41.0).
              chronic tracheobronchitis (J42).
              tracheobronchitis NOS (J40).

J20.0 Acute bronchitis due to Mycoplasma pneumoniae.

J20.1 Acute bronchitis due to Haemophilus influenzae.

It is incorrect to assign code J20 alone. A fourth digit is required to identify the underlying cause of disease, for example, acute bronchitis due to Haemophilus influenzae (J20.1).

EXAMPLES
C08 Malignant neoplasm of other and unspecified major salivary glands.

> **Includes:** malignant neoplasm of salivary ducts.
> Use additional code to identify:
>> alcohol abuse and dependence (F10).
>> exposure to environmental tobacco smoke (Z77.22).
>> exposure to tobacco smoke in the perinatal period (P96.81).
>> history of tobacco use (Z87.891).
>> occupational exposure to environmental tobacco smoke (Z57.31).
>> tobacco dependence (F17).
>> tobacco use (Z72.0).

> **Excludes1:** malignant neoplasms of specified minor salivary glands which are
>> classified according to their anatomical location.

> **Excludes2:** malignant neoplasms of minor salivary glands NOS (C06.9)
>> malignant neoplasm of parotid gland (C07).

C08.0 Malignant neoplasm of submandibular gland.
> Malignant neoplasm of submaxillary gland.

C08.1 Malignant neoplasm of sublingual gland.

Category C08 classifies malignant neoplasms of other and unspecified major salivary glands. A fourth digit must be added to identify the specific gland, such as code C08.1.

CHECKPOINT 4.1

Using the Tabular List of the ICD-10-CM, determine whether the following codes are coded to their highest level of specificity. If not, identify which digit(s) are missing.

C4A.1 _____

I10 _____

I69.81 _____

M80.051 _____

S30.1 _____

Coding Decisions for Signs, Symptoms, and Integral Conditions

Coders are required to make decisions about whether to include aspects of the patient's diagnosis that are not clear-cut. Points 4 to 6 of the General Coding Guidelines explain how to proceed.

Signs and Symptoms
A diagnosis is not always readily established for a patient's condition. Often a series of workups, tests, and examinations during follow-up visits is required before the physician determines a diagnosis. During this process, signs and symptoms, rather than an uncertain diagnosis, are reported for reimbursement of service fees.

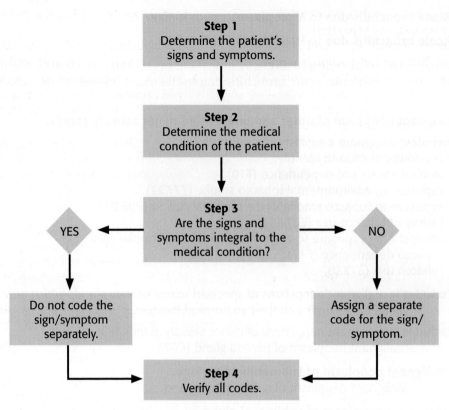

Step 1
Determine the patient's signs and symptoms.

↓

Step 2
Determine the medical condition of the patient.

↓

Step 3
Are the signs and symptoms integral to the medical condition?

YES ←   → NO

↓   ↓

Do not code the sign/symptom separately.   Assign a separate code for the sign/symptom.

Step 4
Verify all codes.

Figure 4.1 Signs and symptoms coding process.

A sign is an objective indication that can be evaluated by the physician, such as weight loss. A symptom is a subjective statement by the patient that cannot be confirmed during an examination, such as pain. In some instances, a sign or symptom may be incorporated and described in the ICD-10 code. For example, code K50.111 describes Crohn's disease of the large intestine with rectal bleeding. The sign of rectal bleeding is included in the code description. Figure 4.1 shows a flowchart that guides the basic process for coding signs and symptoms.

■ CASE SCENARIO

DIAGNOSTIC STATEMENT: A 55-year-old male presents with vague epigastric pain and weight loss. He has not been eating well. He denies nausea, vomiting, changes in bowel habit or blood in stool. Physical examination revealed no abdominal tenderness.

PRIMARY DIAGNOSIS: R10.13, abdominal pain, epigastric region

COEXISTING CONDITION: R63.4, abnormal loss of weight

Point 4 of the General Coding Guidelines states:

Codes that describe symptoms and signs, as opposed to diagnoses, are acceptable for reporting purposes when a related definitive diagnosis has not been established (confirmed) by the provider.

Some examples of signs are fever, tachycardia, and seizure. Symptoms such as abdominal pain, headache, and chest pain are also reported in Chapter 18 of ICD-10-CM. More specific guidelines are based on whether a sign or symptom is integral to a disease process.

Conditions That Are an Integral Part of a Disease Process

Point 5 of the General Coding Guidelines (see Box 4.1) covers conditions that are an integral part of a disease process—certain signs and symptoms that are always seen in patients with the disease.

The coding rule states that codes for signs and symptoms that are integral to the d[...] should not be assigned separately.

Consider the typical signs and symptoms of pneumonia. Objective and measur[...] pneumonia include the patient's temperature (fever). Symptoms (subjective an[...] measured) include difficulty breathing (dyspnea). A patient with pneumonia mig[...] signs of fever and cough and the symptom of difficulty breathing. This guideline e[...] the coder would code only pneumonia, because the signs and symptoms are integr[...] monia and not separately reportable.

To decide how to handle a case, the coder determines whether the sign or symp[...] be routinely present in all cases of the disease. If so, it would not be coded separately. In correct coding language, we would say that cough, fever, and dyspnea are integral to pneumonia, so only pneumonia would be reported.

Conditions That Are Not an Integral Part of a Disease Process

In contrast to the guideline covering integral conditions, point 6 of the General Coding Guidelines states that "additional signs and symptoms that may not be associated routinely with a disease process should be coded when present." For example, a patient may have cirrhosis of the liver and the symptom of ascites. Because ascites is not routinely associated with cirrhosis, it would be reported in addition to the code for cirrhosis. Another example of a symptom that is not integral to the disease process is a coma. A coma is not routinely associated with a stroke. If a patient suffering from a stroke goes into a coma, the coma code would be reported in addition to the code for stroke.

Determining Signs, Symptoms, and Integral Conditions

How can a coder determine whether a sign or symptom is integral to the disease process? This knowledge can be obtained through the study of disease and pathophysiology. Online coding resources can also be used to research a disease process. Another option is to refer to the AHA's *Coding Clinic*® guidelines, which often discuss signs and symptoms of specific diseases and conditions.

EXAMPLE

Abdominal ascites is not integral to *non-alcoholic* cirrhosis of the liver; therefore, both codes should be reported. The liver cirrhosis (K74.60) would be listed first because this is the underlying cause of the symptom abdominal ascites (R18.8).

EXAMPLE

Abdominal ascites (sign) is included in the combination code K70.31 if associated with *alcoholic* cirrhosis, therefore only one code is assigned that includes the underlying cause and sign of ascites.

Use your coding resources to determine whether a sign or symptom is integral to a disease or condition.

EXAMPLE

Chest pain is often a symptom that occasions a visit to the doctor. If the cause of the chest pain is a myocardial infarction, the symptom of chest pain would not be reported separately because chest pain is integral to a myocardial infarction. If the chest pain was due to anxiety, the symptom of chest pain would be reported, because chest pain is not integral to the underlying anxiety.

For the following diagnostic statements, identify the sign or symptom and whether the sign or symptom is integral to the underlying disease.

1. Subdural hemorrhage resulting in a comatose state _____

2. Shortness of breath due to pulmonary embolism _____

3. Hematuria caused by bladder cancer _____

4. Acute stroke with aphasia and neurogenic dysphagia _____

5. Left wrist pain due to recent fracture _____

Code the following diagnostic statements using ICD-10-CM.

6. Acute gastritis, with hemorrhage _____

7. Closed fracture of the left wrist, initial episode of care, with wrist pain _____

8. Acute idiopathic pancreatitis with abdominal ascites _____

9. Acute asthma exacerbation with hypoxia _____

10. Urinary tract infection with dysuria _____

Multiple Coding for a Single Condition

In some instances, two codes are required to fully classify a medical condition and an associated manifestation or underlying cause of disease. The conventions in ICD-10-CM help the coder understand when it is appropriate to assign two codes for one condition. The "use additional code note" and "code first" conventions instruct the coder to assign more than one code. Their application reflects different circumstances for reporting two codes.

Use Additional Code Note

The "use additional code" notes found in the Tabular List identify codes that are not part of etiology and manifestation pairs. In these cases, a secondary code is used to fully describe the condition. For example, for infections not included in Chapter 1 of the ICD-10-CM Tabular List, a secondary code may be required to identify the bacterial organism causing the infection.

EXAMPLE
N39.0 Urinary tract infection, site not specified.
    Use additional code (B95–B97), to identify infectious agent.

    Excludes1: candidiasis of urinary tract (B37.4-).
            neonatal urinary tract infection (P39.3).
            urinary tract infection of specified site, such as:
                cystitis (N30.-).
                urethritis (N34.-).

The example shows a "use additional code" note requiring the coder to also report the organism causing the infection of the kidney. To code the specific organism causing the infection, the main term *infection* or the name of the organism (Streptococcus) is located in the Index. Reporting the condition of Urinary tract infection due to *Streptococcus B* requires reporting two codes: N39.0 (urinary tract infection) and B95.1 (streptococcal B infection). Hint: When reporting the additional organism code, use the main term **Infection**, subterm, *as cause of disease classified elsewhere.*

Code, If Applicable, Any Causal Condition First Note

The *Official Guidelines* use the notation "Code first underlying condition, if known" to instruct the coder to report two codes if documentation supports the known underlying condition of a disease. The underlying condition, or causal condition, is the medical illness that brought on the documented disease. The code for the underlying condition, when known, is listed first. In the example below, the notation is located at the subcategory level of code F48.2. Therefore, if the Pseudobulbar affect was due to multiple sclerosis, the code for multiple sclerosis (G35) would be sequenced first, followed by the code for the Pseudobulbar affect (F48.2). The code for multiple sclerosis is reported only if known as the underlying cause.

EXAMPLE
F48.2 Pseudobulbar affect.
> Involuntary emotional expression disorder.
>
> **Code first** underlying cause, if known, such as:
> > amyotrophic lateral sclerosis (G12.21).
> > multiple sclerosis (G35).
> > sequelae of cerebrovascular disease (I69.-).
> > sequelae of traumatic intracranial injury (S06.-).

Code First Note
The "code first" notes are also used when there is an underlying cause. When a "code first" note and an underlying condition are both present, the underlying condition code must be listed first.

EXAMPLE
M02 Postinfective and reactive arthropathies.
> **Code first** underlying disease, such as:
> > congenital syphilis [Clutton's joints] (A50.5).
> > enteritis due to Yersinia enterocolitica (A04.6).
> > infective endocarditis (I33.0).
> > viral hepatitis (B15–B19).

The "code first" note appears at code M02, postinfective and reactive arthropathies. When assigning the code for postinfective and reactive arthropathy, the coder should first code any underlying condition that is documented, such as associated viral hepatitis (B15–B19). In coding reactive arthropathy due to acute viral hepatitis, the coder reports both codes B17.9 and M02.

CHECKPOINT 4.3

Code the following diagnostic statements using ICD-10-CM.

1. Acute cystitis with hematuria due to pseudomonas infection _____

2. Autonomic dysreflexia due to fecal impaction _____

3. Benign prostatic hypertrophy with urinary obstruction and urinary frequency _____

4. Prolapsed posterior vaginal wall with fecal incontinence _____

5. Septic shock due to *E. coli* sepsis with acute hypoxic respiratory failure _____

6. Diabetes due to chronic pancreatitis _____

7. Pseudobulbar affect caused by amyotrophic lateral sclerosis _____

Acute and Chronic Conditions

Point 8 of the General Coding Guidelines explains:

> If the same condition is described as both acute (subacute) and chronic, and separate subentries exist in the Index at the same indentation level, code both and sequence the acute (subacute) code first.

This guideline instructs the coder to look carefully at the indentation level to determine whether two codes should be assigned when the condition is both acute (subacute) and chronic. An acute illness or condition is one that has severe symptoms and a short duration, whereas a chronic illness or condition has a long duration. *Acute* can also refer to a sudden exacerbation of a chronic condition.

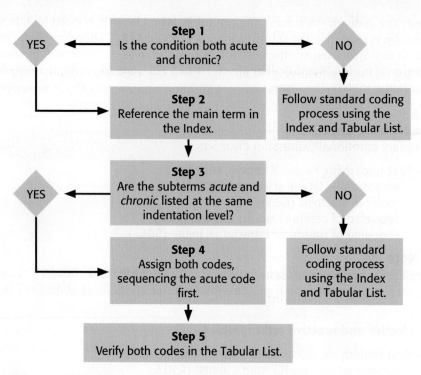

Figure 4.2 Acute and chronic conditions coding process.

EXAMPLE
Pancreatitis K85.90

  acute K85.90
  chronic K86.1

When coding acute and chronic pancreatitis, as in the example above, both subterms, *acute* and *chronic*, are located at the same indentation level. Therefore, both codes K85.90 and K86.1 would be assigned if the patient had both conditions. The acute condition code should be listed first, followed by the code for the chronic condition. The basic coding process for acute and chronic conditions is shown in Figure 4.2.

Combination Codes

As explained in point 9 of the General Coding Guidelines (see Box 4.1), a combination code is one code that classifies:

- Two diagnoses or
- A diagnosis with an associated manifestation
- A diagnosis with an associated complication
- A diagnosis with an associated sign or symptom

Codes that combine two conditions are located in the Index and have subterms. Subterms such as "due to" or "and" or "with" combine two disorders to classify both conditions using one code. These combination codes reflect conditions that are often associated together clinically. For example, if a patient has the diagnoses of diverticulosis with bleeding, code K57.91 classifies both conditions using one code.

When a combination code reflects both a disease and its manifestation, the subterm *with* often appears. For example, for pneumonia *with* lung abscess, code J85.1 identifies the disease pneumonia with the associated manifestation.

An example of a combination code that classifies a diagnosis and an associated complication is a postoperative pneumothorax, where code Z98.3 indicates that the pneumothorax is a post-op complication.

When documentation supports a relationship between two conditions, or there is an assumed relationship with the subterm "with," multiple codes should not be used if a combination code clearly identifies all elements. If the combination code lacks the necessary specificity in describing the manifestation or complication, an additional code should be reported. Remember that the terms "with," "and," or "due to" assume a relationship between both conditions when both are present, and this often results in a combination code.

EXAMPLE
Documentation states the following diagnoses: Type 2 diabetes and mononeuropathy. Report combination code E11.41. The coder assumes that the mononeuropathy is associated with the Type 2 diabetes because of the term "with" in the combination code.

CHECKPOINT 4.4

Code the following diagnostic statements using ICD-10-CM.

1. Acute and chronic cystitis _____

2. Acute and chronic cholecystitis _____

3. Acute appendicitis with perforation _____

4. Postoperative hematoma of circulatory system following cardiac catheterization _____

5. Chronic bronchitis due to tobacco smoking _____

6. Type I diabetes, cataract left eye _____

Sequelae (Late Effects)

According to ICD-10-CM, a sequela (late effect) is "the residual effect (condition produced) after the acute phase of an illness or injury has terminated." Based on point 10 of the General Coding Guidelines (see Box 4.1), a late effect has no time limit for reporting. A late effect may develop very soon after or much later than the acute phase of an illness or injury. For example, a patient may have a residual condition, such as paralysis (residual) from a previous stroke (cause of the residual condition, no longer present), and this paralysis could be present very soon after the stroke. On the other hand, a patient may not develop a residual condition from an accident, such as a nonunion of a fracture, until much later. Terms often used to describe sequelae include *old, previous, due to previous, malunion,* and *nonunion.* The code for the acute phase of an illness or injury that led to the late effect is never used with a code for the sequelae.

Coding of a sequelae generally requires two codes, with the code for the condition or nature of the sequelae (code the condition/residual) listed first, followed by the code for the sequelae (code using the main term *sequelae*). One exception to using two codes involves cases in which the injury code includes a seventh-character extension identifying the sequelae such as sequelae of skull fracture (code only fracture, skull, sequelae, code S02.91xS). Additional coding guidelines for sequelae of cerebrovascular disease and sequelae of pregnancy, childbirth, and the puerperium are discussed later in the text.

> ● Do not use the code for the acute phase of an illness or injury that led to the late effect. Report a code for the sequelae of that illness or injury.

CHECKPOINT 4.5

Underline the residual condition in the following diagnostic statements, then code using ICD-10-CM.

1. Painful scar due to old burn injury, left leg _____

2. Leg paralysis due to previous poliomyelitis _____

3. Sequelae of hyperalimentation _____

4. Normal pressure hydrocephalus due to previous encephalitis _____

5. Malunion of displaced left tibial pilon fracture (traumatic) _____

Impending or Threatened Conditions

As explained in point 11 of the General Coding Guidelines (see Box 4.1), if an impending or threatened condition documented sometime during the patient's stay has actually occurred by the time of discharge, it should be coded as a confirmed diagnosis.

When the medical condition that is noted as "impending" or "threatened" did not occur, the coder should reference those terms as main terms in the Index. There may be a specific code for that impending or threatened condition. If so, assign the code after verifying it in the Tabular List.

> **EXAMPLE**
> **Impending**
>
> coronary syndrome   I20.0
> delirium tremens   F10.239
> myocardial infarction I20.0

An impending myocardial infarction would be reported using code I20.0.

If, on the other hand, the subterm *impending* or *threatened* is not listed, report only the medical condition that exists at the time. Do not report a code for the condition that was noted as impending or threatened because this condition has not yet occurred.

CHECKPOINT 4.6

Code the following diagnostic statements using ICD-10-CM.

1. Threatened abortion _____

2. Impending delirium tremens _____

3. Impending gangrene of the right heel due to stage 4 decubitus ulcer _____

4. Impending respiratory failure due to chronic obstructive pulmonary disease (COPD) exacerbation

    _____

5. Impending myocardial infarction _____

Reporting the Same Diagnosis Code More Than Once

As explained in point 12 of the General Coding Guidelines (see Box 4.1), for cases in which a bilateral condition exists and there are no distinct codes identifying laterality, only one ICD-10-CM diagnosis code should be reported. For example, a ureteral calculus on the left and right would be reported using code N20.1 once, because there is no specific code for a bilateral ureteral calculus. If two different conditions are classified with the same ICD-10-CM diagnosis code, the code is reported once.

Laterality

As explained in point 13 of the General Coding Guidelines (see Box 4.1), for cases in which a bilateral site is classified, the final character of the codes in ICD-10-CM indicates laterality. If the documentation does not indicate left, right, or bilateral, then an unspecified side code is assigned. In some instances a code for "bilateral" is not available in ICD-10-CM and in those cases two codes would be assigned, one for the right and one for the left. For example, a female has bilateral breast cancer. The codes assigned would be C50.911 (malignant neoplasm, right breast) and C50.912 (malignant neoplasm, left breast). If the patient has the condition on both sides, the bilateral code should be assigned. If the condition has resolved on one side, then report only the side with the condition still present. For example: a patient presents for treatment of a left senile cataract, but has a cataract in both eyes. Report the code for bilateral cataracts. If the patient presents for treatment of the right cataract after treatment and correction of the left cataract, report the code for cataract of the right eye only.

Documentation for BMI, Depth of Non-Pressure Ulcers, Pressure Ulcer Stages, Coma Scale, and NIH Stroke Scale

As explained in point 14 of the General Coding Guidelines (see Box 4.1), documentation used to report body mass index, stage of pressure ulcer, coma scale or NIH stroke scale (NIHSS) can be obtained "from clinicians who are not the patient's provider (i.e., physician or other qualified health-care practitioner legally accountable for establishing the patient's diagnosis)." Note that "the associated diagnosis (such as overweight, obesity, or pressure ulcer) must be documented by the patient's provider." For example, the attending physician documents adult morbid obesity and the patient's nutritionist documents the BMI as 42. The codes assigned would be E66.01 and Z68.41. Another example would be a decubitus ulcer (pressure ulcer) of the left heel documented by the physician with nursing stating the ulcer was stage 2. The code assigned would be L89.622. If provider and nursing documentation of BMI or pressure ulcer stage conflicts, the coder should clarify the information with the provider. Often, a written physician query is used for clarification.

Syndromes

As explained in point 15 of the General Coding Guidelines (see Box 4.1), when coding a syndrome follow the Index. When guidance is not provided in the Index, the codes assigned should reflect the manifestations of the Syndrome. For example, when coding Syndrome of inappropriate secretion of antidiuretic hormone (SIADH), the code E22.2 is assigned.

Complications of Care

As explained in point 16 of the General Coding Guidelines (see Box 4.1), provider documentation must support a "relationship between the condition and the care or procedure" in order for a complication code to be assigned. A true cause-and-effect relationship between the care or procedure and the medical condition must be stated. The use of the term "postoperative" is often used to state a cause-and-effect relationship. For example, postoperative ileus would be classified as a complication of care. Be aware, however, that not all conditions that arise after a procedure are complications.

> Query the provider for clarification if a cause-and-effect relationship is not clearly documented.

SELECTION OF PRINCIPAL DIAGNOSIS/ADDITIONAL DIAGNOSES FOR THE INPATIENT SETTING

[handwritten: Coding for Impatient is specialized (more training Req.)]

[handwritten: $ codes for inpatient based on diagnosis]

Inpatient care is an enormous health cost, amounting to nearly $800 billion for 39 million hospital stays, according to recent data. Many patients, particularly elderly or very ill patients, do not have only one diagnosis or condition. According to the Centers for Medicare and Medicaid Services (CMS), almost a quarter of Medicare beneficiaries (usually adults age 65 or over) have five or more chronic conditions. When these patients are admitted for hospital treatment, in many cases, documentation for a single visit covers multiple conditions, health-care factors, and circumstances. For example, an admission to the hospital to evaluate a patient with chest pain, hypertension, and diabetes requires many ICD-10-CM diagnosis codes. These inpatient coding guidelines also apply to other settings to include short term care, long term care, psychiatric hospitals, home health agencies, rehab facilities, nursing homes, and all hospice care. In other words, these guidelines apply to all non-outpatient services. How do coders decide which code is listed first? Sections II and III of the *Official Guidelines* help the coder make this determination. These sections are reprinted in Box 4.2 for your reference.

In the inpatient setting, the first listed diagnosis code is the principal diagnosis code for the encounter. The Uniform Hospital Discharge Data Set (UHDDS) guidelines state that the principal diagnosis is "that condition established after study to be chiefly responsible for occasioning the admission of the patient to the hospital for care."

Section II. Selection of Principal Diagnosis

The circumstances of inpatient admission always govern the selection of principal diagnosis. The principal diagnosis is defined in the Uniform Hospital Discharge Data Set (UHDDS) as "that condition established after study to be chiefly responsible for occasioning the admission of the patient to the hospital for care."

The UHDDS definitions are used by hospitals to report inpatient data elements in a standardized manner. These data elements and their definitions can be found in the July 31, 1985, Federal Register (Vol. 50, No, 147), pp. 31038–40.

Since that time the application of the UHDDS definitions has been expanded to include all non-outpatient settings (acute care, short term, long term care and psychiatric hospitals; home health agencies; rehab facilities; nursing homes, etc.). The UHDDS definitions also apply to hospice services (all levels of care).

In determining principal diagnosis, coding conventions in the ICD-10-CM, the Tabular List and Alphabetic Index take precedence over these official coding guidelines. *(See Section I.A., Conventions for the ICD-10-CM.)*

The importance of consistent, complete documentation in the medical record cannot be overemphasized. Without such documentation the application of all coding guidelines is a difficult, if not impossible, task.

A. Codes for Symptoms, Signs, and Ill-Defined Conditions

Codes for symptoms, signs, and ill-defined conditions from Chapter 18 are not to be used as principal diagnosis when a related definitive diagnosis has been established.

B. Two or More Interrelated Conditions, Each Potentially Meeting the Definition for Principal Diagnosis.

When there are two or more interrelated conditions (such as diseases in the same ICD-10-CM chapter or manifestations characteristically associated with a certain disease) potentially meeting the definition of principal diagnosis, either condition may be sequenced first, unless the circumstances of the admission, the therapy provided, the Tabular List, or the Alphabetic Index indicate otherwise.

C. Two or More Diagnoses That Equally Meet the Definition for Principal Diagnosis

In the unusual instance when two or more diagnoses equally meet the criteria for principal diagnosis as determined by the circumstances of admission, diagnostic workup and/or therapy provided, and the Alphabetic Index, Tabular List, or another coding guidelines does not provide sequencing direction, any one of the diagnoses may be sequenced first.

D. Two or More Comparative or Contrasting Conditions

In those rare instances when two or more contrasting or comparative diagnoses are documented as "either/or" (or similar terminology), they are coded as if the diagnoses were confirmed and the diagnoses are sequenced according to the circumstances of the admission. If no further determination can be made as to which diagnosis should be principal, either diagnosis may be sequenced first.

E. A Symptom(s) Followed by Contrasting/Comparative Diagnoses

GUIDELINE HAS BEEN DELETED EFFECTIVE OCTOBER 1, 2014

F. Original Treatment Plan Not Carried Out

Sequence as the principal diagnosis the condition, which after study occasioned the admission to the hospital, even though treatment may not have been carried out due to unforeseen circumstances.

G. Complications of Surgery and Other Medical Care

When the admission is for treatment of a complication resulting from surgery or other medical care, the complication code is sequenced as the principal diagnosis. If the complication is classified to the T80–T88 series and the code lacks the necessary specificity in describing the complication, an additional code for the specific complication should be assigned.

H. Uncertain Diagnosis

If the diagnosis documented at the time of discharge is qualified as "probable," "suspected," "likely," "questionable," "possible," or "still to be ruled out," or other similar terms indicating uncertainty, code the condition as if it existed or was established. The bases for these guidelines are the diagnostic workup, arrangements for further workup or observation, and initial therapeutic approach that correspond most closely with the established diagnosis.

Note: This guideline is applicable only to inpatient admissions to short-term, acute, long-term care and psychiatric hospitals.

I. Admission From Observation Unit
1. Admission Following Medical Observation
When a patient is admitted to an observation unit for a medical condition, which either worsens or does not improve, and is subsequently admitted as an inpatient of the same hospital for this same medical condition, the principal diagnosis would be the medical condition which led to the hospital admission.

2. Admission Following Post-Operative Observation
When a patient is admitted to an observation unit to monitor a condition (or complication) that develops following outpatient surgery, and then is subsequently admitted as an inpatient of the same hospital, hospitals should apply the Uniform Hospital Discharge Data Set (UHDDS) definition of principal diagnosis as "that condition established after study to be chiefly responsible for occasioning the admission of the patient to the hospital for care."

J. Admission from Outpatient Surgery
When a patient receives surgery in the hospital's outpatient surgery department and is subsequently admitted for continuing inpatient care at the same hospital, the following guidelines should be followed in selecting the principal diagnosis for the inpatient admission:
- If the reason for the inpatient admission is a complication, assign the complication as the principal diagnosis.
- If no complication, or other condition, is documented as the reason for the inpatient admission, assign the reason for the outpatient surgery as the principal diagnosis.
- If the reason for the inpatient admission is another condition unrelated to the surgery, assign the unrelated condition as the principal diagnosis.

K. Admissions/Encounters for Rehabilitation
When the purpose for the admission/encounter is rehabilitation, sequence first the code for the condition for which the service is being performed. For example, for an admission/encounter for rehabilitation for right-sided dominant hemiplegia following a cerebrovascular infarction, report code I69.351, Hemiplegia and hemiparesis following cerebral infarction affecting right dominant side, as the first-listed or principal diagnosis.

If the condition for which the rehabilitation service is no longer present, report the appropriate aftercare code as the first-listed or principal diagnosis, unless the rehabilitation service is being provided following an injury. For rehabilitation services following active treatment of an injury, assign the injury code with the appropriate seventh character for subsequent encounter as the first-listed or principal diagnosis. For example, if a patient with severe degenerative osteoarthritis of the hip, underwent hip replacement and the current encounter/admission is for rehabilitation, report code Z47.1, Aftercare following joint replacement surgery, as the first-listed or principal diagnosis. If the patient requires rehabilitation post hip replacement for right intertrochanteric femur fracture, report code S72.141D, Displaced intertrochanteric fracture of right femur, subsequent encounter for closed fracture with routine healing, as the first-listed or principal diagnosis.

See Section I.C.21.c.7, Factors influencing health states and contact with health services, Aftercare. See Section I.C.19.a for additional information about the use of 7th characters for injury codes.

Section III. Reporting Additional Diagnoses
GENERAL RULES FOR OTHER (ADDITIONAL) DIAGNOSES
For reporting purposes the definition for "other diagnoses" is interpreted as additional conditions that affect patient care in terms of requiring

> clinical evaluation; or
> therapeutic treatment; or
> diagnostic procedures; or
> extended length of hospital stay; or
> increased nursing care and/or monitoring.

The UHDDS item #11-b defines Other Diagnoses as "all conditions that coexist at the time of admission, that develop subsequently, or that affect the treatment received and/or the length of stay. Diagnoses that relate to an earlier episode which have no bearing on the current hospital stay are to be excluded." UHDDS definitions apply to inpatients in acute care, short-term, long-term care and

Continued

BOX 4.2 *Continued*

psychiatric hospital setting. The UHDDS definitions are used by acute care short-term hospitals to report inpatient data elements in a standardized manner. These data elements and their definitions can be found in the July 31, 1985, Federal Register (Vol. 50, No, 147), pp. 31038–40.

Since that time the application of the UHDDS definitions has been expanded to include all non-outpatient settings (acute care, short term, long term care and psychiatric hospitals; home health agencies; rehab facilities; nursing homes, etc.). The UHDDS definitions also apply to hospice services (all levels of care).

The following guidelines are to be applied in designating "other diagnoses" when neither the Alphabetic Index nor the Tabular List in ICD-10-CM provide direction. The listing of the diagnoses in the patient record is the responsibility of the attending provider.

A. Previous Conditions
If the provider has included a diagnosis in the final diagnostic statement, such as the discharge summary or the face sheet, it should ordinarily be coded. Some providers include in the diagnostic statement resolved conditions or diagnoses and status-post procedures from previous admission that have no bearing on the current stay. Such conditions are not to be reported and are coded only if required by hospital policy.

However, history codes (categories Z80–Z87) may be used as secondary codes if the historical condition or family history has an impact on current care or influences treatment.

B. Abnormal Findings
Abnormal findings (laboratory, x-ray, pathologic, and other diagnostic results) are not coded and re-ported unless the provider indicates their clinical significance. If the findings are outside the normal range and the attending provider has ordered other tests to evaluate the condition or prescribed treatment, it is appropriate to ask the provider whether the abnormal finding should be added.
Note: This differs from the coding practices in the outpatient setting for coding encounters for diag-nostic tests that have been interpreted by a provider.

C. Uncertain Diagnosis
If the diagnosis documented at the time of discharge is qualified as "probable," "suspected," "likely," "questionable," "possible," or "still to be ruled out" or other similar terms indicating uncertainty, code the condition as if it existed or was established. The bases for these guidelines are the diag-nostic workup, arrangements for further workup or observation, and initial therapeutic approach that correspond most closely with the established diagnosis.
Note: This guideline is applicable only to inpatient admissions to short-term, acute, long-term care, and psychiatric hospitals.

This section covers the ways in which the circumstances of inpatient admission govern the selection of the principal diagnosis. The coder considers the circumstances of admission as mean-ing the reason for admission, after study. Specific guidelines explain the unique rules for selecting the principal diagnosis in different circumstances, such as when two or more conditions meet the definition of principal diagnosis and when a symptom is listed as the principal diagnosis by the attending physician. Other guidelines address selection of the principal diagnosis when a patient is admitted from observation or from an ambulatory surgery unit. Still others determine which conditions should be reported as additional or secondary diagnoses. Coders who understand and can apply these specific guidelines when assigning ICD-10-CM codes for inpatient visits will be correct, consistent, accurate, and complete in their code assignments.

The Uniform Hospital Discharge Data Set (UHDDS)

doesn't apply to outpatient

The UHDDS is a common core of data. This standardized minimum data set is applied to the inpatient setting (acute care, short-term, long-term care, and psychiatric hospitals; home health agencies; rehab facilities; nursing homes, and all levels of hospice care). The goal of UHDDS data collection is to obtain uniform comparable discharge data on all inpa-tients. A list of all data elements appears in Table 4.1.

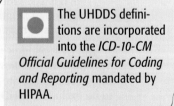
The UHDDS defini-tions are incorporated into the *ICD-10-CM Official Guidelines for Coding and Reporting* mandated by HIPAA.

Table 4.1 Uniform Hospital Discharge Data Set Definitions*

DATA ELEMENT	DESCRIPTION
Personal Identification	A unique number identifying the patient, applicable to the individual regardless of health-care source or third-party arrangement
Date of Birth	Month, day, year
Sex	Male or female
Race and Ethnicity	Race (1) American Indian/Eskimo/Aleut (2) Asian or Pacific Islander (3) Black (4) White (5) Other race (6) Unknown Ethnicity (1) Spanish/Hispanic origin (2) Not of Spanish/Hispanic origin (3) Unknown
Residence	Usual residence, full address, and zip code; nine-digit zip code if available
Hospital Identification	NPI* (a unique institutional number across data systems)
Admission Date	Month, day, and year of admission
Type of Admission	Scheduled: an arrangement with the admissions office at least 24 hours before the admission Unscheduled: all other admissions
Discharge Date	Month, day, and year of discharge
Physician Identification—Attending	National Provider Identifier (NPI)*
Physician Identification—Operating	The NPI* for the clinician who performed the principal procedure
Other Diagnoses	All conditions that coexist at the time of admission, or develop subsequently, that affect the treatment received and/or the length of stay; diagnoses that relate to an earlier episode that have no bearing on the current hospital stay are to be excluded. Code conditions that affect patient care in terms of requiring: Clinical evaluation Therapeutic treatment Diagnostic procedures Extended length of hospital stay Increased nursing care Monitoring
External Causes of Injury Code	The ICD10-CM code for the external cause of an injury, poisoning, or adverse effect
Birth Weight of Newborns	The specific birth weight of the newborn, preferably recorded in grams
Procedures and Dates	All significant procedures are to be reported. A significant procedure is one that (1) Is surgical in nature (2) Carries a procedural risk (3) Carries an anesthetic risk (4) Requires specialized training Surgery includes incision, excision, amputation, introduction, destruction, suture, and manipulation. The date must be reported for each significant procedure.

Continued

Table 4.1 Continued

DATA ELEMENT	DESCRIPTION
	When more than one procedure is reported, the principal procedure is to be designated. In determining which of several procedures is principal, the following criteria apply: The principal procedure is one that was performed for definitive treatment rather than for diagnostic or exploratory purposes, or was necessary to take care of a complication. If two procedures appear to be principal, the one most related to the principal diagnosis should be selected as the principal procedure.
Disposition of Patient	Home, nursing facility, other health-care facility, left against medical advice, expired.
Expected Sources of Payment	Primary source: the primary source that is expected to be responsible for the largest percentage of the patient's current bill
	Other source(s): other sources, if any, that are expected to be responsible for a portion of the patient's current bill; more than one can be identified
Total Charges	All charges billed by the hospital for this hospitalization; professional charges for individual patient care by physicians are excluded

*UPIN has been updated to NPI to reflect current practice.
Source: www.cdc.gov/nchs/data/ncvhs/nchvs92.pdf

The data elements can be categorized into the following:

- Patient identification
- Provider information
- Clinical information about the patient's episode of care
- Financial information

Coders are most concerned about the clinical information regarding the patient's episode of care. These data elements and their definitions drive the coding process in the inpatient setting. Based on applying the documentation guidelines, coders correctly select the principal diagnosis, the principal procedure, and secondary diagnoses.

Documentation in the Inpatient Setting

The patient care flow and clinical documentation in the medical record provide the foundation for ICD-10-CM code assignment. To uncover all relevant diagnostic information, coders review the entire medical record from admission through discharge when coding an inpatient visit. Deciphering the content of the record can help the coder understand the documentation, which ultimately is required for accurate code assignment. The flowchart in Figure 4.3 outlines the physician-documented components of the inpatient medical record that develop as the inpatient visit progresses and then ends.

The flow begins with the medical orders written by the admitting physician. Admission—the formal acceptance by the hospital of a patient—can be either a scheduled admission, in which arrangements have been made prior to the patient's appearing, or a nonscheduled admission, such as via the emergency department. The patient's information is summarized on a *face sheet*, also called an *inpatient admission form*, or using an electronic program to record the data.

> The connection between documentation and coding is essential. A service that is not documented cannot be coded—and cannot be billed.

Admitted patients are then housed appropriately and treated by the medical staff. The attending physician—the medical professional who supervises the patient's care

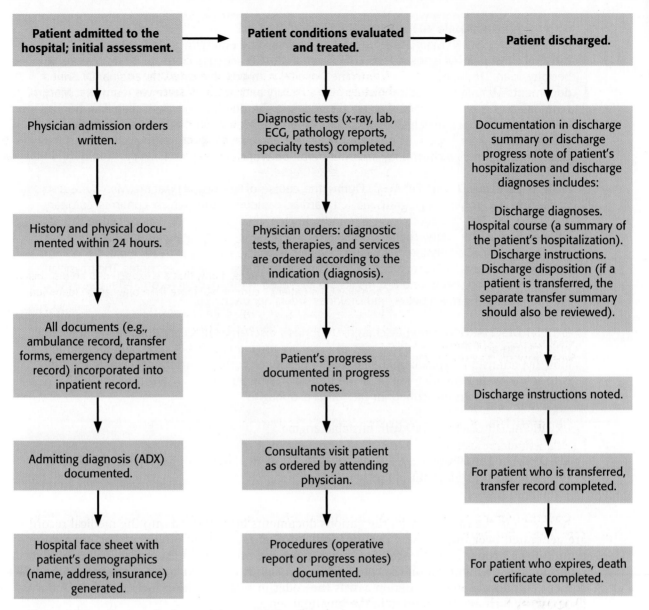

Figure 4.3 Inpatient medical record documentation flowchart.

during hospitalization—directs the medical work that needs to be done to evaluate and treat the patient's conditions.

Following treatment, the patient is released, or discharged, from the hospital. The documentation must contain a discharge summary (or progress note) of the patient's medical condition and disposition or arrangements, indicating whether the patient is returning home, is moving to another facility (such as a rehabilitation facility), or has died.

The discharge summary is typically the best place to begin the coding process because this document contains a recap of the entire hospitalization (that is, hospital course), summarizing the reason for admission and the tests, medications, and services provided.

The easiest way to grasp the concept of medical record documentation flow is to look at a case scenario.

As shown in the case scenario, the various documents incorporated into the medical record are generated over the course of an inpatient hospitalization. The physician documentation found in the history and physical, discharge summary, progress notes, orders, and operative report include the information the coder needs to assign ICD-10-CM codes. Understanding the content and flow of documentation assists the coder in selecting the principal and secondary diagnoses that should be reported in the inpatient setting.

Section II: Selection of the Principal Diagnosis in the Inpatient Setting

The UHDDS defines the principal diagnosis for the inpatient setting as "that condition established after study to be chiefly responsible for occasioning the admission of the patient to the hospital for care." For example, a patient is admitted with unstable angina, but a diagnostic cardiac catheterization with coronary angiography (a diagnostic procedure) shows that the principal diagnosis is coronary artery disease.

The basic coding rules and conventions for determining principal diagnosis in the ICD-10-CM Tabular List take precedence over the *Official Guidelines*. As shown in Figure 4.4, the process involves applying the rules and conventions before the guidelines.

The guidelines in the following sections apply to the selection of the principal diagnosis in the various presenting situations encountered by coders.

> The publication AHA *Coding Clinic®* is a resource for when queries are appropriate. It contains numerous examples of the correct way to write a query about a specific coding situation without appearing to "lead" the physician.

Conventions over rule guidelines

Codes for Symptoms, Signs, and Ill-Defined Conditions

As stated in Section IIA of the *ICD-10-CM Official Guidelines for Coding and Reporting*, "Codes for symptoms, signs, and ill-defined conditions from Chapter 18 are not to be used as principal diagnosis when a related definitive diagnosis has been established." The codes in Chapter 18 of ICD-10-CM range from R00 to R99 and include such diagnoses as fever, dizziness, visual hallucinations, and aphasia. If the related definitive diagnosis has been identified, the symptom code should not be sequenced first. A code that is sequenced first is listed first. Only one code can be sequenced as the principal diagnosis.

> ■ **CASE SCENARIO**
> A patient presents with fever and cough, and if further study and documentation support the diagnosis of pneumonia, the code for pneumonia is sequenced first. Because the basic coding guidelines show that the symptoms of fever and cough are integral to pneumonia, these symptoms are not reported separately. Code J18.9 is reported.

Sometimes incomplete or inconsistent documentation requires a *physician query*, a written communication from the coder asking the physician for clarification. For example, a physician may document chest pain as a principal diagnosis, but an upper endoscopy is positive for gastric ulcer. The physician should be queried about the definitive diagnosis that is causing the chest pain. In this instance, the coder may think that the ulcer is causing the chest pain and may report the symptom of chest pain as the principal diagnosis (R07.9). However, the query results may support the principal diagnosis of gastric ulcer as the cause of chest pain, and the principal diagnosis would be reported as K25.9.

There are many resources that help the coder with the query process. The coder should not lead the provider to specific diagnosis, rather the coder should request clarification and specificity.

> **INTERNET RESOURCE: Article "Physician Query Process: Part 1: Physician Query Basics and When to Query"**
> https://www.libmaneducation.com/physician-query-process-part-1 -physician-query-basics-and-when-to-query/

Two or More Interrelated Conditions, Each Potentially Meeting the Definition for Principal Diagnosis
According to the *Official Guidelines*:

> When there are two or more interrelated conditions (such as diseases in the same ICD-10-CM chapter or manifestations characteristically associated with a certain disease) potentially meeting the definition of principal diagnosis, either condition may be sequenced first, unless the circumstances of the admission, the therapy provided, the Tabular List, or the Index indicate otherwise.

Step 1:
Review the complete inpatient medical record.

↓

Step 2:
Abstract the diagnoses and procedures to be coded based on physician documentation.

↓

Step 3:
Assign the correct ICD-10-CM diagnosis and procedures codes, following the ICD-10-CM rules and conventions.

↓

Step 4:
Sequence the codes based on UHDDS definitions and ICD-10-CM *Official Guidelines.*

↓

Step 5:
Assign the present on admission indicators for each diagnosis code.

↓

Step 6:
Calculate the DRG for the inpatient hospitalization.

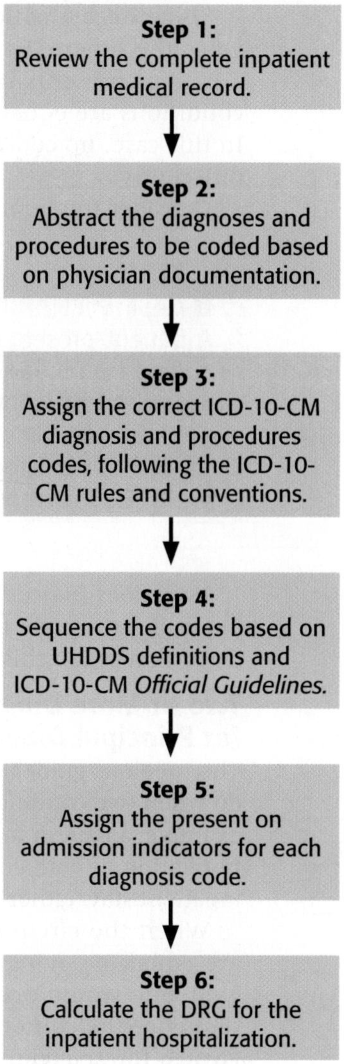

Figure 4.4 Inpatient coding process.

CHECKPOINT 4.7

Identify the sign/symptom and definitive diagnosis for each of the following diagnostic statements.

	Sign/Symptom	Diagnosis
1. Abdominal pain due to gastritis	_____	_____
2. Hematuria due to renal calculus	_____	_____
3. Cerebrovascular accident (CVA) with aphasia	_____	_____
4. Sprained knee with pain	_____	_____
5. Cirrhosis of the liver with ascites	_____	_____

Sometimes a patient is admitted because of interrelated conditions. One condition aggravates the other. For example, congestive heart failure can be related to atrial fibrillation. If a patient presents in atrial fibrillation (I48.0) and congestive heart failure (I50.9) and the conditions are equally treated, both conditions should be coded, sequencing either code first. In this case, no coding convention (such as code first guideline) directs the coder to sequence differently.

Consider this example of interrelated conditions:

■ **CASE SCENARIO**

A patient presents with bleeding esophageal varices and active cirrhosis of the liver. The coding instruction of "code first underlying disease" requires the code for the cirrhosis be reported first followed by the code for bleeding esophageal varices. So even though these are interrelated conditions that equally meet the definition of principal diagnosis, the code for cirrhosis is listed first because the ICD-10-CM Index indicates sequencing. Codes assigned are K74.60 (cirrhosis of the liver) and I85.11 (bleeding esophageal varices).

How does the coder decide which code to sequence first when either code can be reported? Typically, the code that results in the highest payment from a payer for the hospitalization is listed first when this guideline applies.

Two or More Diagnoses That Equally Meet the Definition for Principal Diagnosis

The previous guideline addresses two conditions that are interrelated, but what should the coder do when two conditions that are not related equally meet the definition of principal diagnosis? For example, a patient presents with exacerbation of chronic obstructive pulmonary disease and atrial fibrillation. If both conditions occasioned the admission and were treated equally throughout the inpatient stay, either diagnosis code could be sequenced first.

When the circumstances of admission and the diagnostic workup and therapy provided are equal for more than one condition, either condition may be listed first. The exception guideline would occur when a coding convention (such as "code first") directs the coder to sequence the conditions in a specific order. The circumstances of inpatient admission always govern the selection of the principal diagnosis, and this guideline applies only in the rare instance when two conditions occasion the admission to the hospital and both conditions are equally treated.

CHECKPOINT 4.8

Indicate whether the following scenarios meet the criteria under which the coder may sequence either code first when two conditions are either related or unrelated.

1. Mary presents to the hospital with chest pain and shortness of breath. Further study confirms both pneumonia and congestive heart failure. Mary is treated equally using medications and respiratory therapy. _____

2. Joseph presents with atrial fibrillation. After admission, he develops syncope due to a medication. _____

3. Pamela is admitted due to epigastric pain. Further evaluation by an upper endoscopy is positive for both gastritis and esophagitis. _____

Two or More Comparative or Contrasting Conditions

Occasionally, documentation supports the presence of two or more comparative or contrasting conditions. In such a case, the documentation indicates that the two diagnoses are comparative, using *either/or* (or similar terminology), and both conditions are coded as if the diagnoses were confirmed. The circumstances of the admission will determine the sequencing of the principal diagnoses. Either diagnosis may be sequenced as the principal diagnosis when no other factor, such as a convention, dictates the sequencing.

> ■ **CASE SCENARIO**
> A patient presents with dizziness. The physician documentation supports the diagnosis of benign positional vertigo versus labrynthitis.

In this case, both conditions are reported, and either can be sequenced first because both the comparative and the contrasting conditions are present. The documentation is worded in this way: The patient has both *this and that condition*, or *either this or that is causing the admission*. The documentation of contrasting and comparative diagnoses requires the coder to choose either condition as the principal diagnosis; either will be correct.

CHECKPOINT 4.9

Code the following diagnostic statements using ICD-10-CM. Also note which guideline applies.

	Codes(s)	Guideline
1. Chest pain due to anxiety and reflux esophagitis	_____	_____
2. Upper GI bleeding due to antral and duodenal ulcer	_____	_____
3. Hypotension versus hypoglycemia	_____	_____
4. Pneumonia versus congestive heart failure	_____	_____
5. Sprain and dislocation of the left knee	_____	_____

Original Treatment Plan Not Carried Out

Sometimes a patient is admitted to the hospital with a specified treatment plan, but the plan may not be carried out for one or more reasons. The ICD-10-CM coding guidelines direct the coder to sequence the principal diagnosis as the condition that after study occasioned the admission. Even though the original treatment plan is not carried out, the reason for admission is still considered the principal diagnosis.

■ **CASE SCENARIOS**

• A patient admitted for coronary artery bypass surgery to treat coronary artery disease develops a fever prior to surgery. The surgery is cancelled, and the patient is discharged. In this case, the coronary artery disease (I25.10) is sequenced as the principal diagnosis, followed by a code for the fever (R50.9) and a code to indicate that the surgery was cancelled due to a contraindication (Z53.09). An ICD-10-CM procedure code is not reported because the surgery was not done.

• A patient is admitted for gastrointestinal bleeding due to diverticulitis (K57.33). The initial treatment plan is for the patient to undergo a sigmoid resection, but the patient decides to postpone the surgery for personal reasons. The principal diagnosis is still the condition that after study occasioned the admission to the hospital—diverticulitis with bleeding. Again, a code for surgery not done is assigned as an additional diagnosis code; in this case, Z53.29 is assigned to reflect the fact that the patient's decision was the reason the surgery was not done.

• The original treatment plan is not carried out, but some other treatment is done: The patient is admitted with a closed intertrochanteric femur fracture after falling from a ladder at home in the garden, and surgical reduction of the fracture is required. When the patient is taken to surgery, the surgeon discovers that the patient needs a metal-on-metal total hip replacement. The ICD-10-CM procedure of total hip replacement is reported and the principal diagnosis remains the fractured femur with additional codes to report fall at home. Codes assigned are S72.142A, W11.xxxA, Y92.017.

Complications of Surgery and Other Medical Care

The *Official Guidelines* state that:

> When the admission is for treatment of a complication resulting from surgery or other medical care, the complication code is sequenced as the principal diagnosis. If the complication is classified to the T80–T88 series and the code lacks the necessary specificity in describing the complication, an additional code for the specific complication should be assigned. (See the ICD-10-CM Tabular List for "use additional code" notes.)

Complications may be difficult to determine, but the coder can look for such documentation as "post-op infection," "post-op hematoma," "hip pain due to loose hip prosthesis," or "infected bypass graft." The complication code identifies the presence of a type of complication, and the use of an additional code where directed classifies the specific complication.

For example, the code N99.840 for the diagnostic statement of hematoma of a genitourinary structure following a genitourinary procedure not only classifies the hematoma but also indicates that the hematoma was a complication specifically associated with the genitourinary system. Only one code is required because the type of complication is specific and is included in the code description. In other instances, a second code is required, such as when a patient has an infected tracheostomy as a complication with cellulitis of the neck. The first listed code is the complication code (J95.02, Infection of tracheostomy stoma). The Tabular List directs the coder to use an additional code to identify the type of infection, so the additional code for neck cellulitis is also reported (L03.221). The complication code is listed first if the reason for admission, as determined after study, is the complication.

The main term *complication* is a good place to start in order to assign a complication code. It is sometimes also possible to find the correct complication code by looking up the type of complication with the subterm *postoperative*.

Documentation of complications may also indicate the need for an additional code from Chapter 20, "External Causes of Morbidity," for complete coding. (As a reminder, these codes are supplementary classifications for the causes of injury, complication, poisoning, and adverse events, and are always sequenced after the condition code.) This data element, as shown earlier in Table 4.1, is a required part of the UHDDS elements if applicable. The codes that describe the external cause of a complication (codes from Chapter 20) can be located in the Index to External Causes under the main term *complication* or *misadventure*.

> ### ■ CASE SCENARIO
>
> A patient had a postoperative hemorrhage in the tonsillar fossa following tonsillectomy. Codes reported would be J95.830 (complication, hemorrhage respiratory system) and the external cause code Y83.6 for the abnormal reaction to the removal of an organ.

CHECKPOINT 4.10

Code the following diagnostic statements using ICD-10-CM, sequencing the code(s) in order. Verify all codes in the Tabular List, and read all coding notes and conventions. Do not assign external cause codes.

1. Post-op urinary retention _____

2. Loosening of a left prosthetic hip joint replacement (sequelae) _____

3. Postoperative seroma of skin of abdominal wall following digestive surgery _____

4. Infected urethral catheter with cystitis, initial encounter _____

5. Mechanical breakdown (complication) of a pacemaker electrode, initial encounter

_____

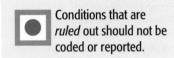

Conditions that are *ruled* out should not be coded or reported.

The Uncertain Diagnosis guideline is applicable only to short-term care, acute care, and long-term care hospice and to psychiatric hospitals. This guideline does not apply to physician service coding regardless of setting.

[handwritten: Inpatient only]

Uncertain Diagnosis

The *Official Guidelines* covering diagnoses that are not definitive state that a condition associated with an uncertain diagnosis should be coded as if it existed or was established if the documented diagnosis at discharge is "probable, suspected, likely, questionable, possible, or still to be ruled out." The reason for coding the possible condition in the inpatient setting is based on the "diagnostic workup, arrangements for further workup or observation, and initial therapeutic approach that correspond most closely with the diagnosis." For example, if documentation states that the discharge diagnosis for an inpatient hospital visit is probable gastroenteritis, the coder assigns the code for gastroenteritis (K52.9).

On the other hand, conditions that are ruled out should not be coded as if they exist. There is a difference between conditions that have been *ruled* out and conditions that remain to be ruled out by a physician; the latter are coded as *rule out* conditions. One letter changes the coding rule drastically. This guideline does not apply to physician services coding regardless of setting. For physician services coding, conditions that are uncertain should not be reported.

EXAMPLES FOR HOSPITAL INPATIENT (NON-PHYSICIAN)

- Nausea and vomiting, gastroenteritis ruled out: only the nausea and vomiting are coded; gastroenteritis was ruled out. Code R11.2 is assigned.

- Nausea and vomiting, rule out gastroenteritis: code the gastroenteritis because conditions that are possible or probable or not ruled out should be coded as if they exist.

Exceptions to this rule are certain illnesses such as multiple sclerosis, AIDS, and epilepsy. If documentation states "possible multiple sclerosis," the coder should discuss the coding with the attending physician. Many physicians are not aware of the coding rule, and reporting these unconfirmed diagnoses may have social or employment ramifications for the patient. Therefore, discussion with the physician is essential.

Admission From Observation Unit

Sometimes a patient is admitted from an observation unit for either medical reasons or following surgery. The guidelines on sequencing the principal diagnosis in these circumstances must be clarified.

Admission Following Medical Observation. The principal diagnosis is the medical condition that led to the hospital admission. Often a patient will present to the observation unit for a condition that needs monitoring, a status referred to as *medical observation*. If that condition does not improve or if it worsens, the patient may require hospital admission. For example, a patient enters observation due to congestive heart failure. Intravenous medications do not improve the patient's condition, and hospital admission is required. The principal diagnosis is reported as congestive heart failure (I50.9).

Admission Following Postoperative Observation. Under various circumstances, a patient may be first admitted to the observation unit for monitoring if a condition or complication occurs following outpatient surgery (a status referred to as *postoperative observation*) and then admitted to the hospital. In this case, the UHDDS definition of principal diagnosis applies: the condition established after study to be chiefly responsible for occasioning the admission to the hospital is the principal diagnosis.

> ■ **CASE SCENARIO**
> A patient is admitted to the observation unit following severe pain from a tonsillectomy. Pain is controlled in the observation unit, but the patient develops a postoperative hemorrhage and requires admission to the hospital. The postoperative hemorrhage is the principal diagnosis because it is chiefly responsible for occasioning the admission. The diagnosis of tonsillitis and the procedure for tonsillectomy are also reported.

Admission From Outpatient Surgery

The *Official Guidelines* provide three scenarios regarding sequencing of the principal diagnosis depending on the circumstances of admission.

Admission From Outpatient Surgery Due to Complication. When a patient who has surgery in the hospital's outpatient surgery department is subsequently admitted because of a complication of surgery, the complication code is sequenced first. The additional codes for the diagnosis and surgery (the ICD-10-PCS) are also reported. An external cause complication code is also reported when the complication code is reported.

> ■ **CASE SCENARIO**
> Mary Jane undergoes inguinal hernia repair. After surgery, she is admitted due to postoperative fever. The principal diagnosis is the post-op fever (R50.82), followed by the diagnosis code for left inguinal hernia (K40.90). The procedure code for hernia repair (ICD-10-PCS) is also reported, along with the external cause code from Chapter 20 to show this was a reaction to a hernia repair (Y83.8).

Admission From Outpatient Surgery With No Complication. "If no complication, or other condition, is documented as the reason for the inpatient admission, assign the reason for the outpatient surgery as the principal diagnosis." This ICD-10-CM guideline applies when there is no complication.

> ■ **CASE SCENARIO**
> Mark is scheduled to undergo a laparoscopic cholecystectomy as an outpatient to treat chronic cholelithiasis. In the outpatient surgery unit, Mark undergoes open cholecystectomy and is admitted to the hospital after surgery for recovery. The principal diagnosis is chronic cholelithiasis (K80.20), and the procedure code for the cholecystectomy (ICD-10-PCS) is also reported for the inpatient stay.

Admission From Outpatient Surgery for an Unrelated Condition. Sometimes, a completely different problem that requires hospital admission arises. "If the reason for the inpatient admission is another condition unrelated to the surgery, assign the unrelated condition as the principal diagnosis."

■ **CASE SCENARIO**

Donna undergoes an outpatient colonoscopy to evaluate anemia. After the surgery, she develops hyperglycemia and her type 2 diabetes mellitus is uncontrolled; this condition requires hospital admission. The principal diagnosis for the inpatient hospital visit is hyperglycemia in a type 2 diabetic (E11.65), and the anemia is coded second (D64.9). The colonoscopy is also reported for the hospital inpatient admission.

> ● The circumstances of admission are critical in assigning the principal diagnosis code for the facility.

Admission/Encounters for Rehabilitation. Reporting diagnosis codes for encounters specifically for rehabilitation depend on whether the condition requiring rehabilitation is still present. If the condition is still present, report that condition. For example, a patient presents to rehabilitation to treat left-sided dominant hemiplegia following a non-traumatic intracerebral hemorrhage, report code I69.152. In this case, the patient still has the medical condition of hemiplegia. In contrast, when the condition for which rehabilitation is no longer present, report the aftercare code first. For example, a patient underwent a left knee joint replacement to treat osteoarthritis and presents for rehabilitation services. Report Aftercare following joint replacement surgery Z47.1 first followed by the additional code to identify the joint replaced (Z96.652). For rehabilitation services following active treatment of an injury, assign the injury code with the subsequent care designation (7th character). For example, a patient requires rehabilitation status post hip replacement for a left intertrochanteric femur fracture, report S72.142D as the first-listed or principal diagnosis.

CHECKPOINT 4.11

Correctly code and sequence the following scenarios using ICD-10-CM.

1. Joe is admitted to the hospital from observation after his unstable angina does not improve with medications. _____

2. Karen is admitted to the hospital due to post-op atelectasis following outpatient bronchoscopy for lung mass. _____

3. After outpatient carotid angiography for syncope, Larry's hypertension is uncontrolled, requiring admission to the hospital. _____

4. Laura is admitted for rehabilitation services following treatment of a right femoral shaft fracture. _____

5. Maxine undergoes cystoscopy with a biopsy for hematuria as an outpatient. She then goes to observation for pain control. In observation, Maxine develops chest pain, which requires her hospitalization. _____

Section III: Reporting Additional Diagnoses

The *Official Guidelines* also indicate which conditions should be reported as secondary diagnoses, meaning other diagnoses. This data element of the UHDDS (see Table 4.1) defines other diagnoses as:

> A comorbidity, which represents "conditions that coexist at the time of admission," or
> a complication, which is a condition that "develops subsequently, or that affects the

treatment received and/or the length of stay. Diagnoses that relate to an earlier episode which have no bearing on the current hospital stay are to be excluded."

The definition of principal diagnosis and reporting of additional diagnoses applies to hospital inpatients and nonoutpatient settings. Nonoutpatient settings are defined by the guidelines to include long-term care, short-term care, psychiatric facilities, home health agencies, and rehabilitation facilities.

General Rules for Other (Additional) Diagnoses

Five key criteria are used in determining whether to report an additional diagnosis or condition. At least one criterion must be met in all cases, but many times one condition may meet one or more criteria. According to the *Official Guidelines*:

> "For reporting purposes the definition for 'other diagnoses' is interpreted as additional conditions that affect patient care in terms of requiring:
>
> 1. clinical evaluation; or
> 2. therapeutic treatment; or
> 3. diagnostic procedures; or
> 4. extended length of hospital stay; or
> 5. increased nursing care and/or monitoring."

 The order for reporting multiple secondary diagnoses is not mandated; however, if there is limited space for reporting, conditions should be reported in the order of their significance, with the most significant condition reported first after the principal diagnosis.

Clinical Evaluation. Many conditions documented by the physician in the inpatient hospital setting may require clinical evaluation. For example, the patient may develop confusion, which requires clinical evaluation from a consultant. Confusion or the underlying cause is reported as an additional or secondary diagnosis.

Physician documentation must support the presence of additional diagnoses.

Therapeutic Treatment. Patients who receive medication for a particular disease are undergoing therapeutic treatment. Physical therapy and speech therapy are also therapeutic treatment, and conditions that require such therapy should be reported.

 REIMBURSEMENT REVIEW

The Medicare Inpatient Prospective Payment System and MS-DRGs

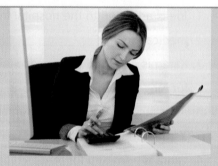

Medicare, by far the largest health plan for hospital reimbursement, pays hospitals for inpatient services based on the Medicare Inpatient Prospective Payment System (IPPS). This system is called *prospective* because rather than paying after the fact, the rate for each service has been set in advance. Rates are established based on Medicare's analysis of how long people are hospitalized, on average, for similar conditions. The length of stay (LOS) is a good predictor of the average use of the hospital's resources and, thus, of the cost of care.

Medicare analyzes and updates a study of all the ICD-10-CM codes—both diagnoses and procedures—that are reported for care during a period of time. Medicare then groups patients into diagnosis-related groups (DRGs). Each DRG number is connected to a dollar amount that is payable for the patients in its category. Patients are assigned a single DRG, which is based on these elements of the UHDDS:

- Diagnoses, principal and other secondary diagnoses
- Significant procedures
- Age, gender, and discharge status

Formerly, each DRG was associated with a single payment rate. In 2008, Medicare adopted a new type of DRG called Medicare Severity DRGs (MS-DRGs) to reflect the different severity

An inpatient receives medication for hypertension throughout a hospitalization. Hypertension is reported as an additional diagnosis.

Diagnostic Procedures. This criterion refers to conditions that require a diagnostic service, including diagnostic blood work, a radiology procedure, or another diagnostic procedure such as a colonoscopy. For example, the condition of anemia requires diagnostic testing to determine the type of anemia. Laboratory test results and physician documentation support a diagnosis of iron-deficiency anemia, so the anemia should be reported as an additional diagnosis.

Extended Length of Hospital Stay. Many circumstances, such as a fever or other complications, can extend a patient's hospital stay. Typically, these conditions develop after admission and may also require clinical evaluation or treatment.

A patient develops a severe headache the evening before his expected discharge. The discharge is cancelled, and the patient undergoes a CAT scan of the brain. Headache is reported as an additional diagnosis because this condition extended the length of stay and also required clinical evaluation.

Increased Nursing Care and/or Monitoring. Many conditions require increased nursing care or monitoring. For example, a patient may be legally blind, a condition that requires increased nursing care and should be reported. A patient may develop hypotension and require increased monitoring of blood pressure; hypotension should be reported as an additional diagnosis.

Because of changing rules from health plans about reimbursement, reporting secondary conditions is increasingly important for the inpatient setting. The Reimbursement Review outlines the key points relating to the effects of secondary codes on payments.

of illness among patients with the same diagnosis. The system better recognizes the severity of illness and the corresponding higher cost of treating Medicare patients with more complex conditions, offset by decreasing payments for other less severely ill patients.

There are 745 DRGs, replacing the former 538. The MS-DRG system increases the importance of listing secondary conditions, because when patients have or develop them, the rate of payment hospitals receive for the hospital stay is increased.

If the secondary diagnosis represents a condition that the patient has at admission, it is called a *comorbidity*. Comorbidities are either conditions that affect a patient's recovery, such as having diabetes mellitus, or another acute illness or injury. If the secondary diagnosis represents a complication that affects the patient's recovery, the length of the hospital stay is increased, logically increasing payment. Complications in this context are those conditions that happen after admission that affect care.

Together, under the UHDDS, the principal diagnosis and the comorbidities/complications are known as the CCs. According to the *Journal of AHIMA* (July/August 2007, p. 18), a base MS-DRG may have three levels of severity:

1. Major CC (MCC)
2. CC
3. Non-CC

To achieve the correct payment level for the hospital stay, coders should code as many secondary conditions as are compliant with the rules for reporting additional diagnoses.

Underline the conditions in the following scenarios that would be reported as additional diagnoses, and identify which criteria for reporting were met (1, 2, 3, 4, and/or 5). *Note:* Your answer may include more than one criterion.

1. Clinical evaluation

2. Therapeutic treatment

3. Diagnostic procedures

4. Extended length of hospital stay

5. Increased nursing care and/or monitoring

Following is an example: Monica is admitted to the hospital for treatment of breast cancer. She is also treated with medication for her <u>hypertension</u> and <u>diabetes</u>. Criterion 2, therapeutic treatment.

1. Joseph develops hypokalemia on the second day of his hospital stay. This condition requires laboratory monitoring and potassium supplements. _____

2. Kevin needs to stay in the hospital one additional day because he becomes dehydrated.

   _____

3. Marlene undergoes an echocardiogram because of a heart murmur heard on examination. The physician documents mitral valve prolapse as the cause of the murmur and prescribes antibiotics prior to surgery. _____

4. Paul becomes dizzy once he is able to get out of bed. The nursing staff is ordered to monitor Paul's blood pressure closely during the next 12 hours because of his dizziness.

   _____

5. After admission, Beth develops chest pain. The chest pain is evaluated by ECG and is treated with nitroglycerin. _____

Additional Guidelines for Other Diagnoses

According to the *Official Guidelines*, the following rules apply to designating other diagnoses when neither the Index nor the Tabular List provides direction.

Previous Conditions. The guidance on previous conditions is as follows:

> If the provider has included a diagnosis in the final diagnostic statement, such as the discharge summary or the face sheet, it should ordinarily be coded. Some providers include in the diagnostic statement resolved conditions or diagnoses and status-post procedures from previous admission that have no bearing on the current stay. Such conditions are not to be reported and are coded only if required by hospital policy.

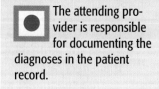

The attending provider is responsible for documenting the diagnoses in the patient record.

■ **CASE SCENARIO**

A physician may document the diagnosis of status post-cholecystectomy on the face sheet. Review of documentation indicates that the cholecystectomy was completed 5 years earlier. No code is assigned for this diagnostic statement.

It is appropriate to assign history codes as secondary codes if the historical condition or family history affects current care or influences treatment.

When coding documented abnormal findings noted as clinically significant, locate these conditions under the main term *findings, abnormal*. This differs from coding outpatient encounters for diagnostic tests that have been interpreted by a provider, such as a chest x-ray with an interpretation of pneumonia.

Abnormal Findings. The attending or treating physician must document clinical significance in order to code abnormal findings (those outside of normal ranges) such as those from laboratory, x-ray, pathology, and other diagnostic results.

If the finding is outside the normal range and the attending provider has ordered other tests to evaluate the condition or has prescribed treatment, it is appropriate to query him or her about whether the abnormal finding should be added. Only the physician can clarify whether abnormal findings should be coded; the coder may not make that determination. If, for example, when reviewing the medical record you notice that the patient's urinalysis is positive for *E. coli* based on urine culture results alone, you should ask the physician whether these results were clinically significant. If you see that a chest x-ray supports the diagnostic impression of COPD, you need provider documentation of clinical significance before you can code the abnormal findings.

Uncertain Diagnoses. As discussed earlier, the rule governing uncertain diagnoses applies for secondary diagnoses as well. If the diagnosis documented at the time of discharge is qualified as probable, suspected, likely, questionable, possible, or still to be ruled out, code the condition as if it existed or has been established. This guideline applies only to short-term care, acute care, long-term care, and psychiatric hospitals.

CHECKPOINT 4.13

Correctly code and sequence the following scenarios using ICD-10-CM.

1. Monica is admitted for acute CVA. After admission, follow-up lab work shows abnormal liver function tests, which are documented and evaluated by the attending physician. The cause of these abnormal findings is not determined. _____

2. The patient is admitted for acute renal failure. The patient had an appendectomy 3 years earlier.
_____

3. Documentation of the discharge diagnoses states the following: congestive heart failure, gouty arthritis, abnormal ECG, history of nicotine dependence. _____

4. Bonnie is admitted for treatment of breast cancer. The face sheet documentation supports the following diagnoses: carcinoma of the left breast (center portion), estrogen receptor positive status, hyponatremia, and possible allergic dermatitis. _____

5. In the outpatient setting, the patient presents to the hospital for an outpatient x-ray due to right ankle pain. Ankle x-ray interpretation by the radiologist supports the diagnosis of osteoarthritis.
_____

PRESENT ON ADMISSION (POA) GUIDELINES

Once the diagnosis codes have been assigned and sequenced, the coder in the inpatient setting must also determine whether each principal and secondary diagnosis, as well as external cause of injury, was present on admission (POA). *Present on admission* means present at the time the order for inpatient admission occurs. Conditions that develop during an outpatient encounter that leads to admission—including in the emergency department, during observation, or during outpatient surgery—are considered present on admission. Whether the condition was present on admission is reported by the use of an indicator, as shown in Table 4.2. The indicator is placed next to each ICD-10-CM diagnosis code reported on a hospital health-care claim. Note that the POA guidelines are a part of the *Official Guidelines*, Appendix I.

> ● The federal requirement to report POA indicators so that Medicare does not pay hospitals for conditions the hospital caused or allowed to develop during an inpatient stay was established in the Deficit Reduction Act of 2005. The *Official Guidelines* added the POA reporting requirements to Appendix I effective the following year.

Table 4.2 POA Indicators

INDICATOR	MEANING	DEFINITION
Y	Yes	Present at the time of inpatient admission.
N	No	Not present at the time of inpatient admission.
U	Unknown	Documentation is insufficient to determine whether the condition is present on admission.
W	Clinically undetermined	Provider is unable to clinically determine whether the condition was present on admission.
———	Blank	If the condition code is on the list of exempt codes, the field is left blank.

Notice that indicators U and W refer to documentation issues or to knowledge about whether the condition was present that the provider was unable to clinically determine. Issues related to inconsistent, missing, conflicting, or unclear documentation must be resolved by the provider.

Leaving the POA field blank is appropriate when an ICD-10-CM diagnosis code that is listed on the POA exempt from reporting list is assigned. Such a code either represents conditions that are always present on admission or does not represent a current disease or injury. For example, normal delivery codes represent conditions that are always present on admission, whereas screening codes and palliative care codes do not represent current diseases. Box 4.3 provides a sample of the codes that are exempt from the POA indicator.

BOX 4.3 Sample of POA Exempt Codes as Referenced in ICD-10-CM Official Coding Guidelines, Appendix I

B90–B94, Sequelae of infectious and parasitic diseases

E64, Sequelae of malnutrition and other nutritional deficiencies

I25.2, Old myocardial infarction

I69, Sequelae of cerebrovascular disease

O09, Supervision of high risk pregnancy

O66.5, Attempted application of vacuum extractor and forceps

O80, Encounter for full-term uncomplicated delivery

O94, Sequelae of complication of pregnancy, childbirth, and the puerperium

P00, Newborn (suspected to be) affected by maternal conditions that may be unrelated to present pregnancy

Q00–Q99, Congenital malformations, deformations and chromosomal abnormalities, except Q53

S00–T88.9, Injury, poisoning and certain other consequences of external causes with 7th character representing subsequent encounter or sequela, except S06 and S63

V00.121, Fall from non-in-line roller-skates

V00.131, Fall from skateboard

V00.141, Fall from scooter (non-motorized)

V00.311, Fall from snowboard

V00.321, Fall from snow-skis

V40–V49, Car occupant injured in transport accident

V80–V89, Other land transport accidents

V90–V94, Water transport accidents

V95–V97, Air and space transport accidents

W03, Other fall on same level due to collision with another person

W09, Fall on and from playground equipment

W15, Fall from cliff

W17.0, Fall into well

W17.1, Fall into storm drain or manhole

W18.01 Striking against sports equipment with subsequent fall

W20.8, Other cause of strike by thrown, projected or falling object

W21, Striking against or struck by sports equipment

W30, Contact with agricultural machinery

W31, Contact with other and unspecified machinery

W32–W34, Accidental handgun discharge and malfunction

W35–W40, Exposure to inanimate mechanical forces

W52, Crushed, pushed or stepped on by crowd or human stampede

W89, Exposure to man-made visible and ultraviolet light

X02, Exposure to controlled fire in building or structure

X03, Exposure to controlled fire, not in building or structure

X04, Exposure to ignition of highly flammable material

X52, Prolonged stay in weightless environment

X71-X83, Intentional self-harm

Y21, Drowning and submersion, undetermined intent

Y22, Handgun discharge, undetermined intent

Y23, Rifle, shotgun and larger firearm discharge, undetermined intent

INTERNET RESOURCES: A list of the hospital acquired conditions that impact payment when the POA is N (no) can be found at https://www.cms.gov/Medicare/Medicare-Fee-for-Service -Payment/HospitalAcqCond/icd10_hacs .html

Some of the guidelines assist the coder in determining whether a condition or external cause (code from Chapter 20) is present on admission.

Conditions Present on Admission—Indicator of Y

The Y (yes) indicator is assigned for any condition that the provider explicitly documents as being present on admission. These may be conditions that were diagnosed prior to admission (such as diabetes) or conditions that were clearly present but not diagnosed until after admission.

Conditions that are possible or probable at the time of discharge are assigned a POA of Y when the diagnosis was suspected at the time of inpatient admission. The coder also assigns a Y for chronic conditions that are present but not diagnosed until after admission. The indicator identifies whether the condition was present at admission, not whether it was diagnosed then.

> **■ CASE SCENARIO**
> Joe presents with chest pain from possible unstable angina. The chest x-ray reveals COPD. Evaluation and testing during hospitalization confirm that Joe has unstable angina due to coronary artery disease and COPD. Treatments are provided, and Joe is discharged. The codes reported are coronary artery disease and unstable angina (I25.110) and COPD (J44.9). The POA indicator for all the codes is Y.

Also assign the POA of Y for external causes of injury that occurred prior to admission. The patient may have fallen out of bed at home, or a patient may have made a suicide attempt prior to admission.

A Y indicator is also assigned for a newborn whose condition developed in utero. This includes conditions that occur during delivery (meconium aspiration, fetal distress). A newborn is not considered to be admitted until after delivery, and congenital conditions are always considered present on admission.

> ● Among the conditions that are not reimbursed by Medicare if they are hospital-stay generated are pressure ulcers, injuries caused by falls, and infections resulting from the prolonged use of catheters in blood vessels or the bladder. Also noted are "serious preventable events" such as leaving a sponge or other object in a patient during surgery and providing a patient with incompatible blood or blood products.

> ● Diagnoses confirmed after admission are considered present on admission if they are documented as suspected or constitute an underlying cause of a symptom present at the time of admission.

Conditions Not Present on Admission—Indicator of N

The POA indicator of N (no) refers to any condition that was not present on admission based on the provider's documentation. If the final diagnosis contains the terms *possible, probable,* or *suspected* and if it was based on symptoms or clinical findings that were not present on admission, the N indicator is assigned.

Assign N for an E code that represents an external cause of injury or poisoning that occurred during inpatient hospitalization. This might be a fall out of bed in the hospital or an adverse reaction to a medication given after admission.

> **■ CASE SCENARIO**
> Maggie is admitted with gastrointestinal bleeding and associated anemia. After a transfusion of red blood cells, she has a transfusion reaction. The code for transfusion reaction is reported with the N indicator because the reaction was not present on admission. The POA indicator for the bleeding and anemia is Y.

Unknown (U) or Undetermined (W) Conditions

When medical record documentation is unclear about whether a condition was present on admission, the indicator U (unknown) is assigned. This indicator is not assigned routinely, because documentation in the medical record should support a more specific indicator of Y or N. If the documentation is unclear, the physician should be queried about whether the condition was present on admission.

If the presence of the condition at admission cannot be determined clinically, the indicator W (undetermined) should be assigned.

Special Circumstances for Assigning POA Indicators

If each code in ICD-10-CM represented just one disease or condition, assignment of a POA indicator might not require an extensive explanation. But ICD-10-CM includes combination codes, acute and chronic conditions, obstetric conditions that indicate complications of pregnancy, and perinatal conditions. These unique facets of ICD-10-CM require additional explanations.

> NOTE: Present on admission indicators are reported on health-care claims for facility inpatient services. The Reimbursement Review on the following pages explains the major points regarding claims and the POA.

POA Indicators for Combination Codes

Combination codes may represent acute exacerbations (such as a COPD exacerbation), complications (such as an ulcer with bleeding), or causal organisms (such as UTI due to *E. coli*). The guidelines instruct the coder to determine whether any part of the combination code was present on admission. If any part of the combination code was *not* present on admission, the N indicator is assigned.

■ CASE SCENARIOS

- If a patient's type 2 diabetes mellitus (E11.9) becomes poorly controlled with hyperglycemia (E11.65) after admission, only code E11.65 is assigned. Because the hyperglycemia portion of the diabetes did not develop until after admission, code E11.65 is assigned the POA indicator N.

- After admission, a patient with a gastric ulcer develops bleeding from the ulcer. Only the combination code for gastric ulcer with hemorrhage (K25.4) is assigned. Because the hemorrhage developed after admission, the N indicator is assigned.

For some codes, acute and chronic or acute exacerbation is not reported. An example is congestive heart failure. The code I50.9 is assigned whether the heart failure is chronic or decompensated (acute exacerbation). Therefore, if the heart failure is present on admission, the indicator is Y even if the heart failure decompensates after admission.

Some combination codes include causative organisms; an example is *E. coli* sepsis (A41.51). For infection codes that include the causal organism, the POA indicator of Y is assigned even if the culture results are determined after admission. Carefully determine whether the infection was present on admission. For example, if a patient presents with sepsis and the culture after admission is positive for *E. coli*, code A41.51 is assigned with the Y indicator.

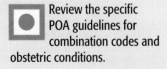

Review the specific POA guidelines for combination codes and obstetric conditions.

Obstetric Conditions

Whether the patient actually delivers during the current hospitalization does not affect the assignment of the POA indicator. The factor that determines the POA assignment is whether the obstetric condition described by the code is present at the time of admission.

If the pregnancy complication or obstetric condition is present on admission, the Y indicator is assigned. This includes such diagnoses as preterm labor and previous cesarean section. The N indicator is assigned when the condition is not present on admission, such as perineal laceration after delivery or postpartum hemorrhage. For an obstetric combination code, if any condition represented by that code is not present on admission, the N indicator is assigned.

■ CASE SCENARIO

Margie presents to the hospital in labor, and the baby is full term. Margie has gestational diabetes (O24.410). After admission, Margie requires a cesarean section due to fetal distress (O77.9). The pregnancy code for gestational diabetes is assigned the Y indicator, and the fetal distress code is assigned the N indicator.

The Hospital Billing Process: Claims and the POA Indicator

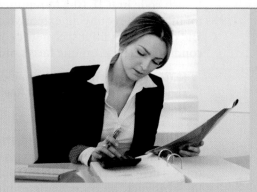

Hospitals submit claims to health plans on behalf of patients, unless the patient is solely responsible for payment. Most hospitals, because they are regulated by HIPAA, send electronic claims, although some may still be using paper claims.

A large percentage of claims are sent to Medicare, and these are transmitted electronically using the HIPAA healthcare claim called the 837I. This electronic data interchange (EDI) form has an *I* at the end for *Institutional*; the corresponding physicians' claim is called 837P (*Professional*). In some situations, a paper claim form called the UB-04 (*uniform billing 2004*), also known as the CMS-1450, is sent. The UB-04 is maintained by the National Uniform Billing Committee.

837I Health-Care Claim Completion

The sections in the 837I require data elements for the billing and the pay-to provider, the subscriber and patient, and the payer, plus claim and service level details. Most of the data elements report the same information as discussed next for the paper claim.

UB-04 Claim Form Completion

The UB-04 claim form shown here has 81 data fields, some of which require multiple entries. The information for the form locators often requires choosing from a list of codes, such as for the type of service. Medicare and private-payer–required fields may be slightly different, and other condition codes or options are often available. The completed form at right shows a claim for a hospital stay of 14 days. Note the ICD-10-CM codes and the POA indicators.

1 GRACE MEMORIAL HOSPITAL	2			3a PAT. CNTL # XX871295			4 TYPE OF BILL
100 MAIN STREET				b. MED. REC. # 7650120			0111
TULSA, OK 74101				5 FED. TAX NO.	6 STATEMENT COVERS PERIOD FROM THROUGH		7
9182367007				07-1282340	033117	041417	

8 PATIENT NAME	a	9 PATIENT ADDRESS	a	201 MAGNOLIA AVE.			
b WILLIAMS, GILBERT, U.		b TULSA			c OK	d 74103	e

10 BIRTHDATE	11 SEX	12 DATE	ADMISSION 13 HR	14 TYPE	15 SRC	16 DHR	17 STAT	18	19	20	21	CONDITION CODES 22	23	24	25	26	27	28	29 ACDT STATE	30
09121920	M	033117	07	1	7	19	01	09												

31 OCCURRENCE CODE / DATE	32 OCCURRENCE CODE / DATE	33 OCCURRENCE CODE / DATE	34 OCCURRENCE CODE / DATE	35 OCCURRENCE SPAN CODE / FROM / THROUGH	36 OCCURRENCE SPAN CODE / FROM / THROUGH	37
18 091285						

38		39 VALUE CODES CODE / AMOUNT	40 VALUE CODES CODE / AMOUNT	41 VALUE CODES CODE / AMOUNT
	a	80 14 00		
	b			
	c			
	d			

42 REV. CD.	43 DESCRIPTION	44 HCPCS / RATE / HIPPS CODE	45 SERV. DATE	46 SERV. UNITS	47 TOTAL CHARGES	48 NON-COVERED CHARGES	49
1 0111	MED-SURG-GY/PVT	72000		13	9,360 00		1
2 0201	ICU/SURGICAL	170100		1	1,701 00		2
3 0230	NURSING INCREM				9,594 00		3
4 0233	NUR INCR/ICU				2,027 00		4
5 0250	PHARMACY				2,579 15		5
6 0260	IV THERAPY				1,545 20		6
7 0270	MED-SUR SUPPLIES				835 90		7
8 0300	LAB				4,942 66		8
9 0301	CHEMISTRY TESTS				125 00		9
10 0320	DX X-RAY			1	433 18		10
11 0340	NUCLEAR MEDICINE			1	784 08		11
12 0350	CT SCAN			1	421 08		12
13 0351	CT SCAN/HEAD			1	1,018 82		13
14 0352	CT SCAN/BODY			4	4,075 28		14
15 0390	BLOOD/ADMIN/STOR				1,008 00		15
16 0410	RESPIRATORY SVC			29	641 56		16
17 0450	EMERG ROOM			2	810 82		17
18 0480	CARDIOLOGY				1,289 86		18
19 0730	EKG/ECG				96 68		19
20 0761	TREATMENT RM				54 45		20
21 0921	PERI VASCUL LAB				804 65		21
23 0001	PAGE 1 OF 1	CREATION DATE 042009	TOTALS ➡		44,148 37		23

50 PAYER NAME	51 HEALTH PLAN ID	52 REL INFO	53 ASG BEN.	54 PRIOR PAYMENTS	55 EST. AMOUNT DUE	56 NPI 1122999665	
A MEDICARE	00308	Y	Y			57 OTHER PRV ID 070089	A
B							B
C							C

58 INSURED'S NAME	59 P.REL	60 INSURED'S UNIQUE ID	61 GROUP NAME	62 INSURANCE GROUP NO.	
A WILLIAMS, GILBERT, U.	18	765452817A			A
B					B
C					C

63 TREATMENT AUTHORIZATION CODES	64 DOCUMENT CONTROL NUMBER	65 EMPLOYER NAME	
A			A
B			B
C			C

66 DX J189	Y C3481	Y C7972	Y J918	Y R590	N J449	Y C771	Y I10	Y J811	Y	68

69 ADMIT DX R069	70 PATIENT REASON DX a. b. c.	71 PPS CODE	72 ECI		73

74 PRINCIPAL PROCEDURE CODE / DATE	a. OTHER PROCEDURE CODE / DATE	b. OTHER PROCEDURE CODE / DATE	75	76 ATTENDING NPI 1022550001	QUAL 1G 58912T
039B00Z 033117	30233N1 040317			LAST FATU FIRST LOUISE	
c. OTHER PROCEDURE CODE / DATE	d. OTHER PROCEDURE CODE / DATE	e. OTHER PROCEDURE CODE / DATE		77 OPERATING NPI 2799906111	QUAL 1G 10340B
				LAST AZODI FIRST ALI	

80 REMARKS	81CC a b3 282N00000X	78 OTHER NPI	QUAL
	b	LAST	FIRST
	c	79 OTHER NPI	QUAL
	d	LAST	FIRST

UB-04 CMS-1450   APPROVED OMB NO. 0938-0997   NUBC™ National Uniform Billing Committee   THE CERTIFICATIONS ON THE REVERSE APPLY TO THIS BILL AND ARE MADE A PART HEREOF.

Assign the present on admission (POA) indicators for all of the diagnoses in the following scenarios.

1. A patient is admitted for a diagnostic workup of syncope. The final diagnosis is Sick Sinus Syndrome, and the patient undergoes pacemaker insertion. _____

2. A patient presents with difficulty breathing. The diagnosis is acute asthma exacerbation.

    _____

3. A patient falls in the emergency department (ED), sustaining a fractured hip. The patient is subsequently admitted due to hip fracture. _____

4. A patient is admitted to the hospital for knee replacement due to osteoarthritis of the knee. After surgery, the patient develops acute blood loss anemia. _____

5. A patient in active labor is admitted. During the stay, a breast abscess is noted when the patient starts breastfeeding the baby. The provider is unable to determine whether the abscess was present on admission. _____

6. A single, live newborn, born in the hospital via cesarean section develops feeding problems after birth. _____

7. A pregnant woman presents to the hospital and undergoes a normal delivery. _____

8. A patient presents with nausea and vomiting. The attending physician documents the discharge diagnosis as possible viral gastroenteritis. _____

9. A patient presents to the ED after a motor vehicle collision. He requires admission due to fractured ribs and a fractured wrist. After admission and surgery, he develops a wound infection.

    _____

10. A homeless patient is admitted with acute renal failure. After admission, the patient develops syncope. The physician documents the diagnoses as acute renal failure and possible cardiogenic syncope. _____

Chapter Summary

1. Section IB, General Coding Guidelines, of the *Official Guidelines for Coding and Reporting* covers basic coding guidelines that all coders must follow in order to accurately assign ICD-10-CM codes. Mistakes in coding can occur if these basic rules are not followed. The rules apply to both the inpatient and outpatient settings and should be used by all health-care providers, including hospitals, physicians, nursing homes, and home health-care agencies.

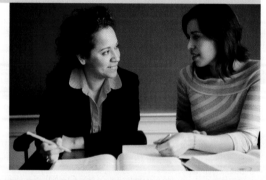

2. Both the Index and the Tabular List should be used for all ICD-10-CM coding. Skipping a step in the coding process can result in coding errors.

3. Always code to the highest level of specificity. This means that if a fourth digit is available for a category (three-digit code), the fourth digit must be assigned, and if a fifth digit is also available, it too must be assigned. ICD-10-CM uses an indented format and conventions to direct the coder to the fourth-, fifth-, sixth-, and seventh-digit levels. Each additional subcategory and seventh-character extension provide a higher level of detail for a particular condition.

4. Conditions that are an integral part of a disease process should not be coded separately. Signs and symptoms that are not integral to the disease process should be reported separately.

5. Multiple codes are often required to report a single condition. Conventions such as *use additional code* and *code also* notations help the coder understand when an additional code is required. Documentation in the medical record must support the use of the additional code.

6. The *Official Guidelines* address the use of combination codes. In a combination code, one code reflects more than one condition. Combination codes can reflect two diseases, a combination of a disease and its underlying cause, or a complication of care.

7. When coding both acute and chronic conditions, the coder must remember to determine whether the subterms *acute* (subacute) and *chronic* are located at the same indentation level. When they are located at the same indentation level, both codes are assigned, and the acute condition code is sequenced first.

8. For sequelae (late effects) coding, the acute condition is no longer present, but a residual condition remains. When coding sequelae, the residual condition (manifestation) is coded first, followed by a code for the cause of the sequelae. The main term *sequelae* is used to locate the code for the cause of the sequelae. Terms in the diagnostic statement such as *old* and *previous* alert the coder that the patient has a sequelae and that sequelae coding rules apply. There are exceptions to the requirement of reporting sequelae with two codes.

9. Impending and threatened conditions should first be coded by looking up the main terms *impending* or *threatened* or by searching for these terms as subterms. If a specific code is not available for an impending or threatened condition, the code for the actual condition should be reported. Typically, documentation of threatened or impending implies that the patient does not actually have the condition but is at risk for developing it.

10. ICD-10-CM diagnosis codes are only reported once. Two codes may be required to report laterality if a bilateral combination code is not available.

11. Documentation used to report body mass index (BMI), Coma Scale, NIH Stroke Scale, and the stage of pressure ulcers can be obtained from clinicians who are not the patient's provider (i.e., physician or other qualified health-care practitioner legally accountable for establishing the patient's diagnosis).

12. A cause-and-effect relationship must be documented in order to assign a code for a complication of care or a complication of a procedure unless the complication is inherent (i.e. colostomy leak).

13. The patient care flow and associated documentation for the inpatient setting begins with hospital admission, where the patient's face sheet with demographics as well as all medical information are compiled; continues during the evaluation and treatment of the patient, supported by appropriate notes; and is completed with the patient's discharge. The documentation in the medical record must support the diagnoses and procedures reported for each patient's hospitalization. Review of the discharge summary, history and physical, progress notes, physician orders, consultations, operative reports, and diagnostic tests is essential in order to assign accurate and complete ICD-10-CM codes. The listing of the diagnoses in the patient record is the responsibility of the attending provider.

14. The Uniform Hospital Discharge Data Set (UHDDS) definitions apply to all nonoutpatient settings. The definitions in the data set are mandated by HIPAA legislation and are incorporated in the *ICD-10-CM Official Guidelines for Coding and Reporting*.

15. The definition of principal diagnosis, which is based on the UHDDS definitions, is "that condition established after study to be chiefly responsible for occasioning the admission of the patient to the hospital for care."

16. Once the diagnosis codes are assigned, their sequencing must be completed. The main rule regarding sequencing of the principal diagnosis codes is that codes for signs and symptoms should not be sequenced first when the underlying condition has been established.

17. (a) When each of two or more interrelated conditions potentially meets the definition of principal diagnosis, either condition can be first listed. If two or more diagnoses equally meet the definition of principal diagnosis, either condition may be sequenced first. If two principal diagnoses are contrasting or comparative in nature, either condition may be sequenced first. (b) If the original treatment plan was not carried out, the definition of principal diagnosis still applies, so the diagnosis after study is first. (c) If the reason for admission is as a complication of medical care, the complication code is sequenced first. Documentation must state that the condition is the result of a procedure or of medical care. In many

instances, an additional code that specifically states the complication is assigned. (d) If a documented diagnosis at discharge is uncertain, probable, suspected, likely, questionable, possible, or still to be ruled out, the condition is coded as if it existed or was established (only for short-term care, acute care, long-term care, and psychiatric hospitals).

18. External cause codes (from Chapter 20) are assigned as appropriate. These codes are often related to complications, such as abnormal reactions to surgery or a medical treatment.

19. For admission following medical observation, the principal diagnosis is the medical condition that leads to the hospital admission; for admission following postoperative observation, the principal diagnosis is that determined after study; and for admission after outpatient surgery, the admission circumstances determine the principal diagnosis.

20. Codes for additional diagnoses, other diagnoses, and secondary diagnoses are not sequenced first. These codes represent other conditions, comorbidities, or complications that affect the current inpatient stay. Abnormal findings from laboratory results, x-rays, pathology reports, and special diagnostic studies cannot be coded without the physician's documentation of their clinical significance. Conditions that are uncertain should also be reported.

21. Once ICD-10-CM codes have been assigned and sequenced, each code must be assigned an indicator that identifies whether the condition was present on admission (POA). The POA reporting requirement applies to inpatient facility coding only. The present on admission indicator represents whether the code was present. Therefore, for a combination code, the entire illness represented by that code must have been present on admission in order to assign an indicator of yes (Y). Other indicators are N (no) if the condition was not present on admission, U if the presence of the condition on admission is unknown, and W if the presence of the condition on admission is clinically undetermined. Some codes are exempt from reporting the POA indicator, in which case the indicator is left blank.

22. The entire inpatient coding process requires review of complete documentation and abstraction of diagnoses and procedures from the patient record. The diagnoses are coded based on the ICD-10-CM *Official Guidelines*. Once all the conditions and procedures have been coded, the codes are sequenced, listing one code as the principal diagnosis and one code as the principal procedure, and all other codes are considered additional. The POA indicators are then assigned for both the principal and secondary diagnoses, including Z codes and external cause codes in some circumstances when not exempt.

Review Questions

Matching

Match the key terms with their definitions.

A. uncertain diagnosis
B. secondary diagnoses
C. abnormal findings
D. CC
E. IPPS

F. integral
G. chapter-specific guidelines
H. code first
I. late effect
J. acute condition

1. __F__ The fact that a symptom is a component part of a disease process

2. __J__ A medical condition that develops suddenly and resolves quickly

3. __G__ A set of rules specific to a chapter in ICD-10-CM

4. __H__ An instructional notation about which code should be listed before another

5. __I__ A circumstance in which a residual condition is present

6. __D__ A comorbidity or complication

7. __A__ Condition that is probable, suspected, likely, questionable, possible, or still to be ruled out

8. __C__ Test results that are outside of normal ranges

9. __B__ Other conditions in addition to the primary condition that are documented, coded, and reported

10. __E__ The Medicare payment system used for inpatients

True or False

Decide whether each statement is true or false.

1. __F__ The *ICD-10-CM Official Guidelines for Coding and Reporting* apply only to the inpatient setting.

2. __T__ The statement "scar from previous burn" would be coded as a sequela.

3. __T__ The coder must verify all codes in the Tabular List.

4. __F__ When coding the presence of a disease that is both acute and chronic, the code for the chronic condition is sequenced first.

5. __T__ The patient has abdominal pain, which represents a symptom.

6. __F__ The UHDDS definitions apply to outpatient visits only.

7. __F__ The coder should review each lab test and x-ray in order to code the results.

8. __F__ All signs and symptoms should be coded.

9. __T__ An external cause code may be required to report complications of a medical or surgical treatment.

10. __F__ A patient is admitted because of urinary incontinence. After admission, the patient develops chest pain. The POA indicator for the chest pain is W.

Multiple Choice

Select the letter that best completes the statement or answers the question.

1. Which codes would be reported for a patient with a seizure disorder from previous viral encephalitis?
   A. G40.909, B94.1
   B. G40.909, B94.8
   C. G40.901, B94.1
   D. G40.901, B94.8

2. Which instruction at code L86 directs the coder to assign a mandatory code for the underlying cause of acquired keratoderma?
   A. Code first the underlying disease
   B. Excludes
   C. Use additional code to identify the underlying disease
   D. None of the above

3. Which codes report the initial episode of a traumatic open fracture, Type I, of the right distal tibia due to collision on the highway with another motor vehicle?
   A. S82.302B, V43.51XA
   B. S82.301A, V43.92XD
   C. S82.301B, V43.92XA
   D. S82.301B, V43.51XA

4. Joseph presented with fever, tachycardia, chest pain, and headache. Which complaint(s) represents a symptom?
   A. Fever
   B. Fever and tachycardia
   C. Chest pain, headache, and tachycardia
   D. Chest pain and headache

5. Which code is reported for type I diabetes, with diabetic ketoacidosis?
   A. E10.10
   B. E10.11
   C. E11.00
   D. E08.10

6. Which documents in the medical record should be reviewed when coding?
   A. Physician progress notes
   B. Physician orders
   C. Discharge summary
   D. All of the above

7. Under which circumstance may a sign or symptom be sequenced as the principal diagnosis?
   A. When the underlying condition is documented
   B. When the sign or symptom is followed by comparative or contrasting conditions
   C. When the underlying cause of the sign or symptom is unknown
   D. Both B and C

8. Which of the following statements represents an uncertain diagnosis?
   A. Myocardial infarction ruled out
   B. Possible myocardial infarction
   C. Myocardial infarction
   D. Chest pain due to myocardial infarction

9. Marlene presents with chest pain. After study, the attending physician determines that the chest pain is due to coronary artery disease. Marlene also has hypertension, which is treated with medication during her stay. What is the principal diagnosis?
   A. Chest pain
   B. Coronary artery disease
   C. Hypertension
   D. Either chest pain or coronary artery disease

10. What should the coder do when documentation supports positive test results, signs and symptoms of a disease, and treatment, but the physician does not document any corresponding diagnosis? (For example, the patient has low potassium levels on lab tests and is treated with supplemental potassium.)
    A. Code the abnormal test results.
    B. Query the physician to seek clarification.
    C. Do not code the lab results.
    D. Code the abnormal test results, and write the diagnosis on the chart.

ICD-10-CM Chapters 1 Through 5: A00–F99

CHAPTER OUTLINE

Certain Infectious and Parasitic Diseases (Chapter 1: A00–B99)

Neoplasms (Chapter 2: C00–D49)

Diseases of the Blood and Blood-Forming Organs and Certain Disorders Involving the Immune Mechanism (Chapter 3: D50–D89)

Endocrine, Nutritional, and Metabolic Diseases (Chapter 4: E00–E89)

Mental, Behavioral, and Neurodevelopmental Disorders (Chapter 5: F01–F99)

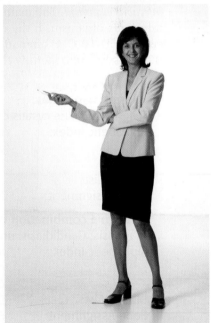

Photodisc/Thinkstock

LEARNING OUTCOMES

After studying this chapter, you should be able to:

1. Describe the general guideline for selecting and sequencing the causes of infectious diseases.
2. List the major points to consider in code selection and assignment for HIV/AIDS.
3. Differentiate among the diagnoses of SIRS and sepsis, identifying the key points for code selection and sequencing for SIRS, sepsis, and severe sepsis.
4. Discuss code selection for septic shock.
5. Describe the coding of methicillin-resistant *Staphylococcus aureus* (MRSA) conditions.
6. Describe the steps in coding for neoplasms.
7. Describe the coding and sequencing of anemias.
8. Discuss the multiple categories of codes for diabetes mellitus and what distinguishes each category.
9. Discuss the coding of diagnoses of mental illness.

Correct code assignment and sequencing of patients' diagnosed or suspected conditions provide the baseline for gathering data to improve treatment and for demonstrating the medical necessity of procedures. By understanding the basic concepts of coding introduced in Part 1, the coder can now code for diseases and conditions from the ICD-10-CM. This chapter will describe the major points to consider in code selection for infectious diseases, neoplasms, illnesses of the blood, endocrine disorders, and mental illness.

CERTAIN INFECTIOUS AND PARASITIC DISEASES (CHAPTER 1: A00–B99)

Infectious and parasitic diseases are an important classification of communicable diseases, those that can be transmitted between people via typical methods, such as through sexual or general body contact. Two major communicable diseases seen in many health-care settings are HIV and AIDS and systemic inflammatory response syndrome (SIRS). HIV is a retrovirus that attacks essential cells in the immune system and is a cause of AIDS (an autoimmune disease that makes patients susceptible to opportunistic infections) and AIDS-related complex (ARC). SIRS is a systemic response to a trauma, infection, or other condition and includes at least two of the following symptoms: tachypnea (fast breathing), tachycardia (fast heartbeat), fever, and/or elevated white blood cells. The categories in Chapter 1 are grouped as shown in Table 5.1.

General Guidance

Often, coding of infectious diseases requires assigning either two codes or a combination code. The goal is to identify both the *infectious site* and the *infectious organism*. The main term *infection* is the place to start to code the infectious organism. If the code for an infection is classified somewhere else in ICD-10-CM, often an additional code from category B95 through B97 is assigned to identify the organism.

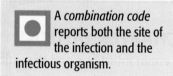 A *combination code* reports both the site of the infection and the infectious organism.

EXAMPLES

• **Assign two codes:**
Diagnosis: Acute cystitis due to pseudomonas

Alphabetic Index:	*Cystitis*	*Infection*
	acute N30.00	pseudomonas as cause of disease classified elsewhere B96.5
Tabular List:	N30 (Use additional code to identify infectious agent)	
Code Assignment:	N30.00 and B96.5	

• **Assign a combination code:**
Diagnosis: Candidiasis, urinary tract

Alphabetic Index:	*Infection*
	candidal (*see Candidiasis*)
	Candidiasis, urogenital site B37.49
Tabular List:	B37.49
Code Assignment:	B37.49

Coders are required to assign codes for infections based on physician statements in documentation rather than on laboratory results alone. If further clarification is needed, a physician query is appropriate. *Query* is the general term for a communication exchange between the physician and the coder. Such communication may follow a well-established protocol in some settings, such as in many inpatient departments.

In general, queries should

Many facilities have specialized staff members called *clinical document improvement specialists* whose job it is to study the documentation process and implement improvements to it by educating physicians on best practices and compliance.

• Be done consistently and without regard to reimbursement.
• Repeat or refer to items in the record that require clarification.
• Be written in an open-ended style so that the physician can answer based on the facts.
• Avoid yes/no or multiple-choice formats and suggestions.

Table 5.1 Organization of ICD-10-CM Chapter 1 Tabular List

BLOCK	BLOCK DESCRIPTION	EXAMPLE(S)
A00–A09	Intestinal infectious diseases	Food poisoning
A15–A19	Tuberculosis	Bacterial infection, usually of the lungs
A20–A28	Certain zoonotic bacterial diseases	Anthrax
A30–A49	Other bacterial diseases	Whooping cough, sepsis
A50–A64	Infections with a predominantly sexual mode of transmission	Syphilis
A65–A69	Other spirochetal diseases	Lyme disease
A70–A74	Other diseases caused by chlamydiae	*Chlamydia* infections
A75–A79	Rickettsioses	Spotted fever
A80–A89	Viral and prion infections of the central nervous system	Rabies, viral meningitis
A90–A99	Arthropod-borne viral fevers and viral hemorrhagic fevers	Yellow fever
B00–B09	Viral infections characterized by skin and mucous membrane lesions	Herpes zoster, measles
B10	Other human herpesviruses	Other herpesvirus encephalitis
B15–B19	Viral hepatitis	Hepatitis A, B, and C
B20	Human immunodeficiency virus (HIV) disease	AIDS
B25–B34	Other viral diseases	Mononucleosis
B35–B49	Mycoses	Candidiasis infections
B50–B64	Protozoal diseases	Toxoplasmosis
B65–B83	Helminthiases	Filariasis
B85–B89	Pediculosis, ascariasis, and other infestations	Scabies
B90–B94	Sequelae of infectious and parasitic diseases	Sequelae of viral hepatitis
B95–B97	Bacterial and viral infectious agents	*H. influenzae* as cause of disease classified elsewhere
B99	Other infectious diseases	Unspecified infectious disease

● Never code from laboratory results alone; review physician documentation as the primary resource, and query the physician as needed.

An example of a situation requiring clarification through the use of a query is documentation on a patient who presents with pneumonia and whose sputum culture is positive for *Staphylococcus aureus*. The diagnostic statement is just pneumonia. The physician should be queried to clarify the significance of this laboratory finding and to determine if there is a relationship to the current pneumonia. An example of a query is shown in Box 5.1.

BOX 5.1 Example of a Coder's Query to a Physician

Dr. B: Documentation in the medical record supports the diagnosis of pneumonia, and sputum culture was positive for *Klebsiella*. Please render an opinion regarding the significance of the positive culture and relationship to the specific type of pneumonia as a diagnosis for this patient. Please document clarification in the medical record.

Human Immunodeficiency Virus (HIV)

The *Official Guideline's Chapter-Specific Coding Guidelines: Certain Infectious and Parasitic Diseases (A00–B99)* cover coding HIV and AIDS infections and illness (see Box 5.2).

Specific coding rules are required in assigning diagnoses codes for both HIV-positive status and for AIDS. The coder must also be familiar with coding for counseling, positive test results alone, and unconfirmed cases. Having HIV-positive serology means that the patient is infected with the HIV virus. To be diagnosed as having AIDS, the patient must exhibit an HIV infection that has compromised the immune system to the extent that an AIDS-related illness (one of multiple illnesses) has occurred.

Overview

Pharmacology comes from the Greek words *pharmacon*, which means "drug," and *logos*, which means "word" or "thought." It is the field of study that seeks to understand how certain chemicals interact with living organisms to produce a change in function. Pharmacologists study the properties, applications, and effects of particular chemicals to determine whether they are beneficial to humans and animals. This work requires intimate knowledge of specific biological systems.

If a substance has medicinal properties, it is considered a *pharmaceutical*. These beneficial substances are used by clinicians to diagnose, prevent, and cure diseases. The safe use of a drug (also known as *medicine* or *medication*) requires sound knowledge of its properties, such as mechanism of action, dose, route of administration, adverse effects, toxicity, and interactions.

Pharmacology is based on science and systematic research rather than on anecdotal information and trial and error. The discovery of many new drugs has revolutionized medical care, and a rational system of laws governing drug-manufacturing processes and distribution has been developed to protect patients. Under current law, the manufacturer of a new drug must provide proof that the drug is both safe and effective before it can be approved for use in the United States.

Related Fields

- Pharmacy deals with preparing and dispensing medicines to the patient as prescribed by a licensed practitioner. The pharmacist also provides information to patients and health professionals.
- *Pharmacognosy* is a term derived from the Greek word *gnosis*, which means "knowledge." It is a branch of pharmacology that deals with the sources of drugs derived from plants and animals. It is also a study of the physical and chemical properties of such substances.
- *Pharmacokinetics* is a term derived from the Greek word *kinesis*, meaning "a movement." It deals with the disposition of drugs in the body, including their absorption, distribution, metabolism, and excretion. Pharmacokinetics provides a basis for determining the dose of a drug and helps determine dosage adjustments in patients with altered physiological and pathological states such as aging and renal or hepatic impairment.

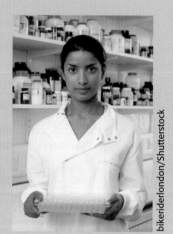
Hospital pharmaceuticals.

- *Pharmacodynamics* (from the Greek *dynamics*, meaning "force") is the study of the physiological and biochemical effects of drugs, the mechanisms of action, and the relationship of drug concentrations in the blood with drug response and duration of action.
- Pharmacogenetics is a relatively new field. It is concerned with genetically mediated variations in drug responses.
- Clinical pharmacology is a branch of pharmacology that deals with the pharmacological effects of drugs in humans. It gives useful data about the potency, safety, effectiveness, and toxicity of new drugs for clinical use.
- The field of biopharmaceutics deals with drug delivery systems and dosage forms. It provides information about how dosage forms can influence the pharmacodynamic and pharmacokinetic properties of a drug.

Drug Nomenclature

Three separate names are assigned to every drug:

1. The *chemical* name is given to the drug based on its chemical structure. This name indicates the precise arrangement of atoms and atomic groups in the drug molecule. Chemical names are too complex and cumbersome to be used in prescriptions.

2. The nonproprietary or generic name is used after a drug is determined to be therapeutically useful. This name is assigned by the United States Adopted Name (USAN) council. These names are used uniformly all over the world by an international agreement moderated by the World Health Organization (WHO). The nonproprietary name is called "official" when it is included in official books such as Indian, British, U.S., or international pharmacopeia.

3. A proprietary, trade, or brand name is selected and registered under patent law by the pharmaceutical company that developed the drug. This name becomes the sole property of the pharmaceutical company. Thus, a nonproprietary drug may be marketed under several proprietary names by different firms.

EXAMPLES

Chemical name	7-chloro-1, 3-dihydro-1-methyl-5-phenyl-2H-1, 4-benzodiazepine-2-one
Nonproprietary name	diazepam
Proprietary name	Valium® (Roche, United States)
	Calmpose® (Ranbaxy, India)

The symbol ® appears at the end of the trade name, indicating that the name is a registered trademark.

Routes of Administration

Pharmaceuticals are prepared in formulations for specific routes of administration. Routes are either *enteral*, meaning any method that involves the gastrointestinal tract, from the mouth through the rectum; or *parenteral,* meaning any other route.

The enteral routes are

- Oral, such as via tablets, capsules, or solutions
- Buccal, in which the tablet is left to dissolve inside the cheek
- Sublingual, in which a tablet or lozenge is dissolved under the tongue
- Rectal, via solutions or suppositories

Common parenteral routes include

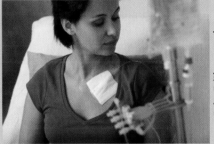

Image Point Fr/Shutterstock

- Intraocular, such as drops in the eye
- Intranasal or inhalation, in which solutions or powders are sprayed or inhaled via the nose
- Intravenous (IV), injection into the vein
- Intramuscular (IM), injection into muscle tissue
- Intradermal, injection into the top layer of skin
- Intrathecal, injection into the spinal column
- Subcutaneous (SC), injection into the subcutaneous layer of the skin

Intravenous administration.

- Dermal administration, such as ointments or creams applied to the skin
- Vaginal administration, such as ointments, creams, or suppositories

Why Coders Study Pharmaceuticals

From a coding perspective, knowledge of medications and their administration assists in

- Coding procedures (e.g., coding of chemotherapy or infusion of thrombolytics)
- Querying clinicians to verify the presence of related diseases based on medical record documentation
- Correctly coding all primary and secondary conditions for appropriate reporting

BOX 5.2 *Official Guidelines*: Human Immunodeficiency Virus (HIV) Infections (A00–B99)

1) **Code Only Confirmed Cases**

   Code only confirmed cases of HIV infection/illness. This is an exception to the hospital inpatient guideline Section II, H.

   In this context, "confirmation" does not require documentation of positive serology or culture for HIV; the provider's diagnostic statement that the patient is HIV positive or has an HIV-related illness is sufficient.

2) **Selection and Sequencing of HIV Codes**

   (a) **Patient admitted for HIV-related condition**

   If a patient is admitted for an HIV-related condition, the principal diagnosis should be B20, Human immunodeficiency virus [HIV] disease, followed by additional diagnosis codes for all reported HIV-related conditions.

   (b) **Patient with HIV disease admitted for unrelated condition**

   If a patient with HIV disease is admitted for an unrelated condition (e.g., a traumatic injury), the code for the unrelated condition (e.g., the nature of injury code) should be the principal diagnosis. Other diagnoses would be B20 followed by additional diagnosis codes for all reported HIV-related conditions.

   (c) **Whether the patient is newly diagnosed**

   Whether the patient is newly diagnosed or has had previous admissions/encounters for HIV conditions is irrelevant to the sequencing decision.

   (d) **Asymptomatic human immunodeficiency virus**

   Z21, Asymptomatic human immunodeficiency virus [HIV] infection status, is to be applied when the patient without any documentation of symptoms is listed as being "HIV positive," "known HIV," "HIV test positive," or similar terminology. Do not use this code if the term "AIDS" is used or if the patient is treated for any HIV-related illness or is described as having any condition(s) resulting from his or her HIV-positive status; use B20 in these cases.

   (e) **Patients with inconclusive HIV serology**

   Patients with inconclusive HIV serology, but no definitive diagnosis or manifestations of the illness, may be assigned code R75, Inconclusive laboratory evidence of human immunodeficiency virus [HIV].

   (f) **Previously diagnosed HIV-related illness**

   Patients with any known prior diagnosis of an HIV-related illness should be coded to B20. Once a patient has developed an HIV-related illness, the patient should always be assigned code B20 on every subsequent admission/encounter. Patients previously diagnosed with any HIV illness (B20) should never be assigned to R75 or Z21, Asymptomatic human immunodeficiency virus [HIV] infection status.

   (g) **HIV infection in pregnancy, childbirth, and the puerperium**

   During pregnancy, childbirth, or the puerperium, a patient admitted (or presenting for a health-care encounter) because of an HIV-related illness should receive a principal diagnosis code of O98.7-, Human immunodeficiency [HIV] disease complicating pregnancy, childbirth, and the puerperium, followed by B20 and the code(s) for the HIV-related illness(es). Codes from Chapter 15 always take sequencing priority.

   Patients with asymptomatic HIV infection status admitted (or presenting for a health-care encounter) during pregnancy, childbirth, or the puerperium should receive codes of O98.7- and Z21.

   (h) **Encounters for testing for HIV**

   If a patient is being seen to determine his or her HIV status, use code Z11.4, Encounter for screening for human immunodeficiency virus [HIV]. Use additional codes for any associated high-risk behavior.

   If a patient with signs or symptoms is being seen for HIV testing, code the signs and symptoms. An additional counseling code Z71.7, Human immunodeficiency virus [HIV] counseling, may be used if counseling is provided during the encounter for the test.

   When a patient returns to be informed of his or her HIV test results and the test result is negative, use code Z71.7, Human immunodeficiency virus [HIV] counseling.

   If the results are positive, see previous guidelines and assign codes as appropriate.

Code Only Confirmed Cases of HIV Infection or Disease

In the general *Official Guidelines*, unconfirmed diagnoses may be reported in the inpatient setting. HIV is an exception to that rule: In both the inpatient and outpatient settings, HIV infection and illness are coded only if the condition is confirmed. In this context, confirmation is the provider's diagnostic statement that the patient is HIV positive or has an HIV-related illness.

EXAMPLES

- Diagnosis: Possible HIV. Do not assign code Z21 or B20 in this case. Code only the signs and symptoms, or query the physician to determine whether the patient has a confirmed case of HIV.

- Diagnosis: HIV symptomatic infection. Assign code B20, not Z21.

Code only *confirmed* cases of HIV. This is an exception to the general rule in the *Official Guidelines* Section II, H. Never assign a code for HIV/AIDS unless the disease is confirmed by the physician's diagnostic statement.

Selection and Sequencing of HIV Codes

The circumstances that occasion the admission to the hospital or reason for the visit will affect the designation of the principal or first-listed diagnosis for inpatient coding. The progression of disease in HIV/AIDS, the complications, and the need for counseling require knowledge of the specific guidelines and, at times, a physician query.

Patient Admitted for HIV-Related Condition. If a patient is admitted for an HIV-related condition (has AIDS), the principal diagnosis should be B20 followed by additional diagnosis codes for all reported HIV-related conditions, such as Kaposi's sarcoma and *Pneumocystis carinii* pneumonia (Box 5.3).

BOX 5.3 Common HIV-Related Illnesses

- *Bacterial diseases* such as tuberculosis (caused by *Mycobacterium tuberculosis*), *Mycobacterium avium* complex disease, bacterial pneumonia, and septicemia ("blood poisoning")
- *Protozoal diseases* such as *Pneumocystis carinii* pneumonia, toxoplasmosis, microsporidiosis, cryptosporidiosis, isosporiasis, and leishmaniasis
- *Fungal diseases* such as candidiasis, cryptococcosis (Cryptococcal meningitis), and penicilliosis
- *Viral diseases* such as those caused by cytomegalovirus, herpes simplex virus, and herpes zoster virus
- *HIV-associated malignancies* such as Kaposi's sarcoma, lymphoma, and squamous cell carcinoma

■ CASE SCENARIO

A patient is admitted due to AIDS-related Kaposi's sarcoma of the stomach. The codes reported are B20 (AIDS) followed by code C46.4 (Kaposi's sarcoma of the stomach).

The underlying cause of the Kaposi's sarcoma (AIDS) is sequenced first.

INTERNET RESOURCE: Information on HIV-Related Conditions and AIDS
https://medlineplus.gov/hivaids.html

Patient With HIV Disease Admitted for Unrelated Condition. A patient with HIV disease may be admitted for an unrelated condition, such as traumatic injury. In that case, the code for the unrelated condition (the nature of injury code) is reported as the principal diagnosis. The HIV/AIDS condition is reported as a secondary diagnosis. Whether the patient is newly diagnosed or has had previous admissions or encounters for HIV conditions is irrelevant in deciding the principal diagnosis.

Patient Has Asymptomatic HIV. The code Z21, asymptomatic human immunodeficiency virus, is assigned when the patient has no documentation of symptoms and when the diagnosis is "HIV positive," "known HIV," "HIV test positive," or the like. If documentation supports the presence of AIDS, Z21 is not reported. It is also not used if the patient is being treated or has been treated for an HIV-related illness or if the patient is described as having any condition resulting from his or her HIV-positive status. In this case, code B20 is reported. In other words, a patient with any known prior diagnosis of HIV-related illness should be coded B20.

Knowledge of the disease process helps the coder understand this guideline. Once a patient develops HIV-related illness (HIV disease or HIV infection), that patient always has AIDS (B20). Thus, a patient with any previous diagnoses of any HIV illness (B20) should never be assigned a code for positive HIV status or inconclusive HIV serology (R75).

EXAMPLES

• Diabetic ketoacidosis (type 1) and HIV-positive status: Report codes E10.10, Z21.

• Diabetic ketoacidosis (type 1) and previous HIV-related pneumonia (pneumonia not currently present): Report codes E10.10, B20.

Patients With Inconclusive HIV Serology. Patients with no definitive diagnosis or manifestation of HIV and an inconclusive HIV serology test are assigned the diagnosis code of R75. To locate this code, start with the main term "Findings, abnormal, without diagnosis" and the subterm "serological." Notice that the positive finding is reported as code Z21, and an inconclusive test is reported as R75 (inconclusive serologic test for human immunodeficiency virus [HIV]).

HIV Infection in Pregnancy, Childbirth, and the Puerperium. Codes from ICD-10-CM Chapter 15 or 16 (pregnancy, childbirth, and the puerperium) always take sequencing priority over codes from other chapters. In other words, a code from Chapter 15 or 16 is sequenced first, followed by a code for the HIV-positive status (Z21) or AIDS (B20) and the related illness. During pregnancy, childbirth, or the puerperium, a patient admitted (or presenting for a health-care encounter) *because* of an HIV-related illness should be assigned a principal diagnosis code of O98.7-. This code is followed by code B20 and the code(s) for the HIV-related illness(es) or the asymptomatic HIV infection status code (Z21).

EXAMPLES

Locate a pregnancy with HIV-positive status code O98.71- in the Index. *(Hint:* See pregnancy complicated by HIV.) Remember that the pregnancy code with HIV infection or illness is sequenced as the principal diagnosis when the inpatient admission was due to the HIV/AIDS. The definition of principal diagnosis still applies.

• Mild hyperemesis gravidarum in the first trimester. The patient is HIV positive. Report codes O21.0, O98.711, Z21.

• Pregnant patient in the third trimester with AIDS-related stomatitis candidiasis. Report codes: O98.713, B37.0, B20.

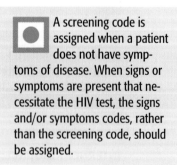

A screening code is assigned when a patient does not have symptoms of disease. When signs or symptoms are present that necessitate the HIV test, the signs and/or symptoms codes, rather than the screening code, should be assigned.

Encounters for Testing for HIV. Many people are tested for HIV annually to determine whether they have the virus, and test results may be negative. Therefore, the code assigned when a patient is tested is the screening for other viral disease code (Z11.4). Sometimes the reason for screening is due to a lifestyle that is high risk for HIV, and an additional code (Z72.5-) can be assigned to identify the high-risk behavior.

Clarify presence of symptomatic HIV infection (AIDS) and associated conditions. Code also any high-risk behavior, if documented.

Some states require the patient to sign a separate authorization that is specific for AIDS before a claim with this diagnosis is transmitted. Billing staff members must verify the requirement with their state medical societies or payers and establish a ruling for the facility or practice.

When results are reported at the return patient visit, the code assignment depends on the actual test results:

- A negative result is reported using the HIV counseling code Z71.7.
- A positive result in a patient without symptoms is reported as Z21; counseling may also be reported as an additional code (Z71.7).
- A positive result in a patient with symptoms is reported as code B20 (AIDS); counseling may also be reported as an additional code.

■ CASE SCENARIOS

- A patient requests screening for HIV during an annual physical: Z11.4. The same patient returns to be informed of the HIV test results, and results are negative. Report code Z71.7.

- A patient undergoes HIV screening due to high-risk heterosexual behavior: Z11.4, Z72.51. Results, received at a second visit, are positive. The patient has no symptoms and is counseled regarding the findings. Report codes Z21, Z72.51, Z71.7.

Pinpoint the Code 5.1 shows an HIV code assignment decision tree.

PINPOINT THE CODE 5.1: HIV

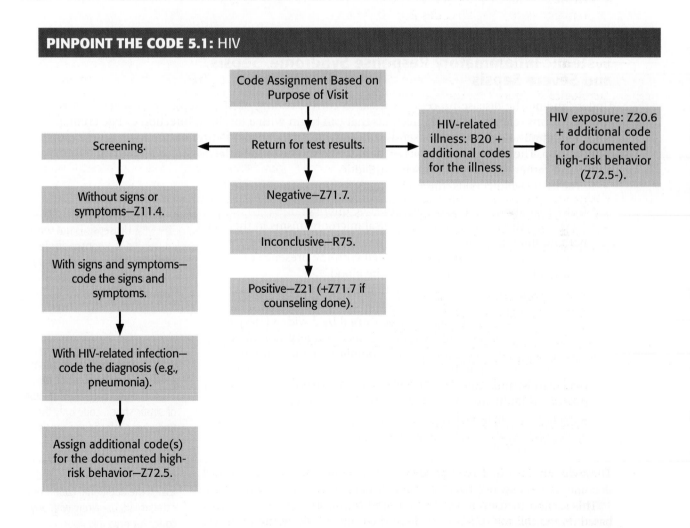

Correctly code and sequence the following statements using ICD-10-CM.

1. HIV-related infection _____

2. HIV positive _____

3. Screening for HIV infection _____

4. *Pneumocystis carinii* pneumonia (PCP), due to HIV infection _____

5. Nonspecific serology of HIV, type 2 _____

6. Asymptomatic HIV infection _____

7. Suspected carrier of HIV infection, counseled during this visit _____

8. Exposure to HIV infection _____

9. AIDS with cytomegaloviral disease _____

10. Pregnancy second trimester with HIV-positive status _____

11. Screening for HIV due to symptoms of headache and night sweats _____

Systemic Inflammatory Response Syndrome, Sepsis, and Severe Sepsis

Understanding the disease process is critical to correct coding of SIRS, sepsis, and severe sepsis. All these terms refer to systemic infections that can begin with a localized infection or bacteremia. Once the immunologic cascade of sepsis starts—which may be in a matter of hours—it is very difficult to stop. The physician attempts to identify the source of the infection in order to treat it with a targeted, rather than a broad-based, antibiotic.

To clarify these infections, the following definitions are important:

- *Urosepsis:* a nonspecific term that must be queried
- *Bacteremia:* the presence of pathological microorganisms in the blood with no findings of illness
- *Septicemia:* a systemic disease associated with the presence of pathological microorganisms or toxins in the blood
- *SIRS:* the body's systemic response to infection, trauma, burns, or other insult with common symptoms of fever, tachypnea, tachycardia, or leukocytosis; SIRS may be caused by a wide variety of conditions, such as trauma, complications of surgery, adrenal insufficiency, pulmonary embolism, a complicated aortic aneurysm, myocardial infarction, hemorrhage, drug overdose, burns, acute pancreatitis, and immunodeficiency (such as AIDS)
  - *Sepsis:* SIRS due to infection; a severe illness caused by overwhelming infection
  - *Severe sepsis:* sepsis with associated organ dysfunction, such as acute renal failure

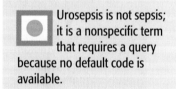 Urosepsis is not sepsis; it is a nonspecific term that requires a query because no default code is available.

When SIRS is documented in the absence of acute organ dysfunction or septic shock, code only the underlying infection of sepsis. Do not report a code from category R65. If severe sepsis is documented, code sepsis and assign the additional code from category R65.2- along with any codes for organ dysfunction.

These definitions can serve the coder as a reference, but medical record documentation may need to be clarified through a query to the physician.

This section focuses on the coding of SIRS, sepsis, and severe sepsis based on the *Official Guideline*. Pinpoint the Code 5.2 shows the decision sequence for sepsis code assignment. Note that the circumstances of admission affect the sequencing of the principal diagnosis.

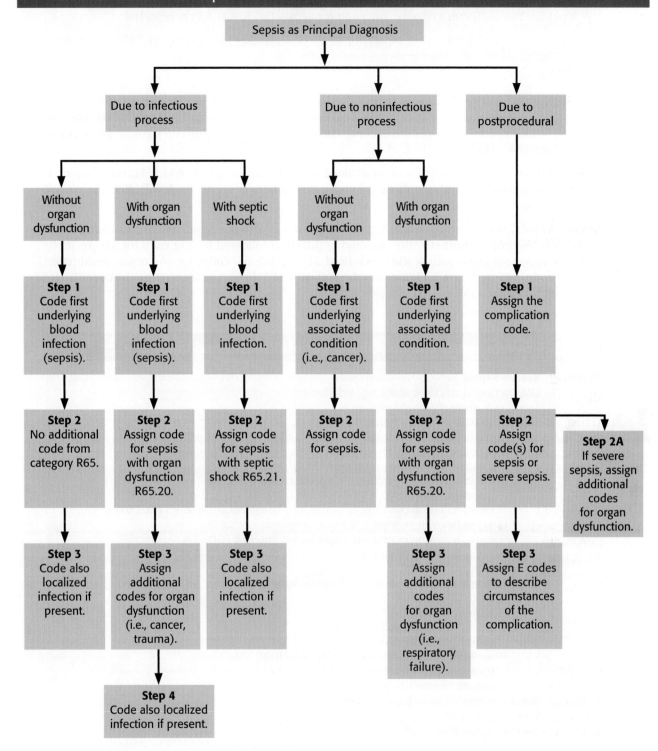

Coding of SIRS, Sepsis, and Severe Sepsis

When coding systemic infections of SIRS, sepsis, and severe sepsis, the coder must determine the underlying cause—either due to an infectious process, a noninfectious process, or a postprocedural infection. The first code assigned represents the underlying cause and additional codes may be required to identify severe sepsis (organ dysfunction) and localized infection.

SIRS. Systemic inflammatory response syndrome due to underlying infection is coded to either sepsis or severe sepsis. Only the code for the underlying infection is required when a diagnosis of SIRS is stated in the absence of severe sepsis or organ dysfunction. Documentation of SIRS in the presence of severe sepsis or organ dysfunction requires at least two codes: first, the underlying infection code followed by, second, the code for severe sepsis (R65.20) or acute organ dysfunction (R65.11).

Sepsis (SIRS). The documentation of sepsis alone results in assigning code A41.9. Further documentation of the specified organism, presence of organ dysfunction, or septic shock will affect the specific code assignment.

Severe Sepsis. When coding severe sepsis, the presence of septic shock will affect code assignment. The first code reported is the underlying infection followed by the code for severe sepsis (R65.20) or severe sepsis with septic shock (R65.21). Additional codes for any organ dysfunction would also be assigned. Box 5.4 illustrates the ICD-10-CM Tabular List instructing the coder to use two codes in the presence of severe sepsis.

BOX 5.4 Severe Sepsis Entry in Tabular List of Diseases and Injuries

R65.2   **Severe Sepsis**
Infection with associated acute organ dysfunction
Sepsis with acute organ dysfunction
Sepsis with multiple organ dysfunction
Systemic inflammatory response syndrome due to infectious process with acute organ dysfunction
Code first underlying infection, such as:
   infection following a procedure (T81.4)
   infections following infusion, transfusion, and therapeutic injection (T80.2-)
   puerperal sepsis (O85)
   sepsis following complete or unspecified spontaneous abortion (O03.87)
   sepsis following ectopic and molar pregnancy (O08.82)
   sepsis following incomplete spontaneous abortion (O03.37)
   sepsis following (induced) termination of pregnancy (O04.87)
   sepsis NOS A41.9
Use additional code to identify specific acute organ dysfunction, such as:
   acute kidney failure (N17.-)
   acute respiratory failure (J96.0-)
   critical illness myopathy (G72.81)
   critical illness polyneuropathy (G62.81)
   disseminated intravascular coagulopathy [DIC] (D65)
   encephalopathy (metabolic) (septic) (G93.41)
   hepatic failure (K72.0-)
R65.20   **Severe Sepsis Without Septic Shock**
Severe sepsis NOS
R65.21   **Severe Sepsis With Septic Shock**

The coder might use a query to clarify the type of infection, the site of infection, the infectious organism, or the presence of severe sepsis and/or organ dysfunction.

Sequencing Sepsis and Severe Sepsis

The *Official Guidelines* on sequencing apply to the coding of sepsis. The circumstances of admission affect the sequencing of the principal diagnosis. Under certain circumstances, the code for systemic infection is listed first, but other circumstances instruct the coder to sequence another code, such as trauma, first. The sequencing guidelines are as follows.

Sequencing of Severe Sepsis. If severe sepsis is present on admission (POA) and meets the definition of principal diagnosis, the underlying systemic infection code should be assigned as the principal diagnosis (such as A41.9), followed by a code from subcategory R65.2. A code from subcategory R65.2 can never be assigned as the principal diagnosis. A code should also be assigned for any localized infection, if present.

■ CASE SCENARIO

A patient is admitted with leukocytosis, fever, tachycardia, and signs of septic shock. Blood cultures are positive for *Staphylococcus aureus*. The diagnosis is severe *Staphylococcus aureus* sepsis with septic shock. Assign codes A41.01, R65.21.

Of course, when sepsis or severe sepsis develops during the visit, all codes for sepsis are sequenced as additional diagnoses.

Unclear Documentation About Whether Sepsis or Severe Sepsis Is Present on Admission. At times, the inpatient coder must query the physician about whether the sepsis or severe sepsis was present on admission. Confirmation of the presence of the disease can require time, because the diagnosis is clinical, not based on test results. Before sequencing the underlying infection as the principal diagnosis, the coder must ensure that the documentation clearly supports the definition of principal diagnosis.

Sepsis or SIRS With Localized Infection

The circumstances of admission assist the inpatient coder in sequencing the principal diagnosis in cases of sepsis or SIRS with localized infection. For example, if a patient presents for localized urinary tract infection (UTI) and sepsis, the code for systemic infection (sepsis) is sequenced first, followed by the code for the localized UTI. If, however, the patient presents with localized infection and sepsis develops after admission, the localized infection code should be sequenced as the principal diagnosis.

■ CASE SCENARIOS

• A patient presents with pneumococcal pneumonia (localized infection) with septic shock. Blood cultures are positive for *Pneumococcus*. The diagnosis of pneumococcal pneumonia, sepsis due to *Pneumococcus*, and septic shock are stated by the physician. Assign codes A40.3, R65.21, J13.

• A patient presents with acute pyelonephritis. After the third hospital day, the patient develops tachycardia, tachypnea, and fever. The physician documents acute pyelonephritis and sepsis. Assign codes N10, A41.9.

Acute Organ Dysfunction That Is Not Clearly Associated With Severe Sepsis

In the presence of acute organ dysfunction, documentation must associate the organ dysfunction with the severe sepsis in order to assign the secondary diagnosis code of R65.20 or R65.21. If the organ dysfunction is related to another medical condition, the codes from subcategory R65.2 should not be reported. A physician query may be required to clarify the relationship between the severe sepsis and organ dysfunction.

EXAMPLES

- Gram-negative sepsis with associated acute respiratory failure with hypoxia. Report codes A41.9, R65.20, J96.01.

- Gram-negative sepsis with acute respiratory failure due to congestive heart failure. Report codes A41.50, J96.00, I50.9.

The presence of septic shock is an exception to this rule because septic shock is always related to severe sepsis. The term *septic shock* refers to circulatory failure associated with severe sepsis; therefore, it represents a type of acute organ dysfunction. For this reason, all cases of septic shock require the codes for systemic infection sequenced first, followed by code R65.2. The code for septic shock cannot be sequenced first; additional codes for other acute organ dysfunctions should also be assigned.

Sepsis and Severe Sepsis Associated With Noninfectious Processes

Many scenarios exist for the reporting of sepsis associated with a noninfectious process. The sequencing of the principal diagnosis depends on the circumstances of admission. Sometimes the noninfectious condition can cause sepsis or infection may result from a noninfectious condition. The following are three scenarios that might apply:

1. A noninfectious process, such as trauma, may lead to an infection, which can result in sepsis or severe sepsis. If sepsis or severe sepsis is documented as associated with a noninfectious condition, such as a burn or serious injury, and this condition meets the definition for principal diagnosis, the code for the noninfectious condition should be sequenced first, followed by the code for the systemic infection and, if present, the code for severe sepsis (subcategory R65.2). Additional codes for any associated acute organ dysfunctions should also be assigned for cases of severe sepsis. If documentation supports SIRS due to noninfectious origin, the additional code from subcategory R65.1 would be assigned. Do not assign a code from both subcategories R65.1 and R65.2 for the same patient as shown in Box 5.5 (Excludes1 note).

BOX 5.5 SIRS Entry in Tabular List

R65   **Symptoms and Signs Specifically Associated with Systemic Inflammation and Infection**

   R65.1   **Systemic inflammatory response syndrome (SIRS) of noninfectious origin**

   Code first underlying condition, such as:

   heatstroke (T67.0)

   injury and trauma (S00–T88)

   Excludes1: sepsis—code to infection

   severe sepsis (R65.2)

R65.10   **Systemic Inflammatory Response Syndrome (SIRS) of Noninfectious Origin without acute organ dysfunction**

   Systemic inflammatory response syndrome (SIRS) NOS

R65.11   **Systemic Inflammatory Response Syndrome (SIRS) of Noninfectious Origin with acute organ dysfunction**

   Use additional code to identify specific acute organ dysfunction, such as:

   acute kidney failure (N17.-)

   acute respiratory failure (J96.0-)

   critical illness myopathy (G72.81)

   critical illness polyneuropathy (G62.81)

   disseminated intravascular coagulopathy [DIC] (D65)

   encephalopathy (metabolic) (septic) (G93.41)

   hepatic failure (K72.0-)

---

2. If the sepsis or severe sepsis meets the definition of principal diagnosis, the systemic infection and sepsis codes should be sequenced before the noninfectious condition.

3. When both the associated noninfectious condition and the sepsis or severe sepsis meet the definition of principal diagnosis, either may be assigned as the principal diagnosis.

Sepsis and Septic Shock Complicating Abortion and Pregnancy

Special sequencing rules apply to reporting sepsis and septic shock complicating abortion, ectopic pregnancy, and molar pregnancy. These conditions are classified to category codes in Chapters 15 and 16 of ICD-10-CM.

Sepsis Due to a Postprocedural Infection

In the unique circumstance of sepsis due to a postprocedural infection, documentation must specifically support a causal relationship between the procedure and the infection. If this is the case, the complication code is sequenced first, followed by the codes for sepsis. The codes for sepsis or severe sepsis would be reported as additional or secondary codes.

EXAMPLES

- Sepsis due to infected vascular catheter, initial episode (*see* Complication, vascular device, infection). Assign codes T82.7xxA (Infection and inflammatory reaction due to other cardiac and vascular devices, implants, and grafts), A41.9 (sepsis).

- Severe sepsis and septic shock from complicated or infected obstetrical wound postpartum. Assign codes O86.0, A41.9, R65.21.

- *Streptococcus*, Group B sepsis due to infected left hip joint prosthesis, initial episode. Assign codes T84.52xA, A40.1.

NOTE: Coding external cause codes in the presence of complications: The use of external cause codes as an additional code when reporting abnormal reactions to a medical device or procedure is covered in Chapter 9 of this text.

Box 5.6 shows the chapter-specific guidelines for septicemia, sepsis, and related conditions from the *Official Guidelines*.

BOX 5.6 *Official Guidelines*: Sepsis, Severe Sepsis, and Septic Shock

1) Coding of Sepsis and Severe Sepsis

(a) Sepsis

For a diagnosis of sepsis, assign the appropriate code for the underlying systemic infection. If the type of infection or causal organism is not further specified, assign code A41.9, Sepsis, unspecified organism.

A code from subcategory R65.2, Severe sepsis, should not be assigned unless severe sepsis or an associated acute organ dysfunction is documented.

(i) Negative or inconclusive blood cultures and sepsis

Negative or inconclusive blood cultures do not preclude a diagnosis of sepsis in patients with clinical evidence of the condition; however, the provider should be queried.

(ii) Urosepsis

The term *urosepsis* is a nonspecific term. It is not to be considered synonymous with sepsis. It has no default code in the Alphabetic Index. Should a provider use this term, he or she must be queried for clarification.

(iii) Sepsis with organ dysfunction

If a patient has sepsis and associated acute organ dysfunction or multiple organ dysfunction (MOD), follow the instructions for coding severe sepsis.

(iv) Acute organ dysfunction that is not clearly associated with the sepsis

If a patient has sepsis and an acute organ dysfunction, but the medical record documentation indicates that the acute organ dysfunction is related to a medical condition other than the sepsis, do not assign a code from subcategory R65.2, Severe sepsis. An acute organ dysfunction must be associated with the sepsis in order to assign the severe sepsis code. If the documentation is not clear as to whether an acute organ dysfunction is related to the sepsis or another medical condition, query the provider.

(b) Severe sepsis

The coding of severe sepsis requires a minimum of two codes: first a code for the underlying systemic infection, followed by a code from subcategory R65.2, Severe sepsis. If the causal organism is not documented, assign code A41.9, Sepsis, unspecified organism, for the infection. Additional code(s) for the associated acute organ dysfunction are also required.

Continued

BOX 5.6 *Continued*

Due to the complex nature of severe sepsis, some cases may require querying the provider prior to assignment of the codes.

2) Septic Shock

(a) Septic shock generally refers to circulatory failure associated with severe sepsis, and therefore, it represents a type of acute organ dysfunction.

For cases of septic shock, the code for the systemic infection should be sequenced first, followed by code R65.21, Severe sepsis with septic shock, or code T81.12, Postprocedural septic shock. Any additional codes for the other acute organ dysfunctions should also be assigned. As noted in the sequencing instructions in the Tabular List, the code for septic shock cannot be assigned as a principal diagnosis.

3) Sequencing of Severe Sepsis

If severe sepsis is present on admission, and meets the definition of principal diagnosis, the underlying systemic infection should be assigned as the principal diagnosis followed by the appropriate code from subcategory R65.2 as required by the sequencing rules in the Tabular List. A code from subcategory R65.2 can never be assigned as a principal diagnosis.

When severe sepsis develops during an encounter (it was not present on admission), the underlying systemic infection and the appropriate code from subcategory R65.2 should be assigned as secondary diagnoses.

Severe sepsis may be present on admission but the diagnosis may not be confirmed until sometime after admission. If the documentation is not clear whether severe sepsis was present on admission, the provider should be queried.

4) Sepsis and Severe Sepsis With a Localized Infection

If the reason for admission is both sepsis or severe sepsis and a localized infection, such as pneumonia or cellulitis, a code(s) for the underlying systemic infection should be assigned first and the code for the localized infection should be assigned as a secondary diagnosis. If the patient has severe sepsis, a code from subcategory R65.2 should also be assigned as a secondary diagnosis. If the patient is admitted with a localized infection, such as pneumonia, and sepsis/severe sepsis doesn't develop until after admission, the localized infection should be assigned first, followed by the appropriate sepsis/severe sepsis codes.

5) Sepsis Due to a Postprocedural Infection

(a) Documentation of causal relationship

As with all postprocedural complications, code assignment is based on the provider's documentation of the relationship between the infection and the procedure.

(b) Sepsis due to a postprocedural infection

For such cases, the postprocedural infection code, such as T80.2, Infections following infusion, transfusion, and therapeutic injection; T81.4, Infection following a procedure; T88.0, Infection following immunization; or O86.0, Infection of obstetric surgical wound, should be coded first, followed by the code for the specific infection. If the patient has severe sepsis, the appropriate code from subcategory R65.2 should also be assigned with the additional code(s) for any acute organ dysfunction.

(c) Postprocedural infection and postprocedural septic shock

In cases where a postprocedural infection has occurred and has resulted in severe sepsis and postprocedural septic shock, the code for the precipitating complication, such as code T81.4, Infection following a procedure, or O86.0, Infection of obstetrical surgical wound, should be coded first followed by code R65.21, Severe sepsis with septic shock, and a code for the systemic infection.

6) Sepsis and Severe Sepsis Associated With a Noninfectious Process (Condition)

In some cases, a noninfectious process (condition), such as trauma, may lead to an infection, which can result in sepsis or severe sepsis. If sepsis or severe sepsis is documented as associated with a noninfectious condition, such as a burn or serious injury, and this condition meets the definition for principal diagnosis, the code for the noninfectious condition should be sequenced first, followed by the code for the resulting infection. If severe sepsis is present, a code from subcategory R65.2 should also be assigned with any associated organ dysfunction(s) codes. It is not necessary to assign a code from subcategory R65.1, Systemic inflammatory response syndrome (SIRS) of noninfectious origin, for these cases.

Methicillin-Resistant *Staphylococcus aureus* (MRSA), Methicillin Susceptible *Staphylococcus aureus* (MSSA), and the Zika Virus

MRSA is a leading cause of serious infection. It is a new staph "superbug" that is resistant to antibiotics and therefore very difficult to treat. MSSA is a condition of being colonized or carrying MSSA or MRSA. Documentation may state a patient is an MSSA "carrier" or "MRSA nasal swab positive." This designation reflects the organism as being present on or in the body, yet no illness may be present.

An organism code is assigned for this infection from the subcategory B95.6 unless a combination code exists. Do not assign a code from subcategory Z16.11, Resistance to penicillins. When a patient is a carrier, a code from subcategory Z22.32 would be assigned. In some instances, both the current infection and carrier status can be reported.

If a patient's MRSA infection develops after admission, the POA indicator MRSA is reported as N. If the patient tests positive for MRSA on admission (Z22.322) and later develops MRSA sepsis, the POA for the positive MRSA *colonization* is Y (condition was present on admission), but N for the MRSA sepsis because the patient did not have a MRSA *infection* at the time of admission.

■ CASE SCENARIO
A patient is MRSA nasal swab positive and has cellulitis of the left leg due to MRSA. Assign codes L03.116, B95.62, Z22.322.

Box 5.7 shows the chapter-specific guidelines for MRSA conditions from the *Official Guidelines*.

EXAMPLE
MRSA sepsis is reported using code A41.02 or MRSA pneumonia, code J15.212. Notice that the site of infection and organism of infection are combined into one code. The code for MRSA infection (B95.62) would not be assigned as an additional code.

Methicillin Resistant *Staphylococcus aureus* (MRSA) Conditions

1) Selection and sequencing of MRSA codes

(a) Combination codes for MRSA infection

When a patient is diagnosed with an infection that is due to methicillin-resistant *Staphylococcus aureus* (MRSA), and that infection has a combination code that includes the causal organism (e.g., sepsis, pneumonia) assign the appropriate combination code for the condition (e.g., code A41.02, Sepsis due to Methicillin-resistant *Staphylococcus aureus* or code J15.212, Pneumonia due to Methicillin resistant *Staphylococcus aureus*). Do not assign code B95.62, Methicillin resistant *Staphylococcus aureus* infection as the cause of diseases classified elsewhere, as an additional code, because the combination code includes the type of infection and the MRSA organism. Do not assign a code from subcategory Z16.11, Resistance to penicillins, as an additional diagnosis.

See Section C.1. for instructions on coding and sequencing of sepsis and severe sepsis.

(b) Other codes for MRSA infection

When there is documentation of a current infection (e.g., wound infection, stitch abscess, urinary tract infection) due to MRSA, and that infection does not have a combination code that includes the causal organism, assign the appropriate code to identify the condition along with code B95.62, Methicillin-resistant *Staphylococcus aureus* infection as the cause of diseases classified elsewhere for the MRSA infection. Do not assign a code from subcategory Z16.11, Resistance to penicillins.

(c) Methicillin susceptible *Staphylococcus aureus* (MSSA) and MRSA colonization

The condition or state of being colonized or carrying MSSA or MRSA is called *colonization* or *carriage*, while an individual person is described as being colonized or being a carrier. Colonization means that MSSA or MRSA is present on or in the body without necessarily causing illness. A positive MRSA colonization test might be documented by the provider as "MRSA screen positive" or "MRSA nasal swab positive."

Assign code Z22.322, Carrier or suspected carrier of methicillin-resistant *Staphylococcus aureus*, for patients documented as having MRSA colonization. Assign code Z22.321, Carrier or suspected carrier of methicillin-susceptible *Staphylococcus aureus*, for a patient *documented* as having MSSA colonization. Colonization is not necessarily indicative of a disease process or as the cause of a specific condition the patient may have unless documented as such by the provider.

(d) MRSA colonization and infection

If a patient is documented as having both MRSA colonization and infection during a hospital admission, code Z22.322, Carrier or suspected carrier of methicillin-resistant *Staphylococcus aureus*, and a code for the MRSA infection may also be assigned.

The Zika virus (A92.5) should only be reported if confirmed as noted in the documentation by the provider. Do not report "possible" or "probable" Zika virus, rather report the signs and symptoms present. The code for exposure to Zika (Z20.828) can also be assigned if appropriate. The mode of transmission of this viral disease does not impact code assignment.

EXAMPLE

Fever and chills with exposure to Zika virus. Documentation states possible Zika Virus. Assign codes R50.9, Z20.828.

Correctly code and sequence the following statements using ICD-10-CM.

1. SIRS due to infectious origin (*Hint:* SIRS due to infection can also be termed *sepsis.*) _____

2. Strep B sepsis _____

3. Gangrenous sepsis _____

4. Acute cellulitis of the abdominal wall due to *Pseudomonas* (*Hint:* To code the organism, look for the main term *infection.*) _____

5. *Streptococcus pneumoniae* sepsis due to stage II decubitus ulcer of the sacrum (*Hint:* This case is an example of a localized infection causing systemic infection.) _____

6. MRSA sepsis with septic shock _____

7. Acute renal failure with tubular necrosis due to severe sepsis _____

8. SIRS due to *Enterobacter*-infected urinary catheter (initial encounter) (*Hint:* SIRS equals sepsis and the infected catheter is a complication.) _____

9. SIRS due to acute pancreatitis (*Hint:* This case is an example of systemic inflammatory response syndrome, not due to infection.) _____

10. Urosepsis, after physician query documentation supports acute candidal cystitis (*Hint:* See the main term *candidiasis.*) _____

11. Peritonsillar abscess due to *Streptococcus*, resistance to penicillin _____

12. Acute upper respiratory infection, MSSA nasal swab positive (*Hint:* See the main term *carrier.*) _____

Answer the following questions on MRSA.

13. The code J14 reflects a combination code: true or false

14. MRSA colonization is the same as MRSA infection: true or false

15. Code acute MRSA pyelonephritis: _____

16. When coding for an additional organism, the coder uses the main term *infection*, subterm for the organism, as the cause of disease classified elsewhere: true or false

NEOPLASMS (CHAPTER 2: C00–D49)

Chapter 2 of ICD-10-CM classifies neoplasms, or tumors, which are growths that arise from normal tissue. Some of these neoplasms are malignant and are thus associated with prevalent diseases such as lung, breast, colon, lymphatic system, ovarian (epithelial), and prostate cancer. The categories in Chapter 2 are grouped as shown in Table 5.2.

Table of Neoplasms in the Alphabetic Index

The Alphabetic Index of ICD-10-CM contains the Table of Neoplasms, which provides codes for neoplasms that are then confirmed in the Tabular List. The Table of Neoplasms lists the anatomical

Common Medications for Infectious and Parasitic Diseases

Infections may result from a variety of organisms and parasites. Antimicrobials, including antibiotics, antivirals, and antifungals, are chemical substances that suppress the growth of microorganisms and may eventually destroy them.

Antibacterials

Antibacterials are agents used to treat bacterial infections. These drugs are prescribed based on the organism causing the infection. Each class of antibiotics has a different mechanism for affecting the microbial agent. Some of the broad classifications include:

- Penicillins
- Cephalosporins
- Carbapenems
- Quinolones
- Tetracyclines
- Macrolides
- Vancomycin
- Aminoglycosides

The table at right lists common brand and generic names of antibacterials.

Antivirals

Antiviral drugs make up a class of medication used specifically for treating viral infections. Like antibiotics, specific antivirals target specific viruses. Most of the antivirals now available are designed to help deal with HIV, herpesviruses (best known for causing cold sores and genital herpes, but actually causing a wide range of diseases), the hepatitis B and C viruses (which can cause liver cancer), and influenza A and B viruses. Almost all antimicrobials, including antivirals, are subject to drug resistance as the pathogens evolve to survive exposure to the treatment.

The table at top left on the following page lists common brand and generic names of antivirals.

Antifungals

An antifungal drug is medication used to treat fungal infections such as athlete's

ANTIBACTERIALS	
TRADE NAME	**GENERIC NAME**
Amikin	amikacin
Amoxil	amoxicillin
Ancef, Kefzol	cefazolin
Augmentin	amoxicillin and potassium clavulanate
Azactam	aztreonam
Bactrim, Septra	sulfamethoxazole and trimethoprim
Biaxin	clarithromycin
Bicillin	penicillin
Ceclor	cefaclor
Ceftin	cefuroxime
Cipro	ciprofloxacin
Cleocin	clindamycin
Ery-Tab	erythromycin
Flagyl	metronidazole
Fortaz, Tazidime, Tazicef	ceftazidime
Garamycin	gentamicin
Keflex	cephalexin
Levaquin	levofloxacin
Macrobid	nitrofurantoin
Nebcin	tobramycin
Pipracil	piperacillin sodium
Primaxin	imipenem-cilastatin
Principen	ampicillin
Rocephin	ceftriaxone
Suprax	cefixime
Ticar	ticarcillin
Timentin	ticarcillin and clavulanate
Unasyn	ampicillin and sulbactam
Vancocin	vancomycin
Vibramycin	doxycycline
Zinacef	cefuroxime
Zithromax	azithromycin
Zosyn	piperacillin and tazobactam
Zymar	gatifloxacin

ANTIVIRALS

TRADE NAME	GENERIC NAME
Combivir	lamivudine and zidovudine
Crixivan	indinavir
Cytovene	ganciclovir
Epivir	lamivudine
Famvir	famciclovir
Flumadine	rimantadine
Foscavir	foscarnet
Hepsera	adefovir
Invirase	saquinavir
Relenza	zanamivir
Rescriptor	delavirdine
Retrovir	zidovudine
Sustiva	efavirenz
Symmetrel	amantadine
Tamiflu	oseltamivir
Valtrex	valacyclovir
Viramune	nevirapine
Virazole	ribavirin
Zovirax	acyclovir

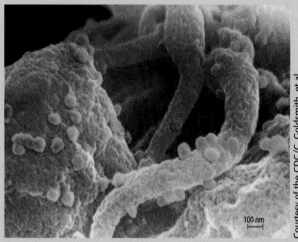

Courtesy of the CDC/C. Goldsmith, et al

False-colored micrograph of HIV-1 (green spheres) on lymphocytes.

foot, ringworm, candidiasis (thrush), and more serious systemic infections such as cryptococcal meningitis.

The table below lists common brand and generic names of antifungals.

ANTIFUNGALS

TRADE NAME	GENERIC NAME
Abelcet	amphotericin b lipid complex
AmBisome	amphotericin b lipid complex
Amphotec	amphotericin b lipid complex
Cancidas	caspofungin
Diflucan	fluconazole
Fungizone	amphotericin b
Grifulvin	griseofulvin
Lamisil	terbinafine
Mycostatin	nystatin
Nizoral	ketoconazole
Sporanox	itraconazole

Table 5.2 Organization of ICD-10-CM Chapter 2 Tabular List

BLOCK	BLOCK DESCRIPTION
C00–C14	Malignant neoplasms of lip, oral cavity, and pharynx
C15–C26	Malignant neoplasms of digestive organs
C30–C39	Malignant neoplasms of respiratory and intrathoracic organs
C40–C41	Malignant neoplasms of bone and articular cartilage
C43–C44	Melanoma and other malignant neoplasms of skin
C45–C49	Malignant neoplasms of mesothelial and soft tissue
C50	Malignant neoplasms of breast
C51–C58	Malignant neoplasms of female genital organs
C60–C63	Malignant neoplasms of male genital organs
C64–C68	Malignant neoplasms of urinary tract
C69–C72	Malignant neoplasms of eye, brain, and other parts of central nervous system
C73–C75	Malignant neoplasms of thyroid and other endocrine glands
C7A	Malignant neuroendocrine tumors
C7B	Secondary neuroendocrine tumors
C76–C80	Malignant neoplasms of ill-defined, other secondary, and unspecified sites
C81–C96	Malignant neoplasms of lymphoid, hematopoietic, and related tissue
D00–D09	In situ neoplasms
D10–D36	Benign neoplasms, except benign neuroendocrine tumors
D3A	Benign neuroendocrine tumors
D37–D48	Neoplasms of uncertain behavior, polycythemia vera, and myelodysplastic syndromes
D49	Neoplasms of unspecified behavior

location in the first column. The next six columns relate to the behavior of the neoplasm, described as:

- One of three types of malignant tumor, each of which is progressive, rapid growing, life threatening, and made of cancerous cells:
  1. **Primary neoplasm:** The tumor that is the encounter's main diagnosis is found at the site of origin.
  2. **Secondary neoplasm:** The tumor that is the encounter's main diagnosis has spread (a condition called *metastasis*) to an additional body site from the original location; called a "seeded" site.
  3. **Carcinoma in situ:** The neoplasm is restricted to one site (it is a noninvasive type); this may also be referred to as *pre-invasive cancer*.
- **Benign neoplasm:** Slow growing, not life threatening, made of normal or near-normal cells.
- **Neoplasm of uncertain behavior:** Neoplastic characteristics; not classifiable when the cells were examined.
- **Neoplasm of unspecified behavior:** No documentation of the nature of the neoplasm; laboratory results pending.

For example, the following entries for a neoplasm sigmoid appear in the Neoplasm Table:

	MALIGNANT PRIMARY	MALIGNANT SECONDARY	CANCER IN SITU	BENIGN	UNCERTAIN BEHAVIOR	UNSPECIFIED
Sigmoid flexure	C18.7	C78.5	D01.0	D12.5	D37.4	D49.0

Basic Coding of Neoplasms

Box 5.8 shows the chapter-specific guidelines for neoplasms. To correctly assign codes for a neoplasm, the site, the morphology, and the behavior of the neoplasm must be documented. The morphology and histology of a neoplasm describe the structure of the tumor.

BOX 5.8 *Official Guideline*: Neoplasms (C00–D49)

General Guidelines

Chapter 2 of the ICD-10-CM contains the codes for most benign and all malignant neoplasms. Certain benign neoplasms, such as prostatic adenomas, may be found in the specific body system chapters. To properly code a neoplasm, it is necessary to determine from the record if the neoplasm is benign, in situ, malignant, or of uncertain histologic behavior. If malignant, any secondary (metastatic) sites should also be determined.

Primary malignant neoplasms overlapping site boundaries

A primary malignant neoplasm that overlaps two or more contiguous (next to each other) sites should be classified to the subcategory/code .8 ('overlapping lesion'), unless the combination is specifically indexed elsewhere. For multiple neoplasms of the same site that are not contiguous, such as tumors in different quadrants of the same breast, codes for each site should be assigned.

Malignant neoplasm of ectopic tissue

Malignant neoplasms of ectopic tissue are to be coded to the site of origin mentioned, e.g., ectopic pancreatic malignant neoplasms involving the stomach are coded to malignant neoplasm of pancreas, unspecified (C25.9).

The neoplasm table in the Alphabetic Index should be referenced first. However, if the histological term is documented, that term should be referenced first, rather than going immediately to the Neoplasm Table, in order to determine which column in the Neoplasm Table is appropriate. For example, if the documentation indicates "adenoma," refer to the term in the Alphabetic Index to review the entries under this term and the instructional note to "see also neoplasm, by site, benign." The table provides the proper code based on the type of neoplasm and the site. It is important to select the proper column in the table that corresponds to the type of neoplasm. The Tabular List should then be referenced to verify that the correct code has been selected from the table and that a more specific site code does not exist.

See Section I.C.21. Factors influencing health status and contact with health services, Status, for information regarding Z15.0, codes for genetic susceptibility to cancer.

a. Treatment Directed at the Malignancy

If the treatment is directed at the malignancy, designate the malignancy as the principal diagnosis.

The only exception to this guideline is if a patient admission/encounter is solely for the administration of chemotherapy, immunotherapy, or external beam radiation therapy, assign the appropriate Z51.-- code as the first-listed or principal diagnosis, and the diagnosis or problem for which the service is being performed as a secondary diagnosis.

b. Treatment of Secondary Site

When a patient is admitted because of a primary neoplasm with metastasis and treatment is directed toward the secondary site only, the secondary neoplasm is designated as the principal diagnosis even though the primary malignancy is still present.

c. Coding and Sequencing of Complications

Coding and sequencing of complications associated with the malignancies or with the therapy thereof are subject to the following guidelines:

1) Anemia associated with malignancy

When admission/encounter is for management of an anemia associated with the malignancy, and the treatment is only for anemia, the appropriate code for the malignancy is sequenced as the principal or first-listed diagnosis followed by the appropriate code for the anemia (such as code D63.0, Anemia in neoplastic disease).

2) Anemia associated with chemotherapy, immunotherapy, and radiation therapy

When the admission/encounter is for management of an anemia associated with an adverse effect of the administration of chemotherapy or immunotherapy and the only treatment is for the anemia, the anemia code is sequenced first followed by the appropriate codes for the neoplasm and the adverse effect (T45.1X5, Adverse effect of antineoplastic and immunosuppressive drugs).

When the admission/encounter is for management of an anemia associated with an adverse effect of radiotherapy, the anemia code should be sequenced first, followed by the appropriate neoplasm code and code Y84.2, Radiological procedure and radiotherapy as the cause of abnormal reaction of the patient, or of later complication, without mention of misadventure at the time of the procedure.

Continued

BOX 5.8 *Continued*

3) Management of dehydration due to the malignancy

When the admission/encounter is for management of dehydration due to the malignancy and only the dehydration is being treated (intravenous rehydration), the dehydration is sequenced first, followed by the code(s) for the malignancy.

4) Treatment of a complication resulting from a surgical procedure

When the admission/encounter is for treatment of a complication resulting from a surgical procedure, designate the complication as the principal or first-listed diagnosis if treatment is directed at resolving the complication.

d. Primary Malignancy Previously Excised

When a primary malignancy has been previously excised or eradicated from its site and there is no further treatment directed to that site and there is no evidence of any existing primary malignancy, a code from category Z85, Personal history of malignant neoplasm, should be used to indicate the former site of the malignancy. Any mention of extension, invasion, or metastasis to another site is coded as a secondary malignant neoplasm to that site. The secondary site may be the principal or first-listed with the Z85 code used as a secondary code.

e. Admissions/Encounters Involving Chemotherapy, Immunotherapy, and Radiation Therapy

1) Episode of care involves surgical removal of neoplasm

When an episode of care involves the surgical removal of a neoplasm, primary or secondary site, followed by adjunct chemotherapy or radiation treatment during the same episode of care, the code for the neoplasm should be assigned as principal or first-listed diagnosis.

2) Patient admission/encounter solely for administration of chemotherapy, immunotherapy, and radiation therapy

If a patient admission/encounter is solely for the administration of chemotherapy, immunotherapy, or radiation therapy assign code Z51.0, Encounter for antineoplastic radiation therapy, or Z51.11, Encounter for antineoplastic chemotherapy, or Z51.12, Encounter for antineoplastic immunotherapy as the first-listed or principal diagnosis. If a patient receives more than one of these therapies during the same admission, more than one of these codes may be assigned, in any sequence.

The malignancy for which the therapy is being administered should be assigned as a secondary diagnosis.

If a patient admission/encounter is for the insertion or implantation of radioactive elements (e.g., brachytherapy), the appropriate code for the malignancy is sequenced as the principal or first-listed diagnosis. Code Z51.0 should not be assigned.

3) Patient admitted for radiation therapy, chemotherapy, or immunotherapy and develops complications

When a patient is admitted for the purpose of radiotherapy, immunotherapy, or chemotherapy and develops complications such as uncontrolled nausea and vomiting or dehydration, the principal or first-listed diagnosis is Z51.0, Encounter for antineoplastic radiation therapy, or Z51.11, Encounter for antineoplastic chemotherapy, or Z51.12, Encounter for antineoplastic immunotherapy followed by any codes for the complications.

When a patient is admitted for the purpose of insertion or implantation of radioactive elements (e.g., brachytherapy) and develops complications such as uncontrolled nausea and vomiting or dehydration, the principal or first-listed diagnosis is the appropriate code for the malignancy followed by any codes for the complications.

f. Admission/Encounter to Determine Extent of Malignancy

When the reason for admission/encounter is to determine the extent of the malignancy, or for a procedure such as paracentesis or thoracentesis, the primary malignancy or appropriate metastatic site is designated as the principal or first-listed diagnosis, even though chemotherapy or radiotherapy is administered.

g. Symptoms, Signs, and Abnormal Findings Listed in Chapter 18 Associated With Neoplasms

Symptoms, signs, and ill-defined conditions listed in Chapter 18 characteristic of, or associated with, an existing primary or secondary site malignancy cannot be used to replace the malignancy as principal or first-listed diagnosis, regardless of the number of admissions or encounters for treatment and care of the neoplasm.

See section I.C.21. Factors influencing health status and contact with health services, Encounter for prophylactic organ removal.

h. Admission/Encounter for Pain Control/Management

See Section I.C.6. for information on coding admission/encounter for pain control/management.

i. Malignancy in two or more noncontiguous sites

A patient may have more than one malignant tumor in the same organ. These tumors may represent different primaries or metastatic disease, depending on the site. Should the documentation be unclear, the provider should be queried as to the status of each tumor so that the correct codes can be assigned.

j. Disseminated Malignant Neoplasm, Unspecified

Code C80.0, Disseminated malignant neoplasm, unspecified, is for use only in those cases where the patient has advanced metastatic disease and no known primary or secondary sites are specified. It should not be used in place of assigning codes for the primary site and all known secondary sites.

k. Malignant Neoplasm Without Specification of Site

Code C80.1, Malignant (primary) neoplasm, unspecified, equates to Cancer, unspecified. This code should only be used when no determination can be made as to the primary site of a malignancy. This code should rarely be used in the inpatient setting.

l. Sequencing of Neoplasm Codes

1) Encounter for treatment of primary malignancy

If the reason for the encounter is for treatment of a primary malignancy, assign the malignancy as the principal/first-listed diagnosis. The primary site is to be sequenced first, followed by any metastatic sites.

2) Encounter for treatment of secondary malignancy

When an encounter is for a primary malignancy with metastasis and treatment is directed toward the metastatic (secondary) site(s) only, the metastatic site(s) is designated as the principal/first-listed diagnosis. The primary malignancy is coded as an additional code.

3) Malignant neoplasm in a pregnant patient

When a pregnant woman has a malignant neoplasm, a code from subcategory O9A.1-, Malignant neoplasm complicating pregnancy, childbirth, and the puerperium, should be sequenced first, followed by the appropriate code from Chapter 2 to indicate the type of neoplasm.

4) Encounter for complication associated with a neoplasm

When an encounter is for management of a complication associated with a neoplasm, such as dehydration, and the treatment is only for the complication, the complication is coded first, followed by the appropriate code(s) for the neoplasm.

The exception to this guideline is anemia. When the admission/encounter is for management of an anemia associated with the malignancy, and the treatment is only for anemia, the appropriate code for the malignancy is sequenced as the principal or first-listed diagnosis followed by code D63.0, Anemia in neoplastic disease.

5) Complication from surgical procedure for treatment of a neoplasm

When an encounter is for treatment of a complication resulting from a surgical procedure performed for the treatment of the neoplasm, designate the complication as the principal/first-listed diagnosis. See the guideline regarding the coding of a current malignancy versus personal history to determine if the code for the neoplasm should also be assigned.

6) Pathologic fracture due to a neoplasm

When an encounter is for a pathological fracture due to a neoplasm, and the focus of treatment is the fracture, a code from subcategory M84.5, Pathological fracture in neoplastic disease, should be sequenced first, followed by the code for the neoplasm.

If the focus of treatment is the neoplasm with an associated pathological fracture, the neoplasm code should be sequenced first, followed by a code from M84.5 for the pathological fracture.

m. Current Malignancy Versus Personal History of Malignancy

When a primary malignancy has been excised but further treatment, such as an additional surgery for the malignancy, radiation therapy, or chemotherapy is directed to that site, the primary malignancy code should be used until treatment is completed.

When a primary malignancy has been previously excised or eradicated from its site, there is no further treatment (of the malignancy) directed to that site, and there is no evidence of any existing primary malignancy, a code from category Z85, Personal history of malignant neoplasm, should be used to indicate the former site of the malignancy.

See Section I.C.21. Factors influencing health status and contact with health services, History (of).

n. Leukemia, Multiple Myeloma, and Malignant Plasma Cell Neoplasms in Remission Versus Personal History

The categories for leukemia, and category C90, Multiple myeloma and malignant plasma cell neoplasms, have codes indicating whether or not the leukemia has achieved remission. There are also codes Z85.6, Personal history of leukemia, and Z85.79, Personal history of other malignant neoplasms of lymphoid, hematopoietic and related tissues. If the documentation is unclear as to whether the leukemia has achieved remission, the provider should be queried.

See Section I.C.21. Factors influencing health status and contact with health services, History (of).

Continued

BOX 5.8 Continued

o. **Aftercare Following Surgery for Neoplasm**
   See Section I.C.21. Factors influencing health status and contact with health services, Aftercare.
p. **Follow-up care for completed treatment of a malignancy**
   See Section I.C.21. Factors influencing health status and contact with health services, Follow-up.
q. **Prophylactic Organ Removal for Prevention of Malignancy**
   See Section I.C. 21, Factors influencing health status and contact with health services, Prophylactic organ removal.
r. **Malignant Neoplasm Associated With Transplanted Organ**
   A malignant neoplasm of a transplanted organ should be coded as a transplant complication. Assign first the appropriate code from category T86.-, Complications of transplanted organs and tissue, followed by code C80.2, Malignant neoplasm associated with transplanted organ. Use an additional code for the specific malignancy.

When the histological type or morphology of neoplasm is documented, that term should be referenced first in the Alphabetic Index. Often the main term and its subterms lead directly to a code, such as adrenal adenoma (D35.00). In other cases, the histological term directs the coder to the Neoplasm Table and a specific column of behavior.

EXAMPLE
Review the entries under the main term *epithelioma* (malignant) from the Alphabetic Index, and look at the instructional note to *"see also* Neoplasm, by site, malignant," instructing the coder to go to the Neoplasm Tab and locate the site of the neoplasm.

Epithelioma (malignant)—*see* also Neoplasm, malignant, by site

- Adenoides cysticum—*see* Neoplasm, skin, benign
- Basal cell—*see* Neoplasm, skin, malignant
- Benign—*see* Neoplasm, benign, by site
- Bowen's—*see* Neoplasm, skin, in situ
- Calcifying, of Malherbe—*see* Neoplasm, skin, benign
- External site—*see* Neoplasm, skin, malignant
- Intraepidermal, Jadassohn—*see* Neoplasm, skin, benign
- Squamous cell—*see* Neoplasm, malignant, by site

> If the neoplasm is malignant, any secondary sites (metastatic) should be determined.

> The term *mass* (or *lump* or *lesion*) should not be regarded as a neoplasm. The Alphabetic Index main term *mass* directs the coder to the site- or organ-specific sections outside Chapter 2.

In this example, notice that, depending on the subterm, the coder is directed to different columns in the Neoplasm Table. For example, a benign epithelioma requires the coder to go to the Neoplasm Table, by site, benign column. If coding a basal cell epithelioma, the coder is directed to go to the Neoplasm Table, skin, malignant. The Tabular List should be referenced to verify correct code assignment as selected from the Neoplasm Table and to determine that a more specific site code does not exist.

INTERNET RESOURCE: American Cancer Society: Types of Tumors
www.cancer.org

What happens when the histological type, as a main term, has no subterms resulting in a specific code? The coder should go back to the main term for the histological type and follow the cross-reference. Consider the term *papillary carcinoma of the lung*. The main term *carcinoma* is the histological type and the subterm is *papillary*. Because there is no cross reference or direction following *papillary*, the coder must return to the main term *carcinoma* for further direction. The coder is then directed to the main term *neoplasm, by site, malignant*.

In this example, if metastasis is not documented, the column for primary neoplasm would be used to assign the code. In the example, papillary cell carcinoma of the lung, code C34.90, would be assigned. If metastasis is documented, the coding guidelines noted in the "Coding Malignant Neoplasms with Metastasis" section apply.

The histological type of neoplasm is most often documented in the pathology report. The term *atypia* means an abnormality in a cell that may be a precancerous indication, depending on the context in which

> If the patient is found to have multiple malignant neoplasms, each can be separately coded as long as the codes do not exactly duplicate one another.

it was diagnosed. *Dysplasia* means an abnormality in the appearance of cells indicative of an early step toward transformation into a neoplasm. This abnormal growth is restricted to the originating system or location. Persistent dysplastic lesions must be removed.

Remember that, in the inpatient setting, the coder cannot code from pathological findings alone; physician documentation of significance is required. The coder may have to query the physician to obtain clarification regarding pathology findings.

Coding Malignant Neoplasms With Metastasis

A malignant neoplasm can metastasize throughout the body. To code for documented metastasis, the Neoplasm Table includes a column headed "Secondary Malignant [Neoplasm]." At least two codes are assigned, one to reflect where the original malignancy started (primary site), and the other to report where the malignancy traveled (secondary site)—which can be more than one site.

EXAMPLES
- Lung cancer left-lower lobe with pulmonary lymph node metastasis (primary site: lung; secondary site: pulmonary lymph node). Assign codes C34.32, C77.1.
- Metastatic brain cancer from the sigmoid colon (primary site: sigmoid colon; secondary site: brain). Assign codes C18.7, C79.31.

The next examples also use two codes, but in these cases one site of malignancy is no longer present or being treated (the documentation reads "history of"), but the second site is still present.

EXAMPLES
- Bone metastasis from previous prostate adenocarcinoma (C79.51) and history of prostate malignancy (Z85.46).
- Axillary lymph node metastasis from resected breast cancer that is no longer present or being treated (C77.3, Z85.3 for Personal history of malignant neoplasm of breast).

The next example includes the location of one site and an unknown secondary site; two codes are still assigned.

EXAMPLE
Liver metastasis from unknown primary site. Assign codes C78.7, C80.1 (neoplasm unknown or specified site).

Documentation can sometimes be vague when it comes to coding neoplasms that have spread. For example, if documentation states *lung metastasis*, the coder cannot be sure that the malignant neoplasm started in the lung (primary) or went to the lung (secondary). But the coder still has to assign two codes because metastasis is documented. When this occurs, the coder refers to the following list of sites that should be coded as secondary only when the documentation of metastasis does not indicate a primary or secondary site:

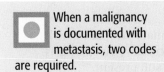
When a malignancy is documented with metastasis, two codes are required.

Bone	Meninges
Brain	Peritoneum
Diaphragm	Pleura
Heart	Retroperitoneum
Liver	Sites classifiable to category 195
Lymph nodes	Spinal cord
Mediastinum	

If one of these sites is mentioned with metastasis, the rule is to code it as a secondary site along with a code for an unknown site.

EXAMPLE
Brain metastasis. Codes are C79.31, C80.1.

Because *brain* is included in the list, it is assumed to be a secondary site (C79.31); the coder then also codes the unspecified primary site (C80.1). This rule applies only when documentation is not clear regarding the primary and secondary malignant sites.

Pinpoint the Code 5.3 shows a neoplasm code assignment decision tree.

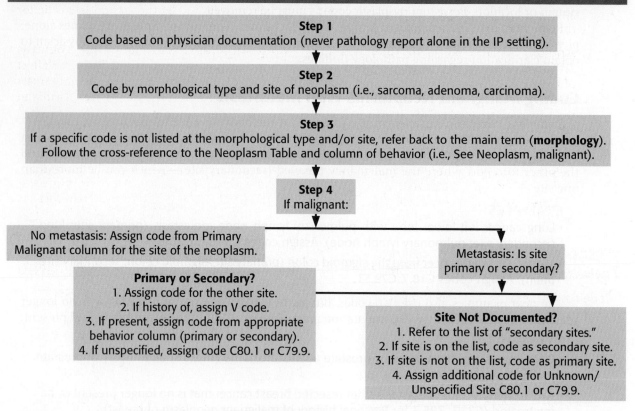

Step 1
Code based on physician documentation (never pathology report alone in the IP setting).

Step 2
Code by morphological type and site of neoplasm (i.e., sarcoma, adenoma, carcinoma).

Step 3
If a specific code is not listed at the morphological type and/or site, refer back to the main term (**morphology**). Follow the cross-reference to the Neoplasm Table and column of behavior (i.e., See Neoplasm, malignant).

Step 4
If malignant:

No metastasis: Assign code from Primary Malignant column for the site of the neoplasm.

Metastasis: Is site primary or secondary?

Primary or Secondary?
1. Assign code for the other site.
2. If history of, assign V code.
3. If present, assign code from appropriate behavior column (primary or secondary).
4. If unspecified, assign code C80.1 or C79.9.

Site Not Documented?
1. Refer to the list of "secondary sites."
2. If site is on the list, code as secondary site.
3. If site is not on the list, code as primary site.
4. Assign additional code for Unknown/Unspecified Site C80.1 or C79.9.

Sequencing of Malignant Neoplasms

As noted previously, the coder must first determine the codes that should be assigned and then sequence them. The terms *primary* and *secondary* referred to in the Neoplasm Table have nothing to do with the principal diagnosis or the secondary diagnosis. Just because a malignant neoplasm originates in the lung (primary) does not mean that the primary malignancy code is sequenced first. The following guidelines apply to sequencing of neoplasms, again based on the circumstances of admission.

Treatment Directed at the Malignancy

The *Official Guidelines* state that "if the treatment is directed at the malignancy, designate the malignancy as the principal diagnosis."

> **EXAMPLE**
> The patient is admitted with cough and abnormal chest x-ray. Bronchoscopy with lung biopsy reveals squamous cell carcinoma of the lung. The code is C34.90.

Treatment of Secondary Site

The *Official Guidelines* state that "when a patient is admitted because of a primary neoplasm with metastasis and treatment is directed toward the secondary site only, the secondary neoplasm is designated as the principal diagnosis even though the primary malignancy is still present."

> ■ **CASE SCENARIO**
> A patient with inoperable right ovarian cancer presents with seizures, headaches, and confusion. The MRI of the brain is positive for brain metastasis. Treatment—drug therapy to control the symptoms of brain metastasis—is begun. The codes are C79.31 and C56.1.

Coding and Sequencing of Complications

The guidelines for treating a patient for complications of a malignancy apply when the encounter or admission is for management of the complication only and treatment is for the complication only. The code for the malignancy is reported as a secondary diagnosis, and the following guidelines apply.

Anemia Associated With Malignancy. The *Official Guidelines* state that when an "admission/encounter is for management of an anemia associated with the malignancy, *and the treatment is only for anemia,*" the appropriate neoplasm code is assigned first followed by the appropriate code for the malignancy-related anemia (D63.0).

Anemia Associated With Chemotherapy, Immunotherapy, and Radiation Therapy. "When the admission/encounter is for management of anemia associated with an adverse effect of the administration of chemotherapy or immunotherapy [or radiotherapy] and the only treatment is for the anemia, the anemia is sequenced first," followed by codes for the neoplasm and the adverse effect code (T45.1x5-).

> ■ **CASE SCENARIO**
> A patient presents with severe weakness due to anemia from previous week's chemotherapy for right breast cancer. She receives 2 units of red blood cells and is discharged. (*Hint:* The code for the adverse effect of chemotherapy is found using the Table of Drugs and Chemicals.) Assign codes D64.81, T45.1x5-, C50.911.

CHECKPOINT 5.3

Code the following statements using ICD-10-CM. Remember to locate the main term for the morphology or histological type first.

1. Fibrous histiocytoma of the right leg _____
2. Endometrial sarcoma _____
3. Left renal cell carcinoma _____
4. Islet cell adenocarcinoma of the pancreas _____
5. Melanoma of the right external ear _____
6. Adenocarcinoma of the areola of the left breast (female) with brain metastasis _____
7. Liver metastasis from gastric adenocarcinoma _____
8. Carcinoma of the lower left lobe of the lung with left pleural metastasis _____
9. History of colon cancer, now with omental metastasis _____
10. Cervical lymph gland metastasis _____

Indicate the primary and secondary sites for the following diagnostic statements.

11. Bladder cancer with pelvic lymph node metastasis
    a. Primary _____
    b. Secondary _____
12. Prostate cancer with bone, brain, and liver metastasis
    a. Primary _____
    b. Secondary _____
13. Cervical lymph node metastasis from laryngeal carcinoma
    a. Primary _____
    b. Secondary _____
14. Lung metastasis from previously resected and treated gallbladder adenocarcinoma
    a. Primary _____
    b. Secondary _____
15. Metastatic endometrial carcinoma
    a. Primary _____
    b. Secondary _____

Common Medications and Treatments for Neoplasms

Chemotherapy

Chemotherapy in its most general sense refers to treatment of disease by chemicals that kill cells, specifically cells of microorganisms or cancer. In popular usage, the term usually refers to antineoplastic drugs used to treat cancer or to the combination of these drugs into a standardized treatment regimen. Each of the several classes of chemotherapy agents has a differing mechanism for use in treating various types of cancer.

The table here lists common brand and generic names for cancer-related antimitotics, antimetabolites, alkylating agents, and antibiotics.

CHEMOTHERAPY DRUGS	
TRADE NAME	**GENERIC NAME**
Adriamycin	doxorubicin
Adrucil	fluorouracil
Alkeran	melphalan
BiCNU	carmustine
Blenoxane	bleomycin
Camptosar	irinotecan
CeeNU	lomustine
Cerubidine	daunorubicin
Cosmegen	dactinomycin
Cytoxan	cyclophosphamide
Fludara	fludarabine
FUDR	floxuridine
Gemzar	gemcitabine
Hycamtin	topotecan
Hydrea	hydroxyurea
Leukeran	chlorambucil
Leustatin	cladribine
Mustargen	mechlorethamine
Mutamycin	mitomycin
Myleran	busulfan
Navelbine	vinorelbine
Neosar	cyclophosphamide
Novantrone	mitoxantrone
Paraplatin	carboplatin
Rheumatrex	methotrexate
Tarabine	cytarabine
Taxol	paclitaxel
Taxotere	docetaxel
Thioplex	thiotepa
Velban	vinblastine
VePesid	etoposide
Vincasar	vincristine
Zanosar	streptozocin

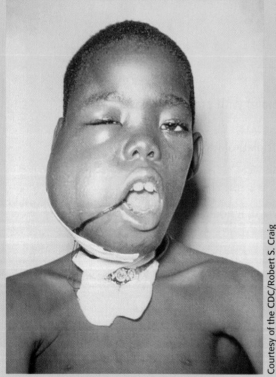

Courtesy of the CDC/Robert S. Craig

Burkitt's lymphoma is often treated with chemotherapy.

■ **CASE SCENARIO**

A male patient presents with severe weakness due to anemia from last week's radiation therapy for sarcoma of the right leg. Assign codes D64.9, Y84.2, C49.21.

Management of Dehydration Due to a Malignancy. When the admission or encounter is to manage dehydration due to a malignancy and/or therapy and only the dehydration is being treated (intravenous rehydration), the dehydration is sequenced first, followed by the codes for the malignancy.

Immunotherapy

Drugs in the immunotherapy category include sex hormones, or hormone-like drugs, that alter the action or production of female or male hormones. They are used to slow the growth of breast, prostate, and endometrial (uterine) cancers, which normally grow in response to natural hormones in the body. These cancer treatment hormones do not work in the same way as do standard chemotherapy drugs. Instead they prevent cancer cells from using the hormone they need to grow, or prevent the body from making the hormone.

The table below lists common brand and generic names.

Radiation Therapy

The goal of radiation therapy is to get enough radiation into the body to kill cancer cells while preventing damage to healthy tissue. There are several ways to do this. Depending on the location, size, and type of cancer, patients may receive one or a combination of techniques.

Radiation therapy can be delivered either externally or internally. In external beam radiation therapy, the radiation oncology team uses a machine to direct high-energy x-rays at the cancer. Internal radiation therapy, or brachytherapy, involves placing radioactive sources (for example, radioactive seeds) inside the body.

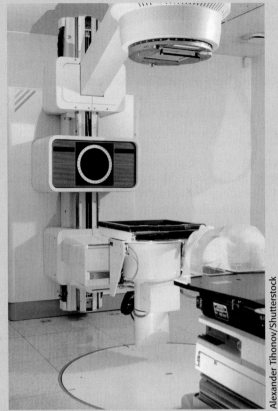

Radiation treatment.

IMMUNOTHERAPHY DRUGS

TRADE NAME	GENERIC NAME
Arimidex	anastrozole
Aromasin	exemestane
Casodex	bicalutamide
Fareston	toremifene
Femara	letrozole
Lupron	leuprolide
Megace	megestrol
Teslac	testolactone
Zoladex	goserelin

■ CASE SCENARIO

A patient presented to the hospital with dehydration from chemotherapy received the day before to treat his right renal cell carcinoma, initial episode. Assign codes E86.0, C64.1, T45.1x5A.

Treatment of a Complication Resulting From a Surgical Procedure. The *Official Guidelines* state that "when the admission/encounter is for treatment of a complication resulting from a surgical procedure, designate the complication as the principal or first-listed diagnosis if treatment is directed at resolving the complication."

Admissions and Encounters Involving Chemotherapy, Immunotherapy, and Radiation Therapy

The circumstances of the admission determine code sequencing when chemotherapy, immunotherapy, or external beam radiation therapy is provided. At times a patient is admitted specifically for the treatment, and at other times the malignancy is detected and then treatment is initiated. According to the guidelines, when the episode of care/admission involves surgical removal of the neoplasm (either a primary or secondary site) followed by adjunct chemotherapy or external beam radiation treatment during the same episode of care, the neoplasm code should be assigned as the principal diagnosis.

When the episode of care/admission is solely for administration of chemotherapy, immunotherapy, or external beam radiation therapy, assign one of these codes as the first-listed or principal diagnosis as appropriate:

- Z51.0, Encounter for antineoplastic radiation therapy
- Z51.11, Encounter for antineoplastic chemotherapy
- Z51.12, Encounter for antineoplastic immunotherapy

A patient may receive more than one of these therapies during the same admission. In that case, multiple codes may be assigned, in any sequence. This sequencing would apply even if the patient developed complications following the therapy during that visit. The code for the complications and the malignancy would be reported as additional diagnoses.

Note that encounters for brachytherapy (placement of radioactive elements) require that the malignancy be reported first, not code Z51.0.

Sequencing Symptoms, Signs, and Ill-Defined Conditions Listed in Chapter 16 Associated With Neoplasms

A patient with a neoplasm may present with symptoms, signs, and ill-defined conditions that are listed in Chapter 16 of ICD-10-CM. When these signs and symptoms are associated with either the primary or secondary site of malignancy, the codes from Chapter 16 cannot be used as the principal diagnosis. A patient may have multiple visits for signs and symptoms of malignancy, but the malignancy is still the principal diagnosis. For example, given a diagnosis of weakness from lung cancer, the principal diagnosis would still be lung cancer (C34.90).

Other conditions associated with malignancy should be coded as secondary diagnoses. For example, if the patient has a large bowel obstruction from ascending colon carcinoma, the carcinoma code (C18.9) would be sequenced first, followed by a code for the large bowel obstruction due to neoplasm (K56.69).

NOTE: The special guidelines regarding the admission for pain control associated with malignancy are covered in the pain management guidelines of this text.

Other Sequencing Issues

The *Official Guidelines* also instruct the coder regarding a few other unique instances pertaining to neoplasms. These include two or more malignancies in noncontiguous sites, disseminated malignant neoplasms, pathological fractures due to neoplasm, and malignant neoplasms in pregnant patients.

Malignancy in Two or More Noncontiguous Sites. When coding malignant neoplasms, *contiguous sites* refers to a malignant tumor overlapping two sites (see Neoplasm, lung, overlapping sites (C34.80)). In some

> When coding follow-up for a malignant neoplasm that is no longer present or being treated, the follow-up codes are used when no recurrence has been found and no symptoms are present. An additional code for history of malignancy is reported as well.

instances a malignant neoplasm has two different, nonoverlapping sites in the same organ. These tumors may represent different primary sites or metastatic disease. To assign the codes correctly for each site, the physician should be queried to determine the status of each tumor.

EXAMPLES

- Female patient with carcinoma of the left breast, upper-outer quadrant and right breast, lower-inner quadrant. Assign codes C50.412, C50.311.

- Male patient was admitted for treatment of carcinoma of the colon in overlapping sites. Assign code C18.8.

Disseminated Malignant Neoplasms, Unspecified. When coding disseminated malignant neoplasms, unspecified, code C80.0 is used only when a patient has advanced metastatic disease and the primary or secondary sites are unknown. The code C80.0 should never be used to replace a code for a site-specific malignancy.

CHECKPOINT 5.4

Code the following statements using ICD-10-CM.

1. Male patient presents with symptoms of obstructive uropathy and urinary retention. Prostate biopsy is positive for adenocarcinoma. _____

2. The same patient is now seen for his second radiation therapy treatment for prostate adenocarcinoma. _____

3. Five months later, this patient presents with weakness and pain in his hip. Bone scan is positive for bone metastasis. (*Hint:* The hip pain code is not reported as the symptom is integral to the bone metastasis.) _____

4. The patient receives additional radiation and chemotherapy for his prostate cancer that is delivered in the outpatient setting. After his chemotherapy, he is extremely dehydrated and requires inpatient services for rehydration. Documentation supports dehydration due to chemotherapy. (*Hint:* Remember to report the code from the Table of Drugs and Chemicals for the adverse effect of chemotherapy [antineoplastic drug].) _____

5. This patient presents with new symptoms of seizures. An MRI of the brain is positive for metastasis from previous prostate cancer. Palliative chemotherapy is given. (*Hint:* Code diagnoses only.) _____

6. Dysphagia from carcinoma of the esophagus _____

7. New pathological fracture of left radius due to osteosarcoma _____

8. Admission for antineoplastic immunotherapy of malignant melanoma of the stomach _____

9. Bowel obstruction due to peritonei carcinomatosis _____

10. Biliary duct obstruction due to metastatic carcinoma of the gallbladder, unknown primary

    _____

11. Pregnancy in the third trimester complicated by newly diagnosed left ovarian cancer _____

12. The patient presents with carcinoma of the middle and third portion of the esophagus (overlapping site). _____

13. The patient presents with anemia related to chronic disease of carcinoma of the uterus. _____

EXAMPLE

Patient presents with disseminated carcinoma. Assign code C80.0.

Pathological Fractures Due to Neoplasm. A pathological fracture is a unique type of fracture caused by disease rather than trauma. In the instances where the underlying disease of a fracture is a neoplasm, the coder would assign codes for both the fracture and the underlying neoplasm. Sequencing of these two codes depends on the circumstances of admission. When the focus of treatment is the fracture, a code from subcategory M84.5 (pathological fracture in neoplastic disease) should be sequenced first. When the focus of treatment is the neoplasm with an associated fracture, the code for the neoplasm should be sequenced first.

> When a malignancy has been removed but further treatment is still directed to that malignancy, the coder should continue to assign the primary malignancy code until treatment is completed. The history of malignancy code(s) is assigned when there is no evidence of any existing malignancy and treatment has been completed.

■ **CASE SCENARIOS**

• A patient with bone metastasis is admitted for treatment of new right femur fracture, initial episode. Patient has history of prostate cancer. Assign codes M84.551A, C79.51, Z85.46.

• A patient presents for further workup of bone metastasis from previous prostate cancer. During workup patient is noted to have a new associated pathological fracture of the rib. Assign codes C79.51, M84.58xA, Z85.46.

Malignant Neoplasm in Pregnant Patient. As discussed earlier, when reporting disease in a pregnant patient, the codes from Chapters 15 and 16 take precedence. The same is true when a pregnant woman has a malignant neoplasm. A code from subcategory O9A.1 should be sequenced first followed by the code to indicate the type of neoplasm.

■ **CASE SCENARIO**

A patient is in her second trimester and carcinoma of the left breast is diagnosed. Assign codes O9A.112, C50.912.

DISEASES OF THE BLOOD AND BLOOD-FORMING ORGANS AND CERTAIN DISORDERS INVOLVING THE IMMUNE MECHANISM (CHAPTER 3: D50–D89)

Codes in this chapter of the ICD-10-CM classify diseases of the blood and blood-forming organs, such as anemia and coagulation defects. When coding diseases of the blood and blood-forming organs, documentation of the specific type of disease is imperative. Currently there are no specific guidelines for the diseases of the blood and blood-forming organs. The categories in Chapter 3 are grouped as shown in Table 5.3.

Table 5.3 Organization of ICD-10-CM Chapter 3 Tabular List

BLOCK	BLOCK DESCRIPTION	EXAMPLES
D50–D53	Nutritional anemias	Iron-deficiency anemia
D55–D59	Hemolytic anemias	Beta thalassemia
D60–D64	Aplastic and other anemias and other bone marrow failure syndromes	Drug-induced aplastic anemia
D65–D69	Coagulation defects, purpura and other hemorrhagic conditions	Hereditary factor IX deficiency
D70–D77	Other disorders of blood and blood-forming organs	Secondary polycythemia
D78 (D78.0)	Intraoperative and postprocedural complications of the spleen	Intraoperative hemorrhage of spleen
D80–D89	Certain disorders involving the immune mechanism	IgE syndrome

Anemia

Anemia refers to any of various conditions marked by deficiency in red blood cells, packed red cell volume, or hemoglobin. These conditions cause fatigue because the body cannot get all the oxygen it needs. Deficiency can occur in many forms and types.

Iron-Deficiency Anemia

Iron-deficiency anemia, the most common type of anemia, is a condition in which the number of healthy blood cells is reduced because of lack of iron. This can result from lack of iron in the diet, poor absorption of iron that is present in the body, or blood loss from internal bleeding, cancer, or heavy menstrual periods, among other conditions. Diagnosis initially is made by complete blood count (CBC); additional diagnostic tests may be done.

This condition is coded to D50.9. If documented as due to blood loss, it is coded to D50.0. Code D62 is reported if the condition is documented as due to acute blood loss.

Anemia of Chronic Disease

Anemia can also result from many chronic illnesses, such as AIDS, malignancy, liver disease, chronic inflammatory diseases, and end-stage renal disease. For example, subcategory D63 has codes for anemia in chronic kidney disease (D63.1), anemia in neoplastic disease (D63.0), and anemia in other chronic illness (D63.8). A code for the chronic disease should also be reported.

Sequencing of these codes depends on the circumstances of admission. If the anemia occasioned the admission to the hospital and this condition meets the definition of principal diagnosis, then the anemia of chronic disease code would be sequenced first.

EXAMPLES

- Anemia due to stage 3 chronic kidney disease. Assign codes D63.1, N18.3.

- Chronic anemia due to male left breast cancer. Assign codes D63.0, C50.122.

When anemia due to malignancy is coded, code D63.0 is assigned unless the anemia is due to antineoplastic therapy (such as chemotherapy). In this case, the specific type of anemia is reported along with the adverse effect code from the Table of Drugs and Chemicals.

EXAMPLE

Acquired hemolytic anemia due to chemotherapy for cancer, unspecified site. Assign codes D59.9, T45.1x5A, C80.1.

Postoperative Anemia

If a patient is documented as having anemia postoperatively but not acute blood loss, code D64.9. If the postoperative anemia is documented as due to acute blood loss, code D62 is assigned. Coders should not use abnormal laboratory findings or blood transfusions alone to report anemia. The coder may query the physician to determine the presence of anemia and the type of anemia (Box 5.9).

BOX 5.9 Example of a Coder's Query to a Physician for Anemia

Dr. A: Please render your opinion regarding a diagnosis related to the decreased hemoglobin noted on laboratory findings the day after surgery and treatment of blood transfusions. If anemia is present, please clarify the type and cause, if known. Please document all clarification in the medical record.

Normally, an expected amount of blood is lost during a surgical procedure. If the documentation does not describe the patient as having anemia or specify that blood loss is a complication of the surgery, do not assign a code for the blood loss.

Sickle-Cell Disease and Sickle-Cell Thalassemia

Sickle-cell disease (also called *hemoglobin SS disease* or *Hb SS*) and sickle-cell thalassemia are inherited blood diseases that affect the body's ability to produce normal hemoglobin. Sickle-cell disease (usually found in people of African descent) is coded to subcategory D57 and is distinguished from thalassemia (usually found in people of Mediterranean descent), which is reduction in hemoglobin resulting in severe anemia, coded to subcategory D57.4. In either condition, when the patient experiences a crisis (sudden pain) in joints or organs, the code for the sickle-cell disease or sickle-cell thalassemia is combined with some syndromes (i.e., Acute chest syndrome code D57.01) or an additional code is assigned for the type of crisis, such as fever (R50.81).

Pancytopenia and Aplastic Anemia

In aplastic anemia (category D61), the bone marrow stops producing new blood cells, and there are too few red blood cells, white blood cells, and platelets. If the patient is documented as having neutropenia (deficiency of white cells) and thromobocytopenia (deficiency of platelets) as well as anemia (deficiency of red cells), the condition is called *pancytopenia* and is coded D61.818.

> Pancytopenia includes the diagnoses of anemia, neutropenia, and thrombocytopenia. Do not separately report the component conditions when code D61.818 is reported.

Blood Loss Anemia

Two codes classify blood loss anemia, acute (D62) and chronic or unspecified (D50.0). To assign codes for anemia due to blood loss, documentation must support the causal relationship.

■ **CASE SCENARIOS**

• A patient presents with gastrointestinal bleeding and has documented anemia. Codes are K92.2, D64.9 (anemia).

• A patient presents with GI bleeding, and documented diagnosis is GI bleeding with associated acute blood loss anemia. Codes are K92.2, D62.

> In the presence of anemia, the specific type of anemia and acuity of the anemia should be documented. The coder may base physician query on treatment of blood transfusions and abnormal lab findings.

The physician may be queried to determine the type, acuity, and cause of anemia in order to assign codes to the highest level of specificity.

CHECKPOINT 5.5

Code the following statements using ICD-10-CM.

1. Hypochromic anemia in chronic illness _____

2. Refractory sideroblastic anemia _____

3. Diverticulitis of the large intestine with hemorrhage, anemia _____

4. Other postoperative anemia _____

5. Acute blood loss anemia _____

6. Hb-C sickle-cell anemia with sickle-cell crisis _____

7. Chest pain syndrome with sickle-cell crisis _____

8. Chronic anemia from end-stage renal disease _____

9. Acute posthemorrhagic anemia _____

10. Microcytic hypochromic anemia _____

ENDOCRINE, NUTRITIONAL, AND METABOLIC DISEASES (CHAPTER 4: E00–E89)

Codes from Chapter 4 include a variety of disorders. The most common disease classified here is diabetes mellitus. Another common condition is clinical obesity, in which excessive accumulation of body fat causes body weight to increase beyond skeletal and physical requirements. Obesity is associated with a number of primary conditions, such as coronary artery disease, gallbladder disease, high cholesterol, hypertension, and type 2 diabetes mellitus. The categories in Chapter 4 are grouped as shown in Table 5.4.

Table 5.4 Organization of ICD-10-CM Chapter 4 Tabular List

BLOCK	BLOCK DESCRIPTION
E00–E07	Disorders of thyroid gland
E08–E13	Diabetes mellitus
E15–E16	Other disorders of glucose regulation and pancreatic internal secretion
E20–E35	Disorders of other endocrine glands
E36	Intraoperative complications of endocrine system
E40–E46	Malnutrition
E50–E64	Other nutritional deficiencies
E65–E68	Overweight, obesity, and other hyperalimentation
E70–E88	Metabolic disorders
E89	Postprocedural endocrine and metabolic complications and disorders, not elsewhere classified

A child may have type 2 diabetes, and an adult may have type 1. Coders should not, however, assume a relationship between the patient's age and the type of DM.

Diabetes Mellitus

The most common condition to code from Chapter 4 is diabetes mellitus (DM), a disorder in the metabolizing of carbohydrates that results in excess glucose in the blood and urine. Millions of people are thought to have undiagnosed diabetes. When left undiagnosed, diabetes can lead to severe complications such as heart disease, stroke, blindness, kidney failure, leg and foot amputation, and death related to pneumonia and flu. Scientific evidence now shows that early detection and treatment of diabetes with diet, physical activity, and medication can prevent or delay much of the illness and complications associated with diabetes.

Coders need to be aware of the different clinical descriptions for the types of diabetes, including type 1, type 2, gestational, and secondary diabetes.

- Patients with **type 1 diabetes mellitus** have lost pancreatic beta cells because of an autoimmune disease and require insulin to survive. Most (but not all) patients with type 1 diabetes develop the condition before reaching puberty, so type 1 diabetes mellitus is also referred to as juvenile diabetes.
- In **type 2 diabetes mellitus,** the pancreatic beta cells are present and do produce insulin. However, there is insulin resistance, so patients may require insulin or other oral agents to reach the insulin level needed to maintain proper glucose (blood sugar) levels. Patients with type 2 diabetes represent over 90% of all diabetics.
- **Gestational diabetes** occurs when pregnant women develop diabetes. Coding the conditions of diabetes complicating pregnancy is covered in Chapter 8 of this text.
- **Secondary diabetes** can develop from numerous other causes, such as congenital, metabolic, or genetic reasons; chronic use of steroids; removal of the pancreas; and chronic pancreatitis.

When the type of diabetes is not documented in the medical record the coder should default to type 2 diabetes, category E11.

Coders should review the *Official Guidelines*, as shown in Box 5.10.

Common Medications and Treatments for Blood Diseases

Blood Transfusions

Blood transfusion is the process of transferring blood or blood-based products from one person into the circulatory system of another person. Blood transfusions can be life saving in some situations, such as in the case of massive blood loss due to trauma, and can be used to replace blood lost during surgery. Blood transfusions may also be used to treat severe anemia or thrombocytopenia caused by a blood disease as well as hemophilia or sickle-cell disease.

Early transfusions used whole blood, but modern medical practice is able to use the components of blood as well, which include packed red blood cells, plasma, and platelets.

Vitamins and Iron

A number of vitamins are used to treat blood disorders:

- Vitamin B_2 (riboflavin) is necessary for red blood cell formation, antibody production, and cellular respiration and growth.
- Vitamin B_9 (folic acid) is needed for energy production and formation of red blood cells; it prevents megaloblastic anemia.
- Vitamin B_{12} (cyanocobalamin) is needed to prevent megaloblastic anemia.
- Vitamin K (phytonadione) is a coenzyme involved in the synthesis of many proteins involved in blood clotting and bone metabolism.

Iron is an integral part of many proteins and enzymes that maintain good health. It is available for human consumption in the forms of ferrous fumarate, ferrous gluconate, and ferrous sulfate. Iron is also available for injection in the form of iron dextran (DexFerrum and INFeD).

Clotting Medications

Coagulation is a complex process by which blood forms clots. It is an important part of hemostasis (the cessation of blood loss from a damaged vessel), whereby a damaged blood vessel wall is covered by a platelet- and fibrin-containing clot to stop bleeding and begin repair. Disorders of coagulation can lead to an increased risk of bleeding (hemorrhage) and/or clotting (thrombosis).

Anticoagulants

Anticoagulants are given to stop thrombosis (inappropriate clotting of blood in the blood vessels). This is useful in primary and secondary prevention of deep venous thrombosis, pulmonary embolism, myocardial infarctions, and strokes in those who are

ANTICOAGULANTS	
TRADE NAME	GENERIC NAME
	heparin
Aggrastat	tirofiban
Aggrenox	dipyridamole, aspirin
Agrylin	anagrelide
Coumadin	warfarin
Fragmin	dalteparin
Integrilin	eptifibatide
Lovenox	enoxaparin
Persantine	dipyridamole
Plavix	clopidogrel
Pletal	cilostazol
ReoPro	abciximab
Ticlid	ticlopidine

predisposed. The anticoagulants table lists common brand and generic names.

Coagulants

Coagulant drugs may be used to assist the body in maintaining hemostasis. They may be administered to dissolve blood clots in situations such as myocardial infarctions and cerebrovascular accidents. The coagulants table lists common brand and generic names.

Hematopoietics

Hematopoietic drugs treat anemia and other blood cell disorders by stimulating the production of blood cells, thereby increasing the number of blood cells in circulation. The hematopoietics table lists common brand and generic names.

COAGULANTS

TRADE NAME	GENERIC NAME
	protamine
Activase	alteplase
Retavase	reteplase
Streptase	streptokinase
TNKase	tenecteplase
Xigris	drotrecogin

HEMATOPOIETICS

TRADE NAME	GENERIC NAME
Aranesp	darbepoetin alfa
Epogen	epoetin alfa
Leukine	sargramostim
Neulasta	pegfilgrastim
Neumega	oprelvekin
Neupogen	filgrastim

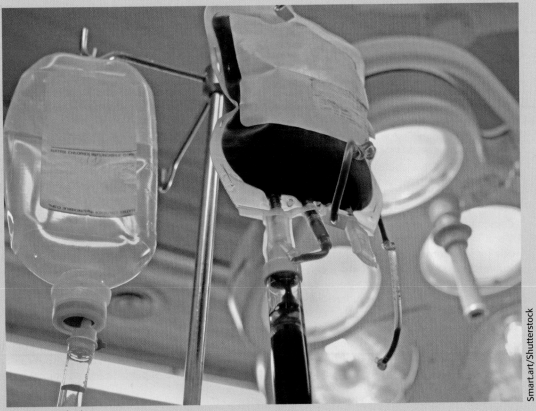

Blood transfusion.

Smart.art/Shutterstock

Coding Guidelines

a. Diabetes Mellitus

The diabetes mellitus codes are combination codes that include the type of diabetes mellitus, the body system affected, and the complications affecting that body system. As many codes within a particular category as are necessary to describe all of the complications of the disease may be used. They should be sequenced based on the reason for a particular encounter. Assign as many codes from categories E08–E13 as needed to identify all of the associated conditions that the patient has.

1) Type of diabetes

The age of a patient is not the sole determining factor, though most type 1 diabetics develop the condition before reaching puberty. For this reason type 1 diabetes mellitus is also referred to as juvenile diabetes.

2) Type of diabetes mellitus not documented

If the type of diabetes mellitus is not documented in the medical record, the default is E11.-, type 2 diabetes mellitus.

3) Diabetes mellitus and the use of insulin and oral hypoglycemics

If the documentation in a medical record does not indicate the type of diabetes but does indicate that the patient uses insulin, code E11.-, type 2 diabetes mellitus, should be assigned. An additional code should be assigned from category Z79 to identify the long-term (current) use of insulin or oral hypoglycemic drugs. If the patient is treated with both oral medications and insulin, only the code for long-term (current) use of insulin should be assigned. Code Z79.4 should not be assigned if insulin is given temporarily to bring a type 2 patient's blood sugar under control during an encounter.

4) Diabetes mellitus in pregnancy and gestational diabetes

See Section I.C.15. Diabetes mellitus in pregnancy.
See Section I.C.15. Gestational (pregnancy induced) diabetes.

5) Complications due to insulin pump malfunction

(a) Underdose of insulin due to insulin pump failure

An underdose of insulin due to an insulin pump failure should be assigned to a code from subcategory T85.6, Mechanical complication of other specified internal and external prosthetic devices, implants and grafts, that specifies the type of pump malfunction, as the principal or first-listed code, followed by code T38.3X6-, Underdosing of insulin and oral hypoglycemic [antidiabetic] drugs. Additional codes for the type of diabetes mellitus and any associated complications due to the underdosing should also be assigned.

(b) Overdose of insulin due to insulin pump failure

The principal or first-listed code for an encounter due to an insulin pump malfunction resulting in an overdose of insulin, should also be T85.6-, Mechanical complication of other specified internal and external prosthetic devices, implants and grafts, followed by code T38.3X1-, Poisoning by insulin and oral hypoglycemic [antidiabetic] drugs, accidental (unintentional).

6) Secondary diabetes mellitus

Codes under categories E08, Diabetes mellitus due to underlying condition, E09, Drug or chemical induced diabetes mellitus, and E13, Other specified diabetes mellitus, identify complications/manifestations associated with secondary diabetes mellitus. Secondary diabetes is always caused by another condition or event (e.g., cystic fibrosis, malignant neoplasm of pancreas, pancreatectomy, adverse effect of drug, or poisoning).

(a) Secondary diabetes mellitus and the use of insulin or hypoglycemic drugs

For patients with secondary diabetes mellitus who routinely use insulin or oral hypoglycemic drugs, an additional code from category Z79 should be assigned to identify the long-term (current) use of insulin or oral hypoglycemic drugs. If the patient is treated with both oral medications and insulin, only the code for long-term (current) use of insulin should be assigned. Code Z79.4 should not be assigned if insulin is given temporarily to bring a type 2 patient's blood sugar under control during an encounter.

(b) Assigning and sequencing secondary diabetes codes and its causes

The sequencing of the secondary diabetes codes in relationship to codes for the cause of the diabetes is based on the Tabular List instructions for categories E08, E09, and E13.

(i) Secondary diabetes mellitus due to pancreatectomy

For postpancreatectomy diabetes mellitus (lack of insulin due to the surgical removal of all or part of the pancreas), assign code E89.1, Postprocedural hypoinsulinemia. Assign a code from category E13 and a code from subcategory Z90.41-, Acquired absence of pancreas, as additional codes.

(ii) Secondary diabetes due to drugs

Secondary diabetes may be caused by an adverse effect of correctly administered medications, poisoning or sequela of poisoning.

See section I.C.19.e for coding of adverse effects and poisoning, and section I.C.20 for external cause code reporting.

Categories E08–E13: Diabetes Mellitus

To correctly code diabetes mellitus, documentation must state

- The type of diabetes or
- The cause of diabetes
- Associated complications or manifestations

The diabetes codes are combination codes that include the type of diabetes, the body system affected, and the associated complications. Many codes within a category (E08–E13) may be assigned to describe all of the complications of the disease. Remember that the convention "with" assumes that the conditions listed are related to diabetes. The sequencing of these codes is based on the reason for the encounter. For example, the subcategories for diabetes type 1 can be determined from the Alphabetic Index as shown in Box 5.11.

BOX 5.11 ICD-10-CM Index to Diseases and Injuries, Main Term Diabetes, Subterm Type 1

Diabetes-Associated Conditions as Noted in the Alphabetic Index

- type 1 E10.9
- - with
- - - amyotrophy E10.44
- - - arthropathy NEC E10.618
- - - autonomic (poly)neuropathy E10.43
- - - cataract E10.36
- - - Charcot's joints E10.610
- - - chronic kidney disease E10.22
- - - circulatory complication NEC E10.59
- - - complication E10.8
- - - - specified NEC E10.69
- - - dermatitis E10.620
- - - foot ulcer E10.621
- - - gangrene E10.52
- - - gastroparesis E10.43
- - - glomerulonephrosis, intracapillary E10.21
- - - glomerulosclerosis, intercapillary E10.21
- - - hyperglycemia E10.65
- - - hypoglycemia E10.649
- - - - with coma E10.641
- - - ketoacidosis E10.10
- - - - with coma E10.11
- - - kidney complications NEC E10.29
- - - Kimmelstiel-Wilson disease E10.21
- - - mononeuropathy E10.41
- - - myasthenia E10.44
- - - necrobiosis lipoidica E10.620
- - - nephropathy E10.21
- - - neuralgia E10.42
- - - neurologic complication NEC E10.49
- - - neuropathic arthropathy E10.610
- - - neuropathy E10.40
- - - ophthalmic complication NEC E10.39

- - - oral complication NEC E10.638
- - - periodontal disease E10.630
- - - peripheral angiopathy E10.51
- - - - with gangrene E10.52
- - - polyneuropathy E10.42
- - - renal complication NEC E10.29
- - - renal tubular degeneration E10.29
- - - retinopathy E10.319
- - - - with macular edema E10.311
- - - - resolved following treatment E10.37
- - - - nonproliferative E10.329
- - - - - with macular edema E10.321
- - - - - mild E10.329
- - - - - - with macular edema E10.321
- - - - - moderate E10.339
- - - - - - with macular edema E10.331
- - - - - severe E10.349
- - - - - - with macular edema E10.341
- - - - proliferative E10.359
- - - - - with
- - - - - - combined traction retinal detachment and rhegmatogenous retinal detachment E10.354
- - - - - - macular edema E10.351
- - - - - - stable proliferative diabetic retinopathy E10.355
- - - - - - traction retinal detachment involving the macula E10.352
- - - - - - traction retinal detachment not involving the macula E10.353
- - - skin complication NEC E10.628
- - - skin ulcer NEC E10.622

EXAMPLES

- Type 1 diabetes with hyperglycemia and diabetic retinopathy. Codes assigned are E10.65, E10.319.

- Diabetes, type 2, nephropathy and chronic left heel ulcer. Codes assigned are E11.21, E11.621, L97.429.

Diabetes Mellitus and the Use of Insulin. As discussed earlier, individuals with type 1 diabetes must use insulin because their bodies do not produce it; individuals with type 2 diabetes may also use insulin or take oral hypoglycemics. Documentation in the medical record may state that the patient uses insulin but not state the type of diabetes. In that case, the coder must assign type 2 diabetes. For patients with type 2 diabetes who routinely use insulin, the code for long-term use of insulin (Z79.4) should be assigned. Code Z79.84 should be assigned for long-term use of hypoglycemics. If the patient requires both long-term insulin and hypoglycemics, report only the long-term insulin use. The codes are not assigned if insulin or hypoglycemics are given temporarily to bring a type 2 patient's blood sugar under control during an encounter.

> INTERNET RESOURCE: Current Information on Managing Diabetes Mellitus
> http://www.diabetes.org/living-with-diabetes/treatment-and-care/

Insulin Pumps

ICD-10-CM contains codes that identify different aspects of insulin pumps, devices used to deliver insulin to patients with DM. Codes for the presence of an insulin pump (Z96.41), insulin pump titration, and counseling and training (Z46.81) are available to identify the specific service or pump status. Complications of these devices can also occur.

> The record documentation may state a condition is a complication of diabetes, or there is an assumed relationship based on the convention "with" in the Index.

Underdose of Insulin Due to Insulin Pump Failure. The *Official Guidelines* indicate that "an underdose of insulin due to an insulin pump failure should be assigned to a code from subcategory T85.6, Mechanical complication of other specified internal and external prosthetic devices, implants and grafts, that specifies the type of pump malfunction, as the principal or first-listed code, followed by T38.3x6-." A code for the types of diabetes and associated complications would also be reported.

> If information regarding an association between DM and a complication/manifestation is not clear, query the physician. Not all conditions often associated with DM are necessarily complications of the disease.

EXAMPLE
Insulin pump failure with insulin underdose in a patient with type 1 DM. Codes are T85.614A, T38.3x6A, E10.9.

Overdose of Insulin Due to Insulin Pump Failure. Similarly, in the case of insulin pump failure resulting in an overdose, the principal code assigned should be code T85.6, Mechanical complication of other specified internal and external prosthetic devices, implants, and grafts. Subsequently, code T38.3x1- is reported for Poisoning by insulin and oral hypoglycemic [antidiabetic] drugs, accidental (unintentional).

EXAMPLE
Insulin overdose due to insulin pump overdose in a patient with type 1 DM. Codes are T85.614A, T38.3x1A, E10.9.

Secondary Diabetes

Secondary diabetes is a diabetic condition that is always caused by an underlying disease process such as cystic fibrosis or a drug or chemical such as steroids. The codes from category E08 (Diabetes mellitus due to underlying condition), E09 (Drug or chemical induced diabetes mellitus), and E13 (Other specified diabetes mellitus) classify complications and manifestations that are associated with secondary diabetes mellitus.

EXAMPLE
Carcinoma of the pancreas with secondary diabetic ketoacidosis. Codes are E08.10, C25.9.

Nutritional Disorders

Conditions grouped under nutritional disorders are not related to diabetes and generally refer to nondiabetic patients. A common diagnosis is obesity. Physician documentation of obesity must be noted in order to assign a code for obesity or, for that matter, for overweight. ICD-10-CM differentiates obesity from morbid obesity. Clinically, morbid obesity is known as *clinically severe obesity*. In this condition, the person weighs more than 100 pounds over the ideal or has a body mass index (BMI) of 35.0 or higher in the presence of one other comorbidity. When assigning a code for obesity, a second code is often assigned to reflect BMI, if known. See the "use additional code" note at category E66 in the ICD-10-CM Tabular List.

Body mass index is defined as the individual's body weight divided by the square of the height. The formula universally used in medicine produces a unit of measure of kilogram per square meter (kg/m²). BMI can also be determined using a BMI chart, which displays BMI as a function of weight and height (Table 5.5). BMI is often calculated by the nutritionist in the inpatient setting. Therefore, it is appropriate to code BMI from nutritionist documentation. However, the diagnosis of obesity cannot be coded unless that condition is documented by the physician, even though the BMI table below indicates the weight status as obesity. In the presence of malnutrition and other nutritional deficiencies, it may be appropriate to assign an additional code for body mass index.

Table 5.5 Body Mass Index

BMI	WEIGHT RANGE	WEIGHT STATUS
18.4 and below	114.0 lbs and below	Underweight
18.5–24.9	114.6–154.3 lb	Normal
25.0–29.9	154.9–185.3 lb	Overweight
30.0–34.9	185.9–216.3 lb	Obese (moderate)
35.0–39.9	216.9–247.2 lb	Obese (severe)
40.0 and above	247.9 lbs and above	Obese (very severe)

EXAMPLES

- The nutrition consultation reports the BMI as 36.0. No code is assigned as obesity was not physician documented. Query the physician for diagnosis of obesity. If documented after the query, both codes for obesity and BMI would be reported.

- The physician documents morbid obesity. Nutrition consultation reports BMI of 45.2. Report codes E66.01, Z68.42.

CHECKPOINT 5.6

Code the following statements using ICD-10-CM. Do not assign procedure codes.

1. Diabetic bilateral proliferative retinopathy _____

2. Type 2 diabetes mellitus and peripheral angiopathy _____

3. Diabetic left foot ulcer due to diabetic neuropathy _____

4. Chronic osteomyelitis of the right femur and diabetes mellitus type 2, with hyperglycemia

   _____

5. Type 2 diabetes with associated Charcot's joint _____

6. Nephropathy with type 2 diabetes mellitus _____

7. Visit for adjustment of an insulin pump titration with type 1 diabetes mellitus _____

8. Insulin overdose due to insulin pump failure in an individual with type 1 diabetes _____

9. Infected insulin pump in an individual with type 1 diabetes (*Hint:* See complication, insulin pump.) _____

10. Insulin underdose resulting in hyperglycemia in an individual with type 1 diabetes _____

11. Diabetes secondary to cystic fibrosis _____

12. Steroid-induced diabetes with diabetic neuropathy _____

13. Severe malnutrition in a 35-year-old patient with a BMI of 18.0 _____

MENTAL, BEHAVIORAL, AND NEURODEVELOPMENTAL DISORDERS (CHAPTER 5: F01–F99)

Codes in Chapter 5 of ICD-10-CM classify the various types of mental disorders, including conditions of drug and alcohol abuse, use, and dependence; dementia; schizophrenic disorders; and mood disturbances. Most psychiatrists use terminology from the *Diagnostic and Statistical Manual of Mental Disorders, Fifth Edition (DSM-V)* of the American Psychiatric Association for diagnoses, but coding follows ICD-10-CM. Box 5.12 outlines the chapter-specific *Official Guidelines* for mental disorders. The categories in Chapter 5 are grouped as shown in Table 5.6.

Pain Disorders Related to Psychological Factors

When pain is documented *exclusively* related to a psychological disorder, the code F45.41 (Pain disorder exclusively related to psychological factors) is assigned. When pain disorders are related to psychological factors (not exclusively related), two codes are required; assign the code for psychological pain with the additional code from category G89 (Pain, not elsewhere classified). Nonpsychological pain category G89 is discussed further in Chapter 7 of this text.

Mental and Behavioral Disorders Due to Psychoactive Substance Use

Classification of psychoactive substance use is classified by use, abuse, or dependence; presence of associated disorders; or remission. Examples of psychoactive substances include alcohol, opioids, cocaine, stimulants, hallucinogens, inhalants, and nicotine.

PHARMACOLOGY CONNECTION

Common Medications Used to Treat Diabetes

Oral Agents

Oral diabetes medications help control blood glucose levels in people whose bodies still produce some insulin (the majority of people with type 2 diabetes). These medications are used in conjunction with specific dietary changes and regular exercise. Several of the medications are used in combination to achieve optimal blood glucose control.

The categories of oral agents include:

- Sulfonylureas
- Meglitinides
- Biguanides
- Thiazolidinediones
- DPP-4 inhibitors
- Alpha-glucosidase inhibitors

The table to the right lists common brand and generic names.

Insulins

Insulin is used medically to treat some forms of diabetes mellitus. Patients with type 1 diabetes mellitus depend on external insulin (most commonly injected subcutaneously) for their survival because the hormone is no longer produced internally. Patients with type 2 diabetes mellitus are insulin resistant,

ORAL AGENTS	
TRADE NAME	**GENERIC NAME**
Actos	pioglitazone
Amaryl	glimepiride
Avandia	rosiglitazone
Byetta	exenatide
DiaBeta	glyburide
Diabinese	chlorpropamide
Glucophage	metformin
Glucotrol	glipizide
Glynase	glyburide
Glyset	miglitol
Januvia	sitagliptin
Micronase	glyburide
Orinase	tolbutamide
Prandin	repaglinide
Precose	acarbose
Starlix	nateglinide
Symlin	pramlintide
Tolinase	tolazamide

The terms *drug addiction* and *drug dependence* indicate chronic physical and mental conditions based on patients' patterns of drug consumption. Drug dependence causes changes in behavior and physiology, including compulsion to take the drug or discomfort in its absence, such as physical signs of withdrawal when the drug is suddenly no longer taken.

When a patient has a drug-taking problem, or takes a drug in excess, but has not reached a stage of dependence, the condition is termed *drug abuse*. Abuse represents the effects of drug use in a maladaptive pattern, which may include detrimental social functioning or physical or mental health. Drug-related conditions include temporary mental disturbance, slurred speech, arguments with family and friends, and difficulty at school or work. Simple drug intoxication is also considered drug abuse.

When reporting psychoactive substance use that is in remission, documentation must specifically state "in remission" by the provider. Psychoactive substance use, abuse and dependence codes are assigned based on a pattern of use in hierarchy. The hierarchy instructs the coder to use one code at the highest pattern of use. For example, the patient has used cocaine and is also cocaine dependent. The coder would assign the code for cocaine dependence only (F14.20). Moderate or severe substance use disorders in early or sustained remission are classified to the appropriate codes for substance dependence in remission. See the *Official Guidelines* in Box 5.12 for the specific hierarchy.

Selection of the Principal Diagnosis

Designation of the principal diagnosis depends on the circumstances of admission or outpatient encounter. As with all other diagnoses, the codes for psychoactive substance use should only be based on provider documentation and when they meet the definition of a reportable diagnosis. (See Section III discussion in Chapter 4.) Many of the codes in this block describe substance-induced complications such as mood disorders, dementia, hallucinations, or sexual dysfunction. Documentation

have relatively low insulin production, or both; some of these patients may eventually require insulin when other medications fail to control blood glucose levels adequately. The table to the left lists representative common trade and generic names for insulin medications.

INSULINS	
TRADE NAME	**GENERIC NAME**
Apidra	insulin glulisine
Exubera	insulin (inhalation)
Humalog	insulin lispro
Humulin (R, N)	insulin, regular and NPH
Lantus	insulin glargine
Levemir	insulin detemir
Novolin (R, N)	insulin, regular and NPH
NovoLog	insulin lispro

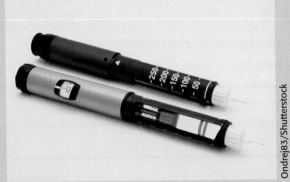

Insulin in two forms.

Ondrej83/Shutterstock

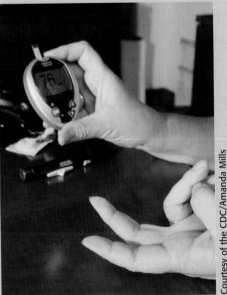

Diabetic monitoring.

Courtesy of the CDC/Amanda Mills

BOX 5.12 Official Guidelines: Mental, Behavioral, and Neurodevelopmental Disorders (F10–F99)

a. Pain Disorders Related to Psychological Factors

Assign code F45.41 for pain that is exclusively related to psychological disorders. As indicated by the Excludes1 note under category G89, a code from category G89 should not be assigned with code F45.41.

Code F45.42, Pain disorders with related psychological factors, should be used with a code from category G89, Pain, not elsewhere classified, if there is documentation of a psychological component for a patient with acute or chronic pain.

See Section I.C.6. Pain.

b. Mental and Behavioral Disorders Due to Psychoactive Substance Use

1. In Remission

Selection of codes for "in remission" for categories F10–F19, Mental and behavioral disorders due to psychoactive substance use (categories F10–F19 with -19, -.21) requires the provider's clinical judgment. The appropriate codes for "in remission" are assigned only on the basis of provider documentation (as defined in the *Official Guidelines for Coding and Reporting*), unless otherwise instructed by the classification.

Mild substance use disorders in early or sustained remission are classified to the appropriate codes for substance abuse in remission, and moderate or severe substance use disorders in early or sustained remission are classified to the appropriate codes for substance dependence in remission.

2. Psychoactive Substance Use, Abuse, and Dependence

When the provider documentation refers to use, abuse, and dependence of the same substance (e.g., alcohol, opioid, cannabis, etc.), only one code should be assigned to identify the pattern of use based on the following hierarchy:

- If both use and abuse are documented, assign only the code for abuse.
- If both abuse and dependence are documented, assign only the code for dependence.
- If use, abuse, and dependence are all documented, assign only the code for dependence.
- If both use and dependence are documented, assign only the code for dependence.

3. Psychoactive Substance Use Disorders

As with all other diagnoses, the codes for psychoactive substance use disorders (F10.9-, F11.9-, F12.9-, F13.9-, F14.9-, F15.9-, F16.9-) should only be assigned based on provider documentation and when they meet the definition of a reportable diagnosis (see Section III, Reporting Additional Diagnoses). The codes are to be used only when the psychoactive substance use is associated with a physical, mental, or behavioral disorder, and such a relationship is documented by the provider.

Table 5.6 Organization of ICD-9-CM Chapter 5 Tabular List

BLOCK	BLOCK DESCRIPTION
F01–F09	Mental disorders due to known physiological conditions
F10–F19	Mental and behavioral disorders due to psychoactive substance use
F20–F29	Schizophrenia, schizotypical, delusional, and other non-mood psychotic disorders
F30–F39	Mood [affective] disorders
F40–F48	Anxiety, dissociative, stress-related, somatoform, and other nonpsychotic mental disorders
F50–F59	Behavioral syndromes associated with physiological disturbances and physical factors
F60–F69	Disorders of adult personality and behavior
F70–F79	Intellectual disabilities
F80–F89	Pervasive and specific developmental disorders
F90–F98	Behavioral and emotional disorders with onset usually occurring in childhood and adolescence
F99	Unspecified mental disorder

must support a relationship between the disorder and the substance use in order to assign those codes. (*Hint:* Code also the blood alcohol level for codes from category F10, if applicable.)

EXAMPLES
- Cocaine withdrawal, initial encounter for treatment with poisoning of undetermined cause. Codes are F14.23, T40.5X4A, F19.939, F14.20.

- Alcohol dependence with alcoholic withdrawal, blood alcohol level of 0.25. Codes are F10.230, Y90.1.

1. If a patient is admitted for detoxification, rehabilitation, or both and there is no identified related organic mental condition, sequence the substance abuse or dependence code as the principal diagnosis.

EXAMPLES
- Alcoholism. Code is F10.20.

- Dependence of analgesics, admitted for rehabilitation. Code is F19.20.

2. If a patient with a diagnosis of alcohol or drug abuse or dependence is admitted because of an unrelated condition, follow the guidelines for the selection of the principal diagnosis.

EXAMPLES
- Acute appendicitis in a patient with alcoholism. Codes are K35.80, F10.20.

- Acute bronchitis in a patient with uncomplicated heroin dependence. Codes are J20.9, F11.20.

3. If a patient with a diagnosis of substance abuse or dependence is admitted for treatment or evaluation of a physical complaint related to such use, follow the directions in the Alphabetic Index for conditions described as due to alcohol or drugs and sequence the combination code. When two codes are required, sequence the physical condition first, followed by the code for abuse or dependence.

EXAMPLES
- Alcoholic cardiomyopathy, alcohol use disorder, severe, in early remission. Codes are I42.6, F10.21.

- Drug-induced sleep disorder, with abuse of sedatives. Code is F13.182.

CHECKPOINT 5.7

Code the following statements using ICD-10-CM.

1. Delirium tremens, alcohol dependence. The patient drinks one pint of vodka per day. _____

2. Alcohol-induced dementia. This alcoholic patient has stopped drinking for 3 years and is known to be in remission. _____

3. Cocaine, cannabis, and heroin dependence. _____

4. Patient admitted for treatment of alcoholic cirrhosis. The patient is intoxicated with a blood alcohol level of 180 mg/100 mL. The patient is alcohol dependent and abuses cocaine twice per month. _____

5. Alcohol and drug abuse. _____

6. Alcohol abuse, admitted for counseling. _____

7. Moderate alcohol use disorder. _____

Common Medications for Mental Disorders

Psychotropic agents—those that affect behavior, psychiatric state, and sleep—treat psychoses and other mental disorders.

Antipsychotics

Antipsychotics (also referred to as *neuroleptics*) are a group of drugs commonly but not exclusively used to treat psychosis, which is typified by schizophrenia. The two classes of antipsychotics, typical and atypical, both tend to block receptors in the brain's dopamine pathways. The antipsychotics table lists common trade and generic names.

Mood-Altering Drugs

Antidepressants are psychiatric medications or other substances (nutrient or herb) used for alleviating depression or altering mood. They may also be used in the treatment of a number of other conditions, including anxiety disorders, bipolar disorder, obsessive-compulsive disorder, and eating disorders, and for chronic pain. Some mood-altering drugs have become known as lifestyle drugs or "mood brighteners." The table lists common trade and generic names of mood-altering drugs.

ANTIPSYCHOTICS	
TRADE NAME	**GENERIC NAME**
Abilify	aripiprazole
Clozaril	clozapine
Etrafon	perphenazine
Geodon	ziprasidone
Haldol	haloperidol
Invega	paliperidone
Loxitane	loxapine
Mellaril	thioridazine
Moban	molindone
Navane	thiothixene
Orap	pimozide
Prolixin	fluphenazine
Risperdal	risperidone
Seroquel	quetiapine
Stelazine	trifluoperazine
Thorazine	chlorpromazine
Zyprexa	olanzapine

Chapter Summary

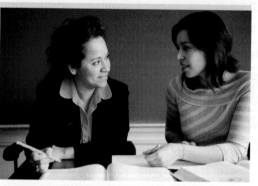

1. Coding of an infectious disease may require only one code to correctly represent the infectious disease and its manifestation, but may also require assigning two codes in order to identify both the infectious disease and its manifestation. Be aware that a code for an infection may be classified elsewhere in ICD-10-CM. Coders are required to assign codes for infections based on the physician documentation, rather than on laboratory results alone.

2. Selection of HIV/AIDS codes depends initially on the reason for the encounter: screening, a return encounter to learn test results, HIV-related illness, and exposure to HIV. Screening codes are selected according to the presence or lack of symptoms. A test result visit is coded according to the nature of the result. HIV illness is coded to B20, with additional code assignment for illnesses. Exposure is coded to Z11.4.

3. SIRS (systemic inflammatory response syndrome) refers to the body's systemic response to infection, trauma, burns, or other insult with common symptoms of fever, tachypnea, tachycardia, or leukocytosis. SIRS may be caused by a wide variety of conditions, such as

MOOD ALTERING	
TRADE NAME	**GENERIC NAME**
Anafranil	clomipramine
Aventyl	nortriptyline
Celexa	citalopram
Cymbalta	duloxetine
Desyrel	trazodone
Effexor	venlafaxine
Elavil	amitriptyline
Lexapro	escitalopram
Nardil	phenelzine
Norpramin	desipramine
Pamelor	nortriptyline
Parnate	tranylcypromine
Paxil	paroxetine
Prozac	fluoxetine
Remeron	mirtazapine
Sinequan	doxepin
Surmontil	trimipramine
Tofranil	imipramine
Wellbutrin	bupropion
Zoloft	sertraline

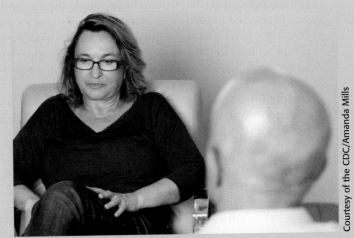

Courtesy of the CDC/Amanda Mills

Psychiatrist with patient.

At times, the medications listed below are used to treat drug abuse and addiction.

DRUG ABUSE AND ADDICTION MEDICATIONS		
PURPOSE	**TRADE NAME**	**GENERIC**
Prevent alcohol use	Depade, ReVia	naltrexone
Curb cocaine desire	Norpramin	desipramine
Narcotic detoxification	Methadone	

trauma, complications of surgery, adrenal insufficiency, pulmonary embolism, a complicated aortic aneurysm, myocardial infarction, hemorrhage, drug overdose, burns, acute pancreatitis, or immunodeficiency (such as AIDS). Sepsis refers to SIRS due to infection; it is a severe illness caused by overwhelming infection.

- The guidelines for SIRS of noninfectious origin require two codes: the first to indicate the origin (trauma, injury, etc.) and a second code to represent SIRS, R65.10 without acute organ dysfunction or R65.11 for SIRS with acute organ dysfunction.
- The guidelines for sepsis indicate that one code will represent the sepsis and its infectious origin. The code categories are A40 and A41. If the origin is unspecified, report A41.9.
- When coding severe sepsis (documentation of sepsis with organ failure or dysfunction), additional codes for organ dysfunctions must be reported. The code for the underlying cause (infection or trauma) is sequenced first, followed by the codes for severe sepsis R65.2X plus codes for specific acute organ dysfunction (such as acute renal failure or acute respiratory failure).

4. *Septic shock* refers to circulatory failure associated with severe sepsis, and therefore it represents a type of acute organ dysfunction. For this reason, all cases of septic shock require the codes for systemic infection to be sequenced first, followed by codes R65.21. The code for septic shock cannot be sequenced first; additional codes for other acute organ dysfunctions should also be assigned.

5. When an infection that is due to MRSA is present and that infection has a combination code that includes the causal organism, that combination code is assigned (Ex. J15.212). When no combination code is available, two codes are required. One code represents the

condition, and code B95.62 is used to identify it as MRSA. Documentation must specifically support the relationship between the MRSA and the condition.

6. Neoplasm code assignment is based on the anatomical location and the behavior of the tumor, which may be malignant (primary site, secondary site, or in situ), benign, uncertain, or unspecified in the documentation. Malignancies are coded according to whether they are primary or secondary. Identify the location, determine its behavior, and refer to the neoplasm table. After determining the potential code, refer to the tabular section of ICD-10-CM to verify its accuracy based on the notes, inclusions, and exclusions as indicated for that code.

7. Coding for DM is represented by five categories of codes and each category has been expanded to contain the manifestation/complication description within that code through the use of fourth and fifth digits. The categories are

E08	DM due to underlying condition
E09	Drug- or chemical-induced DM
E10	Type 1 DM
E11	Type 2 DM
E13	Other specified DM

8. Codes for anemias present in chronic illness are available for anemia in chronic kidney disease (D63.1), anemia in neoplastic disease (D63.0), and anemia in other chronic illness (D63.8). Each of these codes includes the instruction to "Code first" the chronic kidney disease, the neoplastic disease, and the other underlying diseases.

9. For diagnoses of mental illness, most psychiatrists use terminology from the *Diagnostic and Statistical Manual of Mental Disorders, Fifth Edition* of the American Psychiatric Association for diagnoses, but coding follows ICD-10-CM. ICD-10-CM has multiple subchapters, categories, and subcategories for mental, behavioral, and neurodevelopmental disorders. Coders must rely on the provider's documentation to correctly identify whether the patient is in remission, has substance abuse vs. substance dependence vs. substance use as reportable diagnoses located in the F10–F19 codes. Pain disorders related to psychological factors are represented by F45.41.

Review Questions

Matching

Match the key terms with their definitions.

A. bacteremia
B. BMI
C. type 1 diabetes
D. secondary diabetes
E. physician query

F. morphology code
G. neoplasm
H. SIRS
I. metastasis
J. methicillin-resistant *Staphylococcus aureus*

1. __H__ Also known as severe sepsis

2. __E__ Process of asking for additional documentation from a physician

3. __J__ Very-difficult-to-treat staph infection

4. __C__ A type of diabetes in which insulin is not produced

5. __A__ Disease described as an infection in the blood

6. __B__ A measurement using height and weight

7. __F__ A code used to identify the histological type and behavior of a neoplasm

8. __I__ Movement of cancer cells to a secondary site

9. __G__ An abnormal growth of cells

10. __D__ A type of diabetes caused by an underlying process

True or False

Decide whether each statement is true or false.

1. __T__ When coding infectious diseases, two codes are always required.

2. __T__ The principal diagnosis for patients admitted with AIDS-related illness is B20.

3. __T__ The coding of sepsis always requires two codes.

4. __T__ When assigning codes for diabetes, the type of diabetes affects code assignment.

5. __T__ The diagnostic statement of "diabetic retinopathy" indicates a causal relationship between the diabetes and retinal disease.

6. __F__ All neoplasms are malignant.

7. __F__ When coding the diagnostic statement "prostate cancer with bone metastasis," the primary site of cancer is the bone.

8. __T__ The physician should be queried when documentation in the nutrition consult states BMI of 40.3 and the diagnosis of obesity is not stated.

9. __F__ Acute blood loss anemia is coded the same as postoperative anemia.

10. __T__ A history of malignant neoplasm code is assigned when the neoplasm is no longer present or being treated.

Multiple Choice

Select the letter that best completes the statement or answers the question.

1. Which of the following affects code assignment for infectious disease?
   A. Site of infection
   B. Infectious agent
   C. Both A and B
   D. Neither A nor B

2. The diagnosis of positive HIV test would be reported as
   A. B20
   B. Z21
   C. Z71.7
   D. R75

3. Which components should be included in a physician query?
   A. Leading questions
   B. Reference to documentation
   C. Request for yes or no answer
   D. Statement indicating reimbursement increase

4. Acute blood loss anemia due to epistaxis. The patient was admitted and treated for anemia with blood transfusions. Epistaxis occurred during hospitalization but did not require packing. Which codes are reported?
   A. R04.0, D62
   B. D62, R04.0
   C. D50.0, R04.0
   D. D50.0, I78.0

5. Hb-SD sickle-cell acute chest syndrome with crisis is coded as
   A. D57.811
   B. D57.01
   C. D57.00
   D. D57.00, R07.89

6. A neoplasm assigned the code C53.9 is
   A. Benign
   B. A secondary malignancy
   C. A primary malignancy
   D. An in situ carcinoma

7. In the diagnosis adenocarcinoma of the pancreas with extension to the duodenum and metastasis to the liver and mesenteric lymph nodes, the primary site is the
   A. Duodenum
   B. Liver
   C. Pancreas
   D. Mesenteric lymph node

8. A female patient was discharged from the hospital with the diagnosis of brain metastasis with unknown primary site. Which code or codes are reported?
   A. C79.31
   B. C79.31, C80.1
   C. C71.9
   D. C79.9, C71.9

9. Type 2 diabetes, Chronic kidney disease, stage 3, long-term insulin use is coded as
   A. E11.22, N18.3, Z79.4
   B. E10.22, N18.9, Z79.4
   C. E11.9, N18.3, Z79.4
   D. E08.9, N18.9

10. Alcoholic induced depression and alcoholic fatty liver is coded as
    A. F10.20, F32.9, K70.0
    B. F10.24, F32.9, K70.0
    C. F10.49, K76.0
    D. F10.24, K70.0

CHAPTER 6

ICD-10-CM Chapters 6 Through 10: G00–J99

CHAPTER OUTLINE

Diseases of the Nervous System (Chapter 6: G00–G99)

Diseases of the Eye and Adnexa (Chapter 7: H00–H59)

Diseases of the Ear and Mastoid Process (Chapter 8: H60–H95)

Diseases of the Circulatory System (Chapter 9: I00–I99)

Diseases of the Respiratory System (Chapter 10: J00–J99)

LEARNING OUTCOMES

After studying this chapter, you should be able to:

1. Describe the general guidelines for coding pain and pain management, differentiating between visits to manage pain and visits to treat the underlying cause of pain.
2. List the major points to consider in code selection and assignment for paralysis and for epilepsy.
3. Classify eye and adnexa disorders based on laterality, type of disease, and severity.
4. Discuss disorders related to the ear and mastoid process.
5. Identify the key points for coding hypertensive disease.
6. Discuss the coding of cerebrovascular disease.
7. Describe the assignment of initial and subsequent codes for acute myocardial infarction.
8. Describe the steps in code assignment for various types of heart failure.
9. Describe the coding and sequencing of chronic obstructive pulmonary disease (COPD) and asthma.
10. Discuss the coding of pneumonia.

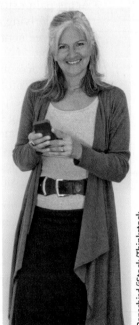

Razerbird/iStock/Thinkstock

C orrect code assignment and sequencing of patients' diagnosed or suspected conditions involving the nervous system, the eye and adnexa, the ear and mastoid process, and the circulatory and respiratory systems are covered in this chapter. The structure and organization of the corresponding ICD-10-CM Tabular List chapters are presented, followed by discussions of code selection and sequencing as instructed by the *Official Guidelines for ICD-10-CM Coding and Reporting*, Section I, Part C.6. The focus is on common code assignment decisions and complex coding scenarios.

DISEASES OF THE NERVOUS SYSTEM (CHAPTER 6: G00–G99)

Disorders of the nervous system include chronic pain, paralysis, and seizure disorders, among many others. The categories in Chapter 6 of ICD-10-CM are grouped as shown in Table 6.1. Box 6.1 presents the applicable guidelines from Section I, Part C, of the *Official Guidelines for Coding and Reporting*.

Pain Management—Category G89

Coding pain and its management requires careful review of the *Official Guidelines* that are covered in this chapter. The reason for the visit, as well as documentation of the type and/or cause of the pain, influences the reporting and sequencing of these codes. Most codes from category G89, "Pain, not elsewhere classified," can be used with codes from other categories and chapters to provide more details about patients' conditions.

Use of Codes From Category G89—General Guidelines
To be assigned from category G89, pain must be documented as one of these conditions:

- Acute pain usually begins suddenly, ranges in severity and duration, and is resolved when the underlying reason is diagnosed and treated.
- Unrelieved acute pain may lead to chronic pain, fairly constant pain that has a much longer duration.
- Post-thoracotomy pain (acute or chronic) is pain other than normal or routine pain following a thoracotomy.
- Postoperative/postprocedural pain (acute or chronic) is pain other than normal or routine pain following surgery or a procedure.
- Neoplasm-related pain is pain related to or associated with cancer.
- Chronic pain syndrome (G89.4) differs from chronic pain. In this condition, which must be specifically documented, the patient has pain that interferes with functioning and causes anger, depression, and anxiety.

If the pain is not specified as one of these conditions (acute or chronic, post-thoracotomy, postprocedural, or neoplasm related), do not assign a code from category G89.

Table 6.1 Organization of ICD-10-CM Chapter 6 Tabular List

BLOCK	BLOCK DESCRIPTION
G00–G09	Inflammatory diseases of the central nervous system
G10–G14	Systemic atrophies primarily affecting the central nervous system
G20–G26	Extrapyramidal and movement disorders
G30–G32	Other degenerative diseases of the nervous system
G35–G37	Demyelinating diseases of the central nervous system
G40–G47	Episodic and paroxysmal disorders
G50–G59	Nerve, nerve root, and plexus disorders
G60–G65	Polyneuropathies and other disorders of the peripheral nervous system
G70–G73	Diseases of myoneural junction and muscle
G80–G83	Cerebral palsy and other paralytic syndromes
G89–G99	Other disorders of the nervous system

The patient presents with acute back pain due to lumbar strain, initial episode. The patient also has chronic low back pain from lumbar spondylosis. Report codes S39.012A, M47.816.

BOX 6.1 *Official Guidelines*: Diseases of the Nervous System (G00–G99)

a. Dominant/Nondominant Side

Codes from category G81, Hemiplegia and hemiparesis, and subcategories, G83.1, Monoplegia of lower limb, G83.2, Monoplegia of upper limb, and G83.3, Monoplegia, unspecified, identify whether the dominant or nondominant side is affected. Should the affected side be documented, but not specified as dominant or nondominant, and the classification system does not indicate a default, code selection is as follows:

• For ambidextrous patients, the default should be dominant.

• If the left side is affected, the default is nondominant.

• If the right side is affected, the default is dominant.

b. Pain—Category G89

1) General coding information

Codes in category G89, Pain, not elsewhere classified, may be used in conjunction with codes from other categories and chapters to provide more detail about acute or chronic pain and neoplasm-related pain, unless otherwise indicated below.

If the pain is not specified as acute or chronic, post-thoracotomy, post-procedural, or neoplasm-related, do not assign codes from category G89.

A code from category G89 should not be assigned if the underlying (definitive) diagnosis is known, unless the reason for the encounter is pain control/management and not management of the underlying condition.

When an admission or encounter is for a procedure aimed at treating the underlying condition (e.g., spinal fusion, kyphoplasty), a code for the underlying condition (e.g., vertebral fracture, spinal stenosis) should be assigned as the principal diagnosis. No code from category G89 should be assigned.

(a) Category G89 codes as principal or first-listed diagnosis

Category G89 codes are acceptable as principal diagnosis or the first-listed code:

• When pain control or pain management is the reason for the admission/encounter (e.g., a patient with displaced intervertebral disc, nerve impingement, and severe back pain presents for injection of steroid into the spinal canal). The underlying cause of the pain should be reported as an additional diagnosis, if known.

• When a patient is admitted for the insertion of a neurostimulator for pain control, assign the appropriate pain code as the principal or first-listed diagnosis. When an admission or encounter is for a procedure aimed at treating the underlying condition and a neurostimulator is inserted for pain control during the same admission/encounter, a code for the underlying condition should be assigned as the principal diagnosis and the appropriate pain code should be assigned as a secondary diagnosis.

(b) Use of category G89 codes in conjunction with site-specific pain codes

(i) Assigning category G89 and site-specific pain codes

Codes from category G89 may be used in conjunction with codes that identify the site of pain (including codes from Chapter 18) if the category G89 code provides additional information. For example, if the code describes the site of the pain, but does not fully describe whether the pain is acute or chronic, then both codes should be assigned.

(ii) Sequencing of category G89 codes with site-specific pain codes

The sequencing of category G89 codes with site-specific pain codes (including Chapter 18 codes), is dependent on the circumstances of the encounter/admission as follows:

• If the encounter is for pain control or pain management, assign the code from Category G89 followed by the code identifying the specific site of pain (e.g., encounter for pain management for acute neck pain from trauma is assigned code G89.11, Acute pain due to trauma, followed by code M54.2, Cervicalgia, to identify the site of pain).

• If the encounter is for any other reason except pain control or pain management, and a related definitive diagnosis has not been established (confirmed) by the provider, assign the code for the specific site of pain first, followed by the appropriate code from category G89.

2) Pain due to devices, implants, and grafts

See Section I.C.19. Pain due to medical devices.

Continued

BOX 6.1 *Continued*

3) Postoperative pain

The provider's documentation should be used to guide the coding of postoperative pain, as well as Section *III. Reporting Additional Diagnoses* and Section *IV. Diagnostic Coding and Reporting in the Outpatient Setting.*

The default for post-thoracotomy and other postoperative pain not specified as acute or chronic is the code for the acute form.

Routine or expected postoperative pain immediately after surgery should not be coded.

(a) Postoperative pain not associated with specific postoperative complication

Postoperative pain not associated with a specific postoperative complication is assigned to the appropriate postoperative pain code in category G89.

(b) Postoperative pain associated with specific postoperative complication

Postoperative pain associated with a specific postoperative complication (such as painful wire sutures) is assigned to the appropriate code(s) found in Chapter 19, Injury, poisoning, and certain other consequences of external causes. If appropriate, use additional code(s) from category G89 to identify acute or chronic pain (G89.18 or G89.28).

4) Chronic pain

Chronic pain is classified to subcategory G89.2. There is no timeframe defining when pain becomes chronic pain. The provider's documentation should be used to guide use of these codes.

5) Neoplasm related pain

Code G89.3 is assigned to pain documented as being related, associated, or due to cancer, primary or secondary malignancy, or tumor. This code is assigned regardless of whether the pain is acute or chronic.

This code may be assigned as the principal or first-listed code when the stated reason for the admission/encounter is documented as pain control/pain management. The underlying neoplasm should be reported as an additional diagnosis.

When the reason for the admission/encounter is management of the neoplasm and the pain associated with the neoplasm is also documented, code G89.3 may be assigned as an additional diagnosis. It is not necessary to assign an additional code for the site of the pain.

See Section I.C.2 for instructions on the sequencing of neoplasms for all other stated reasons for the admission/encounter (except for pain control/pain management).

6) Chronic pain syndrome

Central pain syndrome (G89.0) and chronic pain syndrome (G89.4) are different from the term "chronic pain," and therefore [these] codes should only be used when the provider has specifically documented this condition.

See Section I.C.5. Pain disorders related to psychological factors.

Sequencing of Codes From Category G89

In certain circumstances, a code from category G89 can be sequenced as the principal diagnosis or first-listed code. In other circumstances, a code from category G89 should not be listed first or should not be reported at all.

Pain Management Visits

When the reason for a visit is for pain control or pain management, such as when a patient with a displaced intervertebral disk, nerve impingement, and severe back pain presents for injection of steroids into the spinal canal, the category G89 code is sequenced first, followed by the code for the underlying cause of the pain, if known.

A pain code from category G89 is not assigned if the underlying (definitive) diagnosis is known, unless the reason for the encounter is pain control or management, not management of the underlying condition.

■ CASE SCENARIOS

- Chronic back pain due to lumbar disk displacement (non-traumatic) in a patient presenting for epidural injection of steroids. Assign codes G89.29, M51.26.

- Chronic back pain due to metastatic bone cancer from the prostate. Patient presents for pain control. Assign codes G89.3, C79.51, C61.

When the encounter is for a procedure aimed at treating the underlying condition, the underlying condition should be assigned as the principal diagnosis. No code from category G89 should be assigned.

These examples show how coders apply the rule that a type of pain must be specified.

Visits to Treat the Underlying Cause of Pain

When the reason for the visit is for a procedure aimed at treating the underlying condition rather than managing the pain (for example, for spinal fusion or kyphoplasty), a code for the underlying condition (such as vertebral fracture or spinal stenosis) should be assigned as the principal diagnosis. A code from category G89 should not be assigned.

> ### ■ CASE SCENARIO
> A patient presents for lumbar fusion to treat degenerative disk disease of the lumbar spine. Code the visit as M51.36.

Insertion of a Neurostimulator

Reporting and sequencing pain codes in conjunction with the insertion of a neurostimulator follows the same pattern. When the reason for the visit is insertion of a neurostimulator for pain control, the code from category G89 is assigned as the first-listed or principal diagnosis. On the other hand, when the encounter or admission is for a procedure that treats the underlying condition causing the pain and the neurostimulator is inserted as an adjunct procedure for pain control, the code for the underlying condition is sequenced first, and a code from G89 is assigned as an additional diagnosis.

Use of Category G89 Codes With Site-Specific Pain Codes

When the site of pain is documented and the code from G89 would provide additional information, it is appropriate to assign a code from G89 as an additional diagnosis.

> ### ■ CASE SCENARIO
> A patient presents with chronic right upper quadrant abdominal pain, unknown cause. Report codes R10.11, G89.29.

Sequencing these codes depends on the reason for the visit. If the encounter is for any reason other than pain control, the code for the underlying cause or condition or for the site of pain would be sequenced first.

> ### ■ CASE SCENARIO
> A patient presents with acute chest pain due to trauma, and the reason for admission is pain control. The codes are G89.11, R07.9.

On the other hand, if the same patient presents with acute chest pain due to trauma and the examination is primarily to determine the cause of chest pain, the codes would be sequenced as R07.9, G89.11. (*Note:* This is assuming the underlying cause is not determined.)

Expected postoperative pain immediately after surgery should not be coded.

Postoperative pain may be reported as the principal or first-listed diagnosis when the stated reason for an encounter is documented as postoperative pain control or management.

Postoperative Pain or Post-Thoracotomy Pain

Whether the postoperative or post-thoracotomy pain is acute or chronic will determine the fourth-digit subcategory code of G89.1 (acute) or G89.2 (chronic).

When the postoperative pain is due to a complication, device, implant, or graft, a code from ICD-10-CM Chapter 19, Injury, Poisoning, and Certain Other Consequences of External Causes (Complications), is assigned as the first code, followed by a code from G89 to identify the acute or chronic pain.

EXAMPLE
Chronic right knee pain due to complication from total knee replacement with evaluation of the joint is coded T84.84xS, G89.28, Z96.651.

PHARMACOLOGY CONNECTION

Common Medications for Treatment of the Nervous System

Anesthesia (General)

General anesthesia is a deep state of sleep where the patient loses consciousness and sensation and usually requires assisted ventilation.

Muscle Relaxants—Adjuncts to Anesthesia

Muscle relaxants are used as an adjunct to general anesthesia to facilitate endotracheal intubation and to provide skeletal muscle relaxation during surgery or mechanical ventilation.

MUSCLE RELAXANTS

TRADE NAME	GENERIC NAME
Anectine	succinylcholine
Mivacron	mivacurium
Nimbex	cisatracurium
Norcuron	vecuronium
Pavulon	pancuronium
Tracrium	atracurium
Zemuron	rocuronium

Anesthesia (Local)

Local anesthesia provides numbness to a small area limited to where local anesthetic is injected.

Anesthesia (Spinal/Epidural)

Regional anesthesia, such as spinal or epidural anesthesia, provides numbness to much larger areas because of the nerve blocks involved.

Anesthesia (MAC) and Conscious Sedation

Monitored anesthesia care (MAC), or conscious sedation, uses sedatives and other agents, but the dosage is low enough that patients remain responsive and breathe without assistance. MAC is often used to supplement local and regional anesthesia, particularly

ANESTHESIA (GENERAL)

TRADE NAME	GENERIC NAME
Alfenta	alfentanil
Amidate	etomidate
Brevital	methohexital
Ethrane	enflurane
Fluothane	halothane
Forane	isoflurane
Ketalar	ketamine
Sublimaze	fentanyl
Sufenta	sufentanil
Suprane	desflurane
Thiopental	pentothal
Ultane	sevoflurane
Ultiva	remifentanil

ANESTHESIA (LOCAL)

TRADE NAME	GENERIC NAME
Carbocaine	mepivacaine
Naropin	ropivacaine
Novocain	procaine
Pontocaine	tetracaine
Xylocaine	lidocaine

ANESTHESIA (SPINAL/EPIDURAL)

TRADE NAME	GENERIC NAME
Carbocaine	mepivacaine
Naropin	ropivacaine
Sensorcaine	bupivacaine
Xylocaine	lidocaine

ANESTHESIA (MAC)

TRADE NAME	GENERIC NAME
Diprivan	propofol
Versed	midazolam

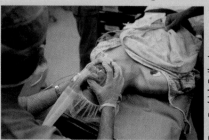

Ryan Rodrick Beiler/Shutterstock.com

Anesthesiologist.

STIMULANTS

TRADE NAME	GENERIC NAME
Adderall	amphetamine mixture
Caffedrine	caffeine
Desoxyn	methamphetamine
Dexedrine	dextroamphetamine
Dopram	doxapram
Focalin	dexmethylphenidate
Provigil	modafinil
Ritalin/ Methylin/ Concerta	methylphenidate

SEDATIVES/HYPNOTICS

TRADE NAME	GENERIC NAME
Ambien	zolpidem
Dalmane	flurazepam
Halcion	triazolam
Lunesta	eszopiclone
ProSom	estazolam
Restoril	temazepam
Rozerem	ramelteon
Sonata	zaleplon

CHOLINESTERASE INHIBITORS

TRADE NAME	GENERIC NAME
Aricept	donepezil
Cognex	tacrine
Exelon	rivastigmine
Razadyne	galantamine

TRANQUILIZERS

TRADE NAME	GENERIC NAME
Amytal	amobarbital
Luminal	phenobarbital
Nembutal	pentobarbital
Seconal	secobarbital

during simple procedures and minor surgery. The purpose of MAC is to provide the patient with anxiety relief, comfort, and safety during uncomfortable procedures. The patient quickly recovers from MAC, and this allows for a timely discharge.

Stimulants
Central nervous system stimulants are used to restore mental alertness or wakefulness. Some are used to treat narcolepsy and attention deficit-hyperactivity disorder (ADHD).

Sedatives/Hypnotics
Sedatives are used to initiate and sustain sleep in patients who have insomnia.

Cholinesterase Inhibitors
These drugs are used in the treatment of dementia in Alzheimer's disease.

Tranquilizers
Tranquilizers depress the central nervous system, resulting in calmness, relaxation, reduction of anxiety, and sleepiness.

Neurotransmitters
These are chemicals that are used to relay, amplify, and modulate signals between a neuron and another cell. Some examples include acetylcholine, norepinephrine, epinephrine, dopamine, and serotonin. These chemicals may be released or inhibited by certain drugs.

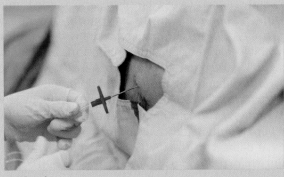

ChaNaWiT/Shutterstock

Epidural.

However, if the reason for the visit is pain control only, the code from category G89 is sequenced first. Postoperative pain that is not associated with a specific complication is assigned to category G89. For example, when a patient is admitted from ambulatory surgery due to acute postoperative pain, the code is G89.18. In this case, the first-listed diagnosis code is the pain, because the reason for the visit was pain control. The condition that required surgery would be reported as an additional diagnosis.

Neoplasm-Related Pain

When coding pain related to cancer, code G89.3 is assigned as the principal diagnosis when documentation supports the reason for the visit as pain control, regardless of whether the pain is acute or chronic. An additional code for the underlying neoplasm should also be assigned.

■ **CASE SCENARIO**

A patient presents for control of severe chronic right upper quadrant pain due to liver metastasis from previous colon cancer. Report codes G89.3, C78.7, Z85.038.

CHECKPOINT 6.1

Code the following pain cases, using ICD-10-CM. Keep sequencing guidelines in mind.

1. Acute postoperative neck pain, admitted for pain control _____

2. Chronic back pain from lumbar stenosis, patient admitted for laminectomy _____

3. Chronic post-thoracotomy pain _____

4. Chronic pain due to bone metastasis, admitted for pain control _____

5. Chronic low back pain _____

Paralysis

Paralysis, the loss of the ability to move voluntarily, is typically caused by damage to the brain or nervous system, especially the spinal cord. Major causes are stroke, trauma, poliomyelitis, amyotrophic lateral sclerosis (ALS), botulism, spina bifida, multiple sclerosis, and Guillain-Barré syndrome. Documentation is the key to assigning an accurate code for paralysis. Often the underlying cause and the type of paralysis are reported with a combination code.

Paralysis may be localized or generalized, or it may follow a certain pattern. For example, localized paralysis occurs in *Bell's palsy,* where one side of the face is paralyzed due to inflammation of the facial nerve on that side. Patients with stroke may be weak throughout their body, referred to as *quadriparesis* (weakness of all four limbs), or have hemiplegia (weakness on one side of the body), or they may have other patterns of paralysis depending on the area of damage in the brain. Lower spinal cord damage from a severe back injury may result in paraplegia (paralysis of the lower torso and legs), while an injury higher up on the spinal cord, such as a neck injury, can cause quadriplegia, complete paralysis of all limbs.

Code Assignment for Hemiplegia

Codes for hemiplegia require specificity regarding paralysis as being on the dominant or nondominant side. A right-handed person is considered right-hand dominant, and a left-handed person is considered left-hand dominant. Therefore, if a left-handed person is paralyzed on the left side, that would be the dominant side. If documentation does not include dominance,

> Codes for hemiplegia, hemiparesis, and monoplegia require specificity of dominant or nondominant side affected. If the classification system does not indicate which side is dominant, the default code selection is as follows:
> - In ambidextrous patients, the default should be the dominant side.
> - If the left side is affected, the default is nondominant side.
> - If the right side is affected, the default is dominant side.

the default code is reported. If no default (unspecified side) code is available, the right-hand side is considered the dominant affected side.

EXAMPLE
Left-sided flaccid hemiplegia in a right-handed patient is coded G81.04.

Paralysis Associated With Cerebrovascular Disease
Transient paralysis is temporary paralysis or paralysis that clears quickly, as often occurs following an acute cerebrovascular accident (CVA, code I63.9). The code for the paralysis is reported as a secondary diagnosis (secondary to the principal diagnosis of acute CVA), as are any other neurological deficits resulting from the CVA.

EXAMPLE
Acute CVA with hemiplegia at discharge is coded I63.9, G81.90.

Sequelae (late effects) of CVA (category I69) can also be used to report hemiplegia from a previous cerebrovascular event. When a patient is admitted for rehabilitation, the functional deficit(s) and/or residuals are reported first followed by a code for the sequelae, unless a combination code is available.

■ CASE SCENARIOS
- A patient visits for therapy to treat dysphagia and hemiplegia (dominant right side) from a previous embolic CVA. Assign codes I69.391, I69.351.

- A patient is admitted to rehabilitation for occupational and physical therapy to treat the sequelae from a previous stroke, which includes right dominant hemiplegia and apraxia. Assign codes I69.351, I69.390.

- A patient is admitted to rehabilitation for left dominant flaccid hemiplegia from a previous traumatic subdural hematoma without loss of consciousness. Assign codes G81.02, S06.5x0S.

If a patient presents with acute cerebrovascular disease (categories I60–I68), it is appropriate to assign an additional code from category I69 (sequelae of cerebrovascular disease) if the patient has both a new CVA and a residual condition from a previous CVA.

Epilepsy and Seizure Disorders

Epilepsy is a chronic neurological disorder characterized by recurrent seizures. Epilepsy should not be confused with a seizure alone; seizures can be caused by numerous other conditions such as fever (a febrile seizure) or alcohol withdrawal. The coder must be careful to distinguish a seizure disorder (coded to epilepsy) from a single seizure (coded as a symptom, R56.9).

A code for epilepsy should not be assigned unless the physician specifically states epilepsy (seizure disorder). Epilepsy is an exception to the rule for coding possible, probable, or suspected (rule-out) conditions in the inpatient setting because of legal and personal ramifications, such as the inability to obtain a driver's license. Therefore, documentation of the diagnosis "possible seizure disorder" should not be coded; instead, the physician should be queried to determine whether the condition actually exists.

> Seizures documented as recurrent are reported with the epilepsy code; therefore, recurrence is not "intractable."

A fourth-digit subcategory identifies the type of epilepsy, such as tonic-clonic intractable epilepsy, code G40.419. A fifth digit identifies whether the epilepsy is "intractable." Intractable epilepsy and/or status epilepticus should not be coded unless the physician documents this specifically in the medical record. In ICD-10-CM, the terms *pharmacoresistant, treatment resistant, refractory,* and *poorly controlled* are equivalent to "intractable."

Code the following statements using ICD-10-CM.

1. Acute cerebral infarction due to embolism of middle cerebral arteries with resulting aphasia

   _____

2. Intraventricular hemorrhage with resulting left lower leg monoplegia in right-handed patient

   _____

3. Acute stroke with neurogenic dysphagia and spastic hemiplegia _____

4. Admission for therapy due to previous cerebral hemorrhage with resulting spastic right-sided hemiplegia in right-handed patient _____

5. Congenital spastic paraplegia _____

6. Symptomatic localized epilepsy with complex partial seizures _____

7. Complex febrile seizure _____

8. Intractable petit mal seizures with status epilepticus _____

9. Seizure disorder _____

10. Grand mal epilepsy, with status epilepticus _____

11. Poorly controlled idiopathic generalized epilepsy _____

DISEASES OF THE EYE AND ADNEXA (CHAPTER 7: H00–H59)

The categories in Chapter 7 of ICD-10-CM are grouped as shown in Table 6.2. Box 6.2 presents the applicable guidelines from Section I, Part C, of the *Official Guidelines for Coding and Reporting.*

Visual Impairment

Blindness

Blindness, the total or partial lack of vision, is coded from category H54, visual impairment. There is overlap in the terminology used in various settings to distinguish profound, moderate, and severe blindness. Total blindness is the complete lack of perception of form and visual light and is clinically recorded as "NLP" (no light perception). For determining benefits in the United States, legal blindness is defined as vision rated as 20/200 or less in the better eye with the best correction possible.

Table 6.2 Organization of ICD-10-CM Chapter 7 Tabular List

BLOCK	BLOCK DESCRIPTION
H00–H05	Disorders of eyelid, lacrimal system, and orbit
H10–H11	Disorders of conjunctiva
H15–H22	Disorders of sclera, cornea, iris, and ciliary body
H25–H28	Disorders of lens
H30–H36	Disorders of choroid and retina
H40–H42	Glaucoma
H43–H44	Disorders of vitreous body and globe
H46–H47	Disorders of optic nerve and visual pathways
H49–H52	Disorders of ocular muscles, binocular movement, accommodation, and refraction
H53–H54	Visual disturbances and blindness
H55–H57	Other disorders of eye and adnexa
H59	Intraoperative and postprocedural complications and disorders of eye and adnexa, not elsewhere classified

a. Glaucoma

1) Assigning glaucoma codes

Assign as many codes from category H40, Glaucoma, as needed to identify the type of glaucoma, the affected eye, and the glaucoma stage.

2) Bilateral glaucoma with same type and stage

When a patient has bilateral glaucoma, both eyes are documented as being the same type and stage, and there is a code for bilateral glaucoma, report only the code for the type of glaucoma, bilateral, with the seventh character for the stage.

When a patient has bilateral glaucoma, both eyes are documented as being the same type and stage, and the classification does not provide a code for bilateral glaucoma (i.e., subcategories H40.10, H40.11, and H40.20), report only one code for the type of glaucoma with the appropriate seventh character for the stage.

3) Bilateral glaucoma stage with different types or stages

When a patient has bilateral glaucoma, each eye is documented as having a different type or stage, and the classification distinguishes laterality, assign the appropriate code for each eye rather than the code for bilateral glaucoma.

When a patient has bilateral glaucoma, each eye is documented as having a different type, and the classification does not distinguish laterality (i.e., subcategories H40.10, H40.11, and H40.20), assign one code for each type of glaucoma with the appropriate seventh character for the stage.

When a patient has bilateral glaucoma, each eye is documented as having the same type but different stage, and the classification does not distinguish laterality (i.e., subcategories H40.10, H40.11, and H40.20), assign a code for the type of glaucoma for each eye with the seventh character for the specific glaucoma stage documented for each eye.

4) Patient admitted with glaucoma and stage evolves during the admission

If a patient is admitted with glaucoma and the stage progresses during the admission, assign the code for highest stage documented.

5) Indeterminate stage glaucoma

Assignment of the seventh character "4" for "indeterminate stage" should be based on the clinical documentation. The seventh character "4" is used when the glaucoma stage cannot be clinically determined. This seventh character should not be confused with the seventh character "0," unspecified, which should be assigned when there is no documentation regarding the stage of the glaucoma.

b. Blindness

If "blindness" or "low vision" of both eyes is documented but the visual impairment category is not documented, assign code H54.3, Unqualified visual loss, both eyes. If "blindness" or "low vision" in one eye is documented but the visual impairment category is not documented, assign a code from H54.6-, Unqualified visual loss, one eye. If "blindness" or "visual loss" is documented without any information about whether one or both eyes are affected, assign code H54.7, Unspecified visual loss.

This means that a legally blind individual with vision correction would have to stand 20 feet (6.1 meters) from an object to see it with the same degree of clarity as a normally sighted person could from 200 feet (61 meters). The chart for this category in the ICD-10-CM Tabular List compares measurements and terms used in the United States and by the World Health Organization (WHO).

EXAMPLE

Legal blindness in both eyes with impairment of the better eye as profound, with lesser eye impairment that is total. The code is H54.8.

The underlying cause of the blindness, such as cataracts, diabetic retinopathy, or glaucoma, should also be reported if present.

Other Common Eye Disorders

Conjunctivitis involves inflammation of the conjunctiva, a mucous membrane that lines the eyelid on the surface of the eyeball. Conjunctivitis coding is based on the cause of the inflammation. The most common form is "pink eye," an acute bacterial condition that is coded H10.029. If documentation records chronic inflammation or the use of topical ointments rather than antibiotics, pink eye is unlikely, and the physician should be queried for clarification. Other causes include allergic reactions, such as an allergy to contact lenses (giant papillary conjunctivitis, code H10.41) and hay fever (vernal conjunctivitis, code H10.44).

A cataract is a clouding of the lens or lens capsule of the eye that prevents light from reaching the retina and causes impaired vision. Cataracts are coded by the zones of the lens involved in decreasing opacity and then by the type, such as congenital, degenerative, traumatic, or secondary. Senile cataract is partial or total lens opacity in patients older than 55 years. If a patient has diabetes and a cataract, the code for diabetic cataract is assigned, unless documentation supports a different cause. This assumed relationship correlates to the convention "with" found in the Index.

Glaucoma refers to increased intraocular pressure (IOP) in the eyeball, which can lead to optic nerve damage and loss of vision. Glaucoma is the leading cause of blindness and has been called the "silent thief of sight," because the loss of vision often occurs gradually over a long period of time. The two main types of glaucoma are primary open-angle glaucoma (POAG), which occurs when the eye's drainage canals become clogged over time; and angle-closure glaucoma, which occurs when the canals are suddenly blocked. POAG and angle-closure glaucoma have multiple stages of disease progression. Each eye may be affected differently, which may result in a different type and/or stage on the left or right eye.

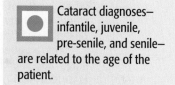 Cataract diagnoses—infantile, juvenile, pre-senile, and senile—are related to the age of the patient.

Assigning Glaucoma Codes

Documentation as to the type of glaucoma, the affected eye, and the stage is critical when assigning codes from category H40. Many codes from this category may be assigned in order to classify the medical condition of the patient.

Bilateral glaucoma with the same type and stage is reported in two ways: If there is a code for bilateral, then report only the code for the type of glaucoma, bilateral, with the seventh character for the stage. The second instance is when there is no code classification designated as bilateral (i.e., subcategories H40.10, H40.11, and H40.20). When this occurs, report only one code for the type of glaucoma with the appropriate seventh character for the stage.

EXAMPLES
- Bilateral primary open-angle glaucoma. Assign code H40.1130.

- Bilateral chronic angle-closure glaucoma. Assign code H40.2230.

When bilateral glaucoma occurs yet each eye has a different type or stage and the classification identifies laterality, a code for each eye is assigned. If laterality is not distinguished, then assign one code for each type of glaucoma with the seventh character for the stage. If the type of glaucoma is the same, yet at different stages, then report a code for the type of glaucoma for each eye with a seventh character for the stage.

 PHARMACOLOGY CONNECTION

Common Medications for the Eye

The agents listed in the table below are used to treat a variety of eye diseases, including glaucoma.

TRADE NAME	GENERIC NAME
Alphagan P	brimonidine
Betagan	levobunolol
Betoptic	betaxolol
Lumigan	bimatoprost
Miochol-E	acetylcholine
Pilocar	pilocarpine
Propine	dipivefrin
Timoptic	timolol
Travatan	travoprost
Trusopt	dorzolamide
Xalatan	latanoprost

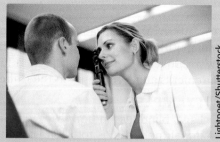

Eye exam.

Lightpoet/Shutterstock

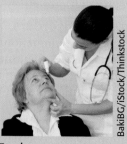

Eyedrops.

BakiBG/iStock/Thinkstock

EXAMPLES
- Secondary glaucoma in the left eye and moderate-stage capsular glaucoma of the right eye. Assign codes H40.52x0, H40.1412.
- Low-tension glaucoma with mild stage of the left eye and moderate stage of the right eye. Assign codes H40.1221, H40.1212.
- Primary open-angle glaucoma, severe stage right eye and moderate stage in the left eye. Assign codes H40.1113, H40.1122

In some instances, the stage of glaucoma progresses during an admission. Always code to the highest stage documented. If the stage is "indeterminate," the seventh character of 4 is used. This refers to a stage that cannot be clinically determined—*not* a stage that is documented as unspecified. When there is no documentation regarding the stage, the unspecified stage, seventh character of 0, is reported.

EXAMPLES
- Secondary glaucoma of the left eye, indeterminate stage. Assign code H40.52x4.
- Secondary glaucoma of the left eye. Assign code H40.52x0.

Glaucoma can be caused by an underlying disorder, and coding conventions direct the coder to report the underlying cause first followed by a code from category H42. It is important that the coder carefully review documentation and the Alphabetic Index when coding glaucoma.

DISEASES OF THE EAR AND MASTOID PROCESS (CHAPTER 8: H60–H95)

Codes from Chapter 8 of ICD-10-CM represent diseases of the ear and mastoid process. Table 6.3 identifies the specific disorders by code block. There are no *Official Guidelines* at this time for coding and reporting diseases of the ear and mastoid process.

Table 6.3 Organization of ICD-10-CM Chapter 8 Tabular List

BLOCK	BLOCK DESCRIPTION
H60–H62	Diseases of external ear
H65–H75	Diseases of middle ear and mastoid
H80–H93	Diseases of inner ear
H90–H94	Other disorders of ear
H95	Intraoperative and postprocedural complications and disorders of ear and mastoid process, not elsewhere classified

These conditions include the diseases of otitis, otosclerosis, labyrinthitis, hearing loss, disorders of the Eustachian tube, tympanic membrane, and mastoid process. Laterality is important in coding these disorders, and the coder must pay close attention to assign additional codes when instructed.

DISEASES OF THE CIRCULATORY SYSTEM (CHAPTER 9: I00–I99)

Disorders of the circulatory system are reported in Chapter 9 of ICD-10-CM unless they are associated with pregnancy or are congenital in nature. The conditions classified in this chapter, such as hypertension, coronary artery disease, congestive heart failure, and stroke, are common among inpatients and in the general public; many are interrelated.

In reporting circulatory conditions (as always), it is imperative to adhere to the notes in the ICD-10-CM Tabular List.

The categories in Chapter 9 of ICD-10-CM are grouped as shown in Table 6.4. Box 6.3 presents the applicable guidelines from Section I, Part C.9, of the *Official Guidelines for Coding and Reporting*. Refer to this table as the various topics are presented.

Hypertensive Disease

Hypertension, persistently elevated arterial blood pressure with a systolic pressure reading of 140 mm Hg, a diastolic pressure at rest of over 90 mm Hg, or both does not cause symptoms in patients, but it can increase their risk of having a stroke, heart failure, or heart attack. Hypertension with no known cause is called *essential hypertension* and is the most common type.

ICD-10-CM classifies hypertension by underlying cause such as heart disease, gestational, secondary, pulmonary, or associated with kidney disease. Table 6.5 summarizes the categories used to classify hypertension.

As Table 6.5 shows, in certain instances the coder can assume that hypertension is related to another disease (in other words, there is a causal relationship—cause and effect—between one disease and another). In other circumstances, a causal relationship must be documented. Specifically, secondary heart disease with hypertension must be documented as causal in order to assign a hypertension code from category I11. A causal relationship is documented as hypertension *due to* renal artery stenosis (stated).

Hypertension With Heart Disease

Hypertensive heart disease is a complication of hypertension in which the heart is affected. Examples are cardiomegaly, cardiovascular disease, myocarditis, and heart failure. As noted in the *Official Guidelines,* heart conditions classified to I50.- or I51.4–I51.9 are assigned to category I11 when a patient has

Table 6.4 Organization of ICD-10-CM Chapter 9 Tabular List

BLOCK	BLOCK DESCRIPTION
I00–I02	Acute rheumatic fever
I05–I09	Chronic rheumatic heart diseases
I10–I15	Hypertensive diseases
I20–I25	Ischemic heart diseases
I26–I28	Pulmonary heart disease and diseases of pulmonary circulation
I30–I52	Other forms of heart disease
I60–I69	Cerebrovascular diseases
I70–I79	Diseases of arteries, arterioles, and capillaries
I80–I89	Diseases of veins, lymphatic vessels, and lymph nodes, not elsewhere classified
I95–I99	Other and unspecified disorders of the circulatory system

a. Hypertension

The classification presumes a causal relationship between hypertension and heart involvement and between hypertension and kidney involvement, as the two conditions are linked by the term "with" in the Alphabetic Index. These conditions should be coded as related even in the absence of provider documentation explicitly linking them, unless the documentation clearly states the conditions are unrelated.

For hypertension and conditions not specifically linked by relational terms such as "with," "associated with" or "due to" in the classification, provider documentation must link the conditions in order to code them as related.

1) Hypertension with heart disease

Hypertension with heart conditions classified to I50.- or I51.4–I51.9, are assigned to a code from category I11, Hypertensive heart disease. Use an additional code from category I50, Heart failure, to identify the type of heart failure in those patients with heart failure.

The same heart conditions (I50.-, I51.4–I51.9) with hypertension are coded separately if the provider has specifically documented a different cause. Sequence according to the circumstances of the admission/encounter.

2) Hypertensive chronic kidney disease

Assign codes from category I12, Hypertensive chronic kidney disease, when both hypertension and a condition classifiable to category N18, Chronic kidney disease (CKD), are present. CKD should not be coded as hypertensive if the physician has specifically documented a different cause.

The appropriate code from category N18 should be used as a secondary code with a code from category I12 to identify the stage of chronic kidney disease.

See Section I.C.14. Chronic kidney disease.

If a patient has hypertensive chronic kidney disease and acute renal failure, an additional code for the acute renal failure is required.

3) Hypertensive heart and chronic kidney disease

Assign codes from combination category I13, Hypertensive heart and chronic kidney disease, when there is hypertension with both heart and kidney involvement. If heart failure is present, assign an additional code from category I50 to identify the type of heart failure.

The appropriate code from category N18, Chronic kidney disease, should be used as a secondary code with a code from category I13 to identify the stage of chronic kidney disease.

See Section I.C.14. Chronic kidney disease.

The codes in category I13, Hypertensive heart and chronic kidney disease, are combination codes that include hypertension, heart disease and chronic kidney disease. The Includes note at I13 specifies that the conditions included at I11 and I12 are included together in I13. If a patient has hypertension, heart disease and chronic kidney disease, then a code from I13 should be used, not individual codes for hypertension, heart disease and chronic kidney disease, or codes from I11 or I12.

4) Hypertensive cerebrovascular disease

For hypertensive cerebrovascular disease, first assign the appropriate code from categories I60–I69, followed by the appropriate hypertension code.

5) Hypertensive retinopathy

Subcategory H35.0, Background retinopathy and retinal vascular changes, should be used with a code from category I10–I15, Hypertensive disease to include the systemic hypertension. The sequencing is based on the reason for the encounter.

6) Hypertension, secondary

Secondary hypertension is due to an underlying condition. Two codes are required: one to identify the underlying etiology and one from category I15 to identify the hypertension. Sequencing of codes is determined by the reason for admission/encounter.

7) Hypertension, transient

Assign code R03.0, Elevated blood pressure reading without diagnosis of hypertension, unless patient has an established diagnosis of hypertension. Assign code O13.-, Gestational [pregnancy-induced] hypertension without significant proteinuria, or O14.-, Pre-eclampsia, for transient hypertension of pregnancy.

8) Hypertension, controlled

This diagnostic statement usually refers to an existing state of hypertension under control by therapy. Assign the appropriate code from categories I10–I15, Hypertensive diseases.

9) Hypertension, uncontrolled

Uncontrolled hypertension may refer to untreated hypertension or hypertension not responding to current therapeutic regimen. In either case, assign the appropriate code from categories I10–I15, Hypertensive diseases.

Continued

BOX 6.3 *Continued*

10) Hypertensive crisis

Assign a code from category I16, Hypertensive crisis, for documented hypertensive urgency, hypertensive emergency or unspecified hypertensive crisis. Code also any identified hypertensive disease (I10–I15). The sequencing is based on the reason for the encounter.

11) Pulmonary hypertension

Pulmonary hypertension is classified to category I27, Other pulmonary heart diseases. For secondary pulmonary hypertension (I27.1, I27.2-), code also any associated conditions or adverse effects of drugs or toxins. The sequencing is based on the reason for the encounter.

b. Atherosclerotic Coronary Artery Disease and Angina

ICD-10-CM has combination codes for atherosclerotic heart disease with angina pectoris. The subcategories for these codes are I25.11, Atherosclerotic heart disease of native coronary artery with angina pectoris, and I25.7, Atherosclerosis of coronary artery bypass graft(s) and coronary artery of transplanted heart with angina pectoris.

When using one of these combination codes, it is not necessary to use an additional code for angina pectoris. A causal relationship can be assumed in a patient with both atherosclerosis and angina pectoris, unless the documentation indicates the angina is due to something other than the atherosclerosis.

If a patient with coronary artery disease is admitted due to an acute myocardial infarction (AMI), the AMI should be sequenced before the coronary artery disease.

See Section I.C.9. Acute myocardial infarction (AMI).

c. Intraoperative and Postprocedural Cerebrovascular Accident

Medical record documentation should clearly specify the cause-and-effect relationship between the medical intervention and the cerebrovascular accident in order to assign a code for intraoperative or postprocedural cerebrovascular accident.

Proper code assignment depends on whether it was an infarction or hemorrhage and whether it occurred intraoperatively or postoperatively. If it was a cerebral hemorrhage, code assignment depends on the type of procedure performed.

d. Sequelae of Cerebrovascular Disease

1) Category I69, sequelae of cerebrovascular disease

Category I69 is used to indicate conditions classifiable to categories I60–I67 as the causes of sequelae (neurologic deficits), themselves classified elsewhere. These "late effects" include neurologic deficits that persist after initial onset of conditions classifiable to categories I60–I67. The neurologic deficits caused by cerebrovascular disease may be present from the onset or may arise at any time after the onset of the condition classifiable to categories I60–I67.

Codes from category I69, Sequelae of cerebrovascular disease, that specify hemiplegia, hemiparesis, and monoplegia identify whether the dominant or nondominant side is affected. Should the affected side be documented, but not specified as dominant or nondominant, and the classification system does not indicate a default, code selection is as follows:

• For ambidextrous patients, the default should be dominant.

• If the left side is affected, the default is nondominant.

• If the right side is affected, the default is dominant.

2) Codes from category I69 with codes from I60–I67

Codes from category I69 may be assigned on a health-care record with codes from I60–I67 if the patient has a current cerebrovascular disease and deficits from an old cerebrovascular disease.

3) Codes from category I69 and personal history of transient ischemic attack (TIA) and cerebral infarction (Z86.73)

Codes from category I69 should not be assigned if the patient does not have neurologic deficits.

See Section I.C.21.4. History (of) for use of personal history codes.

e. Acute Myocardial Infarction (AMI)

1) ST elevation myocardial infarction (STEMI) and non-ST elevation myocardial infarction (NSTEMI)

The ICD-10-CM codes for Type 1 acute myocardial infarction (AMI) identify the site, such as anterolateral wall or true posterior wall. Subcategories I21.0–I21.2 and code I21.3 are used for Type 1 ST elevation myocardial infarction (STEMI). Code I21.4, Non-ST elevation (NSTEMI) myocardial infarction, is used for Type 1 non-ST elevation myocardial infarction (NSTEMI) and nontransmural MIs.

If Type 1 NSTEMI evolves to STEMI, assign the STEMI code. If Type 1 STEMI converts to NSTEMI due to thrombolytic therapy, it is still coded as STEMI.

For encounters occurring while the myocardial infarction is equal to, or less than, four weeks old, including transfers to another acute setting or a postacute setting, and the myocardial infarction meets the definition for "other diagnoses" (see Section III, Reporting Additional Diagnoses), codes from category I21 may continue to be reported. For encounters after the 4 week time frame and the patient is still receiving care related to the myocardial infarction, the appropriate aftercare code should be assigned, rather than a code from category I21. For old or healed myocardial infarctions not requiring further care, code I25.2, Old myocardial infarction, may be assigned.

2) Acute myocardial infarction, unspecified

Code I21.9, Acute myocardial infarction, unspecified, is the default for unspecified acute myocardial infarction. If only STEMI or transmural MI without the site is documented, assign code I21.3, ST elevation (STEMI) myocardial infarction of unspecified site.

3) AMI documented as nontransmural or subendocardial but site provided

If an AMI is documented as nontransmural or subendocardial, but the site is provided, it is still coded as a subendocardial AMI.

See Section I.C.21.3 for information on coding status post administration of tPA (Tissue Plasminogen Activator) in a different facility within the last 24 hours.

4) Subsequent acute myocardial infarction

A code from category I22, Subsequent ST elevation (STEMI) and non-ST elevation (NSTEMI) myocardial infarction, is to be used when a patient who has suffered a type 1 or unspecified AMI has a new AMI within the 4-week timeframe of the initial AMI. A code from category I22 must be used in conjunction with a code from category I21. The sequencing of the I22 and I21 codes depends on the circumstances of the encounter.

Do not assign code I22 for subsequent myocardial infarctions other than type 1 or unspecified. For subsequent type 2 AMI assign only code I21.A1. For subsequent type 4 or type 5 AMI, assign only code I21.A9.

5) Other types of myocardial infarction

The ICD-10-CM provides codes for different types of myocardial infarction. Type 1 myocardial infarctions are assigned to codes I21.0–I21.4. Type 2 myocardial infarction, and myocardial infarction due to demand ischemia or secondary to ischemic balance, is assigned to code I21.A1, Myocardial infarction type 2 with a code for the underlying cause. Do not assign code I24.8, Other forms of acute ischemic heart disease for the demand ischemia. Sequencing of type 2 AMI or the underlying cause is dependent on the circumstances of admission. When a type 2 AMI code is described as NSTEMI or STEMI, only assign code I21.A1. Codes I21.01–I21.4 should only be assigned for type 1 AMIs.

Acute myocardial infarctions type 3, 4a, 4b, 4c, and 5 are assigned to code I21.A9, Other myocardial infarction type.

The "Code also" and "Code first" notes should be followed related to complications, and for coding of postprocedural myocardial infarctions during or following cardiac surgery.

Table 6.5 Hypertensive Disease Categories

	HYPERTENSIVE HEART DISEASE	HYPERTENSIVE RENAL DISEASE	HYPERTENSIVE HEART DISEASE AND RENAL DISEASE	SECONDARY HYPERTENSION
HYPERTENSION I10	**I11**	**I12**	**I13**	**I15**
No related condition documented.	Causal relationship assumed with codes from I50.-, I51.4–I51.9 due to hypertension.	Causal relationship assumed when reported with codes from categories N18 due to hypertension.	Causal relationship assumed with codes from I50.-, I51.4–I51.9 with assumed renal disease with hypertension. OR any condition classifiable with categories I11 and I12.	Hypertension due to other disease.
Code hypertension only.	Use an additional code for heart failure if known (I50.-).	Code also the chronic kidney disease (N18.-).	Code also the chronic kidney disease (N18.-) and heart failure (I50.-).	Code the underlying condition first.

For inpatient coding of the principal diagnosis, sequencing of the codes depends on the circumstances of admission and the after-study reason for the encounter.

hypertension and a condition classified to subcategories I50.-, I51.4–I51.9 (Box 6.4). There is a presumed relationship between these conditions as the two conditions are linked by the term "with" in the Index. When reporting hypertensive heart disease and congestive heart failure, more than one code may be assigned depending on whether it is congestive heart failure with diastolic and systolic heart failure and acute or chronic or both. Therefore, a code for hypertensive heart disease (I11) would always be assigned for a patient with hypertension and congestive heart failure.

BOX 6.4 Hypertension With Heart Disease Listing From the Index

Hypertension, hypertensive (accelerated) (benign) (essential) (idiopathic) (malignant) (systemic) I10
    with heart involvement (conditions in I50.-, or I51.4–I51.9 due to hypertension) -*see* Hypertension, heart
    kidney involvement—*see* Hypertension, kidney

EXAMPLES
- Hypertensive myocarditis. Code as I11.9.
- Hypertension and cardiomyopathy. Code as I10, I42.9 (no causal relationship documented, so code separately).
- Congestive heart failure due to hypertension. Code as I11.0, I50.9.
- Hypertension and cardiomegaly. Code as I11.9, I51.7.
- Hypertension, chronic systolic heart failure. Code as I11.0, I50.22.

Hypertensive Chronic Kidney Disease

When a patient has chronic kidney disease, renal failure, or renal sclerosis (categories N18) and hypertension, the hypertension should be reported using category I12 instead of category I10 because there is an assumed causal relationship between hypertension and the chronic kidney disease (CKD). Category I12 requires a fourth digit, which classifies the associated stage of renal disease as follows:

0 with CKD stage V or end-stage renal disease
9 with CKD stage I through stage IV, or unspecified

Two codes are required when reporting chronic kidney disease (category N18) with hypertension (category I12).

EXAMPLE
Hypertensive chronic kidney disease, stage III, is coded I12.9, N18.3.

Because there is an assumed relationship between chronic kidney disease and hypertension, no cause-and-effect relationship must be documented. The presence of *acute* renal disease—rather than chronic renal disease—is reported separately as acute renal failure, N17.9 Acute renal failure (ARF). Hyperkalemia, which is excessive potassium in the blood, is often associated with acute renal failure.

EXAMPLES
- Hypertension, chronic renal failure, is coded as I12.9, N18.9.
- End-stage renal disease with hypertension is coded as I12.0, N18.6.
- Hypertensive renal disease is coded as I12.9, N18.9.
- Acute renal failure with stage V renal disease, hypertension, is coded as N17.9, I12.0, N18.5.

Hypertensive Heart Disease and Chronic Kidney Disease

Category I13 (hypertensive heart disease and chronic kidney disease) includes combination codes that are assigned when both chronic kidney disease (N18) and heart disease with (I50.-, or I51.4–154.9) hypertension or hypertensive heart disease are stated in the diagnosis (Box 6.5). Table 6.5 describes the causal relationship between heart disease and hypertensive heart disease, with an assumed causal relationship with chronic kidney disease. Remember that the Index directs the coder to report hypertensive heart disease and kidney disease in the presence of conditions classified to I50.-, or I54.1–I51.9 and CKD (N18). Only when documentation specifically states that these conditions are not related should they be coded separately and the hypertension code I10 assigned. The Tabular List contains "Excludes Notes" and "Code also notes" to remind the coder of these guidelines.

I51 Complications and ill-defined descriptions of heart disease
    Excludes1: any condition in I51.4-I51.9 due to hypertension (I11.-)
                  any condition in I51.4-I51.9 due to hypertension and chronic kidney disease (I13.-)
                  heart disease specified as rheumatic (I00–I09)

EXAMPLES
- Hypertensive heart and chronic renal disease. Code as I13.10, N18.9.
- Congestive heart failure (CHF) due to hypertension with chronic end-stage renal failure. Code as I13.2, I50.9, N18.6.

- Hypertension, end-stage renal disease, chronic diastolic heart failure. Code as I13.2 N18.6, I50.32.

Secondary Hypertension

Hypertension can also be caused by other diseases, such as renal artery stenosis. In this case, a code for secondary hypertension is reported along with the code for the underlying cause. The sequencing is determined by the circumstances of admission.

 One of the most common mistakes coders make is assigning code I10 (unspecified essential hypertension) instead of R03.0 when they see high blood pressure documented.

EXAMPLE

Hypertension due to renal artery stenosis is coded as I15.1, I70.1.

Hypertension—Controlled or Uncontrolled

Documentation of *controlled* or *uncontrolled* hypertension represents the patient's response to current therapy and does not affect code assignment. A code from categories I10–I15 is assigned based on the presence of other documented conditions (renal failure, secondary hypertension). Always code to the type of hypertension.

Hypertensive Crisis

Hypertensive crisis can present as hypertensive urgency or hypertensive emergency (A systolic reading of 180 mm HG or higher or a diastolic reading of 110 mm HG or higher for more than one blood pressure reading). Hypertensive emergency exists when blood pressure reaches levels showing organ damage, whereas hypertensive urgency does not support associated organ damage. A separate category I16 identifies the presence of hypertensive crisis, urgency or emergency. An additional code from categories I10–I15 would be assigned.

CHF, codes from I150.- or codes I51.4–I51.9, and CKD should not be coded as hypertensive if the physician has specifically documented a different cause.

EXAMPLE

Hypertensive emergency, hypertension, Stage 3 is coded as I16.1, I12.9, N18.3.

Elevated Blood Pressure and Transient Hypertension

Code R03.0 is assigned when a patient has an elevated blood pressure reading but has not been diagnosed with hypertension or transient hypertension. Transient hypertension in pregnancy is assigned to O14.

CHECKPOINT 6.4

Code the following statements using ICD-10-CM.

1. Elevated blood pressure without a diagnosis of hypertension _____

2. Hypertensive carditis _____

3. Hypertensive urgency, hypertensive chronic diastolic heart failure_____

4. Hypertension due to ureteral calculus _____

5. Chronic renal failure, stage 3, hypertension _____

6. Hypertensive cardiomegaly with acute renal failure with tubular necrosis _____

7. Hypertensive emergency with acute renal failure. Patient has hypertension and CKD stage IV.

_____

Cerebrovascular Infarction, Stroke, Cerebrovascular Accident (CVA)

The terms *cerebrovascular accident (CVA)* and *stroke* both refer to cerebral infarction (sudden loss of oxygen supply to the brain, caused by either a blockage or a hemorrhage), which is classified to code I63.9. Other cerebrovascular diseases that can result in an infarction include carotid stenosis, thrombosis, and cerebral embolism. These conditions cause narrowing and decreased blood flow in the cerebral arteries or veins. A thrombosis is a blood clot inside a blood vessel. An embolism is an obstruction in a blood vessel due to a blood clot or other foreign matter. These clots can lodge in any area of the body and result in decreased blood flow. For example, a patient might develop a pulmonary embolism or a cerebral embolism. When these conditions are present, additional documentation is required to identify the presence of an associated infarction and the specific vessel occluded.

Common Medications for Diseases of the Circulatory System

Epinephrine

Epinephrine is used to relieve respiratory distress due to bronchospasm, to provide rapid relief of hypersensitivity reactions to drugs and other allergens, and to prolong the action of anesthetics.

Vasodilators

Vasodilators are used to relax vascular smooth muscles; the drugs result in dilation of peripheral arteries and veins. This dilation promotes peripheral pooling of blood and decreases venous return to the heart. This action reduces blood pressure on the heart. The dilation of coronary vessels results in increased blood flow to heart muscle and relieves angina.

Medications for Hypertension

The major categories of drugs used to treat hypertension are

- ACE inhibitors and ARB blockers
- Beta blockers
- Calcium channel blockers
- Diuretics

ACE Inhibitors and ARB Blockers

Angiotensin-converting enzyme (ACE) inhibitors and angiotensin II receptor blockers (ARBs) work by causing relaxation of smooth muscles in arteries and veins, which results in vasodilation resulting in decreased blood pressure.

Beta Blockers

Beta blockers (beta adrenergic blocking agents) are used to decrease blood pressure and treat cardiac arrhythmias.

Calcium Channel Blockers

Calcium channel blockers cause relaxation of smooth muscles in arteries and veins, which results in vasodilation resulting in decreased blood pressure.

EPINEPHRINE	
TRADE	GENERIC NAME
Adrenalin	epinephrine

VASODILATORS	
TRADE NAME	GENERIC NAME
Apresoline	hydralazine
Imdur	isosorbide
Nitro-Bid/Nitrostat	nitroglycerin
Vasodilan	isoxsuprine

ACE INHIBITORS AND ARB BLOCKERS	
TRADE NAME	GENERIC NAME
Accupril	quinapril
Altace	ramipril
Atacand	candesartan
Avapro	irbesartan
Benicar	olmesartan
Capoten	captopril
Cozaar	losartan
Diovan	valsartan
Lotensin	benazepril
Mavik	trandolapril
Micardis	telmisartan
Monopril	fosinopril
Tekturna	aliskiren
Univasc	moexipril
Vasotec	enalapril
Zestril/Prinivil	lisinopril

CALCIUM CHANNEL BLOCKERS	
TRADE NAME	GENERIC NAME
Calan	verapamil
Cardene	nicardipine
Cardizem/Tiazac	diltiazem
DynaCirc	isradipine
Nimotop	nimodipine
Norvasc	amlodipine
Plendil	felodipine
Procardia	nifedipine
Sular	nisoldipine

BETA BLOCKERS	
TRADE NAME	GENERIC NAME
Betapace	sotalol
Blocadren	timolol
Brevibloc	esmolol
Coreg	carvedilol
Corgard	nadolol
Inderal	propranolol
Lopressor	metoprolol
Sectral	acebutolol
Tenormin	atenolol
Trandate	labetalol
Visken	pindolol

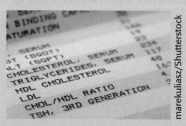

marekuliasz/Shutterstock

Blood cholesterol level test results.

DIURETICS

TRADE NAME	GENERIC NAME
Aldactone	spironolactone
Bumex	bumetanide
Demadex	torsemide
Diuril	chlorothiazide
HydroDIURIL	hydrochlorothiazide
Hygroton	chlorthalidone
Lasix	furosemide
Midamor	amiloride
Zaroxolyn	metolazone

ANTICOAGULANTS

TRADE NAME	GENERIC NAME
	heparin
Arixtra	fondaparinux
Coumadin	warfarin
Fragmin	dalteparin
Innohep	tinzaparin
Lovenox	enoxaparin

STATINS

TRADE NAME	GENERIC NAME
Crestor	rosuvastatin
Lescol	fluvastatin
Lipitor	atorvastatin
Pravachol	pravastatin
Zocor	simvastatin

PLATELET INHIBITORS

TRADE NAME	GENERIC NAME
Aggrastat	tirofiban
Aggrenox	dipyridamole/aspirin
Agrylin	anagrelide
Integrilin	eptifibatide
Persantine	dipyridamole
Plavix	clopidogrel
Pletal	cilostazol
ReoPro	abciximab
Ticlid	ticlopidine

Diuretics

Diuretics work in the kidney and cause the body to excrete more urine. This results in reduced overall body water. This is important in reducing blood pressure and treating pulmonary edema in patients with congestive heart failure.

Anticoagulants

These agents are used to decrease the body's ability to clot blood. This can be important in patients who are at risk for developing blood clots or have a coagulation disorder.

Statins

Statins decrease cholesterol and are also referred to as *lipid-lowering agents*.

Platelet Inhibitors

Platelet inhibitors reduce platelet aggregation, which is part of the coagulation process. These drugs are important for patients who are at risk for developing clots, such as a patient who has had a coronary stent placed.

Thrombolytics

Thrombolytic agents are used to dissolve clots that have caused myocardial infarction or stroke.

THROMBOLYTICS

TRADE NAME	GENERIC NAME
Activase	alteplase
Retavase	reteplase
Streptase	streptokinase
TNKase	tenecteplase
Xigris	drotrecogin

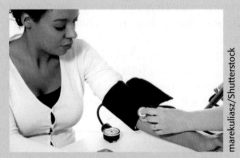

marekuliasz/Shutterstock

Measuring blood pressure.

It may be appropriate to query the physician for further specificity regarding the presence of acute infarction and site of occlusion when documentation is only noted on a CT scan or magnetic resonance imaging (MRI). When a CVA results from another cerebrovascular disease, both should be coded unless combination codes are available.

EXAMPLES

- Cerebral embolism with infarction is coded I63.40, while cerebral embolism is coded I66.9.
- Carotid artery dissection with CVA is coded I77.71, I63.9.

Postoperative and Intraoperative Cerebrovascular Accident

For a code representing intraoperative and postoperative CVA to be assigned, the record must state that the CVA was a result of medical intervention (a post-op complication). The cause-and-effect relationship between the medical intervention and the CVA/hemorrhage must be clearly documented. Proper code assignment depends on whether it was an infarction or hemorrhage and whether it occurred intraoperatively or postoperatively. An additional code may be required to specify the specific disorder. If a cerebral hemorrhage occurred as a complication of a procedure, the code assignment depends on the type of procedure performed.

EXAMPLE

Postoperative CVA due to coronary artery bypass graft for coronary artery disease of the native vessel. Report codes I97.190, I63.9, I25.10 (*see complication circulatory postprocedural*).

Sequelae of Cerebrovascular Disease

Category I69 classifies late effects of cerebrovascular disease, conditions that result from a previous condition classifiable to categories I60–I67. These neurological deficits may arise later or may be present at the initial onset of the disease. It is appropriate to assign multiple codes from category I69 to represent all the neurological deficits. If the neurological deficit from a previous CVA is the reason for admission, the code from category I69 can be sequenced as the principal diagnosis.

EXAMPLE

Recurrent seizures due to previous stroke is coded I69.398, G40.89.

Notice that in this case two codes are required, because the sequelae code I69.398 reports other sequelae of a stroke and an additional code is used to report the specific residual condition of seizure (see "use additional code" note at code I69.398).

It is appropriate to assign a code from category I69 with a code for a current cerebrovascular disease. A patient who has a residual effect from a previous CVA (category I69) may develop a new CVA or infarction (categories I60–I67). When a patient has a history of a CVA or a transient ischemic attack (TIA) with no residual effects, the history code is assigned (Z86.73).

Acute Myocardial Infarction

Acute myocardial infarction (AMI), which is sudden partial or total reduction in the blood supply to the heart, is classified to category I21, with the fourth digit representing the type of infarction and the fifth digit representing the site of infarction. Documentation of the type of myocardial infarction is necessary in order to assign a code from category I21. Type 2 myocardial infarction and myocardial infarction due to demand ischemia is assigned to code I21.A1. If documentation supports a type 3, 4a, 4b, 4c, or 5, the code for other myocardial infarction types I21.A9 is assigned. An acute myocardial infarction is equal to or less than 4 weeks old. The category includes transfers to another acute setting or post-acute setting and the patient requires continued care. The acute myocardial infarction within 4 weeks should be reported when the criteria for an additional diagnosis is met. Remember to follow the "Code also" and "Code first" notes to report additional codes and sequence correctly.

Assignment of the Fourth Digit

Myocardial infarctions that show an ST segment change on an electrocardiogram (ECG) are referred to as *ST elevation myocardial infarctions (STEMIs)*. Codes I21.0–I21.2 specify sites that equate to STEMIs. If a patient has an ST elevation myocardial infarction without a specific site, the code I21.3 (unspecified STEMIs) is assigned. Myocardial infarctions that do not show an ST segment change on an ECG are referred to as *non-ST elevation myocardial infarctions (NSTEMIs)* and are coded to I21.4. These infarctions may also be termed *nontransmural* or *subendocardial* myocardial infarctions. Even if the site of a transmural infarction is stated, the code

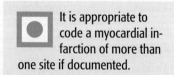
It is appropriate to code a myocardial infarction of more than one site if documented.

I21.4 would still be assigned. Codes reported are based on the type of infarction. Therefore, a type 2 STEMI is assigned code I21.A1 as codes I21.01–I21.4 can only be assigned for type 1 acute myocardial infarctions.

Abnormal ECGs or elevated cardiac enzymes do not qualify for assignment of these infarction codes (query the physician about the cause of these abnormalities), because other conditions can cause ST elevation or abnormal cardiac enzymes.

Sometimes a NSTEMI evolves to a STEMI; in such a case, only the STEMI is coded. The opposite can also be true; a STEMI can convert to a NSTEMI due to thrombolytic therapy. In this case also, only the STEMI is coded. Note that *thrombolytic therapy* refers to the administration of such drugs as streptokinase and reteplase.

Subsequent Acute Myocardial Infarction

A code from category I22, Subsequent ST elevation (STEMI) and non-ST elevation (NSTEMI) myocardial infarction, is to be used when a patient has suffered an acute MI and has a new acute MI within the 4-week timeframe of the initial acute MI. When this occurs, codes from category I21 and from category I22 (subsequent MI) are used with the sequencing depending on the circumstances of the encounter. For example, a patient presents with an acute STEMI of the anterior wall, and 3 days after admission the same patient develops an acute STEMI of the lateral wall. Report code I21.09 for the initial MI and I22.8 for the subsequent lateral wall MI.

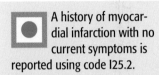
A history of myocardial infarction with no current symptoms is reported using code I25.2.

CHECKPOINT 6.5

Code the following statements using ICD-10-CM.

1. Anterior cerebral artery embolism with infarction and convulsions _____

2. Old (sequelae) cerebral embolism with infarction with residual ataxia _____

3. Left-sided carotid artery stenosis with infarction _____

4. A ruptured cerebral aneurysm _____

5. History of TIA _____

6. Acute ST elevation myocardial infarction of the anterior wall _____

7. Acute subendocardial myocardial infarction _____

8. Admission to skilled nursing facility 2 weeks after treatment of nontransmural myocardial infarction, and patient requires continued treatment _____

9. Admission to Hospital B for inferior wall STEMI 2 weeks after treatment of an acute ST elevated lateral wall myocardial infarction _____

10. Postmyocardial infarction syndrome _____

Coronary Artery Disease and Angina

Combination codes are used to report atherosclerotic heart disease (ASHD)—coronary artery disease (CAD)—with angina pectoris. Coronary artery disease, which is also termed *arteriosclerotic heart disease,* is the condition in which arteriosclerotic plaque lines the walls of the coronary arteries. The relationship between the underlying coronary artery disease and the angina is assumed unless documentation states that the angina is a result of something else. Patients with CAD who develop an acute MI require reporting of both conditions with the MI sequenced first.

The codes for atherosclerotic CAD require knowledge of the location of the disease. The subcategories associated with I25 indicate heart disease of the native coronary arteries, of coronary artery bypass grafts, and coronary arteries of a transplanted heart. If a patient has never had a coronary artery bypass graft (CABG) surgery or a heart transplant (and if this is documented), it is assumed that the CAD is in the native vessel. A coronary artery bypass graft is the procedure in which the blocked coronary vessel is bypassed with a graft in order to restore blood flow to the heart tissue. Without a previous bypass, the CAD can only be found in the patient's native vessels because no bypass vessels would be present.

EXAMPLE
CAD of native coronary artery and arterial bypass is coded I25.10, I25.810.

Documentation of the atherosclerosis of a bypass graft incorporates the type of bypass (arterial or venous, autologous or nonautologous) and associated angina spasm or ischemic chest pain. Combination codes are used to report multiple aspects of the disease.

EXAMPLE
Atherosclerotic coronary artery disease of autologous arterial bypass graft with unstable angina pectoris. Report code I25.720.

PINPOINT THE CODE 6.1: Congestive Heart Failure Code Assignment

Diastolic →	**Step 1** Determine acuity.
	Acute: I50.31 Chronic: I50.32 Acute on chronic: I50.33 Unspecified: I50.30
Systolic →	**Step 1** Determine acuity.
	Acute: I50.21 Chronic: I50.22 Acute on chronic: I50.23 Unspecified: I50.20
Combined diastolic with systolic →	**Step 1** Determine acuity.
	Acute: I50.41 Chronic: I50.42 Acute on chronic: I50.43 Unspecified: I50.40
Rheumatic in nature (in presence of rheumatic heart disease) →	**Step 1** Assign code: I09.81. → **Step 2** Assign additional code for type of heart failure.
With hypertensive heart disease without hypertensive renal disease →	**Step 1** Assign code: I11.0. → **Step 2** Assign additional code for type of heart failure.
With hypertensive heart and chronic kidney disease →	**Step 1** See Hypertension, cardiorenal, with heart failure: I13.0. → **Step 2** Assign additional code for type of heart failure. → **Step 3** Assign additional code for chronic kidney disease if documented.

Heart Failure

> All codes for heart failure include any associated pulmonary edema; no additional code is assigned.

Hypertension, obesity, alcohol consumption, valvular damage, and genetic predisposition may contribute to *heart failure*, a serious condition in more than 5 million Americans. In patients with heart failure, the muscle of the heart fails to pump blood through the circulatory system. This results in decreased blood flow to the kidneys, causing the kidneys to retain water and sodium. The water retained by the kidneys enters the blood circulation, accumulating in the lungs, abdominal organs, and lower extremities. The results of ECGs, Holter monitor tests (ambulatory ECGs), echocardiograms, stress tests, and chest x-rays determine the nature of the heart muscle's illness.

Heart failure can be left sided, right sided, diastolic, systolic, rheumatic, congestive, or combined. The type determines the coding (Pinpoint the Code 6.1). *Congestive heart failure* refers to decreased efficiency of the heart's output, causing fluid collection in the lungs. Systolic heart failure (codes I50.20–I50.23), also referred to as *dilated cardiomyopathy*, results when the left ventricle is weakened and cannot put out a sufficient volume of blood. This is more common than diastolic heart failure (I50.30–I50.33), which happens when the heart muscle is either overgrown or stiffened, also affecting adequate blood flow. A patient may have both systolic and diastolic heart failure combined, which is reported using codes I50.40 to I50.43.

> Heart failure is not the same as cardiac arrest, which is the cessation of normal heartbeat, also known as asystole.

All components are reported when coding heart failure. For example, recall that hypertensive heart failure requires one code for the hypertensive heart disease with heart failure and one or more additional codes to identify the specific type of heart failure (category I50).

> Physicians must describe heart failure as systolic, diastolic, or both on every admission or visit to show specificity of the disease. This may impact reimbursement.

Often, the acute exacerbation or decompensated heart failure (failure to maintain normal circulation; worsening) is the reason for an admission. If that is the case, the code for the heart failure is sequenced first, followed by a code for the underlying cause. Rheumatic heart failure is reported when the patient has a rheumatic heart condition such as aortic valve stenosis with mitral insufficiency (I08.0). Therefore, when a patient with aortic valve stenosis with mitral insufficiency reports to the hospital for heart failure, codes I01.8, I08.0 are assigned. The coder does not assume that the congestive heart failure is rheumatic in nature unless directed by the ICD-10-CM Alphabetic Index or the physician statement that the heart failure is rheumatic. Please remember to follow the code-first instructions at category I50.

> The term *acute on chronic* in coding heart failure means that a patient has a chronic heart condition and has also experienced a sudden serious exacerbation of the problem.

CHECKPOINT 6.6

Code the following statements using ICD-10-CM.

1. Coronary artery disease of an autologous vein bypass graft _____

2. Unstable angina due to CAD (no previous history of coronary artery bypass graft or surgery)

   _____

3. Patient is admitted with impending myocardial infarction due to CAD of an autologous arterial

   bypass. The patient had an MI 5 years ago. _____

4. Patient presents with coronary arteriosclerosis due to lipid-rich plaque _____

5. Rheumatic congestive heart failure _____

6. Acute on chronic diastolic and systolic congestive heart failure _____

7. Ischemic cardiomyopathy with acute congestive heart failure _____

8. Congestive heart failure with tricuspid regurgitation _____

9. Aortic and mitral insufficiency with rheumatic chronic diastolic congestive heart failure _____

DISEASES OF THE RESPIRATORY SYSTEM (CHAPTER 10: J00–J99)

Disorders of the respiratory system are classified to ICD-10-CM Chapter 10. The categories in Chapter 10 of the ICD-10-CM are grouped as shown in Table 6.6. Box 6.6 presents the applicable guidelines from Section I, Part C, of the *Official Guidelines for Coding and Reporting.*

Table 6.6 Organization of ICD-10-CM Chapter 10 Tabular List

BLOCK	BLOCK DESCRIPTION
J00–J06	Acute upper respiratory infections
J09–J18	Influenza and pneumonia
J20–J22	Other acute lower respiratory infections
J30–J39	Other diseases of upper respiratory tract
J40–J47	Chronic lower respiratory diseases
J60–J70	Lung diseases due to external agents
J80–J84	Other respiratory diseases principally affecting the interstitium
J85–J86	Suppurative and necrotic conditions of the lower respiratory tract
J90–J94	Other diseases of the pleura
J95	Intraoperative and postprocedural complications and disorders of respiratory system, not elsewhere classified
J96–J99	Other diseases of the respiratory system

Chronic Obstructive Pulmonary Disease

Chronic obstructive pulmonary disease (COPD) is a general term for unspecified chronic obstructive lung conditions that make it difficult for patients to exhale normally. It includes diseases such as chronic bronchitis, emphysema, and asthma, rather than being a separate disease entity. Due to the variations in the way these conditions are documented, code selection requires careful review of the specific conditions. When documented by a physician, COPD should be reported in all instances, because COPD is a chronic condition that will always affect patient care.

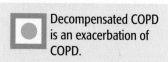
Decompensated COPD is an exacerbation of COPD.

COPD and its forms can exacerbate (or decompensate), which in essence is an acute on chronic condition. Two codes are used to report COPD and asthma according to the "code also" note at category J44 (COPD). Note, however, that an infection superimposed on a chronic condition is not the same as an exacerbation, although the infection may trigger an exacerbation.

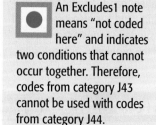
An Excludes1 note means "not coded here" and indicates two conditions that cannot occur together. Therefore, codes from category J43 cannot be used with codes from category J44.

EXAMPLES

- Acute bronchitis with COPD exacerbation is coded J44.0, J44.1, J20.9.

- Acute COPD exacerbation with pneumonia is coded J44.1, J44.0, J18.9 (the infection—pneumonia—is reported separately along with COPD with acute lower respiratory infection).

Acute Exacerbation of Asthma and Status Asthmaticus

In ICD-10-CM reporting of asthma requires documentation of the severity of the asthma (mild, moderate, severe). The fifth digits for asthma include classification for the presence of exacerbation or status asthmaticus. An acute exacerbation of asthma occurs when there is an increased severity of asthma symptoms. Status asthmaticus is more severe than asthma exacerbation because it involves a failure to respond to medication and therapy administered during an asthma attack, a potentially life-threatening condition. When a patient has acute asthma, with any type of COPD or with acute bronchitis, and status asthmaticus, the status asthmaticus should be sequenced first and supersedes any type of COPD or bronchitis. COPD with unspecified asthma, without status asthmaticus, is reported with code J44.9. No additional code for unspecified asthma is required. Sequencing is dependent on the circumstances of the visit.

a. Chronic Obstructive Pulmonary Disease (COPD) and Asthma

1) Acute exacerbation of chronic obstructive bronchitis and asthma

The codes in categories J44 and J45 distinguish between uncomplicated cases and those in acute exacerbation. An acute exacerbation is a worsening or a decompensation of a chronic condition. An acute exacerbation is not equivalent to an infection superimposed on a chronic condition, though an exacerbation may be triggered by an infection.

b. Acute Respiratory Failure

1) Acute respiratory failure as principal diagnosis

A code from subcategory J96.0, Acute respiratory failure, or subcategory J96.2, Acute and chronic respiratory failure, may be assigned as a principal diagnosis when it is the condition established after study to be chiefly responsible for occasioning the admission to the hospital, and the selection is supported by the Alphabetic Index and Tabular List. However, chapter-specific coding guidelines (such as obstetrics, poisoning, HIV, newborn) that provide sequencing direction take precedence.

2) Acute respiratory failure as secondary diagnosis

Respiratory failure may be listed as a secondary diagnosis if it occurs after admission or if it is present on admission, but does not meet the definition of principal diagnosis.

3) Sequencing of acute respiratory failure and another acute condition

When a patient is admitted with respiratory failure and another acute condition (e.g., myocardial infarction, cerebrovascular accident, aspiration pneumonia), the principal diagnosis will not be the same in every situation. This applies whether the other acute condition is a respiratory or nonrespiratory condition. Selection of the principal diagnosis depends on the circumstances of admission. If both the respiratory failure and the other acute condition are equally responsible for occasioning the admission to the hospital, and there are no chapter-specific sequencing rules, the guideline regarding two or more diagnoses that equally meet the definition for principal diagnosis (Section II, Part C.) may be applied in these situations. If the documentation is not clear as to whether acute respiratory failure and another condition are equally responsible for occasioning the admission, query the provider for clarification.

c. Influenza Due to Certain Identified Influenza Viruses

Code only confirmed cases of influenza due to certain identified influenza viruses (category J09) and due to other identified influenza virus (category J10). This is an exception to the hospital inpatient guideline Section II, H (Uncertain Diagnosis). In this context, "confirmation" does not require documentation of positive laboratory testing specific for avian or other novel influenza A or other identified influenza virus. However, coding should be based on the provider's diagnostic statement that the patient has avian influenza or other novel influenza A for category J09, or has another particular identified strain of influenza, such as H1N1 or H3N2, but not identified as novel or variant, for category J10.

If the provider records use the terms "suspected" or "possible" or "probable" regarding avian influenza, novel influenza, or other identified influenza, then the appropriate influenza code from category J11, Influenza due to unidentified influenza virus, should be assigned. A code from category J09, Influenza due to certain identified influenza viruses, should not be assigned nor should a code from category J10, Influenza due to other identified influenza virus.

d. Ventilator-Associated Pneumonia

1) Documentation of ventilator-associated pneumonia

As with all procedural or postprocedural complications, code assignment is based on the provider's documentation of the relationship between the condition and the procedure.

Code J95.851, Ventilator-associated pneumonia, should be assigned only when the provider has documented ventilator-associated pneumonia (VAP). An additional code to identify the organism (e.g., *Pseudomonas aeruginosa*, code B96.5) should also be assigned. Do not assign an additional code from categories J12–J18 to identify the type of pneumonia.

Code J95.851 should not be assigned for cases where the patient has pneumonia and is on a mechanical ventilator and the provider has not specifically stated that the pneumonia is ventilator-associated pneumonia. If the documentation is unclear as to whether the patient has a pneumonia that is a complication attributable to the mechanical ventilator, query the provider.

2) Ventilator-associated pneumonia develops after admission

A patient may be admitted with one type of pneumonia (e.g., code J13, Pneumonia due to *Streptococcus* pneumonia) and subsequently develop VAP. In this instance, the principal diagnosis would be the appropriate code from categories J12–J18 for the pneumonia diagnosed at the time of admission. Code J95.851, Ventilator-associated pneumonia, would be assigned as an additional diagnosis when the provider has also documented the presence of ventilator-associated pneumonia.

PHARMACOLOGY CONNECTION

Common Medications and Treatments for Diseases of the Respiratory System

Oxygen
Uptake of oxygen from the air is the essential purpose of respiration, so oxygen supplementation is used in medicine. Oxygen therapy is used to treat emphysema, pneumonia, some heart disorders, and any disease that impairs the body's ability to take up and use gaseous oxygen.

Mechanical Ventilation
In medicine, mechanical ventilation is a method to mechanically assist or replace spontaneous breathing when patients cannot do so on their own, and must be done so after invasive intubation with an endotracheal or tracheostomy tube through which air is directly delivered. In many cases, mechanical ventilation is used in acute settings such as in the ICU for a short period of time during a serious illness.

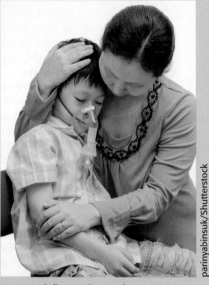

Oxygen delivery via mask.

parinyabinsuk/Shutterstock

CPAP
Continuous positive airway pressure (CPAP) is a very useful treatment involving a machine that improves the movement of air into the lungs. CPAP machines are used mainly by patients for the treatment of sleep apnea at home. CPAP delivers a stream of compressed air via a hose to a nasal pillow, nose mask, or full-face mask. This air pressure keeps the airway open. This method can also be used when transitioning a patient off of ventilation to room air.

BiPAP
Bilevel positive airway pressure (BiPAP) is a similar mechanism to CPAP; however, the air pressures can be set for one pressure for inhalations and another for exhalations. These settings allow patients to get more air in and out of the lungs without the natural muscular effort usually needed to do so.

Bronchodilators
Bronchodilators are agents used to relax airways and relieve reversible bronchospasm associated with acute and chronic bronchial asthma, bronchitis, emphysema, and other obstructive pulmonary diseases.

BRONCHODILATORS	
TRADE NAME	**GENERIC NAME**
Atrovent	ipratropium
Lufyllin	dyphylline
Proventil, Ventolin	albuterol
Serevent	salmeterol
Spiriva	tiotropium
Theo-Dur	theophylline
Xopenex	levalbuterol

Antitussives and Decongestants

Antitussives, medications used to suppress the urge to cough, include the generic drugs codeine and dextromethorphan. Decongestants provide temporary relief of nasal congestion due to colds or allergy. Common medications include Sudafed (pseudoephedrine) and Sudafed PE (phenylephrine).

Corticosteroids

Corticosteroids are very potent anti-inflammatory agents often used to decrease inflammation of the respiratory passages.

CORTICOSTEROIDS	
TRADE NAME	**GENERIC NAME**
Celestone	betamethasone
Cortef	hydrocortisone
Decadron	dexamethasone
Florinef	fludrocortisone
Medrol	methylprednisolone
Prelone	prednisolone

Mucolytics and Expectorants

Mucolytics are agents used to decrease the viscosity of mucous secretions in chronic obstructive pulmonary diseases including cystic fibrosis. Common medications include acetylcysteine (Mucomyst) and dornase (Pulmozyme). Expectorants help loosen phlegm and thin bronchial secretions to rid the bronchial passageways of bothersome mucus, drain bronchial tubes, or make coughs more productive. Common brand names are Robitussin and Mucinex (generic guaifenesin).

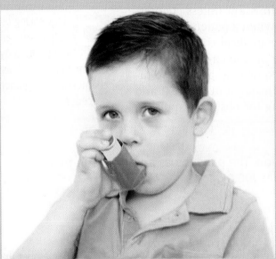

smikeymikey1 /Shutterstock

Albuterol bronchodilator.

Code the following statements using ICD-10-CM.

1. COPD with hypoxemia _____

2. COPD with emphysema _____

3. COPD exacerbation with emphysema _____

4. Acute exacerbation of moderate, persistent asthma, status asthmaticus _____

5. Bronchiolitis due to respiratory syncytial virus (RSV) _____

6. COPD with asthma exacerbation _____

7. Acute asthmatic bronchitis _____

Acute Respiratory Failure

There are two levels of respiratory failure, acute and chronic. Acute respiratory failure, in which the lungs suddenly fail to function, can be caused by a variety of medical conditions such as pneumonia, sepsis, myocardial infarction, stroke, complication of surgery, or poisoning. Respiratory failure codes also classify the presence of hypercapnia or hypoxia. A code from category J96 is reported as an additional (secondary) diagnosis if it occurs after admission or if it was present on admission but does not meet the definition of principal diagnosis.

The code for acute respiratory failure should be assigned as the principal diagnosis based on the circumstances of admission unless chapter-specific coding guidelines state otherwise. Thus, when a patient is admitted with acute respiratory failure due to another medical condition, the determination of the principal diagnosis is based on the circumstance of admission. The chapter-specific exceptions to sequencing acute respiratory failure as the principal diagnosis are found throughout this text and take precedence. These guidelines include coding for obstetrics, poisonings, HIV, newborns, and severe sepsis.

> Hypoxemia (R09.02) is integral to acute respiratory failure and should not be reported separately. Hypoxemia is reported separately with other respiratory conditions.

> Sequencing of acute respiratory failure is determined by the circumstance of admission, and chapter-specific guidelines take precedence.

EXAMPLE

Acute respiratory failure with COPD exacerbation. The patient was admitted due to acute respiratory failure with hypoxemia. Assign codes J96.01, J44.1.

Pneumonia

Pneumonia is infection or inflammation of lung tissue caused by a variety of organisms, including bacteria, viruses, parasites, and others. Pneumonia caused by aspiration, postoperative complications, bacteria, viruses, and influenza are examples of different types of pneumonia. Symptoms of pneumonia include fever, cough, sputum production, chest pain, shortness of breath, headache, and weakness. Diagnostic tests include chest x-ray, bronchoscopy, and blood and sputum cultures; other procedures include lung biopsies.

The coding of pneumonia relies on the type of pneumonia. The major categories are:

> Remember that it is inappropriate for coders to assume a causal organism on the basis of laboratory, radiology, or medication records alone. All codes must be based on physician documentation, such as by the patient's pulmonologist, and abnormal findings require physician documentation of clinical significance.

J12　Viral pneumonia
J13　Pneumococcal (lobar) pneumonia
J14　*Haemophilus influenzae* pneumonia
J15　Other bacterial pneumonia
J16　Pneumonia due to other specified organisms
J17　Pneumonia in diseases classified elsewhere
J18　Pneumonia, unspecified organism

> Pneumonia is not an acute exacerbation of COPD. When the two conditions occur together, both are coded.

Pneumonitis due to inhaling solids and liquids is coded from category J69, and additional pneumonia codes are found in Chapter 1 of ICD-10-CM.

EXAMPLES

• *Haemophilus influenzae* pneumonia is coded J14.

• Aspiration pneumonia due to inhalation of food is coded J69.0.

If a patient develops multiple types of pneumonia, two codes may be assigned.

> If the record does not document the organism causing pneumonia, as in more than half of cases, code J18.9 is assigned.

> ■ **CASE SCENARIO**
> A patient presents with food aspiration pneumonia and sputum cultures support *Pseudomonas* pneumonia as well. Report codes J69.0 for food aspiration pneumonia with J15.1 for *Pseudomonas* pneumonia.

If the pneumonia is postobstructive pneumonia, the code for pneumonia is reported with a code for the obstructive process, such as in the case of postobstructive pneumonia due to carcinoma of the lung—codes J18.9, C34.90. The sequencing depends on the circumstance of admission/visit.

Be careful when coding bacterial pneumonia. For example, if the physician documents mixed bacterial pneumonia, the specific bacterium is not documented, so code J15.9 is reported.

Pneumonia with COPD is considered COPD with acute lower respiratory infection. In this case the COPD code J44.0 is listed first followed by the code for the pneumonia (J18.9).

CHECKPOINT 6.8

Code the following statements using ICD-10-CM.

1. Acute respiratory failure due to pneumonia _____

2. Hypercapnia with acute respiratory failure due to cerebral embolism with infarction _____

3. Severe sepsis with septic shock and acute respiratory failure _____

4. Patient admitted with COPD exacerbation and developed acute hypoxic respiratory failure after admission _____

5. COPD with acute pneumonia with exacerbation of moderate persistent asthma _____

6. Aspiration pneumonia with hypoxemia _____

7. Pneumonia in candidiasis _____

8. Bacterial pneumonia due to *Streptococcus* group B and Serratia _____

9. Bronchiolitis obliterans with organizing pneumonia (BOOP) _____

10. Pneumonia with COPD _____

Chapter Summary

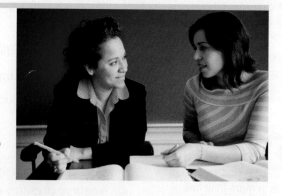

1. Codes in category G89, Pain, are used with other ICD-10-CM codes to provide more detail about pain. If the pain is not specified as acute or chronic, it cannot be coded from category G89, except for post-thoracotomy pain, postoperative pain, neoplasm-related pain, and central pain syndrome. Pain codes are not assigned if the underlying (definitive) diagnosis is known, unless the reason for the encounter is pain control or management rather than management of the underlying condition.

2. Documentation is essential to assign an accurate code for paralysis and monoplegia. Often, the underlying cause and type of paralysis are reported with a combination code. Codes for hemiplegia and monoplegia classify whether the paralysis is on the dominant or nondominant side.

3. A code for epilepsy should not be assigned unless the physician specifically states epilepsy (seizure disorder). Documentation must be specific regarding status epilepticus as well. Terms equivalent to *intractable* are *poorly controlled*, *refractory*, or *pharmacoresistant*. Epilepsy is an exception to the rule for coding possible, probable, or suspected (rule-out) conditions in the inpatient setting.

4. Codes for glaucoma record documentation of laterality, type of glaucoma, and severity. When reporting the presence of bilateral glaucoma, two codes may be required when the type or severity of the disease is not the same in both eyes.

5. Hypertension codes are determined by the underlying cause of the disease. When the cause of hypertension is unknown, this is considered essential hypertension (I10). When hypertension is related to certain heart conditions, the codes from category I11 are assigned. There is an assumed relationship between conditions classified to I50.-, or I51.4–I51.9 and hypertension as directed in the Index. When reporting hypertensive heart failure, use an additional code from category I50 to identify the type of heart failure. If documentation supports a different cause of heart conditions I50.-, or I51.4–I51.9 or CKD, code the conditions separately and report hypertension using code I10. Sequence according to the circumstances of the admission/encounter. When coding hypertension with chronic kidney disease, there is an assumed causal relationship. In this case, a code for the hypertension category I12 is assigned with an additional code for the stage of the chronic kidney disease (N18). When a patient has hypertensive heart disease and renal disease, a code from category I13 is assigned with additional codes to identify the specific kidney disease and heart disease. Two codes are needed for secondary hypertension: one to identify the underlying etiology and the other from category I15 to identify the hypertension. Transient hypertension and the condition stated as elevated blood pressure are coded R03.0.

6. The terms *stroke* and *CVA* are often used interchangeably to refer to a *cerebral infarction*, and all three terms are indexed to the default code I63.9. Other codes are available to classify cerebral infarctions due to occlusive disease such as an embolism. The specific vessel occluded may also affect code assignment along with the presence of an infarction.

7. AMI is classified to category I21, with the fourth digit representing the type or site of infarction and the fifth digit representing the underlying vessel involved.

8. Determining code assignment for general heart failure begins with identifying the type—systolic, diastolic, rheumatic, or other—with consideration of the acuity.

9. COPD, a general syndrome, can include obstructive chronic bronchitis, emphysema, and asthma. The codes for chronic obstructive bronchitis and asthma distinguish between uncomplicated cases and those in acute exacerbation. Due to the overlapping nature of the

conditions that make up COPD and asthma, code selection must be based on the conditions as documented. When selecting the correct code for the documented type of COPD and asthma, it is essential to first review the Index and then to verify the code in the Tabular List, following the many instructional notes under the different COPD subcategories and codes.

10. The coding of pneumonia relies on the type of pneumonia selected from the six available categories. If a patient develops multiple types of pneumonia, multiple codes may be assigned.

Review Questions

Matching

Match the key terms with their definitions.

A. systolic heart failure
B. end-stage renal disease
C. diastolic heart failure
D. status asthmaticus
E. chronic pain

F. acute on chronic
G. acute myocardial infarction
H. causal relationship
I. hypertensive emergency
J. unstable angina

1. Cause and effect H J

2. Pre-infarction heart pain

3. _C_ Condition in which the heart muscle is either overgrown or stiffened, drastically reducing blood flow

4. _I_ Sudden, severe elevation of blood pressure in which the patient typically suffers organ damage or even death

5. _E_ Long-term pain

6. _A_ Condition in which the left ventricle of the heart is weakened and cannot put out a sufficient volume of blood

7. _G_ Sudden partial or total reduction in the blood supply to the heart

8. _B_ Renal disease stage requiring transplantation or dialysis

9. _D_ Patient's failure to respond to therapy administered during an asthmatic episode

10. _F_ Description of sudden serious exacerbation of a patient's chronic condition

True or False

Decide whether each statement is true or false.

1. _T_ A causal relationship between hypertension must be documented in order to assign codes for chronic hypertensive kidney disease.

2. _T_ A patient would have native CAD if he or she never had a coronary artery bypass graft (CABG).

3. _F_ The correct code assignment for rheumatic CHF is I09.81.

4. _T_ Hyperkalemia is one condition that can be associated with acute renal failure.

5. _T_ A woman presented with acute COPD exacerbation with status asthmaticus. The principal diagnosis should be COPD failure.

6. _T_ Coding of COPD and coding of emphysema result in the assignment of two codes.

7. _T_ Glaucoma of different stages in both eyes always requires two codes.

8. _T_ If a patient has a cerebral embolism, the individual is assumed to have had a cerebral infarction.

9. ___F___ If a patient is right handed and hemiplegia is noted on the left-hand side, this patient has dominant-sided hemiplegia.

10. ___T___ The sequencing of acute respiratory failure depends on chapter-specific guidelines.

Multiple Choice

Select the letter that best completes the statement or answers the question.

1. Carotid artery stenosis is coded as
   A. I65.21
   B. I63.139
   C. I65.29
   D. I65.1

2. Acute brainstem hemorrhagic CVA. Aphasia resolved, and hemiplegia on the left side remained. The codes are
   A. I61.3, R47.01, G81.94
   B. I61.3, I69.120
   C. I61.9, R47.01, I69.159
   D. I61.3, I69.120, R69.154

3. Acute bronchitis with COPD and hypoxemia is coded as
   A. J20.9, R09.02
   B. J44.0, R09.02
   C. J44.0, J20.9, R09.02
   D. J20.9

4. Pre-senile nuclear cataract is coded as
   A. H26.039
   B. H26.009
   C. H25.10
   D. Q12.0

5. What is the correct code(s) for bilateral open-angle glaucoma, mild stage in left eye and mild stage in right eye?
   A. H40.213
   B. H40.10x1
   C. H40.212, H40.211
   D. H40.10x0

6. Coronary artery disease, status post–coronary artery angioplasty. The patient has chronic total occlusion of the native coronary vessel. The codes are
   A. I25.110, I25.82
   B. I25.10, I25.83, Z98.61
   C. I25.119, I25.83, Z98.61
   D. I25.10, I25.82, Z98.61

7. Arteriosclerosis of autologous vein bypass with unstable angina is coded as
   A. I25.701
   B. I25.710
   C. I20.0
   D. I25.720

8. Sequelae of cerebral infarction to include dysarthria, cognitive deficits, and convulsions are coded as
   A. I69.322, I69.31, I69.398, R56.9
   B. I69.822, I69.81, I69.898, R56.9
   C. I69.322, I69.31, I69.398
   D. I69.90, R47.1, R41.89, R56.9

9. The condition of varicose veins of the left lower leg with ulcer and inflammation is coded as
   A. I83.229, L97.909
   B. I83.228
   C. I83.92, L97.929
   D. I83.229, L97.929

10. Food aspiration pneumonia with methicillin-resistant *Staphylococcus aureus* (MRSA) pneumonia is coded as
    A. J69.1, J15.211
    B. P24.31, J15.212
    C. J69.0, J15.212
    D. J69.0, J15.20

CHAPTER 7

ICD-10-CM Chapters 11 Through 14: K00–N99

CHAPTER OUTLINE

Diseases of the Digestive System (Chapter 11: K00–K95)

Diseases of the Skin and Subcutaneous Tissue
(Chapter 12: L00–L99)

Diseases of the Musculoskeletal System and Connective Tissue
(Chapter 13: M00–M99)

Diseases of the Genitourinary System (Chapter 14: N00–N99)

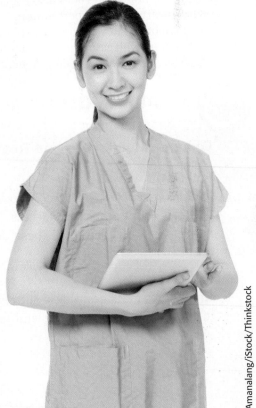

LEARNING OUTCOMES

After studying this chapter, you should be able to:

1. Describe the general points relating to coding for digestive system disorders.
2. Differentiate coding digestive disorders with and without hemorrhage.
3. Discuss the correct coding and sequencing for cellulitis.
4. Describe the coding rules that apply to complications that have caused cellulitis and to gangrenous cellulitis.
5. Describe the coding rules that apply to ischemic ulcers and to venous stasis ulcers.
6. List and briefly define stages of pressure ulcers.
7. Discuss the coding and sequencing of pathological fractures.
8. Describe the coding of osteomyelitis, and explain the unique rule for coding coexisting diabetes and osteomyelitis.
9. Discuss fourth-digit code assignment and sequencing for chronic kidney disease.
10. Identify the key coding guidelines for urinary tract infections and genitourinary disorders.

Amanalang/iStock/Thinkstock

Correct code assignment and sequencing of patients' diseases and conditions involving the integumentary, musculoskeletal, and genitourinary systems are covered in this chapter.

The structure and organization of the corresponding ICD-10-CM Tabular List chapters are presented, followed by discussions of code selection and sequencing as instructed by the *ICD-10-CM Official Guidelines for Coding and Reporting*, Section I, Part C. Once again, the focus is on common code assignment decisions and complex coding scenarios.

DISEASES OF THE DIGESTIVE SYSTEM (CHAPTER 11: K00–K95)

Disorders of the digestive system are classified in ICD-10-CM Chapter 11. Codes are listed according to anatomical location, beginning with the oral cavity and continuing through the intestines. Correct coding requires knowledge of the disease process as well as careful attention to combination codes and excludes notes. The categories in Chapter 11 of ICD-10-CM are grouped as shown in Table 7.1. There are presently no chapter-specific *Official Guidelines* for digestive conditions.

Gastrointestinal Hemorrhage Associated With Digestive Disorders

Gastrointestinal (GI) hemorrhage, bleeding in the intestinal tract, can present in a variety of forms, including hematochezia (passage of blood in the feces), occult bleeding, melena, and hematemesis. Bleeding can occur in the upper or lower GI tract. Causes of GI bleeding are most commonly ulcers, diverticulitis, hemorrhoids, angiodysplasia (also called *arteriovenous malformation*, AVM), and gastritis. Combination codes also code the underlying cause of the bleeding and/or complications such as obstruction and perforation.

It is important to clarify the use of codes K92.2 (GI bleeding), K92.1 (melena), and R19.5 (occult blood in stool) with gastrointestinal disorders. Usage is limited to cases where GI bleeding is documented but no site or cause of bleeding is identified. The code for GI hemorrhage, rectal bleeding, or occult

PHARMACOLOGY CONNECTION

Common Medications and Treatments for Diseases of the Digestive System

Antacids

Antacids (also called H_2 *blockers*) block histamine at the receptors on the gastric parietal cells. This action results in decreased acid secretion. These drugs are used to treat peptic ulcer disease.

Proton Pump Inhibitors

These drugs block gastric acid secretion and are used to treat peptic ulcer disease and gastroesophageal reflux disease (GERD).

ANTACIDS	
TRADE NAME	**GENERIC NAME**
Aciphex	rabeprazole
Axid	nizatidine
Pepcid	famotidine
Tagamet	cimetidine
Zantac	ranitidine

PROTON PUMP INHIBITORS	
TRADE NAME	**GENERIC NAME**
Nexium	esomeprazole
Prevacid	lansoprazole
Prilosec	omeprazole
Protonix	pantoprazole

Table 7.1 Organization of ICD–10–CM Chapter 11 Tabular List

BLOCK	BLOCK DESCRIPTION
K00–K14	Diseases of oral cavity and salivary glands
K20–K31	Diseases of esophagus, stomach, and duodenum
K35–K38	Diseases of appendix
K40–K46	Hernia
K50–K52	Noninfective enteritis and colitis
K55–K64	Other diseases of intestines
K65–K68	Diseases of peritoneum and retroperitoneum
K70–K77	Diseases of liver
K80–K87	Diseases of gallbladder, biliary tract, and pancreas
K90–K95	Other diseases of the digestive system

blood in the stool, should be assigned when the underlying cause of the bleeding is not identified or a combination code is not available. The combination codes for a GI lesion with hemorrhage are assigned only when the physician documents a causal relationship between the lesion and hemorrhage.

EXAMPLE
GI bleeding with unknown source and acute gastritis is coded K92.2, K29.00.

Notice that a causal relationship is not documented. In contrast, if the physician documents acute GI bleeding due to acute gastritis, code K29.01 is assigned. In this case, the causal relationship is documented.

Endoscopic examination of the digestive system can result in multiple findings such as polyps, diverticulosis, hemorrhoids, esophagitis, gastritis, and other lesions. Therefore, the physician must state the source of bleeding in order to report the combination codes. A physician query may be appropriate if the patient has GI bleeding, a causal relationship is not documented, and diagnostic tests are positive for GI lesion.

Antidiarrheals
Antidiarrheal medications decrease intestinal motility and/or absorb increased intestinal secretions associated with diarrhea.

Nutraceuticals
The term *nutraceuticals* refers to extracts of foods claimed to have a medicinal effect on human health. These are usually contained in a medicinal format such as a capsule, tablet, or powder in a prescribed dose. Very few of these products have sufficient scientific evidence proving health benefits to consumers; therefore, few have U.S. Food and Drug Administration (FDA) approval for making health claims on product labels. Common generics include antioxidants, grape seed extract, and omega-3 fatty acids.

Antiflatulence Agents
Antiflatulence agents are used to relieve painful symptoms (pressure, bloating, and discomfort) of excess gas in the stomach and intestines.

ANTIDIARRHEALS

TRADE NAME	GENERIC NAME
Imodium	loperamide
Kaopectate, Pepto-Bismol	bismuth subsalicylate
Lomotil, Lonox	diphenoxylate; atropine

ANTIFLATULENCE AGENTS

TRADE NAME	GENERIC NAME
CharcoCaps	charcoal
Phazyme, Mylicon, Gas-X	simethicone

Code the following cases using ICD-10-CM.

1. The patient presented with rectal bleeding. A colonoscopy is positive for second-degree bleeding internal hemorrhoids and non-bleeding sigmoid diverticulosis. _____

2. Acute large and small intestine diverticulitis with hemorrhage _____

3. Arteriovenous malformation (angiodysplasia) of the duodenum with hemorrhage _____

4. Rectal bleeding, negative colonoscopy in a patient with alcoholic gastritis _____

5. Acute gastric ulcer with hemorrhage and perforation _____

6. Melena due to chronic duodenal ulcer _____

7. Bleeding esophageal varices _____

8. Positive Hemoccult fecal occult blood test (blood in stool) with negative endoscopic studies (*Hint:* See main term *occult.*) _____

9. Upper GI bleeding due to Barrett's esophagus _____

10. Diverticulosis, internal hemorrhoids, and upper GI bleeding, with cause of GI bleeding undetermined _____

Diseases of the Biliary System

Disorders such as cholelithiasis, pancreatitis, and liver disease constitute some of the diseases in the biliary system. Often one disorder (such as cholelithiasis) can trigger a related disease (such as pancreatitis). Coding biliary system disorders requires careful reading of all cross-references, includes notes, and excludes notes, and the use of combination codes.

Cholecystitis (inflammation of the gallbladder) is often associated with calculi (stones) in the gallbladder (cholelithiasis) or bile ducts (choledocholithiasis). Using combination codes and coding both acute and chronic conditions at the same indentation are some of the rules that apply to these conditions.

EXAMPLES
- Acute and chronic cholecystitis is assigned code K81.2.
- Acute and chronic cholecystitis with cholelithiasis is coded K80.12 (the combination code is used).
- Acute and chronic cholecystitis with choledocholithiasis is reported as K80.46.
- Acute and chronic cholecystitis with cholelithiasis and choledocholithiasis is coded K80.66.
- Chronic cholecystitis with choledocholithiasis and cholelithiasis is coded K80.64.

The presence of a stone (calculus) does not mean the presence of obstruction; documentation of obstruction is required before assigning the combination code "with obstruction." Please note that the associated condition of cholangitis is also considered in the combination codes for gallbladder and bile duct disease. For example, choledocholithiasis with acute cholangitis would be coded as K80.32.

Related conditions, such as pancreatitis, should also be reported when documented. The sequencing of the codes depends on the circumstances of admission.

Liver Cirrhosis and Hepatitis

Cirrhosis of the liver can be the underlying cause of hepatic encephalopathy. When a patient is admitted with hepatic encephalopathy associated with liver disease, the code for encephalopathy is sequenced first, followed by a code for the underlying liver disease.

Hepatitis can be acute or chronic, can be caused by a virus (type A, B, C, D, or E), or can be infectious, toxic, or alcoholic. When coding hepatitis, particularly viral hepatitis, documentation is the key to code assignment. Clarification regarding the stage of disease (acute, chronic, in remission, or history of) will determine code assignment. A physician query may be required to obtain clarification.

EXAMPLES
- Acute hepatitis C with hepatic coma. Code B17.11 is reported.
- Chronic hepatitis C. Code B18.2 is reported.
- History of hepatitis C. Code Z86.19 is reported.
- Hepatitis C in remission. Code B18.2 is reported (*see* Hepatitis, C [viral], Chronic).

Hernias of the Abdominal Cavity

Assigning accurate codes for hernias requires knowledge of the location and the type of hernia as well as careful review of subterms and the presence of associated complications such as gangrene or obstruction. For example, inguinal hernias require review of the medical record to determine whether a hernia is unilateral, bilateral, and/or recurrent. The following example highlights the importance of type and location of hernia.

EXAMPLE
Ventral incisional hernia with obstruction is coded K43.0.

CHECKPOINT 7.2

Code the following statements using ICD-10-CM.

1. Alcoholic cirrhosis of the liver (patient has alcoholism) _____

2. History of hepatitis B _____

3. Chronic hepatitis C _____

4. Acute hepatic encephalopathy with liver cirrhosis _____

5. Acute liver failure with alcoholic hepatitis (patient abuses alcohol) _____

6. Left, recurrent, incarcerated inguinal hernia _____

7. Paraumbilical hernia with gangrene _____

8. Recurrent abdominal wall hernia _____

9. Strangulated incisional hernia _____

10. Bilateral femoral hernia with gangrene _____

An entire chapter or section in the Tabular List may be subject to an Excludes1 or Excludes2 note, based on the note's location. For example, the first section in this chapter (categories L00–L08) begins with a note excluding certain skin infections that are classified in Chapter 1.

Note when coding hernias, the subterm "incarcerated" directs the coder to "*see also* Hernia by site, with obstruction." An incarcerated ventral incision hernia would also be reported K43.0.

DISEASES OF THE SKIN AND SUBCUTANEOUS TISSUE (CHAPTER 12: L00–L99)

Many conditions reported using codes from Chapter 12 of ICD-10-CM do not require hospital admission, so coders often assign these codes for physician office visits and hospital outpatient services. For example, acne, dermatitis, skin lesions, rosacea, melanoma, and abscesses are reported using this range of codes. Other conditions classified in this chapter, such as cellulitis, severe pressure ulcers, and ischemic ulcers, do require hospitalization. The focus of instruction is on the more severe conditions reported in the skin and subcutaneous tissue chapter of ICD-10-CM.

The categories in Chapter 12 of ICD-10-CM are grouped as shown in Table 7.2. The guidelines from Section I, Part C, of the *Official Guidelines for Coding and Reporting* for Chapter 12 are shown in Box 7.1.

Table 7.2 Organization of ICD–10–CM Chapter 12 Tabular List

BLOCK	BLOCK DESCRIPTION
L00–L08	Infections of skin and subcutaneous tissue
L10–L14	Bullous disorders
L20–L30	Dermatitis and eczema
L40–L45	Papulosquamous disorders
L49–L54	Urticaria and erythema
L55–L59	Radiation-related disorders of the skin and subcutaneous tissue
L60–L75	Disorders of skin appendages
L76	Intraoperative and postprocedural complications of skin and subcutaneous tissue
L80–L99	Other disorders of the skin and subcutaneous tissue

Cellulitis

Cellulitis is an infection of the deep subcutaneous tissue of the skin. Cellulitis, lymphangitis, and abscess are reported separately unless the code book cross-reference instructs the coder to report a combination code. For example "Lymphangitis with cellulitis"—code by site under Cellulitis. An abscess of the skin is coded separately by specific body site. These conditions can be caused by normal skin flora or bacteria, and cellulitis often occurs where the skin has been broken, such as by cracks in the skin, cuts, blisters, burns, insect bites, surgical wounds, or sites of intravenous catheter insertion. Cellulitis is primarily treated with appropriate antibiotics. Signs and symptoms of cellulitis include redness, swelling, pain, and heat in the infected area. Redness and swelling of a wound do not automatically mean that the patient has cellulitis. There are two important coding considerations:

1. Cellulitis reflects an infection; thus, the infectious organism should be reported as well (see the "use additional code" note at block L00–L08).
2. Cellulitis is often associated with another condition, such as a burn, wound, or ulcer, so the inpatient coder must determine the first-listed or principal diagnosis when both conditions are present.

When cellulitis is associated with an ulcer, an open wound, or a burn, the sequencing of the codes depends on the circumstances of admission/visit. If the wound or burn is minimal, or slightly treated, and the reason for the admission/visit is progression of infection to cellulitis, the cellulitis is sequenced first. If, however, the patient is seen primarily for treatment of the wound, ulcer, or burn, the cellulitis is reported as an additional diagnosis.

BOX 7.1 *Official Guidelines*: Diseases of the Skin and Subcutaneous Tissue (L00–L99)

a. Pressure Ulcer Stage Codes
 1) Pressure ulcer stages
 Codes from category L89, Pressure ulcer, are combination codes that identify the site of the pressure ulcer as well as the stage of the ulcer.
 The ICD-10-CM classifies pressure ulcer stages based on severity, which is designated by stages 1–4, unspecified stage and unstageable.
 Assign as many codes from category L89 as needed to identify all the pressure ulcers the patient has, if applicable.
 2) Unstageable pressure ulcers
 Assignment of the code for unstageable pressure ulcer (L89.–0) should be based on the clinical documentation. These codes are used for pressure ulcers whose stage cannot be clinically determined

(e.g., the ulcer is covered by eschar or has been treated with a skin or muscle graft) and pressure ulcers that are documented as deep tissue injury but not documented as due to trauma. This code should not be confused with the codes for unspecified stage (L89.–9). When there is no documentation regarding the stage of the pressure ulcer, assign the appropriate code for unspecified stage (L89.–9).

3) Documented pressure ulcer stage
Assignment of the pressure ulcer stage code should be guided by clinical documentation of the stage or documentation of the terms found in the Alphabetic Index. For clinical terms describing the stage that are not found in the Alphabetic Index, and when there is no documentation of the stage, the provider should be queried.

4) Patients admitted with pressure ulcers documented as healed
No code is assigned if the documentation states that the pressure ulcer is completely healed.

5) Patients admitted with pressure ulcers documented as healing
Pressure ulcers described as healing should be assigned the appropriate pressure ulcer stage code based on the documentation in the medical record. If the documentation does not provide information about the stage of the healing pressure ulcer, assign the appropriate code for unspecified stage.

If the documentation is unclear as to whether the patient has a current (new) pressure ulcer or if the patient is being treated for a healing pressure ulcer, query the provider.

For ulcers that were present on admission but healed at the time of discharge, assign the code for the site and stage of the pressure ulcer at the time of admission.

6) Patient admitted with pressure ulcer evolving into another stage during the admission
If a patient is admitted to an inpatient hospital with a pressure ulcer at one stage and it progresses to a higher stage, two separate codes should be assigned: one code for the site and stage of the ulcer on admission and a second code for the same ulcer site and the highest stage reported during the stay.

b. Non-Pressure Chronic Ulcers
1) Patients admitted with non-pressure ulcers documented as healed.
No code is assigned if the documentation states that the non-pressure ulcer is completely healed.

2) Patients admitted with non-pressure ulcers documented as healing
Non-pressure ulcers described as healing should be assigned the appropriate non-pressure ulcer code based on the documentation in the medical record. If the documentation does not provide information about the severity of the healing non-pressure ulcer, assign the appropriate code for unspecified severity.

If the documentation is unclear as to whether the patient has a current (new) non-pressure ulcer or if the patient is being treated for a healing non-pressure ulcer, query the provider.

For ulcers that were present on admission but healed at the time of discharge, assign the code for the site and severity of the non-pressure ulcer at the time of admission.

3) Patient admitted with non-pressure ulcer that progresses to another severity level during the admission.
If a patient is admitted to an inpatient hospital with a non-pressure ulcer at one severity level and it progresses to a higher severity level, two separate codes should be assigned: one code for the site and severity level of the ulcer on admission and a second code for the same ulcer site and the highest severity level reported during the stay.

■ **CASE SCENARIOS**
• A patient sustained a laceration to the left index finger (initial episode) and was developing *Streptococcus* cellulitis of the entire finger. The patient was treated with debridement, and antibiotics were given for the cellulitis. Code first the wound of the left index finger, then code cellulitis of the left finger. Report codes S61.211A, L03.012, B95.5.

• The same patient presented with worsening *Streptococcus* cellulitis of the left index finger requiring intravenous antibiotics. The wound was still present and infected, but no treatment was necessary. Code first the cellulitis followed by the wound of the finger (don't forget to code the infectious organism). Report codes L03.012, S61.211A, B95.5.

Cellulitis Associated With a Complication

Cellulitis may develop as a complication from a postoperative wound infection or may be a result of stoma leakage or an infected intravenous catheter site. In these instances, the complication code is sequenced first, followed by a code for the cellulitis, and then a code for the organism causing the infection, if documented.

EXAMPLES
• Cellulitis of the chest wall due to postoperative wound infection is coded (initial episode) T81.4xxA, L03.313.

- Cellulitis of the abdominal wall due to leakage from percutaneous endoscopic gastronomy (PEG) tube is coded K94.22, L03.311.
- *Staphylococcus* cellulitis of the right forearm due to infection from peripherally inserted central catheter (PICC) is coded T82.7xxA, L03.113, B95.8.

Exception for Gangrenous Cellulitis

Gangrenous cellulitis represents death of tissue, which is known as gangrene, and a code for cellulitis (L03) is *not* assigned. Instead, the code for gangrene—located in Chapter 18, Symptoms, Signs, and Abnormal Clinical and Laboratory Findings, Not Elsewhere Classified—is assigned. The underlying cause of the gangrene is reported first, followed by a code for the gangrene.

EXAMPLE
An open wound of the left thigh, initial episode, with gangrenous cellulitis is coded S71.102A, I96.

Cellulitis of Other Areas

Specific codes are reported when cellulitis is documented for sites other than the skin, so codes from categories L03 are not assigned.

EXAMPLES
- Cellulitis of anal and rectal region (K61.-).
- Cellulitis of external auditory canal (H60.1-).
- Cellulitis of eyelid (H00.03-).
- Cellulitis of female external genital organs (N76.4).
- Cellulitis of lacrimal apparatus (H04.3-).
- Cellulitis of male external genital organs (N48.22, N49.-).
- Cellulitis of mouth (K12.2).
- Cellulitis of nose (J34.0).
- Eosinophilic cellulitis (Wells syndrome) (L98.3).
- Febrile neutrophilic dermatosis (Sweet syndrome) (L98.2).
- Lymphangitis (chronic) (subacute) (I89.1).

In these cases, the infectious organism—if documented—is also coded.

CHECKPOINT 7.3

Code the following statements using ICD-10-CM.

1. Group B streptococcus cellulitis of the face _____

2. Open wound of the right lesser toe with cellulitis of the right toe (initial episode) _____

3. Acute lymphangitis of the skin of the jaw _____

4. Gangrenous cellulitis of a left ankle wound (initial episode) _____

5. Cellulitis of the right shoulder due to postoperative wound infection (initial encounter) _____

Skin Ulcers

Skin ulcers—small, open wounds due to infection, inflammation, or pressure—can be caused by many conditions. Diabetes, peripheral vascular disease, venous stasis, varicose veins, or pressure can all cause a skin ulcer. Skin ulcers are often associated with cellulitis as well. The trick in coding these conditions is to look at documentation for the cause of the ulcer and to code all conditions present. The coder may have to assign many codes, depending on the location, severity, cause, and associated infection. When the severity of a non-pressure ulcer progresses, two ulcer codes are reported to represent both levels of involvement for that site. In the outpatient setting, as an ulcer changes in severity, the code reported should reflect that change. For example: The patient presents as an inpatient with a right heel ulcer with skin breakdown (L97.411), which progresses to exposure of the fat layer (L97.412). Both codes are reported as the severity worsened during hospitalization.

Ischemic Ulcers

Ischemia means lack of blood flow to an area. An ischemic ulcer is a result of lack of blood flow to the skin. This condition may be a result of diabetic peripheral vascular disease, arteriosclerotic vascular disease, or stasis dermatitis with or without varicose veins. Typically, an ischemic ulcer is reported with a code for the underlying cause and a code for the ulcer itself (category L97). The additional digits for category L97 report the site and depth of the ulcer.

EXAMPLES

- Arteriosclerosis of the left lower leg with ulcer is coded I70.248, L97.929.
- Type 2 diabetic skin ulcer of the right heel with bone involvement is coded E11.621, L97.416.

Note that the ulcer code is sequenced as secondary, and the underlying cause is reported first. This sequencing is correct based on the *Official Guidelines* and the use of additional code conventions. The code for the ulcer is the additional code and is thus reported second.

When a patient has a chronic ischemic ulcer and cellulitis, both conditions should be reported. A chronic ischemic ulcer is reported using a code from category L97 only, and the cellulitis is reported separately. Sequencing depends on the circumstance of the admission/visit.

When the ischemic ulcer is related to a diabetic complication, two codes are assigned. Two codes are used to report the diabetes and the complication (e.g., type 2 diabetic ulcer of left heel is coded as E11.621 and L97.429). When associated with diabetes, the ulcer code (L97) is reported as a secondary diagnosis code only. If a patient also has cellulitis, the code for cellulitis is reported separately; sequencing depends on the circumstances of admission, as always.

EXAMPLES

- Type 1 diabetic with ulcer and cellulitis of the left heel. Patient was seen for acute cellulitis. Report codes E10.61, L03.116, E10.621, L97.429.
- Type 1 diabetic neuropathy with diabetic ulcer of the left heel and associated cellulitis. Patient was seen for treatment of the ulcer that involved muscle necrosis. Report codes E10.621, L97.423, E10.40, L03.116.

Venous Stasis Ulcers

Venous stasis ulcers represent a chronic venous insufficiency often due to varicose veins. In the absence of varicose veins, the code I87.2 should be reported. See the ICD-10-CM Alphabetic Index under the main term *Ulcer, stasis (varix, leg with ulcer)*. An additional code from ICD-10-CM for the ulcer site and severity (L97.-) is also reported as indicated by the "use additional code" note. If the patient has venous stasis with varicose veins and an ulcer, a code from category I83 is assigned with an additional code to identify the severity of the ulcer (L97.-).

EXAMPLES

- Infected venous stasis ulcer with skin breakdown of the right shin in a patient with varicose veins is coded I83.008, L97.901.
- Venous stasis ulcer of the left calf in a patient with no varicose veins is coded I87.2, L97.229.

Stage III and IV pressure ulcers are major complications and co-morbidities (MCCs) under the Inpatient Prospective Payment System (IPPS). The Centers for Medicare and Medicaid Services (CMS) considers pressure ulcers preventable and does not provide additional payment for inpatient services for hospital-acquired (not present on admission) stage III or IV pressure ulcers.

Pressure Ulcers

A condition often associated with inpatient or long-term care, pressure ulcers are also referred to as *decubitus ulcers, bedsores,* or *pressure sores.* Pressure ulcers are areas of damaged skin caused by staying in one position for too long. They commonly form where bones are close to skin, such as the ankles, back, elbows, heels, and hips. A person who is bedridden, uses a wheelchair, or is unable to change position is at risk. Pressure sores can cause serious infections, some of which are life threatening. They can be prevented by keeping skin clean and dry, changing position every 2 hours, and using pillows and products that relieve pressure.

Pressure ulcers can be treated in a variety of ways, including debridement and excision with a replacement skin flap or graft. The stage of the pressure ulcer might determine the treatment methodology. See the Internet Resource below for a resource that expands on stage and treatment of these specific types of ulcers.

INTERNET RESOURCES: Information on Pressure Ulcers
www.nlm.nih.gov/medlineplus/pressuresores.html

Staging Pressure Ulcers. Reporting a pressure ulcer requires a code from category L89 that classifies the location and stage of the ulcer. In ICD-10-CM, pressure ulcer stages are based on severity, assigning stages I through IV, unspecified stage, and stageable.

Codes for staging are based on the depth of the wound (see Fig. 7.1). For this reason, it is important that the coder understand the different stages of pressure ulcers as defined by the National Pressure Ulcer Advisory Panel and described as follows:

- *Stage I:* A stage I pressure ulcer is an observable pressure-related alteration of intact skin whose indicators, as compared to an adjacent or opposite area on the body, may include changes in skin temperature (warmth or coolness), tissue consistency (firm or boggy feel), and/or sensation (pain or itching). The ulcer appears as a defined area of persistent redness in lightly pigmented skin, whereas in darker skin tones, the ulcer may appear with persistent red, blue, or purple hues.
- *Stage II:* A stage II pressure ulcer is characterized by partial-thickness skin loss involving epidermis, dermis, or both. The ulcer is superficial and presents clinically as an abrasion, blister, or shallow crater.
- *Stage III:* A stage III pressure ulcer is defined as full-thickness skin loss involving damage to, or necrosis of, subcutaneous tissue that may extend down to, but not through, underlying fascia. The ulcer presents clinically as a deep crater with or without undermining of adjacent tissue. Note that the bridge of the nose, ear, occiput, and malleolus do not have subcutaneous tissue, so stage III ulcers in these locations can be shallow.
- *Stage IV:* A stage IV pressure ulcer involves full-thickness skin loss with extensive destruction, tissue necrosis, or damage to muscle, bone, or supporting structures (such as tendon, joint, or capsule). Undermining and sinus tracts also may be associated with stage IV pressure ulcers.
- *Unstageable:* In some situations, the pressure ulcer may be documented as unstageable, meaning that it is not clinically possible to determine the stage due to some circumstance such as prior treatment with a skin flap or graft or coverage with scar tissue.
- *Unspecified stage:* No documentation regarding the stage of the pressure ulcer is available. Assign the code for unspecified stage.

Documentation of the presence of a pressure ulcer is often noted by a team of skin care nurses and other health-care providers in the inpatient setting. However, in order to report a code for a pressure ulcer, the physician must document its presence (site or location). The stage can be

> ⬛● The National Pressure Ulcer Advisory Panel (NPUAP) staging system has been adopted by the Pressure Ulcer Guidelines Panel and is published in the AHRQ pressure ulcer clinical practice guidelines.

> ⬛● *Do not* confuse these codes with the unspecified stage code from (L89.–9). This code is assigned when there is no documentation indicating the stage of the pressure ulcer.

> ⬛● The stage of a pressure ulcer can be documented by level of tissue loss. For example: stage II; partial-thickness skin loss involving epidermis and/or dermis.

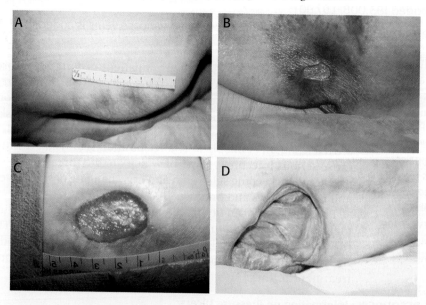

Figure 7.1 Pressure ulcers. A. Stage I, B. Stage II, C. Stage III, C. Stage IV. (From Eagle, S. *Diseases in a Flash! An Interactive, Flash-Card Approach*, F.A. Davis Company, Philadelphia, 2012, p. 117, with permission)

reported using documentation by other clinical staff members (such as the skin care team, resident, or nurse). If the documentation regarding the stage is conflicting, the patient's attending provider should be queried. This is critical for reporting accurate codes.

The unique problem in coding pressure ulcers is to recognize the documentation that specifically states the type of ulcer. For example, a patient might have diabetes with peripheral vascular disease and a pressure ulcer. The patient's diabetic condition does not automatically mean that the patient's ulcer is diabetic only. In other words, not all ulcers in people with diabetes are diabetic ulcers.

> **■ CASE SCENARIO**
> A patient presents with diabetic peripheral angiopathy with stage III decubitus ulcer of the right heel. The ulcer was the reason for admission. Codes L89.613, E11.51 are reported.

Coding Bilateral and Multiple Pressure Ulcers. If they are the same stage, bilateral pressure ulcers—such as those on both heels—are assigned one code. If bilateral pressure ulcers each have a different stage, one code is assigned for each site and stage. If the same pressure ulcer site has an increase in stage during an inpatient stay, code both stages. Report for the ulcer and stage on admission and an additional code for the second stage. Those pressure ulcers that are healed during the admission are reported only for the stage on admission.

> Review the documentation carefully; no code is assigned for *healed* pressure ulcers, while *healing* pressure ulcers are reported.

EXAMPLE
Stage I pressure ulcer of the left heel on admission which progresses to stage II on the third hospital day. Report codes L89.621 and L89.622

EXAMPLE
Stage III decubitus ulcer of the left elbow and stage II decubitus ulcer of the right elbow. Report codes L89.023, L89.012.

If a patient has more than one pressure ulcer located at different anatomical sites, such as heel, elbow, and shoulder, and each is at a different stage, codes are assigned for each pressure ulcer's site and stage.

> If a patient's pressure ulcer worsens during admission, assign codes for the stage on admission and the highest stage during that visit.

EXAMPLE
Decubitus ulcer of the left elbow, stage II, and decubitus ulcer of the right hip, stage III, are coded L89.022 and L89.213.

Present on Admission Coding of Pressure Ulcers. In the inpatient setting, it is essential to assign the present on admission (POA) indicator for decubitus ulcers correctly. If there is any doubt about the presence or stage of a decubitus ulcer, the physician should be queried for clarification.

> **■ CASE SCENARIO**
> Stage III decubitus ulcer of the buttock documented by skin care team on the third hospital day: Query physician for documentation of the decubitus ulcer, and query for presence on admission. "Dear Dr. X: The clinical care specialist documented the presence of a stage III pressure ulcer of the buttock. If you concur with this condition, please document in the progress notes/discharge summary the presence of this disease. If present, document whether the ulcer was present on admission."

CHECKPOINT 7.4

Code the following statements using ICD-10-CM.

1. Type 2 diabetic ulcer of the left foot _____

2. Chronic ischemic ulcer of the left calf with bone necrosis _____

3. Venous stasis ulcer in a patient without varicose veins _____

4. Stage II decubitus ulcer of the buttock (left) _____

5. Type 1 diabetic ulcer of the left midfoot due to diabetic neuropathy _____

PHARMACOLOGY CONNECTION

Common Medications for Diseases of the Skin and Subcutaneous Tissue

Steroids

Topical steroids are used to treat dermatitis and reduce inflammation.

Antifungals

Antifungal agents are used to treat fungal infections such as ringworm.

STEROIDS	
TRADE NAME	GENERIC NAME
Aclovate	alclometasone
Diprolene	betamethasone
Elocon	mometasone
Halog	halcinonide
Hytone	hydrocortisone
Lidex	fluocinonide
Temovate	clobetasol

ANTIFUNGALS	
TRADE NAME	GENERIC NAME
Abelcet	amphotericin b lipid complex
AmBisome	amphotericin b lipid complex
Amphotec	amphotericin b lipid complex
Cancidas	caspofungin
Diflucan	fluconazole
Fungizone	amphotericin b
Grifulvin	griseofulvin
Lamisil	terbinafine
Lotrimin	clotrimazole
Micatin	miconazole
Mycostatin	nystatin
Naftin	naftifine
Nizoral	ketoconazole
Spectazole	econazole

DISEASES OF THE MUSCULOSKELETAL SYSTEM AND CONNECTIVE TISSUE (CHAPTER 13: M00–M99)

Codes in Chapter 13 of ICD-10-CM classify conditions of the bones and joints—arthropathies (joint disorders), dorsopathies (back disorders), rheumatism, and other diseases. Unique coding guidelines apply when reporting pathological fractures with aftercare, stress fractures, and osteomyelitis from this chapter. Musculoskeletal conditions often result from trauma and are reported with codes from Chapter 19 (S00–T88). However, bone, joint, or muscle conditions that are the result of a healed injury (e.g., nonunion) or those that are recurrent are reported with codes from Chapter 13. If it is difficult to determine from the documentation in the medical record whether a condition is from acute trauma (Chapter 19) or is recurrent or healed, query the provider.

The categories in Chapter 13 of ICD-10-CM are grouped as shown in Table 7.3. The guidelines from Section I, Part C, of the *Official Guidelines for Coding and Reporting* for Chapter 13 are shown in Box 7.2.

Codes from this chapter of ICD-10-CM may require a seventh character to identify the course of treatment. For example, a seventh character A is for use as long as the patient is receiving treatment. Examples of active treatment are surgical treatment, emergency department encounter, and evaluation and treatment by a new physician. Seventh character D is to be used for encounters after the patient has completed active treatment. Additional seventh characters may also be available to identify encounters for treatment of problems associated with a fracture (e.g., malunion). Classifying laterality will also be important for diseases of the musculoskeletal system.

Arthritis

Coders address two main kinds of arthritis, osteoarthritis and rheumatoid arthritis. Osteoarthrosis, commonly called *arthritis* or *osteoarthritis (OA)*, is a type of arthritis characterized by deterioration of the

Retinoids

Compounds called *retinoids* are used for treatment of acne vulgaris.

RETINOIDS	
TRADE NAME	**GENERIC NAME**
Accutane	isotretinoin
Differin	adapalene
Panretin	alitretinoin
Retin-A	tretinoin
Soriatane	acitretin
Tazorac	tazarotene

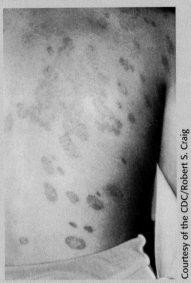

Ringworm is treated with an antifungal.

Courtesy of the CDC/Robert S. Craig

Table 7.3 Organization of ICD–10–CM Chapter 13 Tabular List

BLOCK	BLOCK DESCRIPTION
M00–M02	Infectious arthropathies
M05–M14	Inflammatory polyarthropathies
M15–M19	Osteoarthritis
M20–M25	Other joint disorders
M26–M27	Dentofacial anomalies (including malocclusion) and other disorders of jaw
M30–M36	Systemic connective tissue disorders
M40–M43	Deforming dorsopathies
M45–M49	Spondylopathies
M50–M54	Other dorsopathies
M60–M63	Disorders of muscles
M65–M67	Disorders of synovium and tendon
M70–M79	Other soft tissue disorders
M80–M85	Disorders of bone density and structure
M86–M90	Other osteopathies
M91–M94	Chondropathies
M95	Other disorders of the musculoskeletal system and connective tissue
M96	Intraoperative and postprocedural complications and disorders of musculo-skeletal system, not elsewhere classified
M99	Biomechanical lesions, not elsewhere classified

BOX 7.2 *Official Guidelines*: Diseases of the Musculoskeletal System and Connecting Tissue (M00–M99)

a. Site and Laterality

Most of the codes within Chapter 13 have site and laterality designations. The site represents the bone, joint, or muscle involved. For some conditions where more than one bone, joint, or muscle is usually involved, such as osteoarthritis, there is a "multiple sites" code available. For categories where no multiple site code is provided and more than one bone, joint, or muscle is involved, multiple codes should be used to indicate the different sites involved.

1) Bone versus joint

For certain conditions, the bone may be affected at the upper or lower end (e.g., avascular necrosis of bone, M87, Osteoporosis, M80, M81). Though the portion of the bone affected may be at the joint, the site designation will be the bone, not the joint.

b. Acute Traumatic versus Chronic or Recurrent Musculoskeletal Conditions

Many musculoskeletal conditions are a result of previous injury or trauma to a site, or are recurrent conditions. Bone, joint, or muscle conditions that are the result of a healed injury are usually found in Chapter 13. Recurrent bone, joint, or muscle conditions are also usually found in Chapter 13. Any current, acute injury should be coded to the appropriate injury code from Chapter 19. Chronic or recurrent conditions should generally be coded with a code from Chapter 13. If it is difficult to determine from the documentation in the record which code is best to describe a condition, query the provider.

c. Coding of Pathological Fractures

The seventh character A is for use as long as the patient is receiving active treatment for the fracture. Examples of active treatment are surgical treatment, emergency department encounter, evaluation, and treatment by a new physician.

7th character D is to be used for encounters after the patient has completed active treatment for the fracture and is receiving routine care for the fracture during the healing or recovery phase. The other 7th characters, listed under each subcategory in the Tabular List, are to be used for subsequent encounters for routine care of fractures during the healing and recovery phase as well as treatment of problems associated with the healing, such as malunions, nonunions, and sequelae.

Care for complications of surgical treatment for fracture repairs during the healing or recovery phase should be coded with the appropriate complication codes.

See Section I.C.19. Coding of traumatic fractures.

d. Osteoporosis

Osteoporosis is a systemic condition, meaning that all bones of the musculoskeletal system are affected. Therefore, site is not a component of the codes under category M81, Osteoporosis without current pathological fracture. The site codes under category M80, Osteoporosis with current pathological fracture, identify the site of the fracture, not the osteoporosis.

1) Osteoporosis without pathological fracture

Category M81, Osteoporosis without current pathological fracture, is for use for patients with osteoporosis who do not currently have a pathological fracture due to the osteoporosis, even if they have had a fracture in the past. For patients with a history of osteoporosis fractures, status code Z87.310, Personal history of (healed) osteoporosis fracture, should follow the code from M81.

2) Osteoporosis with current pathological fracture

Category M80, Osteoporosis with current pathological fracture, is for patients who have a current pathological fracture at the time of an encounter. The codes under M80 identify the site of the fracture. A code from category M80, not a traumatic fracture code, should be used for any patient with known osteoporosis who suffers a fracture, even if the patient had a minor fall or trauma, if that fall or trauma would not usually break a normal, healthy bone.

---

cartilage in movable joints and vertebrae. Two categories are classified in block M15–M19, primary and secondary. *Primary OA* (idiopathic) affects the apophyseal joints (joints with bony or nodular ends) of the spine, knee, hip, and certain small joints of the hands and feet. Either a generalized or a localized condition may be documented. *Secondary OA* is due to some injury (post-traumatic) or disease process (secondary) and affects only the joints of one area. Osteoarthritis is assumed primary unless otherwise stated.

■ CASE SCENARIOS

• A patient presents with post-traumatic degenerative joint disease of both knees. Code M17.2 is assigned.

• A patient has localized, primary OA of the left knee. Code M17.12 is assigned.

Rheumatoid arthritis (RA) is a chronic autoimmune disease characterized by pain, inflammation, and stiffness in the joints, muscles, or connective tissue. It may also affect the heart and lungs. Assignment of codes for RA depends on the type (juvenile, seronegative, seropositive) and presence of associated manifestations (e.g., myopathy, heart or lung involvement). When an associated manifestation is documented, a combination code reflects both the type and site of RA and the manifestation.

Pathological Fractures

A pathological fracture is a fracture that is sustained due to bone illness, rather than a fracture due to trauma. Patients with bone metastasis, severe osteoporosis, or osteoarthritis may suffer fractures because of weakened bone.

> If a patient presents with a traumatic fracture, report the condition using a code from ICD-10-CM Chapter 19. If documentation is unclear, query the provider.

In some instances, a minor trauma may cause a fracture in a patient with a pathological disease. If the fracture is due to trauma, a code from the pathological fracture category is *not* assigned. However, when minor trauma results in a fracture due to a pathological disease, the pathological fracture code, rather than the traumatic code, is assigned. For example, if the bone is already weakened due to osteoporosis, a slight fall may cause a hip fracture (fracture of the upper part of the femur) in an elderly patient. If there is any question about whether the fracture is pathological or traumatic, the physician should be queried.

Sequencing depends on the circumstance of admission/visit, but if the patient presents due to a pathological fracture, the fracture code is sequenced first, followed by a code for the underlying disease.

EXAMPLE
Pathological fracture of the left femur due to bone metastasis; patient has history of prostate cancer. Codes M84.452A, C40.22, Z85.46 are reported.

Aftercare of Pathological Fracture

The seventh character for the pathological fracture codes identifies aftercare for fracture treatment and is noted as routine healing. A code from category Z48 (Orthopedic Aftercare) is *not* assigned for fracture aftercare; rather the acute injury code is assigned with the appropriate seventh character for routine healing. A healed fracture (history of fracture) is reported using codes from category Z87, which is discussed later in this text (see Chapter 9).

EXAMPLE
Healing pathological fracture of the left femur due to bone metastasis; patient has history of prostate cancer. Codes M84.452D, C40.22, Z85.46 are reported.

> Malunions and nonunions of pathological fractures are reported using the malunion or nonunion code–seventh character associated with the fracture site.

Complications of Treatment of Pathological Fractures

Complications of treatment of pathologic fractures with artificial materials such as prosthetics and mechanical devices are coded as *complications* from ICD-10-CM Chapter 19, Injury and Poisoning, categories T80–T88, Complications of surgical and medical care, not elsewhere classified. Thus, fracture of a prosthetic joint replacement of the knee used to treat a previous pathologic fracture would be reported using the complication code T84.01–. Chapter 9 of this text covers complications due to failure of prosthetic or mechanical devices used to treat pathological fractures.

Stress Fractures

Stress fractures, also known as *stress reactions*, are caused by repetitive injuries or by overuse, which can cause movement of the bone. Other causes of stress fractures include increased physical stress or intensity of activity, poor equipment, or impact on poor surfaces. Stress fractures are more common in such bones as the spine, femur, lower leg bones, and foot bones. Stress fractures are also classified to Chapter 13 of ICD-10-CM.

The codes for stress fractures align with the common types of stress fractures:

M84.36-	Stress fracture of tibia or fibula
M84.34-	Stress fracture of the metatarsals
M48.4-	Stress fracture of vertebra

PHARMACOLOGY CONNECTION

Common Medications for Conditions of the Musculoskeletal System and Connective Tissue

Analgesics

Analgesics are drugs used to relieve pain. Opioid analgesics are used for moderate to severe pain, but they can be addictive.

Salicylates

Salicylates are drugs used to reduce inflammation and reduce associated pain.

ANALGESICS	
TRADE NAME	GENERIC NAME
	codeine
Darvon*	propoxyphene
Demerol*	meperidine
Dilaudid*	hydromorphone
Dolophine*	methadone
MS Contin, Oramorph*	morphine
Opana*	oxymorphone
OxyContin*	oxycodone
Tylenol	acetaminophen
Ultram*	tramadol
*Opioid agents.	

SALICYLATES	
TRADE NAME	GENERIC NAME
aspirin	acetylsalicylic acid
Dolobid	diflunisal
Salsitab	salsalate

■ **CASE SCENARIO**

A karate instructor saw the physician for pain in the ankle and was diagnosed with a stress fracture of the right fibula. Code M84.363A is reported.

CHECKPOINT 7.5

Code the following statements using ICD-10-CM.

1. Pathological fracture of the left distal radius due to postmenopausal osteoporosis, initial encounter _____

2. Fracture of the distal right tibia due to chronic osteomyelitis, initial encounter _____

3. Nonunion of pathologic fracture of right humerus _____

4. Aftercare of healing pathological fracture of the left femur _____

5. Traumatic arthritis of the left ankle _____

Osteomyelitis

Osteomyelitis is an infection of the bone. The infection can be acute, subacute, hematogenous, and/or chronic. The code assignment for osteomyelitis from category M86 is dependent on the type, location, and acuity (acute, subacute, hematogenous, and/or chronic).

NSAIDs

NSAIDs are used to reduce inflammation and associated pain.

Corticosteroids

Corticosteroids are potent anti-inflammatory drugs.

NSAIDs

TRADE NAME	GENERIC NAME
Clinoril	sulindac
Daypro	oxaprozin
Feldene	piroxicam
Indocin	indomethacin
Mobic	meloxicam
Motrin	ibuprofen
Nalfon	fenoprofen
Naprosyn/Anaprox	naproxen
Voltaren/Cataflam	diclofenac

CORTICOSTEROIDS

TRADE NAME	GENERIC NAME
Celestone	betamethasone
Cortef	hydrocortisone
Decadron	dexamethasone
Florinef	fludrocortisone
Medrol	methylprednisolone
Prelone	prednisolone

Many conditions can cause osteomyelitis (e.g., skin ulcers, decubitus ulcers, and other infections). In these cases, both conditions are reported, and the sequencing depends on the circumstances of admission. Additional codes are also assigned for major osseous defects and the infectious agent.

■ **CASE SCENARIOS**
- A patient presents with acute osteomyelitis of the left calcaneus due to stage IV decubitus ulcer of the left heel. Assign codes M86.172, L89.624.

- A patient presented with chronic osteomyelitis of the left calcaneus, and now presents with new decubitus ulcer stage II of the left heel requiring IV antibiotics and debridement. Assign codes L89.622, M86.572.

CHECKPOINT 7.6

Code the following statements using ICD-10-CM.

1. Acute osteomyelitis of the mandible _____

2. Subacute osteomyelitis of the right radius _____

3. Osteomyelitis of the toe due to typhoid _____

4. Sclerosing, nonsuppurative osteomyelitis of the hip _____

5. Chronic osteomyelitis of the left third toe with draining sinus _____

Documentation of the specific acuity of osteomyelitis must be completed by the physician. Therefore, this aspect of osteomyelitis cannot be coded based on pathology results and diagnostic x-rays alone. If the specific type of osteomyelitis is documented on a bone scan (e.g., acute osteomyelitis of the tibia) and the physician documents osteomyelitis alone, the physician should be queried for documentation to support the specific type or acuity of the osteomyelitis.

DISEASES OF THE GENITOURINARY SYSTEM (CHAPTER 14: N00–N99)

Disorders of the genitourinary (GI) system are classified in ICD-10-CM Chapter 14. These include diseases of the male and female genitourinary (GU) systems, such as infections of the genital tract, renal disease, conditions of the prostate, and problems with the cervix, vulva, and breast. Genitourinary diseases encompass diseases such as renal failure, female genital prolapse, and benign prostatic hypertrophy. Many of these disorders require careful review of coding conventions such as "code also," "use additional code," and "code underlying condition first" notes.

The categories in Chapter 14 of the ICD-10-CM are grouped as shown in Table 7.4. Box 7.3 presents the applicable guidelines from Section I, Part C, of the *Official Guidelines*.

Table 7.4 Organization of ICD-10-CM Chapter 10 Tabular List

BLOCK	BLOCK DESCRIPTION
N00–N08	Glomerular diseases
N10–N16	Renal tubulo-interstitial diseases
N17–N19	Acute kidney failure and chronic kidney disease
N20–N23	Urolithiasis
N25–N29	Other disorders of kidney and ureter
N30–N39	Other diseases of the urinary system
N40–N53	Diseases of male genital organs
N60–N65	Disorders of breast
N70–N77	Inflammatory diseases of female pelvic organs
N80–N98	Noninflammatory disorders of female genital tract
N99	Intraoperative and postprocedural complications and disorders of genitourinary system, not elsewhere classified

Chronic Kidney Disease and Renal Failure

Kidney disease is the ninth leading cause of death in the United States. Nearly 26 million people are afflicted with chronic kidney disease (CKD), which includes conditions that damage the kidneys and decrease their ability to keep people healthy; another 20 million are at risk of developing it. When kidney disease worsens, it results in buildup of wastes in the blood, possibly resulting in complications such as high blood pressure, anemia, and nerve damage. Chronic kidney disease may be caused by diabetes, hypertension, or other disorders. If kidney disease progresses, the patient may develop chronic kidney failure and may require renal dialysis or renal transplant. End-stage renal disease (ESRD), or loss of kidney function, caused by either CKD or acute renal failure results in around 67,000 deaths each year in the United States. ESRD is reported as stage 6 in ICD-10-CM.

Coding of CKD depends on the associated complications and the stage of disease. Measurement of the glomerular filtration rate (GFR) is the accepted test of the level of kidney function, and its results determine the stage of kidney disease. The National Kidney Foundation identifies five stages of chronic kidney disease, as illustrated in Figure 7.2. Additional information regarding CKD can be found at the website listed below.

INTERNET RESOURCE: Kidney Disease
www.kidney.org/kidneydisease

a. **Chronic Kidney Disease**
   1) **Stages of chronic kidney disease (CKD)**
      The ICD-10-CM classifies CKD based on severity. The severity of CKD is designated by stages 1–5. Stage 2, code N18.2, equates to mild CKD; stage 3, code N18.3, equates to moderate CKD; and stage 4, code N18.4, equates to severe CKD. Code N18.6, End-stage renal disease (ESRD), is assigned when the provider has documented ESRD.
      If both a stage of CKD and ESRD are documented, assign code N18.6 only.
   2) **Chronic kidney disease and kidney transplant status**
      Patients who have undergone kidney transplant may still have some form of chronic kidney disease (CKD), because the kidney transplant may not fully restore kidney function. Therefore, the presence of CKD alone does not constitute a transplant complication. Assign the appropriate N18 code for the patient's stage of CKD and code Z94.0, Kidney transplant status. If a transplant complication such as failure or rejection or other transplant complication is documented, see Section I.C.19.g for information on coding complications of a kidney transplant. If the documentation is unclear as to whether the patient has a complication of the transplant, query the provider.
   3) **Chronic kidney disease with other conditions**
      Patients with CKD may also suffer from other serious conditions, most commonly diabetes mellitus and hypertension. The sequencing of the CKD code in relationship to codes for other contributing conditions is based on the conventions in the Tabular List.
      See I.C.9. Hypertensive chronic kidney disease.
      See I.C.19. Chronic kidney disease and kidney transplant complications.

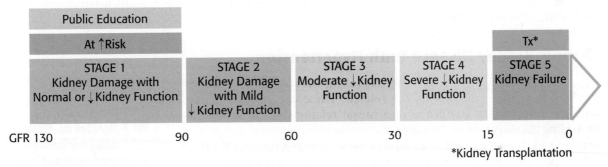

Figure 7.2 Five stages of chronic kidney disease.

For a patient on renal dialysis, an additional code, Z99.2 (renal dialysis status), is assigned.

Code the highest stage of CKD. The code for CKD stage 5 with end-stage renal disease is N18.6.

These five stages correlate exactly with the ICD-10-CM codes for CKD. As noted in the Tabular List, CKD is reported using codes from category N18 (Table 7.5). The third digit classifies the stage of disease.

This background material will help the coder understand the disease process. But remember that the coder cannot code from lab results (in this case, GFR) alone. If the physician does not document the stage of disease, the lab results may be the basis for a physician query. If the physician uses an outdated term such as *renal failure* or *renal insufficiency* without clarifying whether the condition is acute or chronic, a query is required. The physician also must document the stage of the disease, the underlying cause or pathology if known, and any manifestations, such as anemia.

Table 7.5 Category N18 Codes

CODE	CKD STAGE
N18.1	Chronic kidney disease, stage 1
N18.2	Chronic kidney disease, stage 2 (mild)
N18.3	Chronic kidney disease, stage 3 (moderate)
N18.4	Chronic kidney disease, stage 4 (severe)
N18.5	Chronic kidney disease, stage 5
N18.6	End stage renal disease
N18.9	Chronic kidney disease, unspecified

Chronic Kidney Disease and Renal Transplant Status

A patient who has undergone a kidney transplant may still have some CKD; the transplanted organ may not restore full renal function. The presence of CKD alone does not constitute a transplant complication. If a transplant complication such as renal failure or rejection is documented, a complication code from category T86 is reported rather than the code for status post-transplant (Z94.0). Complication codes, external cause codes, and Z codes are covered in depth in Chapter 9 of this text.

EXAMPLES

• Stage IV CKD, status post–renal transplant, is coded N18.4, Z94.0.

• Acute renal failure due to transplant rejection is coded T86.11, N17.9, Y83.0.

If documentation is unclear in terms of whether a complication is present, a physician query for clarification is appropriate.

Chronic Kidney Disease With Hypertension

Often, the guidelines direct the coder regarding documentation requirements when coding conditions are related. These are guidelines that require the physician to document a causal relationship for a particular coding combination to be assigned. For the genitourinary chapter of ICD-10-CM, however, coders are instructed to *assume* a cause-and-effect relationship between CKD and hypertension. Also, as noted earlier, when hypertension is paired with conditions that would be coded from category N18 (CKD), the hypertension code changes to a combination code from category I12 or I13 (hypertensive heart and/or chronic kidney disease). All patients with hypertensive kidney disease have both hypertension and some stage of CKD. The appropriate code for hypertensive kidney disease is sequenced first, followed by a secondary code indicating the stage of CKD from category N18. The codes from category I12 or I13 are combination codes that include hypertension, heart disease, and/or chronic kidney disease. A decision tree for making these coding decisions is provided in Pinpoint the Code 7.1.

Remember: The physician must state a causal relationship between hypertension and heart disease. Patients with hypertensive heart disease and CKD would have a code assigned for hypertension, cardiorenal.

The section on category I12, Hypertensive chronic kidney disease, in the Tabular List includes instructions on the use of the additional CKD codes (Box 7.4).

BOX 7.4 Category I12 From ICD-10-CM

I12   Hypertensive chronic kidney disease.

Includes: any condition in N18 and N26—due to hypertension.
arteriosclerosis of kidney.
arteriosclerotic nephritis (chronic) (interstitial).
hypertensive nephropathy.
nephrosclerosis.

Excludes1: hypertension due to kidney disease (I15.0, I15.1).
renovascular hypertension (I15.0).
secondary hypertension (I15.-).

Excludes2: acute kidney failure (N17.-).

I12.0 Hypertensive chronic kidney disease with stage 5 chronic kidney disease or end stage renal disease.
Use additional code to identify the stage of chronic kidney disease (N18.5, N18.6).

I12.9 Hypertensive chronic kidney disease with stage 1 through stage 4 chronic kidney disease, or unspecified chronic kidney disease.
Hypertensive chronic kidney disease NOS.
Hypertensive renal disease NOS.
Use additional code to identify the stage of chronic kidney disease (N18.1–N18.4, N18.9).

PINPOINT THE CODE 7.1: CKD and Hypertension

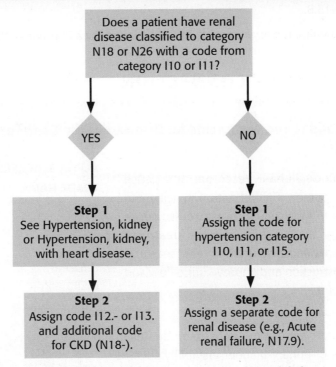

The third digit for category N18 identifies the presence of renal failure. CKD stages 5 and 6 qualify as renal failure. Thus, when reporting code I12.0 (hypertensive renal disease with renal failure), the CKD code would be either N18.5 (stage 5) or N18.6 (end stage). If the stage of CKD is not documented or if CKD is in stages 1 through 4, the hypertensive renal disease is assigned code I12.9.

EXAMPLES

• Hypertension and CKD is coded I12.9, N18.9.

• Hypertensive renal disease, stage 3, is coded I12.9, N18.3.

• End-stage renal disease, hypertension, is coded I12.0, N18.6.

Acute Renal Failure

Acute renal failure (ARF) is the sudden loss of kidney function that occurs when the kidneys do not filter waste from the blood. It is clinically defined as a greater than 50% decrease in GFR over a period of hours or days. It may result from a drastic drop in blood pressure, blockage of blood vessels to the kidneys, or obstructed urine flow.

The assumed association between renal disease and hypertension does not apply to ARF. It applies only to renal disease classified to categories N18. ARF is classified to category N17.

There is no linkage of hypertensive renal disease and acute renal failure, and both conditions are reported.

EXAMPLE
Acute and chronic renal failure, hypertension, is coded N17.9, I12.9, N18.9.

Acute renal failure can also result from dehydration or other disorders such as benign prostatic hypertrophy. Renal failure is a progression of renal insufficiency in which renal function is further impaired. The physician uses more than just an abnormal lab finding to diagnose renal failure; renal failure includes both clinical findings and abnormal lab results (blood urea nitrogen [BUN], creatinine). Documentation might include elevated BUN, creatinine or decreased creatinine clearance, and progression of clinical disorders of hyperkalemia, acidemia, and uremia. While laboratory results alone are not enough to assign a diagnosis of renal failure, a physician query may be appropriate to clarify the presence or absence of the disease given these results.

When coding ARF with other conditions, all sequencing rules apply.

EXAMPLES
• Acute renal failure due to dehydration is coded N17.9, E86.0.

• Acute renal failure due to benign prostatic hypertrophy with obstructive uropathy is coded N17.9, N40.1, N13.8.

Note: In these examples, the acute renal failure occasioned the admission/visit.

PHARMACOLOGY CONNECTION

Common Medications and Treatments for Diseases of the Genitourinary System

Alpha Blockers
Alpha blockers block alpha-1 receptors and cause smooth muscle relaxation. This relaxation in veins and arteries will result in lower blood pressure. However, the primary use for these agents is in the treatment of BPH. These agents decrease urethral resistance and may relieve the obstruction and improve urine flow and other BPH symptoms.

ALPHA BLOCKERS	
TRADE NAME	GENERIC NAME
Cardura	doxazosin
Flomax	tamsulosin
Hytrin	terazosin
Uroxatral	alfuzosin

Anticholinergics
Anticholinergic agents are bladder antispasmodics used to treat symptoms of urinary bladder instability such as dysuria, urgency, nocturia, frequency, and incontinence.

ANTICHOLINERGICS	
TRADE NAME	GENERIC NAME
Detrol	tolterodine
Ditropan	oxybutynin
Enablex	darifenacin
Sanctura	trospium
VESIcare	solifenacin

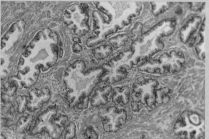

Courtesy of the CDC/Dr. Edwin P. Ewing, Jr.

Prostate cancer cells.

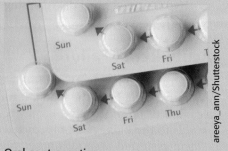

areeya_ann/Shutterstock

Oral contraceptives.

Urinary Calculi

Stones, or calculi, can cause disease, infection, obstruction, and complications in the urinary system. They can be located in the kidney (nephrolithiasis), ureter, and bladder. From a coding perspective, it is important to understand that the conditions *associated with* the calculi (such as hydronephrosis, pyelonephritis, and other infections) should be considered in code assignment. Combination codes are used to report these additional conditions. In the presence of infection, an additional code to identify the infectious agent is also assigned.

EXAMPLES

- Documentation supports the presence of a left ureteral calculus with obstructive hydronephrosis. The combination code N13.2 is assigned.

- Documentation supports the presence of left ureteral calculus with acute *E. coli* pyelonephritis and obstructive hydronephrosis. The codes N13.6 and B96.20 are assigned.

On the other hand, conditions *attributed to* renal calculi (such as hematuria or dysuria) should not be reported separately, because they are integral to the calculi.

EXAMPLES

- Hematuria and urinary retention due to bladder calculi. Report codes N21.0, R33.8.

- Impacted renal calculi with hematuria and acute pyelonephritis. Report code N20.0.

- Bilateral ureteral calculi with dysuria. Report code N20.1.

Oral Contraceptives

Oral contraceptives are combinations of female hormones that are used for contraception.

Hormones

Synthetic female sex hormones are used as replacements, often after female menopause.

HORMONES

TRADE NAME	GENERIC NAME
Climara	estradiol
Megace	megestrol
Menest	esterified estrogens
Ogen	estropipate
Premarin	conjugated estrogens
Provera	medroxyprogesterone

ORAL CONTRACEPTIVES

TRADE NAME	GENERIC NAME
Apri	desogestrel and ethinyl estradiol
Aviane	levonorgestrel and ethinyl estradiol
Balziva	norethindrone and ethinyl estradiol
Cryselle	norgestrel and ethinyl estradiol
Fem con	norethindrone and ethinyl estradiol
Kariva	desogestrel and ethinyl estradiol
Lo Estrin 24 Fe	norethindrone and ethinyl estradiol
Lo/Ovral	norgestrel and ethinyl estradiol
Ortho Evra	norelgestromin and ethinyl estradiol
TriNessa	norgestimate and ethinyl estradiol
Yasmin	drospirenone and ethinyl estradiol

Benign Prostatic Hypertrophy

Benign prostatic hypertrophy (BPH), or prostatic hyperplasia, is noncancerous enlargement of the prostate and requires careful attention to the "code also" notes in the Tabular List. When the enlarged prostate includes lower urinary tract symptoms, the additional symptoms should be reported.

EXAMPLE
The codes used to report benign prostatic hypertrophy with urinary frequency are N40.1 (BPH with urinary symptoms) and R35.0 (urinary frequency).

Treatment for BPH is often a prostatectomy, and pathology results may support the presence of microscopic foci of carcinoma. The coder also has to be careful to apply the Uniform Hospital Discharge Data Set (UHDDS) definition of principal diagnosis when pathology results support such findings. In most cases, the reason for admission to the hospital is for treatment of BPH, so the code for BPH is sequenced first. In the presence of physician documentation supporting carcinoma of the prostate, the carcinoma should be reported as a secondary diagnosis, because the condition may affect future care.

Genital Prolapse

Genital prolapse, meaning prolapse of the uterine or vaginal wall, can result from a variety of causes. Pelvic floor relaxation can result from childbearing, removal of the uterus, obesity, or postmenopausal atrophy. The different types of prolapse include vaginal prolapse and uterine prolapse.

Vaginal prolapse is classified to the specific type of prolapse (see category N81):

- *Cystocele:* a protrusion of the bladder into the vagina
- *Urethrocele:* a protrusion of the urethra into the vaginal canal
- *Rectocele:* a bulge into the vagina due to prolapse of the rectum through the rectovaginal septum
- *Perineocele:* a hernia between the rectum and vagina
- *Cystourethrocele:* a protrusion of the urethra and bladder into the vagina

Uterine prolapse is classified using code N81.2 unless it is combined with a vaginal prolapse (see Prolapse, ureterovaginal). When both a uterine and a vaginal prolapse are present, the coder must consider whether the prolapse is complete or incomplete. The coder must be aware of combination codes and cross-references when coding genital prolapse.

EXAMPLES
- Rectocele with female urinary stress incontinence is coded N81.6, N39.3.

- Incomplete uterine prolapse with rectocele and mixed urinary incontinence is coded N81.2, N39.46.

Urinary Tract Infections

Urinary tract infection (UTI) is a generic term used to describe an infection in an unspecified site of the urinary system. Specific sites of infection have specific names, such as infection in the urethra, which is termed *urethritis*. The code for UTI (N39.0) should be assigned only when the specific site of urinary infection is not documented. If UTI is documented along with a specific site of urinary infection (cystitis, pyelonephritis, or urethritis), the code for UTI is not assigned. Remember to code the causative organism if documented (see "code also" notes).

Urinary infections can be caused by postoperative complications or urinary catheters. When a specific complication causes the UTI, the complication code is sequenced first. For example, a postoperative UTI is reported using codes N99.89, N39.0, Y83.1, and an additional code for the causative organism if known. Note that the presence of a UTI in a patient who has had surgery or a catheter does not mean the UTI is a complication. A causal relationship between the medical service and UTI must be documented in order for the complication codes to be assigned (see Chapter 9).

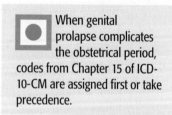
When genital prolapse complicates the obstetrical period, codes from Chapter 15 of ICD-10-CM are assigned first or take precedence.

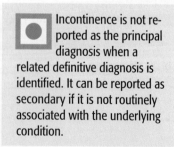
Incontinence is not reported as the principal diagnosis when a related definitive diagnosis is identified. It can be reported as secondary if it is not routinely associated with the underlying condition.

Some patients have recurrent or chronic UTIs without current symptoms. These patients often receive prophylactic antibiotics. In this case, a current acute UTI is not present, and the UTI code is not assigned. Reporting chronic UTI requires the code assignment of Z87.440 (personal history of UTI) along with code Z79.2 (long-term use of antibiotics) when the patient is taking prophylactic antibiotics.

Remember, the coder cannot code from lab results alone, but positive urine culture results are an indication of the need for a physician query.

CHECKPOINT 7.7

Code the following statements using ICD-10-CM.

1. Benign hypertension, end-stage renal disease; patient is on renal dialysis _____

2. Person with type 1 diabetes with CKD stage 4 _____

3. Acute renal failure due to obstructive uropathy from prostatic hyperplasia _____

4. Cystocele and rectocele with stress urinary incontinence _____

5. Chronic renal failure, hypertension _____

6. Hematuria due to calculus of the bladder _____

7. Adenofibromatous hypertrophy of the prostate with urinary frequency, and urinary hesitancy

   _____

8. Acute renal failure, dehydration, and hyperkalemia _____

9. Acute pyelonephritis due to ureteral calculus with hydronephrosis _____

10. Urethral stricture _____

11. Solitary renal cyst _____

12. Phimosis _____

13. Monilial cystitis (*Hint:* Monilial infection is coded to candidiasis.) _____

14. Endometriosis of the fallopian tubes and ovaries _____

15. Infertility due to adhesions of the fallopian tubes _____

16. Acute pelvic inflammatory disease due to *Staphylococcus* _____

17. Encysted hydrocele _____

18. Premenopausal menorrhagia _____

19. Male bladder prolapsed _____

20. Kinking of the ureter _____

21. UTI with acute pyelonephritis _____

22. Acute cystitis due to *E. coli* _____

23. Chronic UTI; patient taking prophylactic antibiotics (*Hint:* Note code as history of UTI and

    long-term use of antibiotics.) _____

24. Acute urethritis due to urethral catheter (*Hint:* See complication due to catheter.) _____

25. Newborn UTI (*Hint:* Code from the chapter containing conditions in the perinatal period.)

    _____

Chapter Summary

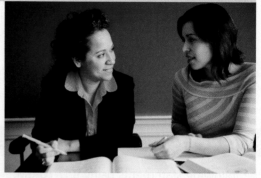

1. Disorders of the digestive system are coded from categories K00–K95. Correct coding requires knowledge of the disease process and paying careful attention to combination codes, excludes notes, and use of fifth digits. Gastrointestinal bleeding, a common condition, is coded according to location. Combination codes are available that code the underlying cause of the bleeding and/or complications such as obstruction or perforation.

2. Cellulitis of the skin may require two codes, one for the condition and the other for its cause. Cellulitis can be present alone or can be a manifestation of another wound. Sequencing of cellulitis is dependent on the circumstances of admission. If the reason for inpatient admission was progression of infection to cellulitis, the cellulitis is sequenced first. If, however, the patient is seen primarily for treatment of a wound, ulcer, or burn, cellulitis is an additional diagnosis. Complications of wounds and postoperative infections can cause cellulitis; the complication code is sequenced first, followed by a code for the cellulitis, then a code for the organism causing the infection, if documented. Gangrenous cellulitis (coded as gangrene) can occur as a complication of diabetes or other vascular disorders; the cause is coded, followed by a gangrene code; the cellulitis is not coded.

3. When coding ischemic and venous stasis ulcers, the underlying disease (ischemia due to atherosclerosis, venous insufficiency) is reported first, with an additional code assigned to report the associated ulcer. The coding convention of "use additional code" reminds the coder to assign both codes.

4. Pressure ulcers are staged according to the severity and depth. Stage I is an observable pressure-related alteration of intact skin. Stage II is characterized by partial-thickness skin loss involving the epidermis, dermis, or both. Stage III is defined as full-thickness skin loss involving damage to, or necrosis of, subcutaneous tissue that may extend down to, but not through, underlying fascia. Stage IV involves full-thickness skin loss with extensive destruction, tissue necrosis, or damage to muscle, bone, or supporting structures.

5. In some instances, a pressure ulcer (decubitus ulcer) is considered unstageable. When documentation is insufficient and the stage is unknown, it is considered an "unspecified" stage. When coding decubitus ulcers, a combination code is assigned to reflect the site of the ulcer and the stage of the ulcer. If the stage of the pressure ulcer at the same site worsens, code the stage on admission and the highest stage for the visit.

6. When coding pathological fractures, the underlying disease must be considered to assign the correct code. An additional code may be required to report the underlying condition when a combination code is not available (see "code also" notes). Pathological fracture codes also require the seventh character to indicate the episode of care (e.g., initial treatment, nonunion). Minor trauma can result in a pathological fracture; the physician should be queried if documentation is unclear.

7. Osteomyelitis is an infection in the bone that can result from a variety of conditions. When osteomyelitis is due to diabetes, both the code for diabetes and the code for osteomyelitis are reported. Osteomyelitis can be acute, subacute, chronic, and/or have an associated draining sinus.

8. ICD-10-CM classifies CKD based on severity, from stages 1 through 5 and ESRD. When both ESRD and a stage of CKD are documented, only code N18.6 is assigned. Patients with CKD may also suffer from other serious conditions, most commonly diabetes mellitus and hypertension. There is an assumed relationship between hypertension and CKD, which requires two codes. The first code identifies hypertensive renal disease (I11); the second code classifies the stage of CKD. The sequencing of the CKD code in relationship to codes for other contributing conditions is based on the conventions in the Tabular List.

9. Coding genitourinary disorders such as female cystocele, rectocele, and/or vaginal prolapse requires additional codes to report related symptoms such as incontinence. Male genitourinary

disorders, such as hypertrophy of the prostate, also require additional codes to report lower urinary tract symptoms such as urinary frequency. Always verify codes in the Tabular List and pay careful attention to conventions that instruct the coder to assign additional codes.

10. *Urinary tract infection* is a broad term for conditions such as pyelonephritis or cystitis that describe the exact site of infection. When coding these infections, recognize that the underlying cause of the infection and the infectious organism impact the code assignment.

Review Questions

Matching

Match the key terms with their definitions.

A. end-stage renal disease
B. cellulitis
C. unstageable
D. stage 3 CKD
E. gangrene
F. hematochezia
G. pressure ulcer

H. ischemic ulcer
I. causal relationship
J. stage III pressure ulcer
K. stress fracture
L. osteomyelitis
M. pathological fracture

1. __A__ Renal disease stage requiring transplantation or dialysis

2. __D__ A form of kidney disease where the GFR is between 30 and 59

3. __F__ Passage of fresh blood in the stool

4. __H__ An ulcer caused by lack of blood flow

5. __I__ Cause and effect

6. __B__ An infection of the skin

7. __C__ A pressure ulcer that cannot be assigned a stage because of the way it presents

8. __E__ The death of tissue

9. __G__ Also called *decubitus ulcer*

10. __M__ A fracture that is due to osteoporosis

11. __J__ Full-thickness skin loss due to pressure

12. __L__ An infection of the bone

13. __K__ A fracture that is due to repetitive injury

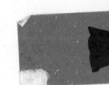

True or False

Decide whether each statement is true or false.

1. _____ A causal relationship between hypertension must be documented in order to assign codes for hypertensive kidney disease.

2. _____ Hyperkalemia is one condition that can be associated with ARF.

3. _____ A patient presented with GI bleeding. Colonoscopy was positive for diverticulosis. The code assigned is diverticulosis with hemorrhage.

4. _____ Documentation of the specific spinal cord disc space (i.e., C3-C4) affects code assignment when reporting primary osteoarthritis of the spine.

5. _____ *Melena* refers to bloody vomitus.

6. _____ The code for stress incontinence should be reported separately when coding vaginal prolapse.

7. _____ There are a total of three different stages of pressure (decubitus) ulcers.

8. _____ If a fracture is due to trauma, a pathological fracture code would not be assigned.

9. _____ In the statement "dysuria due to possible urinary tract infection," the infection code would be assigned as the primary diagnosis in the outpatient setting.

10. _____ Two codes are required to report a stage II pressure ulcer.

11. _____ When coding a venous stasis ulcer of the calf (no mention of varicose vein), only one code is assigned.

Multiple Choice

Select the letter that best completes the statement or answers the question.

1. Vaginal prolapse with rectocele is coded as
   A. N81.10, N81.6
   B. N81.12, N81.6
   C. N81.2
   D. N81.12, N81.2

2. Arteriosclerotic peripheral vascular disease with left heel ulcer is coded as
   A. I70.244
   B. I70.744, L97.429
   C. I70.244, L97.429
   D. L97.429

3. Hematuria due to renal calculus with hydronephrosis is coded as
   A. N13.2, R31.9
   B. N20.0, N13.30
   C. N20.0
   D. N13.2

4. Angiodysplasia of the large intestine with hemorrhage is coded as
   A. K55.20
   B. K31.811
   C. K55.21
   D. K31.819

5. Bleeding esophageal varices with related cirrhosis of liver and chronic hepatitis C is coded as
   A. K74.60, I85.11, B18.2
   B. I85.11, B19.20
   C. K74.60, B18.2
   D. I85.11, K74.60, B19.20

6. Acute cholecystitis with cholelithiasis and choledocholithiasis is coded as
   A. K81.0, K80.50, K80.20
   B. K80.42
   C. K80.00
   D. K80.62

7. Decubitus ulcer of the sacrum, stage III, with gangrene. The patient also had cellulitis with lymphangitis of the left lower shin. What are the correct codes?
   A. L89.153, L03.116
   B. L89.153, I96, L03.116, I89.1
   C. L89.152, I96, L03.116
   D. I96, L03.116, I89.1

8. Herniated disc, C5-C6 with radiculopathy is coded as
   A. M50.12
   B. M50.022
   C. M50.10
   D. M50.11

CHAPTER 8

ICD-10-CM Chapters 15 Through 17: O00–Q99

CHAPTER OUTLINE

Pregnancy, Childbirth, and the Puerperium (Chapter 15: O00–O9A)

Certain Conditions Originating in the Perinatal Period
  (Chapter 16: P00–P96)

Congenital Malformations, Deformations, and Chromosomal
Abnormalities (Chapter 17: Q00–Q99)

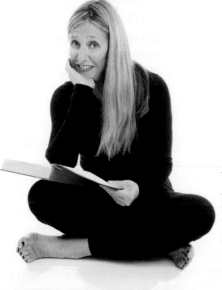

Jrwasserman/iStock/Thinkstock

LEARNING OUTCOMES

After studying this chapter, you should be able to:

1. Define the period of time associated with the process of pregnancy and childbirth indicated by the terms *antepartum, postpartum*, and *peripartum*.
2. Identify the correct use of the final character, which classifies trimester.
3. Assign the seventh character for fetus identification in certain categories.
4. Sequence obstetrical diagnoses based on official reporting guidelines.
5. Discuss code assignment for a normal delivery.
6. Describe the purpose and correct assignment of outcome of delivery codes.
7. Differentiate preexisting conditions versus conditions due to the pregnancy.
8. Discuss the correct coding of conditions that affect the mother, such as HIV infection in pregnancy and diabetes related to pregnancy.
9. Discuss the coding of a pregnancy with an abortive outcome.
10. Explain the criterion of implications for future health-care needs in coding perinatal conditions.
11. Discuss coding of community-acquired conditions in the perinatal period.
12. Describe the coding guidelines for perinatal conditions resulting from maternal factors.
13. Compare and contrast codes for maternal and newborn conditions.
14. Describe the correct assignment of codes for congenital conditions.

Correct code assignment and sequencing of patients' complications involving pregnancy and childbirth, congenital anomalies, and perinatal period–related conditions require careful review of the guidelines because these conditions have sequencing priority over other codes from other chapters. The structure and organization of the corresponding ICD-10-CM Tabular List chapters are presented, followed by discussions of code selection and sequencing as instructed by the *ICD-10-CM Official Guidelines for Coding and Reporting,* Section I, Part C, 15–17. The focus is on common code assignment decisions and complex coding scenarios.

PREGNANCY, CHILDBIRTH, AND THE PUERPERIUM (CHAPTER 15: O00–O9A)

Complications can occur during pregnancy, childbirth, and the puerperium. *Pregnancy* is the period from conception to delivery; *childbirth* refers to the birth of the child and delivery of the placenta; and the *puerperium* is the period immediately after childbirth and continuing up to the time the uterus returns to normal size, usually defined as 42 days. These conditions are coded from ICD-10-CM Chapter 15.

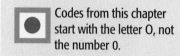

Codes from this chapter start with the letter O, not the number 0.

> **INTERNET RESOURCE:** The stages of pregnancy by trimester
> http://www.womenshealth.gov/pregnancy/you-are-pregnant/stages-of-pregnancy.html

The categories in Chapter 15 of ICD-10-CM are grouped as shown in Table 8.1. Box 8.1 presents the applicable guidelines from Section I, Part C, for Chapter 15 of the *Official Guidelines.*

General Guidelines

Codes from ICD-10-CM Chapter 15 are assigned only to a maternal record, never to a newborn record. An important additional code note from this chapter instructs the coder to report an additional code from category Z3A.-, weeks of gestation, to identify the specific week of pregnancy at the time of the maternal visit. A maternal record represents a patient who is in the obstetrical period, the time span between conception and 6 weeks after delivery. A code representing a complication of pregnancy or delivery can be assigned for service beyond the obstetrical period when the complication is still pregnancy related.

> ■ **CASE SCENARIO**
> A patient receives treatment for postpartum depression 8 weeks after delivery. A code from Chapter 15 should be assigned, even though the obstetrical period has ended.

Codes from Chapter 15 have sequencing priority over codes from other chapters. The rationale for this guideline is that the provider's treatment decisions are based on how the treatments will affect the baby and patient during the entire obstetrical period. Often codes from other chapters are assigned as additional codes to provide further detail. When pregnancy is incidental to the encounter, the code Z33.1 is assigned rather than a code from Chapter 15.

Table 8.1 Organization of ICD-10-CM Chapter 15 Tabular List

BLOCK	BLOCK DESCRIPTION
O00–O08	Pregnancy with abortive outcome
O09	Supervision of high-risk pregnancy
O10–O16	Edema, proteinuria, and hypertensive disorders in pregnancy, childbirth, and the puerperium
O20–O29	Other maternal disorders predominantly related to pregnancy
O30–O48	Maternal care related to the fetus and amniotic cavity and possible delivery problems
O60–O77	Complications of labor and delivery
O80–O82	Encounter for delivery
O85–O92	Complications predominantly related to the puerperium
O94–O9A	Other obstetric conditions, not elsewhere classified

A pregnant patient presents to the emergency department due to a right ring finger laceration. The pregnancy is considered incidental to the laceration. The laceration code S61.214A is reported first, and Z33.1 (incidental pregnancy) is reported as an additional code.

BOX 8.1 *Official Guidelines*: Pregnancy, Childbirth, and the Puerperium (O00–O99)

a. General Rules for Obstetric Cases

1) Codes from Chapter 15 and sequencing priority

Obstetric cases require codes from Chapter 15, codes in the range O00–O9A, Pregnancy, Childbirth, and the Puerperium. Chapter 15 codes have sequencing priority over codes from other chapters. Additional codes from other chapters may be used in conjunction with Chapter 15 codes to further specify conditions. Should the provider document that the pregnancy is incidental to the encounter, then code Z33.1, Pregnant state, incidental, should be used in place of any Chapter 15 codes. It is the provider's responsibility to state that the condition being treated is not affecting the pregnancy.

2) Chapter 15 codes used only on the maternal record

Chapter 15 codes are to be used only on the maternal record, never on the record of the newborn.

3) Final character for trimester

The majority of codes in Chapter 15 have a final character indicating the trimester of pregnancy. The timeframes for the trimesters are indicated at the beginning of the chapter. If trimester is not a component of a code it is because the condition always occurs in a specific trimester, or the concept of trimester of pregnancy is not applicable. Certain codes have characters for only certain trimesters because the condition does not occur in all trimesters, but it may occur in more than just one.

Assignment of the final character for trimester should be based on the provider's documentation of the trimester (or number of weeks) for the current admission/encounter. This applies to the assignment of trimester for pre-existing conditions as well as those that develop during or are due to the pregnancy. The provider's documentation of the number of weeks may be used to assign the appropriate code identifying the trimester.

Whenever delivery occurs during the current admission, and there is an "in childbirth" option for the obstetric complication being coded, the "in childbirth" code should be assigned.

4) Selection of trimester for inpatient admissions that encompass more than one trimester

In instances when a patient is admitted to a hospital for complications of pregnancy during one trimester and remains in the hospital into a subsequent trimester, the trimester character for the antepartum complication code should be assigned on the basis of the trimester when the complication developed, not the trimester of the discharge. If the condition developed prior to the current admission/encounter or represents a pre-existing condition, the trimester character for the trimester at the time of the admission/encounter should be assigned.

5) Unspecified trimester

Each category that includes codes for trimester has a code for "unspecified trimester." The "unspecified trimester" code should rarely be used, such as when the documentation in the record is insufficient to determine the trimester and it is not possible to obtain clarification.

6) 7th character for fetus identification

Where applicable, a 7th character is to be assigned for certain categories (O31, O32, O33.3– O33.6, O35, O36, O40, O41, O60.1, O60.2, O64, and O69) to identify the fetus for which the complication code applies. Assign 7th character "0":

- For single gestations
- When the documentation in the record is insufficient to determine the fetus affected and it is not possible to obtain clarification.
- When it is not possible to clinically determine which fetus is affected.

b. Selection of OB Principal or First-Listed Diagnosis

1) Routine outpatient prenatal visits

For routine outpatient prenatal visits when no complications are present, a code from category Z34, Encounter for supervision of normal pregnancy, should be used as the first-listed diagnosis. These codes should not be used in conjunction with Chapter 15 codes.

2) Supervision of high-risk pregnancy

Codes from category O09, Supervision of high-risk pregnancy, are intended for use only during the prenatal period. For complications during the labor or delivery episode as a result of a high-risk pregnancy, assign the applicable complication codes from Chapter 15. If there are no complications during the labor or delivery episode, assign code O80, Encounter for full-term uncomplicated delivery.

Continued

BOX 8.1 *Continued*

For routine prenatal outpatient visits for patients with high-risk pregnancies, a code from category O09, Supervision of high-risk pregnancy, should be used as the first-listed diagnosis. Secondary chapter 15 codes may be used in conjunction with these codes if appropriate.

3) Episodes when no delivery occurs

In episodes when no delivery occurs, the principal diagnosis should correspond to the principal complication of the pregnancy which necessitated the encounter. Should more than one complication exist, all of which are treated or monitored, any of the complications codes may be sequenced first.

4) When a delivery occurs

When an obstetric patient is admitted and delivers during that admission, the condition that prompted the admission should be sequenced as the principal diagnosis. If multiple conditions prompted the admission, sequence the one most related to the delivery as the principal diagnosis. A code for any complication of the delivery should be assigned as an additional diagnosis. In cases of cesarean delivery, if the patient was admitted with a condition that resulted in the performance of a cesarean procedure, that condition should be selected as the principal diagnosis. If the reason for the admission was unrelated to the condition resulting in the cesarean delivery, the condition related to the reason for the admission should be selected as the principal diagnosis.

5) Outcome of delivery

A code from category Z37, Outcome of delivery, should be included on every maternal record when a delivery has occurred. These codes are not to be used on subsequent records or on the newborn record.

c. Pre-Existing Conditions Versus Conditions Due to the Pregnancy

Certain categories in Chapter 15 distinguish between conditions of the mother that existed prior to pregnancy (pre-existing) and those that are a direct result of pregnancy. When assigning codes from Chapter 15, it is important to assess if a condition was pre-existing prior to pregnancy or developed during or due to the pregnancy in order to assign the correct code.

Categories that do not distinguish between pre-existing and pregnancy-related conditions may be used for either. It is acceptable to use codes specifically for the puerperium with codes complicating pregnancy and childbirth if a condition arises postpartum during the delivery encounter.

d. Pre-Existing Hypertension in Pregnancy

Category O10, Pre-existing hypertension complicating pregnancy, childbirth, and the puerperium, includes codes for hypertensive heart and hypertensive chronic kidney disease. When assigning one of the O10 codes that includes hypertensive heart disease or hypertensive chronic kidney disease, it is necessary to add a secondary code from the appropriate hypertension category to specify the type of heart failure or chronic kidney disease.

See Section I.C.9. Hypertension.

e. Fetal Conditions Affecting the Management of the Mother

1) Codes from categories O35 and O36

Codes from categories O35, Maternal care for known or suspected fetal abnormality and damage, and O36, Maternal care for other fetal problems, are assigned only when the fetal condition is actually responsible for modifying the management of the mother, i.e., by requiring diagnostic studies, additional observation, special care, or termination of pregnancy. The fact that the fetal condition exists does not justify assigning a code from this series to the mother's record.

2) In utero surgery

In cases when surgery is performed on the fetus, a diagnosis code from category O35, Maternal care for known or suspected fetal abnormality and damage, should be assigned identifying the fetal condition. Assign the appropriate procedure code for the procedure performed.

No code from Chapter 16, the perinatal codes, should be used on the mother's record to identify fetal conditions. Surgery performed in utero on a fetus is still to be coded as an obstetric encounter.

f. HIV Infection in Pregnancy, Childbirth, and the Puerperium

During pregnancy, childbirth, or the puerperium, a patient admitted because of an HIV-related illness should receive a principal diagnosis from subcategory O98.7–, Human immunodeficiency [HIV] disease complicating pregnancy, childbirth and the puerperium, followed by the code(s) for the HIV-related illness(es).

Patients with asymptomatic HIV infection status admitted during pregnancy, childbirth, or the puerperium should receive codes of O98.7– and Z21, Asymptomatic human immunodeficiency virus [HIV] infection status.

g. Diabetes Mellitus in Pregnancy

Diabetes mellitus is a significant complicating factor in pregnancy. Pregnant women who are diabetic should be assigned a code from category O24, Diabetes mellitus in pregnancy, childbirth, and the puerperium, first, followed by the appropriate diabetes code(s) (E08–E13) from Chapter 4.

h. Long-Term Use of Insulin and Oral Hypoglycemics

See section I.C.4.a.3 for information on the long-term use of insulin and oral hypoglycemic.

i. Gestational (Pregnancy Induced) Diabetes

Gestational (pregnancy induced) diabetes can occur during the second and third trimester of pregnancy in women who were not diabetic prior to pregnancy. Gestational diabetes can cause complications in the pregnancy similar to those of pre-existing diabetes mellitus. It also puts the woman at greater risk of developing diabetes after the pregnancy. Codes for gestational diabetes are in subcategory O24.4, Gestational diabetes mellitus. No other code from category O24, Diabetes mellitus in pregnancy, childbirth, and the puerperium, should be used with a code from O24.4.

The codes under subcategory O24.4 include diet controlled, insulin controlled, and controlled by oral hypoglycemic drugs. If a patient with gestational diabetes is treated with both diet and insulin, only the code for insulin-controlled is required. If a patient with gestational diabetes is treated with both diet and oral hypoglycemic medications, only the code for "controlled by oral hypoglycemic drugs" is required. Code Z79.4, Long-term (current) use of insulin or code Z79.84, Long-term (current) use of oral hypoglycemic drugs, should not be assigned with codes from subcategory O24.4.

An abnormal glucose tolerance in pregnancy is assigned a code from subcategory O99.81, Abnormal glucose complicating pregnancy, childbirth, and the puerperium.

j. Sepsis and Septic Shock Complicating Abortion, Pregnancy, Childbirth, and the Puerperium

When assigning a Chapter 15 code for sepsis complicating abortion, pregnancy, childbirth, and the puerperium, a code for the specific type of infection should be assigned as an additional diagnosis. If severe sepsis is present, a code from subcategory R65.2, Severe sepsis, and code(s) for associated organ dysfunction(s) should also be assigned as additional diagnoses.

k. Puerperal Sepsis

Code O85, Puerperal sepsis, should be assigned with a secondary code to identify the causal organism (e.g., for a bacterial infection, assign a code from category B95–B96, Bacterial infections in conditions classified elsewhere). A code from category A40, Streptococcal sepsis, or A41, Other sepsis, should not be used for puerperal sepsis. If applicable, use additional codes to identify severe sepsis (R65.2–) and any associated acute organ dysfunction.

l. Alcohol and Tobacco Use during Pregnancy, Childbirth, and the Puerperium

1) Alcohol use during pregnancy, childbirth, and the puerperium

Codes under subcategory O99.31, Alcohol use complicating pregnancy, childbirth, and the puerperium, should be assigned for any pregnancy case when a mother uses alcohol during the pregnancy or postpartum. A secondary code from category F10, Alcohol related disorders, should also be assigned to identify manifestations of the alcohol use.

2) Tobacco use during pregnancy, childbirth, and the puerperium

Codes under subcategory O99.33, Smoking (tobacco) complicating pregnancy, childbirth, and the puerperium, should be assigned for any pregnancy case when a mother uses any type of tobacco product during the pregnancy or postpartum. A secondary code from category F17, Nicotine dependence, should also be assigned to identify the type of nicotine dependence.

m. Poisoning, Toxic Effects, Adverse Effects and Underdosing in a Pregnant Patient

A code from subcategory O9A.2, Injury, poisoning and certain other consequences of external causes complicating pregnancy, childbirth, and the puerperium, should be sequenced first, followed by the appropriate injury, poisoning, toxic effect, adverse effect or underdosing code, and then the additional code(s) that specifies the condition caused by the poisoning, toxic effect, adverse effect or underdosing. *See Section I.C.19. Adverse effects, poisoning, underdosing and toxic effects.*

n. Normal Delivery, Code O80

1) Encounter for full-term uncomplicated delivery

Code O80 should be assigned when a woman is admitted for a full-term normal delivery and delivers a single, healthy infant without any complications antepartum, during the delivery, or postpartum during the delivery episode. Code O80 is always a principal diagnosis. It is not to be used if any other code from Chapter 15 is needed to describe a current complication of the antenatal, delivery, or perinatal period. Additional codes from other chapters may be used with code O80 if they are not related to or are in any way complicating the pregnancy.

2) Uncomplicated delivery with resolved antepartum complication

Code O80 may be used if the patient had a complication at some point during the pregnancy, but the complication is not present at the time of the admission for delivery.

3) Outcome of delivery for O80

Z37.0, Single live birth, is the only outcome of delivery code appropriate for use with O80.

o. The Peripartum and Postpartum Periods

1) Peripartum and postpartum periods

The postpartum period begins immediately after delivery and continues for six weeks following delivery. The peripartum period is defined as the last month of pregnancy to five months postpartum.

2) Peripartum and postpartum complication

A postpartum complication is any complication occurring within the six-week period.

Continued

BOX 8.1 *Continued*

3) Pregnancy-related complications after 6-week period

Chapter 15 codes may also be used to describe pregnancy-related complications after the peripartum or postpartum period if the provider documents that a condition is pregnancy related.

4) Admission for routine postpartum care following delivery outside hospital

When the mother delivers outside the hospital prior to admission and is admitted for routine postpartum care and no complications are noted, code Z39.0, Encounter for care and examination of mother immediately after delivery, should be assigned as the principal diagnosis.

5) Pregnancy-associated cardiomyopathy

Pregnancy-associated cardiomyopathy, code O90.3, is unique in that it may be diagnosed in the third trimester of pregnancy but may continue to progress months after delivery. For this reason, it is referred to as peripartum cardiomyopathy. Code O90.3 is only for use when the cardiomyopathy develops as a result of pregnancy in a woman who did not have pre-existing heart disease.

p. Code O94, Sequelae of Complication of Pregnancy, Childbirth, and the Puerperium

1) Code O94

Code O94, Sequelae of complication of pregnancy, childbirth, and the puerperium, is for use in those cases when an initial complication of a pregnancy develops sequelae requiring care or treatment at a future date.

2) After the initial postpartum period

This code may be used at any time after the initial postpartum period.

3) Sequencing of code O94

This code, like all sequelae codes, is to be sequenced following the code describing the sequelae of the complication.

q. Termination of Pregnancy and Spontaneous Abortions

1) Abortion with liveborn fetus

When an attempted termination of pregnancy results in a liveborn fetus, assign code Z33.2, Encounter for elective termination of pregnancy, and a code from category Z37, Outcome of delivery.

2) Retained products of conception following an abortion

Subsequent encounters for retained products of conception following a spontaneous abortion or elective termination of pregnancy, without complications are assigned the appropriate code from category O03.4, Incomplete spontaneous, abortion without complication, or codes O07.4, Failed attempted termination of pregnancy without complication and Z33.2, Encounter for elective termination of pregnancy. This advice is appropriate even when the patient was discharged previously with a discharge diagnosis of complete abortion. If the patient has a specific complication associated with the spontaneous abortion or elective termination of pregnancy in addition to retained products of conception, assign the appropriate complication in category O03 or O07 instead of code O03.4 or O07.4.

3) Complications leading to abortion

Codes from Chapter 15 may be used as additional codes to identify any documented complications of the pregnancy in conjunction with codes in categories in O04, O07, and O08.

r. Abuse in a Pregnant Patient

For suspected or confirmed cases of abuse of a pregnant patient, a code(s) from subcategories O9A.3, Physical abuse complicating pregnancy, childbirth, and the puerperium, O9A.4, Sexual abuse complicating pregnancy, childbirth, and the puerperium, and O9A.5, Psychological abuse complicating pregnancy, childbirth, and the puerperium, should be sequenced first, followed by the appropriate codes (if applicable) to identify any associated current injury due to physical abuse, sexual abuse, and the perpetrator of abuse.

See Section I.C.19. Adult and child abuse, neglect and other maltreatment.

The physician is responsible for documenting that a pregnancy is incidental to another condition. (*Obstetrical complications* are conditions that affect the management of the pregnancy or are exacerbated by it.) In fact, most conditions aggravate or have an impact on a pregnancy, or a pregnancy aggravates or has an impact on a condition, and in these cases, a code from Chapter 15 is assigned. Only when the physician documentation supports *no* relationship between the conditions can the incidental codes be used.

> ■ To find codes from Chapter 15, research the main terms *pregnancy* or *delivery*, or the subterms *complicating pregnancy, childbirth,* or *puerperium* under specific conditions, such as diabetes, in the Alphabetic Index of ICD-10-CM.

■ CASE SCENARIOS

• A patient is 6 weeks pregnant and has known hypothyroidism. Report codes O99.281, Z3A.01, E03.9.

Childbirth and Conditions Related to Pregnancy

Coding conditions that are related to pregnancy as well as to childbirth require an understanding of the terms that cover the pregnancy and birth process.

Antepartum, Postpartum, and Peripartum Periods

The antepartum period is the time span between conception and delivery of the placenta. Conditions arising antepartum include delivery of the infant, lacerations during delivery, and cord entanglements. Conditions that are postpartum arise immediately following delivery of the placenta and continue for 6 weeks, such as postpartum hemorrhage and anemia. The peripartum period is the time span from the last month of pregnancy to 5 months postpartum.

Final Character for Trimester

Most of the codes in Chapter 15 require a final character to indicate the trimester of pregnancy. The trimesters are counted from the first day of the last menstrual period and are defined as follows:

First trimester: less than 14 weeks 0 days
Second trimester: 14 weeks 0 days to less than 28 weeks 0 days
Third trimester: 28 weeks 0 days until delivery

For example, a patient who is noted to be at 12 weeks 3/7 is 12 weeks and 3 days pregnant, or in the first trimester. For inpatient visits, the trimester upon admission is assigned for the obstetrical conditions, unless the hospitalization extends over two trimesters and a complication develops.

When no choice is provided for classifying the trimester, it is because the condition reported always occurs in a specific trimester. Thus, the trimester is inherent in the code.

When *delivery* occurs during the current admission and there is an "in childbirth" option for the obstetrical complication being coded, the "in childbirth" code should be assigned rather than the code for the complication and the trimester. For example, for a patient with preexisting diabetes mellitus, type 2, who is undelivered at 30 weeks, codes O24.113, E11.9, and Z3A.30 would be reported. For a patient with preexisting diabetes mellitus, type 2 who is admitted and delivers at 38 weeks, codes O24.12 (preexisting diabetes mellitus, type 2, *in childbirth*), E11.9 (diabetes, type 2), and Z3A.38 (38 weeks of gestation) would be reported.

In some instances, patients are hospitalized for longer periods of time, and complications that begin in one trimester extend to a subsequent trimester when the patient remains in the hospital. In this situation, the trimester character should reflect the trimester when the complication developed. If the condition developed prior to the current visit or represents a preexisting condition, the trimester character for the trimester at the time of the visit is assigned.

Seventh Character for Fetus Identification

The seventh character for certain categories classifies to which fetus the complication code applies. These categories are O31, O32, O33.3–O33.6,

O35, O36, O40, O41, O60.1, O60.2, O64, and O69. The seventh character is defined at the category level. The seventh character of 0 (zero) is assigned for the following conditions:

1. For single gestations
2. When documentation of the fetus affected is insufficient and cannot be clarified
3. When it is clinically not possible to determine which fetus is affected

An example of this seventh character code is "Twin pregnancy complicated by breech presentation of fetus #1," code O32.1xx1.

CHECKPOINT 8.1

Identify the trimester represented in the following cases.

1. The patient is 34 weeks pregnant. _____

2. The patient is 12 weeks pregnant. _____

3. The patient is 14 weeks 3/7 pregnant. _____

4. The patient was admitted in the third trimester and developed gestational diabetes at 26 weeks requiring oral hypoglycemics. _____

5. The patient was admitted at 27 weeks with pregnancy-induced hypertension and was discharged during the 29th week. _____

Please answer the following questions:

6. Which trimester character should rarely be used? _____

7. Is the trimester character assigned when there is an "in childbirth" option? _____

8. Code O33.6xx2 reflects a multiple gestation pregnancy with a problem with the second fetus. True or false? _____

9. When reporting code O33.5xx, what is the seventh character assigned for a single newborn? _____

10. What is the seventh character assigned when it is not clinically possible to determine the fetus affected when assigning code O40.3xx? _____

Selection of the Principal Diagnosis

The coder always assigns the principal diagnosis based on the Uniform Hospital Discharge Data Set (UHDDS) definitions discussed throughout this text. Some specific guidelines based on issues related to pregnancy have been developed to help in the coding decision. These include routine prenatal visits and visits for episodes when delivery does or does not occur.

Routine Outpatient Prenatal Visits

The reporting of the first-listed diagnosis for a routine outpatient prenatal visit depends on the absence or presence of high risk. A routine outpatient prenatal visit is classified from category Z34. Additional codes from Chapter 15 should not be used in conjunction with this category.

Routine, uncomplicated prenatal visits should be reported with the principal diagnosis of Z34.0-, Supervision of normal first pregnancy (primigravida), or Z34.9-, Supervision of other normal pregnancy (multigravida). These codes are also used as the admitting diagnosis (not the principal diagnosis) for patients admitted for delivery. To determine whether the patient is primigravida or multigravida, review of the obstetrical history for previous deliveries is helpful.

In instances of a routine outpatient visit in patients with high-risk situations or prenatal visits due to pregnancy complications, codes Z34.0- and Z34.9- are not assigned. The codes for Supervision of high-risk pregnancy (category O09) is sequenced first followed by the code(s) for the high-risk condition from Chapter 15. The code from category O09 is sequenced first during high-risk prenatal care visits.

When the visit is for labor or delivery, and the complication is present, report the code from Chapter 15 that represents the complication. If there are no complications during the labor and delivery visit, then assign code O08 for routine uncomplicated delivery. For instance, elderly primigravida, also known as *advanced maternal age (AMA)*, is considered a high-risk pregnancy because the mother will be 35 years of age or older at the expected date of delivery (code O09.511).

EXAMPLES
- The outpatient visit for normal first pregnancy during the 1st trimester is coded Z34.01.

- The outpatient visit during the 18th week of pregnancy with high-risk pregnancy due to history of preterm labor is coded O09.211, Z3A.18.

- The outpatient visit for urinary tract infection (UTI) during the 14 weeks 3/7 pregnancy is coded O23.92, Z3A.14, N39.0.

- The outpatient visit during the eighth week for high-risk pregnancy due to a young primigravida who also has gestational diabetes is coded O09.611, O24.419, Z3A.08.

When No Delivery Occurs in the Inpatient Setting
The principal diagnosis for an episode in which no delivery occurs should be the condition or pregnancy complication that necessitated the encounter. If more than one pregnancy complication was treated and monitored, either complication code may be sequenced first.

> **■ CASE SCENARIO**
> A patient presents at 24 weeks with premature labor and mild preeclampsia and does not deliver. Codes O60.02, O14.02, Z3A.24 are reported. Either obstetrical code can be sequenced first.

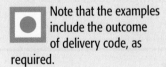
A pregnant woman who does not have a history of hypertension but develops it during the course of pregnancy can acquire preeclampsia, or pregnancy-induced hypertension. This condition must be treated to avoid abruptio placentae (premature separation of the placenta from the uterine wall, which may cause massive internal hemorrhage), acute renal failure, and intrauterine growth restrictions for the fetus.

Note that the examples include the outcome of delivery code, as required.

When Delivery Occurs
Selection of the principal diagnosis for encounters in which delivery occurs can depend on the type of delivery and any complications. When an obstetric patient requires admission, the principal diagnosis rule applies. In other words, the condition which prompts the admission should be listed first. In the instance where multiple conditions require admission, then sequence the condition most closely related to the delivery first.

When the patient delivers via cesarean section, the principal diagnosis should be the condition necessitating the cesarean delivery unless the reason for admission was an unrelated condition resulting in cesarean delivery.

> **■ CASE SCENARIOS**
> - A patient presents at full term (40 weeks), single gestation, and requires cesarean section for cephalopelvic disproportion. Codes O33.9, Z3A.40, Z37.0 are assigned.
>
> - A patient presents at 38 2/7 weeks with oligohydramnios and requires induction of labor. Cesarean section is required after a failed trial of labor due to fetal bradycardia. The codes assigned are O41.03x0, O36.833, Z3A.38, Z37.0 (notice that the reason for admission was oligohydramnios, code O41.03x0).

Outcome of Delivery
On every episode in which a delivery occurs, the mother's coded data must include an outcome of delivery code from category Z37. An outcome of delivery code (found in the Alphabetic Index under the main term *Outcome*) must be reported only once for the visit in which the delivery occurred. Verify the coding by making sure that an outcome of delivery code is reported as a secondary diagnosis for maternal cases with the principal diagnosis of O80 (normal delivery) or Chapter 15 codes with the designation "in childbirth."

Normal delivery at 29 weeks in a patient with a family history of congenital anomalies is coded O80, Z82.79, Z37.0, Z3A.39.

The outcome of delivery code Z37.0 is the only secondary diagnosis code that can be assigned with code O80 (normal delivery of a full-term liveborn infant). Other Z codes relating to the patient's history may be assigned, as in the example, where Z82.79 is assigned to indicate a family history of congenital anomalies.

Preexisting Conditions Versus Conditions Due to Pregnancy

Certain categories in Chapter 15 require the coder to differentiate whether a condition existed prior to pregnancy (preexisting) or was a direct result of pregnancy (developed during pregnancy). Other categories may not distinguish when the condition developed. Other codes are available to identify obstetrical conditions that are present postpartum (in the puerperium)—for example:

- Preexisting diabetes mellitus, type 2, in the 38th week (not delivered) is assigned codes O24.113, E11.9, Z3A.38.
- Preexisting diabetes mellitus, type 2, in the 38th week, (delivered) is assigned codes O24.12, E11.9, Z3A.38, Z37.0.
- Preexisting diabetes mellitus, type 2, treated postpartum is assigned codes O24.13, E11.9.

NOTE: A Z3A category code is not required because the pregnancy is completed.

Preexisting hypertension in pregnancy is classified as category O10. This includes codes for hypertensive heart disease and hypertensive chronic and kidney disease. An additional code is required from the hypertension category when certain hypertension and pregnancy (O10) codes are reported. For example, when a patient with preexisting hypertension and hypertensive chronic kidney disease, stage 2, delivers a single liveborn baby at 38 weeks, the codes assigned are O10.22, I12.9, N18.2, Z3A.38, Z37.0.

CHECKPOINT 8.2

Code the following statements using ICD-10-CM.

1. The patient presents to the hospital during the 12th week due to insulin-controlled gestational diabetes. _____

2. The patient delivers a single liveborn infant at 39 weeks. The patient has preexisting hypertension. _____

3. The patient presents with chorioamnionitis at 37 weeks and delivers a single liveborn infant. _____

4. The patient presents for a routine outpatient prenatal visit at 13 weeks during a normal first pregnancy. _____

5. The patient presents to the physician office during her first pregnancy for a routine high-risk prenatal visit. The patient is high risk because of her age of 40 (elderly primigravida). Her visit is during week 22. _____

Fetal Conditions Affecting Management of the Mother

Sometimes a fetal condition requires the mother to undergo specific treatment, diagnostic services, or monitoring or to terminate the pregnancy. For example, the fetus may have a chromosomal abnormality or a malformation that requires special services or surgery in utero. Codes from categories O35 and O36 (conditions arising in the child during the perinatal period) should be assigned on the mother's record. The fact that a fetal condition is present does not justify including that condition on the record of the mother's encounter. Only when the fetal condition affects the management of the mother should these codes be

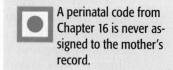
A perinatal code from Chapter 16 is never assigned to the mother's record.

reported. Category O35 is used when surgery is performed on the fetus, and this code identifies the fetal condition.

> ■ **CASE SCENARIO**
> A patient in the 26th week of pregnancy presents for induction of labor with delivery due to fetal distress detected at an outpatient encounter. Codes O36.8920, Z3A.26, Z37.0 are assigned.

HIV Infection

During the obstetrical period, reporting of an HIV infection requires the use of code O98.7-. An additional code for the HIV status (asymptomatic HIV infection) should also have the code Z21 reported. In patients with HIV-related disease (AIDS), additional codes for the HIV disease are also reported. Code O98.7- is reported first with the additional code B20.

> ■ **CASE SCENARIO**
> An HIV-positive patient admitted at full term delivers a normal newborn at 39 weeks. Report codes O98.72, Z21, Z3A.39, Z37.0.

Diabetes Mellitus in Pregnancy

Diabetes mellitus can occur before pregnancy or can result from pregnancy (gestational diabetes). In either instance, the diabetes is a complicating factor in the pregnancy. The code for gestational diabetes is O24.4-. No code from category E10 or E11 is assigned and code includes the type of control. For example, gestational diabetes in pregnancy with diet control is assigned code O24.410 with an additional code for weeks of gestation.

A gestational diabetes code should never be assigned for a patient who had preexisting diabetes—that is, diabetes that was diagnosed before the pregnancy. For such a patient, assign a code from subcategory O24 (preexisting diabetes mellitus) and an additional code for the type of diabetes from category E10 or E11. For example, a patient presents to the physician office at 29 weeks and has type 2 diabetes requiring oral hypoglycemic medications, the codes assigned are O24.113, E11.9, Z79.84, Z3A.29.

An abnormal glucose tolerance test is assigned a code from subcategory O99.81-. This represents an abnormal glucose test without a diagnosis of diabetes mellitus being established.

Sepsis Complicating Abortion, Pregnancy, Childbirth, and the Puerperium

These types of sepsis codes vary depending on when the sepsis occurred (e.g., during labor or following an abortion). An additional code is assigned for the specific type of infection; in cases of severe sepsis, a third code (R65.2-) is also reported. When coding puerperal sepsis, code O85, an additional code is required to identify the organism from category B95 or B96. Do not assign a code from category A40 or A41.

> ■ **CASE SCENARIO**
> A patient presents with severe streptococcus sepsis during labor at 37 weeks. Report codes O75.3, R65.20, B95.5, Z3A.37, Z37.0.

Alcohol and Tobacco Use During the Obstetrical Period

Again we prioritize the code that combines the pregnancy with the associated alcohol or tobacco use by reporting a code from Chapter 15. In this case, codes from O99.3- represent the alcohol and/or tobacco use during the obstetrical period. The coder must assign an additional code to identify the alcohol use and related manifestations or the tobacco use or dependence. Smoking should be assigned for any pregnancy case when a mother uses any type of tobacco product during the obstetrical period.

Normal Delivery

When a patient presents for delivery and the conditions for a normal delivery are met, the normal delivery code, O80, is assigned. A normal delivery has taken place when a woman is admitted for a full-term normal delivery, a single healthy infant is born, no antepartum complications are present, no delivery complications arise, and no postpartum complications occur during the delivery episode (admission). Code O80 is also assigned if an antepartum complication that has resolved is not present at the time of the admission for delivery.

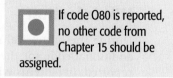 If code O80 is reported, no other code from Chapter 15 should be assigned.

Code O80 is always the principal diagnosis. Additional codes from other ICD-10-CM chapters may be assigned with this code if the diseases are not in any way related to the pregnancy or causing a complication of pregnancy. The only additional codes appropriate with O80 are outcome of delivery Z37.0 (single liveborn) and weeks of gestation Z3A.37–Z3A.40.

Postpartum Complications

Complications arising within the 6 weeks immediately following delivery are considered postpartum complications. Any complications after the 6-week period require physician documentation that they are pregnancy related; these conditions should also be reported as a postpartum complication. Routine postpartum visits are reported using code Z39.0 when a patient is admitted immediately after delivery without complications. Pregnancy-associated cardiomyopathy (O90.3) is a unique condition usually diagnosed in the third trimester and can continue into the postpartum period. For this reason, only code O90.3 is assigned for women who develop this condition during pregnancy. No preexisting heart disease should be present when assigning code O90.3.

Code Z39.0 represents postpartum care and observation in uncomplicated cases. If the mother delivered outside the hospital and had a complication of pregnancy, the complication code is reported instead of observation code Z39.0.

Present on Admission Reporting for Obstetrical Conditions When Reporting Hospital Inpatient Services

Whether the patient delivers during the current hospitalization does not affect assignment of the present-on-admission (POA) indicator. The determining factor for POA assignment is whether the pregnancy complication or obstetrical condition described by the code is present at the time of admission. According to the *Official Guidelines:*

Many commonly reported principal diagnoses—such as first-, second-, and third-degree lacerations with delivery; abnormal fetal heart rate with delivery; primary uterine inertia with delivery; and complicated labor and delivery—are not present on admission, so they carry POA indicator N even if listed first.

- If the pregnancy complication or obstetrical condition is present on admission (e.g., the patient is admitted in preterm labor), assign indicator Y.
- If the pregnancy complication or obstetrical condition is not present on admission (e.g., second-degree laceration during delivery, postpartum hemorrhage that occurs during current hospitalization, fetal distress that develops after admission), assign indicator N.

Code the following statements using ICD-10-CM (no need to report weeks of gestation or outcome of delivery).

1. A mother delivers a single liveborn infant at 39 weeks. The mother has gestational diabetes controlled with diet and is dependent on cigarettes. _____

2. The patient who is HIV positive presents for a routine high-risk antepartum visit at 12 weeks. _____

3. A mother presents to the office due to a single gestation fetal chromosomal abnormality at 25 weeks. _____

4. A mother presents full term at 39 weeks and delivers (in childbirth) a single liveborn infant. Her pregnancy was complicated by preexisting type 2 diabetes that requires long-term insulin use. _____

5. A patient presents with sepsis complicating the postpartum period. _____

6. A patient experiences a normal delivery of a single liveborn at 39 weeks. _____

7. A patient was treated for a urinary tract infection during the 12th week of pregnancy. This resolved, and the patient was admitted at 40 weeks when she delivered a single liveborn infant without complications. _____

8. A patient returns to the hospital 2 weeks postpartum for breast engorgement. _____

9. A patient delivered her full-term newborn at home and presents immediately after delivery for routine postpartum care. _____

10. A patient presents at 38 weeks and requires induction of labor due to pregnancy-associated cardiomyopathy. She delivers a single liveborn infant. _____

- If the obstetrical code includes more than one diagnosis and any of the diagnoses identified by the code were not present on admission, assign indicator N, such as category O11, preexisting hypertension with preeclampsia.
- If the obstetrical code includes information that is not a diagnosis, do not consider that information in the POA determination.

Contraceptive Management and Sterilization

Patients who deliver may request contraceptive management or sterilization after delivery. The diagnosis codes representing the reason for these services are reported using the appropriate Z codes.

■ **CASE SCENARIOS**
- During the inpatient hospitalization, the patient requests tubal ligation for sterilization. Diagnosis code Z30.2 is assigned as an additional diagnosis.

- After delivery, the patient requests Depo-Provera for contraceptive management. Code Z30.8 is assigned.

Termination of Pregnancy and Spontaneous Abortions

An abortion is the removal or expulsion of an embryo or fetus from the uterus, resulting in or caused by its death. A missed abortion occurs when the embryo or fetus has died but a miscarriage has not yet occurred. It is also referred to as a *delayed miscarriage*. Spontaneous abortion, commonly

PHARMACOLOGY CONNECTION

Common Medications Relating to Pregnancy, Childbirth, and the Puerperium

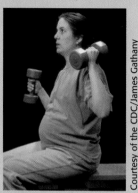

Patient in the obstetrical period.

Courtesy of the CDC/James Gathany

Tocolytics

Tocolytic agents are medications used to suppress contractions associated with premature labor.

Induction of Labor

The agents shown in the accompanying table are typical of those used to stimulate contractions and induce labor.

TOCOLYTICS	
TRADE NAME	**GENERIC NAME**
Brethine	terbutaline
Epsom Salt	magnesium sulfate
Yutopar	ritodrine

INDUCTION OF LABOR	
TRADE NAME	**GENERIC NAME**
Cervidil	dinoprostone
Cytotec	misoprostol
Pitocin	oxytocin

called *miscarriage*, occurs from natural causes. Induced abortion is the removal or expulsion of an embryo or fetus by medical, surgical, or other means at any point during human pregnancy for therapeutic or elective reasons.

When abortions are being coded, the type and presence of complications have an impact on code assignment. When an attempted termination of pregnancy results in a liveborn fetus, the principal diagnosis code is Z33.2, Encounter for elective termination of pregnancy, followed by a code for the outcome of delivery (Z37.0). When the abortion is elective (Z33.2) and the resulting retained products of conception require care, the additional code O07.4 is assigned to indicate a failed attempted termination of pregnancy. In some instances, retained products of conception follow a spontaneous abortion, which is reported using a code from category O03.4 if there is no complication. When there is a complication leading to an abortion, additional codes from Chapter 15 are assigned to represent the specific complication instead of O03.4 or O07.4.

CHECKPOINT 8.4

Code the following statements using ICD-10-CM. Do not assign the additional code for weeks of gestation for these questions.

1. The patient presents with spontaneous incomplete abortion complicated by hemorrhage. _____

2. The patient presents 1 week after a complete spontaneous abortion with defibrination syndrome. _____

3. The patient presents with retained products of conception following a spontaneous abortion.

_____

4. The patient presents with a missed abortion. _____

5. The patient presents with an elective abortion complicated by pelvic peritonitis. _____

6. The patient experiences a spontaneous abortion due to premature rupture of membranes at 15 weeks. _____

7. The patient presents with a failed complete abortion with acute renal failure. _____

8. The patient has an elective termination of pregnancy. _____

CERTAIN CONDITIONS ORIGINATING IN THE PERINATAL PERIOD (CHAPTER 16: P00–P96)

Codes in Chapter 16 of ICD-10-CM classify conditions that are in the perinatal period, the period from shortly before birth until 28 days following delivery of the fetus or of the newborn infant. The baby is considered a neonate up to 28 days after birth. These codes from Chapter 16 are assigned only to conditions of the neonate, not of the mother. (Codes for conditions that affect the management of the mother's pregnancy are in ICD-10-CM Chapter 15.) When the hospitalization is for the birth of the baby, the newborn's record is assigned a principal diagnosis code from category Z38. A code from this category is assigned only once: at the newborn's time of birth. Codes from category Z38 are never used on the mother's record. Category Z38 classifies the place of birth, the type of delivery, and whether it is a single infant or multiple infants (e.g., twins, triplets). For example, a single liveborn infant delivered in the hospital via cesarean section is assigned code Z38.01. If a newborn is transferred, the receiving facility does not assign a code from category Z38.

The categories in Chapter 16 of ICD-10-CM are grouped as shown in Table 8.2. Box 8.2 presents the applicable guidelines from Section I, Part C, of the *Official Guidelines*. Refer to this box as the various topics are presented.

Table 8.2 Organization of ICD-10-CM Chapter 16 Tabular List

BLOCK	BLOCK DESCRIPTION
P00–P04	Newborn affected by maternal factors and by complications of pregnancy, labor, and delivery
P05–P08	Disorders of newborn related to length of gestation and fetal growth
P09	Abnormal findings on neonatal screening
P10–P15	Birth trauma
P19–P29	Respiratory and cardiovascular disorders specific to the perinatal period
P35–P39	Infections specific to the perinatal period
P50–P61	Hemorrhagic and hematological disorders of newborn
P70–P74	Transitory endocrine and metabolic disorders specific to newborn
P76–P78	Digestive system disorders of newborn
P80–P83	Conditions involving the integument and temperature regulation of newborn
P84	Other problems with newborn
P90–P96	Other disorders originating in the perinatal period

BOX 8.2 *Official Guidelines*: Certain Conditions Originating in the Perinatal Period (P00–P99)

The perinatal period is defined as before birth through the 28th day following birth. The following guidelines are provided for reporting purposes.

a. General Perinatal Rules

1) Use of Chapter 16 codes

Codes in this chapter are never for use on the maternal record. Codes from Chapter 15, the obstetric chapter, are never permitted on the newborn record. Chapter 16 codes may be used throughout the life of the patient if the condition is still present.

2) Principal diagnosis for birth record

When coding the birth episode in a newborn record, assign a code from category Z38, Liveborn infants according to place of birth and type of delivery, as the principal diagnosis. A code from category Z38 is assigned only once, to a newborn at the time of birth. If a newborn is transferred to another institution, a code from category Z38 should not be used at the receiving hospital.

A code from category Z38 is used only on the newborn record, not on the mother's record.

3) Use of codes from other chapters with codes from Chapter 16

Codes from other chapters may be used with codes from Chapter 16 if the codes from the other chapters provide more specific detail. Codes for signs and symptoms may be assigned when a definitive diagnosis has not been established. If the reason for the encounter is a perinatal condition, the code from Chapter 16 should be sequenced first.

Continued

BOX 8.2 *Continued*

4) Use of Chapter 16 codes after the perinatal period

Should a condition originate in the perinatal period, and continue throughout the life of the patient, the perinatal code should continue to be used regardless of the patient's age.

5) Birth process or community-acquired conditions

If a newborn has a condition that may be either due to the birth process or community acquired and the documentation does not indicate which it is, the default is due to the birth process and the code from Chapter 16 should be used. If the condition is community acquired, a code from Chapter 16 should not be assigned.

6) Code all clinically significant conditions

All clinically significant conditions noted on routine newborn examination should be coded. A condition is clinically significant if it requires:

• Clinical evaluation; or
• Therapeutic treatment; or
• Diagnostic procedures; or
• Extended length of hospital stay; or
• Increased nursing care and/or monitoring; or
• Has implications for future health-care needs

Note: The perinatal guidelines listed above are the same as the general coding guidelines for "additional diagnoses," except for the final point regarding implications for future health-care needs. Codes should be assigned for conditions that have been specified by the provider as having implications for future health-care needs.

b. Observation and Evaluation of Newborns for Suspected Conditions Not Found

1) Use of Z05 codes

Assign a code from category Z05, Observation and evaluation of newborns and infants for suspected conditions ruled out, to identify those instances when a healthy newborn is evaluated for a suspected condition that is determined after study not to be present. Do not use a code from category Z05 when the patient has identified signs or symptoms of a suspected problem; in such cases code the sign or symptom.

2) Z05 on other than the birth record

A code from category Z05 may also be assigned as a principal or first-listed code for readmissions or encounters when the code from category Z38 code no longer applies. Codes from category Z05 are for use only for healthy newborns and infants for which no condition after study is found to be present.

3) Z05 on a birth record

A code from category Z05 is to be used as a secondary code after the code from category Z38, Live-born infants according to place of birth and type of delivery.

c. Coding Additional Perinatal Diagnoses

1) Assigning codes for conditions that require treatment

Assign codes for conditions that require treatment or further investigation, prolong the length of stay, or require resource utilization.

2) Codes for conditions specified as having implications for future health-care needs

Assign codes for conditions that have been specified by the provider as having implications for future health-care needs.

Note: This guideline should not be used for adult patients.

d. Prematurity and Fetal Growth Retardation

Providers utilize different criteria in determining prematurity. A code for prematurity should not be assigned unless it is documented. Assignment of codes in categories P05, Disorders of newborn related to slow fetal growth and fetal malnutrition, and P07, Disorders of newborn related to short gestation and low birth weight, not elsewhere classified, should be based on the recorded birth weight and estimated gestational age. Codes from category P05 should not be assigned with codes from category P07.

When both birth weight and gestational age are available, two codes from category P07 should be assigned, with the code for birth weight sequenced before the code for gestational age.

A code from P05 and codes from P07.2 and P07.3 may be used to specify weeks of gestation as documented by the provider in the record.

e. Low Birth Weight and Immaturity Status

Codes from category P07, Disorders of newborn related to short gestation and low birth weight, not elsewhere classified, are for use for a child or adult who was premature or had a low birth weight as a newborn and this is affecting the patient's current health status.

See Section I.C.21. Factors influencing health status and contact with health services, Status.

f. Bacterial Sepsis of Newborn

Category P36, Bacterial sepsis of newborn, includes congenital sepsis. If a perinate is documented as having sepsis without documentation of congenital or community acquired, the default is congenital and a code from category P36 should be assigned. If the P36 code includes the causal organism, an additional code from category B95, Streptococcus, Staphylococcus, and Enterococcus as the cause of diseases classified elsewhere, or B96, Other bacterial agents as the cause of diseases classified elsewhere, should not be assigned. If the P36 code does not include the causal organism, assign an additional code from category B96. If applicable, use additional codes to identify severe sepsis (R65.2-) and any associated acute organ dysfunction.

g. Stillbirth
Code P95, Stillbirth, is only for use in institutions that maintain separate records for stillbirths. No other code should be used with P95. Code P95 should not be used on the mother's record.

General Reporting Guidelines

Chapter 16 codes for perinatal conditions are never assigned on the mother's record or as maternal data. (As stated earlier, all maternal conditions or fetal conditions affecting the mother are reported using codes from Chapter 15.) Codes from Chapter 16 represent conditions that arise in the perinatal period. These codes may be assigned throughout a patient's life if the condition continues to be present. Remember that these codes are assigned on the newborn record, never on the maternal record.

Principal Diagnosis for Birth Record
The principal diagnosis for birth record is a code from category Z38. This code is assigned once, at the time of birth. Codes from category Z38 are never assigned on the mother's record.

Use of Codes From Other Chapters With Codes From Chapter 16
Codes from other chapters are used with codes from Chapter 16 to provide specific detail. Codes from other chapters may also be assigned when a definitive diagnosis has not been established. When codes from Chapter 16 and other chapters are assigned on the same record and the reason for the encounter is for the perinatal condition (not the birth), the code from Chapter 16 is sequenced first.

> **EXAMPLE**
> Congenital congestive heart failure and diarrhea with unknown cause is coded P29.0, R19.7.

Use of Chapter 16 Codes After the Perinatal Period
A condition that originates in the perinatal period and continues throughout the life of the patient should be coded as a perinatal condition. The patient age has no impact on code assignment under these circumstances. As noted in the example for congenital congestive heart failure, the patient will require the code P29.0 throughout his or her life.

Birth Process and Community-Acquired Conditions
Sometimes a medical condition arises in the perinatal period that is not related to the birth process. For example, a newborn who is 14 days old may develop a urinary tract infection (UTI) at home. The UTI is unrelated to the birth and is considered a community-acquired condition. A community-acquired condition arising in the perinatal period should not be coded from Chapter 16.

Conditions that arise due to the birth process should always be assigned to Chapter 16 regardless of the patient's age. If documentation is unclear and the circumstances are unknown, the coder should default to the codes for perinatal conditions (those arising in the perinatal period) and assign a code from Chapter 16.

EXAMPLES
- A newborn UTI at birth is coded P39.3.
- A UTI in a 3-week-old infant that is community acquired is coded N39.0.
- A UTI in a 3-week-old infant (default to Chapter 16) is coded P39.3.

A code assignment decision tree for perinatal conditions is presented in Pinpoint the Code 8.1.

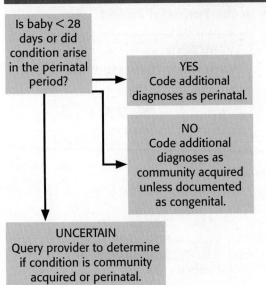

PINPOINT THE CODE 8.1: Perinatal Conditions Code Assignment

Is baby < 28 days or did condition arise in the perinatal period?

→ YES
Code additional diagnoses as perinatal.

→ NO
Code additional diagnoses as community acquired unless documented as congenital.

UNCERTAIN
Query provider to determine if condition is community acquired or perinatal.

Code All Clinically Significant Conditions

The rules for coding perinatal conditions are different from the rules for nonperinatal conditions. Although they are similar, there is one additional criterion that, if met, means that a condition can be coded. This criterion states that a condition that has implications for future health-care needs should be reported. Therefore, the inclusive list of criteria, according to the *Official Guidelines*, for reporting an additional diagnosis is as follows:

A condition is clinically significant and should be reported if it requires:

- Clinical evaluation or
- Therapeutic treatment or
- Diagnostic procedures or
- Extended length of hospital stay or
- Increased nursing care and/or monitoring or
- Has implications for future health-care needs

As is evident, other than the addition of the last criterion, these guidelines are the same as those for coding all other inpatient conditions. Codes from the perinatal chapter should not be assigned unless the provider has established a definitive diagnosis. These criteria apply to all diagnoses, both principal and secondary.

> ■ **CASE SCENARIO**
> A single newborn (born in the hospital via cesarean delivery) is noted to have a seizure after birth. Codes Z38.01, P90 are reported.

> ● The criteria for significant conditions arising in the perinatal period do not apply to adults.

Observation and Evaluation of Newborns for Suspected Conditions Not Found

Category Z05 reflect suspected conditions that are not related to a maternal condition. The code from category Z05 is assigned when the condition is ruled out. However, if the newborn presents with signs and symptoms of the condition, report the signs or symptoms, not a code from category Z05. The code from category Z05 is listed as a secondary diagnosis when the reason for admission is birth. Example: After birth, the newborn develops fever, and sepsis is ruled out. Report the newborn code from category Z38 and secondary diagnosis for fever as the symptom was present. A code from Z05 would not be assigned. On the other hand, if the newborn was ruled out for a congenital anomaly in the absence of signs or symptoms, the newborn code from Z38 is assigned with a secondary diagnosis of Z05.41.

PHARMACOLOGY CONNECTION

Common Medications for Treatment of Conditions in the Perinatal Period

Surfactant

Surfactants are agents used to prevent respiratory distress syndrome (RDS) in premature infants at high risk for RDS. They may also be used to treat premature infants who develop RDS or hyaline membrane disease.

Caffeine Therapy

Caffeine is used to treat apnea of prematurity. Premature infants have lungs that are not fully developed, and caffeine helps stimulate their breathing.

Nitric Oxide

Nitric oxide gas is used in premature babies to reduce pressure on the lungs when mechanical ventilation is required.

SURFACTANTS	
TRADE NAME	**GENERIC NAME**
Curosurf	poractant alfa
Infasurf	calfactant
Survanta	beractant

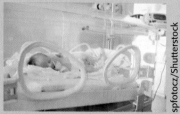

Preemie.

spfotocz/Shutterstock

In other instances, Z05 may be listed first if the newborn or infant code from category Z38 no longer applies. The Z05 is assigned to reflect a healthy newborn or infant encounter in which no condition, after study, is present. No signs or symptoms related to a condition would be present.

Prematurity and Fetal Growth Retardation

Two categories in ICD-10-CM are used to report prematurity and associated weeks of gestation. Physician documentation is required to assign these codes, because providers use different criteria to determine prematurity, which is generally defined as birth at fewer than 37 weeks after conception. The five broad factors in determining prematurity are (1) infant's gestational age, (2) infant's gender, (3) whether the infant was exposed to antenatal corticosteroids, (4) whether the infant is a single or multiple birth, and (5) infant's birth weight. Category P07 codes are assigned based on recorded birth weight and reported gestational age. Codes for weeks of gestation (P07.2) are not assigned on every newborn's chart. Remember that both weeks of gestation (P07.2) and newborn weight (P07.0 or P07.1) must be documented to assign these codes correctly.

Newborns are not considered to be admitted until after birth. Any condition present at birth or that developed in utero (including injury that occurred during delivery) is considered present on admission and should be reported with the POA indicator of Y.

The second category used to report disorders of newborn-related length of gestation and fetal growth is category P05. Codes from category P05 should not be assigned with codes from category P07. P07 category codes are for use with a child or adult whose prematurity or low birth weight as a newborn is affecting the patient's current health status. For example, a patient was born at 27 weeks, and this prematurity is still affecting the child at 2 years old. The appropriate code to assign is from category P07.

EXAMPLES

- A premature infant is born via vaginal delivery at 34 weeks and 1,765 grams. Codes Z38.00, P07.17, P07.37 are reported.

- A small-for-gestational-age newborn is delivered via cesarean section. Birth weight is 1,256 grams. Codes Z38.01, P05.15 are reported.

Bacterial Sepsis of Newborn

Bacterial sepsis of newborn is category P36, which includes congenital sepsis. Without documentation as to whether the sepsis is congenital or community acquired, the coder should default to the congenital category (P36). Sometimes the code from category P36 includes the classification of the causal organism. If the organism is not classified as a combination code, an additional code from category B96 should be assigned as well. In the presence of severe sepsis, the code from category R65.2- is reported along with the codes for any associated organ dysfunction. For example, for a newborn who is admitted at 3 weeks for treatment of severe *E. coli* sepsis with acute respiratory failure, the coder would assign codes P36.4, R65.20, J96.00.

Stillbirth

The stillbirth code, P95, is assigned only in facilities that maintain a separate record for stillbirths. Do not assign the stillbirth code to the mother's record.

Maternal Causes of Perinatal Mortality

In some instances, the mother's conditions can have an impact on the fetus or newborn. In other instances, the mother's conditions may be present but do not affect the newborn or fetus. Codes for the mother's conditions should not be assigned to the newborn record unless the maternal conditions affect the newborn or fetus. The coder should use the main term *newborn*, with the subterm "affected by" to locate these conditions.

■ **CASE SCENARIOS**
The mother may have abused cocaine during pregnancy.

- If the newborn infant tests positive for cocaine, assign code P04.41 in addition to the newborn code from Z38. (See Newborn, affected by cocaine.)

- If the newborn tests negative for cocaine and has no condition related to maternal drug use, assign only the newborn code from category Z38.

Code the following cases using ICD-10-CM.

1. A single full-term liveborn infant was born via cesarean section in the hospital. _____

2. Twin A was born vaginally at 33 weeks; mate was also liveborn. Twin A weighed 2,181 grams and was born from a mother with diabetes. Diabetes in the baby was ruled out. _____

3. Twenty-day-old infant presents with urinary tract infection due to *Escherichia coli* (*E. coli*). _____

4. Newborn health check, physician office visit. _____

5. Baby was transferred to hospital B due to hyaline membrane disease after being delivered via cesarean section at hospital A. _____

6. Newborn (vaginal delivery in hospital) evaluated for sepsis, not found. Mother was septic. _____

7. Newborn (vaginal delivery in hospital) evaluated for sepsis, with fever; sepsis was not found. _____

8. Large-for-gestational-age newborn was born via cesarean section with transitory tachypnea. _____

9. A newborn presents to the office and is fussy according to the mom who suspects gastroenteritis. The provider states healthy newborn, gastrointestinal disorder ruled out. _____

CONGENITAL MALFORMATIONS, DEFORMATIONS, AND CHROMOSOMAL ABNORMALITIES (CHAPTER 17: Q00–Q99)

Chapter 17 covers codes for congenital anomalies, malformations, and diseases that exist at birth. Unlike acquired disorders, congenital conditions are either hereditary or a result of influencing factors during gestation.

Although congenital anomalies are defined as existing at birth, they do not always immediately affect the patient. For example, normal human beings have 33 vertebrae, but a person without the normal number may be asymptomatic. Patients with dominant polycystic disease may not experience impaired function until adulthood. The classifications for congenital anomalies thus are not related to patients' ages.

When coding a congenital anomaly, the coder must ensure that the entire condition is coded. For example, some codes specifically state the congenital anomaly and its manifestations; in other words, the code has an inherent component.

For the birth admission, the code for a newborn (category Z38) is sequenced first, followed by a code for any congenital anomaly. The categories in Chapter 17 of ICD-10-CM are grouped as shown in Table 8.3. Box 8.3 presents the applicable guidelines from Section I, Part C, of the *Official Guidelines*.

Congenital malformations are also known as *birth defects* or *anomalies*. When coding these conditions, there is often a distinct subterm that denotes the condition as "congenital." The ICD-10-CM coding system differentiates diseases that are congenital from those that are acquired. For example, congenital renal cyst is reported as Q61.00 and acquired renal cysts are reported as N27.1. If a condition is documented as congenital, then the condition cannot be considered acquired. There is no time frame or age restriction on reporting a disease or disorder as congenital.

Table 8.3 Organization of ICD-10-CM Chapter 17 Tabular List

BLOCK	BLOCK DESCRIPTION
Q00–Q07	Congenital malformations of the nervous system
Q10–Q18	Congenital malformations of eye, ear, face, and neck
Q20–Q28	Congenital malformations of the circulatory system
Q30–Q34	Congenital malformations of the respiratory system
Q35–Q37	Cleft lip and cleft palate
Q38–Q45	Other congenital malformations of the digestive system
Q50–Q56	Congenital malformations of genital organs
Q60–Q64	Congenital malformations of the urinary system
Q65–Q79	Congenital malformations and deformations of the musculoskeletal system
Q80–Q89	Other congenital malformations
Q90–Q99	Chromosomal abnormalities, not elsewhere classified

BOX 8.3 *Official Guidelines*: Congenital Malformations, Deformations, and Chromosomal Abnormalities (Q00–Q99)

Assign an appropriate code(s) from categories Q00–Q99, Congenital malformations, deformations, and chromosomal abnormalities, when a malformation/deformation or chromosomal abnormality is documented. A malformation/deformation/or chromosomal abnormality may be the principal/first-listed diagnosis on a record or a secondary diagnosis.

When a malformation/deformation/or chromosomal abnormality does not have a unique code assignment, assign additional code(s) for any manifestations that may be present.

When the code assignment specifically identifies the malformation/deformation/or chromosomal abnormality, manifestations that are an inherent component of the anomaly should not be coded separately. Additional codes should be assigned for manifestations that are not an inherent component.

Codes from Chapter 17 may be used throughout the life of the patient. If a congenital malformation or deformity has been corrected, a personal history code should be used to identify the history of the malformation or deformity. Although present at birth, malformation/deformation/or chromosomal abnormality may not be identified until later in life. Whenever the condition is diagnosed by the physician, it is appropriate to assign a code from codes Q00–Q99. For the birth admission, the appropriate code from category Z38, Liveborn infants, according to place of birth and type of delivery, should be sequenced as the principal diagnosis, followed by any congenital anomaly codes, Q00–Q99.

INTERNET RESOURCE: The following web site provides facts regarding congenital anomalies and their causes.
http://www.who.int/mediacentre/factsheets/fs370/en

CHECKPOINT 8.6

Code the following cases using ICD-10-CM.

1. Renal artery anomaly _____

2. The patient with ductus arteriosus with atrial tachycardia _____

3. Bilateral cleft palate with unilateral cleft lip _____

4. Single newborn born via vaginal delivery in the hospital with esophageal atresia _____

5. Congenital hydrocephalus with lumbar spina bifida _____

Chapter Summary

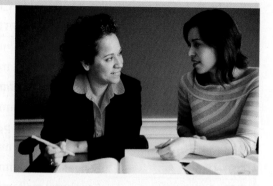

1. The assignment of pregnancy complication codes requires knowledge of these definitions: *antepartum period,* the time span between conception and delivery of the placenta; *postpartum,* the period immediately following delivery of the placenta and continuing for 6 weeks; and *peripartum,* the time span from the last month of pregnancy to 5 months postpartum.

2. Normal delivery from a coding perspective means that there were no complications associated with delivery, either those aggravated by pregnancy or those that aggravate the pregnancy. Normal delivery is assigned ICD-10-CM code O80.

3. Outcome of delivery codes (Z37.-) are assigned as additional codes on the maternal record for every encounter in which a baby was born (liveborn or stillborn).

4. Specific guidelines are present for coding conditions of the mother, such as HIV, diabetes, and fetal conditions that affect the mother. The pregnancy complication code is sequenced first, followed by a code for the specific condition.

5. Pregnancies with abortive outcomes are classified by the type of abortion (attempted, spontaneous, missed) and whether the products of conception have been completely or partially expulsed (incomplete). Complications of abortions are also reported; code assignment is based on the type of complication and whether it arose during the encounter or on a subsequent visit.

6. When a baby is born, two medical records are created: one for the mother and one for the baby. The documentation for the baby reflects newborn conditions, and codes from Chapter 16 of ICD-10-CM are assigned along with the newborn codes for the delivery (category Z38). The maternal record contains codes only from ICD-10-CM Chapter 15. When a delivery occurs, a code from category Z37 should be reported on the maternal record as an additional code to identify the outcome of delivery. Coders should be careful not to assign maternal codes for the baby or vice versa.

7. The criteria for reporting additional diagnoses is unique for newborns. Conditions that have implications for future health-care needs should also be reported.

8. Some conditions that arise in the perinatal period (birth to 28 days of life) are community acquired or otherwise not related to the birth. Code assignment depends on documentation; if the condition is community acquired, do not assign a code from Chapter 16. If the condition is not stated as community acquired, the coder should default to codes for perinatal conditions.

9. Categories P00 to P04 represent conditions that were caused by a maternal condition suspected or confirmed in the perinatal period. Codes from these categories are assigned when the baby has no symptoms, but a workup for a suspected condition is done. In some circumstances, the mother has a condition that may not affect the baby (such as diabetes). Only when documentation supports an effect on the baby of the mother's condition is the condition (present or suspected) reported for the newborn.

10. Codes for prematurity and fetal growth retardation are assigned only when documented. Fetal weight and gestation are considered in the accurate assignment of these codes.

11. Congenital anomalies (conditions people are born with) may be reported throughout a person's life. Some congenital conditions are not detected until later in life, and code assignment is not age related.

Review Questions

Matching

Match the key terms with their definitions.

A. antepartum period
B. obstetrical period
C. congenital anomaly
D. peripartum
E. elderly primigravida

F. perinatal period
G. abortion
H. prematurity
I. primigravida
J. postpartum

1. __C__ Condition that a child is born with
2. __J__ Period from delivery of placenta to 6 weeks after birth
3. __E__ A patient who is 35 years old at the time of delivery of her infant
4. __F__ Period from birth to 28 days
5. __B__ Period from conception to 6 weeks after birth
6. __A__ Period from conception through complete delivery
7. __D__ Period from last month of pregnancy to 5 months postpartum
8. __G__ Termination of pregnancy
9. __H__ Period of birth to 37 weeks
I 10. __I__ First pregnancy

True or False

Decide whether each statement is true or false.

1. _____ According to the ICD-10-CM classifications, all abortions are considered legal abortions.

2. _____ A code from category Z38 can be assigned only on a newborn record.

3. _____ A code from category Z38 can be assigned only once and is always the principal diagnosis when a baby is born alive.

4. _____ It is appropriate to assign code O80 with a pregnancy complication code.

5. _____ An outcome of delivery code should be assigned on the mother's record for an encounter in which the baby is born.

6. _____ An additional code for weeks of gestation is assigned for all newborns delivered.

7. _____ A code from the congenital anomalies chapter can be assigned, if appropriate, regardless of patient age.

8. _____ Code Z34.91 is assigned for a routine prenatal visit in the first trimester.

9. _____ A baby who exhibits any sign of life is considered a liveborn.

10. _____ Codes from the perinatal chapter are for mothers and their babies.

Multiple Choice

Select the letter that best completes the statement or answers the question.

1. Incomplete spontaneous abortion with severe sepsis and acute kidney failure is coded
   A. O07.37, R65.20, N17.9
   B. O03.37, R65.20
   C. O03.37, R65.20, N17.9
   D. O03.37, N17.9

2. One week after a legal abortion, the patient now presents for a visit with a laceration of the bladder. This is coded
   A. O04.84
   B. O07.34
   C. O03.84
   D. O03.34

3. Which of the following code pairs could be assigned for the same encounter?
   A. O80, Z37.2
   B. O80, Z37.0
   C. P05.06, P07.16
   D. O24.013, O24.02

4. Which of the following main terms would *not* be used to code a mother's record?
   A. Pregnancy
   B. Delivery
   C. Outcome
   D. Newborn

5. A single premature newborn is born via vaginal delivery at 35 weeks of gestation. The newborn weight is 2,323 grams. Which of these codes would be reported?
   A. O80, Z37.0, P07.38
   B. Z38.00, P07.18
   C. Z38.00, P07.18, P07.38
   D. Z38.01, P07.18, P07.38

6. A full-term newborn was delivered via cesarean section two weeks ago. The newborn is now admitted with neonatal jaundice and feeding problems. Which of these codes would be reported?
   A. P59.3, P92.8
   B. Z38.01, P59.9, P92.9
   C. P59.9, P92.9
   D. Z38.01, P55.9, P92.9

7. A 23-year-old female presents with premature rupture of membranes (PROM) and delivers a single liveborn infant at 39 weeks of gestation. The mother has morbid obesity with BMI of 45 and smoked cigarettes (dependence throughout her pregnancy). Which of these codes would be reported?
   A. O42.92, O99.214, E66.01, Z68.42, O99.334, F17.210, Z37.0, Z3A.39
   B. O42.92, O99.213, E66.01, Z68.42, O99.333, F17.210, Z37.0, Z3A.39
   C. O42.90, O99.214, E66.9, Z68.42, O99.334, Z37.0, Z2A.39
   D. Z38.00, O42.92, O99.213, O99.333, F17.210, Z2A.39

8. A 20-year-old female presented in labor at 38 weeks. Cesarean section was required due to obstructed labor from compound presentation for this twin pregnancy. Diachorionic/diamniotic twin girls were born alive. Which of these codes would be reported?
   A. O64.5xx9, O30.043, Z37.2, Z3A.38
   B. O64.5xx0, O30.043, Z37.2, Z3A.38
   C. O64.5xx0, Z37.0, Z3A.338
   D. O64.5xx9, Z37.0, Z3A.38

9. A 34-year-old female delivers a single liveborn at 34 weeks of gestation. The patient develops breast engorgement after delivery. Which of these codes would be reported?
   A. O60.2xx0, Z37.0, O92.79, Z3A.34
   B. O60.14x0, O92.79, Z3A.34
   C. O60.10x0, Z37.1, O92.79, Z3A.34
   D. O60.14x0, Z37.0, O92.79, Z3A.34

10. A 30-year-old female presents for repeat low transverse cesarean section at 37 weeks of gestation and delivers a single liveborn girl. The mother also has an elective sterilization during this visit. Which of these codes would be reported?
    A. O80, Z30.2, Z37.0, Z3A.37
    B. O34.211, Z30.2, Z37.0, Z3A.37
    C. O34.211, Z37.0, Z3A.37
    D. O34.211, Z30.2, Z38.00, Z3A.37

CHAPTER 9

ICD-10-CM Chapters 18 Through 21: R00–Z99

CHAPTER OUTLINE

Symptoms, Signs, and Abnormal Clinical and Laboratory Findings, Not Elsewhere Classified (Chapter 18: R00–R99)

Injury, Poisoning, and Certain Other Consequences of External Causes (Chapter 19: S00–T88)

External Causes of Morbidity (Chapter 20: V00–Y99)

Factors Influencing Health Status and Contact With Health Services (Chapter 21: Z00–Z99)

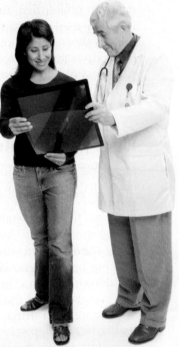

LEARNING OUTCOMES

After studying this chapter, you should be able to:

1. Differentiate between the coding rules for integral and nonintegral signs and symptoms.
2. Describe the difference in the way signs and symptoms are reported in the inpatient setting versus the outpatient setting.
3. Discuss general guidelines for coding injuries.
4. Compare the assignment of codes for acute versus healing fractures.
5. Describe the steps for coding burns, and explain when multiple codes are needed.
6. Discuss the coding of adverse effects.
7. Define poisoning as used in ICD-10-CM coding, and describe the steps for coding this condition.
8. Define toxic effects as used in ICD-10-CM, and describe the steps for coding these events.
9. Discuss general guidelines for coding complications of care.
10. Discuss the assignment of external cause codes for inpatient (facility) coding.
11. Describe the purpose, categories, and assignment of Z codes.

This chapter covers the ICD-10-CM chapters involving symptoms, signs, and abnormal clinical and laboratory findings, not elsewhere classified; injury, poisoning, and certain other consequences of external causes; external causes of morbidity; and factors influencing health status and contact with health services. Also presented is the correct use of the Table of Drugs and Chemicals.

The structure and organization of the corresponding ICD-10-CM Tabular List chapters are presented, followed by discussions of code selection and sequencing as instructed by the *ICD-10-CM Official Guidelines for Coding and Reporting*, Section I, Part C. Once again, the focus is on common code assignment decisions and complex coding scenarios.

SYMPTOMS, SIGNS, AND ABNORMAL CLINICAL AND LABORATORY FINDINGS, NOT ELSEWHERE CLASSIFIED (CHAPTER 18: R00–R99)

Codes in Chapter 18 of the ICD-10-CM classify patients' signs, symptoms, and ill-defined conditions for which definitive diagnoses have not been made. A sign is an objective indication that can be evaluated by the physician, such as weight loss. A symptom is a subjective statement made by the patient that cannot be confirmed during an examination, such as pain.

Codes from this chapter describe many, but not all, signs and symptoms. Signs and symptoms that point to a probable diagnosis are classified in the appropriate chapter in ICD-10-CM. For example, the symptom of shortness of breath is reported as R06.02 (Chapter 18), but the sign of melena (K92.1) is classified to Chapter 11, Diseases of the Digestive System. No matter what chapter the sign or symptom is classified to, the guidelines still apply.

Codes that describe signs or symptoms are acceptable when a related definitive diagnosis has *not* been established. In other words, the *Official Guidelines* state that a code from Chapter 18 is not to be used when a related definitive diagnosis has been established. For example, if the diagnosis is shortness of breath due to pneumonia, the code is J18.9; the symptom code of shortness of breath is not reported because the definitive diagnosis of pneumonia, which encompasses the shortness of breath symptom, has been established.

The categories in Chapter 18 of ICD-10-CM are grouped as shown in Table 9.1. Guidelines from Section I, Part C, of the *Official Guidelines* for Chapter 18 are given in Box 9.1.

Signs and Symptoms That Are Integral to the Disease Process

Signs and symptoms that are integral to the underlying disease process should not be reported as additional diagnoses, according to the *Official Guidelines*. This means that in the earlier example of shortness of breath due to pneumonia, the shortness of breath is not coded because the definitive diagnosis has been established *and* the symptom of shortness of breath is integral to pneumonia.

The student may ask, "How do I know which symptoms are integral to each disease?" If the coder is not certain whether a sign or symptom is typical or associated routinely with a disease that has been diagnosed, then the coder should research the disease process in order to make the determination. The coder may be instructed in the Tabular List to code associated signs and symptoms and the instructions should be followed. For example, code N40.1, enlargement of prostate with urinary symptoms, instructs the coder to add the urinary symptoms. Coders regularly ask themselves whether a patient with a disease typically has a documented sign or symptom. For example, does a patient with pneumonia usually have shortness of breath? The answer is yes, so the symptom of shortness of breath is integral to the pneumonia and is not reported separately.

Signs and Symptoms That Are Not Integral to the Disease Process

Other signs and symptoms are not integral (not associated routinely) to the disease process. For example, coma is reported using code R40.20. Because comatose is a status, it is not integral to any underlying condition. In other words, what condition would typically always include a comatose state? Is a coma integral to a stroke? The answer is that a coma is not integral to any condition; the sign of a coma should be coded.

Table 9.1 Organization of ICD-10-CM Chapter 18 Tabular List

BLOCK	BLOCK DESCRIPTION
R00–R09	Symptoms and signs involving the circulatory and respiratory systems
R10–R19	Symptoms and signs involving the digestive system and abdomen
R20–R23	Symptoms and signs involving the skin and subcutaneous tissue
R25–R29	Symptoms and signs involving the nervous and musculoskeletal systems
R30–R39	Symptoms and signs involving the genitourinary system
R40–R46	Symptoms and signs involving cognition, perception, emotional state, and behavior
R47–R49	Symptoms and signs involving speech and voice
R50–R69	General symptoms and signs
R70–R79	Abnormal findings on examination of blood, without diagnosis
R80–R82	Abnormal findings on examination of urine, without diagnosis
R83–R89	Abnormal findings on examination of other body fluids, substances, and tissues, without diagnosis
R90–R94	Abnormal findings on diagnostic imaging and in function studies, without diagnosis
R97	Abnormal tumor markers
R99	Ill-defined and unknown cause of mortality

BOX 9.1 *Official Guidelines:* Symptoms, Signs, and Abnormal Findings (R00–R99)

Chapter 18 includes symptoms, signs, abnormal results of clinical or other investigative procedures, and ill-defined conditions regarding which no diagnosis classifiable elsewhere is recorded. Signs and symptoms that point to a specific diagnosis have been assigned to a category in other chapters of the classification.

a. Use of Symptom Codes
Codes that describe symptoms and signs are acceptable for reporting purposes when a related definitive diagnosis has not been established (confirmed) by the provider.

b. Use of a Symptom Code with a Definitive Diagnosis Code
Codes for signs and symptoms may be reported in addition to a related definitive diagnosis when the sign or symptom is not routinely associated with that diagnosis, such as the various signs and symptoms associated with complex syndromes. The definitive diagnosis code should be sequenced before the symptom code.

Signs or symptoms that are associated routinely with a disease process should not be assigned as additional codes, unless otherwise instructed by the classification.

c. Combination Codes That Include Symptoms
ICD-10-CM contains a number of combination codes that identify both the definitive diagnosis and common symptoms of that diagnosis. When using one of these combination codes, an additional code should not be assigned for the symptom.

d. Repeated Falls
Code R29.6, Repeated falls, is for use for encounters when a patient has recently fallen and the reason for the fall is being investigated.

Code Z91.81, History of falling, is for use when a patient has fallen in the past and is at risk for future falls. When appropriate, both codes R29.6 and Z91.81 may be assigned together.

e. Coma Scale
The coma scale codes (R40.2-) can be used in conjunction with traumatic brain injury codes, acute cerebrovascular disease or sequelae of cerebrovascular disease codes. These codes are primarily for use by trauma registries, but they may be used in any setting where this information is collected. The coma scale may also be used to assess the status of the central nervous system for other non-trauma conditions, such as monitoring patients in the intensive care unit regardless of medical condition. The coma scale codes should be sequenced after the diagnosis code(s).

These codes, one from each subcategory, are needed to complete the scale. The 7th character indicates when the scale was recorded. The 7th character should match for all three codes.

At a minimum, report the initial score documented on presentation at your facility. This may be a score from the emergency medicine technician (EMT) or in the emergency department. If desired, a facility may choose to capture multiple coma scale scores.

Continued

BOX 9.1 *Continued*

Assign code R40.24, Glasgow coma scale, total score, when only the total score is documented in the medical record and not the individual score(s).

f. Functional Quadriplegia

GUIDELINE HAS BEEN DELETED EFFECTIVE OCTOBER 1, 2017

g. SIRS Due to Non-Infectious Process

The systemic inflammatory response syndrome (SIRS) can develop as a result of certain non-infectious disease processes, such as trauma, malignant neoplasm, or pancreatitis. When SIRS is documented with a noninfectious condition, and no subsequent infection is documented, the code for the underlying condition, such as an injury, should be assigned, followed by code R65.10, Systemic inflammatory response syndrome (SIRS) of non-infectious origin without acute organ dysfunction, or code R65.11, Systemic inflammatory response syndrome (SIRS) of non-infectious origin with acute organ dysfunction. If an associated acute organ dysfunction is documented, the appropriate code(s) for the specific type of organ dysfunction(s) should be assigned in addition to code R65.11. If acute organ dysfunction is documented, but it cannot be determined if the acute organ dysfunction is associated with SIRS or due to another condition (e.g., directly due to the trauma), the provider should be queried.

h. Death NOS

Code R99, Ill-defined and unknown cause of mortality, is only for use in the very limited circumstance when a patient who has already died is brought into an emergency department or other healthcare facility and is pronounced dead upon arrival. It does not represent the discharge disposition of death.

i. NIHSS Stroke Scale

The NIH stroke scale (NIHSS) codes (R29.7- -) can be used in conjunction with acute stroke codes (I63) to identify the patient's neurological status and the severity of the stroke. The stroke scale codes should be sequenced after the acute stroke diagnosis code(s).

At a minimum, report the initial score documented. If desired, a facility may choose to capture multiple stroke scale scores.

See Section I.B.14. for information concerning the medical record documentation that may be used for assignment of the NIHSS codes.

CHECKPOINT 9.1

Which of the following signs and symptoms are integral to the underlying condition?

1. _____ Chest pain due to myocardial infarction

2. _____ Abdominal pain due to gastric ulcer

3. _____ Dysuria due to renal calculus

4. _____ Dyspnea due to lung cancer

5. _____ Fever due to sepsis

Outpatient and Inpatient Coding

The setting, either inpatient or outpatient, affects the coding of signs and symptoms.

Signs and Symptoms in the Inpatient Setting

Per the *Official Guidelines,* remember that in the acute inpatient setting, conditions that are suspected, possible, or probable are reported as if they exist. Therefore, a diagnostic statement of abdominal pain probably due to acute gastritis requires reporting of the gastritis alone (K29.70). The coder bases the coding on the diagnosis of abdominal pain due to gastritis. The symptom of abdominal pain is integral to gastritis, so it is not reported separately.

EXAMPLES

- Diagnosis: Chest pain probably due to costochondritis. Code costochondritis; do not assign the Chapter 18 code for chest pain because it is integral and thus implicit in the diagnosis.

- Diagnosis: Chest pain probably due to angina. Code the angina; do not code chest pain because it is implicit or integral to the diagnosis of angina.

- Diagnosis: Ascites probably due to alcoholic cirrhosis of the liver. Code the cirrhosis, followed by the code from Chapter 18 for ascites, because patients with cirrhosis do not necessarily have ascites, and the presence of ascites may modify the treatment given. Ascites is not integral to cirrhosis; therefore, it should be reported separately.

Sign and symptom codes for unscheduled hospital outpatient services are reported on the UB-04/837I claim form, in the fields designated as "reason for visit," in addition to the first-listed diagnosis code to support the claim. For example, the ED documentation is nausea, vomiting, and diarrhea due to acute gastroenteritis. The first-listed diagnosis is K29.00 (acute gastroenteritis). The reason for visit code fields can be used to report the signs and symptoms: R11.2 (nausea and vomiting) and R19.7 (diarrhea).

Signs and Symptoms in the Outpatient Setting

Conditions that are possible, probable, or suspected are not coded in the outpatient setting, whether the visit is to the hospital emergency department (ED), physician office, or ambulatory center. In the outpatient setting, codes are assigned for the condition documented at the highest level of certainty established at the time of visit. Thus, a diagnosis of shortness of breath possibly due to pneumonia requires reporting only the shortness of breath, which is the established condition at the time of service.

EXAMPLES

- Diagnosis: Ascites probably due to alcoholic cirrhosis. Code only the ascites.

- Diagnosis: Nausea, vomiting, and diarrhea due to suspected gastroenteritis. Code only the signs and symptoms of nausea, vomiting, and diarrhea.

- Diagnosis: Chest pain due to possible angina. Report the code for chest pain only.

INTERNET RESOURCE: Symptom Checker: Symptoms and Signs A–Z
http://www.medicinenet.com/symptoms_and_signs/article.htm#introView

Combination Codes That Include Symptoms

ICD-10 often uses combination codes to report an underlying condition and an associated condition. When these combination codes are available, the symptom is not reported separately. For example, regional enteritis, the disease, with rectal bleeding, the symptom, is reported using code K50.911 (regional enteritis with rectal bleeding).

Sequencing of Signs and Symptoms as the Principal Diagnosis in the Inpatient Setting

A code for a sign or symptom may be reported as the principal diagnosis in the inpatient setting. This is the exception rather than the rule in the inpatient setting, because the underlying condition causing the symptom is usually determined or suspected and can thus be assigned a code. In rare instances, however, it is appropriate to sequence a symptom code as the principal diagnosis:

1. Underlying cause of symptoms is undetermined.
   a. Patient is discharged prior to determination.
   b. Workup is negative: underlying cause is unknown.
2. The patient is an outpatient at the time the possible condition is documented.

An example is when the patient is transferred to another facility, leaves the hospital against medical advice, or expires before the underlying cause is determined.

EXAMPLE
Chest pain and positive EKG (electrocardiogram); patient is transferred to a cardiac hospital. Codes R07.9, R94.31 are reported.

A symptom can be the principal diagnosis when a suspected condition is ruled out. In this case, only the symptom code can be reported.

EXAMPLE
Chest pain, myocardial infarction ruled out, is coded R07.9.

Best practice is for coders to take note of an inpatient encounter that results in a symptom as a principal diagnosis. Review the record to ensure that the principal diagnosis is correct and the underlying condition has not been documented. The coder may query the physician to determine the underlying cause in the inpatient setting. When multiple symptoms occasion the admission and the underlying cause has not been determined, each symptom is reported separately. The sequencing depends on the circumstance of admission. If all conditions equally meet the definition of principal diagnosis, any symptom may be sequenced first.

EXAMPLE

Hematuria and flank pain, undetermined etiology, is coded with both R31.9 (hematuria) and R10.9 (flank pain). Either code can be reported first.

Coma Scale

Coma scale codes, R40.2-, are used as additional codes with the underlying cause sequenced first. Diseases or injuries that can result in a comatose state are traumatic brain injuries, skull fractures, cerebrovascular accidents, or other cerebrovascular disease. Review of the Tabular List assists the coder in assigning these codes; the seventh character classifies the time or place the coma scale was reported (Box 9.2). The initial score documented on presentation should always be reported. A facility may capture multiple coma scale scores if desired. Many trauma hospitals elect to report multiple coma scores for their trauma registry.

BOX 9.2 Tabular List R40.2-

Coma
Code first any associated:
> coma in fracture of skull (S02.-)
> coma in intracranial injury (S06.-)

The appropriate 7th character is to be added to each code from subcategory R40.21-, R40.22-, R40.23-:
- 0 - unspecified time
- 1 - in the field [EMT or ambulance]
- 2 - at arrival to emergency department
- 3 - at hospital admission
- 4 - 24 hours or more after hospital admission

Note: A code from each subcategory is required to complete the coma scale.

There are three coma scale subcategories to reflect eyes open, best verbal response, and best motor response. When reporting a coma, a code from each subcategory is required to complete the coma scale. The seventh character must match for all three codes and reflect the point in time at which the scale was measured. For example, patient presents with acute CVA and coma. Documentation at arrival to the ED states the patient has eyes open to sound, no verbal response, and obeys commands. The codes reported are

1. Cerebrovascular accident I63.9
2. Eyes open to sound R40.2132
3. No verbal response R40.2212
4. Obeys commands R40.2362

The NIH stroke scale (NIHSS) is a tool to quantify stroke impairment levels. There are 11 items which are scored for abilities such as level of consciousness, visual field test, motor drift, etc. The total score is reported using a code from subcategory R29.7-. The NIHSS score is reported as an additional code for those patients with a stroke (I63-). The patient's neurological status and severity of stroke may change over the course of care, thus the NIHSS code may be reported more than once if the facility chooses. The NIH stroke scale code is reported as an additional diagnosis.

EXAMPLE

The patient was admitted with a cerebral infarction due to thrombosis of bilateral carotid arteries with a NIHSS score of 25. Report codes I63.033 and R29.725.

Code the following cases using ICD-10-CM.

1. Abnormal coagulation profile _____

2. Chronic fatigue syndrome _____

3. Hospital ED (outpatient): chest pain probably due to angina versus gastroesophageal reflux

   _____

4. Physician office: fever, cough, and shortness of breath probably related to pneumonia _____

5. Coma secondary to acute subdural hemorrhage; at hospital admission coma scale reflected eyes open to pain, no verbal response, and patient responds with flexion withdrawal _____

6. Hospital ED (outpatient): cardiac arrest, possible acute myocardial infarction as the cause

   _____

7. Hospital inpatient: cardiac arrest, possible acute myocardial infarction as the cause; patient expired 8 hours after admission _____

8. Abdominal pain due to gastritis and hernia _____

9. Hydronephrosis due to obstructing renal calculus _____

10. Fever and leukocytosis, infection ruled out _____

INJURY, POISONING, AND CERTAIN OTHER CONSEQUENCES OF EXTERNAL CAUSES (CHAPTER 19: S00–T88)

Many patients require medical care for initial and healing injuries such as fractures, dislocations, sprains, wound, burns, and poisonings. All of these events are coded from Chapter 19 of the ICD-10-CM. To handle the broad category of injuries, coders need to understand the specific guidelines that focus on multiple injuries, the specific types of injuries, and the extensive use of combination codes for injuries. Similarly, the rules for coding burns and poisoning are important for coders to know. The seventh character that is used for most of the categories in this chapter requires and represents the episode of care. The categories in Chapter 19 of ICD-10-CM are grouped as shown in Table 9.2.

In the hospital setting, external cause codes are required as additional codes to describe the circumstances and place of the injury.

Injuries, Fractures, Dislocations, Sprains and Strains, and Wounds

A large number of the codes in Chapter 19 are used to code the broad classifications of *injuries,* which include fractures, dislocations, sprains and strains, and wounds. Box 9.3 presents the applicable guidelines from Section I, Part C, of the *Official Guidelines.*

Code Assignment

A separate code for each injury is assigned unless a combination code is available that better suits the situation that is documented. For multiple injuries, a combination code may also be available for assignment, although more specific codes are generally preferable.

Different seventh characters for each injury code are assigned when an injury is in active treatment, a healing phase, or when there is a sequela of the injury.

Application of Seventh Characters in Chapter 19

The seventh character assigned to most injuries identifies the episode of care for that injury. For example, a patient sustains a fractured wrist and presents to the ED; this is the initial encounter.

Table 9.2 Organization of ICD-10-CM Chapter 19 Tabular List

BLOCK	BLOCK DESCRIPTION
S00–S09	Injuries to the head
S10–S19	Injuries to the neck
S20–S29	Injuries to the thorax
S30–S39	Injuries to the abdomen, lower back, lumbar spine, pelvis, and external genitals
S40–S49	Injuries to the shoulder and upper arm
S50–S59	Injuries to the elbow and forearm
S60–S69	Injuries to the wrist, hand, and fingers
S70–S79	Injuries to the hip and thigh
S80–S89	Injuries to the knee and lower leg
S90–S99	Injuries to the ankle and foot
T07	Injuries involving multiple body regions
T14	Injury of unspecified body region
T15–T19	Effects of foreign body entering through natural orifice
T20–T32	Burns and corrosions
T20–T25	Burns and corrosions of external body surface, specified site
T26–T28	Burns and corrosions confined to eye and internal organs
T30–T32	Burns and corrosions multiple and unspecified body regions
T33–T34	Frostbite
T36–T50	Poisoning by, adverse effect of, and underdosing of drugs, medicaments, and biological substances
T51–T65	Toxic effects of substances chiefly nonmedicinal as to source
T66–T78	Other and unspecified effects of external causes
T79	Certain early complications of trauma
T80–T88	Complications of surgical and medical care, not elsewhere classified

BOX 9.3 *Official Guidelines:* Injury, Poisoning, and Certain Other Consequences of External Causes (S00–T88)

a. Application of 7th Characters in Chapter 19

Most categories in Chapter 19 have a 7th character requirement for each applicable code. Most categories in this chapter have three 7th character values (with the exception of fractures): A, initial encounter, D, subsequent encounter and S, sequela. Categories for traumatic fractures have additional 7th character values. While the patient may be seen by a new or different provider over the course of treatment for an injury, assignment of the 7th character is based on whether the patient is undergoing active treatment and not whether the provider is seeing the patient for the first time.

For complication codes, active treatment refers to treatment for the condition described by the code, even though it may be related to an earlier precipitating problem. For example, code T84.50XA, Infection and inflammatory reaction due to unspecified internal joint prosthesis, initial encounter, is used when active treatment is provided for the infection, even though the condition relates to the prosthetic device, implant or graft that was placed at a previous encounter.

7th character "A", initial encounter is used for each encounter where the patient is receiving active treatment for the condition.

7th character "D" subsequent encounter is used for encounters after the patient has completed active treatment of the condition and is receiving routine care for the condition during the healing or recovery phase.

The aftercare Z codes should not be used for aftercare for conditions such as injuries or poisonings, where 7th characters are provided to identify subsequent care. For example, for aftercare of an injury, assign the acute injury code with the 7th character "D" (subsequent encounter).

7th character "S," sequela, is for use for complications or conditions that arise as a direct result of a condition, such as scar formation after a burn. The scars are sequelae of the burn. When using

7th character "S," it is necessary to use both the injury code that precipitated the sequela and the code for the sequela itself. The "S" is added only to the injury code, not the sequela code. The 7th character "S" identifies the injury responsible for the sequela. The specific type of sequela (e.g., scar) is sequenced first, followed by the injury code.

b. Coding of Injuries

When coding injuries, assign separate codes for each injury unless a combination code is provided, in which case the combination code is assigned. Codes from category T07, Unspecified multiple injuries, should not be assigned in the inpatient setting unless information for a more specific code is not available. Traumatic injury codes (S00–V86) are not to be used for normal, healing surgical wounds or to identify complications of surgical wounds.

The code for the most serious injury, as determined by the provider and the focus of treatment, is sequenced first.

1) Superficial injuries

Superficial injuries such as abrasions or contusions are not coded when associated with more severe injuries of the same site.

2) Primary injury with damage to nerves/blood vessels

When a primary injury results in minor damage to peripheral nerves or blood vessels, the primary injury is sequenced first with additional code(s) for injuries to nerves and spinal cord (such as category S04), and/or injury to blood vessels (such as category S15). When the primary injury is to the blood vessels or nerves, that injury should be sequenced first.

c. Coding of Traumatic Fractures

The principles of multiple coding of injuries should be followed in coding fractures. Fractures of specified sites are coded individually by site in accordance with both the provisions within categories S02, S12, S22, S32, S42, S49, S52, S59, S62, S72, S79, S82, S89, S92 and the level of detail furnished by medical record content.

A fracture not indicated as open or closed should be coded to closed. A fracture not indicated whether displaced or not displaced should be coded to displaced.

More specific guidelines are as follows:

1) Initial versus subsequent encounter for fractures

Traumatic fractures are coded using the appropriate 7th character for initial encounter (A, B, C) for each encounter where the patient is receiving active treatment for the fracture. Examples of active treatment are: surgical treatment, emergency department encounter, and evaluation and treatment by a new physician. The appropriate 7th character for initial encounter should also be assigned for a patient who delayed seeking treatment for the fracture or nonunion.

Fractures are coded using the appropriate 7th character for subsequent care for encounters after the patient has completed active treatment of the fracture and is receiving routine care for the fracture during the healing or recovery phase. Examples of fracture aftercare are: cast change or removal, removal of external or internal fixation device, medication adjustment, and follow-up visits following fracture treatment.

Care for complications of surgical treatment for fracture repairs during the healing or recovery phase should be coded with the appropriate complication codes.

Care of complications of fractures, such as malunion and nonunion, should be reported with the appropriate 7th character for subsequent care with nonunion (K, M, N,) or subsequent care with malunion (P, Q, R).

Malunion/nonunion: The appropriate 7th character for initial encounter should also be assigned for a patient who delayed seeking treatment for the fracture or nonunion.

The open fracture designations in the assignment of the 7th character for fractures of the forearm, femur and lower leg, including ankle are based on the Gustilo open fracture classification. When the Gustilo classification type is not specified for an open fracture, the 7th character for open fracture type I or II should be assigned (B, E, H, M, Q).

A code from category M80, not a traumatic fracture code, should be used for any patient with known osteoporosis who suffers a fracture, even if the patient had a minor fall or trauma, if that fall or trauma would not usually break a normal, healthy bone.

See Section I.C.13. Osteoporosis.

The aftercare Z codes should not be used for aftercare for traumatic fractures. For aftercare of a traumatic fracture, assign the acute fracture code with the appropriate 7th character.

2) Multiple fractures sequencing

Multiple fractures are sequenced in accordance with the severity of the fracture.

During the episode of treatment, the patient may return to his or her orthopedist for routine care during recovery or healing. A year later, the patient may develop a late effect or sequela from that same injury. The seventh character is used to classify the different points of care for this injury. Separate codes are not used; rather, unique seventh characters that describe the entire episode are used. The descriptions of some of these seventh characters are noted below and are also in the *Official Guidelines* (see Box 9.3). It is important to remember that these seventh characters must always be the last digit in the code. The place holder ("x") is used when the subcategory code ends at the fourth or fifth digit. For example, S123.4xxA is the format you might use when reporting an injury code where the subcategory includes four digits only, but a seventh character is required.

Summary of Guidelines for Seventh Characters From Chapter 19. As stated in the *Official Guidelines*:

Seventh character "A," initial encounter, is used while the patient is receiving active treatment for the condition.

Seventh character "D," subsequent encounter, is used for encounters after the patient has received active treatment of the condition and is receiving routine care for the condition during the healing or recovery phase (i.e., cast change, routine follow-up).

Seventh character "S," sequela, is used for complications or conditions that arise as a direct result of a condition, such as scar formation after a burn. When using seventh character "S," it is necessary to use both the injury code that precipitated the sequela and the code for the sequela itself. The "S" is added only to the injury code, not the sequela code.

Sequencing of Injury Codes

"The code for the most serious injury, as determined by the provider and the focus of treatment, is sequenced first." This guideline is stated in the *Official Guidelines*, so it is a firm rule. If there is uncertainty as to which injury is the "most serious," then the physician should be queried.

Coding of Traumatic Fractures

Traumatic fractures—a break in a bone—are coded using the fracture code while the patient is receiving active treatment for the fracture, such as surgical treatment, an ED encounter, and evaluation and treatment by a new physician. Traumatic fractures are classified by site of fracture, displacement, and type of fracture. A fracture not indicated as open or closed is classified as closed. A displaced fracture is one in which the bone is out of alignment. A fracture not indicated as displaced or not displaced should be coded as displaced.

It is imperative for the coder to recognize the type of fracture (impacted, spiral, greenstick, etc.) in order to assign an accurate code. Both the medical record and radiology reports often specifically locate the fracture, helping the coder assign the most appropriate code.

INTERNET RESOURCE: CDC NCHS Injury Data and Resources
www.cdc.gov/nchs/injury.htm

Guidelines for Traumatic (Acute) Fractures. Fracture coding follows the principles of coding of injuries, with these additional points:

- Fractures of specified sites are coded individually by site.

EXAMPLE
Fracture of the shaft and base of the second metacarpal, left hand. Initial episode is coded S62.341A, S62.351A.

- Combination categories for multiple fractures are provided for use when there is insufficient detail in the medical record (such as when a trauma case is transferred to another hospital), when the reporting form limits the number of codes that can be used in reporting pertinent clinical data, or when there is insufficient specificity at the fourth- or fifth-digit level.

EXAMPLE
Multiple fractures of the lower end of the femur. Initial episode is coded S72.499A.

- Multiple unilateral or bilateral fractures of same bone(s) that have the same three-digit category but are classified to different fourth- or fifth-digit subdivisions (bone part) are coded individually by site.

If a primary injury results in minor damage to peripheral nerves or blood vessels, the primary injury is sequenced first, with one or more additional code(s) for the nerve or blood vessel injuries. When the primary injury is to the blood vessels or nerves, that injury should be sequenced first.

Superficial injuries such as abrasions or contusions are not coded when associated with more severe injuries of the same site.

If the fracture is not indicated as displaced or nondisplaced, code it as displaced. Code assignment is also based on the type of fracture (greenstick, spiral, etc.) for some fractures. X-ray results may be helpful to determine the type and location of fractures.

Handwritten notes:

Example

⊞ T34.521 — A
🔲 T34.1 _ _ _ — D
         ↑↑   S
      place-
      holder

EXAMPLES

- Initial episode of care for fracture of the left shaft of the humerus and fracture of the right distal end of the humerus is coded S42.302A and S42.401A.

- Traumatic spiral fracture, displaced, bilateral shaft of the humerus, is coded S42.341A (right) and S42.342A (left).

  - For sequencing, when multiple fractures are present, the coder must determine, based on the severity of the fractures, which fracture code is sequenced first. This is usually handled by a request to the provider to sequence the fracture diagnoses in order of severity. Note that this would apply when the most severe injuries are fractures, and another, more severe injury does not exist.

■ CASE SCENARIO

A patient presents after car accident with open fracture of the left femur, closed fracture of the left wrist. The femur fracture is more severe and thus is sequenced first. Codes S72.92xB, S62.102A are assigned.

Acute Fracture Coding Versus Healing Fractures and Complications. The above rules apply to *acute fractures* and *healing fractures treated previously, complication of fractures or sequela* after initial care.

After initial treatment of fractures, the same fracture code is assigned with a revised seventh character to reflect the healing/routine services, a complication (i.e., malunion) or sequela.

CHECKPOINT 9.3

Code the following cases using ICD-10-CM. (Do not assign external cause of injury codes at this point.)

1. Traumatic hemothorax with three left rib fractures (initial episode of care) _____
2. Subdural hematoma with occipital skull fracture, loss of consciousness for 45 minutes (initial episode of care) _____
3. Subcapital traumatic fracture of the left femur (initial episode of care) _____
4. Blister of the right hand (initial episode of care) _____
5. Initial episode of treatment for Grade II liver laceration (moderate) _____
6. Traumatic bucket-handle tear of left medial meniscus (initial episode of care) _____
7. Compound bimalleolar fracture of the left ankle and fracture of multiple nasal bones (initial episode of care) _____
8. Nonunion of traumatic greenstick fracture of right ulnar shaft _____
9. Delayed healing fracture of the facial bone _____
10. Insect bite of the right leg (initial episode of care) _____
11. Laceration of the lip and scalp; left ring finger laceration with embedded glass in the wound (subsequent encounter) _____

Burns

Burn coding is governed by specific rules, as shown in Box 9.4, the excerpted guidelines from the *Official Guidelines*.

BOX 9.4 *Official Guidelines:* Burns and Corrosions

The ICD-10-CM makes a distinction between burns and corrosions. The burn codes are for thermal burns, except sunburns, that come from a heat source, such as a fire or hot appliance. The burn codes are also for burns resulting from electricity and radiation. Corrosions are burns due to chemicals. The guidelines are the same for burns and corrosions.

Current burns (T20–T25) are classified by depth, by extent, and by agent (X code). Burns are classified by depth as first degree (erythema), second degree (blistering), and third degree (full-thickness involvement). Burns of the eye and internal organs (T26–T28) are classified by site, but not by degree.

1) **Sequencing of Burn and Related Condition Codes**
   Sequence first the code that reflects the highest degree of burn when more than one burn is present.
   a. When the reason for the admission or encounter is for treatment of external multiple burns, sequence first the code that reflects the burn of the highest degree.
   b. When a patient has both internal and external burns, the circumstances of admission govern the selection of the principal diagnosis or first-listed diagnosis.
   c. When a patient is admitted for burn injuries and other related conditions such as smoke inhalation and/or respiratory failure, the circumstances of admission govern the selection of the principal or first-listed diagnosis.

2) **Burns of the Same Local Site**
   Classify burns of the same local site (three-character category level, T20–T28) but of different degrees to the subcategory identifying the highest degree recorded in the diagnosis.

3) **Non-Healing Burns**
   Non-healing burns are coded as acute burns.
   Necrosis of burned skin should be coded as a non-healed burn.

4) **Infected Burn**
   For any documented infected burn site, use an additional code for the infection.

5) **Assign Separate Codes for Each Burn Site**
   When coding burns, assign separate codes for each burn site. Category T30, Burn and corrosion, body region unspecified, is extremely vague and should rarely be used.

6) **Burns and Corrosions Classified According to Extent of Body Surface Involved**
   Assign codes from category T31, Burns classified according to extent of body surface involved, or T32, Corrosions classified according to extent of body surface involved, when the site of the burn is not specified or when there is a need for additional data. It is advisable to use category T31 as additional coding when needed to provide data for evaluating burn mortality, such as that needed by burn units. It is also advisable to use category T31 as an additional code for reporting purposes when there is mention of a third-degree burn involving 20 percent or more of the body surface.

   Categories T31 and T32 are based on the classic "rule of nines" in estimating body surface involved: head and neck are assigned nine percent, each arm nine percent, each leg 18 percent, the anterior trunk 18 percent, posterior trunk 18 percent, and genitalia one percent. Providers may change these percentage assignments where necessary to accommodate infants and children who have proportionately larger heads than adults, and patients who have large buttocks, thighs, or abdomen that involve burns.

7) **Encounters for Treatment of Sequelae of Burns**
   Encounters for the treatment of the late effects of burns or corrosions (i.e., scars or joint contractures) should be coded with a burn or corrosion code with the 7th character "S" for sequela.

8) **Sequelae with a Late Effect Code and Current Burn**
   When appropriate, both a code for a current burn or corrosion with 7th character "A" or "D" and a burn or corrosion code with 7th character "S" may be assigned on the same record (when both a current burn and sequelae of an old burn exist). Burns and corrosions do not heal at the same rate and a current healing wound may still exist with sequela of a healed burn or corrosion.

9) **Use of an External Cause Code with Burns and Corrosions**
   An external cause code should be used with burns and corrosions to identify the source and intent of the burn, as well as the place where it occurred.

The general guideline is that burns require two codes: a code for the burn's body site and severity, and a second code for its extent. In the hospital setting, a third code—an external cause code—is required for the circumstance that caused the injury. Burn documentation should therefore provide the site, depth, extent, and circumstance.

The depths of burns are classified as follows:

- First degree, in which the epidermis—top layer of skin—is affected (referred to as *erythema*)
- Second degree, with *blistering*
- Third degree, with *full-thickness involvement*

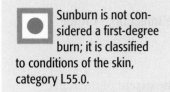 Sunburn is not considered a first-degree burn; it is classified to conditions of the skin, category L55.0.

The depths of burns at the same local site can often be mixed. When different degrees of burns are present and classified to the same subcategory, code the highest degree of burn for that site.

> ### ■ CASE SCENARIO
> A patient has both a second- and a third-degree burn of the back of the hand. In this case, the coder should assign *only* the code that reflects the highest degree of burn for the same site: code T23.369A, T31.0 (extent < 10%).

When a patient has multiple burn sites, each site of a burn should be coded separately. Category T30.0 (Burn of unspecified body region, unspecified degree) is used only if the exact locations of the burns are not documented. Documentation (site, extent, and circumstance) in the medical record should include the details of the burn(s) in order to assign specific codes.

EXAMPLE
Second-degree burns of the right thigh and right forearm (12%) are coded T22.211A, T24.211A, T31.10 (extent).

Sequencing of Burn and Related Condition Codes
As has been emphasized throughout this text, the principal diagnosis depends on the circumstances of admission. When the reason for the admission or encounter is a patient's burns, the following sequencing rules apply:

- *More than one burn present:* Sequence the code for the highest degree of burn first when more than one burn is present.

EXAMPLE
Third-degree burn of the foot (2%), and second-degree burn of the ankle (2%) are coded T25.329A, T25.219A, T31.10.

- *Internal and external burns:* When a patient has both internal and external burns, both are coded. The circumstances of admission will determine the selection of the principal diagnosis.

EXAMPLE
Burn of the intestine and third-degree burn of the chin (2%). Patient admitted for debridement of facial burn. Assign codes T20.33xA, T28.2xxA, T31.10.

- *Burn injuries with other related conditions:* When a patient is admitted for a burn and another related condition such as smoke inhalation and/or respiratory failure, again, the circumstances of admission determine the principal diagnosis.

EXAMPLE
Patient admitted with smoke inhalation. Patient also sustained a second-degree burn of the ear (1%). Assign codes T59.813A, T20.219A, T31.0.

As always, the circumstances of admission determine the sequencing of inpatient diagnoses when multiple injuries and burns are present.

Nonhealing Burns and Infected Burns
Nonhealing burns are coded as acute (current) burns. Documentation may describe first the treatment of an initial burn and then a subsequent visit for a burn that is nonhealing. In this instance, the second visit for the nonhealing burn would require the burn code to be classified as an acute burn. This rule also applies to *necrosis* (tissue death) of a nonhealing burn; so necrosis of burned skin should be coded as a non-healed burn.

EXAMPLE
Necrosis of third-degree burn of the scalp (8%) is coded T20.35xA, T31.0.

An *infected* burn requires two codes: one code for the burn site and an additional code that classifies the infection (infected burn, code T79.8xxA). Remember that the code for the infected burn is an additional code, and that the burn site code is sequenced first.

Infected first-degree burn of the left palm is coded T23.152A, L08.9 (see Infection, skin for site of infection).

Extent of Burns

After classifying burns by site and depth, the next component for coding is the extent of the burn, classified from categories T31 and T32. A code from this category must be assigned as an additional code. Codes from categories T31 and T32 can also be used when documentation includes the extent of burn only, and no additional information regarding about the site is available.

The extent of burn code is typically assigned when the record mentions a third-degree burn involving 20% or more of the body surface. Burn units may also use these codes for data collection purposes.

The fourth digit in categories T31 and T32 classify the extent of body surface burned, known as the *total body surface area (TBSA)*. The fifth digit in these categories classifies the extent of body surface of third-degree burn only. This concept is best explained by an example:

EXAMPLE

Code T31.41 is assigned when 40% of body surface is burned, with 10% at third degree: T31.41. The fourth digit 4 reflects the TBSA (40%), and the fifth digit of 1 reflects the extent of third-degree burns (10%).

As illustrated in Figure 9.1, the rule of nines is used to estimate the percentage of body surface. For adults, this rule assigns a percentage of body surface to body areas as follows:

Head and neck: 9%
Each arm: 9%
Each leg: 18%
Anterior trunk: 18%
Posterior trunk: 18%
Genitalia: 1%

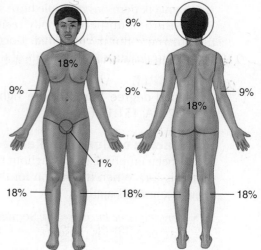

Figure 9.1 The rule of nines for calculating TBSA.

(From Thompson, G. *Understanding Anatomy & Physiology: A Visual, Auditory, Interactive Approach*, F.A. Davis Company, 2013.)

These estimates may change where necessary to accommodate infants and children who have proportionately larger heads than adults and patients who have large buttocks, thighs, or abdomens with burns. The coder may need to query the physician to determine the extent of burn before assigning a code from category T31.

Late Effects of Burns With a Current Burn

For late effects of burns, such as a scar or joint contracture, the coder must follow these rules:

1. Code first the residual condition (sequelae).
2. Code the late effect of burn code (look up the main term *"Late"* in the Alphabetic Index).
3. Assign a late effect external cause code (inpatient coding requirement).

> ■ **CASE SCENARIO**
> A patient presents with painful cicatrix (scar) of the right forearm from a second-degree burn sustained 6 months ago. She burned her arm accidentally while boiling water. Assign codes L90.5, T22.211S, Y33.xxxS.

Some patients have multiple burns that heal at different rates. In such a case, a patient may present with both a current burn and a late effect of a burn during the same encounter.

> ● Remember that codes from category T31 are used as additional codes unless documentation states extent of burn only, which is indeed rare.

> ● Remember that a *late effect* is the residual condition produced at any point in time after the acute phase of an illness or injury is over.

> ● The codes that reflect the circumstances of an injury or poisoning known as external cause codes are discussed in detail later in this chapter.

CHECKPOINT 9.4

Code the following cases using ICD-10-CM. (Do not assign external cause codes. Assign the extent of burn code when documented.)

1. Sunburn of the face _____

2. Burn with blisters of the right buttock _____

3. Bee sting with cellulitis of the right hand _____

4. Full-thickness infected burn of the left ear _____

5. Second- and third-degree burns of the left foot _____

6. Second-degree burns of the chin, cheek, and head _____

7. Accidental acid chemical burn of the left cornea _____

8. Inhalation burn of the left lung _____

9. First-degree burn of the left knee with third-degree burns of both legs _____

10. Second-degree burns of the left hand and third-degree burns of both arms; total extent of the burns is 20%, 18% third-degree burns _____

11. Painful scar contracture from previous burn of the back _____

Adverse Effects, Poisoning, and Toxic Effects

The *Official Guidelines* contain instructions for coding adverse effects, poisoning, and toxic effects, as shown in Box 9.5.

BOX 9.5 *Official Guidelines:* Adverse Effects, Poisoning, Underdosing, and Toxic Effects (T36–T65)

Codes in categories T36–T65 are combination codes that include the substance that was taken as well as the intent. No additional external cause code is required for poisonings, toxic effects, adverse effects, and underdosing codes.

1) **Do Not Code Directly from the Table of Drugs**
   Do not code directly from the Table of Drugs and Chemicals. Always refer back to the Tabular List.
2) **Use as Many Codes as Necessary to Describe**
   Use as many codes as necessary to describe completely all drugs, medicinal or biological substances.
3) **If the Same Code Would Describe the Causative Agent**
   If the same code would describe the causative agent for more than one adverse reaction, poisoning, toxic effect, or underdosing, assign the code only once.
4) **If Two or More Drugs, Medicinal or Biological Substances**
   If two or more drugs, medicinal or biological substances are reported, code each individually unless a combination code is listed in the Table of Drugs and Chemicals.
5) **The Occurrence of Drug Toxicity Is Classified in ICD-10-CM as Follows:**
   (a) **Adverse effect**
      When coding an adverse effect of a drug that has been correctly prescribed and properly administered, assign the appropriate code for the nature of the adverse effect followed by the appropriate code for the adverse effect of the drug (T36–T50). The code for the drug should
      Continued

BOX 9.5 *Continued*

have a 5th or 6th character "5" (for example T36.0X5-). Examples of the nature of an adverse effect are tachycardia, delirium, gastrointestinal hemorrhaging, vomiting, hypokalemia, hepatitis, renal failure, or respiratory failure.

(b) Poisoning

When coding a poisoning or reaction to the improper use of a medication (e.g., overdose, wrong substance given or taken in error, wrong route of administration), first assign the appropriate code from categories T36–T50. The poisoning codes have an associated intent as their 5th or 6th character (accidental, intentional self-harm, assault and undetermined). If the intent of the poisoning is unknown or unspecified, code the intent as accidental intent. The undetermined intent is only for use if the documentation in the record specifies that the intent cannot be determined. Use additional code(s) for all manifestations of poisonings.

If there is also a diagnosis of abuse or dependence of the substance, the abuse or dependence is assigned as an additional code.

Examples of poisoning include:

(i) Error was made in drug prescription

Errors made in drug prescription or in the administration of the drug by provider, nurse, patient, or other person.

(ii) Overdose of a drug intentionally taken

If an overdose of a drug was intentionally taken or administered and resulted in drug toxicity, it would be coded as a poisoning.

(iii) Nonprescribed drug taken with correctly prescribed and properly administered drug

If a nonprescribed drug or medicinal agent was taken in combination with a correctly prescribed and properly administered drug, any drug toxicity or other reaction resulting from the interaction of the two drugs would be classified as a poisoning.

(iv) Interaction of drug(s) and alcohol

When a reaction results from the interaction of a drug(s) and alcohol, this would be classified as poisoning.

See Section I.C.4. if poisoning is the result of insulin pump malfunctions.

(c) Underdosing

Underdosing refers to taking less of a medication than is prescribed by a provider or a manufacturer's instruction. For underdosing, assign the code from categories T36–T50 (fifth or sixth character "6").

Codes for underdosing should never be assigned as principal or first-listed codes. If a patient has a relapse or exacerbation of the medical condition for which the drug is prescribed because of the reduction in dose, then the medical condition itself should be coded.

Noncompliance (Z91.12-, Z91.13-) or complication of care (Y63.6–Y63.9) codes are to be used with an underdosing code to indicate intent, if known.

(d) Toxic effects

When a harmful substance is ingested or comes in contact with a person, this is classified as a toxic effect. The toxic effect codes are in categories T51–T65.

Toxic effect codes have an associated intent: accidental, intentional self-harm, assault, and undetermined.

f. Adult and Child Abuse, Neglect, and Other Maltreatment

Sequence first the appropriate code from categories T74.- (Adult and child abuse, neglect, and other maltreatment, confirmed) or T76.- (Adult and child abuse, neglect, and other maltreatment, suspected) for abuse, neglect, and other maltreatment, followed by any accompanying mental health or injury code(s).

If the documentation in the medical record states abuse or neglect it is coded as confirmed (T74.-). It is coded as suspected if it is documented as suspected (T76.-).

For cases of confirmed abuse or neglect an external cause code from the assault section (X92–Y09) should be added to identify the cause of any physical injuries. A perpetrator code (Y07) should be added when the perpetrator of the abuse is known. For suspected cases of abuse or neglect, do not report external cause or perpetrator code.

If a suspected case of abuse, neglect, or mistreatment is ruled out during an encounter, code Z04.71, Encounter for examination and observation following alleged physical adult abuse, ruled out, or code Z04.72, Encounter for examination and observation following alleged child physical abuse, ruled out, should be used, not a code from T76.

If a suspected case of alleged rape or sexual abuse is ruled out during an encounter code Z04.41, Encounter for examination and observation following alleged adult rape or code Z04.42, Encounter for examination and observation following alleged child rape, should be used, not a code from T76.

See Section I.C.15. Abuse in a pregnant patient.

The Table of Drugs and Chemicals following the Alphabetic Index lists the agents alphabetically, and columns identify the circumstance in which the drug or chemical was used. Use the table first to point to a code that you verify in the Tabular List under categories T36–T50.

Assigning codes for adverse effects, poisonings, underdosing, and toxic effects requires the use of the Table of Drugs and Chemicals that follows the general Alphabetic Index to Diseases and Injuries in ICD-10-CM.

It is critical for the coder to differentiate between an *adverse effect* and a *poisoning* in order to assign the correct codes. The major differences are summarized in Table 9.3. From a health-care perspective, drugs, medicinals, and biological substances may cause toxic reactions. These include prescription medications, over-the-counter medications, alcohol, and gases (to name just a few). Underdosing is defined as taking less of a medication than prescribed. The Table of Drugs and Chemicals has a distinct column when these circumstances result in illness. Sequelae or late effects of poisonings, adverse effects, and underdosing are reported using the seventh character of "S."

Table 9.3 Comparison of Poisoning and Adverse Effects

	POISONING	ADVERSE EFFECT
Definition	Drug or medicinal substance is not prescribed or taken correctly.	Drug or medicinal substance is prescribed and taken correctly.
Example documentation	Patient took 30 Lortab in suicide attempt.	Patient developed a skin rash after taking Lortab as prescribed.
Example coding	1. Assign the poisoning code from the Table of Drugs and Chemicals based on the substance or substances taken. 2. Assign the code for the effect(s) of the substance(s).	1. Assign a code for the adverse effect (i.e., drug rash, tachycardia, hemorrhage, or syncope). 2. Assign the code from the Adverse Effect column of the Table of Drugs and Chemicals.

Adverse Effects Versus Poisoning

An adverse effect is defined as a patient's negative reaction to a drug that is *correctly prescribed and administered*. Adverse effects of medicinal substances can result in toxicity, synergistic reactions, side effects, and idiosyncratic reactions. These effects may be due to differences among patients (i.e., age, disease, genetics) and drug-related factors (i.e., type of drug; route of administration; or dosage, especially common for the medications warfarin, insulin, and digoxin).

Coding an adverse effect requires two codes, the first for the nature of the reaction, and the second from the Adverse Effect column of the Table of Drugs and Chemicals to identify the causative substance of the effect.

Poisoning occurs when prescribed substances are taken (ingested) *incorrectly*. This may occur if the prescription itself is incorrect or as a result of a medication error by the provider, nurse, patient (who may have taken an incorrect amount or otherwise not followed the prescription's instructions), or other person. Poisoning is coded from the T36–T50 categories.

Some unique scenarios can occur that are also classified as poisonings:

- Nonprescribed drug taken with correctly prescribed and properly administered drug
- Interaction of drug(s) and alcohol

Poisoning can also occur when a *nonprescribed* substance (a drug or medicinal agent) is taken along with a correctly prescribed and properly administered drug. The interaction of the two drugs can cause drug toxicity or other reactions. Only when documentation states "undetermined" circumstances is the code from the column "Poisoning Undetermined" assigned.

■ **CASE SCENARIO**

A patient accidentally takes 800 mg of Motrin (as prescribed) with 400 mg of Advil (ibuprofen), which results in GI bleeding. Assign codes T39.311A, K92.9.

Common Medications for Injuries and Poisoning

Activated Charcoal

Activated charcoal (brand name: Actidose) is an agent used to bind ingested toxins and prevent their absorption.

Syrup of Ipecac

Syrup of ipecac is used to induce vomiting and empty the stomach of ingested toxins and prevent absorption.

Acetylcysteine

Acetylcysteine (brand names: Mucomyst, Acetadote) is used to treat acetaminophen overdose or poisoning.

If two different drugs were taken in combination incorrectly (one prescribed and one not prescribed), then two poisoning codes would be used. See Pinpoint the Code 9.1, which delineates the decision process to differentiate a poisoning from an adverse effect.

■ **CASE SCENARIO**

A patient took 800 mg of Advil PM with a prescribed antidepressant in a suicide attempt. The patient became lethargic. Assign codes T39.312A, T43.202A.

Any medicinal substance taken with alcohol that causes the patient to be ill is also considered a poisoning, and should be coded as such. The poisoning codes for both substances are assigned.

■ **CASE SCENARIO**

A patient takes antidepressants as prescribed with a "nightcap" of a vodka martini, which results in a seizure. The circumstances are not stated and codes T43.201A, T51.0x1A are assigned. Assume accidental circumstances unless otherwise notified.

PINPOINT THE CODE 9.1: Poisoning

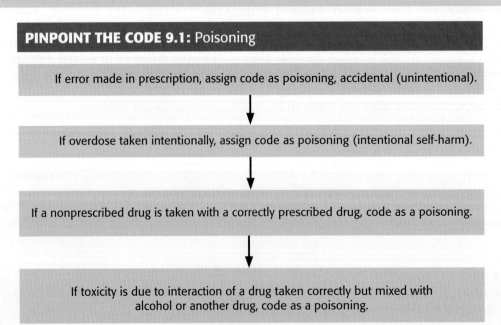

If error made in prescription, assign code as poisoning, accidental (unintentional).

↓

If overdose taken intentionally, assign code as poisoning (intentional self-harm).

↓

If a nonprescribed drug is taken with a correctly prescribed drug, code as a poisoning.

↓

If toxicity is due to interaction of a drug taken correctly but mixed with alcohol or another drug, code as a poisoning.

Flumazenil

Flumazenil (brand name: Romazicon) is used to treat benzodiazepine overdose or poisoning.

Pralidoxime

Pralidoxime (brand name: Protopam) is used to treat organophosphate poisoning.

Burn Treatments (Silvadene)

Silvadene (generic: silver sulfadiazine) is used to prevent wound sepsis in patients with second- and third-degree burns.

Sequencing of Poisoning

When coding a poisoning or reaction to the improper use of a medication (e.g., such as a wrong dose, wrong substance, or wrong route of administration), the poisoning code is sequenced first, followed by a code for the manifestation. Additional codes for drug abuse or dependence are assigned as additional codes when supported by documentation.

Drug toxicity is an overdose of a drug that was intentionally or accidentally taken or administered. This condition is coded as a poisoning (T51–T65 series).

Note that a toxic effect of a drug taken correctly is coded based on rules for coding adverse effects.

■ **CASE SCENARIO**

A patient accidentally takes an antidepressant as prescribed with a vodka martini, which results in a seizure. The patient is alcohol dependent. Assign codes T51.0x1A, T42.6x1A, R56.9, F10.20.

Toxic Effects and Drug Toxicity

A toxic effect (categories T51–T65) can occur when a harmful substance (i.e., chemical or drug) is taken or the patient comes in contact with a chemical or drug (i.e., such as by inhalation).

For toxic effects coding, the code from the table is sequenced first and includes the associated intent, followed by a code that reflects the manifestation of the toxic effect (the result).

■ **CASE SCENARIO**

A patient experienced toxic effect of natural gas when accidentally inhaled because of gas leak. Patient is hypoxic. Assign codes T59.2x1A, R09.02.

Code the following cases using ICD-10-CM.

1. Drug rash from taking penicillin as prescribed. _____

2. Wife took her husband's oxycodone by mistake, and as a result of the drug she developed nausea and vomiting. _____

3. Burns of the esophagus from accidentally swallowing bleach. _____

4. Gastrointestinal bleeding from mixing aspirin with naproxen. The physician did not prescribe either drug. _____

5. Mild mental retardation from previous suicide attempt. The patient took an overdose of fentanyl. _____

6. Abnormal coagulation profile due to Coumadin taken as prescribed. _____

7. Suicide attempt. The patient took 30 Percodan tablets with 1 pint of whiskey. _____

8. A baby accidentally swallowed cleaning detergent. _____

9. Carbon monoxide poisoning from car exhaust (car not in transit) in a suicide attempt. Patient had resulting acute respiratory failure. _____

10. Neutropenia due to chemotherapy. _____

Complications of Care

Provider documentation must support a relationship between the medical condition and the procedure to assign a complication of care code. In the medical record, this relationship is documented as "postoperative," "intraoperative," or "due to." Postoperative (post-op) hemorrhage is a complication of care. The statement "cellulitis due to vascular catheter" is also considered a complication of care.

Many different types of complications can occur. For example, complications can be mechanical (loosening or breaking of a part), infectious, a condition that causes pain, thrombosis, or due to a device malfunction or a misadventure (medical error). If documentation is unclear, the physician should be queried regarding the relationship of the medical condition and medical care. Box 9.6 presents the *Official Guidelines* for general coding of complications of care.

■ **CASE SCENARIO**
A patient develops a urinary tract infection after bladder surgery, but the infection may not be a postoperative complication, requiring a query.

Assigning Codes for Complication of Care

The main term *Complication* in the Alphabetic Index is often the right place to start when looking up complications of care for coding. In other instances, the subterm *postoperative* can lead the coder to the correct complication code.

Some complication codes include both the condition present and the presence of a complication and only one code is required.

EXAMPLE

Postoperative hematoma of the skin following dermatologic procedure (L76.31) is a combination code that reflects the exact postoperative complication.

On the other hand, the Tabular List may instruct the coder to assign an additional code to specify the exact condition that results from the medical care:

BOX 9.6 *Official Guidelines:* Complications of Care

1) General Guidelines for Complications of Care
  (a) Documentation of complications of care
    See Section I.B.16. for information on documentation of complications of care.

2) Pain Due to Medical Devices
  Pain associated with devices, implants or grafts left in a surgical site (for example, painful hip prosthesis) is assigned to the appropriate code(s) found in Chapter 19, Injury, poisoning, and certain other consequences of external causes. Specific codes for pain due to medical devices are found in the T code section of the ICD-10-CM. Use additional code(s) from category G89 to identify acute or chronic pain due to presence of the device, implant or graft (G89.18 or G89.28).

3) Transplant Complications
  (a) Transplant complications other than kidney
    Codes under category T86, Complications of transplanted organs and tissues, are for use for both complications and rejection of transplanted organs. A transplant complication code is only assigned if the complication affects the function of the transplanted organ. Two codes are required to fully describe a transplant complication: the appropriate code from category T86 and a secondary code that identifies the complication.
      Pre-existing conditions or conditions that develop after the transplant are not coded as complications unless they affect the function of the transplanted organs.
      See I.C.21. for transplant organ removal status.
      See I.C.2. for malignant neoplasm associated with transplanted organ.
  (b) Kidney transplant complications
    Patients who have undergone kidney transplant may still have some form of chronic kidney disease (CKD) because the kidney transplant may not fully restore kidney function. Code T86.1- should be assigned for documented complications of a kidney transplant, such as transplant failure or rejection or other transplant complication. Code T86.1- should not be assigned for post kidney transplant patients who have CKD unless a transplant complication such as transplant failure or rejection is documented. If the documentation is unclear as to whether the patient has a complication of the transplant, query the provider.
      Conditions that affect the function of the transplanted kidney, other than CKD, should be assigned a code from subcategory T86.1, Complications of transplanted organ, kidney, and a secondary code that identifies the complication.
      For patients with CKD following a kidney transplant, but who do not have a complication such as failure or rejection, *see Section I.C.14, Chronic kidney disease and kidney transplant status.*

4) Complication Codes That Include the External Cause
  As with certain other T codes, some of the complications of care codes have the external cause included in the code. The code includes the nature of the complication as well as the type of procedure that caused the complication. No external cause code indicating the type of procedure is necessary for these codes.

5) Complications of Care Codes within the Body System Chapters
  Intraoperative and postprocedural complication codes are found within the body system chapters with codes specific to the organs and structures of that body system. These codes should be sequenced first, followed by a code(s) for the specific complication, if applicable.

EXAMPLE
Post-op urinary retention. Assign codes N99.89, R33.9.

Finally, note that most complications may require an additional external cause code to reflect the type of surgery causing the complication. This additional code may also explain the circumstances of the complication (inpatient setting required only). The associated external cause codes that reflect complications of care are found in the ICD-10-CM External Cause of Injuries Index under the main terms *Complication Reaction, abnormal,* or *misadventure.*

EXAMPLES
• Post-op wound infection following appendectomy is coded T81.4xxA, Y83.6.

• Intraoperative atrial fibrillation during coronary artery bypass surgery is coded I97.790, I48.91, Y83.2.

When coding complications, the coder must pay attention to "Excludes" and "Use additional code" notes. There are many of these conventions throughout the complication of care code section.

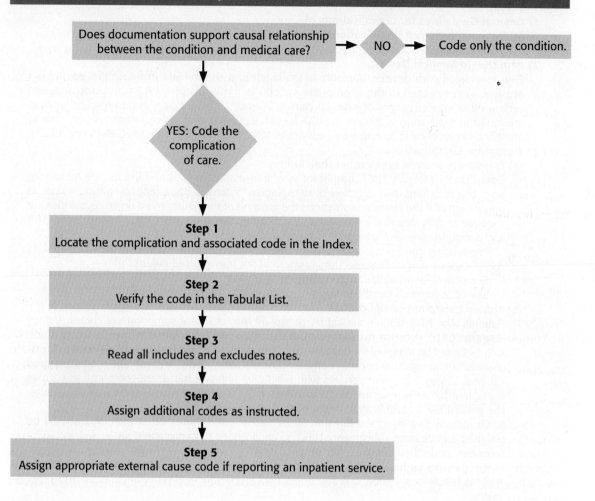

Does documentation support causal relationship between the condition and medical care? → **NO** → Code only the condition.

YES: Code the complication of care.

Step 1
Locate the complication and associated code in the Index.

Step 2
Verify the code in the Tabular List.

Step 3
Read all includes and excludes notes.

Step 4
Assign additional codes as instructed.

Step 5
Assign appropriate external cause code if reporting an inpatient service.

EXAMPLE

A postoperative wound infection (code T81.4XXA) excludes an infection due to an implanted device, infection due to infusion, or a postoperative obstetrical wound. An additional code is assigned to identify the infection.

Some complications are classified in other sections of ICD-10-CM.

EXAMPLE

A malfunctioning colostomy is reported using code K94.03.

To understand complication coding thoroughly, study the decision tree in Pinpoint the Code 9.2 and then review the following coded scenarios:

EXAMPLES

- Infected central venous catheter is coded T80.219A, Y84.8.

- Intraoperative cardiac arrest—patient undergoing amputation is coded I97.711, Y83.5.

- Paracolostomy hernia is coded K43.5.

- Postoperative ileus following colon resection with anastomosis is coded K91.89, K56.7, Y83.2.

- Blood transfusion reaction is coded T80.92xA, Y84.8.

- Accidental laceration of the bladder during hysterectomy is coded N99.71, Y83.6.

- Coronary stent thrombosis is coded T82.867A, Y83.1.

- Periprosthetic fracture, status post–left knee replacement is coded M97.12xA, Z96.652, Y83.1.

As you can see, these statements support a causal relationship between the medical care and the medical condition. In some instances, the complication code includes the presence of a complication and the medical condition, and in other cases additional codes are required to classify the complete condition.

Transplant Complications

The *Official Guidelines* provide instructions for nonkidney transplants and for kidney transplant complications.

Complications Other Than Kidney Transplants

The specific category for complications of transplanted organs (T86) is used to classify a transplant complication or transplant rejection other than for a kidney transplant. The transplant complication code is only assigned if the complication affects the function of the transplanted organ. Thus two codes are required: one code to reflect the complication (T86.8x) and an additional code to reflect the specific complication (i.e., such as infection).

Sometimes the patient has a preexisting condition, or a condition develops after transplant. Again, the complication code would only be assigned if the preexisting condition affects the function of the transplanted organ. For a malignant neoplasm of a transplanted organ, the complication code is sequenced first, followed by code C80.2 (malignant neoplasm associated with transplanted organ), and a third code to specify the malignancy.

> ### EXAMPLE
> For renal cell carcinoma of a transplanted kidney, assign codes T86.10, C80.2, C64.9, Y83.0.

As we have seen in many instances throughout ICD-10-CM, there is an exception to this rule. The following coding guidelines are specific to chronic kidney disease in patients with a kidney transplant.

Chronic Kidney Disease and Kidney Transplant Complications

There is an exception to the complication rule specific to chronic kidney disease (CKD) after a kidney transplant. A new kidney may not fully restore renal function, so CKD may still be present after a kidney transplant. Therefore, the presence of CKD alone does not constitute a transplant complication. In these instances, assign the appropriate N18 code for the patient's stage of CKD and code Z94.0 (status post–renal transplant).

The complication code for a renal transplant in the presence of CKD is only assigned when documentation supports rejection of the transplanted kidney, transplant failure, or a specific transplant complication.

If documentation regarding the presence of a transplant complication is unclear, the provider should be queried. In the presence of transplant failure, or rejection, a code from subcategory T86.1 should be assigned first followed by an additional code for the complication.

Code the following cases using ICD-10-CM and include external cause codes where appropriate.

1. Postoperative wound infection with abdominal wall cellulitis; the patient recently underwent colon resection with anastomosis _____

2. Infected arteriovenous fistula used for renal dialysis with end-stage CKD_____

3. Chronic pain due to internal orthopedic fixation device (nail) _____

4. Malfunctioning insulin pump in an individual with type 1 diabetes, with resulting underdosing _____

5. Dislocation of prosthetic right knee _____

6. Postoperative pulmonary embolism following knee replacement _____

7. Ulcer of large intestinal anastomosis _____

8. Postoperative seroma; patient underwent hernia repair _____

9. Sponge (foreign body) accidentally left in abdominal cavity after gastric bypass surgery _____

10. Renal transplant rejection resulting in CKD, stage 5 _____

11. Ventilator-associated *Klebsiella* pneumonia _____

12. *Staphylococcal aureus* infection of left lower leg amputation stump _____

EXTERNAL CAUSES OF MORBIDITY (CHAPTER 20: V00–Y99)

External cause codes classify the specifics of an injury and poisoning regarding the cause, the intent, the place, the activity, and patient status. These codes explain the circumstances of injuries resulting from environmental events such as falls, fires, transportation accidents, accidental poisoning by a drug or other substance, and adverse effects. This information is used for injury research and prevention.

The categories in Chapter 20 of ICD-10-CM are grouped as shown in Table 9.4. Box 9.7 presents the instructions from the *Official Guidelines*. These guidelines apply for the coding and collection of external cause codes from records in hospitals, outpatient clinics, EDs, other ambulatory care settings and provider offices, and nonacute care settings, except when other specific guidelines apply.

Table 9.4 Organization of ICD-10-CM Chapter 20 Tabular List

BLOCK	BLOCK DESCRIPTION
V00–X58	Accidents
V00–V99	Transport accidents
V00–V09	Pedestrian injured in transport accident
V10–V19	Pedal cycle rider injured in transport accident
V20–V29	Motorcycle rider injured in transport accident
V30–V39	Occupant of three-wheeled motor vehicle injured in transport accident
V40–V49	Car occupant injured in transport accident
V50–V59	Occupant of pick-up truck or van injured in transport accident
V60-V69	Occupant of heavy transport vehicle injured in transport accident
V70–V79	Bus occupant injured in transport accident
V80-V89	Other land transport accidents
V90–V94	Water transport accidents
V95–V97	Air and space transport accidents
V98–V99	Other and unspecified transport accidents
W00–X58	Other external causes of accidental injury
W00–W19	Slipping, tripping, stumbling, and falls
W20–W49	Exposure to inanimate mechanical forces
W50–W64	Exposure to animate mechanical forces
W65–W74	Accidental nontransport drowning and submersion
W85–W99	Exposure to electric current, radiation, and extreme ambient temperature and pressure
X00–X08	Exposure to smoke, fire, and flames
X10–X19	Contact with heat and hot substances
X30–X39	Exposure to forces of nature
X52–X58	Accidental exposure to other specified factors
X71–X83	Intentional self-harm
X92–Y08	Assault
Y21–Y33	Event of undetermined intent
Y35–Y38	Legal intervention, operations of war, military operations, and terrorism
Y62–Y84	Complications of medical and surgical care
Y62–Y69	Misadventures to patients during surgical and medical care
Y70–Y82	Medical devices associated with adverse incidents in diagnostic and therapeutic use
Y83–Y84	Surgical and other medical procedures as the cause of abnormal reaction of the patient, or of labor complication, without mention of misadventure at the time of the procedure
Y90–Y99	Supplementary factors related to causes of morbidity classified elsewhere

BOX 9.7 *Official Guidelines:* Injury, Poisoning, and Certain Other Consequences of External Causes (S00–T88)

External cause codes are intended to provide data for injury research and evaluation of injury prevention strategies. These codes capture how the injury or health condition happened (cause), the intent (unintentional or accidental; or intentional, such as suicide or assault), the place where the event occurred, the activity of the patient at the time of the event, and the person's status (e.g., civilian, military).

a. General External Cause Coding Guidelines

1) Used with any code in the range of A00.0–T88.9, Z00–Z99

An external cause code may be used with any code in the range of A00.0–T88.9, Z00–Z99, classification that is a health condition due to an external cause. Though they are most applicable to injuries, they are also valid for use with such things as infections or diseases due to an external source, and other health conditions, such as a heart attack that occurs during strenuous physical activity.

2) External cause code used for length of treatment

Assign the external cause code, with the appropriate 7th character (initial encounter, subsequent encounter, or sequelae) for each encounter for which the injury or condition is being treated.

3) Use the full range of external cause codes

Use the full range of external cause codes to completely describe the cause, the intent, the place of occurrence, and if applicable, the activity of the patient at the time of the event, and the patient's status, for all injuries, and other health conditions due to an external cause.

4) Assign as many external cause codes as necessary

Assign as many external cause codes as necessary to fully explain each cause. If only one external code can be recorded, assign the code most related to the principal diagnosis.

5) The selection of the appropriate external cause code

The selection of the appropriate external cause code is guided by the Alphabetic Index of External Causes and by Inclusion and Exclusion notes in the Tabular List.

6) External cause code can never be a principal diagnosis

An external cause code can never be a principal (first-listed) diagnosis.

7) Combination external cause codes

Certain of the external cause codes are combination codes that identify sequential events that result in an injury, such as a fall which results in striking against an object. The injury may be due to either event or both. The combination external cause code used should correspond to the sequence of events regardless of which caused the most serious injury.

8) No external cause code needed in certain circumstances

No external cause code from Chapter 20 is needed if the external cause and intent are included in a code from another chapter (e.g., T36.0X1-, Poisoning by penicillins, accidental (unintentional)).

b. Place of Occurrence Guideline

Codes from category Y92, Place of occurrence of the external cause, are secondary codes for use after other external cause codes to identify the location of the patient at the time of injury or other condition.

A place of occurrence code is used only once, at the initial encounter for treatment. No 7th characters are used for Y92. Only one code from Y92 should be recorded on a medical record. A place of occurrence code should be used in conjunction with an activity code, Y93.

Do not use place of occurrence code Y92.9 if the place is not stated or is not applicable.

c. Activity Code

Assign a code from category Y93, Activity code, to describe the activity of the patient at the time the injury or other health condition occurred.

An activity code is used only once, at the initial encounter for treatment. Only one code from Y93 should be recorded on a medical record. An activity code should be used in conjunction with a place of occurrence code, Y92.

The activity codes are not applicable to poisonings, adverse effects, misadventures, or sequelae.

Do not assign Y93.9, Unspecified activity, if the activity is not stated.

A code from category Y93 is appropriate for use with external cause and intent codes if identifying the activity provides additional information about the event.

d. Place of Occurrence, Activity, and Status Codes Used with Other External Cause Code

When applicable, place of occurrence, activity, and external cause status codes are sequenced after the main external cause code(s). Regardless of the number of external cause codes assigned, there should be only one place of occurrence code, one activity code, and one external cause status code assigned to an encounter.

e. If the Reporting Format Limits the Number of External Cause Codes

If the reporting format limits the number of external cause codes that can be used in reporting clinical data, report the code for the cause/intent most related to the principal diagnosis. If the format permits capture of additional external cause codes, the cause/intent, including medical misadventures, of the additional events should be reported rather than the codes for place, activity, or external status.

f. Multiple External Cause Coding Guidelines

More than one external cause code is required to fully describe the external cause of an illness or injury. The assignment of external cause codes should be sequenced in the following priority:

If two or more events cause separate injuries, an external cause code should be assigned for each cause. The first-listed external cause code will be selected in the following order:

External codes for child and adult abuse take priority over all other external cause codes.
See Section I.C.19, Child and Adult abuse guidelines.

External cause codes for terrorism events take priority over all other external cause codes except child and adult abuse.

External cause codes for cataclysmic events take priority over all other external cause codes except child and adult abuse and terrorism.

External cause codes for transport accidents take priority over all other external cause codes except cataclysmic events, child and adult abuse, and terrorism.

Activity and external cause status codes are assigned following all causal (intent) external cause codes.

The first-listed external cause code should correspond to the cause of the most serious diagnosis due to an assault, accident, or self-harm, following the order of hierarchy listed above.

g. Child and Adult Abuse Guideline

Adult and child abuse, neglect, and maltreatment are classified as assault. Any of the assault codes may be used to indicate the external cause of any injury resulting from the confirmed abuse.

For confirmed cases of abuse, neglect, and maltreatment, when the perpetrator is known, a code from Y07, Perpetrator of maltreatment and neglect, should accompany any other assault codes.
See Section I.C.19, Adult and child abuse, neglect, and other maltreatment.

h. Unknown or Undetermined Intent Guideline

If the intent (accident, self-harm, assault) of the cause of an injury or other condition is unknown or unspecified, code the intent as accidental intent. All transport accident categories assume accidental intent.

1) Use of undetermined intent

External cause codes for events of undetermined intent are only for use if the documentation in the record specifies that the intent cannot be determined.

i. Sequelae (Late Effects) of External Cause Guidelines

1) Sequelae external cause codes

Sequelae are reported using the external cause code with the 7th character "S" for sequela. These codes should be used with any report of a late effect or sequela resulting from a previous injury.

2) Sequelae external cause code with a related current injury

A sequelae external cause code should never be used with a related current nature of injury code.

3) Use of sequelae external cause codes for subsequent visits

Use a late effect external cause code for subsequent visits when a late effect of the initial injury is being treated. Do not use a late effect external cause code for subsequent visits for follow-up care (e.g., to assess healing, to receive rehabilitative therapy) of the injury when no late effect of the injury has been documented.

j. Terrorism Guidelines

1) Cause of injury identified by the federal government (FBI) as terrorism

When the cause of an injury is identified by the federal government (FBI) as terrorism, the first-listed external cause code should be a code from category Y38, Terrorism. The definition of terrorism employed by the FBI is found at the inclusion note at the beginning of category Y38. Use additional code for place of occurrence (Y92.-). More than one Y38 code may be assigned if the injury is the result of more than one mechanism of terrorism.

2) Cause of an injury is suspected to be the result of terrorism

When the cause of an injury is suspected to be the result of terrorism a code from category Y38 should not be assigned. Suspected cases should be classified as assault.

3) Code Y38.9, Terrorism, secondary effects

Assign code Y38.9, Terrorism, secondary effects, for conditions occurring subsequent to the terrorist event. This code should not be assigned for conditions that are due to the initial terrorist act.

It is acceptable to assign code Y38.9 with another code from Y38 if there is an injury due to the initial terrorist event and an injury that is a subsequent result of the terrorist event.

k. External Cause Status

A code from category Y99, External cause status, should be assigned whenever any other external cause code is assigned for an encounter, including an activity code, except for the events noted below. Assign a code from category Y99, External cause status, to indicate the work status of the person at the time the event occurred. The status code indicates whether the event occurred during military activity, whether a non-military person was at work, whether an individual including a student or volunteer was involved in a non-work activity at the time of the causal event.

A code from Y99, External cause status, should be assigned, when applicable, with other external cause codes, such as transport accidents and falls. The external cause status codes are not applicable to poisonings, adverse effects, misadventures or late effects.

Do not assign a code from category Y99 if no other external cause codes (cause, activity) are applicable for the encounter.

An external cause status code is used only once, at the initial encounter for treatment. Only one code from Y99 should be recorded on a medical record.

Do not assign code Y99.9, Unspecified external cause status, if the status is not stated.

General External Cause Coding Guidelines

External cause codes, or codes that describe external causes, are a supplemental classification system. They are assigned as an additional diagnosis with any code from A00.0–T88.9 or Z00–Z99. These codes are applicable to injuries, but they may be assigned when an external service causes disease in the hospital setting. However, their use is considered voluntary in the physician setting, that is, for physician services. External cause codes explain the circumstances and location of injuries, poisonings, and adverse effects. The guidelines address reporting as follows:

Place of occurrence
Adverse effects of drugs, medicinal and biological substances
Multiple causes
Child and adult abuse
Unknown, suspected, or undetermined causes
Late effects
Misadventures and complications of care
Terrorism

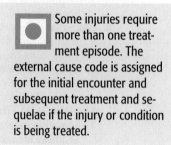

An external cause code can never be reported as a principal diagnosis.

As coders know, external cause codes are never reported first. Therefore, they can be used as secondary codes with any code in the ICD-10-CM, although they are not usually reported with Z codes, because external cause codes describe circumstances of injury or adverse effects, neither of which requires a Z code. The first-listed code reflects the exact injury, poisoning, or adverse effect, followed by the external cause code to explain the circumstances and location (i.e., such as home, street, public building).

Some injuries require more than one treatment episode. The external cause code is assigned for the initial encounter and subsequent treatment and sequelae if the injury or condition is being treated.

Full Range of External Cause Codes

Given a particular set of circumstances surrounding an injury, poisoning, adverse effect, or late effect of an injury or a poisoning, more than one external cause code may be assigned to completely describe the cause, the intent, and the place of occurrence, if applicable. If there is space for only one external cause code to be recorded, assign the external cause code most related to the principal diagnosis. When space permits, at least one external cause code from each category (cause, intent, place) if possible should be reported. The limitation may occur primarily due to reporting space.

The UB-04/837I claim allows a facility to report a defined number of diagnosis codes, so the number of external cause codes—considered supplemental diagnoses—that can be reported may be limited.

Place of Occurrence Guideline

Codes from category Y92 are secondary codes used to report the *place of occurrence* for injuries, poisonings, or other conditions. This type of code describes where the event took place and is used once at the initial encounter. If the place of occurrence is not stated or not applicable, do NOT use Y92.9 (Unspecified place). Some state reporting systems require a place of occurrence, even if unlisted, so the coder should check with the state requirements. Officially, however, according to the guidelines, Y92.9 should not be assigned. Some external cause codes that describe the circumstance of the accident include the place. Two examples illustrate both scenarios:

EXAMPLES
- Code W21.89xA, which describes being struck accidentally in sports without a fall, can be reported with code Y92.838, Accident occurring at place of recreation and sport.

- Code V49.88xA describes a car occupant being injured in another type of specified transport accident. No additional place of occurrence code would need to be assigned.

Activity Codes

These codes describe the activity of the patient at the time an injury or health condition occurred and are assigned from category Y93. These codes are reported once, at the initial encounter and are assigned in conjunction with a code from category Y92 for the place of occurrence. When the activity is unspecified, code Y93.9 should not be assigned.

External Cause Status

Codes for category Y99, external cause status, are used as additional codes with any other external cause code. This category classifies the work status of the patient at the time of the event.

Assign external cause status codes once at the initial encounter for treatment. The unspecified external cause status code Y99.9 is not assigned if the status is not stated.

Multiple-Cause Coding Guidelines

In some instances, a patient may have been involved in two or more events that cause separate injuries. In this case, multiple external cause codes would be assigned (at least for each cause). The following hierarchy assists the coder in selecting the first-listed external cause code in these situations:

1. External cause codes for child and adult abuse take priority over all other external cause codes.
2. External cause codes for terrorism events take priority over all other external cause codes except child and adult abuse.
3. External cause codes for cataclysmic events take priority over all other external cause codes except child and adult abuse and terrorism.
4. External cause codes for transport accidents take priority over all other external cause codes except cataclysmic events, child and adult abuse, and terrorism.
5. The first-listed external cause code should correspond to the cause of the most serious diagnosis due to an assault, accident, or self-harm, following the order of hierarchy listed above.

Adult and Child Abuse, Neglect, and Other Maltreatment

For instances of adult and child abuse, neglect, and other maltreatment, the code for the abuse (from category T76) is reported first, followed by a code for the specific injury or mental health disorder. The "use additional code" notes in the Tabular List assist the coder in completely coding these cases. In cases where no injuries or signs or symptoms are present, the code for the abuse is still reported, followed by the external cause codes for the nature of abuse and the perpetrator. The external cause code that denotes the perpetrator is assigned second, with the external cause code for the mechanism of injury sequenced first. This guideline is stated in the *Official Guidelines* notes on external cause codes (Section C.19.ef.). Confirmed (T74) or suspected (T76) cases of abuse, neglect, or maltreatment are reported versus those ruled out.

Unknown or Undetermined Intent Guideline

In some cases, the intent of an injury or poisoning is unknown or suspect. For example, a patient who has serious injuries may be unable to describe the circumstances, or a patient may refuse to describe the circumstances, such as shot in the street. In these instances, the coder must follow these guidelines to select an external cause code:

1. *Intent unknown:* If the intent (accident, self-harm, assault) of the cause of an injury or poisoning is stated as unknown or unspecified, code the intent as undetermined.

2. *Intent suspect or questionable:* If the intent (accident, self-harm, assault) of the cause of an injury is unknown or unspecified, without specific documentation, code the intent as undetermined.

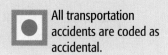 All transportation accidents are coded as accidental.

■ **CASE SCENARIO**
Police brought the patient to the hospital with a gunshot wound to the face. The circumstances were not stated. Assign codes S09.93xA, Y24.9xxA.

The external cause code for the mechanism of injury is reported throughout the episodes of care using the appropriate seventh character.

Terrorism Guidelines

The external cause codes for terrorism are only assigned when the cause of injury is identified by the federal government (specifically, the FBI) as terrorism (Y38). In these cases, the terrorism external cause code is the *first-listed and only external cause* code assigned. The FBI defines terrorism as "injuries resulting from the unlawful use of force or violence against persons or property to intimidate or coerce a Government, the civilian population, or any segment thereof, in furtherance of political or social objective."

EXAMPLE
Second-degree burn of the arm due to terrorist bombing is coded T22.20xA, Y38.2x2A.

Injuries or poisonings suspected to be due to terrorism do not meet the guidelines for terrorism, and a code from category Y38 should not be assigned. External cause code assignment in these cases is reported as an assault or based on documentation of intent and mechanism.

CHECKPOINT 9.7

Define the following using the definitions located in the beginning of Chapter 20 in the Tabular List.

1. Tricycle: _____

2. Rowboat: _____

3. Interurban streetcar: _____

4. Bulldozer: _____

5. Person riding a skateboard: _____

Assign only external cause codes to the following.

6. Fall from tree at home in yard _____

7. Kicked by horse in the barn while horseback riding _____

8. Fall from baseball stadium steps _____

9. Struck in the head by falling object at work (in factory) _____

10. Child neglect (did not feed child) by father, unintentional _____

11. Fall from ATV motor vehicle (driver) _____

12. Burned by fall into bonfire at beach _____

13. Hand cut by lawn mower blade at apartment building residence _____

14. Cut by electric knife at grocery store while preparing food as an employee _____

15. Bicyclist hit by car in traffic, bicyclist injured (initial encounter) _____

FACTORS INFLUENCING HEALTH STATUS AND CONTACT WITH HEALTH SERVICES (CHAPTER 21: Z00–Z99)

Chapter 21 of ICD-10-CM contains the Z codes, which help coders complete coding scenarios by providing the reasons for many common visits to health-care providers. They identify encounters for reasons other than illness or injury. The categories of Z codes are grouped as shown in Table 9.5.

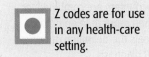

Z codes are for use in any health-care setting.

Not all Z codes can be sequenced first. Some Z codes can be sequenced first or second, whereas others may only be first or only be second.

Most people have received health-care services when they are not ill. Examples are a visit for an immunization, a screening because of a family history of colon cancer, or a visit because of an exposure to a virus, but with no disease present. The Z codes are considered diagnosis codes that classify encounters for circumstances other than a disease or injury. In other words, this supplementary classification is provided to classify occasions when circumstances other than a disease or injury (codes A00–T88) are recorded as a diagnosis or problem. These circumstances include:

- A person who is not currently sick encounters the health services for some specific reason, such as to act as an organ donor; to receive prophylactic care, such as inoculations or health screenings; or to receive counseling on health-related issues.
- A person with a resolving or chronic condition encounters the health-care systems for specific aftercare or treatment such as dialysis for renal disease, chemotherapy, or a cast change.
- Circumstances or problems influencing a person's health status are not in themselves a current illness or injury.
- A newborn's diagnosis reflects birth status.
- A maternity encounter for delivery includes the outcome of delivery.

Table 9.5 Organization of ICD-10-CM Chapter 21 Tabular List

BLOCK	BLOCK DESCRIPTION
Z00–Z13	Persons encountering health services for examinations
Z14–Z15	Genetic carrier and genetic susceptibility to disease
Z16	Resistance to antimicrobial drugs
Z17	Estrogen receptor status
Z18	Retained foreign body fragments
Z20–Z28	Persons with potential health hazards related to communicable diseases
Z30–Z39	Persons encountering health services in circumstances related to reproduction
Z40–Z53	Encounters for other specific health care
Z55–Z65	Persons with potential health hazards related to socioeconomic and psychosocial circumstances
Z66	Do not resuscitate status
Z67	Blood type
Z68	Body mass index (BMI)
Z69–Z76	Persons encountering health services in other circumstances
Z77–Z99	Persons with potential health hazards related to family and personal history and certain conditions influencing health status

Sequencing Z Codes

A Z code can be used as either a first-listed code (the principal diagnosis code in the inpatient setting) or a secondary code, depending on the particular code and, for facility coding, on the circumstances of the encounter. Some Z codes can only be used as the principal diagnosis or first-listed diagnosis, as laid out in the *Official Guidelines* Section I.C.21.c.16. For example, codes from category Z38, liveborn infants, can only be used as a principal or first-listed diagnosis.

It is important to remember that Z codes are diagnosis codes. In some instances, the Z code (diagnosis codes) classifies the reason for the encounter (e.g., admission for chemotherapy). A corresponding procedure code (either an ICD-10-PCS procedure code for inpatient coding or a CPT/HCPCS code for the physician setting) accompanies the Z code to describe the procedure actually performed.

EXAMPLES

- Admission for chemotherapy in a female patient with right breast cancer is coded Z51.11, C50.911 (diagnoses). The procedure codes for chemotherapy are also assigned.

- Outpatient visit for prophylactic vaccination/inoculation against measles, mumps, and rubella (MMR) is coded Z23. The procedure codes for the inoculation and the substance injected would also be assigned.

Common main terms in the Alphabetic Index that result in Z code assignment are as follows:

Admission for	Donor	Observation
Aftercare	Encounter for	Outcome of Delivery
Attention To	Examination	Prophylactic
Checking of	Exposure	Removal
Checkup	Fitting of	Replacement
Chemotherapy	Follow-up	Screening
Convalescence Carrier	History of	Status Post
Counseling	Newborn	Vaccination

Categories of Z Codes

In discussing the Z code guidelines, it is best to look at the *Official Guidelines*, as summarized in the part that describes these categories.

Contact/With, Exposure To, or Carrier of Infectious Disease

Categories Z20, Z22, and Z77 indicate contact with expected exposure to communicable diseases (Z20), carriers of infectious disease (Z22), or contact and suspected exposure hazardous to health (Z77). These circumstances can occur when the patient has had contact with or exposure to an infected individual and/or carries the infection but no signs, symptoms, or disease are present. There is a potential health risk for these patients, and the Z codes classify that risk.

EXAMPLES

- Patient visit after being exposed to rabies: Z20.3

- Hepatitis B carrier: Z22.51

Inoculations and Vaccinations

Codes from category Z23 are used to classify services related to inoculations and vaccinations. These codes indicate that a patient is being seen to receive a prophylactic inoculation against a disease, again when no disease is present. The Z code is the reason for the visit, and these codes would have a corresponding procedure code that represents the service itself, but the Z code is the reason for the visit. These codes can be used as secondary diagnoses when inoculation or vaccination is accompanied by another reason for the visit or takes place during a routine preventive visit.

EXAMPLES

- Routine newborn visit (25 days old), measles-mumps-rubella vaccine provided. Assign codes Z00.111, Z23.

- Office visit for routine influenza vaccine is coded Z23.

Status

Status Z codes indicate that a patient has the sequelae (residuals; conditions following as a consequence) of a past disease or condition. These Z codes do not reflect sequelae of an injury because these would be reported using a seventh character for the episode of care. The Z codes are used because they give additional information regarding the status of the patient that can impact care.

EXAMPLE

The presence of a prosthetic or device is represented by a status code.

It is important to note that the use of Z codes does reflect a current status, not a history of a previous condition. A history of a previous condition indicates that the patient no longer has the condition at all. Use of the status Z codes is limited to reflecting status only. In the presence of related disease, the status code is not assigned.

EXAMPLE

Code Z94.1, Heart transplant status, should not be used with code T86.20, Unspecified complication of transplanted heart. The status code does not provide additional information; rather, the complication code already indicates that the patient is status post–heart transplant.

Table 9.6 lists the Z code categories from the *Official Guidelines* that reflect a patient's status:

Table 9.6 Status Z Codes

CODE	STATUS
Z14	Genetic carrier Genetic carrier status indicates that a person carries a gene associated with a particular disease that may be passed to offspring who may develop that disease. The person does not have the disease and is not at risk of developing the disease.
Z15	Genetic susceptibility to disease Genetic susceptibility indicates that a person has a gene that increases the risk of that person developing the disease. Codes from category Z15 should not be used as principal or first-listed codes. If the patient has the condition to which he/she is susceptible, and that condition is the reason for the encounter, the code for the current condition should be sequenced first. If the patient is being seen for follow-up after completed treatment for this condition, and the condition no longer exists, a follow-up code should be sequenced first, followed by the appropriate personal history and genetic susceptibility codes. If the purpose of the encounter is genetic counseling associated with procreative management, code Z31.5, Encounter for genetic counseling, should be assigned as the first-listed code, followed by a code from category Z15. Additional codes should be assigned for any applicable family or personal history.
Z16	Resistance to antimicrobial drugs This code indicates that a patient has a condition that is resistant to antimicrobial drug treatment. Sequence the infection code first.
Z17	Estrogen receptor status
Z18	Retained foreign body fragments
Z19	Hormone sensitivity malignancy status
Z21	Asymptomatic HIV infection status This code indicates that a patient has tested positive for HIV but has manifested no signs or symptoms of the disease.
Z22	Carrier of infectious disease Carrier status indicates that a person harbors the specific organisms of a disease without manifest symptoms and is capable of transmitting the infection.

Continued

Table 9.6 *Continued*

CODE	STATUS
Z28.3	Underimmunization status
Z33.1	Pregnant state, incidental
	This code is a secondary code only for use when the pregnancy is in no way complicating the reason for the visit. Otherwise, a code from the obstetrical chapter is required.
Z66	Do not resuscitate
	This code may be used when it is documented by the provider that a patient is on do-not-resuscitate status at any time during the stay.
Z67	Blood type
Z68	Body mass index (BMI)
Z74.01	Bed confinement status
Z76.82	Awaiting organ transplant status
Z78	Other specified health status
	Code Z78.1, Physical restraint status, may be used when it is documented by the provider that a patient has been put in restraints during the current encounter. Please note that this code should not be reported when it is documented by the provider that a patient is temporarily restrained during a procedure.
Z79	Long-term (current) drug therapy
	Codes from this category indicate a patient's continuous use of a prescribed drug (including such things as aspirin therapy) for the long-term treatment of a condition or for prophylactic use. It is not for use for patients who have addictions to drugs. This subcategory is not for use of medications for detoxification or maintenance programs to prevent withdrawal symptoms in patients with drug dependence (e.g., methadone maintenance for opiate dependence). Assign the appropriate code for the drug dependence instead.
	Assign a code from Z79 if the patient is receiving a medication for an extended period as a prophylactic measure (such as for the prevention of deep vein thrombosis) or as treatment of a chronic condition (such as arthritis) or a disease requiring a lengthy course of treatment (such as cancer). Do not assign a code from category Z79 for medication being administered for a brief period of time to treat an acute illness or injury (such as a course of antibiotics to treat acute bronchitis).
Z88	Allergy status to drugs, medicaments, and biological substances
	Except: Z88.9, Allergy status to unspecified drugs, medicaments, and biological substances status
Z89	Acquired absence of limb
Z90	Acquired absence of organs, not elsewhere classified
Z91.0-	Allergy status, other than to drugs and biological substances
Z92.82	Status post administration of tPA (rtPA) in a different facility within the last 24 hours prior to admission to a current facility
	Assign code Z92.82, Status post administration of tPA (rtPA) in a different facility within the last 24 hours prior to admission to current facility, as a secondary diagnosis when a patient is received by transfer into a facility and documentation indicates they were administered tissue plasminogen activator (tPA) within the last 24 hours prior to admission to the current facility.
	This guideline applies even if the patient is still receiving the tPA at the time they are received into the current facility.
	The appropriate code for the condition for which the tPA was administered (such as cerebrovascular disease or myocardial infarction) should be assigned first.
	Code Z92.82 is only applicable to the receiving facility record and not to the transferring facility record.
Z93	Artificial opening status
Z94	Transplanted organ and tissue status
Z95	Presence of cardiac and vascular implants and grafts
Z96	Presence of other functional implants
Z97	Presence of other devices

Z98	Other postprocedural states
	Assign code Z98.85, Transplanted organ removal status, to indicate that a transplanted organ has been previously removed. This code should not be assigned for the encounter in which the transplanted organ is removed. The complication necessitating removal of the transplant organ should be assigned for that encounter.
	See Section I.C19. for information on the coding of organ transplant complications.
Z99	Dependence on enabling machines and devices, not elsewhere classified
	Note: Categories Z89–Z90 and Z93–Z99 are for use only if there are no complications or malfunctions of the organ or tissue replaced, the amputation site, or the equipment on which the patient is dependent.

History (of)

The history Z codes reflect the patient's own history as well as family history. *History* implies that the medical condition no longer exists and that no treatment is being provided for it, but that it merits continued monitoring.

EXAMPLE

History of colon cancer (Z85.038). The cancer is no longer present and is no longer being treated, but there is a potential for recurrence that requires monitoring.

History Z codes can be used with other Z codes that represent follow-up services or screening services.

EXAMPLES

• Screening colonoscopy in patient with history of colon cancer, no recurrence found, is coded Z12.11, Z85.038.

• Follow-up colon resection due to colon cancer is coded Z08, Z85.038.

Personal history Z codes are coded within categories Z87–Z92. Family history Z codes, used when a patient has a family member(s) who has had a particular disease that causes the patient to be at higher risk of also contracting the disease, are coded within categories Z80–Z84.

Screening

Screening is defined as testing for disease or disease precursors in a seemingly well individual for early detection and treatment. Depending on patient risk factors (e.g., age, gender), certain screenings are recommended, such as routine mammograms in women over 50. The screening Z codes are assigned for these encounters. In the presence of signs or symptoms of a suspected condition, the screening codes are not assigned; rather, the presenting signs and symptom codes are assigned.

When a medical condition is discovered during the screening examination, the condition found should also be reported as a secondary diagnosis.

EXAMPLE

Colon cancer screening via colonoscopy. Colonoscopy was positive for diverticulosis of large intestine. Assign codes Z12.11, K57.30 (plus the appropriate procedure code for the colonoscopy using the appropriate procedure code).

Observation

Observation Z codes (Z03, Z04, and Z05) are used in limited circumstances. They represent observation for a suspected condition that is ruled out. Again, no disease exists. These codes are not used when signs or symptoms related to the suspected condition are documented. These codes can be assigned as a principal diagnosis only, unless assigned for a liveborn infant, or when the observation services are unrelated to the suspected condition being observed. For encounters for expected fetal conditions that are inconclusive following testing, assign the appropriate code from category O35, O36, O40, or O41.

The observation Z code categories:

Z03 Encounter for medical observation for suspected diseases and conditions ruled out

Z04 Encounter for examination and observation for other reasons

Except: Z04.9, Encounter for examination and observation for unspecified reason

Z05 Encounter for observation and evaluation of newborn for suspected diseases and conditions ruled out

EXAMPLES

• Single live newborn (vaginal delivery), observation for suspected newborn sepsis ruled out is coded Z38.00, Z05.1.

• Observation for suspected maternal oligohydramnios, condition not found, is coded Z03.71.

Aftercare

Continuation of care during the healing and recovery phase of an illness is termed *aftercare*. To use one of the aftercare codes, the initial treatment of the disease or injury must have been performed at an earlier encounter. The aftercare Z code categories are listed in Table 9.7.

Table 9.7 Aftercare Z Codes

CODE	AFTERCARE TREATMENT
Z42	Encounter for plastic and reconstructive surgery following medical procedure or healed injury
Z43	Encounter for attention to artificial openings
Z44	Encounter for fitting and adjustment of external prosthetic device
Z45	Encounter for adjustment and management of implanted device
Z46	Encounter for fitting and adjustment of other devices
Z47	Orthopedic aftercare
Z48	Encounter for other postprocedural aftercare
Z49	Encounter for care involving renal dialysis
Z51	Encounter for other aftercare and medical care

If the current treatment is being carried out for an injury or disease, the code for the specific disease or injury is assigned rather than the Z code for aftercare. Exceptions to this rule include the following:

• Z51.0, Encounter for antineoplastic radiation therapy
• Z51.1, Encounter for antineoplastic chemotherapy and immunotherapy

These codes are always listed first, followed by the diagnosis code for the neoplasm. When both radiotherapy and chemotherapy are the reasons for the admission, then either code may be sequenced first.

EXAMPLE

Patient admitted solely for chemotherapy to treat right lung cancer. Assign codes Z51.11, C34.91.

Of course, if aftercare for one condition is provided, and a separate unique condition exists, the aftercare code can be sequenced as an additional diagnosis. Aftercare codes should be used in conjunction with other diagnosis codes to provide more detail on the specifics of an aftercare encounter visit, unless otherwise directed by the classification.

Follow-Up

Follow-up Z codes are assigned when treatment of a disease is completed yet continuing surveillance is required (Table 9.8). In other words, the disease that is being "followed up on" is no longer present. Follow-up codes should not be confused with aftercare codes or injury codes in which the seventh character represents the encounter for ongoing care of a healing condition.

 Z codes should NOT be used for aftercare for injuries.

Continuing surveillance is often required for certain conditions, and the follow-up codes are assigned for this surveillance. The coder must be careful in these instances and ensure the following:

1. Avoid confusing these codes with aftercare services (current treatment for a healing condition).
2. When recurrence of a disease or a new condition is found during surveillance, the illness or condition (illness) found should be reported, not the follow-up Z code.

3. Follow-up codes are often used with history codes to provide a full picture of the healed condition and its treatment. The follow-up code is sequenced first, followed by the history code.

Table 9.8 Follow-Up Z Codes

CODE	FOLLOW-UP TREATMENT
Z08	Encounter for follow-up examination after completed treatment for malignant neoplasm
Z09	Encounter for follow-up examination after completed treatment for conditions other than malignant neoplasm
Z39	Encounter for maternal postpartum care and examination

■ CASE SCENARIOS

- A patient presents for follow-up cystoscopy due to history of bladder cancer treated 1 year ago by fulguration. Assign codes Z08, Z85.51 (plus procedure code for cystoscopy).

- A patient presents for follow-up colonoscopy due to excision of sigmoid polyps excised 1 year ago. A new polyp is found. Assign code D12.5 (plus the colonoscopy/polypectomy procedure code).

Donor

A special category, Z52, is used to assign services for living individuals who are donating blood or other tissues. Only the donor for others would have services reported using category Z52. Self-donations or cadaveric donations would not be reported using these codes.

■ CASE SCENARIO

A mother presents to donate her kidney to her child. Code Z52.4 is assigned.

Counseling

Certain Z codes represent visits for specified services, as is the case for the counseling Z codes (Table 9.9). This type of counseling code is used when counseling a patient or family member who receives assistance in the aftermath of illness or when support is required. Counseling can be provided for contraceptive management, genetics, family circumstances, and dietary and other situations. Many medical situations exist in which it is not necessary to use a counseling code because the diagnosis code includes a counseling component. Counseling codes should not be reported when counseling is integral to the service.

The counseling Z code categories are as follows:

Table 9.9 Counseling Z Codes

CODE	COUNSELING SERVICE
Z30.0-	Encounter for general counseling and advice on contraception
Z31.5	Encounter for procreative genetic counseling
Z31.6-	Encounter for general counseling and advice on procreation
Z32.2	Encounter for childbirth instruction
Z32.3	Encounter for childcare instruction
Z69	Encounter for mental health services for victim and perpetrator of abuse
Z70	Counseling related to sexual attitude, behavior, and orientation
Z71	Persons encountering health services for other counseling and medical advice, not elsewhere classified
Z76.81	Expectant mother prebirth pediatrician visit

EXAMPLES

- Contraceptive management counseling is coded Z30.09.

- Counseling for surgical options for a patient with colon cancer is coded C18.9. (No counseling code is assigned because counseling is integral.)

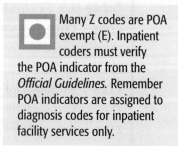

See Chapter 8 of this text regarding the use of codes for obstetrical conditions. A brief review is provided here as well.

Obstetrics and Related Conditions

In pregnancy, Z codes are assigned only when a complication of the obstetrical period is not present. If a complication is present, then the code from the obstetrics chapter (Chapter 15) is assigned, rather than a Z code for pregnant state. The Z codes Z34.0-, Supervision of normal first pregnancy, and Z34.8-, Supervision of other normal pregnancy, are always first-listed and are not to be used with any other code from the obstetrics chapter. These codes are also used as the admitting diagnosis when a patient presents for delivery.

Z code categories for obstetrical and reproductive services are listed in Table 9.10.

Table 9.10 Obstetrical and Reproductive Services

CODE	SERVICE
Z30	Encounter for contraceptive management
Z31	Encounter for procreative management
Z32.2	Encounter for childbirth instruction
Z32.3	Encounter for childcare instruction
Z33	Pregnant state
Z34	Encounter for supervision of normal pregnancy
Z36	Encounter for antenatal screening of mother
Z3A	Weeks of gestation
Z37	Outcome of delivery
Z39	Encounter for maternal postpartum care and examination
Z76.81	Expectant mother prebirth pediatrician visit

Category Z37 is assigned on the mother's chart to report the outcome of delivery. This code must be reported as an additional code when the encounter results in a delivery. Additional Z codes for family planning, contraceptive management, and counseling can also be assigned for the visit as a secondary diagnosis as well when the visit is for delivery. When an outpatient visit may be for contraceptive management alone, the Z code can be sequenced first.

Routine and Administrative Examinations

Sometimes we visit health-care providers for routine visits, school physicals, preoperative examinations, or routine health checks. The routine and administrative examinations Z codes classify these services (Table 9.11). These codes should not be used if the examination is for diagnosis of a suspected condition or for treatment purposes. In these cases, the diagnosis code is reported.

In some instances, a diagnosis or condition is discovered during a routine examination. When this occurs, the routine examination Z code is assigned first, followed by a code for the condition or disease found. Preexisting and chronic conditions and history codes may also be included as additional codes as long as the examination is for administrative purposes and not focused on any particular condition.

Many Z codes are POA exempt (E). Inpatient coders must verify the POA indicator from the *Official Guidelines*. Remember POA indicators are assigned to diagnosis codes for inpatient facility services only.

Preoperative examination Z codes are assigned when a patient is being cleared for surgery and no treatment is given. An additional code for the condition that requires surgery should also be reported along with comorbid conditions that are evaluated.

■ **CASE SCENARIO**
Preoperative cardiac examination for patient scheduled for an inguinal hernia repair. The patient has hypertension and hypercholesterolemia. Codes Z01.810, I10, E78.00 are reported.

Table 9.11 Routine Examinations

CODE	EXAMINATION
Z00	Encounter for general examination without complaint, suspected or reported diagnosis
Z01	Encounter for other special examination without complaint, suspected or reported diagnosis
Z02	Encounter for administrative examination
	Excerpt: Z02.9, Encounter for administrative examinations, unspecified
Z32.0-	Encounter for pregnancy test

Pinpoint the Code 9.3 illustrates a decision tree for Z codes.

PINPOINT THE CODE 9.3: Z Code

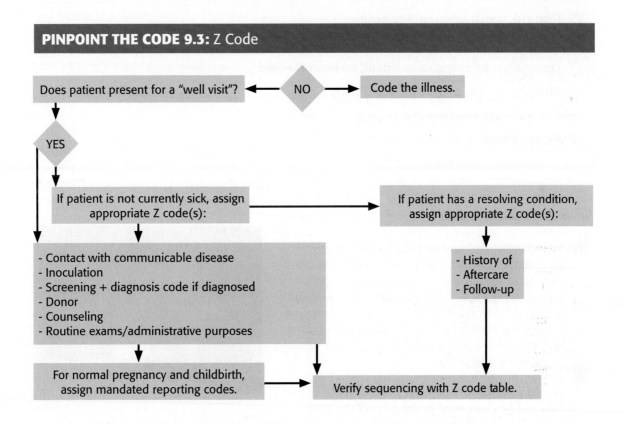

Code the following cases using ICD-10-CM.

1. Exposure to venereal disease _____

2. Group B streptococcus carrier _____

3. Vaccination not carried out because of acute illness _____

4. Family history of coronary artery disease _____

5. Insufficient prenatal care, patient in third trimester _____

6. Status post–bone marrow transplant _____

7. Attention to colostomy _____

8. Awaiting heart transplant _____

9. Prophylactic breast removal; family history of breast cancer _____

10. Admission for routine pacemaker pulse generator change _____

11. Aftercare following traumatic fracture of the left humerus _____

12. Visit for dressing change _____

13. Admission for removal of vascular catheter, no complications _____

14. Hospice care (palliative care) for patient with end-stage congestive heart failure _____

15. High-risk sexual behavior, HIV positive _____

16. Visit for preemployment exam _____

17. Observation following car accident; no injuries noted _____

18. Body mass index of 35.4 (adult), obesity _____

19. Visit for routine hearing test _____

20. Kidney donor _____

Chapter Summary

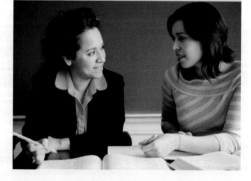

1. Reporting of sign and symptom codes requires knowledge of the disease process. The term *integral* indicates that a sign or symptom is typically present with a specific disease process. Signs and symptoms that are integral to the disease process are not reported separately. Signs and symptoms that are not integral to the disease process should be reported separately.

2. It is common for signs and symptoms to be reported for outpatient services, because the workup may not be completed at the time of the visit. Conditions documented as possible in the outpatient setting cannot be coded; only the farthest extent of the disease at the time of the visit can be reported. In the inpatient setting, signs and symptoms on admission are evaluated, and often an underlying cause is determined. Therefore, the coder is less likely to report numerous signs and symptoms in the inpatient setting.

3. Each injury, whether it is a single injury or one of multiple injuries, is assigned a separate code unless a combination code is available that better suits the situation that is documented. Superficial injuries associated with more severe wounds at the same site are not coded separately. Fractures are coded according to location, whether they are displaced or nondisplaced, and episode of care.

4. During healing, fractures or complications of care are coded with the appropriate fracture and appropriate seventh character to reflect the episode of care.

5. The general guideline is that burns require two codes: a code for the burn's body site and severity, and a second code for its extent. Extent refers to the total amount of body surface involved. Calculating the extent follows the rule of nines.

6. An adverse effect is defined as a patient's negative reaction to a drug correctly prescribed and administered. Reporting an adverse effect requires two codes, the first for the nature of the reaction, and an external cause of morbidity code from the Table of Drugs and Chemicals to identify the causative substance for an adverse effect of drugs, medicinal or biological substances, correctly prescribed and properly administered.

7. Poisoning occurs when prescribed substances are taken (ingested) incorrectly. This may occur if the prescription itself is incorrect or if a medication error has been made by the provider, nurse, patient, or other person. It may also occur when the prescribed substance interacts with another nonprescribed ingested substance or with alcohol, causing the patient to become ill. Poisoning is coded from the Table of Drugs and Chemicals and is reported first. The manifestation of poisoning is reported as an additional code.

8. A toxic effect can occur when a harmful substance is taken or the patient comes in contact with a toxic chemical or drug (i.e., such as by inhalation). The poisoning code is sequenced first, followed by a code that reflects the manifestation of the toxic effect (the result).

9. For a condition to be classified as a complication, documentation must state a causal relationship between the condition and the medical care or procedure. To code a condition as a complication of a transplanted organ, the function of the transplanted organ must be affected. Two codes are required to report transplant complications, the appropriate code for the complication and a secondary code that identifies the specific effect. The rules for kidney transplants are different. A patient with CKD may still have some form of CKD after a transplant, because the transplant may not fully restore kidney function. This type of CKD is not a complication. If a complication such as transplant failure or rejection is documented, then the kidney transplant complication code is assigned.

10. External cause codes represent a supplementary classification for providing further information about injuries resulting from environmental events such as falls, fires, transportation accidents, accidental poisoning by a drug or other substances, and adverse effects. Coding of external causes requires use of a separate alphabetic index. The reporting of external cause codes is required for all facility services. In the nonfacility setting (i.e., physician), external cause code reporting is optional. Guidelines apply to assigning and sequencing codes for place of occurrence; activity and patient status; multiple causes; child and adult abuse; unknown, suspected, or undetermined causes; and terrorism. External cause codes are never the first-listed diagnosis codes.

11. Z codes are used to report encounters for healthy patients or to denote factors that can influence health, such as family history of colon cancer. There are 15 categories, including Z codes for visits relating to contact with or exposure to communicable diseases; inoculations and vaccinations; status; history; screening; observation; aftercare; follow-up; donors; counseling; obstetrics and related conditions; newborns, infants, and children; routine and administrative examinations; miscellaneous categories; and nonspecific categories. Whether a particular Z code can be the first-listed or principal code is governed by Section I.C.21.c.16 of the *Official Guidelines*.

Matching

Match the key terms with their definitions.

A. screening Z code
B. observation Z code
C. poisoning
D. counseling Z code
E. adverse effect
F. displaced
G. external cause code

H. status Z code
I. fracture aftercare
J. history Z code
K. sign
L. symptom
M. pathological fracture
N. stress fracture

1. _____ Type of code that reports testing for disease in a seemingly well individual

2. _____ A subjective condition the patient reports, such as abdominal pain

3. _____ Type of code used when a patient or family member receives assistance in the aftermath of an illness or injury

4. _____ Type of code indicating that a patient has the sequelae of a past disease or condition

5. _____ A fracture that is due to repetitive injury

6. _____ Patient's negative reaction to a drug correctly prescribed and administered

7. _____ Occurs when prescribed substances are taken (ingested) incorrectly

8. _____ Bone break in which the bone ends are not aligned

9. _____ Cast changes, cast removal, removal of fixation devices, medication adjustment, or any follow-up visits

10. _____ A fracture that is due to osteoporosis

11. _____ A code that can never be used first

12. _____ Type of code that is assigned when a suspected condition is ruled out

13. _____ Type of code that reports that a medical condition no longer exists and that no treatment is being provided for it, but that it merits continued monitoring

14. _____ An objective condition, such as a fever

True or False

Decide whether each statement is true or false.

1. __F__ Mixing alcohol with prescribed medication is considered an adverse reaction.

2. __T__ When sequencing injury codes, the most severe injury is sequenced first.

3. __T__ Follow-up codes are assigned for the second visit when a disease is treated.

4. __T__ An encounter for radiation therapy Z code is always a secondary code.

5. __F__ A screening code is assigned for a patient presenting with signs and symptoms of the disease.

6. __T__ When reporting burn codes, report only the highest degree of burn for the same anatomical site.

7. __T__ Routine and administrative examination codes are assigned for routine visits, school physicals, preoperative examinations, or routine health checks.

8. __T__ A code for rehabilitation is assigned as a secondary code when the encounter is for rehabilitation.

9. __F__ The diagnosis of prosthetic fracture is considered a complication.

10. __T__ A patient history code is assigned when the medical condition no longer exists or is no longer under treatment.

11. __T__ The seventh character "D" is used to describe a fracture that is healing for which treatment was provided previously.

12. __F__ A symptom code can never be the principal diagnosis.

13. __T__ If a fracture is due to trauma, a pathological fracture code would not be assigned.

14. __F__ In the statement "dysuria due to possible urinary tract infection," the infection code would be assigned as the primary diagnosis in the outpatient setting.

15. __T__ Weakness is a symptom that is integral to anemia.

16. __T__ A symptom code may be the principal diagnosis when the cause of the symptom is unknown.

Multiple Choice

Select the letter that best completes the statement or answers the question.

1. Which of the following code pairs reflects a follow-up colonoscopy in a patient with a history of colon cancer, no recurrence found?
   A. Z08, Z85.038
   B. Z85.038, Z08
   C. Z08, Z80.0
   D. Z12.11, Z85.038

2. Status post–motor vehicle accident, initial observation for suspected head injury, none found, is coded
   A. Z04.1, S09.90xA
   B. Z04.3
   C. S09.90xA
   D. Z04.1

3. Initial treatment was for a compound sub-capital fracture of the left femur. The patient also sustained a laceration of the left eyebrow after tripping and falling on the carpet at her house in the bedroom. Which codes are reported?
   A. S72.011A, S01.111A, W18.09xxA, Y92.019
   B. S72.012A, S01.112A, W18.09xxA, Y92.003
   C. M84.452, S01.110A, W22.8xxA, Y92.003
   D. S72.012A, S01.112A, W22.8xxA, Y92.042

4. Patient with right lung cancer was admitted for chemotherapy. How is this coded?
   A. C34.90, Z51.11
   B. Z51.11, C34.91
   C. Z51.11
   D. C34.91

5. Patient accidentally took Tegretol as prescribed and then drank three martinis, which resulted in a syncopal episode. Which codes are reported?
   A. T42.1x1A, R55
   B. T42.1x1A, T51.0x1A
   C. T42.1x1A, T51.0x1A, R55
   D. R55, T42.1x4A

6. Postoperative ileus following resection of colon with anastomosis is coded
   A. K91.89, Y83.6
   B. K56.7, Y83.6,
   C. K91.870, Y83.2
   D. K91.89, K56.7, Y83.2

7. Acute chest pain due to gastroesophageal reflux and anxiety is coded
   A. R07.9, K21.9, F41.9
   B. K21.9, F41.9
   C. K21.9, F41.9, R07.9
   D. F41.9, K21.9, R07.9

8. Epigastric pain due to gastritis is coded
   A. K29.00
   B. K29.70
   C. R10.13, K29.70
   D. K29.70, R10.13

9. Routine child health check is coded
   A. Z02.89
   B. Z00.121
   C. Z00.129
   D. Z00.00

10. Physician office visit with diagnosis of dyspnea, shortness of breath, rule out pneumonia, is coded
    A. J18.9
    B. R06.00, R06.02, J18.9
    C. J18.9, R06.00, R06.02
    D. R06.00, R06.03

11. Initial care for fracture of the second lumbar vertebra secondary to idiopathic osteoporosis is coded
    A. M80.88xA
    B. M81.8, M80.88xA
    C. M80.88xA, M81.8
    D. S32.029A, M81.8

12. Initial treatment for infected urinary catheter causing acute *E. coli* pyelonephritis is coded
    A. N10, B96.20
    B. T83.51xA, N10, B96.20, Y84.6
    C. T83.51xA, N10, Y84.6
    D. N10, T83.51xA, Y84.6

13. Initial encounter is for a patient with infected puncture wound of the left ring finger with cellulitis due to pseudomonas. Patient has a history of breast cancer. Which codes are reported?
    A. S61.235A, A49.8, L03.012, Z85.3
    B. S61.235A, L03.012, Z85.3
    C. L03.012, B96.5, Z85.3
    D. S61.235A, L03.012, B96.5, Z85.3

14. Initial aftercare is provided for nonunion of left tibial shaft fracture with ankle pain. Patient was a driver in a car when the car collided with a bus. Report codes
    A. S82.202K
    B. S82.200K
    C. S82.202K, V49.9xxA
    D. S82.202A, V44.9xxA

15. Underdosing of Lasix resulting in acute on chronic diastolic congestive heart failure is coded
    A. T50.1x6A, I50.31
    B. T50.1x6A, I50.33
    C. T50.1x5A, I50.33
    D. T50.1x6A, I50.9

CHAPTER 10

ICD-10-CM Outpatient Coding Guidelines

CHAPTER OUTLINE

Basic Coding Guidelines for Outpatient Settings

Selection of First-Listed Diagnosis

Reporting Secondary Diagnoses and External Cause Codes in Outpatient Settings

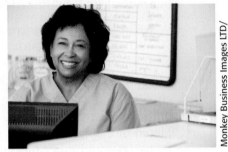

Monkey Business Images LTD/Monkey Business/Thinkstock

LEARNING OUTCOMES

After studying this chapter, you should be able to:

1. Define the outpatient settings to which Section IV of the *Official Guidelines* applies.
2. Define the term *first-listed diagnosis* as it relates to the outpatient setting.
3. Apply diagnosis code sequencing rules for a variety of outpatient encounters, such as outpatient procedures/ambulatory surgeries, observation stays, and encounters for circumstances other than disease or injury.
4. Apply ICD-10-CM coding guidelines to outpatient visits when patients receive only diagnostic services, therapeutic services, or preoperative examinations.
5. Understand the coding and sequencing guidelines for routine outpatient prenatal visits.
6. Compare and contrast coding for uncertain conditions in the outpatient and inpatient settings.
7. Apply outpatient coding guidelines for emergency department visits.
8. Understand how chronic diseases and coexisting conditions are coded in the outpatient setting.
9. Understand guidelines regarding reporting of additional diagnoses and External Cause codes in the outpatient setting.
10. Based on diagnostic statements, correctly assign diagnosis codes for the outpatient setting.

The majority of health-care patients' visits are to outpatient settings. A typical year involves more than a million physician office visits, nearly 100 million visits to hospital outpatient departments, and well over a million emergency department (ED) visits. These numbers compare with about 35 million inpatient hospital discharges, not counting normal newborn discharges. Therefore, correct outpatient diagnostic coding is vital for both professional and facility billing.

Assigning ICD-10-CM diagnosis codes in outpatient settings requires knowledge of specific official guidelines. This chapter introduces information outpatient coders must understand, starting with the definition of an outpatient and moving to the guidelines that apply to each type of outpatient service. In many cases, these guidelines are different from inpatient guidelines. For example, the Uniform Hospital Discharge Data Set (UHDDS) definition of *principal diagnosis* does not apply in the outpatient setting, because the workup of the patient's condition typically occurs over a series of visits rather than during a single hospital inpatient stay.

These unique guidelines, however, build on the basic rules and conventions for assigning diagnosis codes using the ICD-10-CM code set, such as coding to the highest level of specificity. This chapter provides the details and guidelines for outpatient diagnostic coding.

BASIC CODING GUIDELINES FOR OUTPATIENT SETTINGS

Box 10.1 presents the outpatient coding guidelines from Section IV of the *ICD-10-CM Official Guidelines for Coding and Reporting*. Like the inpatient guidelines, these outpatient guidelines have been developed and approved by the cooperating parties. They are approved for use by hospitals and physicians in coding and reporting diagnoses for both facility-based outpatient services and *all* physician services. ICD-10-CM conventions and general guidelines apply to assigning these codes, but outpatient diagnostic coding differs from inpatient coding in three ways:

1. The definition of *principal diagnosis*
2. The coding of inconclusive diagnoses
3. Reporting from diagnostic test results (x-ray, pathology, etc.)

The definition of *principal diagnosis*—the diagnosis arrived at after study—in the UHDDS does not apply in any outpatient setting. In the outpatient setting, the study of a patient's disease is not always completed in a single visit. The patient may make many visits and have many tests and other procedures before the diagnosis is determined. Therefore, the phrase "after study," which defines the principal diagnosis for a hospital inpatient stay, does not apply in outpatient settings. In the outpatient setting, the term *first-listed diagnosis/condition* is used to identify the code that is listed first on the claim.

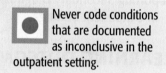

Never code conditions that are documented as inconclusive in the outpatient setting.

In addition, inconclusive conditions—those that are documented as possible, probable, or suspected—are not assigned codes in outpatient settings. Instead, the coder assigns codes to the condition, sign, or symptom that is known at the time of the visit. For example, if the documentation states "cough, rule out pneumonia," the outpatient coder codes the diagnosis of cough only; the inconclusive diagnosis of pneumonia is not reported. The coding guidelines stating that codes for inconclusive diagnoses apply to inpatient reporting only.

Another difference between coding diagnoses in the outpatient setting versus the inpatient setting is the guideline regarding coding of diagnostic test results. In the outpatient setting, the coder can code from physician-interpreted test results such as radiology or pathology reports. For example, the pre-op and post-op diagnoses state breast mass, and pathological findings state adenocarcinoma of the breast. The outpatient code for adenocarcinoma would be reported based on the pathology results.

Definition of Outpatient Visit

Because Section IV of the *Official Guidelines* applies only to outpatient visits, it is important to understand that an outpatient *visit* or *encounter*—the terms are used interchangeably—is one in which the patient is not formally admitted to a facility. Such a visit occurs in an outpatient setting that is either a hospital-based or -owned facility or a freestanding facility. Hospital-based facility outpatient services are the responsibility of the hospital-based facility and take place in EDs, ambulatory surgery units, observation units, clinics (a distinct part of a facility or a separate facility used

BOX 10.1 *Official Guidelines:* Diagnostic Coding and Reporting Guidelines for Outpatient Services

These coding guidelines for outpatient diagnoses have been approved for use by hospitals/providers in coding and reporting hospital-based outpatient services and provider-based office visits. Guidelines in Section I, Conventions, general coding guidelines and chapter-specific guidelines, should also be applied for outpatient services and office visits.

The terms *encounter* and *visit* are often used interchangeably in describing outpatient service contacts and, therefore, appear together in these guidelines without distinguishing one from the other.

Though the conventions and general guidelines apply to all settings, coding guidelines for outpatient and provider reporting of diagnoses will vary in a number of instances from those for inpatient diagnoses, recognizing that: The Uniform Hospital Discharge Data Set (UHDDS) definition of principal diagnosis does not apply to hospital-based outpatient services and provider-based office visits.

Coding guidelines for inconclusive diagnoses (probable, suspected, rule out, etc.) were developed for inpatient reporting and do not apply to outpatients.

a. Selection of First-Listed Condition

In the outpatient setting, the term *first-listed diagnosis* is used in lieu of *principal diagnosis.*

In determining the first-listed diagnosis, the coding conventions of ICD-10-CM, as well as the general and disease-specific guidelines, take precedence over the outpatient guidelines.

Diagnoses often are not established at the time of the initial encounter/visit. It may take two or more visits before the diagnosis is confirmed.

The most critical rule involves beginning the search for the correct code assignment through the Alphabetic Index. Never begin searching initially in the Tabular List as this will lead to coding errors.

1) Outpatient Surgery

When a patient presents for outpatient surgery (same-day surgery), code the reason for the surgery as the first-listed diagnosis (reason for the encounter), even if the surgery is not performed due to a contraindication.

2) Observation Stay

When a patient is admitted for observation for a medical condition, assign a code for the medical condition as the first-listed diagnosis.

When a patient presents for outpatient surgery and develops complications requiring admission to observation, code the reason for the surgery as the first-reported diagnosis (reason for the encounter), followed by codes for the complications as secondary diagnoses.

b. Codes from A00.0 Through T88.9, Z00–Z99

The appropriate code(s) from A00.0 through T88.9, Z00–Z99 must be used to identify diagnoses, symptoms, conditions, problems, complaints, or other reason(s) for the encounter/visit.

c. Accurate Reporting of ICD-10-CM Diagnosis Codes

For accurate reporting of ICD-10-CM diagnosis codes, the documentation should describe the patient's condition, using terminology that includes specific diagnoses as well as symptoms, problems, or reasons for the encounter. There are ICD-10-CM codes to describe all of these.

d. Codes That Describe Symptoms and Signs

Codes that describe symptoms and signs, as opposed to diagnoses, are acceptable for reporting purposes when a diagnosis has not been established (confirmed) by the provider. Chapter 18 of ICD-10-CM, Symptoms, Signs, and Abnormal Clinical and Laboratory Findings, Not Elsewhere Classified (codes R00–R99), contains many, but not all, codes for symptoms.

e. Encounters for Circumstances Other Than a Disease or Injury

ICD-10-CM provides codes to deal with encounters for circumstances other than a disease or injury. The Factors Influencing Health Status and Contact with Health Services codes (Z00–Z99) are provided to deal with occasions when circumstances other than a disease or injury are recorded as diagnoses or problems.
See Section I.C.21. Factors influencing health status and contact with health services.

f. Level of Detail in Coding

1) ICD-10-CM codes with *3, 4, 5, 6, or 7 characters*

ICD-10-CM is composed of codes with 3, 4, 5, 6, or 7 characters. Codes with three characters are included in ICD-10-CM as the heading of a category of codes that may be further subdivided by the use of 4th, 5th, 6th, or 7th characters to provide greater specificity.

2) Use of full number of *characters* required for a code

A three-character code is to be used only if it is not further subdivided. A code is invalid if it has not been coded to the full number of characters required for that code, including the 7th character, if applicable.

g. ICD-10-CM Code for the Diagnosis, Condition, Problem, or Other Reason for Encounter/Visit

List first the ICD-10-CM code for the diagnosis, condition, problem, or other reason for encounter/visit shown in the medical record to be chiefly responsible for the services provided. List additional

Continued

BOX 10.1 *Continued*

codes that describe any coexisting conditions. In some cases, the first-listed diagnosis may be a symptom when a diagnosis has not been established (confirmed) by the physician.

h. Uncertain Diagnosis

Do not code diagnoses documented as "probable," "suspected," "questionable," "rule out," or "working diagnosis" or other similar terms indicating uncertainty. Rather, code the condition(s) to the highest degree of certainty for that encounter/visit, such as symptoms, signs, abnormal test results, or other reason for the visit.

Note: This differs from the coding practices used by short-term care, acute care, long-term care, and psychiatric hospitals.

i. Chronic Diseases

Chronic diseases treated on an ongoing basis may be coded and reported as many times as the patient receives treatment and care for the condition(s).

j. Code All Documented Conditions That Coexist

Code all documented conditions that coexist at the time of the encounter/visit and require or affect patient care treatment or management. Do not code conditions that were previously treated and no longer exist. However, history codes (categories Z80–Z87) may be used as secondary codes if the historical condition or family history has an impact on current care or influences treatment.

k. Patients Receiving Diagnostic Services Only

For patients receiving diagnostic services only during an encounter/visit, sequence first the diagnosis, condition, problem, or other reason for encounter/visit shown in the medical record to be chiefly responsible for the outpatient services provided during the encounter/visit. Codes for other diagnoses (e.g., chronic conditions) may be sequenced as additional diagnoses.

For encounters for routine laboratory/radiology testing in the absence of any signs, symptoms, or associated diagnosis, assign Z01.89, *Encounter for other specified special examinations*. If routine testing is performed during the same encounter as a test to evaluate a sign, symptom, or diagnosis, it is appropriate to assign both the Z code and the code describing the reason for the non-routine test.

For outpatient encounters for diagnostic tests that have been interpreted by a physician and for which the final report is available at the time of coding, code any confirmed or definitive diagnosis(es) documented in the interpretation. Do not code related signs and symptoms as additional diagnoses.

Note: This differs from the coding practice in the hospital inpatient setting regarding abnormal findings on test results.

l. Patients Receiving Therapeutic Services Only

For patients receiving therapeutic services only during an encounter/visit, sequence first the diagnosis, condition, problem, or other reason for encounter/visit shown in the medical record to be chiefly responsible for the outpatient services provided during the encounter/visit. Codes for other diagnoses (e.g., chronic conditions) may be sequenced as additional diagnoses.

The only exception to this rule is that when the primary reason for the admission/encounter is chemotherapy or radiation therapy, the appropriate Z code for the service is listed first, and the diagnosis or problem for which the service is being performed is listed second.

m. Patients Receiving Preoperative Evaluations Only

For patients receiving preoperative evaluations only, sequence first a code from subcategory Z01.81, *Encounter for pre-procedural examinations, to describe the pre-op consultations*. Assign a code for the condition to describe the reason for the surgery as an additional diagnosis. Code also any findings related to the pre-op evaluation.

n. Ambulatory Surgery

For ambulatory surgery, code the diagnosis for which the surgery was performed. If the postoperative diagnosis is known to be different from the preoperative diagnosis at the time the diagnosis is confirmed, select the postoperative diagnosis for coding, because it is the most definitive.

o. Routine Outpatient Prenatal Visits

See Section I.C.15. Routine outpatient prenatal visits.

p. Encounters for General Medical Examinations With Abnormal Findings

The subcategories for encounters for general medical examinations, Z00.0-, and encounter for routine child health examination, Z00.12-, provide codes for with and without abnormal findings. Should a general medical examination result in an abnormal finding, the code for general medical examination with abnormal finding should be assigned as the first-listed diagnosis. An examination with abnormal findings refers to a condition/diagnosis that is newly identified or a change in severity of a chronic condition (such as uncontrolled hypertension, or an acute exacerbation of chronic obstructive pulmonary disease) during a routine physical examination. A secondary code for the abnormal finding should also be coded.

q. Encounters for Routine Health Screenings

See Section I.C.21. Factors influencing health status and contact with health services, Screening.

only to provide outpatient physician services), or specialized units such as physical therapy and cardiac catheterization units. A patient coming to the hospital for diagnostic testing who is not admitted is also considered a hospital outpatient.

A freestanding facility provides services in which a hospital has no responsibility. Outpatient services that are freestanding take place in physician offices, public health clinics, urgent care centers, diagnostic centers, etc.

This distinction is important primarily because of Medicare billing requirements; the two different settings are required to submit different types of health-care claims. The facility outpatient claim is the 837I electronic claim or its paper-based equivalent, the CMS-1450; non-hospital providers submit the 837P (P for professional) or its paper-based equivalent, the CMS-1500. The reason for different claim formats is that hospitals are paid for outpatient services based on different sets of fees, as explained in the accompanying Reimbursement Review of the Medicare Outpatient Prospective Payment System.

INTERNET RESOURCE: Outpatient Prospective Payment System
www.cms.hhs.gov/HospitalOutpatientPPS

The facility outpatient claim requires reporting the patient's reason for visit for unscheduled outpatient visits, such as those to emergency departments. The patient's reason-for-visit code represents the ICD-10-CM diagnosis code for the condition the patient indicated as the reason for the visit to the provider, if applicable—in other words, the patient's chief complaint or reason for the encounter. For example, a patient presents to the ED for nausea and vomiting, diarrhea, and fever. The ED doctor evaluates the patient and determines the diagnosis of viral gastroenteritis. The reason-for-visit codes would be reported as nausea and vomiting, diarrhea, and fever, and the primary or first-listed diagnosis would be viral gastroenteritis.

CHECKPOINT 10.1

Indicate whether the diagnostic coding for the following patient services would follow the inpatient or outpatient guidelines.

1. A patient presents to the hospital ED for a wrist sprain and goes home. _____

2. A patient visits the physician's office for an annual physical. _____

3. A patient is transferred from the hospital to a nursing home after being in the hospital for

   3 days. _____

4. A patient stays in the psychiatric unit at the hospital for 30 days. _____

5. A patient receives physical and occupational therapy in the outpatient clinic for 2 hours. _____

6. A patient has a cataract removed in the ambulatory surgery center. _____

7. A patient goes to the hospital laboratory to have blood drawn to determine cholesterol level. _____

8. A patient is admitted to the hospital and dies the same day. _____

9. A patient goes from the ED to the observation unit due to asthma. _____

10. A patient visits the orthopedic clinic to have a cast removed. _____

The Medicare Outpatient Prospective Payment System

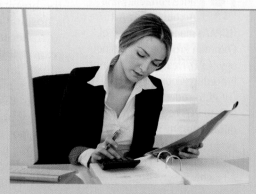

Paralleling the Medicare Inpatient Prospective Payment System (IPPS) for hospital inpatient services is the Medicare Outpatient Prospective Payment System (OPPS), which is maintained by the Centers for Medicare and Medicaid Services (CMS). As with IPPS, under the OPPS system, rates are also established based on Medicare's analysis of similar outpatient medical services and procedures. The OPPS was implemented in 2000 to establish a prospective payment system for hospital-provided ambulatory procedures.

OPPS applies to covered hospital outpatient services furnished by all hospitals participating in the Medicare program. Certain services—physical, occupational, and speech therapies; orthotic and prosthetic devices; erythropoietin for patients with end-stage renal disease; durable medical equipment; ambulance; and clinical laboratory services—are paid under other schedules, not OPPS.

Medicare analyzes and updates the reported costs for procedures and then groups them into ambulatory payment classifications (APCs). The APCs each categorize clinically similar services that require comparable resources. Each APC number is assigned a relative weight that is connected to a dollar amount that is payable. The payment rate for a new technology APC is set at the midpoint of its average cost.

Level of Detail in Coding

The guidelines requiring the greatest detail in coding apply in the outpatient setting. The use of a fourth, fifth, or sixth digit provides greater specificity regarding site, etiology, or manifestation of disease. Therefore, a three-digit code is used only when that category is not further subdivided. The coder should apply the highest number of digits available—no more and no fewer.

Guidelines for Code Selection

The ICD-10-CM code set is used to identify the symptoms, problems, complaints, diagnoses, or other documented reasons for an outpatient visit. Reasons for outpatient visits include:

- Chest pain (symptom)
- Exposure to tuberculosis (problem)
- Palpitations (complaint)
- Diabetes mellitus (diagnosis)
- Well-child visit (other reason)

All these reasons for the encounter can be coded from ICD-10-CM, following the general process shown in Figure 10.1.

Symptoms and Signs

Often, the reason for an outpatient encounter is that the patient presents with a sign or symptom. ICD-10-CM codes that describe symptoms and signs, rather than diagnoses, are acceptable for

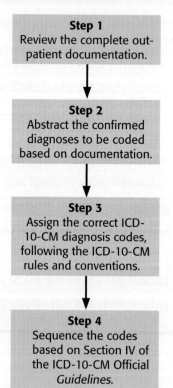

Step 1
Review the complete outpatient documentation.

↓

Step 2
Abstract the confirmed diagnoses to be coded based on documentation.

↓

Step 3
Assign the correct ICD-10-CM diagnosis codes, following the ICD-10-CM rules and conventions.

↓

Step 4
Sequence the codes based on Section IV of the ICD-10-CM Official *Guidelines*.

Figure 10.1 The outpatient coding process.

Within each APC, integral items and services are packaged with the primary service and not paid separately. Examples are routine supplies, anesthesia, recovery room services, and most implants. A hospital may receive multiple APC payments for a single visit when multiple services have been performed during that encounter. Examples of separately paid services are

- Blood and blood products
- Surgical and diagnostic procedures
- Some observation services
- Clinic and ED visits
- Some drugs, biologicals, and radiopharmaceuticals

The APCs are based on the procedural coding system called *CPT*. CPT codes are the HIPAA-mandated procedure codes that are assigned by coders to each medical and surgical outpatient procedure. The CPT codes must be reported for outpatient services in place of ICD-10-PCS codes. The ICD-10-CM diagnosis codes, however, continue in the outpatient setting to show the medical necessity of the services provided during the encounter.

OPPS APC status indicators are used to show what procedures are paid under the system. For example, a status indicator of *A* means that the procedure is paid. But some procedures are typically provided *only* in the inpatient setting, and so CMS does not pay for them under the OPPS. CMS publishes a list of these procedures, to be followed for correct claim completion; these have a status indicator of C.

reporting purposes when the provider has not established (confirmed) a diagnosis. The code range in ICD-10-CM Chapter 18, Symptoms, Signs, and Abnormal Clinical and Laboratory Findings (R00–R99), contains most of the codes for symptoms; others are located in system-specific chapters. For example, the symptom of chest pain (R07.9) is located in Chapter 18, whereas the symptom of ankle pain (M25.579) is located in Chapter 13, Diseases of the Musculoskeletal System and Connective Tissue.

Circumstances Other Than Disease or Injury (Z Codes)

Chapter 21, Factors Influencing Health Status and Contact With Health Services, provides codes to classify outpatient encounters for circumstances other than diseases and injuries. In such cases, the reason for the visit is not recorded as a diagnosis or a problem (sign or symptom). For example, when a patient visits the physician's office for an annual vaccination or for cancer screening, the codes from this chapter are assigned.

CHECKPOINT 10.2

Code the following cases using ICD-10-CM for outpatient encounters, keeping the outpatient coding guidelines in mind.

1. Shortness of breath and fever, with possible pneumonia _____

2. Screening for malignant neoplasm of the colon _____

3. Visit for poliomyelitis vaccination _____

4. Nausea and vomiting _____

5. Well-child examination _____

SELECTION OF FIRST-LISTED DIAGNOSIS

In outpatient settings, diagnoses may not be established at the time of an encounter. For this reason, the definition of the principal diagnosis does not apply in the outpatient setting. In its place is the term *first-listed diagnosis*.

These are the outpatient coder's guidelines:

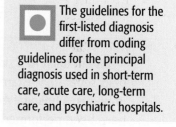

The guidelines for the first-listed diagnosis differ from coding guidelines for the principal diagnosis used in short-term care, acute care, long-term care, and psychiatric hospitals.

- If just one diagnosis is provided, the code for that condition is reported.
- If a definite condition is not documented, the code for the *patient's chief complaint* and/or symptom is reported.
- If multiple diagnoses can be assigned as the reasons for the encounter, all are coded.

REIMBURSEMENT REVIEW

Outpatient Claims: Hospital (Institutional) Billing

When a patient receives outpatient care at a facility or facility-owned place of service, the facility is permitted to bill for its part of the services (the room, supplies, etc.), and the physician bills for his or her part (the surgical or other procedural work). For example, a patient visit to a same-day surgery unit for a procedure on a bunion is billed by two entities: (1) the hospital outpatient facility and (2) the physician.

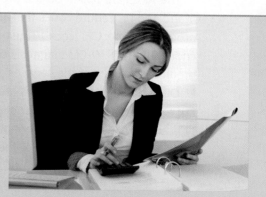

The CMS-1450 paper claim or the 837I electronic claim format is utilized for both inpatient and outpatient facility services. Although not required, some facilities choose to voluntarily report ICD-10-PCS procedure codes for outpatient services.

The CMS 1500 shown in this box illustrates the professional bill for the patient above who underwent bunion surgery. Please note the filed number on the claim, which would contain the following information:

a. Diagnosis reported in ICD-10: Field 21, indicator 0, code A M20.11
b. Procedure reported in CPT/HCPCS: Field 24D
c. Modifier RT (right): Field 24D
d. Diagnosis pointer: Value of A (pointing to the diagnosis of bunion, M20.11)

Locate the distinct fields on the claim to identify the total number of diagnoses that can be reported (12) and the number of CPT/HCPCS codes (6).

In the last situation, which diagnosis should be listed first? The main sequencing guideline for all scheduled outpatient visits is that the first-listed diagnosis is the diagnosis, condition, problem, or other reason for the encounter that is shown in the medical record to be chiefly responsible for the services provided.

Note, however, that the general ICD-10-CM rules and conventions, as well as the general and disease-specific guidelines, take precedence over the outpatient guidelines. For example, conventions such as "code first underlying disease" determine the sequencing of codes for certain diagnoses, overriding an instruction in Section IV of the *Official Guidelines*.

There are specific guidelines for determining the first-listed diagnosis codes for the following outpatient cases:

Remember that the Index to Diseases and Injuries drives the code assignment, with verification of codes completed using the Tabular List.

- Outpatient procedures and ambulatory surgery
- Observation services
- Diagnostic services
- Therapeutic services

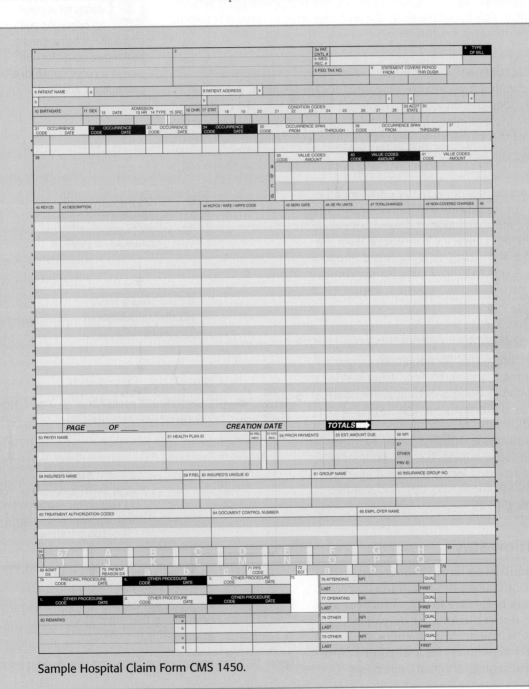

Sample Hospital Claim Form CMS 1450.

- Preoperative evaluations
- Routine outpatient prenatal care
- Uncertain diagnoses
- ED visits

Outpatient Procedures and Ambulatory Surgery

Typically, an outpatient procedure is one that is completed outside of an operating room. Examples include an outpatient colonoscopy or an outpatient cardiac catheterization. These procedures are typically performed in a specialty unit specifically designed to perform them, such as a cardiac catheterization laboratory. Patients having an ambulatory surgery, also called *same-day surgery,* typically receive services in an operating room or surgical suite. For example, cataract extraction, rotator cuff repair, and laparoscopic cholecystectomy are considered ambulatory surgeries.

When a patient presents for an outpatient procedure or ambulatory surgery, the reason for the procedure or surgery is the first-listed diagnosis, unless the preoperative diagnosis and the postoperative diagnosis are different. If this happens, then the postoperative diagnosis is coded, because it is the most definitive.

> By definition, POA stands for *present on admission* and so would not be reported on health-care claims for outpatient services, for which a patient is not admitted.

■ CASE SCENARIO

A patient with a preoperative diagnosis of skin lesion of the cheek (L98.9) undergoes an excision. After the lesion is excised and analyzed by the pathologist, documentation confirms basal cell carcinoma of the cheek (C44.399). Only the basal cell carcinoma is reported.

If the procedure is not actually performed because of a contraindication, the reason for the visit code is still listed first, followed by a code to represent the cancelled procedure from the category Z53. If the surgery is cancelled due to a contraindication (Z53.09), a code for the contraindication would also be reported. Figure 10.2 explains the code assignment process.

■ CASE SCENARIO

A patient presented to outpatient surgery for a coronary angiogram due to unstable angina. After conscious sedation, the staff noted a cardiac arrhythmia. The surgery was cancelled because of the contraindication of cardiac arrhythmia. The first-listed diagnosis is the unstable angina (I20.0). Additional codes are reported for surgery not done due to contraindication (Z53.09) and cardiac arrhythmia (I49.9).

Observation Stay

Some circumstances surrounding outpatient observation care affect the first-listed diagnosis. A patient may begin care in one outpatient area and receive services in another outpatient area. For example, a patient may present to the ambulatory surgery department for a scheduled procedure and then require observation services.

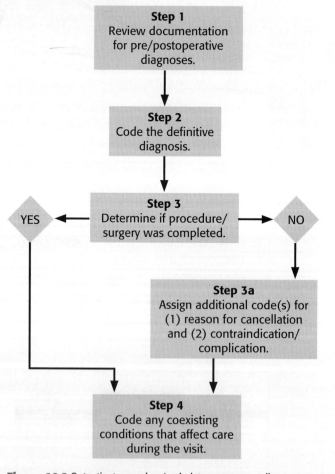

Figure 10.2 Outpatient procedure/ambulatory surgery coding process.

The *Official Guidelines* state that when a patient is admitted for observation due to a medical condition, a code for that medical condition should be the first-listed diagnosis. For example, a patient may be placed in the observation unit because of acute asthma exacerbation (J45.901). Also, when a patient presents for an outpatient procedure or ambulatory surgery and then develops complications that require admission for observation, the surgical diagnosis code is the first-reported diagnosis. This primary diagnosis code is followed by the codes for the complications as secondary diagnoses.

■ **CASE SCENARIO**
A patient presents to ambulatory surgery for elective laparoscopic gallbladder removal due to chronic cholecystitis. After surgery, he develops chest pain that requires observation services. First-listed diagnosis: chronic cholecystitis (K81.1); secondary diagnosis: chest pain (R07.9).

Diagnostic Services

Patients may present for procedures that assist the physician in making a diagnosis. Such diagnostic services include many types of laboratory/pathology tests, radiology procedures, and diagnostic surgical procedures such as biopsies. Patients may or may not have signs or symptoms relating to the conditions for which they are tested. For diagnostic services, the first-listed code is the diagnosis, condition, problem, or other reason shown in the medical record to be chiefly responsible for the diagnostic services provided during the encounter. Codes for other diagnoses may be sequenced as additional codes.

As noted in the *Official Guidelines*, codes from the category representing special investigations and examinations (Section I.C.18.d, paragraph 13)—specifically, codes Z00–Z02 and Z32.0—may be used as the first-listed diagnoses when the reason for the visit is routine testing in the absence of signs, symptoms, and associated diagnoses. If routine testing is performed at the same time as a test to evaluate a sign, symptom, or medical condition, both the Z code and the code describing the reason for the nonroutine test are reported.

When a physician orders hospital-based outpatient services for a Medicare patient, Medicare's Conditions of Participation for Hospitals require a diagnosis for the outpatient tests and procedures. If the diagnosis is not documented and signed by the ordering physician, the hospital staff should contact the physician for clarification.

■ **CASE SCENARIOS**
- A patient presents to the outpatient radiology center for a routine chest x-ray as part of a general medical exam. Code Z00.00 is reported.

- A patient presents for a routine pre-op laboratory test and also undergoes an MRI of the back due to back pain. Both the code for routine lab work (Z01.812) and the code for back pain (M54.9) are reported.

Code signs and symptoms for laboratory services that are read by a technician but not confirmed by a physician. Code the definitive diagnosis of the physician-radiologist who reads the films for radiology services.

The information that is available to the coder affects the assignment of ICD-10-CM codes for diagnostic services. If diagnostic tests have been interpreted by a physician and a definitive diagnosis has been documented in the final report, the coder may report the condition that has been confirmed. If the final report is not available, the coder may code only for the condition that is certain at the point of coding.

■ **CASE SCENARIO**
A patient presents to the hospital outpatient department for a scheduled echocardiogram because of a heart murmur. The results support the presence of mitral valve prolapse based on physician interpretation. If this fact is available at the time of coding, the first-listed diagnosis is the definitive diagnosis of mitral valve prolapse (I34.1). However, if results are not available at the time of coding, the diagnosis of heart murmur (R01.1) is reported.

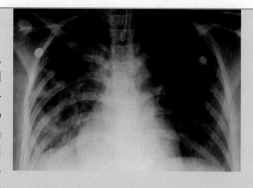

The Musculoskeletal System

The musculoskeletal system includes the muscles, bones, and joints. Diseases of the musculoskeletal system can occur as a result of congenital abnormalities, injuries, or inflammation, or they may be due to or associated with another disease or condition, such as arthritis associated with diabetes. Musculoskeletal diseases include *arthropathy, injuries* (most commonly fractures, sprains, and strains), and *degenerative* diseases (e.g., muscular dystrophy and osteoporosis). In addition, other musculoskeletal diseases are hereditary (e.g., gout), and some are conditions of unknown origin (e.g., a ganglion).

Arthritis or Arthropathy

Arthritis is the leading cause of disability in the United States. The terms *arthritis* and *arthropathy* refer to any inflammation of a joint. It can be *acute* (severe, sudden, and of short duration), *chronic* (occurring over a long period of time), or *subacute* (somewhere between acute and chronic; often with no symptoms). Arthritis is often *due to* or *associated with* another condition including diabetes, gout, rheumatoid arthritis, and infection. Arthritis is subclassified as site specified (e.g., in the hand), as site unspecified, or as occurring in multiple sites. *Rheumatoid arthritis* is a chronic autoimmune disorder and is sometimes confused with *rheumatism*, a general term for any condition causing discomfort to the muscles, joints, tendons, or bones.

Injuries

Injuries to the musculoskeletal system are a common result of many traumas, such as automobile accidents. Falls are a leading cause of death for people over 65 years of age, usually because of the resulting hip fractures. Other fractures occur over all age groups. A dislocation can occur with or without a fracture and may be further classified as *simple, recurrent, open, closed, subluxation* (partial dislocation), or *articulation* (occurring at a joint). Less traumatic

---

■ CASE SCENARIO

A patient presents to the ED after sustaining an injury to her left wrist, and her wrist is x-rayed. Before the radiologist interprets the x-ray, the patient is discharged from the ED with the diagnosis of wrist sprain. After review of the x-ray results, the radiologist documents a diagnosis of wrist fracture. In this case, however, the ED coder must assign the code for the condition that was known at the time of discharge. Therefore, the facility reports left wrist sprain (S63.502A).

Therapeutic Services

Patients may receive only therapeutic services—the many procedures done to treat conditions and injuries—during outpatient visits. For these visits, as for diagnostic services, the ICD-10-CM code reported first represents the diagnosis, condition, problem, or other reason for the encounter that the medical record shows is chiefly responsible for the outpatient services provided.

■ CASE SCENARIO

A patient presents to the dermatologist's office to have a skin lesion removed from her back. Following removal, the lesion is sent for analysis. The pathology report is returned with a diagnosis of squamous cell carcinoma of the back. The first-listed diagnosis is squamous cell carcinoma of the back (C44.599).

injuries, such as *carpal tunnel syndrome, sprains,* and *strains,* can require medical intervention, including pain management.

Fractures occur at specific or at multiple sites. They are categorized in various ways. First, they are classified based on how they occur: *adduction* (an abnormal turning inward), *abduction* (an abnormal turning outward), *avulsion* (a forcible tearing away), *compression* (resulting from a force pressing on a bone), *crush* (caused by a crushing blow), *dislocation* (movement away from a normal location), *oblique* (at an angle), *separation* (with displacement), *open* (with broken skin), or *closed* (covered by unbroken skin). Closed fractures and open fractures are further divided into types. Some closed fractures are *greenstick* (broken on one side only) and *Colles* (characteristic deformity of the wrist as a result of a fracture). Examples of open fractures are *compound* (with the broken bone protruding through the skin) and *missile* (caused by something projected into the bone from an outside source).

Strains and sprains occur in joints, ligaments, muscles, and tendons. Strains result from overstretching or overexertion. Sprains result from overstraining or wrenching (without fracturing).

> Related signs and symptoms (those that are integral) should not be coded as additional diagnoses when the underlying condition is documented in physician-interpreted diagnostic test results.

> Coding from physician-interpreted diagnostic services applies in the out-patient setting only. This differs from the coding practice regarding abnormal findings on test results in hospital inpatient settings.

Degenerative Diseases

Some degenerative diseases are genetically linked (e.g., Duchenne's muscular dystrophy and some forms of osteoporosis). Others result from other diseases or conditions or have unknown causes. *Osteoporosis* (loss of bone density) is usually categorized as *generalized* (occurring in various parts of the body). It is further divided into types, such as *postmenopausal* and *drug induced. Osteopenia* is a reduction in bone mass that is less severe than osteoporosis. Fractures due to bone disorders such as osteoporosis are *pathological* fractures rather than traumatic ones.

In this example, the therapeutic service of skin lesion removal was performed. By waiting for the pathologist's interpretation, the coder was able to report the diagnosis of squamous cell carcinoma. If the diagnosis had been reported before receipt of the pathology findings, the diagnosis of skin lesion would have been reported (L98.9). There is no code to report admission for surgery; rather, the reason for the therapeutic services should be reported first.

There is an exception to the general rule for sequencing therapeutic services. When the primary reason for the visit is a specialized service such as chemotherapy, radiation therapy, renal dialysis, or rehabilitation, the appropriate code for the service is the first-listed ICD-10-CM code. The diagnosis or problem for which the patient requires the specialized service is reported as a secondary diagnosis.

■ CASE SCENARIO

A patient presents to the hospital outpatient unit for chemotherapy. He is receiving chemotherapy for his sigmoid colon cancer. The first-listed diagnosis is encounter for chemotherapy (Z51.11), followed by the code for sigmoid colon cancer (C18.7).

In this example, the patient presented for a specialized service (chemotherapy). Therefore, the encounter for chemotherapy code is sequenced first, followed by the code that represents the problem (sigmoid colon cancer) that required the service.

The Integumentary System

Diseases of the skin can be categorized as *infections of the skin and subcutaneous tissue, other inflammations and conditions,* and *diseases of specific parts of the integumentary system.* In addition, ICD-10-CM provides categories for other types of skin disorders such as *ulcers* and *urticaria.* Skin lesions may be indicative of a disease process (e.g., cancer) or may be from an injury (e.g., burns and scars).

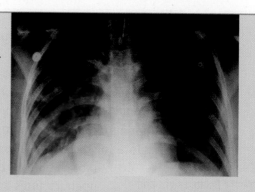

Infections of the Skin and Subcutaneous Tissue

Infections of the skin—especially a *carbuncle* (localized inflammation of subcutaneous tissue with suppuration), a *furuncle* (pus-filled staphylococcal infection), and *cellulitis* (inflammation of the deep subcutaneous tissue)—are usually categorized by location (e.g., cellulitis of the face or trunk or a carbuncle of the neck). Localized bacterial infections of tissue are called *abscesses.* Abscesses occur in the skin or elsewhere in the body. *Impetigo* is an infectious skin disease categorized as *bullous* (having blisters), *circinate* (having circular lesions), *contagiosa* (acutely contagious), *neonatorum* (occurring in a newborn), or *simplex* (common and localized). *Pyoderma* is a bacterial skin infection with pus-filled lesions.

Other Skin Inflammations and Conditions

Dermatitis is a general term for inflammation of the skin. It is categorized in many ways, including *allergic* (caused by an allergy), *contact* (caused by contact with something, such as a chemical), *occupational* (work related), or *venenata* (caused by something poisonous). Dermatitis is further subdivided into specific causes or locations, such as *due to solar radiation* (sunburn) or *diaper rash* (located underneath a diaper). It can also be due to allergies (e.g., to food or drugs). Some serious types of dermatitis, such as *pemphigus* (a chronic, blistering skin disease), can

Preoperative Evaluations

Some outpatient encounters occur because the patient needs to be cleared for surgery. When a patient receives a preoperative evaluation encounter for preprocedural examinations only, a code from category Z01.81 (other specified examinations) is sequenced first. The coder also assigns additional codes that describe the reason for the surgery along with any findings related to the preoperative evaluation.

> ■ CASE SCENARIO
> A patient presents to his primary doctor for a preoperative evaluation prior to his scheduled inguinal hernia repair. During the exam, the physician also notes hypertension. The first-listed code is Z01.818 (preoperative examination), followed by the secondary diagnosis codes of K40.90 (inguinal hernia) and I10 (hypertension).

Routine Outpatient Prenatal Visits

The guideline for prenatal visits applies when a patient's prenatal visit occurs and no complications are present. Under these circumstances, the first-listed diagnosis is reported using supervision of normal pregnancy, code Z34.90. If the patient has a complication of pregnancy, these codes are not reported.

be fatal. *Erythematous conditions* (redness of the skin) may be *generalized* or may be due to specific conditions such as *lupus* or *rosacea. Psoriasis,* a chronic inflammatory skin disease, is sometimes associated with inflammatory arthritis.

Pruritus is a general term for itching. Pruritus may be categorized according to location, such as the ear or genital area. *Eczema* is an inflammation of the skin accompanied by itching. It is classified in a number of ways, including *acute, chronic,* and *allergic.* It may also be categorized by location (*external ear*), cause (*contact*), or other (*infantile*).

Skin Diseases of Specific Parts of the Integumentary System

Diseases of the hair commonly include *alopecia* (baldness) and *hirsutism* (excess hair growth). Diseases of the nails include *ingrowing nail, onychia* (inflammation of the matrix of the nail), and *paronychia* (inflammation of the skin bordering the nail). The *sebaceous glands* (oil-producing glands) are responsible for *acne,* the most common variety of which is *acne vulgaris.* They also produce *sebaceous cysts, seborrhea* (an excessive discharge of sebum), and *seborrheic dermatitis* or *dandruff.* Disorders of the sweat glands include *anhidrosis* (lack of the ability to sweat), *prickly heat* (a rash produced by sweating), and *hyperhidrosis* (overproduction of sweat).

Ulcers and Urticaria

Ulcers of the skin can occur on any part of the body. *Decubitus ulcers, pressure sores,* or *bedsores* are divided into stages depending on the severity of the skin damage. In stage 1, the skin is warm, firm, or stretched. The other stages indicate the depth of the ulcer; in the last stage, the ulcer has reached the bone. Other skin ulcers are categorized by location, such as *ulcer of ankle.* These ulcers may be caused by other underlying conditions, such as arteriosclerosis.

Urticaria are commonly known as *hives.* They are categorized by type (e.g., *giant*) or cause (e.g., *allergic urticaria*). They may also be *unspecified.*

■ CASE SCENARIOS

• A female patient presents to her obstetrician's practice for her routine fourth-month prenatal visit. This is her first pregnancy. The first-listed diagnosis is Z34.02.

• A female patient who is pregnant with twins presents to her obstetrician's practice for a prenatal visit in her fifth month. The first-listed diagnosis is twin pregnancy, antepartum, code O30.002.

Uncertain Diagnoses

In the outpatient setting, uncertain diagnoses—those documented as probable, suspected, questionable, rule out, or working diagnoses—are not coded. Only the condition to the highest degree of certainty for that visit is assigned a code. The code may represent a symptom, sign, abnormal test result, or other reason for the visit.

Emergency Department Visits

The guidelines for first-listed diagnosis apply to ED visits. The first-listed diagnosis is the diagnosis, condition, problem, or other reason for the encounter shown in the medical record to be chiefly responsible for the services provided. However, ED visits are unscheduled outpatient visits. Thus, the patient's reason-for-visit codes should also be reported by the hospital. Reporting both diagnosis codes provides a clear picture of the presenting problems and of the medical necessity of the procedures that were performed. The ED physician does not report reason-for-visit codes.

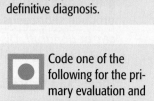

Code signs and symptoms unless a physician confirms a definitive diagnosis.

Code one of the following for the primary evaluation and management service that the physician's documentation supports: the diagnosis of the ED physician, signs and symptoms, or the definitive diagnosis.

For example, a patient may present with chest pain (patient's reason for visit), yet after an ECG, chest x-ray, and laboratory studies, the ED physician documents the diagnosis of gastroesophageal reflux. If the patient's reason for visit of chest pain (R07.9) is not reported, the medical necessity of the ECG, chest x-ray, and blood work may not be met. Thus, the first-listed diagnosis code in this case is the physician's diagnosis after evaluation and management of the patient. The hospital would also report the patient's reason-for-visit diagnosis codes to reflect the initial complaints of the patient.

Note that the reporting of the chest pain does *not* contradict previous explanations, for two reasons. First, chest pain is not integral to gastroesophageal reflux, which is often diagnosed in patients who do not have that symptom. Second, without the listing of chest pain, the medical necessity of the ED visit is not correctly presented to the third-party payer.

Code the diagnoses for the following outpatient case scenarios. Sequence the first-listed diagnosis code first using the outpatient coding guidelines.

1. A patient presents to the outpatient department for a cholecystogram with the diagnosis of possible gallstone. The radiologist interprets the cholecystogram and lists the diagnosis of cholelithiasis. _____

2. At the time of a visit to a physician's office, the documented diagnosis is epigastric pain, nausea, and vomiting, rule out gastritis. _____

3. A patient presents to the outpatient department for a screening colonoscopy for malignancy. The colonoscopy reveals the finding of external hemorrhoids. _____

4. A patient has had right shoulder pain for months. His physician documents the presence of a chronic rotator cuff tear. The patient now presents for rotator cuff repair in the hospital ambulatory surgery department. After surgery, he requires observation services for chest pain.

   _____

5. A patient presents at the ED with chest pain, fever, and shortness of breath. After an ECG, blood work, and chest x-ray, the ED physician documents the diagnosis of pneumonia.
   A. Which code or codes are reported by the hospital as the reason(s) for the visit? _____
   B. Which code is reported as the first-listed condition? _____

6. A patient presents for coronary angiography due to an abnormal stress test. After the angiography, postoperative documentation supports coronary artery disease of the native coronary arteries. What is the code for the first-listed condition? _____

7. A patient visits her obstetrician for prenatal care in the sixth month. This is her second pregnancy with no complications. _____

8. A patient presents to the hospital outpatient department for a barium enema due to lower GI bleeding. The barium enema is normal. _____

9. A patient presents to the hospital outpatient laboratory for a thyroid hormone level test. The patient has hypothyroidism, according to the physician order. _____

10. A patient presents to the outpatient surgery center for treatment of ureteral calculus. After preparation for surgery, he develops noncardiac chest pain, which requires the cancellation of surgery. _____

REPORTING SECONDARY DIAGNOSES AND EXTERNAL CAUSE CODES IN OUTPATIENT SETTINGS

Not only must the coder identify the first-listed diagnosis for an outpatient visit, but other diagnoses (secondary diagnoses) should also be reported as appropriate. The following guidelines cover which chronic conditions and coexisting conditions should be reported in addition to the first-listed diagnosis. Information about external cause codes, also required to be reported, if applicable, are also provided.

Chronic Diseases

Chronic diseases, such as hypertension, diabetes mellitus, and osteoarthritis, persist over a long period of time. Chronic diseases that are treated on an on-going basis may be coded and reported as many times as the patient receives treatment and care for them. For example, a patient may require regular fingerstick glucose testing for diabetes mellitus, so diabetes mellitus would be reported for each visit in which the patient receives the treatment or care.

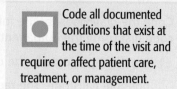
Code all documented conditions that exist at the time of the visit and require or affect patient care, treatment, or management.

Coexisting Conditions

All documented conditions that coexist at the time of the encounter *and* require or affect patient care, treatment, or management should be coded. Conditions that were previously treated and no longer exist or no longer affect treatment or patient management should not be reported. History codes may be used as secondary codes if the historical condition or family history has an effect on current care or influences treatment. For example, a patient may present for a screening colonos-copy (Z12.11) due to family history of colon cancer (Z80.0). In this case, the secondary diagnosis of family history of colon cancer affects the patient care, because this is the reason for the patient screening. Other codes reflecting a patient's status may also be reported if that status has an effect on current care or influences treatment.

■ CASE SCENARIOS

- A patient visits his doctor for evaluation of cough, fever, and shortness of breath. He has previously been diagnosed with hypertension and diabetes. During the office visit, his blood pressure is measured, and his fingerstick glucose is normal. The diagnosis of acute bronchitis is documented along with the diagnoses of diabetes mellitus (type 2) and hypertension. The codes reported are J20.9 (acute bronchitis), E11.9 (diabetes mellitus), and I10 (hypertension).

- A patient presents to her doctor for evaluation of ear pain. She was treated for a urinary tract infection (UTI) 3 months earlier. Physician documentation for this visit states the diagnoses as acute otitis media and history of UTI. The correct code is H66.91 (acute otitis media) only. The code for UTI is not reported, because the UTI is no longer present and does not affect the current care and treatment.

External Cause Codes

As with inpatient ICD-10-CM coding, in the outpatient setting external cause codes (known as E codes) are strongly suggested. In some states, external cause codes are required for outpatient hospital services report-ing. Also, some payers require external cause codes regardless of setting. Table 10.1 summarizes this requirement and provides an overview of the differences in procedural coding, billing, and Medicare payment system for hospital inpatient, hospital outpatient, and physician services.

Do not code conditions that were previously treated and no longer exist or that do not affect the patient's care.

Table 10.1 Comparison of Coding, Billing, and Payment Methods

	HOSPITAL INPATIENT	HOSPITAL OUTPATIENT	ALL PHYSICIAN SERVICES
Diagnosis codes	ICD-10-CM	ICD-10-CM	ICD-10-CM
Procedure codes	ICD-10-PCS	CPT/HCPCS ICD-10-PCS (optional)	CPT/HCPCS
Billing form	837I or UB-04	837I or UB-04	837P or CMS-1500
Medicare payment	Medicare Severity Diagnosis Related Group (MS-DRG)	APC	Resource-based relative value scale (RBRVS)

Assign the appropriate ICD-10-CM diagnosis codes for the following case scenarios.

1. A patient presents to the hospital for chemotherapy to treat his cancer of the cecum. He has a family history of colon cancer. _____

2. A patient presents to the ED and is evaluated and treated for acute cystitis. She is also currently being treated for chronic gout. _____

3. A patient sees the dermatologist due to a painful scar. Complete exam also reveals rosacea and seborrheic keratosis. Medications are ordered, and the patient is to return for excision of the scar the next week. _____

4. A patient visits his physician every 3 months due to his type 2 diabetic polyneuropathy. During each visit, his other chronic conditions are evaluated. These include osteoarthritis of the lumbar spine, benign hypertension, and asthma. _____

5. A patient sees her cardiologist for preoperative clearance for laparoscopic vaginal hysterectomy due to menometrorrhagia. The cardiologist examines the patient and clears her for surgery. Documentation supports the presence of native coronary artery disease and congestive heart failure as cardiac conditions. _____

Chapter Summary

1. An outpatient is a patient who is not admitted to an acute care facility, short-term hospital, or any other inpatient setting; outpatients receive care from a facility and typically return home the same day. Examples of outpatient encounters include visits to an ED, ambulatory surgery center, urgent care center, physician office, radiology center, and physical therapist.

2. The first-listed diagnosis refers to the diagnosis code that is listed first for outpatient encounters. The rules and definition for principal diagnosis for the inpatient setting *do not apply to outpatients*. In the outpatient setting, the first-listed diagnosis is the reason for the visit, whether it is for a medical condition, screening, well visit, routine testing, immunization, or other reason. Uncertain or ill-defined conditions—those that are possible, probable, or suspected—are never coded; instead, the signs and symptoms are the basis for code assignment, because often at the time of the encounter a definitive diagnosis is not yet known.

3. Sequencing of the first-listed diagnosis in the outpatient setting encompasses many different scenarios. An ambulatory surgery visit or an observation stay often has a documented diagnosis of a disease or injury. Other outpatient visits require the use of Chapter 21 (Factors Influencing Health Status codes) for reporting the first-listed diagnosis.

4. When a patient presents as an outpatient and receives special diagnostic services, therapeutic services, preoperative exams, or routine prenatal visits, a code from Chapter 21 (Factors Influencing Health Status) may be the first-listed diagnosis. In these cases, a special diagnostic service such as a screening colonoscopy may be the first-listed diagnosis. Other examples include a well-child visit or routine chest x-ray.

5. The first-listed diagnosis reported for routine prenatal visits should be for supervision of pregnancy. These codes are used only if there are *no* pregnancy complications. In the presence of complications, the complication codes would be assigned and supervision codes would not be reported.

6. Conditions that are documented as uncertain (possible, probable, suspected, or rule out) should not be reported in the outpatient setting. Instead, the condition(s) reported should be the condition that is known at the time of the visit. Remember that the opposite is true in the inpatient setting, where these uncertain conditions are coded.

7. Emergency department visits are considered unscheduled visits; therefore, the reason-for-visit codes on form UB-04 used for facility coding only, and should be reported in addition to the first-listed diagnosis.

8. Chronic or coexisting conditions are also reported for outpatient encounters when these conditions impact the outpatient care. These conditions may impact outpatient care in many ways, such as requiring evaluation or treatment in addition to the first-listed diagnosis (e.g., diabetes, hypertension) or these conditions may influence care (e.g., family history of cancer). Conditions that are not currently present or do not impact care should not reported.

9. Additional diagnoses (i.e., secondary diagnoses) should be reported in the outpatient setting. These additional diagnoses represent chronic diseases and coexisting conditions that require or affect patient care treatment or management. External cause codes are also reported as applicable.

10. The entire outpatient coding process is similar to that followed for inpatient coding, with three major exceptions: the selection of the first-listed diagnosis based on the reason for the patient's visit, the assignment of codes for symptoms and signs to ill-defined or uncertain conditions, and physician-interpreted report results used to report diagnoses.

Review Questions

Matching

A. OPPS APC status indicator
B. ambulatory surgery
C. APC
D. patient's reason for visit
E. visit

F. freestanding facility
G. history codes
H. therapeutic services
I. coexisting condition
J. hospital-based facility

Match the key terms with their definitions.

1. __C__ The payment group in the Medicare Facility Outpatient Prospective Payment System

2. __F__ A facility not owned or managed by a hospital

3. __G__ Codes representing factors influencing health status

4. __J__ A facility owned or managed by a hospital

5. __D__ ICD-10-CM code assigned to the patient's chief complaint

6. __A__ Letter connected to a code that shows whether the procedure is payable under the OPPS APC system

7. __B__ Services performed for an outpatient in an operating room

8. __E__ Another term for *encounter*

9. __H__ Special services provided to treat a patient

10. __I__ Documented conditions that are present at the time of the visit that require or affect patient care, treatment, or management

True or False

Decide whether each statement is true or false.

1. __F__ The UHDDS definition of *principal diagnosis* applies to the outpatient setting.

2. __✗__ An interpretation by a radiologist of an x-ray can be used to assign a diagnosis code in the Emergency Department.

3. __F__ Signs and symptoms codes are never used in the outpatient setting.

4. __T__ A patient goes to get a lab test. This is considered an outpatient visit.

5. __F__ A visit to an observation unit in a hospital is always reported with an "admit for observation" code as the first-listed diagnosis.

6. __F__ In the diagnostic statement "chest pain due to suspected coronary artery disease," the primary diagnosis in the outpatient setting is coronary artery disease.

7. __T__ Chronic conditions that have no bearing on the current outpatient visit should not be reported.

8. __T__ When a patient presents to the physician's office for an annual physical without abnormal findings, the diagnosis code of Z00.00 is reported.

9. __F__ There is no difference in coding rules for a hospital inpatient visit and for a hospital outpatient visit.

10. __T__ The hospital completes the 837P or CMS-1500 form when providing services to a patient who undergoes an upper endoscopy in the outpatient unit.

Multiple Choice

Select the letter that best completes the statement or answers the question.

1. Which of the following is considered an outpatient visit?
   A. A two-day stay in a hospital intensive care unit
   B. A hospital emergency department visit
   C. A baby born in the hospital
   D. All of the above

2. Which is an example of a diagnostic procedure in the outpatient setting?
   A. Colonoscopy
   B. Appendectomy
   C. Cataract extraction
   D. Coronary stent insertion

3. Which of the following represents a symptom?
   A. Pneumonia
   B. Syncope
   C. Diverticulosis
   D. Peripheral vascular disease

4. Which of the following would be reported for a patient visit to the physician's office with a diagnosis of abdominal pain probably due to gastroenteritis?
   A. R10.9
   B. K52.9
   C. A04.9, R10.9
   D. K52.9, R10.9

5. A patient presents to the ambulatory surgery unit for left inguinal hernia repair. After surgery, the patient goes to observation for acute postoperative pain due to surgery. Which codes would be reported?
   A. K40.90, G89.18, R52
   B. K40.91, R52
   C. K40.90, G89.18
   D. R52, K40.90

6. A patient presents to the physician's office for an influenza vaccination. Which of the following would be reported?
   A. Z23
   B. Z23, Z00.01
   C. Z00.00, Z23
   D. None of the above

7. For the visit in Question 6, which coding system would be used to report the flu shot?
   A. ICD-10-CM
   B. CPT
   C. UB-04
   D. APC

8. What should the coder do when documentation in an ED record states, "injury to the wrist, rule out fracture," and the radiologist interprets the x-ray with the diagnosis of wrist fracture?
   A. Code only the wrist fracture.
   B. Query the ED physician to seek clarification.
   C. Code the wrist injury.
   D. Report both the wrist injury and wrist fracture codes.

9. If a patient who is pregnant with her third child presents to the physician's office for a routine obstetrical exam in the second trimester, what code(s) would be reported?
   A. Z34.02
   B. Z34.82
   C. O80
   D. Z34.82, O80

10. If a pediatric patient presents to the pediatrician's office for evaluation of obesity and the physician documents obesity with body mass index of the 90th percentile, which codes would be reported?
    A. E66.9, Z68.33
    B. E66.01, Z68.23
    C. E66.01, Z68.53
    D. E66.9, Z68.53

ICD-10-PCS Overview and Format

CHAPTER OUTLINE

History and Purpose of ICD-10-PCS

ICD-10 PCS Basics

ICD-10-PCS Basic Coding Process

ICD-10-PCS Format and Structure

ICD-10-PCS Code Tables

ICD-10-PCS Coding Simulation

LEARNING OUTCOMES

After studying this chapter, you should be able to:

1. Briefly discuss the background and history of ICD-10-PCS.
2. Discuss the importance of the *ICD-10-PCS Official Guidelines for Coding and Reporting.*
3. Describe the organization, content, and structure of ICD-10-PCS.
4. Interpret the conventions used in ICD-10-PCS.
5. Define the seven characters of an ICD-10-PCS procedure code.
6. List the basic process of assigning ICD-10-PCS codes.
7. Identify online coding resources used to assist in the assignment of accurate ICD-10-PCS codes.
8. Use online resources to assign ICD-10-PCS codes.

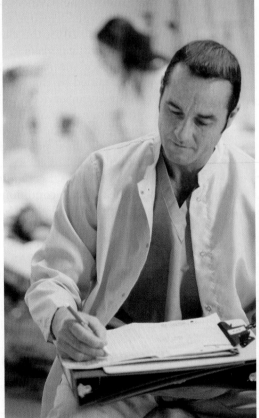

Standard procedure codes represent both therapeutic and diagnostic procedures used to treat or diagnose diseases, injuries, or conditions that affect health. In the health-care setting, different classification systems and nomenclatures are used to report procedures depending on the provider and setting of the medical service. In the outpatient setting, the code sets used to assign procedure codes are the Current Procedural Terminology (CPT) and Healthcare Common Procedure Coding System (HCPCS) code sets. Nonhospital providers also use CPT and HCPCS codes to report procedures performed regardless of the setting. These code sets are discussed in Chapters 12 to 30 in this text.

Hospitals use the *International Classification of Diseases, 10th Revision, Procedure Coding System* (ICD-10-PCS) only when reporting hospital inpatient procedure services. It replaced ICD-9-CM, Volume 3 effective October 1, 2015. Some hospitals elect to report an ICD-10-PCS code for outpatient procedures on a voluntary basis for internal data collection purposes. Use of the ICD-10-PCS code set is limited to inpatient diagnostic and therapeutic procedures for hospital inpatients. The codes reported are important for health-care reimbursement, research, quality measurement, and management decisions, and they must be accurate. Knowledge of medical terminology, anatomy and physiology, and current coding guidelines is essential to assign all ICD-10-PCS procedure codes accurately and sequence those codes in the correct order. Resources that can help ensure accuracy when coding include printed and electronic codebooks with useful enhancements, medical dictionaries, drug references, and national guidelines.

HISTORY AND PURPOSE OF ICD-10-PCS

October 1, 2015, was the effective start date for use of the ICD-10-PCS code set. This code set is used to collect data, determine payment, and support the electronic health record for all acute hospital inpatient procedures performed in the United States.

Prior to October 1, 2015, the classification system used to record all procedures for all acute hospital inpatient hospital visits in the United States was the *International Classification of Diseases, Ninth Revision, Clinical Modification, Volume 3*, called *ICD-9-CM, Volume 3*. The ICD-9-CM coding system was maintained by the National Center for Health Statistics (NCHS) and the Centers for Medicare and Medicaid Services (CMS), both of which are departments of the federal Department of Health and Human Services. This change in inpatient hospital procedure coding resulted in a change in code format. The *ICD-9-CM, Volume 3* procedure codes were three to four numeric characters with a decimal point whereas the format of ICD-10-PCS codes is seven-character alphanumeric codes.

The ICD-10-PCS code set is required because the new ICD-10-CM classifies only disease, injuries, and other health-care conditions. The new ICD-10-PCS code set was developed by 3M Health Information Systems in 1993 for CMS. ICD-10-PCS was originally published in 1998 and has been updated annually since that time. Remember: This ICD-10-PCS coding system is used to classify *inpatient* procedures reported by hospitals; it is mandated by the Health Insurance Portability and Accountability Act of 1996 (HIPAA) and replaces Volume 3 of ICD-9-CM.

The new ICD-10-PCS classification system was created to meet the demands for multiple uses of electronically coded data. ICD-10-PCS was designed to enable each code to have a standard structure and be descriptive yet flexible enough to accommodate future needs. Nevertheless, the process of coding still requires documentation review and use of an Index and/or Code Tables.

ICD-10-PCS Changes in 2018

The ICD-10-CM code set does not include a procedural coding system. Therefore, annual changes to the code set are published separately by CMS. The changes in ICD-10-PCD 2017 to ICD-10-PCS 2018 include 3,562 new codes, 1,821 revised codes, and 646 deleted codes. These changes are primarily in the medical and surgical section and simplify body part values and correct clinical discrepancies.

> **INTERNET RESOURCE: CMS ICD-10-PCS (2018)**
> **Details of all changes effective October 1, 2017 are available on the Centers for Medicare & Medicaid Services (CMS) website.**
> **https://www.cms.gov/Medicare/Coding/ICD10/2018-ICD-10-PCS-and-GEMs.html**

Identify which coding system (A–D) is described in the following statements.

    A. ICD-10-PCS

    B. ICD-9-CM Volume 3

    C. ICD-10-CM

    D. CPT

1. Classifies hospital inpatient procedures prior to October 1, 2015 ___

2. Classifies hospital outpatient and physician procedures ___

3. Used to classify hospital inpatient procedures effective October 1, 2015 ___

4. Developed by 3M and published in 1998 ___

5. Used to report diagnoses, injuries, and medical conditions beginning October 1, 2015 ___

6. Maintained by NCHS ___

7. Uses a three- or four-digit numeric format ___

8. Uses a flexible table format ___

9. Contains seven alphanumeric characters ___

10. Classifies external causes of disease effective October 1, 2015 ___

NOTE: Use ICD-10-PCS for *inpatient* procedures, and use CPT (covered in Chapters 12 to 30) for coding *outpatient* procedures. Hospitals may choose to report ICD-10-PCS procedures for outpatient visits for reporting purposes only.

ICD-10-PCS BASICS

This section is designed to provide an overview of ICD-10-PCS basics rather than in-depth instruction for ICD-10-PCS. Effective in 2018, there are 78,705 codes in ICD-10-PCS, which suggests the use of a supplemental text to present all the details of this procedural coding system. Later in this chapter, a simulation is provided that uses the ICD-10-PCS files from CMS at https://www.cms.gov/Medicare/Coding/ICD10/Index.html. This website provides an electronic ICD-10-PCS code book and the resources summarized in this basic instruction.

ICD-10-PCS References

Reference Manual

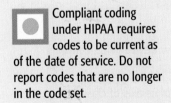

Compliant coding under HIPAA requires codes to be current as of the date of service. Do not report codes that are no longer in the code set.

The ICD-10-PCS *Reference Manual* describes in detail the history of ICD-10-PCS; the code structure, design, and organization of the coding system; and offers a detailed discussion of many procedures the code set contains. This document is the primary resource for coding instructions and clarifications for coding using ICD-10-PCS. The coder should keep the *Reference Manual* available when using ICD-10-PCS in order to follow the coding rules for each section. The introductory pages in the manual supplement the instruction in this text. The *Reference Manual* was published with the October 2016 references and is organized into four chapters and contains two appendices:

1. ICD-10-PCS Overview
2. Provides a device and substance classification section
3. Procedures in the Medical and Surgical-Related sections

4. Procedures in the Ancillary Sections
5. Appendix A: ICD-10-PCS Definitions
6. Appendix B: ICD-10-PCS Device and Substance Classification

INTERNET RESOURCE: ICD-10-PCS Resources
www.cms.gov/medicare/coding/ICD10/2016-ICD-10-PCS-and-GEMS.html

ICD-10-PCS Official Guidelines

The HIPAA rules, in addition to mandating the ICD-10-PCS code set, also require the use of the *ICD-10-PCS Official Guidelines for Coding and Reporting (Official Guidelines)* when codes are selected. The guidelines assist in standardizing the assignment of ICD-10-PCS codes for all users. For example, they include the rules for selecting the principal procedure when a patient has more than one surgical operation and assist coders in understanding the basic rules of code selection. The *Official Guidelines* also include a description of the conventions that outline the characteristics and unique terms used.

Box 11.1 lists the conventions outlined in the first part of the *Official Guidelines*.

AHA Coding Clinic® for ICD-10-CM/PCS

AHA Coding Clinic® for ICD-10-CM/PCS is published by the American Hospital Association (AHA). The AHA's central office handles all ICD-10 coding-related issues and works with NCHS and CMS to maintain the integrity of the coding system. *AHA Coding Clinic* provides advice on coding certain procedures in ICD-10.

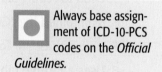 Always base assignment of ICD-10-PCS codes on the *Official Guidelines.*

AHA Coding Clinic® is published quarterly, or as needed, and can be purchased from the AHA. The coding advice is approved by CMS for Medicare reimbursement and is also accepted by many other payers.

INTERNET RESOURCE: *AHA Coding Clinic® for ICD-10-CM/PCS*
www.ahacentraloffice.org

BOX 11.1 ICD-10-PCS *Official Guidelines:* A. Conventions

A1
ICD-10-PCS codes are composed of seven characters. Each character is an axis of classification that specifies information about the procedure performed. Within a defined code range, a character specifies the same type of information in that axis of classification.
Example: The fifth axis of classification specifies the approach in sections 0 through 4 and 7 through 9 of the system.
A2
One of 34 possible values can be assigned to each axis of classification in the seven-character code: they are the numbers 0 through 9 and the alphabet (except I and O because they are easily confused with the numbers 1 and 0). The number of unique values used in an axis of classification differs as needed.
Example: Where the fifth axis of classification specifies the approach, seven different approach values are currently used to specify the approach.
A3
The valid values for an axis of classification can be added to as needed.
Example: If a significantly distinct type of device is used in a new procedure, a new device value can be added to the system.
A4
As with words in their context, the meaning of any single value is a combination of its axis of classification and any preceding values on which it may be dependent.
Example: The meaning of a body part value in the Medical and Surgical section is always dependent on the body system value. The body part value 0 in the Central Nervous body system specifies Brain and the body part value 0 in the Peripheral Nervous body system specifies Cervical Plexus.
A5
As the system is expanded to become increasingly detailed, over time more values will depend on preceding values for their meaning.

Continued

BOX 11.1 *Continued*

Example: In the Lower Joints body system, the device value 3 in the root operation. Insertion specifies Infusion Device and the device value 3 in the root operation. Replacement specifies Ceramic Synthetic Substitute.

A6

The purpose of the alphabetic index is to locate the appropriate table that contains all information necessary to construct a procedure code. The PCS Tables should always be consulted to find the most appropriate valid code.

A7

It is not required to consult the index first before proceeding to the tables to complete the code. A valid code may be chosen directly from the tables.

A8

All seven characters must be specified to be a valid code. If the documentation is incomplete for coding purposes, the physician should be queried for the necessary information.

A9

Within a PCS table, valid codes include all combinations of choices in characters 4 through 7 contained in the same row of the table.

A10

"And," when used in a code description, means "and/or."

Example: Lower Arm and Wrist Muscle means lower arm and/or wrist muscle.

A11

Many of the terms used to construct PCS codes are defined within the system. It is the coder's responsibility to determine which documentation in the medical record equates to the PCS definitions. The physician is not expected to use the terms used in PCS code descriptions, nor is the coder required to query the physician when the correlation between the documentation and the defined PCS terms is clear.

CHECKPOINT 11.2

Answer the following questions.

1. When was ICD-10-PCS implemented? _Oct. 1 2015_

2. Which legislation mandates the use of ICD-10-PCS? _HIPPA_

3. Who is required to use ICD-10-PCS codes? _inpatient procedures in hospitals_

4. Which ICD-10-PCS resource contains the conventions? _offical Guidelines_

5. How many ICD-10-PCS procedure codes effective October 1, 2017 are there? _78 705_

_____

Matching

Match the resource to the following statements:

A. *Official Guidelines*: Conventions   D. *AHA Coding Clinic for ICD-10-CM/PCS*

B. *Reference Manual*   E. Device key

C. *Official Guidelines*: Selection of Principal Procedures

6. _____ Contains articles offering practical information to improve data quality

7. _____ Provides the primary source for coding instructions and clarification

8. _____ Provides a device and substance classification

9. _____ Contains the rules for principal procedure selection

10. _____ Instructs the coder that the same row of an ICD-10-PCS table must be used to assign a valid code

ICD-10-PCS BASIC CODING PROCESS

Procedure coding requires knowledge of the format of each ICD-10-PCS section and of the conventions and rules each uses to assist the coder in finding different types of procedure codes, such as surgical codes, diagnostic services or procedures, or obstetrical services. A codebook is the source of the codes; the *Official Guidelines* are the source of the conventions and rules. There are additional conventions that guide the coder in the basic coding process. These include the correct use of the Index, the use of main terms, the use of cross-references, and the use of the tables.

An ICD-10-PCS codebook has two sections:

1. *Index:* The Index is organized alphabetically by main terms.
2. *Code Tables:* These tables are organized by section (first character). Then, within each first character, the numerical values are followed by the alphabetic values.

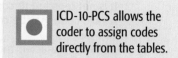 ICD-10-PCS allows the coder to assign codes directly from the tables.

Appendices may be supplied that include the root operations definitions, the Body Part key, and/or the Device key table. These appendices are dependent on the publisher of the codebook.

The coding process starts with looking up words. Thus, the ICD-10-PCS Index, which contains surgical terms, is used first. Remember, the conventions do allow for the coder to assign codes directly from the tables; however, most coders begin in the Index. Using a surgical main term and sub-term in the Index results in either a partial code, which must be completed by using the Code Table or a complete code, which must be verified in the Code Table.

ICD-10-PCS FORMAT AND STRUCTURE

ICD-10-PCS represents an improvement over ICD-9-CM, Volume 3, with regard to specificity and comprehensiveness. The 17 sections in ICD-10-PCS are categorized as either medical and surgical or ancillary (Table 11.1). All codes in ICD-10-PCS have a structure that begins with the general type of procedure (the section determines the first character) and develops into a specific code

Table 11.1 Medical-, Surgical-, and Ancillary-Related Sections

1ST MEDICAL/SURGICAL CHARACTER	SECTION
0	Medical and Surgical
1	Obstetrics
2	Placement
3	Administration
4	Measurement and Monitoring
5	Extracorporeal Assistance and Performance
6	Extracorporeal Therapies
7	Osteopathic
8	Other Procedures
9	Chiropractic
1ST ANCILLARY CHARACTER	**SECTION**
B	Imaging
C	Nuclear Medicine
D	Radiation Therapy
F	Physical Rehabilitation and Diagnostic Audiology
G	Mental Health
H	Substance Abuse Treatment
X	New Technology

built of six additional components. Each component is called a *character,* and has a distinctive meaning, and each character is represented by a value. The system is multi-axial; that is, each character has the same meaning within a section. We discuss these meanings in more detail later.

Coding in ICD-10-PCS is a process rather than just a matter of looking up a defined, fixed code from the Index. A code is built by adding values for each character based on tables within a particular section, body system, and root operation. The rules outlined in the *Official Guidelines* and *Reference Manual* are important to the construction of a code.

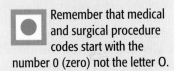

Remember that medical and surgical procedure codes start with the number 0 (zero) not the letter O.

The character value can be a letter or number, for a total of 34 possible values for each character space. The possible values for an ICD-10-PCS code are the numbers 0 to 9 and the letters A to Z, except I and O. This range allows for expansion of the coding system. Codes are derived by choosing a specific value for each of the seven characters. The meaning of each value in a specific character space depends on the procedure performed and the components of that procedure. A complete PCS code might look like this: 0DBN8ZX (colonoscopy with a biopsy of the sigmoid colon).

ICD-10-PCS Index

The ICD-10-PCS Index directs the coder to the appropriate table that contains the additional information necessary to build or construct the complete procedure code. The Index is organized alphabetically by main terms, words that describe common procedures, anatomical sites, or a device. The main terms most often represent the value of the third character. For example, in the Medical and Surgical section of ICD-10-PCS, the third character represents the root operation. The root operation *Excision* is a main term in the Index. Another example of a main term in the Index is the name of a device, such as *Pacemaker.*

Other examples of main terms are *Introduction* (root type), *Appendectomy* (procedure name), *Femoral Artery* (body part), and *Hancock Bioprosthesis* (device).

Subterms are used to provide further clarification and detail surrounding the main term. Box 11.2 provides an example of an ICD-10-PCS index entry. The indented format helps coders see that the word *Left* refers specifically to Acetabulum, which refers to the main term *Repair.* It is important to observe this pattern of indention.

> **BOX 11.2 Example of an ICD-10-PCS Index Entry**
>
> **Repair**
> Abdominal Wall 0WQF
> Acetabulum
>   Left 0QQ5
>   Right 0QQ4

Only a portion of the code is referenced in the Index. Typically, the Index provides the first three or four values of the code; therefore, the coder must determine the required additional character values from the tables. Always verify code assignment in the tables. Another example from the Index is shown in Box 11.3. The main term for the device, Bone Anchored Hearing Device, lists the first three character values of the code for the insertion of a bone-anchored hearing device.

> **BOX 11.3 Example of the First Three Characters in an Index Entry**
>
> Bone Anchored Hearing Device
>   *use* Hearing Device, Bone Conduction in 09H
>   *use* Hearing Device in Head and Facial Bones

Cross-References Used in the Index

> **BOX 11.4 Example of the Cross-Reference *See* Index Entry**
>
> **Cholecystectomy**
>   *see* Excision, Gallbladder 0FB4
>   *see* Resection, Gallbladder 0FT4

The two remaining official conventions pertinent to the Index are the cross-references *see* and *use.* The term *see* used as a cross-reference directs the coder to the root operations that are possible and includes valid tables that can be used based on the objective of the procedure. For example, Box 11.4 shows the cross-reference *see* when looking up the main term *Cholecystectomy.* Depending on the intent of the procedure, the coder should see the root operation *Excision* and table 0FB4 or Resection table 0FT4.

The second cross-reference in ICD-10-PCS is the word *use* (Box 11.5). This term instructs the coder based on anatomical sites in the Body Part key and the device terms from the Device key. The ICD-10-PCS codebook contains an appendix for both of these keys in addition to listing these terms in the Index. For example, the main term *Greater Trochanter* (body part) instructs the coder to *use* (1) Upper Femur, Right or (2) Upper Femur, Left.

The codebook provides two references to assist the coder in using ICD-10-PCS terminology: the Body Part Key and the Device Key. The Body Part Key is used to identify anatomical sites and their classification in PCS. For example, the body part platysma muscle is classified in PCS as a neck muscle. The Device Key provides a cross-reference that gives a PCS description for a specific device term. An example from the Device Key is a bone bank bone graft: This is classified as a nonautologous tissue substitute. The word *use* is noted in the Index to direct the user to these keys. The Index may include the PCS definition, but it does not direct the user to a cross-reference or specific table; instead, it provides guidance to selecting a particular value. For example, in Box 11.6, the Body Part Key value is in the Index. The coder would assign the body part of muscle, upper arm, for the biceps brachii muscle.

Box 11.7 depicts a page from the ICD-10-PCS Index. Identify the main terms, cross-references and *use* conventions. For example, the main term Gastrectomy directs the coder to see Resection for a total gastrectomy. When reporting a procedure on the gastrocnemius muscle, the coder should use the body part lower leg muscle. The Index also provides the first few characters of the ICD-10-PCS code. The completion of the code requires use of the appropriate table. For example, the coder would reference the code for Gait training (F07) in the table to complete the code.

BOX 11.5 Example of the Cross-Reference *Use* Index Entry

Index Entry
Greater Trochanter
 use Upper Femur, Right
 use Upper Femur, Left

BOX 11.6 Example of the Body Part Key

Biceps brachii muscle
 use Muscle, Upper Arm, Right
 use Muscle, Upper Arm, Left

BOX 11.7 Example From ICD-10-PCS Index, 2017

Gait training *see* Motor Treatment, Rehabilitation F07
Galea aponeurotica *use* Subcutaneous Tissue and Fascia, Scalp
GammaTile™ *use* Radioactive element, Cesium-131 Collagen Implant in 00H
Ganglion impar (ganglion of Walther) *use* Sacral Sympathetic Nerve
Ganglionectomy
 Destruction of lesion *see* Destruction
 Excision of lesion *see* Excision
Gasserian ganglion *use* Trigeminal Nerve
Gastrectomy
 Partial *see* Excision, Stomach 0DB6
 Total *see* Resection, Stomach 0DT6
 Vertical (sleeve) *see* Excision, Stomach 0DB6
Gastric electrical stimulation (GES) lead *use* Stimulator Lead in Gastrointestinal System
Gastric lymph node *use* Lymphatic, Aortic
Gastric pacemaker lead *use* Stimulator Lead in Gastrointestinal System
Gastric plexus *use* Abdominal Sympathetic Nerve
Gastrocnemius muscle
 use Lower Leg Muscle, Right
 use Lower Leg Muscle, Left
Gastrocolic ligament *use* Greater Omentum
Gastrocolic omentum *use* Greater Omentum
Gastrocolostomy
 see Bypass, Gastrointestinal System 0D1
 see Drainage, Gastrointestinal System 0D9
Gastroduodenal artery *use* Hepatic Artery
Gastroduodenectomy
 see Excision, Gastrointestinal System 0DB
 see Resection, Gastrointestinal System 0DT

Continued

BOX 11.7 *Continued*

Gastroduodenoscopy 0DJ08ZZ
Gastroenteroplasty
   see Repair, Gastrointestinal System 0DQ
   see Supplement, Gastrointestinal System 0DU
Gastroenterostomy
   see Bypass, Gastrointestinal System 0D1
   see Drainage, Gastrointestinal System 0D9
Gastroesophageal (GE) junction *use* Esophagogastric Junction
Gastrogastrostomy
   see Bypass, Stomach 0D16
   see Drainage, Stomach 0D96
Gastrohepatic omentum *use* Lesser Omentum
Gastrojejunostomy
   see Bypass, Stomach 0D16
   see Drainage, Stomach 0D96

CHECKPOINT 11.3

Answer the following questions.

1. How many possible values are there for each character in ICD-10-PCS? _____

2. Which character values are not used in ICD-10-PCS? _____

3. The first character value of B in an ICD-10-PCS code represents which section? _____

4. What is the main term in Box 11.2? _____

5. What is the term used in ICD-10-PCS that directs the coder to an alternative main term?

   _____

Using Box 11.7 (ICD-10-PCS Sample Index), answer the following questions.

6. Which body part should be reported for the gastric plexus? _____

7. What are the first characters of the ICD-10-PCS code for a sleeve gastrectomy? _____

8. What is the ICD-10-PCS code for a gastroduodenoscopy? _____

9. A gastric pacemaker lead is considered what type of device in ICD-10-PCS? _____

10. Which two cross-references are used to code a gastrojejunostomy? _____

ICD-10-PCS CODE TABLES

> Within a PCS Code Table, the coder must choose values from the same row. Never cross rows.

Code Tables must be used to assign an ICD-10-PCS code. The first three characters of a code define each table. The first character of PCS codes is determined by the section; within each section, the second and third characters comprise the table. Once the first three characters have been determined, the coder must reference the Code Tables. Think of this as building a code. Each table contains columns that list the possible last four characters of codes and rows that provide valid values for each character. The coder must stay in a row to assign valid combinations for characters 4 to 7. For example, Figure 11.1 shows the first three characters as 0DB (Medical and Surgical section, Procedure of the GI system with an excision). If the coder chose the fourth character of 6 (stomach), the row across represents the five valid approaches associated with a stomach excision procedure. No device is applicable. Notice that the last character value, 3 (the qualifier), can be assigned only with the fourth character body part value of 6 (stomach) in the second row. Figure 11.2 shows the table used to assign the code for reattachment of the right elbow (0XMB0ZZ).

Section	0	Medical and Surgical			
Body System	D	Gastrointestinal System			
Operation	B	Excision: Cutting out or off, without replacement, a portion of a body part			

Body Part	Approach	Device	Qualifier
1 Esophagus, Upper 2 Esophagus, Middle 3 Esophagus, Lower 4 Esophagogastric Junction 5 Esophagus 7 Stomach, Pylorus 8 Small Intestine 9 Duodenum A Jejunum B Ileum C Ileocecal Valve E Large Intestine F Large Intestine, Right H Cecum J Appendix K Ascending Colon P Rectum	0 Open 3 Percutaneous 4 Percutaneous Endoscopic 7 Via Natural or Artificial Opening 8 Via Natural or Artificial Opening Endoscopic	Z No Device	X Diagnostic Z No Qualifier
6 Stomach	0 Open 3 Percutaneous 4 Percutaneous Endoscopic 7 Via Natural or Artificial Opening 8 Via Natural or Artificial Opening Endoscopic	Z No Device	3 Vertical X Diagnostic Z No Qualifier
G Large Intestine, Left L Transverse Colon M Descending Colon N Sigmoid Colon	0 Open 3 Percutaneous 4 Percutaneous Endoscopic 7 Via Natural or Artificial Opening 8 Via Natural or Artificial Opening Endoscopic X External	Z No Device	X Diagnostic Z No Qualifier

Figure 11.1 Table from the Medical and Surgical section.

Section	0	Medical and Surgical			
Body System	X	Anatomical Regions, Upper Extremities			
Operation	M	Reattachment: Putting back in or on all or a portion of a separated body part to its normal location or other suitable location			

Body Part	Approach	Device	Qualifier
0 Forequarter, Right 1 Forequarter, Left 2 Shoulder Region, Right 3 Shoulder Region, Left 4 Axilla, Right 5 Axilla, Left 6 Upper Extremity, Right 7 Upper Extremity, Left 8 Upper Arm, Right 9 Upper Arm, Left B Elbow Region, Right C Elbow Region, Left D Lower Arm, Right F Lower Arm, Left G Wrist Region, Right H Wrist Region, Left J Hand, Right K Hand, Left L Thumb, Right M Thumb, Left N Index Finger, Right P Index Finger, Left Q Middle Finger, Right R Middle Finger, Left S Ring Finger, Right T Ring Finger, Left V Little Finger, Right W Little Finger, Left	0 Open	Z No Device	Z No Qualifier

Figure 11.2 PCS Code table for upper extremity reattachment.

Section	B	Imaging
Body System	N	Skull and Facial Bones
Type	2	Computerized Tomography (CT Scan): Computer reformatted digital display of multiplanar images developed from the capture of multiple exposures of external ionizing radiation

Body Part	Contrast	Qualifier	Qualifier
0 Skull 3 Orbits, Bilateral 5 Facial Bones 6 Mandible 9 Temporomandibular Joints, Bilateral F Temporal Bones	0 High Osmolar 1 Low Osmolar Y Other Contrast Z None	Z None	Z None

Figure 11.3 PCD Code table from the Imaging section.

Figure 11.3 is another example of the table structure from the Imaging section of ICD-10-PCS. Notice that the fourth through seventh characters have different meanings from those of the Medical and Surgical section. The coder would still follow the guidelines for code assignment based on the table format, which requires assigning values for each character based on column and row structure.

Remember: There are many Code Tables that are used to construct a code. The first three characters define which table to use, and the possible values for each of the remaining characters are listed in the same row of the table. All seven characters must be specified to form a valid code. Note the following when using the ICD-10-PCS tables:

1. There may be multiple tables for the first three characters.
2. Some tables cover multiple pages.
3. The same value of the fourth character may be in several rows.
4. The order of the tables is 001–0YW, then 102–10Y, and so on.

For example, using Figure 11.1 the valid code 0DB58ZX represents an upper endoscopy with a diagnostic biopsy of the esophagus.

For the purposes of this introduction to ICD-10-PCS, we will focus on the specific guidelines and table structure of the Medical and Surgical section of ICD-10-PCS. To delineate the structure of codes in this section, the coder must understand the seven characters represented in a Medical and Surgical procedure code:

CHARACTER	1	2	3	4	5	6	7
	Section	Body System	Root Operation	Body Part	Approach	Device	Qualifier

Character 1 for procedures classified to the ICD-10-PCS identifies the section. Medical and Surgical section codes always start with a 0 (zero). Codes are then constructed character by character, with the second character representing the Body System. The Body System (character 2) is broken down into 31 values. For example, the value of 1 is the peripheral nervous system, and a value of V is the male reproductive system. The numeric values are followed by alphabetic values. The Code Tables are ordered by the value of the character. These first two characters are easier to classify than the third character, which represents the Root Operation.

The Root Operation identifies the objective of the procedure. There are 31 Root Operations in ICD-10-PCS. In the Code Tables, the Root Operation and its definition are noted. It is the combination of these first three characters that determines the table used to construct the remainder of the code. The surgeon is not expected to change documentation to reflect these distinct root operations; rather, the coder's responsibility is to determine what documentation in the medical record equates to the PCS definition. For example, if the physician documents "excisional biopsy," the coder can independently correlate that to the Root Operation of excision without seeking further clarification. The full list of Root Operations is shown in Table 11.2. (This chapter provides a brief overview of ICD-10-PCS. Further instruction is needed to apply the concepts of Root Operations and code construction for characters 3 to 7.)

Table 11.2 Root Operations

ROOT OPERATION	WHAT OPERATION DOES	OBJECTIVE OF PROCEDURE	PROCEDURE SITE	EXAMPLE
Excision	Takes out some/all of a body part	Cutting out/off without replacement	Some of a body part	Breast lumpectomy
Resection	Takes out some/all of a body part	Cutting out/off without replacement	All of a body part	Total mastectomy
Detachment	Takes out some/all of a body part	Cutting out/off without replacement	Extremity only, any level	Amputation above elbow
Destruction	Takes out some/all of a body part	Eradicating without replacement	Some/all of a body part	Fulguration of endometrium
Extraction	Takes out some/all of a body part	Pulling out or off without replacement	Some/all of a body part	Suction D&C
Drainage	Takes out solids/fluids/gases from a body part	Taking/letting out fluids/gases	Within a body part	Incision and drainage
Extirpation	Takes out solids/fluids/gases from a body part	Taking/cutting out solid matter	Within a body part	Thrombectomy
Fragmentation	Takes out solids/fluids/gases from a body part	Breaking solid matter into pieces	Within a body part	Lithotripsy
Division	Involves cutting or separation only	Cutting into/separating a body part	Within a body part	Neurotomy
Release	Involves cutting or separation only	Freeing a body part from constraint	Around a body part	Adhesiolysis
Transplantation	Puts in/puts back or moves some/all of a body part	Putting in a living body part from a person/animal	Some/all of a body part	Kidney transplant
Reattachment	Puts in/puts back or moves some/all of a body part	Putting back a detached body part	Some/all of a body part	Reattach severed finger
Transfer	Puts in/puts back or moves some/all of a body part	Moving, to function for a similar body part	Some/all of a body part	Skin transfer flap
Reposition	Puts in/puts back or moves some/all of a body part	Moving to normal or suitable location	Some/all of a body part	Move undescended testicle
Restriction	Alters the diameter/route of a tubular body part	Partially closing orifice/lumen	Tubular body part	Gastroesophageal fundoplication
Occlusion	Alters the diameter/route of a tubular body part	Completely closing orifice/lumen	Tubular body part	Fallopian tube ligation
Dilation	Alters the diameter/route of a tubular body part	Expanding orifice/lumen	Tubular body part	Percutaneous transluminal coronary angioplasty (PTCA)
Bypass	Alters the diameter/route of a tubular body part	Altering route of passage	Tubular body part	Coronary artery bypass graft (CABG)
Insertion	Always involves a device	Putting in nonbiological device	In/on a body part	Central line insertion

Continued

Table 11.2 Continued

ROOT OPERATION	WHAT OPERATION DOES	OBJECTIVE OF PROCEDURE	PROCEDURE SITE	EXAMPLE
Replacement	Always involves a device	Putting in device that replaces a body part	Some/all of a body part	Total hip replacement
Supplement	Always involves a device	Putting in device that reinforces or augments a body part	In/on a body part	Abdominal wall herniorrhaphy using
Change	Always involves a device	Exchanging device without cutting/puncturing	In/on a body part	Drainage tube change
Removal	Always involves a device	Taking out a device	In/on a body part	Central line removal
Revision	Always involves a device	Correcting a malfunctioning/displaced device	In/on a body part	Revision of pacemaker insertion
Inspection	Involves examination only	Visual/manual exploration	Some/all of a body part	Diagnostic cystoscopy
Map	Involves examination only	Locating electrical impulses/functional areas	Brain/cardiac conduction mechanism	Cardiac mapping
Repair	Includes other repairs	Restoring body part to its normal structure	Some/all of a body part	Suture laceration
Control	Includes other repairs	Stopping/attempting to stop postprocedural bleed	Anatomical region	Postprostatectomy bleeding
Fusion	Includes other objectives	Rendering joint immobile	Joint	Spinal fusion
Alteration	Includes other objectives	Modifying body part for cosmetic purposes without affecting function	Some/all of a body part	Face lift
Creation	Includes other objectives	Making new structure for sex change operation	Perineum	Artificial vagina/penis

The fourth character represents the Body Part. This is the anatomical site of the body system on which the procedure was performed. For example, the respiratory system (second character value) has the body part of lower lung lobe, right. The urinary system has the body part bladder.

Character 5 represents the surgical Approach: open (0), percutaneous (3), percutaneous endoscopic (4), via natural or artificial opening (7), via natural or artificial opening endoscopic (8), via natural or artificial opening with percutaneous endoscopic assistance (F), and external (X). The approach comprises three components: (1) the access location, (2) the method, and (3) the type of instrumentation. For example, a laparoscopic approach is classified as percutaneous endoscopic (4). A colonoscopy would be reported using the approach value of 8, which is "via natural or artificial opening endoscopic."

The Device, character 6, is used to identify a device that remains after a procedure is completed. There are four types of devices: grafts and prostheses, implants, simple or mechanical appliances, and electronic appliances. The Device key discussed earlier is used to determine the value for this character. An example is a percutaneous insertion of a pacemaker lead in the right ventricle; the code 02HK3JZ would have a value of J in the sixth-character position to represent the Device.

The Qualifier is character 7. It identifies some characteristic of the procedure. For example, in reporting a total hip replacement, the 7th character qualifier classifies whether cement was used during the procedure.

CHECKPOINT 11.4

Based on the code structure of ICD-10-PCS, identify the meaning of each character space in the ICD-10-PCS code.

1. First: _____
2. Second: _____
3. Third: _____
4. Fourth: _____
5. Fifth: _____
6. Sixth: _____
7. Seventh: _____

True or False

8. _____ Medical and surgical procedure codes have a first character of 0.

9. _____ T83.4567 is a valid ICD-10-PCS code.

10. _____ The character 8 is used as a value for the operative approach.

11. _____ The letter B represents the section for imaging.

12. _____ The first three characters of a code define the table.

Match the root operation with the appropriate definition.

A. dilation   F. extirpation

B. excision   G. removal

C. resection   H. restriction

D. inspection   I. supplement

E. repair   J. fragmentation

13. _____ Restoring a body part to its normal anatomical structure or function

14. _____ Cutting out or off, without replacement, all of a body part

15. _____ Cutting out or off, without replacement, a portion of a body part

16. _____ Putting in or on biological or synthetic material that physically reinforces a body part

17. _____ Expanding an orifice or lumen of a tubular body part

18. _____ Taking out or off a device from a body part from an abnormal physical constraint

19. _____ Visually exploring a body part

20. _____ Partially closing an orifice or the lumen of a tubular body part

21. _____ Taking or cutting out solid matter from a body part

22. _____ Breaking solid matter in a body part into pieces

Use Boxes 11.2 to 11.6 and Figures 11.1 to 11.3 to answer the following questions.

23. What are the first four characters in the code for repair of the left acetabulum? _____

24. What is the ICD-10-PCS classification for the body part left upper femur? _____

25. What is the value for the percutaneous approach in table 0DB? _____

26. What is the code for a CT scan of the mandible using low osmolar contrast? _____

27. What main term would be used to find the table 0XM? _____

ICD-10-PCS CODING SIMULATION

The instructions that follow provide the basic steps for assigning an ICD-10-PCS code using the CMS codebook. Keep in mind that this basic instruction is only a precursor to the in-depth instruction required for an inpatient coder to be fully adept in ICD-10-PCS coding.

All ICD-10-PCS references are available on the CMS website: the complete code set (Index and Code Tables), the *Official Guidelines*, the *Reference Manual*, and GEMs. We will use this website to practice ICD-10-PCS coding.

INTERNET RESOURCE: Center for Medicare and Medicaid Services
https://www.cms.gov/Medicare/Coding/ICD10/2018-ICD-10-PCS-and-GEMs.html

Code Tables and Index

This section gives you a screen-shot guide to using the Code Tables and Index. The ICD-10-PCS Index and Code Tables files are located on the CMS website. You can use this file as a codebook to find the main term in the Index and then develop the complete procedure code using the Table. To view the Index and Code Tables, use the steps that follow to access a list of download options for ICD-10-PCS.

1. Visit https://www.cms.gov/Medicare/Coding/ICD10/2018-ICD-10-PCS-and-GEMs.html (Fig. 11.4)

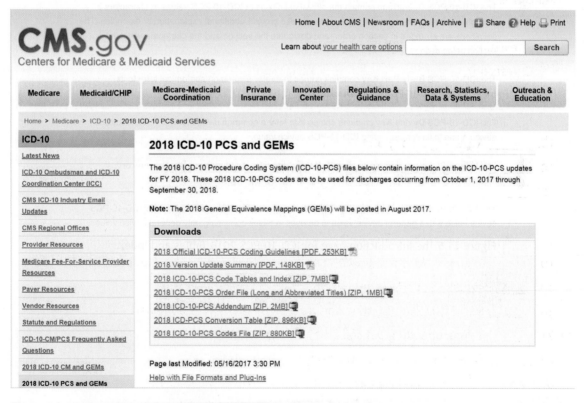

Figure 11.4 Screen shot of the CMS.gov 2018 ICD-10 PCS and GEMs home page.

2. Click "2018 ICD-10-PCS Code Tables and Index [ZIP, 5MB]." Download and save the folder. You will then have a list of files to choose from. Open the PDF file titled pcs_2018.
3. Moving forward in this section, we will be working with this file, so be sure to save it in an easily accessible location.

As we proceed, when practicing with the online code set, use the following scenario throughout this first coding example: colonoscopy with a biopsy of the cecum. A biopsy is the root operation Excision.

Example 1

Now that you have opened and saved the online code set, you are ready to begin coding. The first page of the Code Tables and Index provides links to the Tables, Index, Definitions, and other Keys as shown below (Fig. 11.5).

1. From the Introduction, choose ICD-10-PCS Index.

ICD-10 Procedure Coding System
(ICD-10-PCS)
2018 Tables and Index

Introduction

The ICD-10-PCS Tables contain all valid codes in table format. The tables are arranged in alphanumeric order, and organized into separate tables according to the first three characters of the seven-character code.

The ICD-10-PCS Index contains entries based on the terms (known as values) used in the ICD-10-PCS Tables, as well as entries based on common procedure terms. Index entries either link directly to a PCS table or refer the user to another index entry.

The ICD-10-PCS Definitions contain the official definitions of ICD-10-PCS values in characters 3 through 7 of the seven-character code, and may also provide additional explanation or examples. The definitions are arranged in section order, and designate the section and the character within the section being defined.

The ICD-10-PCS Body Part Key contains entries that refer a common anatomical term to its corresponding ICD-10-PCS body part value(s).

The ICD-10-PCS Device Key contains entries that refer a common device term or manufacturer's device name to its corresponding ICD-10-PCS device value.

The ICD-10-PCS Substance Key contains entries that refer a common substance name or manufacturer's substance name to its corresponding ICD-10-PCS substance value.

The ICD-10-PCS Device Aggregation Table contains entries that correlate a specific ICD-10-PCS device value with a general device value to be used in tables containing only general device values.

Figure 11.5 The Introduction page for ICD-10-PCS 2018 Tables and Index.

2. To gain access to the main term Excision in the Index, select E "E-Luminexx through EXtreme" (Fig. 11.6). Scroll through the pages to find the main term Excision, subterm Cecum.

Index

Back to Top

3	3f
A	Abdominal through Axillary
B	BAK/C® through Bypass
C	Caesarean through Cystourethroplasty
D	DBS through Dynesys®
E	E-Luminexx™ through EXtreme
F	Face through Fusion
G	Gait through Guidance
H	Hallux through Hysterotrachelorrhaphy
I	IABP through Itrel
J	Jejunal through Jugular
K	Kappa through Kuntscher
L	Labia through Lysis
M	Macula through Myringotomy
N	Nail through Nutrition
O	Obliteration through Oxygenation
P	Pacemaker through Pyramidalis
Q	Quadrangular through Quarantine
R	Radial through Rupture
S	Sacral through Systemic
T	Takedown through Tympanotomy
U	Ulnar through Uvulotomy
V	Vaccination through Vulvectomy
W	WALLSTENT® through Wiring
X	X-ray through XLIF®
Y	Yoga
Z	Z-plasty through Zyvox

Figure 11.6 ICD-10-PCS Index.

3. At Excision, Cecum, click on ODBH to link to the table (Fig. 11.7).

Carpal
Left **OPBN**
Right **OPBM**
Cecum **ODBH**
Cerebellum **00BC**

Figure 11.7 Index entry for Excision, Cecum

4. Using the table shown in Figure 11.8, finish building the ICD-10-PCS code for the colonoscopy with biopsy of the cecum. The coding path is shown using red arrows on the figure below. (*Hint:* A biopsy is always considered a diagnostic procedure according to the *Reference Manual.*)
5. The correct code for a colonoscopy with biopsy of the cecum is 0DBH8ZX.

Section	0	Medical and Surgical
Body System	D	Gastrointestinal System
Operation	B	Excision: Cutting out or off, without replacement, a portion of a body part

Body Part	Approach	Device	Qualifier
1 Esophagus, Upper 2 Esophagus, Middle 3 Esophagus, Lower 4 Esophagogastric Junction 5 Esophagus 7 Stomach, Pylorus 8 Small Intestine 9 Duodenum A Jejunum B Ileum C Ileocecal Valve E Large Intestine F Large Intestine, Right H Cecum ◄— J Appendix K Ascending Colon P Rectum	0 Open 3 Percutaneous 4 Percutaneous Endoscopic 7 Via Natural or Artificial Opening 8 Via Natural or Artificial Opening Endoscopic ◄———	Z No Device ◄—	X Diagnostic ◄— Z No Qualifier
6 Stomach	0 Open 3 Percutaneous 4 Percutaneous Endoscopic 7 Via Natural or Artificial Opening 8 Via Natural or Artificial Opening Endoscopic	Z No Device	3 Vertical X Diagnostic Z No Qualifier
G Large Intestine, Left L Transverse Colon M Descending Colon N Sigmoid Colon	0 Open 3 Percutaneous 4 Percutaneous Endoscopic 7 Via Natural or Artificial Opening 8 Via Natural or Artificial Opening Endoscopic X External	Z No Device	X Diagnostic Z No Qualifier

Figure 11.8 Table for Medical and Surgery, Gastrointestinal System, Excision.

Example 2

Our next example illustrates that it is not always necessary to use the Index to code. You can code a colonoscopy with a biopsy of the cecum starting from the Medical and Surgical section and continue building the code by knowing the body system and the root operation.

1. Access the ICD-10-PCS code set from the CMS website as instructed earlier.
2. From the Introduction, click on the ICD-10-PCS Tables link.
3. Choose the Medical and Surgical section (0) from the Table of Contents.
4. Click "Gastrointestinal System (Fig. 11.9)."
5. Then click "Excision (Fig. 11.10)."

6. Once you choose "Excision" (0DB) you will link to the table shown in Fig. 11.8 and then build the code for a colonoscopy with biopsy of the cecum, which as noted previously is 0DBN8ZX.

Medical and Surgical

00	Central Nervous System and Cranial Nerves
01	Peripheral Nervous System
02	Heart and Great Vessels
03	Upper Arteries
04	Lower Arteries
05	Upper Veins
06	Lower Veins
07	Lymphatic and Hemic Systems
08	Eye
09	Ear, Nose, Sinus
0B	Respiratory System
0C	Mouth and Throat
0D	Gastrointestinal System
0F	Hepatobiliary System and Pancreas
0G	Endocrine System
0H	Skin and Breast
0J	Subcutaneous Tissue and Fascia
0K	Muscles
0L	Tendons
0M	Bursae and Ligaments
0N	Head and Facial Bones
0P	Upper Bones
0Q	Lower Bones
0R	Upper Joints
0S	Lower Joints
0T	Urinary System
0U	Female Reproductive System
0V	Male Reproductive System
0W	Anatomical Regions, General
0X	Anatomical Regions, Upper Extremities
0Y	Anatomical Regions, Lower Extremities

Figure 11.9 Medical and Surgery Index.

Gastrointestinal System

0D1	Bypass
0D2	Change
0D5	Destruction
0D7	Dilation
0D8	Division
0D9	Drainage
0DB	Excision
0DC	Extirpation
0DD	Extraction
0DF	Fragmentation
0DH	Insertion
0DJ	Inspection
0DL	Occlusion
0DM	Reattachment
0DN	Release
0DP	Removal
0DQ	Repair
0DR	Replacement
0DS	Reposition
0DT	Resection
0DU	Supplement
0DV	Restriction
0DW	Revision
0DX	Transfer
0DY	Transplantation

Figure 11.10 Gastrointestinal Index.

NOTE: To navigate back to the first page of the Code Tables and Index, click "Back to Top" in the upper-right-hand corner of the page.

Example 3

This example uses the Tables section of ICD-10-PCS. We can code a delivery using the Obstetrics section. The scenario is a normal spontaneous delivery of a single newborn.

1. Access the ICD-10-PCS code set from the CMS website as instructed earlier.
2. From the Introduction, choose ICD-10-PCS Tables.
3. Click "Obstetrics" (1).
4. Click "Pregnancy" to access the list shown in Figure 11.11.
5. Choose "10E Delivery." You will link to the table shown in Fig. 11.12. Then build the code for a normal spontaneous delivery, which is coded 10E0XZZ.

Obstetrics

102	Change
109	Drainage
10A	Abortion
10D	Extraction
10E	Delivery
10H	Insertion
10J	Inspection
10P	Removal
10Q	Repair
10S	Reposition
10T	Resection
10Y	Transplantation

Figure 11.11 Medical and Surgery, Obstetrics Index.

10E

Back to Top

Section	1	Obstetrics			
Body System	0	Pregnancy			
Operation	E	Delivery: Assisting the passage of the products of conception from the genital canal			

Body Part	Approach	Device	Qualifier
0 Products of Conception	**X** External	**Z** No Device	**Z** No Qualifier

Figure 11.12 Obstetrics, Delivery.

More Examples

Using the online code set, code the following examples:

1. Open appendectomy (*Hint:* Main term Appendectomy, *see* Resection): 0DTJ0ZZ.
2. Total left hip replacement using a ceramic synthetic substitute prosthesis, without bone cement (*Hint:* Main term Replacement, Hip, Left): 0SRB03A.

3. Mechanical traction of entire right leg (*Hint:* Main term Traction, Extremity, Lower, Right): 2W6LX0Z.

Remember that ICD-10-PCS is for hospital inpatient coding only and replaces Volume 3 of ICD-9. Surgeons are not expected to change their documentation to accommodate the root operation definitions in PCS; rather, the coder must interpret the guidelines and resources combined with physician documentation to accurately assign codes.

Chapter Summary

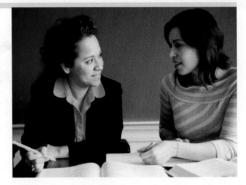

1. ICD-10-PCS is maintained by the CMS. This coding system replaces ICD-9-CM, Volume 3, and is used for hospital inpatient coding of procedures. This code set contains more than 70,000 codes and is updated annually in October.

2. To use ICD-10-PCS accurately and consistently, all health-care providers must follow the national guidelines for its use. ICD-10-PCS guidelines are published in the *ICD-10-PCS Official Guidelines for Coding and Reporting* and the *Reference Manual.* HIPAA legislation mandated their use effective October 1, 2015. The guidelines address basic coding steps, conventions, sequencing, and chapter-specific guidelines. National guidelines provide coders with consistent, comprehensive instructions on the use of ICD-10-PCS.

3. The structure and content of ICD-10-PCS are completely different from ICD-9-CM, Volume 3. All codes are built using a table consisting of columns and rows. All ICD-10-PCS codes must contain seven characters. Each character space has defined values depending on the table.

4. Conventions, or rules of coding, are specific to the use of ICD-10-PCS. For example, one of 34 values is possible for each axis of clarification in a seven-character code. Possible values are the numbers 0 to 9 and letters A to Z, except I and O. Another convention states that the meaning of any single value of a character is dependent on the preceding values in a particular table. It is imperative to understand and apply these conventions in order to assign codes accurately.

5. To delineate the structure of codes in this section, the coder must understand the seven characters represented in a Medical and Surgical procedure code:

Character 1	Medical and Surgical Section (0)
Character 2	Body System
Character 3	Root Operation
Character 4	Body Part
Character 5	Approach
Character 6	Device
Character 7	Qualifier

6. The basic coding process begins with a review of complete medical documentation and abstraction of procedures performed. Each procedure is coded either by identifying the main term representing the intent of the procedure or by direct access to a table. The main term is one word that describes the intent of the procedure, a device, or a body part that the coder uses to find in the Index. For example, the procedure hip replacement requires the coder to look up the main term, Replacement. Indented subterms are used to provide specificity in coding a procedure. Once the first three or four characters of a code have been located in the Index, the remaining characters are assigned using a table. All conventions and instructions must be followed for accuracy in coding.

7. Having the resources to assign ICD-10-PCS codes accurately is essential. Access to national coding guidelines, published coding advice, medical dictionaries, and medical Internet sites and use of encoders are some of the resources coders use to keep current with medical practice, understand medical documentation, and assign accurate codes. The best way to keep up to date on ICD-10-PCS code changes is to use the Internet. The website for ICD-10-PCS resources (www.cms.gov/Medicare/Coding/ICD10/2018-ICD-10-PCS-and-GEMs.html) contains the latest information on ICD-10-PCS codes. This website also includes the crosswalk tool from old codes to new codes, called *GEMs*, and official coding resources.

Review Questions

Matching

Match the key terms with their definitions using the ICD-10-PCS Body Part Key and Device Key. (*Hint:* Access these files from the downloaded PCS code book, page 1, Introduction)

A. Physiomesh (tm) flexible composite mesh
B. stent, intraluminal
C. medical canthus
D. cubital nerve
E. hip joint liner

F. lap-band
G. otic ganglion
H. ischium
I. trifecta valve
J. pinna

1. _____ Intraluminal device

2. _____ Head and neck sympathetic nerves

3. _____ Ulnar nerve

4. _____ Zooplastic tissue in heart and great vessels

5. _____ Liner in lower joints

6. _____ External ear

7. _____ Synthetic substitute

8. _____ Lower eyelid

9. _____ Pelvic bone

10. _____ Extraluminal device

Multiple Choice

Select the letter that best completes the statement or answers the question. Use the ICD-10-PCS online tools when necessary.

1. Which of the following describes the structure of ICD-10-PCS?
   A. Multi-axial
   B. Based on disease process
   C. Limited in expansion capabilities
   D. Allows for use of letters only

2. How many possible values are there for each character in an ICD-10-PCS code?
   A. 16
   B. 36
   C. 26
   D. 34

3. Which of the following is an invalid code?
   A. 06H033T
   B. 06H233Z
   C. 06H003T
   D. 06H14DZ

4. Which of the following is an invalid code?
   A. 3E0F37Z
   B. 3E0F87Z
   C. 3E0F03D
   D. 3E0F3SF

5. Which of the following root operations describes the taking or cutting out of solid matter from a body part?
   A. Drainage
   B. Extirpation
   C. Excision
   D. Removal

6. Posterior lumbar fusion (posterior approach, anterior column) of L2–L4 with insertion of CAGES-style interbody fusion devices and use of morphogenic bone graft would be coded
   A. 0SG00AJ, 0SG00AJ
   B. 0SG10A0
   C. 0SG30AJ
   D. 0SG10AJ

7. Colonoscopy with a biopsy of the sigmoid and cecum would be coded
   A. 0DBG7ZX
   B. 0DBH8ZX, 0DBN8ZX
   C. 0DBH8ZZ, 0DBN8ZZ
   D. 0DBH4ZX, 0DBN4ZZ

8. Percutaneous left renal biopsy followed by open wedge resection of the left kidney would be coded
   A. 0TB13ZZ
   B. 0TB13ZZ, 0TB10ZZ
   C. 0TB10ZZ
   D. 0TB13ZX, 0TB10ZZ

9. Percutaneous endoscopic coronary angioplasty (dilation) of the left anterior descending and left circumflex arteries with insertion of two drug-eluting stents would be coded
   A. 02713DZ
   B. 027245Z
   C. 027145Z
   D. 027044Z, 027044Z

10. Percutaneous needle core biopsy of the left and right breast would be coded
    (*Hint:* See excision, and a biopsy is considered diagnostic.)
    A. 0HBV3ZX
    B. 0HBT3ZX, 0HBU3ZX
    C. 0HBV0ZZ
    D. 0HBV3ZZ

11. Laparoscopic cholecystectomy followed by total open cholecystectomy (converted procedure) would be coded
    A. 0FJ44ZZ
    B. 0FT44ZZ
    C. 0FT44ZZ, 0FJ44ZZ
    D. 0FT40ZZ, 0FJ44ZZ

12. Right ankle joint amputation would be coded
    A. 0Y9K00Z
    B. 0Y6M0Z0
    C. 0Y6M0Z9
    D. 0Y6N0Z0

13. Laser destruction of four warts on the left hand and two warts on the right hand would be coded
    A. 0H5GXZD, 0H5FXZD
    B. 0H5GXZZ, 0H5FXZZ
    C. 0HBGXZX, 0HBFXZX
    D. 0HDGXZZ, 0HDFXZZ

14. Laparoscopy with ablation of endometriosis of the endometrium and endometriosis of bilateral fallopian tubes would be coded
    (*Hint:* Laparoscopy is a percutaneous endoscopic approach)
    A. 0U5B3ZZ, 0U573ZZ
    B. 0U5B4ZZ, 0U574ZZ
    C. 0U558ZZ, 0U68ZZ
    D. 0U5B8ZZ, 0U578ZZ

15. Endoscopic lithotripsy of left and right ureteral calculus would be coded
    A. 0TF38ZZ, 0TF48ZZ
    B. 0TC68ZZ, 0TC78ZZ
    C. 0TF64ZZ, 0TF74ZZ
    D. 0TF68ZZ, 0TF78ZZ

PART III

CPT and HCPCS Coding

CHAPTER 12

CPT Basics

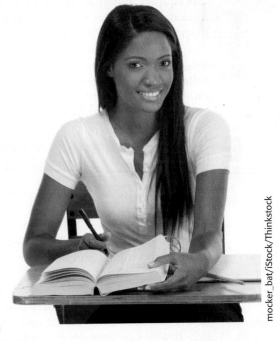

mocker_bat/iStock/Thinkstock

CHAPTER OUTLINE

History and Purpose of CPT

CPT Organization and Content

CPT Punctuation and Symbols

CPT Modifiers

CPT Updates

A Review: ICD-10-CM and CPT Comparison

How to Assign CPT Codes and Modifiers

CPT Coding Resources

LEARNING OUTCOMES

After studying this chapter, you should be able to:

1. Describe several uses of data collected from health-care claims.
2. Explain the purpose of the CPT code set.
3. Identify the medical settings in which CPT is used.
4. Describe the content and organization of CPT.
5. Identify the meaning of the symbols, format, and punctuation used in CPT.
6. Discuss the purpose and use of CPT modifiers—distinguishing among CPT professional, HCPCS, and facility modifiers.
7. Recognize the importance of using current codes and discuss ways to stay current.
8. Compare and contrast the ICD-10-CM and CPT code sets.
9. Recognize when an unlisted code is required and identify the purpose and parts of a special report.
10. Demonstrate various ways of finding a CPT code in the Index.
11. List the nine steps to accurately assign CPT codes and append appropriate modifiers.
12. List CPT coding resources and references.

Procedural coding is a required process performed by both physicians and facilities to receive proper reimbursement for therapeutic and diagnostic services provided. Physicians and facilities use procedure codes to account for outpatient medical, surgical, and diagnostic services provided. To receive reimbursement from payers, these codes, along with ICD-10 diagnosis codes that show why the procedures were medically necessary, are reported on health-care claims.

The United States uses several coding and classification systems to document and report health-care encounters and services. Regardless of the medical setting, accurate coding and adherence to coding guidelines are paramount. The *International Classification of Diseases, Tenth Revision, Clinical Modification* (ICD-10-CM) is used to report diagnoses in all health-care settings. The *International Classification of Diseases, Tenth Revision, Procedure Coding System* (ICD-10-PCS) is used to report inpatient procedures only and is not utilized to report procedures outside the inpatient setting. Physician professional charges, procedures, and services provided to inpatients (patients formally admitted to the hospital) are reported with Current Procedural Terminology (CPT) procedure codes, not ICD-10-PCS. The Healthcare Common Procedure Coding System (HCPCS) is used to report *services* rendered to Medicare and Medicaid recipients and to describe supplies dispensed to patients, regardless of their insurance type. HCPCS is the only coding system available that incorporates codes for supplies, implants, and equipment provided to a patient. This coding system is used to report supplies or equipment provided to any patient, regardless of insurance carrier. HCPCS is discussed in detail in Chapter 30 of this text.

This chapter discusses the CPT coding system and establishes a foundation in CPT coding by introducing the format and organization of the CPT manual and explaining procedural coding fundamentals and guidelines. A thorough understanding of the organization of the CPT code set and of the printed manual in which it appears is the logical starting point. CPT is further discussed in subsequent chapters of this text, where the student will apply concepts learned in this chapter and build on them, adding body system chapter-specific guidelines.

Coders must realize the impact of code assignments. Codes reported, whether accurately or inaccurately, affect data collection, statistics, reimbursement, and ultimately may trigger fraud, waste, and abuse audits. Coders must be made aware that the codes they report have a greater long-term impact than just the immediate payment to the facility or physician. Claims data are collected that affect national coverage determinations, national fee schedule reimbursement rates, physician profiling and contract negotiations, and physician report cards published online. The report cards grade and rank physicians utilizing data collected from claims submitted to carriers for payment.

Various private and government agencies use data collected on diagnosis and procedure codes to establish practice guidelines for the delivery of the best possible care for patients and create payment policies and reimbursement methodologies for different sites of service. Medical researchers track various treatment plans for patients with similar diagnoses; compare variables such as place of service, cause of illness or injury, symptoms, drugs used, and courses of treatments; and evaluate patient outcomes. This process is referred to as *data mining*. Data mining entails taking large volumes of medical and pharmaceutical claims data, loading the data into a database, looking for patterns and trends, and using this information to build data models. This type of analysis requires vast data stores and sophisticated algorithms to detect unknown patterns and identify providers or patients who fall outside of a normal pattern of care. Data analysis has become increasingly important because financial pressures have heightened the need for health-care organizations to make timely decisions based on the analysis of clinical and financial data. For example, data mining can help health-care insurers detect fraud and abuse and assist insurers and physicians in identifying effective medical and surgical treatments and proven overall best practices whereby the patient outcome is best and the health-care services are most affordable. For instance, this type of analysis has shown that a patient who has had a heart attack can reduce the risk of another attack by taking a class of drugs called *beta blockers*. The results are shared with participating physicians and payers so that best practices can be implemented.

One of the key features of data mining is the predictive modeling concept, which allows predictions to be made about whether a specific event will happen. Insights gained from data mining can drive down the costs of medical, surgical, and pharmaceutical supplies and services, increase revenues for both facilities and providers, and improve operating efficiency while maintaining a high level of patient care. As a case in point, several data elements collected on a group of individuals, such as gender, age, weight, body mass index (BMI), hip-to-waist ratio, smoking status, family history of diabetes, and number of exercise events per week, are used to predict the likelihood that an individual will develop diabetes. The predictive model will show how these factors increase the risk of developing the disease. The knowledge gained from this study will result in intervention with high-risk individuals based on this model.

In 2004, Medicare implemented a system to track patients enrolled in Medicare HMO (Advantage) plans and measure the severity of their illnesses. This system, the Hierarchical Condition Categories (HCC) model, measures the disease burden of a Medicare Advantage plan to adjust capitation payments to these private health-care plans for the health expenditure (the cost) risk of their enrollees. In simple terms, the sicker the patient base, the more money Medicare compensates the health plan. It all boils down to the data collection process and correct coding and reporting of all diagnoses and procedures, which always points back to the physician's office and the medical record documentation. The important point here is that coding influences decisions made at the national and international levels.

In health-care practices, physicians, medical coders, or outside billing companies assign diagnosis, procedure, and supply codes. Some practices employ coders who also perform the billing function using many titles: medical billing specialist, certified coder, or insurance specialists, to name a few. Most medical offices share the coding function; physicians and/or coding staff assign procedure codes and the coding or billing staff assign diagnosis codes. The office router or encounter form commonly lists frequently used diagnosis and procedure codes for ease of reporting; however, these lists are not exhaustive and often are not updated in a timely manner with code changes. A coder in this setting likely assigns modifiers, in addition to diagnoses to support medical necessity and checks for code accuracy (i.e., missing digits). In facilities, the Health Information Management (HIM) department (also called the *Medical Record Department*) employs coders who specialize in inpatient and outpatient medical and surgical facility coding and perform all aspects of the coding function for the facility.

HISTORY AND PURPOSE OF CPT

CPT is a coding nomenclature or catalog system that allows descriptions of medical procedures to be translated from words to numbers. The CPT code set is based on the various types of professional services performed by physicians and other health-care professionals such as physician's assistants; nurses; physical, occupational, and speech therapists; chiropractors; and dietitians. CPT codes cover thousands of professional services, from office visits to surgery, radiology, laboratory and pathology, anesthesiology, and other medical procedures.

CPT Background

CPT was developed in 1966 and is currently maintained by the American Medical Association (AMA). According to the AMA, "the purpose of a CPT coding system is to provide a uniform language that accurately describes medical, surgical, and diagnostic services and provides a means for reliable nationwide communication among physicians, patients, and insurance carriers." CPT was first widely used in 1983 when the Centers for Medicare and Medicaid Services (CMS; then called HCFA, or Health Care Financing Administration) decided to require it for Medicare and Medicaid claims.

Medicare developed an Outpatient Prospective Payment System (OPPS) to reimburse facilities for emergency department and outpatient facility visits. In August 2000, as part of the Medicare OPPS, ambulatory payment classifications (APCs) were imposed that require facilities to report CPT codes for services rendered in outpatient departments to reflect the volume and intensity of resources utilized by the facility in providing patient care. Up until this point, CPT codes were used for professional services only. Now they are used in all outpatient settings by doctors and hospitals to report services, but never by facilities to report facility charges for *inpatient* services.

INTERNET RESOURCE: AMA
www.ama-assn.org

CMS next combined CPT with HCPCS (pronounced "hick-picks")—commonly referred to as *supply codes*—to make a multilevel coding system for reporting services, procedures, and supplies to Medicare, Medicaid, and other government insurance beneficiaries. Now, under the Health Insurance Portability and Accountability Act (HIPAA), these codes may be reported to all payers for drugs, supplies, implants, and services. HCPCS coding is discussed in detail in Chapter 30 of this text.

• CPT is the mandated code set for physician procedures under HIPAA.
• HCPCS is the mandated code set for supplies under HIPAA.

HCPCS Level I is the CPT code set printed in the AMA's CPT manual. HCPCS Level II codes are maintained by the federal government and are printed in commercial printers' HCPCS books. Level II codes are used to report supplies, drugs, and some services that are not in CPT. Officially, then, CPT is the first part of HCPCS, and the supply/drug/equipment codes and codes for other services are the second part. Most people, though, refer to the codes in the CPT manual as *CPT codes* and the Level II codes as *HCPCS codes*.

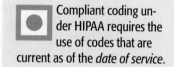
Compliant coding under HIPAA requires the use of codes that are current as of the *date of service*.

CPT Today

CPT codes provide a way to precisely report procedures performed without sending lengthy operative reports or written descriptions to payers. Health-care claims are usually sent electronically and processed for payment decisions. The use of CPT codes reduces the need for a payer to manually process claims, thus increasing administrative efficiency. For this reason, the U.S. Department of Health and Human Services designated CPT as the nationally accepted HIPAA standard code set for physician and other health-care professional services.

The information represented by CPT codes is used for many purposes, including:

- Reimbursing physicians' professional services at all types of locations (office, inpatient, nursing home) and for outpatient facility services
- Trending services provided to patients nationally
- Future planning from many perspectives, such as budgeting, policy development, and resource allocation by payers, providers, and the government
- Benchmarking against similar facilities, practices, and geographic locations on cost of providing services, availability of services, and the like
- Measuring patient outcomes and quality of care by providers nationwide

To be included in the CPT code set, a procedure or service must meet the following conditions:

- It must be commonly performed by many physicians across the country.
- It must be consistent with mainstream medical practice.
- It must be approved by the AMA CPT Editorial Panel. The panel is made up of physicians and representatives from several organizations, such as CMS, the American Health Information Management Association (AHIMA), and the American Hospital Association (AHA). Panel members decide whether to implement additions, deletions, or changes submitted by payers, medical associations, and physicians. The AMA CPT Advisory Committee consists of individuals chosen by their peers (nominated) to represent each clinical specialty. Their responsibility is to answer questions from the editorial panel about a code and/or revisions to a code. They serve as the technical and specialty experts working in the field.

CPT ORGANIZATION AND CONTENT

The printed CPT code set in the CPT manual is arranged, with the exception of the Evaluation and Management (E/M) section, in numerical order. As shown in Box 12.1, the manual begins with an introduction followed by six sections of Category I codes, which are the major part of the manual; one section each of Category II and Category III codes; and the appendices. The Index, located at the back of the CPT manual, lists terms and abbreviations in alphabetical order.

The CPT Code

Each CPT code is a unique code followed by a descriptor of the service. There are more than 8,000 CPT codes, and no two are the same. At times one descriptor may be very close in wording to another, but there are always clear differences in definitions, so each code descriptor must be read in its entirety. One word or a punctuation mark can change the meaning of the entire code.

As you read the following description of the CPT sections, look at the sample CPT entries provided in Figure 12.1. Every CPT code is five digits long. Symbols and notes in parentheses, called *parenthetical notes,* are instructions for the coder to follow when assigning codes from the manual. References are made under particular codes to provide resources to read before proceeding with code assignment. The meanings of the symbols are discussed later in this chapter.

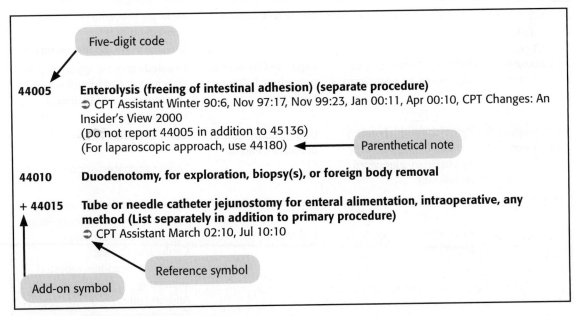

Figure 12.1 Example of CPT codes in the CPT manual.

The CPT *Introduction*

The introductory information at the beginning of CPT provides insights and rules used in the CPT code set. It also gives instructions on using the CPT manual, explanations of key terms, editorial notations, and information on tapes and disks available as resources. This information should be read carefully, because it supplies useful background.

Category I Codes: Six Sections

Category I codes are permanent CPT codes. There are six sections of Category I codes in the CPT manual: Evaluation and Management (E/M), Anesthesia, Surgery, Radiology, Pathology and Laboratory, and Medicine. Each of these sections has its own section guidelines that appear in the beginning with definitions of terms, explanation of notes that appear around codes, and other related information. Each section also has subheadings and subsections with special instructions throughout. For example, at the end of each subsection there is a code called an *unlisted code* that can be used when there is no CPT code to reflect the exact procedure performed. See Table 12.1 for an overview of these six sections.

Table 12.1 CPT Category I Code Sections

SECTION	DEFINITION OF CODES	STRUCTURE	KEY GUIDELINES
Evaluation and Management	Physician or other qualified health-care professional services that are performed to determine the best course for patient care	Organized by place and/or type of service	New/established patients; other definitions Unlisted services, special reports Selecting an E/M service level
Anesthesia	Anesthesia services by or supervised by a physician; includes general, regional, and local anesthesia	Organized by body site	Time based Services covered (bundled) in codes Unlisted services; special reports Qualifying circumstances codes
Surgery	Surgical procedures performed by physicians	Organized by body system and then body site, followed by procedural groups	Surgical package definition Follow-up care definition Add-on codes Separate procedures Subsection notes Unlisted services; special reports
Radiology	Radiology services by or supervised by a physician	Organized by type of procedure, followed by body site	Unlisted services; special reports Supervision and interpretation (professional and technical components)
Pathology and Laboratory	Pathology and laboratory services by physicians or by physician-supervised technicians	Organized by type of procedure Panels	Complete procedure Unlisted services; special reports
Medicine	Evaluation, therapeutic, and diagnostic procedures by or supervised by a physician	Organized by type of service or procedure and specialty	Subsection notes (Vaccines, Psychotherapy, End-Stage Renal Disease, Ophthalmology, Cardiovascular, etc.) Multiple procedures reported separately Add-on codes Separate procedures Unlisted services; special reports Supplied materials

Evaluation and Management Section

The codes in the Evaluation and Management (E/M) section cover physician and other qualified health-care provider services that are performed to determine the best course for patient care. Although the numbers are out of order—ranging from 99201 through 99499—the E/M codes are listed first in CPT because they are used so often by all types of physicians and midlevel qualified health-care providers. Often called the *cognitive* codes, the E/M codes cover the complex process a physician or qualified health-care provider uses to gather and analyze information about a patient's illness and to make decisions about the patient's condition and the best treatment or course of management. If services other than the physician or qualified health-care provider exam and interview are performed, they may be reported separately by utilizing a code from another section of the CPT manual. Codes for the actual treatment or diagnostic test—such as surgical procedures, labwork, and vaccines—are covered in the CPT sections that follow the E/M codes, such as the Surgery, Pathology and Laboratory, and Medicine sections. E/M coding is discussed in Chapters 13 and 14 of this text.

Anesthesia Section

The codes in the Anesthesia section are used to report anesthesia services performed by a physician or certified registered nurse anesthetist (CRNA), or anesthesia services supervised by a physician. These services include general and regional anesthesia and supplementation of local anesthesia. Each anesthesia code includes the complete usual services of an anesthesiologist:

- Usual preoperative visits for evaluation and planning
- Care during the procedure, such as administering fluid or blood, placing monitoring devices or IV lines, laryngoscopy, interpreting lab data, and nerve stimulation
- Routine postoperative care

Anesthesia codes are covered in Chapter 15 of this text.

Surgery Section

The Surgery section is divided into each of the body systems (Integumentary, Musculoskeletal, Respiratory, Cardiovascular, Digestive, Urinary, Male/Female, Nervous, Eye/Ocular Adnexa, and Auditory). Surgery section codes are used for the many hundreds of surgical procedures performed by physicians or qualified health-care providers. This is the largest procedure code section, with codes ranging from 10021 to 69990. The Surgery section has codes for significant procedures, such as incision, excision, repair, manipulation, amputation, endoscopy, destruction, suturing, and introductions.

In each body system subsection, codes are grouped to make locating them easier, such as under related anatomical, procedural, condition, or descriptor subheadings (Box 12.2). The AMA tries to maintain the same order in each of the body system subsections to promote consistency. Headings are arranged from head to toe and from least invasive to most invasive; for example, moving from incision, excision, introduction, removal of foreign body, and repair to destruction.

> **BOX 12.2 Example of Subsection Format in the Surgery Section**
>
> **Section:** Surgery
> **Subsection/Category:** Musculoskeletal
> **Subcategory:** Leg and Ankle Joint
> **Heading:** Incision
> **Procedure:** Incision and drainage, leg or ankle; deep abscess or hematoma

Surgical Package. In the Surgery section, the grouping of related work under a single procedure code is called a surgical package. The surgical code includes all the usual services in addition to the operation itself:

> CPT includes procedures that carry the name of the person who developed the particular surgical approach or service, such as a McBride bunionectomy.

- After the decision for surgery, one related E/M encounter on the day before or on the day of the procedure
- The operation: preparing the patient for surgery, including injection of anesthesia by the surgeon (local infiltration, metacarpal/metatarsal/digital block, or topical anesthesia), and performing the operation, including normal additional procedures, such as debridement (cleansing of a wound)
- Immediate postoperative care, including dictating operative notes and talking with the family and other physicians

- Writing orders
- Evaluating the patient in the postanesthesia recovery area
- Typical postoperative follow-up care

EXAMPLE

Procedural statement: Procedure conducted 2 weeks ago in office to correct hallux valgus (bunion) on left foot; local nerve block administered, correction by simple exostectomy. Saw patient in office today for routine follow-up; complete healing.

Code: 99024 Postoperative follow-up visit.
Code: 28292 was reported 2 weeks ago when the surgery was performed.

The surgical package is a payment concept; payers assign a fee to a surgical package code that reimburses all the services provided under it for a specified period of time called the *postoperative period* or *global period*. Visits relating to the surgery are not paid in addition to the fee for the surgical package. Typically, the postoperative period is 10 days for minor procedures and 90 days for major surgery.

Postoperative Days

Postoperative days or global days are assigned to codes based on whether the procedures are major or minor in surgical nature. Major surgery is classified as such because of the complexity of the operation, inherent surgical risks, and postoperative recovery time. This type of surgery is conducted in an operating room and involves general anesthesia, opening into the great cavities of the body, severe hemorrhage risk, and/or requires special anatomical knowledge and manipulative skills. Minor surgeries typically require local or conscious sedation, do not require respiratory assistance, and involve minimal postoperative recovery time. The Medicare Physician Fee Schedule located on the CMS website (www.cms.gov/ under *Medicare Fee-for-Service Payment, Physician Fee Schedule, then PFS Relative Value Files*) includes a Global Days column to indicate whether the procedure is a 10-day or 90-day procedure.

Services Not Included

Two types of services are not included in surgical package codes. These services are billed separately and are reimbursed in addition to the surgical package fee:

1. Complications or recurrences that arise after therapeutic surgical procedures
2. Care for the condition for which a diagnostic surgical procedure is performed. Routine follow-up care included in the code refers only to care related to recovery from the diagnostic procedure itself, not the condition. For example, a diagnostic colonoscopy was performed to examine a growth in the patient's colon. An office visit after the surgery to evaluate the patient for chemotherapy because the tumor is cancerous is billed separately; it is not included as a postoperative visit.

Separate Procedures. In some cases, the phrase *separate procedure* follows a code descriptor. If a procedure is labeled a separate procedure, CPT explains that it can be reported if it was performed alone, for a specific purpose, and independent of any other related service provided. If it is performed as a component part of a larger procedure, it is not billed separately. For example, for an exploratory laparotomy (code 49000) with repair of the inferior mesenteric artery (code 35221), only 35221 would be reported, because 49000 is a designated separate procedure.

Radiology Section

The codes in the Radiology section are used to report radiological services performed by or supervised by a physician. Radiology codes follow the same types of guidelines noted in the Surgery section. For example, some radiology codes are identified as separate procedure codes. These codes are usually part of a larger, more complex procedure and should not be reported as separate codes unless the procedure was done independently.

Most radiology services are performed and billed by radiologists working in hospital or clinic settings. Most medical practices do not have radiology equipment and instead refer patients to these specialists. In many cases, the radiologist performs both the technical (capturing the image) and the professional (interpreting the image) components. Codes are selected based on body part and the number and type of views. Radiology, pathology and laboratory, and medicine codes are covered in Chapters 27, 28, and 29, respectively, of this text.

Pathology and Laboratory Sections

The codes in the Pathology and Laboratory sections cover services provided by physicians or by technicians under the supervision of physicians. A complete procedure includes:

- Ordering the test
- Taking and handling the sample
- Performing the actual test
- Analyzing and reporting on the test results

Medicine Section

The Medicine section contains codes for the many types of evaluation, therapeutic, and diagnostic procedures that physicians and other health-care professionals perform. (Codes for the Evaluation and Management section described earlier in the chapter, 99201 to 99499, actually fall at the end of this section numerically, but the AMA puts them in the first section of CPT because they are the most frequently used codes.) They include procedures and services provided by family practice physicians or other qualified health-care professionals, such as immunizations, therapeutic injections, wound care management, and medication therapy management services. The services of many specialists, such as allergists, cardiologists, physical therapists, neurologists, ophthalmologists, and psychiatrists, are also covered in the Medicine section. Some Medicine section codes are for services used to support diagnosis and treatment, such as rehabilitation, occupational therapy, and nutrition therapy, whereas others are strictly diagnostic tests, such as neuromuscular testing and EKGs/EEGs.

CHECKPOINT 12.1

Locate each term in the CPT Index, and then indicate which type of term it is—an abbreviation, an anatomical site, an eponym, or a procedure. Record the codes that are listed for it. The first one is completed as an example.

1. Epstein-Barr virus	Eponym	86663–86665
2. Evisceration	_____	_____
3. ETOH	_____	_____
4. Nasolacrimal duct	_____	_____
5. Myringotomy	_____	_____
6. Tetralogy of Fallot	_____	_____

Category II Codes

Category II codes were created by the AMA to track physician or other qualified health-care professional performance in measuring and monitoring patient care. The codes were created to facilitate collection and reporting of data on evidence-based performance measures at the time of service, rather than as a result of a labor-intensive retrospective chart review. These alpha numeric codes (four digits and one alpha character) capture services such as prenatal care, smoking cessation counseling, and tracking of chronic conditions. These codes typically describe services that are included in an E/M service; therefore, the Category II codes do not have relative value units (RVUs). These types of services, while not directly billable, improve the quality of care and treatment of patients. For example, a number of services are related to watching for problems due to a patient's diabetes mellitus or coronary artery disease (CAD). The use of the Category II codes is expected to decrease the time spent abstracting a record and to decrease the time spent by physicians and other qualified health-care professionals on chart review to confirm that the measures were performed. For example, if you are tracking hemoglobin A1C levels in patients with diabetes in a practice, reporting code 3044F,

Most recent hemoglobin A1C (HbA1C) level less than 7.0% (DM)[2,4], or 3046F, Most recent hemoglobin A1C level greater than 9.0% (DM)[4], in addition to the E/M code, will allow you to do this through coding and report generation rather than through chart review. Category II codes are a quick way to note that these important services were done; they take the place of a lengthy documentation process. An appendix to CPT describes the meanings of the codes.

EXAMPLE
2001F *Weight recorded (PAG)[1].*

NOTE: You may be wondering what the superscript numbers that follow the Category II code descriptions are. These correspond to the listing in the front matter of the Category II code introduction and reference the entity that developed the code.

These codes are optional—that is, they are not required for correct coding. They are not directly reimbursed, but if the insurance carrier has pay-for-performance (P4P) measures that reward physicians or other qualified health-care professionals for providing such care, they can be integral to receiving a higher level of payment under insurance participation contracts. Providers are compensated or rewarded for specific performance results rather than simply for time worked or key components documented. Health-care P4P programs reward hospitals, physician practices, and other providers with financial and nonfinancial incentives based on performance on select measures. These performance measures can cover various aspects of health-care delivery: clinical excellence and improved safety, efficiency, patient experience, and health information technology (HIT) adoption. Sponsors of P4P programs typically include government agencies and health insurance plans.

Category II codes are released annually with the general CPT code set and published twice a year, January 1 and July 1, on the AMA website.

> The most current listing, along with guidelines and forms for submitting code change proposals for Category II codes, is at www.ama-assn.org/go/CPT.

Category III Codes

Category III codes were introduced in CPT in 2002. These alphanumeric codes (four digits and a *T*) are located immediately after the Category II codes and before the appendices. They are used to report emerging technologies, services, and procedures that do not have CPT codes assigned.

These codes allow researchers to track emerging technology services. To be assigned a Category III code, CPT does not require that the new procedure must be Food and Drug Administration (FDA) approved and performed by many health-care professionals in clinical practice in multiple locations as it does with Category I codes. If a Category III code is being widely used, the AMA may advance it to the permanent CPT Category I level. In this case, CPT will contain a cross-reference pointing to the location of the advanced code.

Category III codes are added by the AMA twice a year and are published on the AMA's website. If a Category III code has not been used after 5 years, it will be archived.

> Not all payers accept these codes. Before submitting a Category III code, check with the payer. If the payer does not accept these codes, report the appropriate unlisted procedure code instead. Category III codes are at www.ama-assn.org/go/CPT.

EXAMPLE
0184T *Excision of rectal tumor, transanal endoscopic microsurgical approach (i.e., TEMS), including muscularis propria (i.e., full thickness).*

Appendices

Appendices, located after the Category III codes, supply important information that can answer many coding questions.

The appendices include the following:

> Become familiar with the appendices, which can assist you in all CPT coding situations.

- *Appendix A—Modifiers:* A listing of modifiers (defined later in this chapter) with descriptions and, in some cases, examples of usage.
- *Appendix B—Summary of Additions, Deletions, and Revisions:* A summary of the codes added, revised, and deleted in the current version.

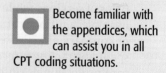

It is a useful list of changes from the prior year's book. This appendix and Appendix M are helpful quick references when updating office computer systems and billing forms.

- *Appendix C—Clinical Examples:* Case examples of the proper use of the codes in the Evaluation and Management section. This is a tool to help coders and physicians or other qualified health-care professionals gauge E/M code level assignment by comparing their current coding situation with similar circumstances and levels.
- *Appendix D—Summary of CPT Add-on Codes:* Supplemental codes for procedures that are commonly done in addition to the primary procedure. These codes are also located throughout the CPT manual (indicated by the + symbol). Offices can use this tool to flag add-on codes in their computer to ensure they will not be reported alone or listed first on claims.
- *Appendix E—Summary of CPT Codes Exempt From Modifier 51:* Codes to which the modifier showing multiple procedures cannot be attached because they already include a multiple descriptor. These appear in the CPT manual (indicated by the ⊘ symbol). Offices can use this appendix to flag these codes in their computer to alert staff that a modifier is not appropriate.
- *Appendix F—Summary of CPT Codes Exempt From Modifier 63:* This appendix is helpful to specialists who perform surgery on infants. These surgery codes are located throughout the CPT codebook and have parenthetical notes beneath them warning not to assign the –63 modifier to the code.
- *Appendix J—Electrodiagnostic Medicine Listing of Sensory, Motor, and Mixed Nerves:* This appendix is referenced when coding nerve conduction studies from the Medicine section.
- *Appendix K—Product Pending FDA Approval:* Denoted by the ⫲ symbol in the Medicine section.
- *Appendix L—Vascular Families:* This appendix is helpful for coding interventional radiology procedures and catheterizations.
- *Appendix M—Renumbered CPT Codes Citation Crosswalk:* Provides a crosswalk (a comparison) between deleted codes and the correct codes that replaced them for the years 2007–2009 only.
- *Appendix N—Summary of Resequenced CPT Codes:* This appendix is helpful when a coder cannot find a routinely used code in the same location as in a previous edition of the CPT manual. The resequenced code is not "renumbered" and the code definitions are not modified, but rather the code is placed in a more appropriate location. Resequenced codes are indicated with a # symbol.
- *Appendix O—Multianalyte Assays With Algorithmic Analyses (MAAA):* This section of CPT codes contains new administrative and Category I codes describing MAAA procedures to aid in accurate reporting of these services. MAAAs are complex and advanced genetic laboratory tests used to identify patients predisposed to a given disease, diagnose whether a patient has a specific disease, determine/define the severity of a disease, and quantify the effectiveness of a particular method of therapy.
- *Appendix P-CPT Codes That May Be Used for Synchronous Telemedicine Services:* The listed CPT codes may be used for reporting synchronous or real-time telemedicine services when modifier –95 is reported with the CPT code. Telemedicine services involve electronic communication using interactive telecommunications equipment, at a minimum, audio and video. These codes are identified by the ★ symbol.

CHECKPOINT 12.2

List the name of the CPT section in which each of the following codes is located.

1. 99212 _____

2. 90389 _____

3. 75630 _____

4. 00820 _____

5. 80055 _____

6. 0071T _____

7. 35180 _____

8. 4000F _____

CPT PUNCTUATION AND SYMBOLS

Several coding symbols and characters are used to direct the coder. It is extremely important to understand what each of the symbols means. The characters are located inside the front cover of the CPT book as well as along the bottom of each two-page layout.

Semicolon (;)

The semicolon (;) is used in CPT to conserve space and to divide the common portion of a code descriptor from the unique portion. It is a way of sorting a long list of procedures that are related. Use of the semicolon avoids repeating the entire code description for each of a related group of codes. The common portion or the main entry (the *root code*) is separated by a semicolon (;) from a unique portion that is indented to make it easier to see. This format indicates that the main entry applies to, and is part of, all indented entry codes that follow.

The semicolon in CPT reads like the word "and." Code descriptions should be read carefully, noting where the semicolon is placed. Both the common portion (before the semicolon) and the descriptor after the semicolon are needed for a complete code description.

EXAMPLES

33533	*Coronary artery bypass, using arterial graft(s); single arterial graft.*
33534	*Two coronary arterial grafts.*

The common portion of CPT code 33533, "Coronary artery bypass, using arterial graft(s);" should be considered part of CPT code 33534. The unique portion is "two coronary arterial grafts." Therefore, the full procedure represented by code 33534 is read as "33534 Coronary artery bypass, using arterial graft(s); two coronary arterial grafts."

> ● If an indented code is selected, only that code must be assigned, not the root code too.

As a general rule, the farther down an indented listing a code is, the more complex it is. At times, more than one code from the related group is reported; most often, however, just one appropriate code is selected.

Bullet (•)

The bullet (•) designates a new code for that year. The bullet is in front of the code. Bullets appear for 1 year only, because they denote new procedures for that year.

Triangle (▲)

The triangle (▲) signifies a revised code, meaning that the descriptor is revised in some way. Some changes may seem small, but the impact on reimbursement may be significant. Approximately 7% of the CPT book changes from year to year. Appendix B lists these changed codes. Like bullets, triangles appear in the current year's CPT manual only, because they denote that the procedure before which they appear has been revised or changed in some way for the new volume of CPT.

Plus Symbol (+)

The plus symbol (+) identifies an add-on code. Add-on codes are considered "additional" codes for procedures carried out along with a primary procedure. The primary procedure is the main procedure performed. It is the most comprehensive, complex in nature, and resource-intensive procedure and is listed first, before all other procedures. Secondary procedures are less extensive or resource intensive and are listed in addition to the primary procedure.

Add-on codes are considered secondary procedures. They cannot be reported alone and must be used with the related base code. Appendix D lists all add-on codes in CPT. Add-on codes often are described with phrases in the code description such as "each additional" or "(List separately in addition to code for primary procedure)." In Figure 12.1, 44010 is the primary procedure and 44015 is the add-on code, as indicated by the plus symbol in front of the code.

EXAMPLES

11200   *Removal of skin tags, multiple fibrocutaneous tags, any area, up to and including 15 lesions.*

+ 11201   *Each additional ten lesions or part thereof. (List separately in addition to code for primary procedure.)*

In parentheses under code 11201, CPT states to use 11201 in conjunction with 11200. Based on this instruction, if more than 15 skin tags were removed, two codes must be reported, 11200 and 11201, in that order. Note the use of "or part thereof" in the description for +11201.

Modifier −51 Exempt (⊘)

The symbol ⊘ indicates that a code cannot be assigned a −51 modifier (modifiers are described later in this chapter). They do not fall under the same payment scheme as other codes that do allow the modifier, meaning these services will be reimbursed at 100% of the allowed or negotiated rate and not receive a multiple procedure reduction. Appendix E lists these in their entirety.

EXAMPLE

⊘ 31500   *Intubation, endotracheal, emergency procedure.*

Facing Triangles (▶◀)

The facing triangle symbol (▶◀) in front of a code indicates that text is new or has been revised from the prior year's edition. The triangles mark the beginning and ending of the new and/or revised text in the guidelines and instruction notes. Many cross-references and additional instructions are located within these symbols. Coders should read this information to ensure proper code assignment.

Lightning Bolt (⚡)

The lightning bolt symbol (⚡) signifies that the code is for a vaccine that is pending FDA approval; all codes with this symbol are located in the Medicine section. Coders cannot report a code that has the symbol. When a vaccine is approved, the symbol is removed from the CPT code listing.

INTERNET RESOURCE: Category I Vaccine Code Updates
www.ama-assn.org/ama/pub/physician-resources/
solutions-managing-your-practice/coding-billing-insurance/
cpt/about-cpt/category-i-vaccine-codes.page

Stay up to date on approval status for vaccine codes with the lightning symbol. These codes are prereleased every 6 months on the AMA website and can be used as soon as they appear.

Pound Sign (#)

The pound sign (#) preceding a code signifies that it has been moved from another section of the CPT manual or resequenced, or a new code has been added and there are no available numbers in that sequence of codes. The existing code is not deleted or renumbered; it is moved to a section of CPT that is more appropriate based on the code's description.

An entry where this code was previously housed directs the coder to the new location.

EXAMPLES

21555 *Excision, tumor, soft tissue of neck or anterior thorax, subcutaneous; less than 3 cm*
21552 *3 cm or greater*
21556 *Excision, tumor, soft tissue of neck or anterior thorax, subfascial; less than 5 cm*

CPT and Professional Fees

Physicians and other qualified health-care professionals bill their services based on fee schedules covering their commonly performed services. For example, in physician practices, physicians establish a list of their usual fees for the CPT codes they frequently perform. The usual fees on the physician's fee schedule are defined as those that they charge to most of their patients most of the time under typical conditions. The typical ranges of physicians' fees nationwide are published in commercial databases, and can be analyzed by physicians and practice managers.

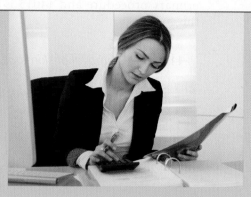

If a physician or other qualified health-care professional bills and is paid the full amount on the fee schedule, this is called a *fee-for-service* payment. Payers, however, do not necessarily pay physicians or other qualified health-care professionals based on the physician's usual fee. Private payers and government payers alike usually negotiate some kind of payment schedule that reduces these amounts. The following are examples of this:

- If the payer is a *health maintenance organization (HMO)*, it may pay the physician a salary, or it may pay on a *capitation* basis. The HMO creates a network of physicians, hospitals, and other providers by employing or negotiating contracts with them. Capitation (from *capit*, Latin for *head*) is a fixed prepayment to a medical provider for all necessary contracted services provided to each patient who is a plan member. The capitated rate, which is called *per member per month*, is a prospective payment—it is paid *before* the patient visit. It covers a specific period of time. The health plan makes the payment whether the patient receives many or no medical services during that specified period. The capitated rate of prepayment, however, covers only services listed on the schedule of benefits for the plan. The provider may bill the patient for any other services.

Star Symbol (★)

The star symbol (★) preceding a code indicates that the code may be reported for telemedicine services when the –95 modifier is reported with the code.

CPT Assistant or *CPT Changes: An Insider's View*

The ➜ symbol appears only in the professional editions of CPT books below the code description. It means that the coder may refer to a specific issue of *CPT Assistant* or *CPT Changes: An Insider's View* for guidance on the code use.

CPT Assistant is designated under HIPAA as required guidance for the use of CPT codes and is published monthly by the AMA. *CPT Changes: An Insider's View* is published annually by the AMA as a tool for understanding changes made to CPT from the previous year.

EXAMPLE

95060 *Ophthalmic mucous membrane tests.*

➜*CPT Assistant Summer 91:16, Jan 13:9.*

- If the payer is another type of health plan called a *preferred provider organization (PPO)*, it usually pays physicians discounted fees under a contract. Physicians, other qualified health-care professionals, hospitals and clinics, and pharmacies contract with the PPO plan to provide care to its insured clients. These medical providers accept the PPO plan's fee schedule and guidelines for its managed medical care. PPOs generally pay participating providers based on a discount from their physician fee schedules, called a *discounted fee-for-service* payment.
- The major government health plan, Medicare, pays most of its participating providers—those who agree to accept its fees in exchange for the benefit of acquiring Medicare beneficiaries as patients—on the basis of a resource-based relative value scale (RBRVS), which is a way of assigning a relative weight to each procedure in a group of related CPT codes that can be converted to a fee. There are three parts to an RBRVS fee:

  1. *The nationally uniform RVU:* The relative value is based on three cost elements—the physician or other qualified health-care professional's work, the practice cost (overhead), and the cost of malpractice insurance.
  2. *A geographic adjustment factor:* A geographic adjustment factor is a number that is used to multiply each relative value element so that it better reflects a geographical area's relative costs.
  3. *A nationally uniform conversion factor:* A uniform conversion factor is a dollar amount used to multiply the relative values to produce a payment amount. It is used by Medicare to make adjustments according to changes in the cost-of-living index.

- Workers' compensation patients often must be charged according to a state-mandated fee schedule.

Whatever payment method is applied, coders assist physicians and other outpatient providers by correctly assigning CPT codes that accurately reflect the services that were provided. Assignment of correct ICD-10-CM codes, of course, is also essential to demonstrate the medical necessity of the procedures.

CHECKPOINT 12.3

Answer the following questions.

1. What is the common portion of code 46760? _____

2. What is the unique portion of code 46942? _____

3. What is the complete code description of 54326? _____

4. If a diagnostic flexible colonoscopy is performed in a physician's endoscopy suite and the physician supplies the IV sedation, is it appropriate to report both code 45378 and code 99152?

_____

5. In the CPT manual you are using, identify three new codes (indicated by a bullet), three revised codes (indicated with a triangle), and three codes with new or revised text (indicated by facing triangles). _____

CPT MODIFIERS

Modifiers are two-digit characters that may be appended to (added to the end of) most CPT codes. Modifiers are used to communicate special circumstances involved with services, telling the payer that the physician or other qualified health-care professional considers the service noted in the code's descriptor to have been changed in some way, but not enough to assign a different CPT code.

Modifier use is described in each of the six major section's guidelines. Some modifiers are associated with a particular medical specialty, such as coding for a physician office, surgical practice, facility, or anesthesia practice. A modifier often increases or decreases the normal payment for the code to which it is attached. For example, the modifier –76, repeat procedure by same physician, is used when the reporting physician repeats a procedure or service after doing the first one. Modifiers are appended to the CPT code by adding a hyphen.

> **EXAMPLE**
> Procedural statement: Physician performed chest x-rays before placing a chest tube and then, after the chest tube was placed, performed a second set of x-rays to verify its position.
>
> 71046–76　　　*Radiologic examination, chest, two views, frontal and lateral; repeat procedure or service by same physician.*

In this example, because an additional x-ray was required, the modifier tells the payer that code 71046 is not a duplicate error, it represents a second, repeat service.

If CPT codes are verbs (such as *examine*, *evaluate*, and *operate*), modifiers can be thought of as adverbs. They further describe an action taken or service provided and the circumstances surrounding that service. Below is a partial list of the uses for the modifiers:

- That a procedure was performed bilaterally (−50)
- That more than one procedure was performed at the same time (−51)
- That a service was performed by more than one physician (e.g., an assistant surgeon participated) or in more than one location (−81, −59)
- That a service or procedure was increased or decreased (−22, −52)
- That only part of a service was performed (−52)
- That unusual events occurred during a procedure or service (−22)
- That a service has two parts or components—a technical component and a professional component (−TC, −26)
- The physical status of a patient for anesthesia administration (P1−P5)

Types of Modifiers

Three basic types of modifiers are used with CPT codes:

1. *CPT modifiers* for professional services
2. *Level I (facility) modifiers* approved for hospital outpatient use
3. *Level II (HCPCS/national) modifiers* (Not all HCPCS modifiers are applicable for use with CPT codes.)

These three types, including the special physical status modifiers that are used only with anesthesia codes and performance measurement modifiers, are described here.

CPT Modifiers

Thirty-one CPT modifiers are approved for use with CPT codes reported for physician or other qualified health-care professional services and procedures. Modifiers are listed on the inside front cover of the CPT manual in the left column. Table 12.2 provides an overview of all modifiers.

Table 12.2 Modifiers: Description and Common Use in Main Text Sections

Modifier Quick Reference Guide

LEGEND

[icon] = Bundling/CCI related

[icon] = Global package

[icon] = Physician E/M code

= Number of surgeons

[icon] = Anesthesia codes

[icon] = Lab

[icon] = Facility-only modifier

[icon] = Special report needed

[icon] = Procedure modifier

[icon] = Radiology

MD = Physician or other qualified health-care professional–only modifier

FINANCIAL IMPACT OF MODIFIER USE

[scissors] = Reimbursement increases.

[icon] = Reimbursement decreases.

[icon] = Required to get claim paid. No change in reimbursement.

[icon] = No change. Explanation only.

DIRECTIONS FOR USE

Find the modifier you are considering assigning. Check to see whether the modifier is appropriate to use in your setting. Also check to see whether the modifier can be appended to the code you are submitting by referencing the symbols on the left.

Modifiers that affect payment are sequenced first.

Modifier	Description	[$]	MD Only	E/M	Anesthesia Provider	Procedure	Radiology	Path/Lab	Global Package	Facility
–22	Increases procedural services	[scissors]	MD	[special report]	[special report]	[scissors][special report]	[radiology][special report]	[lab]		
–23	Unusual anesthesia	[bundling]	MD		[anesthesia]					
–24	Unrelated E/M service during post-op	[bundling]	MD	[E/M]					[global]	
–25	Significant separately identifiable E/M service	[bundling]		[E/M]					[global][bundling]	[facility]
–26	Professional component	[decreases]	MD	[E/M]			[radiology]	[lab]	[bundling]	
–32	Mandated services	[bundling][no change]	MD	[E/M]	[anesthesia]	[scissors]	[radiology]	[lab]		
–33	Preventive services	[bundling]	MD	[E/M]		[E/M]				
–47	Anesthesia by surgeon	[scissors][no change]	MD			Surgeon only				
–50	Bilateral procedure	[scissors]				[scissors]	[radiology]			[facility]
–51	Multiple procedures	[decreases]	MD		[E/M]	[scissors]	[radiology]			
–52	Reduced services	[decreases]		[E/M]		[scissors]	[radiology]	[lab]		[facility]
–53	Discontinued procedure	[decreases]	MD		[E/M]	[scissors]	[radiology]	[lab]		
–54	Surgical care only	[decreases]	MD			[scissors]			[global]	
–55	Post-op management only	[decreases]	MD	[E/M]					[global]	

Continued

Table 12.2 *Continued*

Modifier	Description	💰	MD Only	E/M	Anesthesia Provider	Procedure	Radiology	Path/Lab	Global Package	Facility
−56	Pre-op management only	[icon]	MD	[hand]					[circle]	
−57	Decision for surgery	[icon]	MD	[hand]					[circle]	
−58	Staged or related procedure	[icon]				[scissors]	[skull]		[circle]	[facility]
−59	Distinct procedural service	[icon]			[hand]	[scissors] [envelope]	[skull]	[mouse]	[icon]	[facility]
−62	Two surgeons	[icon]	MD			[scissors] # [envelope]	[skull]			
−63	Procedure performed on infants <4 kg	[scissors]	MD			[scissors] (not skin)				
−66	Surgical team	[icon]	MD			[envelope] [scissors] #				
−73	Discontinued outpatient procedure prior to anesthesia	[icon]				[scissors]				[facility]
−74	Discontinued outpatient procedure after anesthesia	[icon]				[scissors]				[facility]
−76	Repeat procedure by same physician	[icon]				[scissors]	[skull]		[circle]	[facility]
−77	Repeat procedure by other physician in practice	[icon]				[scissors]	[skull]		[circle]	[facility]
−78	Unplanned return to OR for related procedure during post-op period	[icon]				[scissors]	[skull]		[circle]	[facility]
−79	Unrelated service by same physician during post-op period	[icon]		[hand]		[scissors]	[skull]		[circle]	[facility]
−80	Assistant surgeon	[icon]	MD			[scissors] # [envelope]	[skull]			
−81	Minimum assistant surgeon	[icon]	MD			[scissors] # [envelope]				
−82	Assistant surgeon—qualified resident not available	[icon]	MD			[scissors] # [envelope]				
−90	Reference outside lab	[icon]	MD					[mouse]		
−91	Repeat clinical diagnostic lab test	[icon]						[mouse]		[facility]
−92	Alternate laboratory platform testing	[icon]	MD					[mouse]		
−95	Synchronous telemedicine service		MD							

Continued

Table 12.2 Continued

Modifier	Description	💰	MD Only	E/M	Anesthesia Provider	Procedure	Radiology	Path/Lab	Global Package	Facility
–96	Habilitative services		MD			✂				
–97	Rehabilitative services		MD			✂				
–99	Multiple modifiers	📄	MD			✂	☠			

Level I (Facility) Modifiers

Fourteen Level I facility modifiers have been approved for use in coding hospital-based outpatient services and procedures. Table 12.3 provides an overview of these modifiers. Note that some are the same as the CPT modifiers, and some are distinct.

Table 12.3 Modifiers Approved for Hospital Outpatient Use

MODIFIER	DESCRIPTION
–25	Significant, separately identifiable E/M service by the same physician on the same day of the procedure or other service
–27	Multiple outpatient hospital E/M encounters on the same date
–33	Preventive Services
–50	Bilateral procedure
–52	Reduced services
–58	Staged or related procedure/service by the same physician during the postoperative period
–59	Distinct procedural service
–73	Discontinued outpatient procedure prior to anesthesia administration
–74	Discontinued outpatient procedure after anesthesia administration
–76	Repeat procedure by same physician
–77	Repeat procedure by another physician
–78	Unplanned return to the operating room for a related procedure during the postoperative period
–79	Unrelated procedure/service by the same physician during the postoperative period
–91	Repeat clinical diagnostic laboratory test

Level II (HCPCS/National) Modifiers

Level II modifiers, which are alphanumeric, are called *HCPCS modifiers*. Some HCPCS Level II modifiers are listed in the front of the CPT manual, with the rest listed in the HCPCS coding book. There are many more HCPCS modifiers than CPT modifiers. HCPCS modifiers are updated annually. They are required specifically when filing claims to government payers such as Medicare and Medicaid but may also be required or accepted by commercial insurance companies. The inside cover of the CPT manual lists the HCPCS modifiers. Table 12.4 summarizes many of the modifiers. HCPCS coding is covered in Chapter 30 of this text.

Level II modifiers are reported with CPT codes on outpatient institutional claims (UB-04/837I) only and never on inpatient claims.

Proper use of Level II modifiers is important to obtain proper reimbursement for services rendered and to remain compliant with coding guidelines and payer policies. Payers look for ways to detect fraud, waste, and abuse, and one of the ways they do this is by tracking and trending modifier use and misuse. Payers monitor modifier usage and may take one of the following actions based on their findings: (1) Modify or create reimbursement policies specific to the use of certain modifiers, (2) deny the claim and request medical record documentation, (3) educate their provider network, or (4) perform an audit of a provider's claims with possible recoupment of monies. Examples of some things they look for during this review are as follows:

- Do all in-office procedures have an E/M with a modifier –25?
- Is the use of modifier –59 high?
- Is modifier –22 used every time a certain procedure is performed?
- Are there numerous denials for inclusive or unbundled procedures or services?
- Is an assistant surgeon utilized for every primary surgeon's case?

Table 12.4 Selected Level II (HCPCS/National) Modifiers

MODIFIER	DESCRIPTION
–AI	Principal physician of record
–BL	Special acquisition of blood and blood products
–CA	Procedure payable in the inpatient setting only when performed emergently on an outpatient who expires prior to admission
–CR	Catastrophic/disaster related
–E1	Upper left eyelid
–E2	Lower left eyelid
–E3	Upper right eyelid
–E4	Lower right eyelid
–FA	Left hand, thumb
–F1	Left hand, second digit
–F2	Left hand, third digit
–F3	Left hand, fourth digit
–F4	Left hand, fifth digit
–F5	Right hand, thumb
–F6	Right hand, second digit
–F7	Right hand, third digit
–F8	Right hand, fourth digit
–F9	Right hand, fifth digit
–FB	Item provided without cost to provider or supplier or full credit received for replaced device
–FC	Partial credit received for replaced device
–GA	Waiver of liability statement on file
–GG	Performance and payment of a screening mammogram and diagnostic mammogram on the same patient, same day
–GH	Diagnostic mammogram converted from screening mammogram on same day
–LC	Left circumflex coronary artery
–LD	Left anterior descending coronary artery
–LM	Left main coronary artery
–LT	Left side (identifies procedures performed on the left side of the body)
–Q0	Investigational clinical service provided in a clinical research study that is an approved study
–Q1	Routine clinical service provided in a clinical research study that is an approved study
–QM	Ambulance service provided under arrangement by a provider of services
–QN	Ambulance service furnished directly by a provider of services
–RC	Right coronary artery
–RI	Ramus intermedius coronary artery
–RT	Right side (identifies procedures performed on the right side of the body)
–TA	Left foot, great toe

Continued

Table 12.4 *Continued*

MODIFIER	DESCRIPTION
–T1	Left foot, second digit
–T2	Left foot, third digit
–T3	Left foot, fourth digit
–T4	Left foot, fifth digit
–T5	Right foot, great toe
–T6	Right foot, second digit
–T7	Right foot, third digit
–T8	Right foot, fourth digit
–T9	Right foot, fifth digit

Proper Use of Modifiers

A coder needs to clearly understand the meaning of each modifier before using it. Not all circumstances or codes warrant a modifier, and modifiers should not be haphazardly assigned, because reimbursement may be affected. For example, if the goal was to indicate that a procedure was unusual or more difficult and the coder put a –52 modifier instead of the –22 modifier, the reimbursement will be reduced.

EXAMPLE
37722–52 indicates that ligation, division, and complete stripping of the long saphenous vein from the saphenofemoral junction to the knee or below was a lesser service than what is described in the CPT code 37722. Code 37722–22 would indicate that a greater service was provided to the patient over and above what is indicated in the code description.

It is also important to note that not all modifiers are available for use with every CPT section's codes:

> Payer policies vary widely on how modifiers are reported, how many are stored in their data vaults, which ones are used to calculate reimbursement, and which ones they accept. Check with each payer for individual policies regarding modifiers.

- Some modifiers apply only to certain sections. For example, the modifier –24, *Unrelated evaluation and management services by the same physician during a postoperative period*, is used only with codes that are located in the Evaluation and Management section, as its descriptor implies. As another example, modifier –23 may only be used with anesthesia codes.
- Add-on codes that begin with a plus sign (+) cannot be modified with –51, multiple procedures, because the add-on code is used to add increments to a primary procedure, so the need for multiple procedures is replaced by procedures added on.
- Codes that begin with ⊘ also cannot be modified with –51, multiple procedures.

Sometimes more than one modifier needs to be reported with a procedure. When sequencing more than two modifiers, the sequence should be from highest to lowest priority. Some insurance plans can only price and pay based on one modifier, or the modifier in the first position on the claim form; therefore, always list the modifier that affects payment first. The use of modifier 99 varies widely when reporting more than two modifiers, and should only be used if reporting four or more modifiers.

Modifier –22, Increased Procedural Service
Modifier –22 is used to indicate that the procedure is more complicated or unusual from the services indicated in the code description. The procedure may have involved increased risk, or the surgeon may have had difficulty performing the surgery or accessing the particular site because of trauma or anatomical malformation, hemorrhage (blood loss over 600 cc), unusual findings (e.g., excessively large surgical specimen), or prolonged cleansing. There may have been a complication that could not be identified by using another CPT code so the –22 modifier will draw attention to this.

To correctly assign this modifier, work and effort need to have been increased by about 30% to 50%. Reimbursement associated with the appropriate use of the –22 modifier will be increased by 20% to 30%. Documentation justifying the use of this modifier must accompany the claim. The –22 modifier is only reported with surgical procedure codes.

EXAMPLE

Excision of a lesion on a patient with morbid obesity in the crease of the neck. The obesity makes it more difficult to reach the lesion so it warrants a modifier. In fact, many procedures on people who are morbidly obese are more difficult to perform because of impaired view and additional tissue to cut through.

Modifier –23, Unusual Anesthesia

Modifier –23 is used when a procedure that normally would not be done under anesthesia required anesthesia. The anesthesiologist is the only physician who would use this modifier. Anesthesia providers use it occasionally when performing procedures on children and on people with severe anxiety or mental retardation who are uncooperative, making it safer and easier to perform the procedure with IV sedation or general anesthesia.

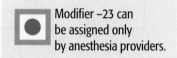
Modifier –23 can be assigned only by anesthesia providers.

EXAMPLE

Patient with mental retardation required anesthesia to perform a CT scan of the head.

Modifier –24, Unrelated Evaluation and Management Service by the Same Physician or Other Qualified Health-Care Professional During a Postoperative Period

At times, a patient is seen for a new or ongoing problem during the postoperative period. If the reason for the visit is to evaluate a condition that is clearly not related to the reason for the surgery, modifier –24 is used so that the visit will be paid. It is not essential that the diagnosis code is different from the surgery code; there are many circumstances when the condition that warranted the surgery is getting worse and requires evaluation.

> ■ **CASE SCENARIO**
>
> A patient is 3 weeks post-op lithotripsy. Patient is now complaining of warts that have appeared on his genital area. Patient is diagnosed with genital herpes. Code: 99212–24.

Modifier –25, Significant, Separately Identifiable E/M Service by the Same Physician or Other Qualified Health-Care Professional on the Same Day of the Procedure or Other Service

Modifier –25 is frequently misused in professional practice, often because it seems to be an easy way to be paid for extra work during a patient encounter. It should be used to report an authentic, separately reportable procedure-type service provided at the same time a valid E/M service is rendered.

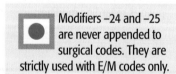
Modifiers –24 and –25 are never appended to surgical codes. They are strictly used with E/M codes only.

Note that both the separately identifiable E/M service and the procedure or other service may be related to the same diagnosis. According to CMS, this modifier is assigned for an E/M service that is above and beyond the procedure performed, that is beyond the usual preoperative and postoperative care associated with the procedure, and that requires all the necessary elements of an E/M service.

> ■ **CASE SCENARIO**
>
> A patient presented with an excoriated lesion, and a biopsy was performed along with the services indicative of the E/M code 99214. This would warrant a –25 modifier. In effect, the E/M service provided the information that a procedure was required. If the lesion was evaluated at a previous session and the patient was returning for only the biopsy, modifier –25 would not be used.

Modifier –26, Professional Component

Modifier –26 is used to report the physician or other qualified health-care professional service or component separately from the facility's services for the technical component of the same service. This modifier alerts the insurance company to pay the physician or other qualified health-care professional for his or her professional services separately from the payment to the facility for its costs to provide the technical service, such as the room and the supplies. An example would be cardiac catheterizations utilizing hospital equipment. The physician or other qualified health-care professional is providing only the professional component of those services.

Modifier –27, Multiple Outpatient Hospital E/M Encounters on the Same Date

Modifier –27 is used in hospital outpatient coding only, where it indicates that more than a single E/M encounter for the same patient was provided within that facility's clinics on the same date of service.

Modifier –32, Preventive Services

Modifier –32 is used when an insurance carrier or outside federal agency requires (*mandates*) that a service be provided. Certain diagnoses may require a second or third opinion from another provider (not a family member's request) before some insurance carriers (not Medicare) will pay for it. Report modifier –32 when a third party such as a workers' compensation payer is requiring E/M services. This modifier alerts the payer that the claim should be paid at its full amount without any charge to the patient.

> ■ **CASE SCENARIO**
>
> A 53-year-old truck driver is being seen in follow-up from an injury on the job. He fell out of his tractor-trailer and fractured his shoulder, requiring repair with prosthesis. His recent evaluation did not demonstrate total inability to use this shoulder. The workers' compensation carrier is requiring an independent evaluation with an orthopedist who specializes in shoulder joint replacements. Based on this evaluation, the carrier may reduce his benefits. The orthopedist will report this work with an appropriate E/M code and a –32 modifier.

Modifier –33, Preventive Services

When reporting preventive services, the CPT code should be appended with the –33 modifier unless the service is inherently preventive and the code description indicates such. For services specifically identified as preventive in the code description, the modifier should not be used. For example, codes that contain the word "screening" or "immunization" would not require the –33 modifier.

> ● Medicare created HCPCS codes for some preventive medicine services and these codes should be utilized instead of the E/M preventive codes when billing services for Medicare beneficiaries.

Modifier –33 is used to identify to insurance companies that the service provided was preventive service under the provision of the Patient Protection and Affordable Care Act (PPACA) and/or state mandate or other federal legislation. Services billed with a –33 modifier are waived from copays, coinsurance, and deductibles. The intent of the modifier is to alert the payer to waive respective patient liability for the preventive service. If multiple preventive medicine services are provided on the same day, the modifier is appended to the codes for each preventive service rendered on that day. This modifier is also used to modify services that were intended to be preventive but were converted to a therapeutic service. The most common example of this is screening colonoscopy (code 45378), which results in a polypectomy (code 45384).

> **EXAMPLE**
>
> Abdominal aortic aneurysm screenings for men and office visits where child obesity screening and counseling are provided would qualify for the use of the –33 modifier.

Services may be identified by appending modifier –33 when the primary purpose of the service is the delivery of an evidence-based service in accordance with a U.S. Preventive Services Task Force (USPSTF) A or B rating in effect and other preventive services identified in preventive services mandates (legislative or regulatory).

A complete list of codes that are classified as either an A or B by the USPSTF is located on its website (www.USPreventiveServicesTaskForce.org).

Modifier –47, Anesthesia by Surgeon

Modifier –47 is used when a regional nerve block or general anesthesia is administered by the surgeon, rather than by anesthesia personnel. It is not used with anesthesia codes; it is only appended to a CPT code for the procedure. Note that this modifier is not accepted by Medicare.

Modifier –50, Bilateral Procedure

Procedures listed in the CPT manual are inherently unilateral unless otherwise stated. The –50 modifier states that the identical procedure was performed bilaterally during the same operative session. The term *bilateral* pertains to paired body organs that are distinctly left or right, such as the left breast and right breast. To use this modifier, the code description may not state "one or both or bilateral" or list the plural form of a body part such as *turbinate(s)*. The modifiers –RT and –LT are not used when modifier –50 applies. Payers typically pay 150% of the regular unilateral charge for a bilateral procedure. Payer guidelines must be checked with respect to reporting –50.

> **EXAMPLE**
>
> The description for CPT code 31231 *Nasal Endoscopy, diagnostic, unilateral or bilateral (separate procedure)*.

In this example, it would be inappropriate to use –50 because the code description includes "bilateral." However, in the following example, the –50 modifier is correctly used to mean that foreign bodies were removed from both ears.

> **EXAMPLE**
>
> 69200–50 *Removal of foreign body of the external auditory canal; without general anesthesia*.

Modifier –51, Multiple Procedures

The –51 modifier is assigned when more than one *surgical* procedure is performed on the *same day* or at the *same operating session* by the *same provider*. The procedures can be performed on the same or different body parts through the same or a different incision.

> **EXAMPLE**
>
> 30000 *Drainage abscess or hematoma, nasal, internal approach* done at the same operative session as 30200 *Injection into turbinate(s), therapeutic* would be reported as 30000, 30200–51.

Modifier –52, Reduced Services

When a procedure is partially reduced or eliminated, modifier –52 is used. This alerts the payer that the service was not completed to the fullest extent, such as when a doctor performs a procedure unilaterally but the code description indicates bilateral. Modifier –52 is also reported when the coder cannot find a procedure code that adequately describes the partially reduced services, when such a code does not exist, or when directed by CPT parenthetical notes. Do not report modifier –52 with time-based codes. Reimbursement is calculated based on the percentage of the procedure that was completed.

> **EXAMPLES**
>
> - Patient with above-the-knee amputation (AKA) had an extremity arterial study (93923). A –52 modifier would be appropriate here because he did not have an entire leg for the study.

 The CMS Medicare Physician Fee Schedule Relative Value File is a good source for determining whether or not to append the –50 modifier. This file is a "go to" resource for coders, billers, auditors, physicians, facilities, and insurance carriers and can be used as a guide for modifier reporting, setting physician pricing for services, determining global days, updating reimbursement tables within computer systems, and much more. This file is located on the CMS website and is free to download (www.cms.gov/ Medicare/Medicare-Fee-for-Service-Payment/PhysicianFee Sched/PFS-Relative-Value-Files .html). Bookmark this site and refer to this file because it is updated quarterly. Refer to the Reimbursement Review later in this chapter for further instruction on this concept.

The most complex or major procedure is listed first because it will receive full reimbursement. The second procedure code with the –51 modifier will receive partial payment (typically 50% of the first amount).

Do not append the –51 modifier to services performed in an outpatient hospital surgery clinic or an ambulatory surgical center. Also do not use it with add-on codes, –51 modifier–exempt codes, or unlisted procedures.

Each payer has its own policy regarding modifiers –52 and –53, often paying half the usual amount. Documentation should accompany the claim.

- On the flip side to the previous example, if the code description includes "unilateral" or "bilateral," do not append modifier –52 when the procedure was only performed on one side.

Modifier –53, Discontinued Procedure

Modifier –53 indicates that a started procedure was terminated for an extenuating circumstance (threat to patient, instrument or equipment failure, hypotension, or the like). It is not used to report elective cancellations before a procedure is started. The modifier applies to surgical procedures only and would never be applied to E/M codes. Reimbursement is calculated based on the percentage of the procedure that was completed. Supporting documentation should be available to describe the following:

- When the procedure was started
- When the procedure was stopped (not just the time but at what point in the scheduled procedure)
- Why the procedure was discontinued
- Percentage of the procedure completed

Global Surgery Modifiers

CPT created a way to submit codes for surgical services in which the same physician did not carry out the entire surgical package. Surgical codes with global periods of greater than 10 days where two or three physicians carried out portions of service are submitted with one of three modifiers: –54, –55, or –56.

Modifier –54, Surgical Care Only. Modifier –54 is used by the surgeon who actually performed the surgery but did not or will not provide the pre-op or post-op care.

Modifier –55, Postoperative Management Only. Modifier –55 is appended to the surgery code to reflect care provided by a physician who did not perform the original surgery.

Modifier –56, Preoperative Management Only. If a physician performs a preoperative evaluation and determines that surgery is necessary but does not perform the actual surgery or post-op follow-up, it would appropriate to append the –56 modifier to the surgical code.

Modifier –57, Decision for Surgery

If during an E/M visit a physician initially decides that surgery is needed, the visit is reimbursable separately from the global package. Using modifier –57 with the appropriate E/M code notifies the payer of this fact and indicates that a surgical claim will follow.

Modifier –58, Staged or Related Procedure or Service by the Same Physician or Other Qualified Health-Care Professional During the Postoperative Period

For the use of modifier –58, the surgeon's medical record should document that a staged procedure was planned during the specified postoperative period for the first procedure code. This modifier should not be used with codes whose definitions already include the word "staged" or language indicating that the surgery or procedure is usually done in multiple sessions. Instead, it is used when a procedure was planned prospectively, was more extensive than the original procedure, or was for therapy following a diagnostic surgical procedure and each of the stages of the procedure was performed by the original surgeon. This modifier is not used to report a problem or complication resulting from the original surgery that required a return to the operating room.

> ■ **CASE SCENARIO**
> A physician performed debridement of a nonhealing wound three times and then performed a skin graft. The physician and patient discussed this course of treatment ahead of time. Each subsequent debridement and the skin graft would have the –58 modifier appended if performed during the post-op period of the original debridement procedure.

Modifier –59, Distinct Procedural Service

Modifier –59 states that two codes that are normally paid under one surgical package were performed as two separate procedures. One procedure has been performed independently of the other or is unrelated to the other. Usually one of the codes is a CPT-designated separate procedure, as explained in this

Medicare Physician Fee Schedule

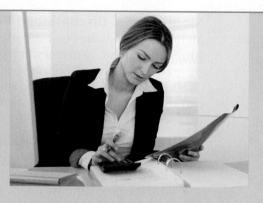

The Medicare Physician Fee Schedule (MPFS) Relative Value File (RVF) contains important reimbursement criteria applied by payers in calculating payment to physicians for services performed in or outside of a facility. Learning how to interpret this document and using the information during the coding and billing process will help offset claim denials and assist the coder/biller in determining proper reimbursement and reporting of services to Medicare. Many commercial plans base their reimbursement policies and fees on the MPFS. Physicians and coders use this document to determine global periods for procedures, modifier requirements, supervision requirements, procedure status indicators, and RVUs to calculate reimbursement, to name a few of its uses.

The MPFS is updated quarterly and available on the CMS website (www.cms.gov/Medicare/Medicare-Fee-for-Service-Payment/PhysicianFeeSched/PFS-Relative-Value-Files.html). Download the most current version of the file located in a compressed .zip format (named RVUxxD, where "xx" denotes the two-digit year of the file you are retrieving). The two main files you will need within this .zip file are "PPRVUxx" (a Microsoft Excel document) and "RVUPUFxx" a (Microsoft Word document). Again, the "xx" denotes the two-digit year of the file you are retrieving. The Word document explains the meanings of the column headers located in the Excel document, essentially functioning as a legend. The Excel document is commonly referred to as the *MPFS* or simply the *Physician Fee Schedule (PFS)* and contains 15,000+ HCPCS/CPT codes that are listed in alphanumerical order by code. The example on the next page shows

instruction from the *CPT Assistant* (July 1999): "When codes designated as separate procedures are carried out independently or considered unrelated or distinct from other procedures/services provided at the same time, they can be reported in addition to the other procedures by appending a –59 modifier."

Modifier –59 is important for receiving payment for both procedures, rather than a reduced fee for the second procedure. The guideline is that if the procedures were done at different sites or organs, a separate incision was made, a separate excision was done, or the doctor was treating a separate injury or lesion, modifier –59 is correct. CMS no longer accepts modifier –59 for pricing claims due to problems with the incorrect usage of this modifier. CMS created four modifiers for use in reporting specific scenarios that meet the specification of a separate and distinct encounter. This is further discussed in Chapter 30.

EXAMPLE

Excision of a benign 2-cm lesion of the right arm (11402) and a 1.5-cm benign lesion of the back (11402–59). Multiple excisions are normally reported with modifier –51, but because both lesions are reported with the same code even though they are on different anatomical sites, the modifier –59 is used to prevent confusion about duplicate billing.

Some payers have policies automatically denying a claim line with the –59 modifier appended if documentation does not accompany the claim. When reporting two or more modifiers on a single claim line, sequence the modifier that has the greatest impact on payment first, followed by the others. Per CMS, modifiers –59 and –51 can be reported on the same claim line. The –59 modifier should be sequenced first because it may override National Correct Coding Initiative (NCCI) edits, which garner the greater impact on payment.

In this example, the procedures are at different sites, so it is acceptable to report the same code twice, appending the –59 modifier to the second use.

the fee schedule column heads that are commonly used in the coding/billing process. Note that this is not a full representation of all columns located within the fee schedule. Most of the columns are self-explanatory; however, some require the use of the legend to understand the meaning of the letter or number indicators. For example, column D, *Status Code*, has 16 status categories A–T, X, and without the accompanying Word file or legend, the user would not know that the "P" refers to bundled or excluded codes.

If a code is missing from this fee schedule, it means that the service is not paid for under the MPFS. Let's briefly review these columns and their meanings.

					FULLY											PHYSICIAN		DIAGNOSTIC
					IMPLEMENTED											SUPERVISION OF		IMAGING
			STATUS	WORK	FACILITY	PCTC	GLOB	PRE	INTRA	POST	MULT	BILAT	ASST	CO-	TEAM	ENDO	DIAGNOSTIC	CALCULATION	FAMILY
HCPCS	MOD	DESCRIPTION	CODE	RVU	TOTAL	IND	DAYS	OP	OP	OP	PROC	SURG	SURG	SURG	SURG	BASE	PROCEDURES	FLAG	INDICATOR

HCPCS contains a listing of HCPCS codes and CPT codes. The *MOD* column is populated with either one of three modifiers or it is blank:

- −26 = professional component
- −TC = technical component
- −53 = separate RVUs and a fee schedule amount for discontinued procedure
- Blank = services other than those with a professional and/or technical component

Some codes will be listed more than once depending on which modifiers apply. Codes with no entry in the *MOD* column (a blank), represent the global service concept and all diagnostic tests. These global services are those that do not have a professional and/or technical component. The one exception is when separate RVUs and fee schedule amounts have been established for procedures that the physician terminated before completion. In this case, the modifier −53 is used.

Modifier −62, Two Surgeons
Modifier −62 is applicable when the procedure required 50% of each surgeon's skill and time if two surgeons were participating in the same procedure. An example is the need for an orthopedist and a neurosurgeon to work together to perform a Harrington rod technique. If two surgeons were operating at the same time but were performing two different procedures, this modifier does not apply.

Modifier −63, Procedure Performed on Infants Less Than 4 Kg
Modifier −63 is used to report services on neonates and infants weighing less than 4 kg. Increased complexity and physician work are associated with this type of patient.

Modifier −66, Surgical Team
Modifier −66 is used mainly in transplant procedures or cases of multiple trauma when the skills of several different surgeons are required.

Modifier −73, Discontinued Outpatient Procedure Prior to Anesthesia Administration
Modifier −73 is reported only by hospital outpatient coders to indicate that a procedure was terminated before anesthesia was administered.

Modifier −74, Discontinued Outpatient Procedure After Anesthesia Administration
Modifier −74 is reported only by hospital outpatient coders to indicate that a procedure was terminated after local or general anesthesia was given. This includes situations in which the patient was in the operating room and anesthesia was started and situations in which sedation was given in the holding area.

Modifier –76, Repeat Procedure or Service by Same Physician or Other Qualified Health-Care Professional

Modifier –76 is used to report a second procedure that had been previously performed on the same day. It is usually used to report the identical service repeated in radiology and the lab, and minor procedures such as repeat blood sugar. Some payers recognize this modifier; others do not.

Modifier –77, Repeat Procedure or Service by Another Physician or Other Qualified Health-Care Professional

At times, a procedure previously performed by another physician must be repeated. For this modifier to be utilized, the identical CPT code (other than a pathology code) must have been previously submitted on a health claim by another physician. The modifier alerts the insurance company that a procedure was performed again by a different physician and that the claim is not a duplicate claim. Medical necessity must be clear.

> ■ **CASE SCENARIO**
>
> A patient was treated in the emergency department (ED) for epistaxis. The physician performed nasal cautery of the left nostril with packing. He submitted CPT code 30901–LT. Later that day, the patient returned to the ED and was seen by a different physician who performed the same procedure. He submitted 30901–LT–77 with a procedure note and letter explaining that the patient was seen earlier in the day by another physician who performed the same service.

Modifier –78, Unplanned Return to the Operating/Procedure Room by the Same Physician or Other Qualified Health-Care Professional Following Initial Procedure for a Related Procedure During the Postoperative Period

Modifier –78 is used when the surgeon must perform additional surgery in the operating room (OR) during the postoperative period for a reason related to the original surgery. A complication such as hemorrhaging, a failed flap or graft, or a hematoma that arose from the original procedure requires a return to the OR. Most payers recognize this as a secondary procedure for a related complication. For this modifier to be used, the patient must be taken back to the OR, not to an examining room. For the second procedure, the physician and facility must bill the code that best describes the procedures performed. If one does not exist, an unlisted procedure is filed. The original surgery code is used only if the identical procedure was carried out a second time. For example, patients with bilateral cataracts routinely have both cataracts removed within 30 to 60 days of each other. There is a 90-day global period assigned to cataract extraction codes so the ophthalmologist should report a –78 modifier along with the respective anatomical modifier (RT or LT) to avoid denial for the same service being performed during the global period.

> ● Do not assign this modifier for code descriptions using words such as "subsequent," "staged," "related," or "redo."

> ● When a code is submitted with the –78 modifier, a new global period does not begin with the date of this service. The global period is determined by the date of service of the original procedure.

> ■ **CASE SCENARIO**
>
> A patient returns for removal of internal fixation 80 days after the initial surgery. The patient had a joint replacement and would like the retained screws removed due to persistent pain and swelling. The doctor submits 20680–78, because the original procedure has a postoperative period of 90 days.

Modifier –79, Unrelated Procedure or Service by the Same Physician or Other Qualified Health-Care Professional During the Postoperative Period

A physician may perform surgical or diagnostic services during the postoperative period of a previous surgery performed by the same doctor for the same patient. The –79 modifier alerts the payer

> CPT modifiers cannot be appended to Category III codes, unlisted codes, or add-on codes. Category II codes have their own set of modifiers—1P, 2P, 3P, and 8P—located in the instructional front matter of the Category II code section and can only be appended to Category II codes.

that the doctor was aware of the postoperative period restrictions, but that this procedure was unrelated to the previous encounter. To use this modifier, both the diagnosis and the procedure must be unrelated to the reason for the original surgery.

> **■ CASE SCENARIO**
> A patient was treated for ulnar nerve entrapment of the right elbow. Sixty days later, the same neurosurgeon also performs a lumbar laminectomy due to a slipped disc. The laminectomy code would be submitted with a –79 modifier.

Modifiers –80, –81, and –82, Assistant Surgeons and Minimum Assistant Surgeons

These modifiers are used to indicate that an assistant was required to perform the surgery (–80). Minimum assistants do no hands-on care (–81). Modifier –82 is used when a surgical resident is not available (usually in teaching hospitals or rural hospitals) or there is no adequate training program for the medical specialty that is needed to perform the procedure. Modifiers –90, –91, and –92 are discussed further in Chapter 28.

Supporting Documentation

When modifiers –22, –23, –24, –25, –52, –53, –59, –76, –77, and –99 are reported, a claim attachment is necessary to describe the situation to the payer. A special report describing the details of the procedure is an example of this documentation; other examples are operative reports and pathology reports. According to CPT, a special report should include the following:

- Nature, extent, and need for the procedure
- Time and effort and equipment used

The following information may also be included:

- Complexity of symptoms
- Final diagnosis
- Pertinent physical findings (sizes, extent, severity)
- Diagnostic and therapeutic procedures
- Concurrent related or unrelated problems
- Required follow-up

Payer Requirements

It is important to know each payer's requirements regarding modifier use. For example, CPT coding modifier information issued by CMS differs from the AMA's coding advice. In addition, not all modifiers are accepted by Medicare (e.g., –32, –47, –63, and –81) or Medicaid. Many other payer-specific modifiers apply to various coding situations, which are spelled out in the corresponding payer provider manual or contract. Coders learn these on the job. Medicaid in particular uses its own approved list of modifiers.

Payers differ on requirements for reporting modifiers, how many modifiers they use to price payment, and the position of the modifier. Some carriers can only price on one modifier in the first position, while others can recognize modifiers in all four positions.

Some carriers will automatically resequence codes on the claim in descending order by RVU, but do not assume that all carriers do this. It is important to place the code with the highest RVU or weight first.

Medicare does not recognize the –51 modifier and automatically reduces the fee for any code not listed first on a claim. Their exception is the codes that are –51 modifier exempt, which are paid at the normal rate.

Accurate reporting of both CPT codes and modifiers is essential for correct coding and maximum appropriate reimbursement, as explained in the Reimbursement Review that follows on the next page.

Outpatient Claims: Physician or Other Qualified Health-Care Professional Billing

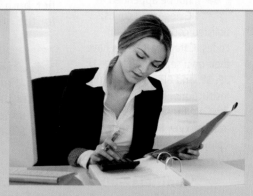

Physicians bill for their professional services. When the place of service is the office or other nonhospital setting, the physician's payment includes an amount that accounts for the provision of the overhead and supplies. When the patient receives outpatient care at a facility or facility-owned place of service, the facility is permitted to bill for its part of the services (the room and so on), and the physician bills for his or her part (the surgical or other procedural work). For example, a patient visit to a same-day surgery unit for a procedure on a bunion is billed by two entities, (1) the hospital outpatient facility and (2) the physician.

Physicians bill their medical services and procedures on the 837P or its paper equivalent, the CMS-1500 claim form. The professional claim format, as shown in Figure 12.2, has two major sections.

Fields 1 through 13 (also referred to as the *demographic information*) contain information about the patient, including:

- The patient's health plan and identification number
- The patient's name, address, date of birth, and telephone number
- Data concerning the patient's employer, additional insurance coverage, and whether the claim involves an accident

The second section, made up of fields 14 through 33, holds the data concerning the particular visit being billed, the dates and services/procedures, and the provider. Note in Figure 12.2 that the health plan is Medicare, the place of service is 11 (for office), and the CPT code is 99203. The related ICD-10-CM codes—essential for establishing the medical necessity of the claim—are R50.9 and R59.9. These codes mean that the patient saw the physician for evaluation of his complaints of fever and 7 swollen glands.

1500

HEALTH INSURANCE CLAIM FORM

APPROVED BY NATIONAL UNIFORM CLAIM COMMITTEE 08/05

PICA | PICA | CARRIER

1. MEDICARE [X] (Medicare #) MEDICAID [ ] (Medicaid #) TRICARE CHAMPUS [ ] (Sponsor's SSN) CHAMPVA [ ] (Member ID#) GROUP HEALTH PLAN [ ] (SSN or ID) FECA BLK LUNG [ ] (SSN) OTHER [ ] (ID)

1a. INSURED'S I.D. NUMBER (For Program in Item 1): 456 22 1234A

2. PATIENT'S NAME (Last Name, First Name, Middle Initial): NAPJER JOHN D

3. PATIENT'S BIRTH DATE MM DD YY: 05 05 1938 SEX M [X] F [ ]

4. INSURED'S NAME (Last Name, First Name, Middle Initial)

5. PATIENT'S ADDRESS (No., Street): 47 CARRIAGE DR

6. PATIENT RELATIONSHIP TO INSURED: Self [X] Spouse [ ] Child [ ] Other [ ]

7. INSURED'S ADDRESS (No., Street)

CITY: CHESHIRE STATE: CO

8. PATIENT STATUS: Single [ ] Married [X] Other [ ]

CITY STATE

ZIP CODE: 80034 TELEPHONE (Include Area Code): (720) 123 5555

Employed [ ] Full-Time Student [ ] Part-Time Student [ ]

ZIP CODE TELEPHONE (INCLUDE AREA CODE) ( )

9. OTHER INSURED'S NAME (Last Name, First Name, Middle Initial)

10. IS PATIENT'S CONDITION RELATED TO:

11. INSURED'S POLICY GROUP OR FECA NUMBER

a. OTHER INSURED'S POLICY OR GROUP NUMBER

a. EMPLOYMENT? (CURRENT OR PREVIOUS) [ ] YES [X] NO

a. INSURED'S DATE OF BIRTH MM DD YY SEX M [ ] F [ ]

b. OTHER INSURED'S DATE OF BIRTH MM DD YY SEX M [ ] F [ ]

b. AUTO ACCIDENT? [ ] YES [X] NO PLACE (State)

b. EMPLOYER'S NAME OR SCHOOL NAME

c. EMPLOYER'S NAME OR SCHOOL NAME

c. OTHER ACCIDENT? [ ] YES [X] NO

c. INSURANCE PLAN NAME OR PROGRAM NAME

d. INSURANCE PLAN NAME OR PROGRAM NAME

10d. RESERVED FOR LOCAL USE

d. IS THERE ANOTHER HEALTH BENEFIT PLAN? [ ] YES [ ] NO *If yes, return to and complete item 9 a-d.*

READ BACK OF FORM BEFORE COMPLETING & SIGNING THIS FORM.

12. PATIENT'S OR AUTHORIZED PERSON'S SIGNATURE I authorize the release of any medical or other information necessary to process this claim. I also request payment of government benefits either to myself or to the party who accepts assignment below.

SIGNED SOF DATE

13. INSURED'S OR AUTHORIZED PERSON'S SIGNATURE I authorize payment of medical benefits to the undersigned physician or supplier for services described below.

SIGNED

PATIENT AND INSURED INFORMATION

14. DATE OF CURRENT: ILLNESS (First symptom) OR INJURY (Accident) OR PREGNANCY(LMP) MM DD YY: 10 01 2008

15. IF PATIENT HAS HAD SAME OR SIMILAR ILLNESS. GIVE FIRST DATE MM DD YY

16. DATES PATIENT UNABLE TO WORK IN CURRENT OCCUPATION FROM MM DD YY TO MM DD YY

17. NAME OF REFERRING PHYSICIAN OR OTHER SOURCE

17a.

17b. NPI

18. HOSPITALIZATION DATES RELATED TO CURRENT SERVICES FROM MM DD YY TO MM DD YY

19. RESERVED FOR LOCAL USE

20. OUTSIDE LAB? [ ] YES [X] NO $ CHARGES

21. DIAGNOSIS OR NATURE OF ILLNESS OR INJURY. (Relate Items 1,2,3 or 4 to Item 24e by Line)

1. 78.06
2. 78.56
3. ___ . ___
4. ___ . ___

22. MEDICAID RESUBMISSION CODE ORIGINAL REF. NO.

23. PRIOR AUTHORIZATION NUMBER

	24. A. DATE(S) OF SERVICE From MM DD YY	To MM DD YY	B. PLACE OF SERVICE	C. EMG	D. PROCEDURES, SERVICES, OR SUPPLIES (Explain Unusual Circumstances) CPT/HCPCS	MODIFIER	E. DIAGNOSIS POINTER	F. $ CHARGES	G. DAYS OR UNITS	H. EPSDT Family Plan	I. ID. QUAL.	J. RENDERING PROVIDER ID. #
1	10 02 2008		11		99203		1,2	95 00	1		NPI	8221238999
2											NPI	
3											NPI	
4											NPI	
5											NPI	
6											NPI	

PHYSICIAN OR SUPPLIER INFORMATION

25. FEDERAL TAX I.D. NUMBER: 123 45 9666 SSN [X] EIN [ ]

26. PATIENT'S ACCOUNT NO.: NAP0123

27. ACCEPT ASSIGNMENT? (For govt. claims, see back) [X] YES [ ] NO

28. TOTAL CHARGE: $ 95 00

29. AMOUNT PAID: $ 0 00

30. BALANCE DUE: $ 95 00

31. SIGNATURE OF PHYSICIAN OR SUPPLIER INCLUDING DEGREES OR CREDENTIALS (I certify that the statements on the reverse apply to this bill and are made a part thereof.)

SIGNED SOF DATE

32. SERVICE FACILITY LOCATION INFORMATION: SAME

a. NPI b.

33. BILLING PROVIDER INFO & PHONE #: (720) 554 1222

CENTER CLINIC
3810 EXECUTIVE BLVD
RAYTOWN CO 80033

a. 4455667788 b.

NUCC Instruction Manual available at: www.nucc.org

Figure 12.2 CMS-1500 health insurance claim form for a fictional patient.

Provide the correct modifier for each of the following descriptions.

1. Multiple modifiers _____

2. Distinct procedural service _____

3. Co-surgery _____

4. Staged procedure _____

5. Assistant surgeon _____

6. Discontinued procedure after sedation was started; service is being reported by a hospital outpatient facility _____

7. Repeat procedure by same physician _____

8. Unusual anesthesia _____

9. Mandated services _____

10. Surgical team _____

CPT UPDATES

New, deleted, and changed CPT codes are released by the AMA in September or October of each year and go into effect every January 1. Category II and Category III codes are updated twice a year, on January 1 and July 1. Why is the CPT code set updated so often? Medicine is always changing rapidly, new technology makes new procedures available, and other procedures need to be more accurately described. The AMA CPT Editorial Panel makes CPT changes its members feel best represent medical practices.

Coders must access the current year's codes to guarantee submission of correct codes and to obtain correct and timely reimbursement. If invalid codes are submitted, reimbursement will be delayed or claims will be denied. Coding managers, office managers, and business offices must be sure to update software programs such as practice management programs (PMP) and charge description masters (CDM) with new and revised codes and must remember to delete old codes to ensure submission of the most accurate and current codes. To stay current, providers can access the AMA's CPT website.

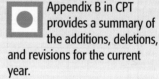 Appendix B in CPT provides a summary of the additions, deletions, and revisions for the current year.

INTERNET RESOURCES: AMA CPT Updates
www.ama-assn.org/go/cpt

Each November, the AMA hosts a CPT symposium just after it releases revisions to CPT codes for the coming year to discuss the changes, the associated rationale, and anticipated impact. Each year when the current version of CPT is published, the AMA also publishes errata that list corrections to the manual. Coders can find the errata at the AMA's CPT website under *CPT Code Information and Education.* Coders should make notes in their CPT books to fix the errors. This may appear cumbersome but it is very important and it takes only a few minutes.

INTERNET RESOURCE: AMA Errata Data
www.ama-assn.org/ama/pub/physician-resources/solutions-managing-your-practice/
coding-billing-insurance/cpt/about-cpt/errata.page

AHIMA and the American Academy of Professional Coders (AAPC) offer many avenues to stay abreast of CPT changes and updates. Each organization offers several opportunities via onsite meetings or webinars to educate coders and physicians on coding, code revisions, and reimbursement methodologies. Each organization publishes professional journals and newsletters to notify members of changes to code sets, regulatory changes, HIPAA, and much more. Both also provide educational seminars, administer coding certification exams, and offer a means of networking with coders. Each posts helpful links to outside organizations and to legislation that affects health care, such as the *Federal Register*, along with many other helpful resources on their websites. Joining these national organizations is paramount and promotes a level of quality and professionalism that cannot be overestimated.

> In 2005, CMS eliminated the grace period historically provided at the beginning of each year for reporting deleted codes. Most payers are following their lead by also not allowing the use of old codes; however, insurance carriers often fall behind in updating their computer systems. Watch for claim denials when submitting new codes during the first quarter of the year.

A REVIEW: ICD-10-CM AND CPT COMPARISON

When first learning to code, initially it is possible to confuse ICD-10 and CPT concepts and conventions. It is important for coders to understand key differences and similarities between the two coding methodologies and recognize when each is appropriate to use. In some courses, ICD-10 is taught before CPT, whereas for others, it is the opposite. Table 12.5 describes the basic differences between the code sets.

Table 12.5 ICD-10 Comparison With CPT

	ICD-10-CM	CPT	ICD-10-PCS
Code length	Diagnosis codes are three to seven characters in length. E and V codes are made up of the letter and three or four digits.	Category I codes are five digits. Category II and Category III codes are four digits and an alphanumeric character.	Seven characters in length: 1st character = section 2nd character = body system 3rd character = root operation 4th character = body part 5th character = approach 6th character = device 7th character = qualifier
Decimal point	Used in diagnosis code after the first three characters	Not used	Not used in procedure codes
Medical settings	ICD-10-CM codes are used in all settings and places of service.	Used by physicians in all outpatient and inpatient settings. Facilities use CPT for all outpatient services and ancillary services captured by the chargemaster (lab, x-ray, etc.) for inpatient visits, but it is never used for inpatient facility reporting or reimbursement.	ICD-10-PCS procedure codes are only used in inpatient hospital facility reporting.
Maintained primarily by	NCHS (ICD-10-CM); CMS (ICD-10-PCS)	AMA	Developed and maintained by CMS
Updated	Annually, October 1	Category I code updates are released October 1 for use effective January 1 of the following year. Category II and III codes are prereleased on the AMA website every 6 months and can be used when they appear.	Annually, October 1
Official coding guideline source	*Coding Clinic* by the AHA	*CPT Assistant* by the AMA	*Coding Clinic* by the AHA
Modifier use	Not applicable for diagnoses	CPT (HCPCS Level I—	Modifiers are built into the

Continued

Table 12.5 *Continued*

	ICD-10-CM	CPT	ICD-10-PCS
		professional and facility) and Level II anatomical	codes with no stand-alone modifier.
Content	Diagnosis and procedure codes	E/M codes and procedure codes only	Inpatient procedures only
Character type	Diagnosis codes are alphanumeric with the first digit being alpha, digits two and three being numeric, and digits four through seven being alpha or numeric.	Primarily numeric. Category II and III codes are alphanumeric.	Alphanumeric

Key: AHA = American Hospital Association, AMA = American Medical Association, CMS = Centers for Medicare and Medicaid Services, CPT = Current Procedural Terminology, NCHS = National Center for Health Statistics

---

CHECKPOINT 12.5

Determine whether the following codes are ICD-10-CM or CPT codes.

1. I10 _____

2. 99283 _____

3. Z85.3 _____

4. W61.01 _____

5. 1002F _____

6. S31.110A _____

7. 19318 _____

8. 0075T _____

HOW TO ASSIGN CPT CODES AND MODIFIERS

To assign CPT codes to procedures or services, follow the process outlined in Pinpoint the Code 12.1 and described in the paragraphs that follow.

Step 1: Review the Complete Medical Documentation

To code for professional services, the coder first reads the documentation, which is made up primarily of reports created by a physician with other supporting medical documents, and determines where the service took place (the place of service) and the health plan (payer), if applicable. For CPT codes to apply, the provider must be a physician or other professional practitioner (not an inpatient facility). These points are checked:

- The patient may be cared for as an outpatient or an inpatient. The patient's age and gender should be verified.
- The place of service may be an office, a facility, or another health-care setting.
- The payer may be a private or self-funded payer, a government payer (Medicare, Medicaid, TRICARE, or CHAMPVA), or a *self-payer*—the term used when the patient is responsible for the bills.

Step 2: Abstract the Medical Procedures That Need Coding

Based on the documentation, the coder sorts out the procedures and other services the patient received. For medical services, the description is carefully noted; for surgeries, the operative report states the procedure that was performed.

PINPOINT THE CODE 12.1: CPT code process

Step 1
Review complete record documentation noting place of service, provider type, and patient.

↓

Step 2
Abstract the procedures that should be coded.

↓

Step 3
Identify all main terms and related terms.

↓

Step 4
Locate these terms in the Index, and follow cross-references.

↓

Step 5
Review the codes, descriptors, and notes.

↓

Step 6
Verify that the code description matches the services.

↓

Step 7
Assign codes for all significant services.

↓

Step 8
Assign applicable modifier(s).

↓

Step 9
Check all possible codes before final selection. Assign HCPCS code, Category III code, or unlisted code for services not located in CPT I or II code listings.

⊙ Never code directly from the CPT Index. The Index is just a way of putting you in the approximate area in the appropriate section.

Step 3: Identify the Main Term and Related Terms

Identify all main terms and related terms for the abstracted procedures. Look for action words or sentences by locating the following:

- Procedure or service (e.g., biopsy, E/M, laparoscopy)
- Organ or body part (e.g., intestines, prostate, bladder)
- Condition or disease being treated (e.g., abscess, varicose veins)
- Common abbreviation (e.g., ECG or CT)
- Eponym (e.g., McBride operation)
- Symptom (e.g., tinnitus)

Step 4: Locate the Terms in the CPT Index

Locate the procedures in the Index at the back of the CPT manual. Locate all main terms (based on the medical terminology in the documentation), accounting for significant procedures or services performed. For each entry, a listing of a code or code range directs the coder to the appropriate heading and procedure code(s) in CPT. Some entries have a "*See*" cross-reference or a "*See also*" to guide the coder to another index entry.

EXAMPLE
Code Range Index Entry.
X-RAY
    Ankle. . . . . .73600–73610.

When a code range is listed, read the code descriptions for all codes within the range indicated in the Index before assigning a final code. Pay very close attention to punctuation (semicolons, colons, parentheses). The recommended procedure is to also read the description of one code above and one code below the selected code to ensure that the selected code accurately reflects what has been done. The goal is to select the most specific code.

Step 5: Review the Codes, Descriptors, and Notes

The next step is to review all possible codes in the CPT section that the index entries point to. It is very important to review any notes provided at the beginning of each subsection or the section guidelines, and to check for notes directly under the code, within the code description, or after the code description. Parenthetical notes are located immediately above or below a code and apply to that code. They give directions to see other code ranges, use add-on codes, and so on. For example, in Figure 12.1, a note below code 44005 directs the coder to 44180 for laparoscopic approach.

Step 6: Verify the Code Against the Documentation

Verify that the code description matches what was performed based on the documentation. At this point, choose the most appropriate code based on the service performed and the documentation provided.

Step 7: Assign Codes for All Significant Services

If two distinct procedures or services were performed, both can be coded. Continue coding until all components of the procedure or service have been accounted for according to the directions in the CPT manual.

> Pay close attention to code descriptions for wording both with and without age-specific notations, the gender of the patient, and punctuation.

Step 8: Assign Modifiers If Appropriate

Correct use of modifiers is critical to compliant coding. Coders ask themselves the following questions when determining whether a modifier is required:

> Remember not to assign –51 modifiers to add-on codes, –51 modifier–exempt codes, or unlisted procedure codes.

- Does the code description for the CPT code I want to assign already include identifiers such as unilateral or bilateral, biopsy(s), staged, or more than one occurrence?
- Will a modifier add more information or clarify any questions regarding the anatomical site (e.g., –LT, –T5)?
- Does CPT include several body parts in one code description? If so, using anatomical modifiers is incorrect because the code does not identify a specific part or side of the body.
- Will a modifier help eliminate the appearance of duplicate billing? Will it clarify that the same procedure was performed at the same time but on a different site?
- Will a modifier eliminate the appearance of incorrectly reporting multiple procedures? Remember that a separate procedure is typically bundled into a more comprehensive procedure in that subsection if it is performed at the same time as a more complex procedure. In this case, a –59 modifier may apply.
- Will a modifier help explain the time frame within which a service was performed?
- Will a modifier help clarify what portion of a service or procedure was performed by an assistant or other care provider?
- Does the situation require the use of more than one modifier? If so, did I follow the proper sequencing of modifiers?

    — CPT modifiers that affects payment are sequenced first (–52, –22, –50, –74, etc.). Any global surgery modifier or a modifier that overrides NCCI would fall into this category.
    — HCPCS Level II anatomical modifiers follow (–T1, –E3, –RT, etc.).
    — Remaining CPT modifiers that do not affect payment follow.

Not all codes require a modifier. Double-check the code description before assigning –50, –51, or any anatomical modifiers. Look for language in the code description such as "both," "bilateral," "each," "single," "multiple," "each additional," "digit," and so on to assist in making a modifier selection.

Step 9: Check All Possibilities Before Final Assignment

Coders will discover that there is no designated CPT code for every procedure or service that may be provided. A procedure's inclusion or exclusion in the book does not indicate whether the AMA supports it. Nor does it mean that a procedure is or is not paid by insurance plans.

Never make a code "fit." A code that is close to the actual procedure should not be used. If a code cannot be found that matches what was done, check the HCPCS code set carefully to see if a code matches the services performed. The code set HCPCS may also have new procedures that are not yet included in CPT. If HCPCS does not include a code that fits, or if the payer does not accept HCPCS codes, next check the Category III code section. Finally, if there is no appropriate code in this section, assign an unlisted procedure code from the appropriate subsection of CPT. The guidelines at the beginning of each CPT section include a complete list of unlisted procedure codes available for use.

> Trying to make an existing code "fit" is incorrect coding and may be classified as fraud.

Avoid submitting unlisted codes without first informing the carrier that an unlisted code will be used. Research the procedure performed and be as specific as possible; submit this information

about the procedure performed in advance, so that the carrier can evaluate how to reimburse the procedure. Most carriers do not pay for unlisted procedure codes and will require the operative report or procedure note to determine payment based on a "similar" service with equivalent work effort.

Coding Example

Using the flowchart in Pinpoint the Code 12.1, what code(s) would you assign to the service described in the following example? Also assign a modifier, if needed. Knowing the site of service will enable you to select the correct modifiers, if needed.

EXAMPLE

Imagine that you are coding for a physician's work (professional service) at an ambulatory surgery center (ASC). The female patient is 57 years old and has Blue Cross and Blue Shield coverage (a private payer). She was admitted to the ambulatory surgery center for a left breast reconstruction with tissue expander insertion.

Step 1: Review the documentation and determine the provider, patient, place, and payer from the case scenario provided in this example. The provider is the physician, and the patient is a 57-year-old female presenting for outpatient surgery. Place of service is an outpatient surgery facility. Blue Cross and Blue Shield is the payer.

Step 2: The procedure is left breast reconstruction with tissue expander insertion.

Step 3: Identify the main term in the procedural statement. There are actually three main terms to choose from: breast, insertion, and reconstruction.

Step 4: Go to the Index and look up the word "breast." Scan the subterms for "reconstruction." You will see many different entries under "reconstruction." You specifically want "reconstruction with tissue expander."

Step 5: Look up the code that you think is correct, checking all notes.

Step 6: Double-check that the description of the code you have selected matches the procedure performed.

Step 7: No additional procedures were documented.

Step 8: Because the procedure was done on the left breast, you would assign an –LT modifier to indicate which breast was operated on.

Step 9: As a check, use another term to verify the code selection. Look up one of the other main terms, *reconstruction*. In this case, *reconstruction* is the main term and *breast* is the subterm. The code range is 19357–19369. Listed under "breast" are the same methods of reconstruction. There doesn't appear to be any alternative code to choose; "with tissue expander" 19357 is a perfect fit.

> Remember that you cannot find a diagnosis code in CPT.

CHECKPOINT 12.6

List all possible index entries for locating the service listed, and then assign the code. The first entry has been completed as an example.

	Index Entry	Code
1. Excision of mucous cyst of a finger	Excision, Mucous cyst	26160
2. Endoscopic biopsy of the nose	_____	_____
3. Laparoscopic meniscectomy of the right knee	_____	_____
4. Drainage of a salivary gland cyst	_____	_____
5. Cystoscopy with fragmentation of ureteral calculus	_____	_____

This scenario is one of many that demonstrates how the same code can be achieved by looking up different words, but always following the correct process.

CPT CODING RESOURCES

The AMA's *CPT Professional Edition* is a more complete codebook than the *Standard Edition* for both beginning and seasoned coders. It has *CPT Assistant* references to expedite researching coding guidelines, along with anatomical and procedural pictures and color-coding to assist in proper code assignment. In the *Professional Edition,* the edges of the pages are color-coded, and thumb tabs also assist in locating sections of the book. Overall, the format of both editions is the same. Subscribing to *CPT Assistant* is highly recommended so that coders can gain access to official coding guidelines published by the AMA. The AMA also publishes the following resources: *CPT Reference of Clinical Examples* and *CPT Changes: An Insider's View.* These further explain the clinical concepts behind each code with common examples and rationales for changes.

Regardless of which specialty or setting a coder works in (physician office, ASC, hospital), several helpful publications are available to the coder. For example, *Anesthesia & Pain Management Coding Alert*, a newsletter published by the Coding Institute, is useful in an anesthesia group practice or a pain management facility. Some publishers provide specialty-specific references and books. For example, Optum publishes a *Coding Illustrated for the Eye* that would be beneficial to an ophthalmologist's practice or the *Coding Companion for OB/GYN* for use by gynecological practices.

> Always be sure to use a current edition of any codebook. Do not code from cheat sheets and superbills.

The Office of the Inspector General recommends that the following resources be available and used by coding and billing staff:

- Medical dictionary
- An anatomy and physiology text or atlas
- Current ICD-10-CM codebook
- Current CPT codebook
- Current HCPCS codebook
- *Physicians' Desk Reference*
- *Merck Manual*
- Contractor's provider manual
- Up-to-date subscription to the *AHA Coding Clinic*
- Up-to-date subscription to the AMA's *CPT Assistant*
- For Medicare billing, the NCCI, which can be accessed online at www.cms.hhs.gov/National CorrectCodInitEd and coverage information online at www.cms.hhs.gov/center/coverage .asp.

You should also become familiar with these additional CPT references:

- General Medicare information at www.cms.hhs.gov
- *Medicare Part B News* on Medicare topics and specialty coders' *Pink Sheets*, published by DecisionHealth, which cover coding and billing topics across many specialties (information online at www.decisionhealth.com)
- AMA's website (www.ama-assn.org), where coders can submit questions for official direction, read responses to frequently asked questions, and read clinical vignettes with official advice on troublesome or confusing topics

Accurate coding is the first step in obtaining the reimbursement that physicians or facilities have earned. Accurate and consistent coding is achieved through a thorough understanding of CPT. Stay informed of changes and updates by reading recommended periodicals and attending seminars to ensure that your coding is accurate and consistent.

Chapter Summary

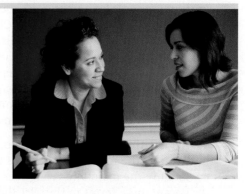

1. Coding affects the financial well-being of every organization and has a direct correlation with how a provider or facility is reimbursed for services. Data collected from coded health-care claims is used for many purposes. It drives many decisions, such as which physician to choose based on quality of care rankings, how much to reimburse for a service, and frequency limitations on services, to name a few. These data are also used to compare providers within the same specialty or geographic location to monitor abusive or fraudulent billing patterns.

2. The CPT code set is used for many purposes. Information gathered from CPT code reporting is used for trending outpatient services, benchmarking services provided, and measuring and improving quality of patient services in addition to being the principal means of communicating with insurance carriers for reimbursement of professional services. CPT provides a system for coding and reporting professional medical and surgical procedures.

3. All outpatient medical and surgical settings are required to report CPT codes for services performed. Facilities report CPT codes for certain procedures. CPT codes are submitted by physicians and select allied health professionals to describe professional services rendered regardless of location or type of service.

4. The content and organization of the CPT printed manual are standardized throughout. The CPT codes are listed in three categories: Category I, Category II, and Category III. The book begins with an introduction followed by six sections of Category I codes, a section of Category II codes, a section of Category III codes, and appendices. The Index is located at the very end of the book. All terms and abbreviations are in alphabetical order.

5. Symbols and punctuation are important features of CPT. Consistently acknowledging symbols and punctuation is important in proper code selection. A legend is located at the bottom of each page with definitions of symbols. Symbols are also described in the introduction. The semicolon (;) is used to conserve space and to identify and divide the common portion of the code from the unique portion. The bullet (•) designates a new code for that year. The triangle (▲) signifies a revised code, meaning that the descriptor is revised in some way. The plus (+) symbol identifies an add-on code. The symbol circle with a backslash (⊘) indicates that a code cannot be assigned a –51 modifier. Facing triangles (▶◀) before a code indicate that the text is new or has been revised from the prior year's edition. The lightning bolt symbol (⚡) signifies that the vaccine code is for a product that is pending FDA approval. The star (★) signifies that the code may be used for telemedicine services.

6. Modifiers are reported along with CPT codes to describe events that modified the procedure or service; they do not change the basic meaning of the code. They are located on the inside cover of the CPT codebook with the full modifier descriptions located in Appendix A of CPT. Modifiers are divided into categories for use by hospitals and by physicians. Modifiers for facilities are listed under the heading "Modifiers Approved for Hospital Outpatient Use." Anatomical modifiers or HCPCS modifiers are also located here under the heading "Level II (HCPCS/National)." Not all codes require modifiers. Procedures performed on fingers, toes, eyelids, and coronary vessels require HCPCS Level II anatomical modifiers. Refer to Tables 12.2 and 12.3 for a thorough review.

7. Always use a current edition of a codebook to ensure use of the most up-to-date codes. Payment will be delayed or claims denied if valid codes are not submitted. Never use outdated coding books.

8. Coders must understand the key differences and similarities of ICD-10-CM and CPT to correctly assign codes in the appropriate setting. ICD-10-CM diagnosis codes are submitted for inpatient, outpatient, facility, and professional claims alike. ICD-10-PCS procedure codes are submitted

by the facility for inpatient procedures only. CPT codes are submitted for all outpatient and inpatient services for a physician's services and outpatient services only for the facility.

9. Do not make a code fit. Assign a HCPCS code, a Category III code, or an unlisted code for services not located in CPT. Unlisted procedure codes are used when a service has no designated Category I, Category II, or Category III code. A special report should be submitted whenever an unlisted code is reported in order to clarify the procedure performed.

10. A CPT code can be found in four ways: By looking for the procedure or service, the organ or other anatomic site, the patient's condition or by synonyms, eponyms and abbreviations.

11. There are nine steps to follow when assigning a CPT code:

   a. Review the complete medical documentation.
   b. Abstract the medical procedures that should be coded.
   c. Identify the main and related terms for the procedures to be coded.
   d. Locate these terms in the CPT Index. Read the descriptions for all codes within the code range.
   e. Review the codes, descriptors, and notes. Follow cross-references located in the Index and respective subsection of CPT. Read the guidelines at the beginning of the chapter and section. Read any instructional notes above or below the code.
   f. Verify that the code description matches the services described in the documentation.
   g. Assign codes for all significant services and distinct procedures.
   h. Assign applicable modifier(s) based on documentation and code description language.
   i. Check all possible sources for hard-to-locate codes; report HCPCS, Category III, or unlisted codes for services when required by the situation.

12. References are tailored to specialties and work settings. Regardless of work setting, all coders should have access to *CPT Assistant;* the current ICD-10-CM, CPT, and HCPCS codebooks; a medical dictionary; Medicare NCCI edits; an anatomy book or body atlas; and Medicare local coverage determinations. The *AHA Coding Clinic* and *Merck Manual* are primarily utilized by hospitals and are an absolute necessity for inpatient coders

Review Questions

Matching

Match the key terms with their definitions.

A. special report
B. significant procedure
C. separate procedure
D. Category III codes
E. surgical package

F. postoperative period
G. Category II codes
H. add-on code
I. unlisted code
J. modifier

1. __B__ A major professional service

2. __D__ Temporary codes for emerging technology, services, and procedures

3. __E__ Procedure code that groups related procedures under a single code

4. __I__ __H__ A service that is not listed in CPT and requires a special report

5. __F__ The period of care following a surgical procedure

6. __G__ CPT codes that are used to track performance measures

7. __A__ __J__ Information that must accompany the reporting of an unlisted code

8. __C__ A procedure usually done as an integral part of a surgical package, but that may be reported if performed alone, or in a separate site, or during a separate session

9. __H__ A secondary procedure that is performed with a primary procedure and that is indicated in CPT by a plus sign (+) next to the code

10. __J__ A two-character addition to a CPT code indicating that special circumstances were involved with a procedure, such as a reduced service or a discontinued procedure

CPT © 2017 American Medical Association, All Rights Reserved.

True or False

Decide whether each statement is true or false.

1. __T__ Inclusion of a code in CPT indicates that it is covered by insurance.

2. __F__ Specific guidelines are found at the end of each section of the CPT manual.

3. __T__ CPT codes listed as "(separate procedure)" must be coded separately from the primary procedure.

4. __T__ The unique portion of a CPT code follows a semicolon.

5. __F__ Codes that begin with "99" are unlisted Medicine section codes.

6. __T__ CPT codes cannot be located in the Index by looking up a diagnosis as the main term.

7. __T__ CPT codes are submitted to insurance companies only for services provided by a physician.

8. __T__ Unlisted procedure codes can never be reported to Medicare.

9. __F__ It is permissible to code directly from the Index in situations where only one code choice is listed.

10. __T__ Modifiers are used to indicate when a procedure was modified and the description changed.

11. __T__ Category III codes are not required for reporting because they are for emerging technology and are considered temporary codes.

12. __T__ Under HIPAA, HCPCS codes are used for all payers.

13. __F__ CPT codes are reported for inpatient procedures only.

14. __F__ All payers recognize all HCPCS Level I and Level II modifiers.

15. __T__ One of the CPT appendices contains clinical examples of the codes in the E/M section.

Multiple Choice

Select the letter that best completes the statement or answers the question.

1. Add-on codes can be identified by the following criteria:
   A. They can never stand alone and must be reported with another service.
   B. The code describes additional anatomical sites where the same procedure is performed.
   C. The code is marked with a • in the codebook.
   D. The code can be used with a −51 modifier.
   E. All of the above.
   F. A and B only.
   G. A, B, and D only.

2. Which of the following is the symbol for a new CPT code?
   A. ★
   B. ⊃
   C. •
   D. ▶◀

3. Which of the following contains a complete list of modifier −51 exempt codes?
   A. Appendix F
   B. Appendix A
   C. Index
   D. Appendix E

4. Review the code range 20526–20610. What is the correct code assignment for injection of a carpometacarpal joint?
   A. 20550
   B. 20600
   C. 20526
   D. 20610

5. Which of the following symbols signifies a revised code?
   A. ▶◀
   B. ⟳
   C. •
   D. ▲

6. Which of the following would be considered a Medicine code?
   A. 99212
   B. 72100
   C. 0126T
   D. 93745

7. What is the correct code assignment for removal of impacted cerumen from both ears?
   A. 69200–50
   B. 69210–50
   C. 69210
   D. 69210–RT, –LT

8. Which modifier would the physician assign to indicate that only a portion of a planned procedure was completed?
   A. –22
   B. –53
   C. –26
   D. –52

9. Additions, deletions, and revisions of codes from the prior year are listed in which appendix?
   A. B
   B. A
   C. M
   D. P

10. Which modifier is assigned to the code for postoperative care only following right inguinal hernia by another surgeon?
    A. –78
    B. –55
    C. –54
    D. –24

CHAPTER 13

CPT: Evaluation and Management Codes

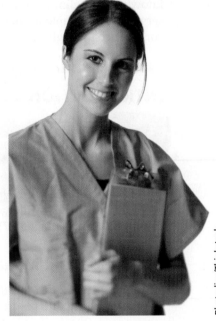

Photodisc/Thinkstock

CHAPTER OUTLINE

LEARNING OUTCOMES

After studying this chapter, you should be able to:

1. Describe the organization of the CPT Evaluation and Management (E/M) section.
2. Discuss the use of the section guidelines as a resource for E/M coding.
3. List five questions that are used to select appropriate E/M code ranges and assign correct codes.
4. State the difference between new and established patients in CPT terms.
5. Discuss the three key components that determine the level of service and list the four levels of each.
6. Describe the process used to determine the level of service for E/M coding, including the part played by the contributing components.
7. Compare and contrast consultations and new patient (referral) E/M services.
8. Discuss the factors that are important in assigning critical care codes.
9. Define *observation* and *standby services*.
10. Assign CPT E/M codes, correctly applying the rules and exceptions for each category of service.

This chapter covers coding services that are a core responsibility of physicians: the services to assess the nature of their patients' conditions and to devise plans to treat them. This work is done by all medical specialties in the multitude of settings where patients are seen, from the practice office to every type of health-care facility. Although these medical services have in common the formal name *evaluation and management*, the time, effort, and training required to perform them varies widely according to the situation. Compare diagnosing an earache for a young, healthy child to assessing the coronary symptoms of an elderly, frail patient. Because the services provided vary so widely, many are paid on a scale that reflects time, effort, and complexity. Medical coders who know the guidelines and payer regulations for accurate, complete, and compliant coding of these services are valuable to their employers. They can improve coding accuracy, reimbursement, and compliance through their coding efforts.

INTRODUCTION TO EVALUATION AND MANAGEMENT CODES

E/M codes represent the physician's *evaluation* of a patient's condition and *management* of a patient's care. First developed in 1992 by the American Medical Association (AMA), E/M codes are used by every type of physician to report patients' encounters for health-related problems. They are considered *cognitive* codes because physicians must gather and analyze information regarding each patient to make a decision about the condition and determine how to manage it. Because they are used so often and so widely, the E/M codes and section guidelines are listed first in the Current Procedural Terminology (CPT).

Evaluation and Management Codes Organization

The E/M section of CPT is divided into categories and subcategories that specifically define the services provided and reported by the physician, as shown in Table 13.1.

Basic Selection Process

Working with E/M codes requires an understanding of the structure of the E/M section. The coder can best accomplish this by studying and answering the following standard set of five questions to locate the correct code range in the E/M categories and then to pick the correct code:

1. Who is the patient?
2. What is the place of service?
3. What is the patient's status?
4. What type of service is being provided?
5. What level of service is being provided?

> To make E/M coding as efficient as possible, familiarize yourself with the E/M section categories and subcategories so that you can research individual codes quickly.

Table 13.1 E/M Categories and Subcategories

CATEGORY	SUBCATEGORY	CODE RANGE
Office or other outpatient services	New patient	99201–99205
	Established patient	99211–99215
Hospital observation services	Discharge services	99217
	Initial services	99218–99220
	Subsequent services	99224–99226
Hospital inpatient services	Initial hospital care	99221–99223
	Subsequent hospital care	99231–99233
	Same-day admission and discharge	99234–99236
	Discharge services	99238–99239
Consultations	Office/outpatient	99241–99245
	Hospital	99251–99255
Emergency department services	New or established patient	99281–99285
	Other emergency services	99288
Critical care services	Time based	99291–99292
Nursing facility services	Initial care	99304–99306
	Subsequent care	99307–99310
	Discharge services	99315–99316
	Other nursing facility services	99318
Domiciliary, rest home, etc.	New patient	99324–99328
	Established patient	99334–99337
	Oversight services	99339–99340
Home services	New patient	99341–99345
	Established patient	99347–99350
Prolonged services	Direct patient contact	99354–99357
	Without direct patient contact	99358–99359
	Prolonged clinical staff services with physician or other qualified health care professional supervision	99415–99416
	Standby services	99360
Case management services	Medical team conferences	99366–99368
Care plan oversight services		99374–99380
Preventive medicine services	New patient	99381–99387
	Established patient	99391–99397
	Counseling risk and behavior change	99401–99429
Non–face-to-face physician services	Telephone services	99441–99443
	On-line medical evaluation	99444
	Interprofessional consultations	99446–99449
Special E/M services		99450–99456
Newborn care services, delivery attendance		99460–99465
Inpatient neonatal and pediatric critical care services	Pediatric critical care transport	99466–99467
	Inpatient neonate critical care	99468–99469
	Inpatient pediatric critical care	99471–99476
	Initial and continuing intensive care	99477–99480
Cognitive assessment and care plan services		99483
Care management services		99490
Transitional care management services		99495–99496
Advance care planning		99497–99498
Other E/M services		99499

Question 1: Who Is the Patient?

In the first step in the E/M coding process, the coder identifies and categorizes the patient. Reviewing the column of subcategories in Table 13.1, the terms *new patient* and *established patient* recur, as do various terms that describe a patient's age and other characteristics.

New Versus Established Patients. Pinpoint the Code 13.1 is a flowchart for distinguishing between a new and an established patient for purposes of E/M coding. A new patient (NP):

- Has not received any professional services from the physician/qualified health-care professional or another physician/qualified health-care professional of the identical specialty and subspecialty who belongs to the same group practice within the past 3 years.

EXAMPLES

- Ms. Jones saw Dr. Abbot 4 years ago and schedules an appointment to be seen by him again. Dr. Abbot will report a new patient code from 99201–99205.
- Ms. Jones saw Dr. Abbot's partner 2 years ago and makes an appointment to see Dr. Abbot. Dr. Abbot's partner is in the same specialty as Dr. Abbot. Dr. Abbot will report an established patient code from 99211–99215.

PINPOINT THE CODE 13.1: New Patient (99201–99205) Versus Established Patient (99211–99215)

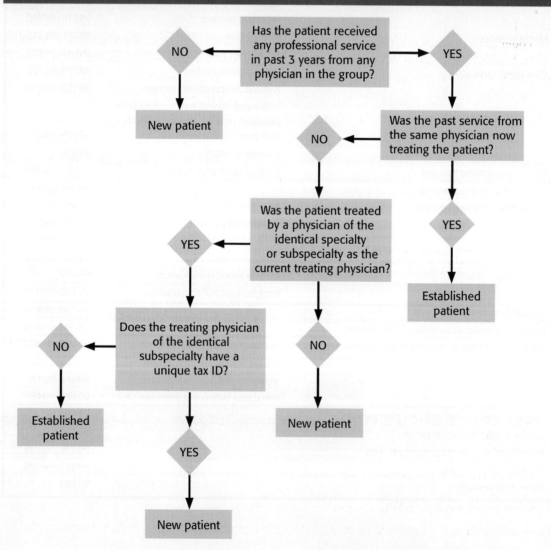

Ms. Jones saw Dr. Abbot's partner, a cardiologist, 2 years ago and makes an appointment to see Dr. Abbot, a gastroenterologist, whom she has not seen in 4 years. Dr. Abbot will report a new patient code from 99201–99205.

In contrast to a new patient is an established patient (EP), a person who either has received professional services from the physician within the past 3 years or has received professional services from another physician of the same specialty and subspecialty who belongs to the same group practice within the past 3 years. There are other scenarios for new versus established patients:

1. *Covering for another physician.* There are times when one physician/qualified health-care professional (QHP) will cover for another physician/QHP seeing patients. That patient encounter is classified as if the patient is seeing his or her own physician/QHP who is not available.

2. *Physicians joining new practices.* As physicians leave their practices to join a new practice, their patients will often move with them. The patients' status with their physician in the new group is the same as if their physician was still with the previous group. If they have been seen within the previous 3 years, they are established patients even though their physician may have a new tax ID number. According to the American Academy of Family Physicians (AAFP) the physician has been providing professional services to the patient within the last 3 years if, regardless of whether or not medical records have been transferred, that patient status remains the same.

Patients Categorized by Age. Often different age categories are important, such as the following:

- Neonate (birth to 28 days)
- Pediatric (29 days to 24 months)
- Adult
- Specific age ranges, such as 40 to 64 years in preventive medicine coding

Question 2: What Is the Place of Service (POS)?

The coder next determines the place of service (POS), which may be a physician office, hospital, nursing facility, or outpatient department of a facility such as an emergency department (ED) or an observation room.

> NOTE: Place of service codes that are generally recognized are listed at the beginning of the CPT book.

Question 3: What Is the Patient's Status?

The patient's status also points to the correct E/M code range by category or subcategory. Is the patient ill or injured? Is the patient critically ill? Does the patient need to be hospitalized? Is the patient presenting for an annual physical? Is the patient being cared for by an outside agency under supervision of the physician?

Question 4: What Type of Service Is Being Provided?

The major types of care shown in Table 13.1 are as follows:

- Initial care for a first visit for a particular problem
- Subsequent care for follow-up visits for a particular problem
- Prolonged care, meaning care provided for extended time periods
- Standby services, during which a physician is ready to provide services as needed

The coder identifies the type of service (care) that the physician provided to further narrow down the possible code range options.

Question 5: What Level of Service Is Being Provided?

Questions 1 through 4 help the coder select the correct range of E/M codes. The final step is to determine the level of service (LOS) that was provided to the patient, which permits choosing the specific code when a range is offered. The possible levels are as follows:

- Problem focused (PF)
- Expanded problem focused (EPF)
- Detailed (DET)
- Comprehensive (COMP)

The level of service is indicated in each of the code descriptions in the CPT E/M section.

Example of Code Selection

The following example is used to show how the coder's E/M questions can narrow the options and select the correct code.

> ### ■ CASE SCENARIO
> A 56-year-old male patient who has never been seen before by the physician has an office visit for left ankle pain caused by a fall.

The coder selects code range 99201–99205 to represent the services provided in *evaluating* the patient's left ankle pain and in determining how to *manage* the patient's condition. The factors used to decide the code range are listed in the accompanying table.

The answers to questions 1 through 4 point to the range of codes from which a code will be picked. This was a *new* (question 1) *adult* (question 1) patient seen in the physician *office* (question 2) for an *injury* (question 3). The care was *initial*, or new (question 4), because

Who is the patient?	New patient, adult
What is the POS?	Office
What is the patient's status?	Injured, in pain
What type of service is being provided?	New, or initial care

the visit was for a new injury. In the next section, picking the level of service, which involves following a specific process, is discussed. If, in this example, the level of service is determined to be detailed, the appropriate code from the new patient code range of 99201–99205 would be 99203.

CHECKPOINT 13.1

Read the following cases and answer the questions.

A 47-year-old patient was seen last month in the physician office for intermittent chest pain. He is seen today in the office to follow up on the results of medication prescribed during last month's visit and to follow up on the chest pain complaint.

1. Who is the patient? _____

2. What is the place of service? _____

3. What is the patient's status? _____

4. What type of service is being provided? _____

A family with a 3-year-old child has moved 200 miles to a new home. The child became ill with a fever, and the parents have contacted a pediatrician so that the child can be evaluated and treated.

5. Who is the patient? _____

6. What is the place of service? _____

7. What is the patient's status? _____

8. What type of service is being provided? _____

DETERMINING THE LEVEL OF SERVICE

Evaluation and management services are considered the foundation of physician services because they are provided by almost every specialty in the medical field. E/M codes represent approximately one-third of all charges reported to third-party payers. Because of the importance of E/M codes, third-party payers, auditors, and government agencies pay close attention to how physicians report them. Each E/M code has its own descriptor and key component requirements. Coders must understand the code distinctions to appropriately report E/M services. Determining the level of service is an essential responsibility of coders.

Selection of the level of service for E/M codes is based on the following E/M components:

- History
- Examination
- Medical decision making
- Counseling
- Coordination of care
- Nature of the presenting problem
- Time

The first three of these components (history, examination, and medical decision making, abbreviated H/E/MDM) are considered the key components in selecting a level of service. The next four components (counseling, coordination of care, nature of presenting problem, and time) are considered contributory components.

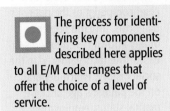 The process for identifying key components described here applies to all E/M code ranges that offer the choice of a level of service.

The example in the previous section indicated a code range of 99201–99205 with a detailed level of service (99203). The physician and/or coder determines the LOS by examining the documentation of the key components of E/M coding (H/E/MDM) and applying the E/M coding guidelines to select a code. For example, the guidelines state that a detailed LOS requires a detailed history, a detailed examination, and low MDM.

The information needed to determine the LOS appears in the code descriptions, provided in Tables 13.2 and 13.3.

Table 13.2 New Patient Codes

CODE	DESCRIPTION
99201	Problem-focused history, problem-focused exam, straightforward MDM
99202	Expanded problem-focused history, expanded problem-focused exam, straightforward MDM
99203	Detailed history, detailed exam, low MDM
99204	Comprehensive history, comprehensive exam, moderate MDM
99205	Comprehensive history, comprehensive exam, high MDM

Note that the three key component requirements for 99204 and 99205 differ only in the MDM.

Table 13.3 Established Patient Codes

CODE	DESCRIPTION
99211	No key components required (code is described later in this chapter)
99212	Problem-focused history, problem-focused exam, straightforward MDM
99213	Expanded problem-focused history, expanded problem-focused exam, low MDM (note the difference from 99202)
99214	Detailed history, detailed exam, moderate MDM (note the difference from 99203)
99215	Comprehensive history, comprehensive exam, high MDM

Step 1: Determine the History Level

The term *history* describes the information that patients communicate to the physician both to explain their illnesses, injuries, and/or symptoms and in response to the physician's questions. History is considered *subjective* information that is provided in the patient's own words. History consists of the history of present illness (HPI), a review of systems (ROS) and past, family, social history (PFSH). To determine the documented level of the history, the following information is required.

Required for problem-focused history:

- Chief complaint (CC)
- Brief *history of the present illness or problem*

Required for expanded problem-focused history:

- Chief complaint
- Brief *history of the present illness or problem*
- Problem-pertinent *system review*

Required for detailed history:

- Chief complaint
- Extended *history of present illness* (HPI) or problem
- Extended *system review* (ROS) (more than just problem pertinent)
- Pertinent **past history, family history,** and/or **social history** (PFSH) directly related to the patient's problem

Required for comprehensive history:

- Chief complaint
- Extended HPI or problem
- Review of all body systems (ROS)
- Complete past, family, and social history (PFSH)

> The third element of history is referred to as *PFSH*, for past, family, and social history. The patient's past history relates to the personal medical history. The family history reviews the medical events in the patient's family. It includes the health status or cause of death of parents, brothers and sisters, and children; specific diseases that are related to the patient's chief complaint or the patient's diagnosis; and the presence of any known hereditary diseases. The facts gathered in the social history, which depend on the patient's age, include marital status, employment, and other factors.

CHECKPOINT 13.2

What differentiates an expanded problem-focused history from a detailed history? List each element, and indicate whether it is different or the same. _____

Step 2: Determine the Examination Level

The term *examination* describes the information a physician collects from examining the patient. The examination is considered *objective*: It is not based on feelings or the patient's interpretation; it is based on factual findings. To determine the level of the examination, the following information is required.

Required for problem-focused (PF) examination:

- Limited exam of affected body area or organ system

Required for expanded problem-focused (EPF) examination:

- Limited exam of affected body area or organ system and other symptomatic or related organ systems

Required for detailed (DET) examination:

- Extended exam of affected body area or organ system and other symptomatic or related organ systems

Required for comprehensive (COM) examination:

- General multisystem exam or complete examination of a single organ system

Step 3: Determine the Medical Decision-Making Level

Medical decision making encompasses the complex process of establishing a diagnosis and determining how to treat or manage the diagnosed condition. Patients present to their physicians with symptoms. It is the physician's role to assess and evaluate those symptoms to determine the correct diagnosis and treatment.

> ■ **CASE SCENARIO**
> A patient presents with a 3-day history of redness in the left eye. There is no trauma or foreign body irritation. The patient also complains of itching and discharge from the left eye. There is no evidence of any changes in the patient's vision.

At this point the physician reviews the patient's history, examines the patient, and then makes a decision about what is wrong with the patient.

For medical decision making, CPT departs from the range of problem focused through comprehensive. Instead, the *level* of MDM can be straightforward, low complexity, moderate complexity, or high complexity. MDM rates how the physician puts all the patient-encounter information together to assess the patient's condition and to plan the treatment of that condition. MDM is often referred to as the *assessment and plan.*

To rate the level of MDM, three measurements are considered:

1. The number of diagnoses or management options
2. The amount of and/or complexity of medical records, tests, and other information (data)
3. The risk of complications, morbidity, and/or mortality (overall risk)

Each of the three measurements is assessed and then put into a level as follows:

Straightforward:

1. Minimal diagnoses or management options
2. Minimal or no data
3. Minimal risk

Low complexity:

1. Limited diagnoses or management options
2. Limited data
3. Low risk

Moderate complexity:

1. Multiple diagnoses or management options
2. Moderate data
3. Moderate risk

High complexity:

1. Extensive diagnoses or management options
2. Extensive data
3. High risk

Table 13.4 lays out the MDM measurements, with the type of decision making listed in the fourth column.

To assign one of the four levels level of MDM, coders will work with three scenarios. First, in the simplest scenario, all three measurements are at the same level. As indicated in Table 13.4, if all three measurements are at the same level, select the type of decision making shown in that row.

> **EXAMPLE**
> A limited number of diagnoses, a limited amount of data reviewed, and low risk equal *low-complexity decision making.*

Second, when two of the three measurements are at the same level and one is at a lower level, disregard the lowest measurement, and base the level of decision making on the remaining two.

> **EXAMPLE**
> Multiple diagnoses, limited data review, and moderate medical decision making equal *moderate complexity.* The lowest measure is disregarded, and the decision-making level is based on the remaining two levels.

Third, when all three measurements are at different levels, disregard the lowest measurement, and base the level of decision making on the remaining two measurements. In this scenario, the lowest of the remaining two measurements controls the level of medical decision making.

Table 13.4 Medical Decision Making

NUMBER OF DIAGNOSES OR MANAGEMENT OPTIONS	AMOUNT AND/OR COMPLEXITY OF DATA TO BE REVIEWED	RISK OF COMPLICATIONS AND/OR MORBIDITY OR MORTALITY	TYPE OF DECISION MAKING
Minimal	Minimal or none	Minimal	Straightforward
Limited	Limited	Low	Low complexity
Multiple	Moderate	Moderate	Moderate complexity
Extensive	Extensive	High	High complexity

EXAMPLE

Multiple diagnoses, extensive data review, and low risk equal *moderate complexity*. The lowest measure is disregarded, and the level of decision making is based on the lowest level of the remaining two measures.

The rule is that two of the three measurements must be at or above that particular level. This is usually phrased as "two of the three must meet or exceed that level."

EXAMPLE

After assessing the patient, the physician determines that there is a *limited* number of diagnoses, which puts a check mark in the low MDM row. The physician has evaluated a *minimal* amount of data, which puts a check mark in the straightforward MDM row, and the overall risk for this patient's problem is *low,* putting another check mark in the low MDM row. The level of MDM that is assigned is low, because the guideline is "two out of three."

Similarly, the number of diagnoses might be *multiple*, the amount of data might be *limited*, and the overall risk might be *high*. In this not-uncommon scenario, using the criterion of "meet or exceed two of the three elements," the level of MDM is moderate. In a case like this, the step-by-step process to assign an MDM level is as follows:

1. Analyze the MDM measurements, and record their levels:

    • Number of diagnoses is *multiple*: moderate MDM
    • Amount of data is *limited*: low MDM
    • Overall risk is *high*: high MDM

2. Drop the lowest measure of MDM, in this case the amount of data (low), and base the overall level of MDM on the remaining two measures using the criterion that the lower of the two measures controls the level of MDM. The MDM is moderate.

Continuing the example of the patient with a red eye:

■ CASE SCENARIO

After reviewing the patient's history and examining the patient, the physician determined that the patient had conjunctivitis of the left eye. The patient is to apply an over-the-counter ophthalmic solution twice a day for 1 week and also apply warm, moist compresses each morning.

The number of diagnoses or management options: *limited*
Amount and/or complexity of data: *none*
The risk of complications, morbidity, mortality: *low*
The MDM level: *low complexity*

INTERNET RESOURCES: Acronyms are important in medical documentation and particularly in E/M coding. Review the following sites for assistance in finding acronyms.
www.medilexicon.com
https://en.wikipedia.org/wiki/List_of_medical_abbreviations

Read the following cases and answer the questions.

The physician determines that there are multiple diagnoses, limited data, and low risk based on the review of the history and performance of the examination.

1. What is the level of MDM? _____

A patient who suffered a hip dislocation presents with leg and hip pain and chronic abdominal pain radiating into the chest. After obtaining the patient's history and performing an examination, the physician reviews an x-ray and blood work that was ordered and determines that the femur was injured in the course of treating the hip dislocation. The patient has been taking too much ibuprofen for the pain and now has gastroesophageal reflux. The physician prescribes physical therapy for the leg problem and medication for the reflux problem.

2. Assess the three measurements of MDM, and give the level of MDM. _____

In summary, follow these steps to select a level of service:

1. Identify the category and subcategory.
2. Review the guidelines for that category and subcategory.
3. Review the code descriptions specific to that category and subcategory.
4. Determine the extent of history documented.
5. Determine the extent of examination documented.
6. Determine the extent of medical decision making documented.
7. Select the appropriate code based on the three key components.

■ CASE SCENARIO

A new patient is being seen by a family practitioner. He mentions that he has begun to develop acne and is very self-conscious. He also has a rash on his leg. His physician obtains an expanded problem-focused history, an EPF exam, and straightforward MDM.

A coder can determine the LOS by using the instructions provided earlier as follows:

1. New patient, adult
2. Patient has not been seen within 3 years
3. Requires three of three key components
4. EPF history
5. EPF exam
6. Straightforward MDM
7. Code that meets the requirements:

   99202: EPF history
   99202: EPF exam
   99202: Straightforward MDM

Working With the Level of Service Requirements

To work with the LOS, coders need to know not only the three key components of E/M services but also which codes require all three key components and which require just two of the three key components. The list provided in Table 13.5 appears in the E/M guidelines in the CPT book and in each code descriptor in the E/M section.

For a code that requires all three key components, the key component at the lowest level controls the level of service. For example, if a physician examining a new patient documented a detailed history, a detailed exam, and straightforward medical decision making, the codes for each key component would be as follows:

For codes that require all three key components, the lowest key component controls the level that is assigned. In other words, the LOS can be no higher than the lowest key component.

Table 13.5 Determining LOS

THREE COMPONENTS	TWO OF THREE COMPONENTS
New patient: 99201–99205	Established patient: 99212–99215
Initial observation care: 99218–99220	
Initial hospital care: 99221–99223	Subsequent hospital care: 99231–99233
Consultations: 99241–99255	
Emergency department: 99281–99285	
Nursing facility initial: 99304–99306	Nursing facility subsequent: 99307–99310
Domiciliary new patient: 99324–99328	Domiciliary established patient: 99334–99337
Home new patient: 99341–99345	Home established patient: 99347–99350

EXAMPLES

99203: Detailed history.
99203: Detailed exam.
99202: Straightforward MDM.

The component at the lowest level—the one that controls the level of service—is MDM, so the coder would report 99202 as the LOS. For the service to have been coded as 99203, the MDM complexity level would have had to be low.

If a code requires only two of the three key components to be used in determining the level of service, disregard the lowest key component, and base the level of service on the remaining two key components, still following the rule that the lowest key component of the remaining two controls the level of service. If the physician documented a detailed history, a detailed exam, and straightforward MDM for an established patient, the codes for the key components would be:

EXAMPLES

99214: Detailed history.
99214: Detailed exam.
99212: Straightforward MDM.

The MDM level is disregarded because it is the lowest key component. Both of the remaining two key components are at the same level, so the service should be reported as 99214.

If, however, the three key components were at different levels for an established patient, the documentation might look like this:

EXAMPLES

99214: Detailed history.
99213: Expanded problem-focused exam.
99212: Straightforward MDM.

The MDM level is disregarded because it is the lowest key component. Of the remaining two key components, the lowest, the exam, controls the level of service, so the service should be reported as 99213.

CHECKPOINT 13.4

Determine the level of service in the following scenario using both new patient and established patient criteria.

Key Components	New Patient LOS	Established Patient LOS
Expanded problem-focused history	_____	_____
Detailed exam	_____	_____
Moderate MDM	_____	_____

The Contributory E/M Components

Counseling, coordination of care, and the nature of the presenting problem are considered *contributory* factors in E/M coding. While they are important, these services do not have to be provided at every patient encounter.

Counseling

The contributory component of counseling is a discussion with a patient and/or family about the following:

- Diagnostic results, impressions, and/or recommended diagnostic studies
- The prognosis
- The risks and benefits of management (treatment) options
- Instructions for management (treatment) and/or follow up
- The importance of compliance with chosen management (treatment) options
- Risk-factor reduction
- Patient and family education

Coordination of Care

The coordination of care component involves a physician's work to coordinate a patient's care with other providers or agencies. For example, a patient may need to be set up with nursing care at home or may need to see other providers for more specific care (for example, a surgeon or physical therapist), or laboratory studies may need to be arranged.

Nature of the Presenting Problem

The nature of the presenting problem is generally the reason for the patient's encounter with a physician. It can be a disease, a condition, an illness, an injury, a symptom, a sign, a finding, or a complaint. There are five types of presenting problems:

1. *Minimal:* The problem may not require the presence of a physician but is provided under a physician's supervision, such as a blood pressure check.
2. *Self-limited or minor:* The problem is transient, will not permanently alter a patient's health status, or has a good prognosis.
3. *Low severity:* The risk of becoming seriously ill (morbidity) without treatment is low; there is little or no risk of mortality without treatment.
4. *Moderate severity*: The risk of morbidity and/or mortality without treatment is moderate.
5. *High severity:* The risk of morbidity without treatment is high, and the risk of mortality without treatment is moderate.

Time

There are two measures of time in E/M coding: (1) face-to-face time, also referred to as *direct time*, and (2) unit/floortime. Direct time is associated with outpatient services and represents the time a physician spends with the patient obtaining the history, providing the examination, and discussing the findings and plan. Unit/floortime represents care provided to the patient in a facility setting (such as a hospital or nursing home) and includes care given at the bedside and services on the unit or floor where the patient is located, such as reviewing the patient's medical record, writing orders, or reviewing films or test results.

As a general guideline, neither face-to-face time nor unit/floortime should be considered a determining E/M component. Time is indicated in the code descriptors merely to represent averages or estimates of time associated with the levels of service. The one exception, however, is discussed in the following section.

Exception to the Key Component Rule: Using Time as the Determining Factor

Counseling and coordination of care are contributory components of E/M services. When one of them dominates (i.e., is more than 50% of) the physician–patient and/or physician–family encounter, time is the key or controlling factor in determining the level of service. The extent of the counseling and/or coordination of care must be documented in the medical record.

■ CASE SCENARIO

For more than a year, a patient has been treated by his nephrologist for kidney disease. At the current E/M encounter, the physician informs the patient that based on previous examinations, lab results, and diagnostic tests, kidney transplant surgery is inevitable and the patient's name is being placed on the transplant list. The patient is upset, and the physician spends

---

30 minutes of the 40-minute visit talking with the patient about the consequences, lifestyle impact, and family issues associated with transplant surgery.

Based on the physician's documentation

- The encounter involved a problem-focused history, a problem-focused exam, and high MDM.
- Based on the key components only, the reportable code would be 99212.
- Based on the facts that the visit totaled 40 minutes and that 30 minutes were spent in counseling, the reportable code would be 99215. Refer to the second paragraph under each E/M code's key components to find the time factor.

> ◼● The time for each E/M code is listed in the paragraphs below each code description.

CHECKPOINT 13.5

Read the following case and answer the questions.

A patient has been treated for diabetes for 4 years and was most recently seen 2 weeks ago. During today's visit, after reviewing lab results and examining the patient, the physician determines that the patient will have to start insulin treatment immediately. The patient is upset because her mother was severely affected by long-term insulin use. The physician discusses the effects of insulin and its impact on lifestyle and health. The exam is EPF, and the MDM is moderate. The physician spends 15 minutes of the 25-minute visit counseling the patient.

1. What is the correct established patient code for the scenario? _____

2. Explain how you determined that level of service. _____

Evaluation and Management Flowchart and Matrix

To apply the E/M selection process, coders need to be familiar with the major categories and subcategories of E/M coding, which are discussed in the remainder of this chapter. Pinpoint the Code 13.2 presents an E/M selection flowchart. Coders should refer also to the E/M matrix in Table 13.6 to review the most common E/M services.

PINPOINT THE CODE 13.2: Evaluation and Management

Step 1
Identify the patient as new or established.

↓

Step 2
Identify the place of service (office, hospital, or other).

↓

Step 3
Identify the patient's status (ill, critically ill, well visit, other).

↓

Step 4
Identify the type of service (initial care, subsequent care, prolonged care, standby, other).

↓

Step 5
Decide if E/M code is based on LOS or other.

Time-based codes: Determine documented time.
↓
Assign E/M code.

LOS-based codes: Determine whether three or two key components are required.
↓
Assign E/M code.

OFFICE OR OTHER OUTPATIENT SERVICES

99201–99205	New patient	Requires all three key components
99211–99215	Established patient	Requires two of three key components

Table 13.6 Key Component Requirements, 99201–99215

	HISTORY	EXAM	MDM
99201	PF	PF	Straightforward
99202	EPF	EPF	Straightforward
99203	DET	DET	Low
99204	COMP	COMP	Moderate
99205	COMP	COMP	High
99211	N/A	N/A	N/A
99212	PF	PF	Straightforward
99213	EPF	EPF	Low
99214	DET	DET	Moderate
99215	COMP	COMP	High

Office or other outpatient services E/M codes represent the services provided to evaluate and manage the care of new or established patients in the physician office or other outpatient facility, such as an emergency department or an ambulatory surgical center. Tables 13.6 and 13.7 provide information on the key component requirements for using these codes.

■ CASE SCENARIO

Ms. Jones recently moved to Detroit and has not yet established herself with a new physician. When her pancreatitis flares up, she makes an appointment with Dr. Abbot. Dr. Abbot obtains a detailed history, does a detailed examination, and, after his assessment of the patient's condition, provides low medical decision making. Dr. Abbot will report code 99203.

Table 13.7 E/M Code Selection Tool: Office Visits

CPT CODES	New Patients					Established Patients				
	99201 NP level 1	99202 NP level 2	99203 NP level 3	99204 NP level 4	99205 NP level 5	99211 EP level 1	99212 EP level 2	99213 EP level 3	99214 EP level 4	99215 EP level 5
Key Components										
History						Minimal				
Problem focused	Y						Y			
Expanded problem focused		Y						Y		
Detailed			Y						Y	
Comprehensive				Y	Y					Y
Examination						Minimal				
Problem focused	Y						Y			
Expanded problem focused		Y						Y		
Detailed			Y						Y	
Comprehensive				Y	Y					Y
Medical decision making						Minimal				
Straightforward	Y	Y					Y			
Low complexity			Y					Y		
Moderate complexity				Y					Y	
High complexity					Y					Y
Number of key components required	3	3	3	3	3	2	2	2	2	2

Professional Services and New or Established Patients

As part of the definition of new and established patients, the AMA has specified that professional services are face-to-face services. Why? Review the following example.

> ### ■ CASE SCENARIO
> A patient with recurrent chest pain is hospitalized by his internist, and electrocardiograms (ECGs) are taken. The hospital contracts with a private cardiologist to review all hospital ECGs. The cardiologist reports the correct CPT for the work of interpreting the tests, but has never seen the patient. This patient later makes an appointment to see this cardiologist—within 3 years of the hospital stay.

Because professional services are defined as face-to-face services, the cardiologist can report a new patient E/M code for the visit. If the definition did not specify a face-to-face service, the record would show that the cardiologist provided a service to the patient, and the E/M service would have to be reported as an established patient E/M code. This would not be appropriate because the cardiologist had not provided any type of E/M service to the patient and consequently does not know anything about him.

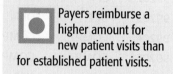 Payers reimburse a higher amount for new patient visits than for established patient visits.

To report the new patient codes 99201–99205, a physician's documentation must meet the criteria for all three key components for the level of service reported. To report the established patient codes 99212–99215, a physician's documentation must meet the criteria for two of the three key components for the level of service reported.

CHECKPOINT 13.6

Read the following case and answer the question.

A patient with long-term hypertension sees her internist. Her previous visit was 2 years ago, and the patient is concerned that her hypertension has escalated since her last visit. The history is detailed, the exam is detailed, and the medical decision making is low. The physician submits a claim for code 99213.

1. Is the claim correct? Explain your answer. _____

Documentation Guidelines

In 1992, the AMA first issued the evaluation and management codes presented in this chapter for determining the level of work associated with E/M services. Before this time, E/M coding was based on conflicting methodologies, for example, using time rather than clinical content to determine the level of service. Subsequently, to make the assignment of the new E/M codes more consistent, the AMA and the Health Care Financing Administration (HCFA; now the Centers for Medicare and Medicaid Services [CMS]) developed code selection guidelines that are now known as the 1995 Documentation Guidelines.

After the 1995 guidelines were in use, physicians from the various medical specialties requested a refinement of the guidelines to more appropriately reflect specialty E/M services. In 1997, the E/M guidelines were refined for single-specialty and multisystem exams. This refinement is referred to as the 1997 Documentation Guidelines. The accompanying Reimbursement Review provides a brief overview of the differences between the two sets of guidelines.

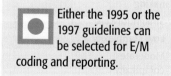 Either the 1995 or the 1997 guidelines can be selected for E/M coding and reporting.

Code 99211: The Exception

As defined in CPT, code 99211 is used for "the evaluation and management of an established patient, which may or may not require the presence of a physician. Usually, the presenting problem(s) are minimal. Typically, 5 minutes are spent performing or supervising these services."

Review both the 1995 general multisystem guidelines and the 1997 specialty-specific guidelines at the following website: www.cms.gov/Outreach-and-Education/Medicare-Learning-Network-MLN/MLNEdWebGuide/EMDOC.html.

Coders will note that no key components are listed as required, making it difficult to know when it is appropriate to report this code. As indicated in the description, a physician does not necessarily have to directly (face to face) provide the service, but the physician must *supervise* the service.

To report 99211, the encounter must be face to face, as follows:

- Do not use the code for telephone calls.
- The code may be used for a blood pressure check.
- The code may be used by a nurse providing a dressing change or removing sutures.
- The code may be used when a patient comes into the office to have a tuberculin test result read.

Some portion of an E/M service must be provided. The code may not be used for patients who come in to pick up prescriptions, nor may it be used when a nurse takes vital signs before the patient's visit with the physician, because those services are included in the physician visit. It also is inappropriate to use the code for services that are represented more accurately by other codes. For example, blood draw services should be billed with code 36415.

REIMBURSEMENT REVIEW

Brief Comparison of the 1995 Documentation Guidelines and the 1997 Documentation Guidelines

1995 GUIDELINES	1997 GUIDELINES
Original guidelines.	Developed in response to specialty physicians' concerns that the 1995 guidelines were inappropriate for their services.

History and medical decision-making criteria are the same for both the 1995 and the 1997 guidelines. The examination criteria differentiate the two sets of guidelines.

1995 EXAM REQUIREMENTS	1997 GENERAL MULTISYSTEM EXAM REQUIREMENTS
Problem Focused	**Problem Focused**
Limited exam of affected body area or organ system	One to five elements identified by a bullet
Expanded Problem Focused	**Expanded Problem Focused**
Limited exam of affected body area or organ system and any other symptomatic or related body area(s)	At least six elements identified by a bullet
Detailed	**Detailed**
Extended exam of affected body area(s) or organ system(s) and any other symptomatic or related body area(s) or organ system(s)	At least two elements identified by a bullet from each of six areas or systems, or at least 12 elements identified by a bullet in two or more areas or systems
Comprehensive	**Comprehensive**
General multisystem exam or complete examination of a single organ system and other symptomatic or related area(s) or system(s)	At least two elements identified by a bullet from each of nine areas or systems

The explanations under the printed 1997 guidelines make reference to bullets, or bulleted items.

Read the following case and answer the questions.

An internal medicine physician sees a patient for stomach pain. The physician documents a brief history and low medical decision making. The physician examines the gastrointestinal system, the respiratory system, and the cardiovascular system.

1. Based on the 1995 guidelines, which system is the symptomatic system and which are the related systems? _____

2. What is the level of service for the exam? _____

HOSPITAL OBSERVATION SERVICES

99217	Observation care discharge	
99218–99220	Initial observation care	Requires all three key components
99224-99226	Subsequent observation care	Requires two of three key components

Hospital observation codes represent the E/M services provided to patients who are in outpatient observation status at the hospital but who have *not* gone through the hospital admission process. If a patient is in another place of service for observation, such as a clinic or a practice office, these codes cannot be reported. Observation care is initiated because the patient needs further evaluation to determine the necessity for additional treatment or admission to the hospital. The physician who placed the patient in observation status is responsible for the patient during the observation period.

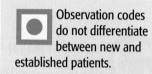

Observation codes do not differentiate between new and established patients.

■ CASE SCENARIO

A physician sees an established patient in the office for stomach pain and rectal bleeding. On examination the physician is not sure the patient is well enough to be at home and sends the patient to the hospital for observation. Later in the day, the physician will see the patient at the hospital to determine whether the patient needs to be admitted, to stay under observation, or to be discharged.

Observation Care Discharge

Code 99217 represents the services provided when a physician discharges a patient from observation care. These services include final examination of the patient, discussion of the hospital stay, instructions for continuing care, and preparation of discharge records.

Initial Observation Care

As shown in Pinpoint the Code 13.3, an observation care code assignment flowchart, codes 99218, 99219, and 99220 represent the initiation of outpatient hospital observation status, the supervision of the care plan for observation, and the performance of required periodic assessments of the patient while in observation care. Level of service is determined according to the criteria in Table 13.8.

Table 13.8 Key Component Requirements, 99218–99220

CODE	HISTORY	EXAM	MDM
99218	DET or COMP	DET or COMP	Straightforward or low
99219	COMP	COMP	Moderate
99220	COMP	COMP	High

> • If a patient is sent for and discharged from observation care on the same day, do not report the observation care codes. Instead, use same-day admission and discharge codes 99234–99236.
> • Do not use the observation care codes to report postoperative recovery services for any surgery that has a specified postoperative period. The postoperative recovery visits are part of the surgical package and are not separately reportable.

Observation status is usually initiated in the physician office or the ED. The patient has not been admitted to the hospital, but has instead been sent to or admitted to observation status at the hospital. The patient does not have to be in a specific observation room or area in order for these codes to be used.

Subsequent Observation Care

Subsequent observation care includes reviewing the medical record, the results of diagnostic studies, and changes in the patient's status related to history, physical condition, and the patient's response to management (Table 13.9). It is important to note that these codes are out of numerical sequence and CPT indicates that status with the pound symbol (#) to the left of the CPT code.

Roll-Up Rule

Observation care codes provide an example of the roll-up rule in coding for E/M services. According to the roll-up rule, if a patient is seen in the office by the physician and is then sent to the hospital for observation on the same day, the only reportable code is an initial observation care code. That code represents all the accumulated services provided to the patient on that day in any location by that physician. These codes start at higher levels of service than most of the E/M codes for exactly that reason.

> **■ CASE SCENARIO**
> A patient is seen in the physician office for chest pain. The physician is not certain that the patient is well enough to go home, nor is he ill enough to be admitted to the hospital. The patient is sent to the hospital for observation. The physician sees the patient at the hospital later in the day and evaluates his condition, deciding to keep the patient under observation care until the next day. The combined documentation from the office visit and observation care indicates a comprehensive history, a comprehensive examination, and moderate medical decision making. In effect, the services provided in the office *roll up* into the observation codes.

Table 13.9 Key Component Requirements, 99224–99226

CODE	HISTORY	EXAM	MDM
99224	PF	PF	Straightforward or low
99225	EPF	EPF	Moderate
99226	DET	DET	High

PINPOINT THE CODE 13.3: Observation Care

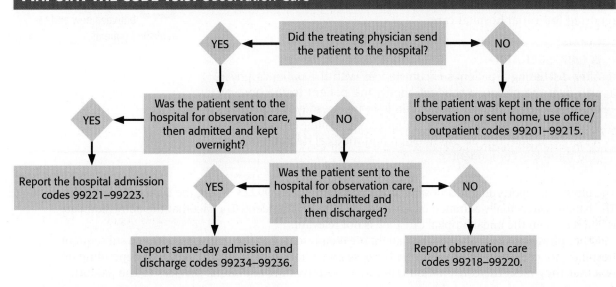

The initial observation care code, 99219, is assigned for the services provided to the patient on the first day. If the patient is discharged from observation care on the second day, the observation care discharge code, 99217, is assigned for that day.

If, after observing the patient at the hospital, the physician determines that he should be admitted to the hospital, all E/M services provided to the patient on the first day will *roll up* into the codes for initial hospital care, 99221–99223, which are covered in the next section.

CHECKPOINT 13.8

Read the following case and answer the question.

A patient sees her cardiologist for follow up of her hypertension and coronary artery disease. The patient reports intermittent chest pain and some dizziness. Based on the patient's symptoms, the cardiologist is not comfortable sending the patient home, but, based on the examination and blood work, the patient's condition is not severe enough for admission to the hospital. The physician sends the patient to the hospital for observation and then subsequently sees the patient later at the hospital in observation and reevaluates her. The cardiologist reports a code from the 99212–99215 category and another code from the 99218–99220 category of codes.

1. Have the correct code categories been used? Explain your answer. _____

HOSPITAL INPATIENT SERVICES

99221–99223	Initial hospital care	Requires all three key components
99231–99233	Subsequent hospital care	Requires two of three key components
99234–99236	Same-day admission and discharge	Requires all three key components
99238–99239	Hospital discharge services	Time based

Hospital inpatient services codes represent E/M services to patients who are admitted to the hospital and are seen by physicians during their hospital stays.

Initial Hospital Care

Initial hospital care codes 99221, 99222, and 99223 (Table 13.10) are used to report the *first* hospital inpatient encounter by the admitting physician. Only the admitting physician can report these codes.

In using these codes, the date of service (DOS) is the date that service is provided, not the date of admission if they differ. This may seem redundant, but there is often confusion about which date should be reported for initial hospital care.

The initial hospital care codes 99221–99223 are reported if the patient is seen in a physician's office and is subsequently admitted to the hospital by the same physician on the same day.

Inpatient service codes do not differentiate between new and established patients.

■ CASE SCENARIO
After discussing a patient's circumstances with the patient's physician over the phone, a resident admits the patient to the hospital on Tuesday evening. The date of admission is Tuesday. The patient's physician visits his patient on Wednesday morning and obtains a history and performs an examination and medical decision making (the three key components).

The physician reports an initial hospital care code from 99221–99223, listing the DOS as Wednesday. The patient was actually admitted on Tuesday evening by a resident. The fact that the admission date is different from the initial hospital care date is not relevant.

Other physicians may also see the patient on Wednesday, but they must use either a subsequent hospital care code (99231–99233) or a hospital consultation code (99251–99255), depending on whether they meet the consultation criteria or are providing additional services to the patient.

Table 13.10 Key Component Requirements, 99221–99233

CODE	HISTORY	EXAM	MDM
99221	DET or COMP	DET or COMP	Straightforward
99222	COMP	COMP	Moderate
99223	COMP	COMP	High
99231	PF	PF	Straightforward or low
99232	EPF	EPF	Moderate
99233	DET	DET	High

Subsequent Hospital Care

Subsequent hospital care codes 99231, 99232, and 99233 (see Table 13.10) are used to report visits by the admitting physician to the patient after the first day. Other physicians may also use these codes for their visits to the patient during a hospital stay.

■ CASE SCENARIO
A patient is admitted by the endocrinologist for uncontrolled diabetes. After the initial hospital care day, it is determined that the patient also needs to be followed for cardiac disease, and the patient's cardiologist sees the patient. Both the endocrinologist and the cardiologist will report subsequent hospital care codes.

Same-Day Admission and Discharge

The codes 99234, 99235, and 99236 represent the services provided to patients who are in observation care or have been admitted to the hospital *and* are discharged on the same date as they were admitted and received the services. These codes require all three key components to select a level of service (Table 13.11).

Table 13.11 Key Component Requirements, 99234–99236

CODE	HISTORY	EXAM	MDM
99234	DET or COMP	DET or COMP	Straightforward or low
99235	COMP	COMP	Moderate
99236	COMP	COMP	High

The roll-up rule applies to same-day services.

Physicians must document time if they intend to report 99239. Without that documentation, the services are reported using 99238.

Hospital Discharge Services

Hospital discharge services are the services provided by the admitting or attending physician on the date of discharge. The codes represent the total amount of time spent by the physician for the patient's final discharge, whether the time is continuous or not. The codes are time based and do not have key component requirements:

99238: 30 minutes or less
99239: More than 30 minutes

The services include final examination of the patient, discussion of the hospital stay, instructions for continuing care with the patient and/or other caregivers, and preparation of discharge records, prescriptions, and referral forms.

Read the following case and answer the question.

A patient is seen in her physician's office, is sent to the hospital for observation, and is discharged from observation care on the same day.

1. What code range would be reported? Explain your answer. _____

CONSULTATIONS

99241–99245	Office/outpatient	Requires all three key components
99251–99255	Hospital	Requires all three key components

Consultation codes (Table 13.12) represent the services of a physician who has been asked to give an opinion or advice on a patient (the consulting physician). The request comes from another physician or another appropriate source, such as a physician's assistant, a nurse-practitioner, a doctor of chiropractic, a physical therapist, an occupational therapist, a speech-language therapist, a psychologist, a social worker, a lawyer, or an insurance company.

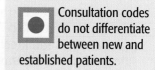 Consultation codes do not differentiate between new and established patients.

■ CASE SCENARIO

A patient has had ongoing chest pain for 3 months. Her family practitioner cannot determine the cause of the pain and is concerned that it may be caused by a cardiac condition that is not appearing on the ECG or other tests. He indicates that the patient should see a cardiologist for an opinion. The cardiologist will report the office consultation codes.

If the family practitioner had decided that the chest pain was cardiac related and had referred his patient to the cardiologist for care, rather than for an opinion, the cardiologist would report the new patient codes 99201–99205 in place of the consultation codes.

Table 13.12 Key Component Requirements, 99241–99255

CODE	HISTORY	EXAM	MDM
Office Consults			
99241	PF	PF	Straightforward
99242	EPF	EPF	Straightforward
99243	DET	DET	Low
99244	COMP	COMP	Moderate
99245	COMP	COMP	High
Hospital Consults			
99251	PF	PF	Straightforward
99252	EPF	EPF	Straightforward
99253	DET	DET	Low
99254	COMP	COMP	Moderate
99255	COMP	COMP	High

Criteria for Coding a Consultation

The following criteria are required for coding a consultation:

- The patient encounter is for an opinion or advice about a specific problem.
- The request is made by a physician or another appropriate source.
- The requesting physician or other appropriate source retains responsibility for managing the care of the patient at the time of the consultation.
- The consultant may initiate diagnostic and/or therapeutic services (for example, a cardiologist may schedule a stress test).
- The written or verbal request for the consultation is documented in the patient's medical record. (Both the physician requesting the consultation and the consulting physician should document the consultation request in the patient's chart.)

- The consultant's findings are in writing and are sent to the requesting physician. For outpatient consultations, this means a letter to the requesting physician. For inpatient consultations, this means a note in the patient's chart.

If, after the initial consultation in the office, the patient is again seen by the consulting physician, that physician will report a code from the 99211–99215 E/M codes for office or outpatient services.

If, after the initial consultation in the hospital, the patient is again seen by the consultant, the consultant will report 99231–99233 E/M codes for subsequent hospital care.

If a consultation is requested by the patient and/or family member, the consultant must use either a new patient code from 99201–99205 or an established patient code from 99211–99215 for the office or outpatient setting, or a subsequent hospital care code from 99231–99233 in the hospital setting.

Referral or Consultation

A consultation is reimbursed at a higher rate than a new patient visit. For this reason, payers demand documentation that supports assigning a consultation code. Distinguishing between a new patient referral and a consultation is problematic for most physicians and coders. Under a referral, the care of the patient is passed by the referring physician to the provider to whom he or she is referred. In contrast, consultants provide an opinion and then return the patient to the requesting doctor's care.

The decision rests with the intention of the requesting physician. Is the requesting physician asking for an opinion about a patient's problem, or is the requesting physician turning the patient over to a new physician to take care of the problem? Often, the requesting physician's intention is not known when the appointment is made. Physicians often say to their patients, "I want you to see this cardiologist so we can get a handle on what's going on." When the patient makes the appointment, his or her status is not clear. Because the second physician must have documentation to support the use of the consultation code, that physician needs to be clear on what service is performed. Often, the two physicians have discussed the patient on the phone, and it is clear that the patient is to be seen in consultation, not as a new patient, but documentation is the key.

Coders may want to use a chart to assist in the determination of whether a patient is being seen as a new patient on referral or for consultation (Table 13.13). Pinpoint The Code 13.4, a flowchart for consultations, is a useful tool.

Table 13.13 Referral Versus Consultation

CONSULTATION	REFERRAL OF A NEW PATIENT
A patient with unresolved lethargy and stomach pain is sent to a gastroenterologist for an opinion on treatment and/or diagnosis.	The internist determines the problem and sends the patient to a gastroenterologist for care of the problem.
The gastroenterologist renders an opinion on the patient's diagnosis after doing tests in the office, prescribes medication, and sends a letter to the internist giving her opinion and advice. The patient's care is still in the hands of the internist.	Gastroenterologist takes over the treatment and care of the patient.

Myths

Several myths about consultation codes cause confusion for physicians and coders. The following are the most prevalent false assumptions:

- A consultant cannot bill a consultation if he or she provides treatment during the visit.
- A physician cannot request a consultation from another physician in the same group.
- A nonphysician practitioner cannot request a consultation.
- If the diagnosis is known, a consultation cannot be reported.
- Consultation codes cannot be used for established patients.

It is important for both physicians and coders to understand these "myths" because they can cause a loss of reimbursement for services that should be coded as consultations.

Preoperative Consultations

Preoperative consultations are a particular type of consultation service. For example, a patient scheduled for surgery may require preoperative clearance before the surgery is performed. Commonly, a surgeon will send the patient to an internist, cardiologist, or other specialist, depending on the planned surgery and the underlying condition that needs evaluation. When a surgeon sends the patient to another physician for preoperative evaluation and clearance, the stage is set for a consultation service. The consultant will see the patient for evaluation before surgery and will provide the surgeon with an opinion about the patient's condition and ability to withstand the surgical procedure, fulfilling the requirement for the three Rs.

> Think of the three Rs when determining whether to use a consultation code: request, render, and respond. These three words summarize the consultation criteria: a request from a physician, a rendering of the service to the patient, and a response by the consultant to the requesting physician.

PINPOINT THE CODE 13.4: Consultation

Did a physician or other appropriate source refer the patient?
- **NO** → Report either the new patient codes 99201–99205 or established patient codes 99211–99215 as appropriate.
- **YES** → Did the referring physician or other appropriate source request opinion or advice on the patient's problem?
  - **NO** → Patient was referred for care of the problem; report new patient codes.
  - **YES** → Did the physician who provided the opinion or advice send a written response to the requesting physician?
    - **NO** → Consultation codes cannot be reported.
    - **YES** → Did the consulting physician document the consultation request in the patient's medical record?
      - **YES** → Report consultation codes.
      - **NO** → Report new patient codes.

CPT © 2017 American Medical Association, All Rights Reserved.

Clinical pathology consultations requested by the attending physician that do not involve the pathologist's examination of the patient are coded in the Pathology and Laboratory section, CPT codes 80500 and 80502. An interpretation of clinically abnormal findings and a written report are required.

■ **CASE SCENARIO**

After performing a cardiac exam for an established patient who is diabetic and hypertensive, the internist sends the patient to a cardiologist. A week later, after performing several tests, the cardiologist determines that the patient needs an angioplasty to clear a blockage in his coronary artery. The cardiologist asks the internist to see the patient for preoperative clearance for surgery. The internist sees the patient, updates a history on the patient, examines him, and determines whether he can proceed with surgery. The internist sends his findings to the cardiologist.

Is this case scenario a consultation for the internist or an established patient visit? To answer, review the following points:

Did the cardiologist ask for the internist's opinion about whether to proceed with the angioplasty procedure?

Did the internist provide the key components?

Did the internist send her findings to the cardiologist?

Does the fact that the patient is already an established patient with the internist mean that a consultation cannot be provided?

Because the answer to all of these questions but the last is yes, the internist provided a preoperative consultation and may report a code from the range 99241–99245.

Medicare's Revisions to Consultation Services

As of 2010, the consultation codes 99241–99255 were no longer recognized for Medicare Part B payment. In place of the consultation codes, CMS increased the work relative value units (RVUs) for new and established office visits and for initial hospital and initial nursing facility visits. Based on the patient's status as new or established in the office/outpatient setting, physicians report codes 99201–99205 or 99212–99215 in place of the consultation codes. In the hospital setting, physicians report the initial hospital care codes 99221–99223 or the subsequent hospital care codes 99231–99233. This information can be found in Medicare's *MLN Matters*, article number MM6740.

Medicare also clarified that the documentation requirements associated with the consultation codes will not be required; however, conventional medical practice indicates that when a physician refers a patient to another physician, the physician accepting the referral should document the request to provide an evaluation for the patient. The same physician should continue to follow appropriate medical documentation standards and communicate the results of an evaluation to the requesting physician.

In an office/outpatient consultation scenario, the consulting physician should not report from the code range 99241–99245. To report this service to Medicare, the consultant should use code range 99201–99205 if the patient is a new patient to the consultant, or code range 99212–99215 if the patient is an established patient to the consultant.

■ **CASE SCENARIO**

A patient has had right leg pain for 2 months and his internist has been unable to resolve the problem. The internist has the patient see an orthopedist for the orthopedist's opinion on what is causing the leg pain and how to treat it. The orthopedist provides a detailed history, detailed examination, and moderate medical decision making. The consultation code would be 99243. The patient has Medicare and the services must be billed according to Medicare's guidelines. The patient is a new patient to the orthopedist and the orthopedist will report code 99203.

Note that the codes 99243 and 99203 require detailed history, detailed exam, and low medical decision making. The example indicates moderate medical decision making, which is a higher level (99244, 99204). These codes require that all three key components be at the levels indicated in the code description; if one key component is at a higher level, it does not change the code selection. Remember, the lowest key component controls the level of service—the coder must report 99243 or 99203.

AI Modifier

In the hospital setting, the attending physician would add the AI modifier to the initial and subsequent hospital care codes 99221–99223/99231–99233 to identify his or her status as the attending physician of record. This clarifies that other physicians using the initial and subsequent hospital care codes instead of the consultation codes (as required by Medicare) are not the attending physician.

■ CASE SCENARIO

A patient is admitted to the hospital on Tuesday by his endocrinologist due to the patient's uncontrolled diabetes. On that same day, the endocrinologist requests a cardiology consultation because of the patient's chest pain and shortness of breath. Based on Medicare's guidelines for consultation coding and the documentation key components, both physicians will report the code range 99221–99223. The endocrinologist will use the AI modifier to identify his status as the admitting physician when reporting his services.

CHECKPOINT 13.10

Are the following cases correctly described as consultations? (Disregard Medicare guidelines.)

1. A family physician has been treating a patient with diabetes and is concerned that the patient may develop diabetic retinopathy. The patient is sent to an ophthalmologist for his opinion. The ophthalmologist examines the patient and sends an opinion on the potential for diabetic retinopathy to the family physician. _____

2. A patient presents with urinary difficulties, and his physician is concerned that the problem may be related to an enlarged prostate. The internist sends the patient to a urologist for an opinion on the cause of the urinary problem and to determine whether the patient is a candidate for surgery. The urologist examines the patient and sends his findings in writing to the internist. _____

3. A patient goes to the ED with severe leg pain. He is seen and evaluated by the ED physician, who suspects muscle deterioration that cannot be explained. The ED physician recommends that the patient see an orthopedist as soon as possible. The patient is able to get an appointment the next day with an orthopedist. _____

4. In case 3, if the orthopedist had seen the patient at the ED and admitted the patient to the hospital, should the consultation code or the admission code be billed? Can both be billed? _____

EMERGENCY DEPARTMENT SERVICES

99281–99285	New or established patient	Requires all three key components
99288	Other emergency services	

Emergency department codes 99281–99285 represent services provided in the ED. CPT specifically defines an emergency department as "an organized hospital-based facility for the provision of unscheduled episodic services to patients who present for immediate medical attention. The facility must be available 24 hours a day." The American College of Emergency Physicians defines emergency services as the following:

Those health care services provided in a hospital emergency department to treat medical conditions of acute onset and sufficient severity that would lead a prudent lay person possessing an average knowledge of medicine and health care to believe that urgent medical care is required to reduce the level of pain, prevent the deterioration of one's condition, and prevent disability and/or death. (American College of Emergency Physicians. Definition of an emergency service. *Ann Emerg Med.* 1991;23:1397)

ED codes have five levels of service; selection of a level requires all three key components (Table 13.14). No time factor is associated with these codes. Generally, ED services are related to unexpected health issues or events that call for prompt, if not immediate, medical attention. ED codes do not differentiate between new and established patients.

Criteria

Emergency department codes are normally reported by the physicians who are assigned to the ED. Other physicians are not precluded from using the ED codes, but they must be aware of the circumstances that will prevent them from doing so.

■ CASE SCENARIO
A patient is brought to the ED for evaluation of his injuries after a motor vehicle accident. The ED physician obtains a history, performs an examination, and determines that the patient may have internal bleeding in the abdomen. A general surgeon is then asked to see the patient.

Table 13.14 Key Component Requirements, 99281–99285

CODE	HISTORY	EXAM	MDM
99281	PF	PF	Straightforward
99282	EPF	EPF	Low
99283	EPF	EPF	Moderate
99284	DET	DET	Moderate
99285	COMP	COMP	High

In this case scenario, the ED physician will report one of the ED codes (99281–99285) for his evaluation of the patient. The general surgeon, depending on the circumstances, will report either an office/outpatient consultation code (99241–99245) or an office/outpatient visit code (99212–99215). Because the ED physician provided E/M services to the patient, the general surgeon would not use the same ED codes.

ED codes are not reported for emergency conditions in the office or other outpatient areas. The codes are based on services performed in the specific location of an ED, not just on the patient's condition.

Physicians providing critical care (discussed in the next section) in the ED may report both the ED and the critical care codes, appending modifier –25 to the critical care code. Note that this is an exception to the roll-up rule.

Physician Direction of Emergency Medical Systems

Code 99288 represents the services of a physician located in the hospital ED or in the critical care department. This physician, who is in two-way voice communication with ambulance or rescue personnel who are *outside* the hospital, directs the ambulance or rescue personnel in providing medical procedures, including but not limited to the following:

- Telemetry of cardiac rhythm
- Cardiac and/or pulmonary resuscitation
- Endotracheal or esophageal airway intubation
- Administration of intravenous fluids
- Administration of intramuscular, intratracheal, or subcutaneous drugs
- Electrical conversion of arrhythmia

It is important to note that Physician Direction of Emergency Medical Systems is not a face-to-face service, it is a voice communication service. The critical care services in the next section are initially face-to-face services that also incorporate non–face-to-face services.

CRITICAL CARE SERVICES

| 99291–+99292 | Critical care services | Time based |

Critical care is the provision of medical care to a critically ill or critically injured patient. Medical care qualifies as critical care only if *both* the illness or injury *and* the treatment being provided meet the critical care requirements. Critical illness or injury impairs one or more vital organ systems, causing a high probability of imminent or life-threatening deterioration in a patient's condition.

Critical care involves high-complexity decision making to assess, manipulate, and support vital system functions, treatment of single or multiple vital organ system failure, and/or prevention of further life-threatening deterioration of a patient's condition. Examples of vital organ system failure include but are not limited to the following:

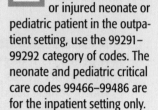

Remember that an add-on code (+) is never reported without its parent code.

- Central nervous system
- Circulatory system
- Renal system
- Hepatic system
- Metabolic system
- Respiratory system
- Shock

Critical care service codes are as follows:

99291: Critical care evaluation and management, first 30 to 74 minutes
+99292: Critical care evaluation and management, each additional 30 minutes

To code for critical care services, it is important to carefully review the extensive guidelines associated with these services. Critical care has its specific definition and included services as well as defined time calculation criteria. The services included in critical care are as follows:

If critical care is provided to a critically ill or injured neonate or pediatric patient in the outpatient setting, use the 99291–99292 category of codes. The neonate and pediatric critical care codes 99466–99486 are for the inpatient setting only.

- Interpretation of cardiac output measurements (93561, 93562)
- Chest X-rays (71045, 71046)
- Pulse oximetry (94760–94762)
- Blood gases (82800–82930)
- Information stored in computers (e.g., ECGs, blood pressures, hematologic data—99090)
- Gastric intubation (43752, 43753)
- Temporary transcutaneous pacing (92953)
- Ventilator management (94002–94004, 94660, 94662)
- Vascular access procedures (36000, 36410, 36415, 36591, 36600)

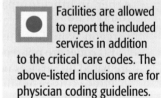

Facilities are allowed to report the included services in addition to the critical care codes. The above-listed inclusions are for physician coding guidelines.

Any services not in the preceding list may be reported in addition to the critical care codes.

Criteria for Critical Care

The criteria for selection are as follows:

- Critical care may be provided on multiple days, even if no changes are made in the treatment rendered, provided that the patient's condition continues to require critical care.
- Critical care codes reflect the total amount of time spent by the physician in providing critical care, even if the time spent is not continuous.
- The physician must devote full attention to the patient and cannot provide services to other patients during the same time period.
- Critical care may be provided in any setting; the patient does not have to be in a specific critical care unit of the hospital. Location does not define critical care services.
- The fact that a patient is in some type of critical care unit does not mean that services are critical care services. Physicians may provide routine care in a critical care unit, in which case they would report the subsequent hospital care codes.

- Services not listed are separately reportable. Examples include bronchoscopy, Swan-Ganz catheter placement, and cardiopulmonary resuscitation.
- Physicians may report other E/M codes in addition to the critical care codes. This is another exception to the roll-up rule.

> **■ CASE SCENARIO**
> A physician sees a patient with heart problems for follow-up care (99231–99233) in the morning. Later in the day, the patient goes into complete heart block, and the physician is called in to stabilize and treat the patient, providing critical care. Both the subsequent hospital care code and the critical care code can be reported using modifier –25 on the critical care codes.

Physician Work Time for Critical Care

Time must be documented to qualify for reporting critical care; doing so is an essential requirement. The following physician work may be included in reporting critical care:

- Caring for the patient at the bedside
- Reviewing test results or studies on the unit or floor
- Discussing the patient's care with other medical staff
- Documenting critical care services in the medical record
- Documenting the patient's clinical condition (an essential requirement)
- Discussing care directly related to the management of the patient on the unit or floor with family members or other decision makers of a patient who cannot participate in discussions

The following physician work *may not* be included in reporting critical care:

- Work that occurs outside the unit or off the floor
- Unrelated work or work that does not directly contribute to the patient's critical care treatment
- Services that are separately reportable from critical care (see above)
- Provision of critical care services that takes less than 30 minutes (use the subsequent hospital care codes 99231–99233 instead)

EXAMPLE

The physician spends 1 hour 10 minutes providing critical care at the patient's bedside. He also spends 20 minutes reviewing films in the radiology department on a separate floor and then 15 minutes documenting the care he provided. The physician would report 99291 and 99292 for 1 hour 25 minutes of critical care. The 20 minutes in the radiology department is not reported as critical care because the physician is not immediately available to the patient.

How to Calculate Critical Care Time

Code 99291 represents the first 30 to 60 minutes. Code 99291 represents the first 30 to 60 minutes and 99292 represents additional time. According to the 15-minute rule, however, the time spent after the first hour must exceed 14 minutes before 99292 can be reported. As a result, code 99291 is used for the first 74 minutes. Code 99292 represents the extra 30-minute block of time beyond the first 74 minutes, up to 104 minutes (99291 and 99292). If the care exceeds 104 minutes, then multiples of code 99292 are reported.

For example, if the physician spent 65 minutes providing critical care, report 99291 because the extra 5 minutes did not meet the 15-minute rule. If the physician spent 80 minutes, report 99291 and 99292 for the additional 20 minutes. The extra time invoked the 15-minute rule. If the physician spent 2 hours providing critical care, report 99291 for the first 60 minutes, and 99292 × 2 for the additional 60 minutes.

TIME SPENT	DESCRIPTION	CODE
30–74 minutes	First 30 minutes through first hour plus 14 minutes	99291
75–104 minutes	First hour plus 14 minutes through additional half hour	99291, 99292
105–134 minutes	First hour and a half plus 14 minutes through additional half hour	99291, 99292 × 2

Critical Care Documentation. When a patient is admitted to a cardiac care unit (CCU), such as for respiratory failure after an acute myocardial infarction with possible renal failure, the physician does a review of systems (ROS) and a medical history (as obtainable). The three key components (H/E/MDM) are not critical care code requirements, so the physician's documentation must focus on the details of clinically appropriate services. The physician is likely to document the following:

- Neurological status
- Peripheral pulses
- Skin examination
- Heart and lung examination
- ECG interpretation
- Cardiac enzymes
- Respiratory examination
- Ventilation management
- Lab results
- Gastrointestinal system examination
- Physician's assessment and plan

CHECKPOINT 13.11

Read the following cases and answer the questions.

1. The physician spent 1 hour and 10 minutes at the patient's bedside providing critical care. He also spent 20 minutes reviewing films on the unit and documenting the care he provided. What code(s) would the physician report?_____

2. In the above case, the physician also performed cardiopulmonary resuscitation (CPR) just prior to the 1 hour and 10 minutes of critical care. Can the physician report the CPR in addition to the critical care? _____

NURSING FACILITY SERVICES

99304–99306	Initial nursing facility care, per day	Requires all three key components
99307–99310	Subsequent nursing facility care, per day	Requires two of three key components
99315–99316	Nursing facility discharge services	Time based
99318	Other nursing facility services	Requires all three key components

E/M codes for nursing facilities, which are organized like other IP codes, are reported for the evaluation and management of patients in nursing facilities, such as a skilled nursing facility (SNF), an intermediate care facility (ICF), or a long-term care facility (LTCF). They are also used for patients in a psychiatric residential treatment center that provides 24-hour group living and that has been therapeutically planned and is professionally staffed. Initial and subsequent nursing facility care codes do not differentiate between new and established patients. Table 13.15 shows the key component requirements for these E/M codes.

Physicians who report the nursing facility codes have a central role in ensuring that all residents receive thorough assessments and that medical plans of care for them have been instituted or revised. Nursing facilities are required to use resident assessment instruments (RAIs), which include the minimum data set (MDS) and resident assessment protocols (RAPs). The MDS is the primary screening and assessment tool, and the RAPs provide identification of potential problems and guidelines for follow-up assessments.

Table 13.15 Key Component Requirements, 99304–99318

CODE	HISTORY	EXAM	MDM
99304	DET or COMP	DET or COMP	Straightforward or low
99305	COMP	COMP	Moderate
99306	COMP	COMP	High
99307	PFPF	Straightforward	
99308	EPF	EPF	Low
99309	DET	DET	Moderate
99310	COMP	COMP	High
99315, 99316	Guidelines for these discharge codes are consistent with those for the hospital discharge services codes 99238 and 99239.		
99318	Represents the annual nursing facility assessment service and is not reported in addition to initial or subsequent nursing facility care codes 99304–99316. The annual assessment is a separate service.		

The roll-up rule applies to these codes with one exception. If the patient was discharged from a hospital (99238 or 99239) or from observation care (99217) on the same date as admission to the nursing facility, both services are separately reportable. Nursing facility codes are per-day codes. The subsequent nursing facility care codes 99307–99310 always include reviewing the results of diagnostic studies and changes in the patient's status.

According to the May 2002 *CPT Assistant*, the nursing home discharge codes can also be used to report services when a physician must pronounce a patient's death as long as the physician performs any of the discharge criteria. The November 2009 *CPT Assistant* newsletter further clarified this for hospital discharge services: "The hospital discharge services codes may be used to report discharge services to patients who die during the hospital stay. The attending physician may be needed to perform the final examination of the patient (to pronounce the patient's death), discuss the hospital stay with family members or others, and prepare the discharge records (such as the discharge summary for the hospital record). However, if the physician is not the discharging physician, there is no CPT code for reviewing the patient's medical record, selecting and preparing the death summary. The selection of the appropriate hospital discharge services code (99238 or 99239) is based on the unit/floor time, which includes establishing and/or reviewing the patient's chart, examining the patient, writing notes and communicating with other professionals and the patient's family. It is important to note, therefore, that there must be unit/floor time, i.e., completion of forms/records in the medical records department or completion of a death certificate in the office is not reported as a discharge service." The *CPT Assistant* newsletter for May 2002 stipulated these same criteria for nursing home discharge.

DOMICILIARY, REST HOME, OR CUSTODIAL CARE SERVICES

99324–99328	New patient	Requires all three key components
99334–99337	Established patient	Requires two of three key components

These codes represent the E/M services provided to patients located in a "facility that provides room, board, and other personal assistance services, generally on a long-term basis" (www.cms.gov/Medicare/Coding/place-of-service-codes/Place_of_Service_Code_Set.html). AMA also includes assisted-living facilities, group homes, custodial care, and intermediate care facilities in this definition; however, to qualify for these codes, the facilities must not include a medical component in their services.

The codes are organized exactly like the new patient and established patient codes for office or other outpatient services. The levels of service of the new patient and established patient codes differ slightly, as shown in Table 13.16.

Table 13.16 Key Component Requirements, 99324–99337

CODE	HISTORY	EXAM	MDM
New Patient			
99324	PF	PF	Straightforward
99325	EPF	EPF	Low
99326	DET	DET	Moderate
99327	COMP	COMP	Moderate
99328	COMP	COMP	High
Established Patient			
99334	PF	PF	Straightforward
99335	EPF	EPF	Low
99336	DET	DET	Moderate
99337	COMP	COMP	Moderate to high

DOMICILIARY, REST HOME, OR HOME CARE PLAN OVERSIGHT SERVICES

99339	Within a calendar month, 15–29 minutes
99340	Within a calendar month, 30 minutes or more

Care plan oversight codes represent the services that physicians provide to patients who are at home or in domiciliary or rest homes (assisted-living facilities), *without* face-to-face contact. These services are comparable to the care plan oversight services in codes 99374–99380 (described later in this chapter), but the patients are not under the care of a home health agency or hospice program. The codes represent the services of the supervising physician who oversees the care of a patient by taking calls or coordinating care with other medical and nonmedical service providers and the patient's family members. The physician is also responsible for developing and/or revising care plans, reviewing reports of patient status, and reviewing laboratory and other studies.

These codes are reported separately from any face-to-face services—such as home, domiciliary, or rest home visits—the physician provides to the patient during the reporting period. They also include the physician's oversight of work or school programs where therapy is provided. The codes are reported per calendar month and represent the services provided during that month.

■ **CASE SCENARIO**
An 80-year-old patient has lived with his children since suffering a stroke 2 years ago. He is now in the early stages of Alzheimer's disease, is increasingly dependent on his children for all aspects of daily living, and has started to become agitated and uncooperative. His children are unable to get him to the physician office for visits. A home visit is made by the physician. During the next month, the physician speaks with the family about the patient's care, assessing progress or lack of progress. The oversight of this patient's care by the physician is necessary to support the caregivers, to avoid hospitalization, and to diminish the patient's potential for delirium.

The selection criteria are as follows:

- Only one physician reports these codes—the supervising physician.
- These codes are reported per calendar month and represent the services provided during that month.
- Do not report these codes unless the patient requires recurrent supervision of his or her therapy/treatment.

- The physician supervision is such that it requires complex and multidisciplinary care modalities, involving regular physician development and/or revision of care plans, review of reports on patient status, and laboratory and other studies.
- The physician supervision will also require communication for the purpose of assessment of the patient, care decisions with health-care professional(s), family member(s), and surrogate decision maker(s).
- The supervising physician will integrate new information into the patient's medical treatment plan, and/or make adjustments to that plan.
- Do not report these codes for patients under the care of a home health agency, in a hospice program, or for nursing facility assessments.

HOME SERVICES

These codes, shown in Table 13.17, represent E/M services provided to patients in their homes. The criteria are the same as those for new and established patients, 99201–99215.

Table 13.17 Key Component Requirements, 99341–99350

CODE	HISTORY	EXAM	MDM
New Patient			
99341	PF	PF	Straightforward
99342	EPF	EPF	Low
99343	DET	DET	Moderate
99344	COMP	COMP	Moderate
99345	COMP	COMP	High
Established Patient			
99347	PF	PF	Straightforward
99348	EPF	EPF	Low
99349	DET	DET	Moderate
99350	COMP	COMP	Moderate to high

PROLONGED SERVICES

+99354	Face-to-face services in office or outpatient setting	First hour
+99355	Each additional 30 minutes	Use with 99354
+99356	Face-to-face services in inpatient setting	First hour
+99357	Each additional 30 minutes	Use with 99356
99358	Non–face-to-face services in office, outpatient, inpatient setting	
+99359	Each additional 30 minutes	Use with 99358

The range of prolonged services codes represents services that go beyond typical service in either the inpatient or outpatient setting. The face-to-face services are all add-on codes and are always reported in addition to other E/M codes. The codes are not based on the three key components; instead, they are time based. They are divided into direct care services, meaning those provided face to face, and nondirect care, which refers to services that are not face to face and are provided either before or after face-to-face patient care was provided and not necessarily on the same day. Prolonged services can be provided in the physician office or outpatient location or in the hospital (inpatient) unit or floor where the patient is located.

- Direct prolonged service: An established patient comes into the physician office reporting chest pain. The patient asks whether the spicy food he has been eating lately could be the cause of the chest pain. An ECG is done, with results comparable to an ECG done 2 months ago. No problem is found. The physician provides a problem-focused history, a detailed exam, and moderate MDM. The patient then mentions some left arm pain. The physician is not comfortable letting the patient go home, so she allows him to remain in one of the examining rooms for the next 4 hours; during that time she evaluates the patient's vital signs and examines him to look for conditions that might indicate the underlying problem. The physician spends 40 minutes providing face-to-face care to the patient in addition to the time spent on the key components of the initial evaluation. Assign codes 99214 and +99354.

- Nondirect prolonged service: An 80-year-old patient with a long history of several complex systemic health problems moves to a new area to be closer to her family. Before the patient's visit, her new physician spends an hour reviewing the medical records sent to him by the patient's previous physician. Assign a new patient code from the 99201–99205 range and 99358.

Criteria

Prolonged service codes are reported once per day, but the time the physician spends with the patient need not be continuous on that day. However, the physician must exceed the typical primary E/M code time by at least an additional 30 minutes (see Table 13.18 for E/M code times). Additional time less than 30 minutes would be included in the primary E/M code and would not be separately reported.

EXAMPLE

The typical time assigned to code 99214 is 25 minutes. If the physician spends a total of 45 minutes in direct care of the patient, the prolonged care codes are not reported (45 minutes – 25 minutes = 20 minutes). The remaining time of 20 minutes does not meet the minimum 30-minute requirement.

Physicians and coders may want to consider the counseling and coordination of care time rule if applicable. When counseling or coordination of care dominates (i.e., uses more than 50% of the time) of the physician and patient and/or family encounter, time *is* the key or controlling factor to determine the level of service. The extent of the counseling or coordination of care must be documented in the medical record. If the total visit time is at the highest level of service (99205 for new patient, 99215 for established patient) *and* the visit continues for an additional 30 minutes or more, report +99354 in addition to 99205, 99215. If the visit continues for less than 30 minutes, report only the E/M code.

The following services are reportable with prolonged service codes 99354 and 99355:

99201–99205:	New patient
99212–99215:	Established patient
99241–99245:	Office/outpatient consultations
99324–99337:	Domiciliary, rest home services
99341–99350:	Home services
90837:	Psychotherapy
90847:	Family psychotherapy

The following services are reportable with the prolonged service codes 99356 and 99357:

99218–99220:	Initial observation care
99221–99223:	Initial hospital care
99224–99226:	Subsequent observation care
99231–99233:	Subsequent hospital care
99234–99236:	Same-day admission and discharge

99251–99255:	Hospital consultations
99304–99310:	Nursing facility care
90837:	Psychotherapy

Some services are not reportable with any prolonged service codes. An example of services that do not have typical times associated with them are 99281–99285: Emergency department.

Do not report codes 99358, 99359 with:

- Care plan oversight codes 99339, 99340, 99374–99380
- Home and outpatient INR monitoring codes 93792, 93793
- Medical team conference codes 99366, 99368
- Online medical evaluation code 99444
- Other non–face-to-face services that have more specific codes and no upper time limit in their code set.

Calculating Time

Use the 15-minute rule to calculate the amount of time to bill for time-based prolonged services:

- After the first hour (99354), 14 minutes must be exceeded to use 99355.
- After the first 1.5 hours (99354, 99355), 14 minutes must be exceeded to use 99355 again.

Table 13.18 illustrates the 15-minute rule. Table 13.19 provides the times associated with E/M codes.

Table 13.18 The 15-Minute Rule for Time-Based Prolonged Services

TIME SPENT	DESCRIPTION	CODE
30–74 minutes	First 30 minutes through first hour plus 14 minutes	99354
75–104 minutes	First hour plus 15 minutes through 1.5 hours plus 14 minutes	99354, 99355
105–134 minutes	First 1.5 hours plus 15 minutes through 2 hours plus 14 minutes	99354, 99355 × 2

Table 13.19 Typical Primary E/M Code Times

CODE	TYPICAL TIME (IN MINUTES)	CODE	TYPICAL TIME (IN MINUTES)
99201	10	99223	70
99202	20	99231	15
99203	30	99232	25
99204	45	99233	35
99205	60	99234	40
99212	10	99235	50
99213	15	99236	55
99214	25	99241	15
99215	40	99242	30
99218	30	99243	40
99219	50	99244	60
99220	70	99245	80
99224	15	99251	20
99225	25	99252	40
99226	35	99253	55
99221	30	99254	80
99222	50	99255	110

Continued

Table 13.19 *Continued*

CODE	TYPICAL TIME (IN MINUTES)	CODE	TYPICAL TIME (IN MINUTES)
99304	25	99335	25
99305	35	99336	40
99306	45	99337	60
99307	10	99341	20
99308	15	99342	30
99309	25	99343	45
99310	35	99344	60
99324	20	99345	75
99325	30	99347	15
99326	45	99348	25
99327	60	99349	40
99328	75	99350	60
99334	15	90837	60

CHECKPOINT 13.12

Indicate whether the following statements are true or false, and explain why.

1. Prolonged services codes are the only codes reported when counseling and coordination of care are greater than 50% of the patient services provided on that day. _____

2. Prolonged services codes are never billed alone. _____

3. Codes 99234–99236 cannot be reported with codes 99356–99357. _____

4. The difference between direct and nondirect services is the place of service. _____

Physician Standby Services

99360	Physician standby service, requiring prolonged physician attendance, each 30 minutes

CPT code 99360 is used for standby services, which are provided when a physician asks another physician to stand by during treatment of a patient. In effect, the standby physician is required to be available in the location of the patient's treatment, immediately ready to provide services that may be needed. For example, the standby physician reports code 99360 when asked to stand by for possible surgery (a surgeon), to analyze a frozen section (a pathologist), to help with a cesarean or high-risk delivery (a pediatrician), or to monitor an electroencephalogram (a neurologist).

EXAMPLE

A cardiologist has scheduled a percutaneous (through the skin) cardiac procedure that may require immediate open-heart surgery if the patient does not respond well. The cardiologist asks a cardiothoracic surgeon to stand by during the cardiac procedure in case her services are required.

The following criteria must be met to use this code:

- The standby physician has no face-to-face contact with the patient.
- The standby physician does not provide care or services to other patients during the standby period; for example, the standby physician does not see other patients who are in the hospital.
- The standby physician is not proctoring another physician (in other words, the physician is not overseeing or monitoring another physician during a procedure).
- If the standby service results in the performance of a procedure subject to a surgical package, the standby physician reports the procedure only, not the standby code.

EXAMPLE

In the preceding example, if the standby physician/surgeon has to perform open-heart surgery such as a coronary artery bypass (CABG), she will report only the CABG code, not the standby code.

- The standby service time must be 30 minutes or longer. Standby service of less than 30 minutes is not reportable.
- To report 99360 more than once, the physician must stand by for a full 30 minutes in addition to the first 30 minutes.

EXAMPLE

If the cardiothoracic surgeon stands by for 1 hour during the cardiologist's procedure, she will report 99360 × 2. If she stands by for 40 minutes during the cardiologist's procedure, she will report 99360 only.

NOTE: Code 99360 is not reported in addition to code 99464, the physician attendance code for newborn care (see the Newborn Care section later in this chapter).

CHECKPOINT 13.13

Read the following case and answer the question.

A neurologist asks a neurosurgeon to stand by during neurological testing performed in the operating room because there is concern about the stability of the patient to withstand the testing, and surgery might be required on an emergency basis. The neurosurgeon stands by for 35 minutes.

1. What is the appropriate code for this service? _____

CASE MANAGEMENT SERVICES

99366–99368	Medical team conferences	Time based

Case management codes represent the services of a physician who is responsible for direct care of a patient but is also in team conferences related to that patient.

Medical Team Conferences

99366	Nonphysician face to face	30 minutes or more
99367	Physician non–face to face	30 minutes or more
99368	Nonphysician non–face to face	30 minutes or more

The team conference codes are used for medical conferences held with an interdisciplinary team of health professionals of different specialties/disciplines, each of whom provides direct care to the patient. The codes differentiate whether or not the patient and/or family are present. To report these codes, the participants must have provided a face-to-face evaluation or treatment of the patient within the previous 60 days. No more than one qualified health-care professional from the same specialty may report these team conference codes.

Physicians do not report the face-to-face codes. If they provide this conference-type service face to face, they report the E/M codes (99212–99215) using time as the controlling factor for the level of service. Because of the requirement that there had to have been a face-to-face service within the prior 60 days, physicians would not report codes 99201–99205.

> ■ **CASE SCENARIO**
> A patient with a mental illness needs to have a brain aneurysm excised. The patient's neurosurgeon meets with the patient's psychiatrist and radiologist to discuss his care.

CARE PLAN OVERSIGHT SERVICES

99374	Home health agency patient, 15–29 minutes
99375	Home health agency patient, 30 minutes or more
99377	Hospice patient, 15–29 minutes
99378	Hospice patient, 30 minutes or more
99379	Nursing facility patient, 15–29 minutes
99380	Nursing facility patient, 30 minutes or more

Care plan oversight codes represent the services that physicians provide to patients who are under the care of a home health agency, hospice, or a nursing facility without face-to-face contact. These services involve overseeing the care of a patient by taking calls from the nurse or agency handling the patient and by reviewing and revising care plans. The codes are reported separately from face-to-face services, such as office or nursing home visits, provided during the reporting period.

> ■ **CASE SCENARIO**
> Ms. Jones is homebound because of uncontrolled diabetes, hypertension, and resulting claudication, making walking far too difficult, if not impossible. Her home health agency nurse visits every 2 days to be sure she is taking care of herself, taking the appropriate medications, exercising correctly, and eating the right foods. At least once every 2 weeks, the agency needs to call her physician to discuss complications caused by noncompliance. The physician reviews the agency's latest written report, her notes from previous phone calls, and the plan of care, and she revises previous orders based on the latest information. The physician reports 99374 if she spends 15 to 29 minutes on these activities in a calendar month or 99375 for 30 minutes or more.

Selection criteria are as follows:

• Only one physician reports these codes—the supervising physician.
• These codes are reported per calendar month and represent the services provided during that month.

- Do not report these codes unless the patient requires recurrent supervision of the therapy/treatment.
- The supervision requires complex and multidisciplinary care modalities, involving regular physician development and/or revision of care plans, review of reports on patient status, and laboratory and other studies; communication for the purpose of assessment of the patient, care decisions with health-care professional(s), family member(s), and surrogate decision maker(s); and integrating new information into the patient's medical treatment plan, and/or making adjustments to that plan.

CHECKPOINT 13.14

Read the following case and answer the question.

A physician is responsible for the care of an 84-year old man with many complex health-care issues, who is currently in a nursing facility. She has seen this patient at the nursing home, and she also takes the calls from the nursing home for required changes in care plans and about lab studies and tests that are required to maintain the patient's health, as well from the patient's daughter, who visits her father daily. The physician discusses treatment with the nurses in charge of her patient's care at the facility on a regular basis. Her office documentation indicates that she has spent 40 minutes on such oversight this month.

1. What code should be reported for this month's time? _____

PREVENTIVE MEDICINE SERVICES

99381–99387	New patient codes for the initial comprehensive preventive medicine service, early childhood (age 1–4 years) through 65 years and older
99391–99397	Established patient codes for the periodic comprehensive preventive medicine service, same age range as the new patient codes
99401–99429	Counseling and/or risk-factor reduction and behavior change intervention

Preventive medicine services codes represent services provided to assess patients' health on a regular basis or to promote their health and prevent illness or injury. This code range is separated from the rest of the E/M code categories, which cover problem-oriented visits.

Codes 99381–99397 are used for patients who present for their annual physicals as either new or established patients. These are age-based codes, and the patient's age generally determines the extent of the services provided. The services include counseling, anticipatory guidance, and risk-factor reduction interventions. (Note that 99401–99429 are reported when the counseling and related services are provided during a separate encounter with the patient.) Other work—such as immunizations, labs, studies, and radiology services—is reported in addition to preventive medicine codes when provided.

The preventive medicine codes are used when patients who are not currently ill present for their annual physicals. It is not unusual for the physician to encounter an abnormality or preexisting condition while performing a preventive medicine service. If the abnormality or preexisting condition is significant enough to require additional work in terms of history, examination, and medical decision making (the three key components), a code from the 99201–99215 (E/M codes for problem-oriented visits) should be reported in addition to the preventive medicine code, and the modifier –25 should be appended to the problem-oriented E/M code.

• A patient who is 55 years of age is seen for his annual physical. He also has significant pain, soreness, redness, and heat in his right extremity. This condition requires the physician to ask additional questions (history) and do an additional examination and evaluation (medical decision making) to determine whether the patient has phlebitis. Both the preventive service code and the problem-oriented service codes will be reported.

• A patient who is 40 years of age is seen for her annual physical. She has had a cough for the past week. An evaluation of the respiratory system is part of preventive medicine services. Although the physician may have to ask some additional questions to resolve the cough, this scenario rarely justifies the use of a problem-oriented code in addition to the preventive medicine code.

Counseling Risk-Factor Reduction

99401–99404	Preventive medicine individual counseling	Time based
99411–99412	Preventive medicine group counseling	Time based

Codes 99401–99404 represent the services provided to patients for promoting health and preventing illness or injury. These services must be provided at a separate encounter, not during the preventive medicine visits represented by codes 99381–99397, which include appropriate counseling.

The type of counseling that is typically provided relates to family problems, diet and exercise, substance abuse, sexual practices, injury prevention, dental health, and diagnostic and laboratory test results that are available at the time of the encounter. These counseling codes are not to be used for patients with symptoms or established illnesses, which are coded with the appropriate problem-oriented office, hospital, or consultation codes.

Behavior Change Intervention

99406–99409	Behavior change interventions, individual	Time based

Codes 99406 and 99407 represent counseling services for smoking and tobacco use cessation. Codes 99408 and 99409 are for alcohol and/or substance abuse screenings and brief intervention services.

■ CASE SCENARIO
A patient falls down the stairs and then goes to the ED. Testing indicates the patient is intoxicated and further review of the patient's record indicates this is his fourth visit in 2 months for injuries related to intoxication. The physician does a detailed screening interview and because of the patient's repeated alcohol injuries an intervention is provided to motivate the patient to decrease or abstain from alcohol.

NON–FACE-TO-FACE PHYSICIAN SERVICES

99441–99443	Telephone services	Time based
99444	Online medical evaluation	

Telephone services are E/M services initiated by an established patient or guardian of a patient. This type of service should not be reported if a previous E/M service occurred within 7 days, or if the call results in a face-to-face service within 24 hours, or if the next available urgent visit appointment occurs during the postoperative period of a previous procedure. The call would be considered as included in those previous or subsequent services.

A patient with diabetes who monitors his blood sugar levels calls his physician to discuss an increase in his levels. The 10-minute discussion determines that the patient has been taking too little medication. The physician asks the patient to increase his medication, monitor his blood sugar levels, and call back if the levels do not go back to normal. The patient was last seen 2 months ago. Report code 99441.

Online medical evaluation services are initiated by an established patient for Internet E/M services and require a permanent storage capability (electronic or printed copy). Report these services only once for the same episode of care during a 7-day period. Again, if an E/M service was performed within the previous 7 days or within the postoperative period of a previous procedure, the online service would be included in those services. Do not report these codes with care plan oversight codes or anticoagulant codes.

SPECIAL EVALUATION AND MANAGEMENT SERVICES

99450	Basic life and/or disability examination	
99455	Work-related or medical disability	Treating physician
99456	Work-related or medical disability	Other than treating physician
99499	Unlisted E/M service	

If other E/M services or CPT procedures are provided on the same date, they can be reported. Attach modifier –25 to the additional code if the provider's documentation supports the use of modifier –25.

These codes represent services provided to establish baseline information before the issuance of life or disability insurance certificates. They are appropriate for any outpatient setting and for either new or established patients. No active management of the patient's problems occurs during the encounter. Note that code 99455 is for the patient's treating physician, whereas code 99456 is for the service provided by another physician.

NEWBORN CARE

Do not report 99455 and 99456 with CPT 99080 for the completion of workers' compensation forms.

99460	Initial care of normal newborn infant—report per day
99461	Initial care of normal newborn in other than hospital or birthing room—report per day
99462	Subsequent hospital care of normal newborn—report per day
99463	Initial care of normal newborn admitted and discharged same date—report per day
99464	Attendance at delivery
99465	Newborn resuscitation

Do not confuse stabilization with standby. The pediatrician is actually present in the delivery room, not elsewhere in the delivery suite.

Newborn care codes represent various services provided to newborns in different settings and include codes for three types of initial care based on the newborn's delivery location or if the newborn was admitted and discharged on the same date. The code for a newborn delivered in the hospital or birthing room includes initiation of diagnostic and treatment programs and preparation of hospital records. If the child is born in a location other than the hospital or birthing room, the code includes the physical examination of the baby and conferences with the parents.

There is only one code for the subsequent care of a newborn, 99462, which is reported each day the physician provides care to a newborn in the hospital. Code 99463, which represents care provided to a newborn assessed and discharged on the same date, is not commonly used now. It is more likely for a newborn to be delivered and to remain in the hospital for more than 1 day. However, when the same-date scenario occurs, the code includes preparation of medical records.

A delivering physician sometimes anticipates a problem for the newborn upon delivery and asks a pediatrician to attend the delivery in order to be immediately available to provide care if necessary. The pediatrician will report code 99464, which covers stabilization, including resuscitation, of the newborn. This code may be reported with code 99460 (initial care of newborn) but not with 99465 (resuscitation of newborn) or for standby services (99360).

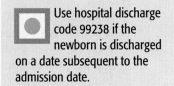

Use hospital discharge code 99238 if the newborn is discharged on a date subsequent to the admission date.

A pediatrician who is not asked to attend the delivery may be called in after the child is born if the child is having trouble breathing (acute inadequate ventilation) or the child's heart is not pumping correctly (inadequate cardiac output). Under these circumstances, the physician will provide positive pressure ventilation and/or chest compression and will report code 99465. Attention should be given to the parenthetical note following code 99465. This note instructs that certain procedures may be provided in the delivery room prior to admission to the neonatal intensive care unit and separately reported if they are required for the resuscitation. Examples are intubation and vascular lines.

CHECKPOINT 13.15

Read the following case and answer the question.

The pediatrician treated the newborn in the hospital after delivery and during the 2 days the baby remained in the hospital after the delivery date.

1. What codes should the pediatrician report for the hospital services? _____

Pediatric Critical Care Patient Transport

99466	Face-to-face transport	First 30–74 minutes
+99467	Add-on code	Each additional 30 minutes
99485	Supervision of care during transport	First 30 minutes
+99486	Add-on code	Each additional 30 minutes

Codes 99466 and 99467 represent the services of a physician who accompanies a critically ill or critically injured pediatric patient 24 months of age or younger during interfacility transport and who provides face-to-face services. The face-to-face care begins when the physician assumes the responsibility for the pediatric patient at the referring hospital or facility, and it ends when the receiving hospital or facility accepts responsibility for the patient's care. The transport must involve 30 minutes or more of service. Critical care services of less than 30 minutes should be reported with other outpatient E/M codes such as 99201–99215.

The critical care guidelines for patient transport are the same as those listed for the neonatal and pediatric critical care services. Watch for the services that are included in the critical care guidelines and are not separately reported.

Codes 99485 and 99486 represent the services of a physician who supervises the care of a 24 months of age or younger patient who is critically ill or critically injured in transport from a referring facility to a receiving facility. The controlling or supervising physician is in two-way communication with the specialized personnel transporting the patient. To report these services, the physician must document the time spent supervising the transport team. The time spent does not have to be continuous and services of less than 15 minutes are not reportable. If another physician is providing face-to-face services during the transport, do not report codes 99485 and 99486.

INPATIENT NEONATAL INTENSIVE CARE SERVICES AND PEDIATRIC AND NEONATAL CRITICAL CARE SERVICES

99468	Initial inpatient neonatal critical care	Per day
99469	Subsequent inpatient neonatal critical care	Per day
99471	Initial inpatient pediatric critical care 29 days–24 months of age	Per day
99472	Subsequent inpatient pediatric critical care 29 days–24 months of age	Per day
99475	Initial inpatient pediatric critical care 2–5 years of age	Per day
99476	Subsequent inpatient pediatric critical care 2–5 years of age	Per day

The critical care guidelines for codes 99291 and 99292 are the same for neonatal and pediatric patients and have the same included services; however, the neonatal and pediatric codes include additional services. The physician cannot report these services separately:

Vascular access procedures:

- Peripheral vessel catheterization (36000)
- Other arterial catheters (36140, 36620)
- Umbilical venous catheters (36510)
- Central vessel catheterization (36555)
- Vascular access procedures (36400, 36405, 36406)
- Vascular punctures (36420, 36600)
- Umbilical arterial catheters (36660)

Airway and ventilation management:

- Endotracheal intubation (31500)
- Ventilatory management (94002–94004)
- Bedside pulmonary function testing (94375)
- Surfactant administration (94610)
- Continuous positive airway pressure (CPAP) (94660)
- Monitoring or interpretation of blood gases or oxygen saturation (94760–94777)
- Car seat evaluation (94780–94781)
- Transfusion of blood components (36430, 36440)
- Oral or nasogastric tube placement (43752)
- Suprapubic bladder aspiration (51100)
- Lumbar puncture (62270)

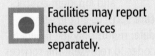

Facilities may report these services separately.

Any services not listed above may be reported separately.

It is important to note that these codes/services are *inpatient* only and are reported *per day;* they are not time-based codes. When services are provided to neonatal and pediatric patients on an outpatient basis (office or emergency department), report codes 99291–99292.

Additional guidelines are associated with the varied circumstances in neonatal and pediatric critical care coding:

- Same physician provides critical care in both the outpatient and inpatient settings on the same day.
  - The outpatient services roll up into the inpatient codes. The physician reports only the inpatient per-day codes.

- Critical care is provided at two separate facilities by two physicians from different groups on the same date of service.
  - The physician at the referring facility reports 99291, 99292.
  - The physician at the receiving facility reports 99468 or 99471 or 99475 based on the patient's age.
- The critically ill or critically injured patient improves and is transferred to a lower level of care to another physician in another group in the same facility.
  - The transferring physician does not report critical care codes; instead report the following:
    - Subsequent hospital care codes 99231–99233 or
    - Time-based critical care codes 99291–99292
  - The choice of codes depends on the patient's condition and the services provided as indicated in critical care guidelines.
  - The receiving physician reports the following:
    - Subsequent continuing intensive care codes 99478–99480 or
    - Subsequent hospital care codes 99231–99233
    - Code choice is based on the patient's condition.
- After receiving normal newborn services (99460, 99461, 99462) or continuing intensive care services (99477–99480) or hospital services (99221–99233), the patient becomes critically ill on the same day and is transferred to the critical care level.
  - The transferring physician will report the following:
    - Time-based critical care codes 99291–99292 or
    - Continuing intensive care services 99477–99480 or
    - Hospital care services 99221–99233 or
    - Normal newborn services 99460, 99461, 99462
  - The receiving physician must be from a different group and report initial or subsequent inpatient neonatal or pediatric critical care codes 99468–99476 based on age and whether or not this is an initial or subsequent admission.
  - If the receiving physician is from the same group, report the initial critical care code 99468 or 99471 or 99475 based on the patient's age.

Inpatient Neonatal Critical Care

Inpatient neonatal critical care codes represent critical care provided to children 28 days of age or younger. On admission for critical care services, report 99468; subsequent days that the neonate remains in critical care are reported with 99469. If readmitted on the same day or stay, report the subsequent care code 99469 for that day and each day following the readmission.

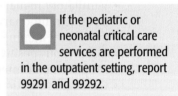

If the pediatric or neonatal critical care services are performed in the outpatient setting, report 99291 and 99292.

The initial day neonatal code 99468 is reportable with other newborn care codes if these services are performed:

- *Attendance at delivery 99464:* For example, if the pediatrician is asked by the obstetrician to attend the delivery and to stabilize the newborn and then admits the newborn to critical care.
- *Newborn resuscitation 99465:* For example, if the pediatrician is called into the delivery room to resuscitate a newborn and then admits the newborn to critical care.
- *Endotracheal intubation (31500) and other resuscitation procedures*, if they are performed as part of the preadmission delivery room care, are a necessary component of the resuscitation, and are not performed in the delivery room as a convenience before admission to the neonatal intensive care unit.

If the physician provides both outpatient and inpatient critical care services on the same date, report only the inpatient codes to represent the services provided in both locations.

Inpatient pediatric critical care codes 99471–99476 represent critical care provided to critically ill or injured children who are 29 days through 5 years of age. They start with the date of admission and go through all subsequent days.

Do not report time-based outpatient critical care codes when the same patient is receiving services on the same day as the per day critical care codes 99468–99476. This guideline applies if the services are provided by the same individual or an individual of the same specialty and same group. The time-based codes may be reported on the same day if the individual is of a different specialty in the same group or a different group.

Initial and Continuing Intensive Care Services

99477	Initial hospital care, neonate	Per day
99478	Subsequent intensive care, recovering very low birth weight Present body weight less than 1,500 grams	Per day
99479	Subsequent intensive care, recovering low birth weight Present body weight 1,500–2,500 grams	Per day
99480	Subsequent intensive care, recovering infant Present body weight 2,501–5,000 grams	Per day

● The inpatient neonatal intensive care services codes include the same procedures that are outlined in the neonatal and pediatric critical care guidelines.

Code 99477 represents the initial day of inpatient care for neonate patients who do not meet the definition of critically ill but who require intensive observation, frequent interventions, and other intensive services. Codes 99478–99480 are for the subsequent day of services providing continuing intensive care to the very low, low, and normal body weight patients who require intensive observation, frequent interventions, and other intensive services. For subsequent care of the sick neonate who weighs more than 5,000 grams, use the subsequent hospital care codes 99231–99233. The reporting physician is the physician who directs the health-care team providing continuing intensive care of these patients.

These are per-day codes, and the types of services that are typically provided include the following:

- Cardiac and respiratory monitoring
- Continuous and/or frequent vital sign monitoring
- Heat maintenance
- Enteral and/or parenteral nutritional adjustments
- Laboratory and oxygen monitoring
- Constant observation by the health-care team

The initial day code 99477 is reportable with modifier –25 if the following newborn care codes are provided:

- *Attendance at delivery 99464:* For example, if the pediatrician is asked by the obstetrician to attend the delivery and to stabilize the newborn and then admits the newborn to continuing intensive care.
- *Newborn resuscitation 99465:* For example, if the pediatrician is called into the delivery room to resuscitate a newborn and then admits the newborn to continuing intensive critical care.
- *Endotracheal intubation (31500) and other resuscitation procedures,* if they are performed as part of the preadmission delivery room care, are a necessary component of the resuscitation and are not performed in the delivery room as a convenience before admission to the neonatal intensive care unit.

This series of continuing intensive care services follows the same guidelines for transferring the patient to a lower level of care as the neonatal and pediatric critical care codes.

■ **CASE SCENARIO**
A 2,550-gram neonate who was suffering from respiratory distress, shock, and cardiac arrhythmia is now recovering but still requires oxygen and is maintained on his central venous catheter, pending full recovery. His pediatrician will attend to and monitor his cardiovascular stability, pulmonary status, and gastrointestinal function. This will require comprehensive evaluations of these organ systems with particular attention to possible infection and atelectasis in the lungs. The child will be visited throughout the day and evening to ensure that he continues to recover. The code is 99480.

COGNITIVE ASSESSMENT AND CARE PLAN SERVICES

These services represented by CPT code 99483 are provided to both new and established patients who are experiencing signs and/or symptoms of cognitive impairment. The evaluation is comprehensive and is required to establish or confirm a diagnosis, etiology and severity for the condition. The evaluation is both medical and psychosocial.

- All required elements must be performed in order to report these codes.
- If any required elements are considered unnecessary for the patient's condition, do not report these codes; report E/M codes instead.
- Code 99483 should not be reported more than once every 180 days.

These services include:

- Cognition relevant history
- Assessment of factors that may contribute to cognitive impairment (e.g., psychoactive medication, chronic pain syndromes, infection, depression, brain disease).

There are many codes that cannot be reported with code 99483, all are noted below code 99483's description.

CARE MANAGEMENT SERVICES

99490	Chronic care management services	Per calendar month
99487	Complex chronic care management services	Per calendar month
99489	Add-on code, each additional 30 minutes —report with code 99487	Per calendar month

Care management services are those provided by clinical staff to patients residing at home, in a domiciliary/rest home, or in an assisted-living facility. The services are provided under the direction of a physician or other QHP and involve the establishment, implementation, revision, or monitoring of the patient's care plan. The services also involve coordination of care with other professionals and agencies, and education of the patient or caregiver regarding the patient's condition, care plan, and prognosis. It is the physician's or QHP's responsibility to oversee these services for all medical conditions, psychosocial needs, and activities of daily living. There are extensive guidelines within the CPT book regarding these services and they must be carefully reviewed.

> CMS considers care management services as bundled into other E/M services provided to these patients. Give attention to the codes that cannot be reported with this group of services.

Codes 99487, 99489, and 99490 are reported only once per calendar month and are time based. The codes are reported by the individual physician or QHP who has assumed the case management role for that patient. These services incorporate face-to-face and non–face-to-face time spent by the clinical staff with patients and/or family, caregivers, other professionals, and agencies. Only one clinical staff member's time may be counted even though others may be involved in the patient's care. When determining the per-month time to report, do not report clinical staff time on a day when the physician or QHP provides an E/M service. CPT indicates many other services that are included in the care management codes and those services should not be reported separately.

Chronic Care Management Services

This specific type of care management service represented by CPT code 99490 is provided to patients with medical and/or psychosocial needs. They have two or more chronic continuous or episodic health problems that will last 12 months or until the patient dies. The health problems these patients have place them at significant risk of death, acute exacerbation, decompensation, or functional decline. The service provided must incorporate establishment, implementation, revision, or monitoring of the care plan. This per-calendar-month reporting process requires at least 20 minutes of time on the part of the clinical staff.

Complex Chronic Care Management Services (CCCM)

The criteria for this specific type of care management service require that the patient needs the coordination of a number of specialties and services due to his or her inability to perform activities of daily living and/or cognitive impairment. The patient will have psychiatric and other medical comorbidities and have social support requirements or difficulty with access to care. The CPT codes are 99487 and +99488 and are reported per calendar month and are based on time.

PSYCHIATRIC COLLABORATIVE CARE MANAGEMENT SERVICE

99492	Requires:	Initial care, first 70 minutes in first calendar month, with required elements
99493	Requires:	Subsequent care, first 60 minutes in a subsequent month, with required elements
+99494	Requires:	For initial or subsequent care, each additional 30 minutes in a calendar month

These services are provided during a calendar month when a patient has a diagnosis of a psychiatric disorder that requires:

- a behavioral health-care assessment
- establishing, implementing, revising, or monitoring a care plan
- provision of brief interventions

The services are provided under the direction of the treating physician or QHP within a calendar month. The episode of care begins when the patient is directed to the behavioral health-care manager and ends under three types of situations:

- attainment of goals
- failure to attain goals
- no continued engagement over a consecutive 6-month calendar period

There are extensive guidelines in CPT and coders should review all of them.

TRANSITIONAL CARE MANAGEMENT SERVICES (TCM)

| 99495 | Requires: | Communication with patient/caregiver within 2 business days of discharge
At least moderate medical decision making
Face-to-face visit within 14 calendar days of discharge |
| 99496 | Requires: | Communication with patient/caregiver within 2 business days of discharge
High medical decision making
Face-to-face visit within 7 calendar days of discharge |

Transitional care management (TCM) services represent transition of care from the inpatient setting to the community setting and apply to established patients whose medical and/or psychosocial problems required moderate- or high-complexity medical decision making during the transition.

Services should address any needed coordination of care provided by multiple disciplines and community service agencies.

Inpatient:

- Partial hospital
- Observation
- Skilled nursing facility

Community setting:

- Home
- Rest home
- Assisted living

Requirements:

- Face-to-face visit within the stated service time
- Interactive contact with the patient or caregiver within 2 business days of discharge based on Monday through Friday except holidays; the interaction can be face to face or telephone or electronic
- Medication reconciliation and management no later than the date of the face-to-face visit
- Medical decision making of at least moderate complexity during the service period
- Report once within 30 days of discharge
- Reported by one physician or QHP who has the care coordination role for that patient

If another physician/QHP provides TCM within the postoperative period of a surgical package, modifier 54 is not required by the physician who performed the procedure.

Watch for the parenthetical notes following the CCCM and TCM codes for "do not report" information.

CMS has accepted the TCM codes with some modifications:

- Codes are allowed for new and established patients, not just established.
- The physician who reports a procedure for a particular patient and that procedure has a defined global period cannot report the TCM codes.
- The same physician can report discharge day management and TCM codes for the same patient; however, CMS will not allow the same physician to report the discharge day management code and TCM-included E/M visit on the same day. To report discharge day management and TCM for the same date, the E/M service that is included in TCM cannot be on the same day.

ADVANCE CARE PLANNING

Advanced care planning services are reported by the physician or other QHP when meeting with the patient, family member, or surrogate. These services represent counseling and discussing advance directives whether or not the legal forms are completed. Use of code 99497 or +99498 means that the patient's problem(s) has not been actively managed. Many other E/M services are included in these codes and should not be reported separately.

Information on CCCC and TCM

These codes include the following:

- Care plan oversight
- Prolonged services without face-to-face contact
- Anticoagulation management
- Medical team conferences
- Education and training
- Telephone services
- End-stage renal disease services
- Online medical evaluation
- Preparation of special reports
- Analysis of data

- Medication therapy management
- CCCC includes TCM provided during same time period
- TCM includes CCCC provided during same time period

INTERNET RESOURCE: The CMS website has a frequently asked questions (FAQs) section for the TCM codes. Go to www.cms.gov and type "transitional care management" into the search box. A drop-down menu will offer you a FAQ option. Review these FAQs for help with this coding area.

GENERAL BEHAVIORAL HEALTH INTEGRATION CARE MANAGEMENT

| 99484 | Requires: | Care management services for behavioral health conditions for at least 20 of clinical staff time |

Other requirements are as follows:

- The services are performed by clinical staff for patients with behavioral health conditions that require care management service. The services are reported by the supervising physician or QHP
- The services may be face-to-face or non–face-to-face and 20 minutes or more within a calendar month.
- A treatment plan need not be comprehensive.

The distinctions between general behavioral integration care management, chronic care management, and psychiatric collaborative care management can be difficult to determine. This fact requires clear understanding of these three areas by reviewing the guidelines in great depth.

MODIFIER –25

No chapter on E/M coding is complete without reference to modifier –25. This modifier is used to represent an E/M service that is significant and separately identifiable from a procedure or another E/M service provided on the same date by the same physician.

All procedures include some E/M services:

- Assessing the site or condition of the problem area
- Explaining the procedure
- Obtaining consent

If the E/M service goes beyond the above criteria, consider using modifier –25 on the E/M service to indicate that the physician has performed a significant and separately identifiable E/M service in addition to what is included in the procedure.

> ■ **CASE SCENARIO**
> A new patient is seen by an orthopedist for knee pain. The physician evaluates the patient, determines the cause of the pain, and determines that a knee injection is a possible treatment for the condition.

The E/M service is significant and separately identifiable from the knee injection, and both the E/M code and the knee injection code will be reported. The –25 modifier is placed on the E/M code.

> ■ **CASE SCENARIO**
> An established patient who saw his physician for ongoing knee pain returns for a knee injection, as the physician suggested at the last visit, because the knee pain stayed the same and no new problems occurred.

At this time, only the knee injection code would be reported. There is no reason for an E/M service that is significant or separately identifiable.

Read the following case and answer the questions.

A dermatologist has been treating a patient for skin lesions. At the patient's fifth visit, the dermatologist explains that the right arm lesion will need to be incised and drained at the next visit unless it resolves from the application of medication. At the next visit, the lesion is unchanged, and the incision and drainage are performed. However, the patient has developed several similar lesions in other body areas. The dermatologist reports an E/M service with modifier −25 and the incision and drainage code.

1. Did the dermatologist report his services correctly? _____

2. Explain why or why not. _____

INTERNET RESOURCE: The Internet can provide insight into coding issues. Below is a link to a Medicare site that answers frequently asked questions (FAQs) about E/M coding (select Resources/Tools, then Medicare FAQs, and scroll down to Evaluation and Management [E/M] Services).
www.connecticutmedicare.com

Chapter Summary

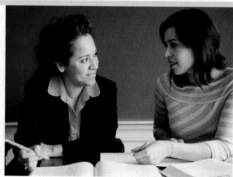

1. The CPT E/M section is organized by categories and subcategories to delineate the CPT coding structure. Categories identify the broadest context of services, such as hospital inpatient services. Subcategories identify the more specific context, such as initial hospital care and subsequent hospital care. This organization allows the coder to identify the place where the service is provided and the type of service provided.

2. The introductory guidelines for each section (such as Observation Care, Critical Care, and Care Plan Oversight) are the coding instructions specific to each section of E/M coding. They provide the rules that control how the listed codes can be applied and whether other codes in the E/M section affect the use of the codes. They also identify whether codes in that section are time based and how to determine time. Also included in the guidelines is information on what services may or may not be included in that code set.

3. The five questions to ask in order to select the appropriate E/M category and the correct codes are:
   a. Who is the patient?
   b. What is the place of service?
   c. What is the patient's status?
   d. What type of service is being provided?
   e. What level of service is being provided?

4. To be classified as a new patient, the individual cannot have received a professional service within 3 years by the physician or another physician of the same specialty in the same group. Established patients have received a professional service within the 3-year period. Professional service means that a face-to-face service was provided by the physician. Some code categories in the E/M section do not differentiate new and established patients; such codes are applicable to both. These include codes for consultations, the ED, and initial and subsequent hospital care.

5. The three key components are history, examination, and medical decision making. Each key component has a level of service that determines the code to be selected. The levels of service are problem focused, expanded problem focused, detailed, and comprehensive. Not all E/M codes have key component requirements.

6. To determine the level of service, first determine the three key component levels: history, examination, and medical decision making. Then review the E/M codes to find out whether they require all three key components to be at the level reported, or if they require only two of the three key components to be at the level reported. The contributory components of counseling and coordination of care will be the determining factors if more than 50% of the time spent during the patient encounter was for counseling and/or coordination of care.

7. Consultations require that a physician request an opinion and/or advice from a consultant and that the consultant render the consultation and then respond in writing to the requesting physician. In the new-patient scenario, the referring physician hands over care of the patient to a different physician for treatment of a specific condition.

8. To assign critical care codes, coders have to know the meaning of "critically ill and/or injured" and of "critical care." Also, coders must know what services are included in critical care. Critical care codes are time based, not based on key components, and coders must know what services may and may not be included in the time determination.

9. Observation care coding requires that the patient be in the hospital under "observation status," and it involves periodic reassessments of the patient by the supervising physician. Patients are placed in "observation status" when their conditions are not severe enough to require admission to the hospital, nor are their conditions stable enough that they can be sent home. To report standby services, the standby is requested by another physician, the service is not face to face, at least 30 minutes are spent in standby, and the standby physician is not providing care or services to other patients during the standby period.

10. To correctly assign codes in the E/M section of CPT, close attention must be paid to the extensive rules and exceptions in each category:
    a. Know which codes require all three or only two of the three key components.
    b. Remember that if more than one E/M service is provided by the same physician to the same patient on the same day, only one E/M code is reported (roll-up rule).
    c. Note the exceptions to the roll-up rule.
    d. Know that some codes are based on the level of service and others are based on time.
    e. There are age-based codes.
    f. Certain codes include other services (for example, critical care).
    g. Certain time-based codes are reported on a per-month basis (for example, care plan oversight).

Review Questions

Matching

Match the key terms with their definitions.

A. admitting physician
B. category
C. chief complaint
D. consultation
E. contributory component
F. direct care
G. new patient
H. observation care
I. preventive medicine
J. roll-up rule

1. _____ Patient's explanation to the physician of why he or she needs to be seen

2. _____ The situation in which a physician provides an opinion or advice on a patient and does not take over the care of the patient

3. _____ Patient who has not been seen by the physician for 3 years

4. _____ Nature of the presenting problem

5. _____ The situation in which a patient is sent to the hospital for care, but is not admitted to the hospital

6. _____ Guideline for a coding situation in which, after being treated in the office, the patient is sent to the hospital to be admitted, and only an admission code is reported for service provided at both locations

7. _____ Type of face-to-face care provided by a physician to a pediatric patient in transport from one facility to another

8. _____ Type of E/M grouping called *office* or *outpatient consultations*

9. _____ Type of care for a patient who is evaluated by a physician without a specific diagnosis, illness, or condition being reported for that evaluation

10. _____ A physician who is allowed to bill the initial hospital care codes 99221–99223

Multiple Choice

Select the letter that best completes the statement or answers the question.

1. Which code is used for the initial office visit of a patient with a 2-day history of lower abdominal pain and occasional vomiting in which the physician obtains a detailed history and detailed examination and does low MDM?
   A. 99204
   B. 99214
   C. 99203
   D. There is not enough information to determine the level of service.

2. An internist asks an endocrinologist to give an opinion on a diabetic patient's bilateral lower extremity neuropathy. In his office, the endocrinologist provides a detailed history, an expanded problem-focused exam, and moderate medical decision making. The endocrinologist writes a letter to the internist indicating his findings. Which code is used?
   A. 99203
   B. 99243
   C. 99242
   D. 99254

3. An established patient has diabetes and hypertension and is morbidly obese. The physician provides an expanded problem-focused history and exam and moderate MDM. Blood work reveals that the patient must start on insulin, and the patient is counseled for 15 minutes regarding the insulin regimen and risks. The total time for the visit is 25 minutes. Which code is used?
   A. 99213
   B. 99214
   C. 99243
   D. 99244

4. An internist sends a patient with long-term back pain to a spine specialist for treatment of the problem. The spine specialist provides an expanded problem-focused history and exam and low MDM. The patient discusses his years of stress-related pain and his dissatisfaction with his previous care. The physician spends a total of 35 minutes with the patient. Which code is used?
   A. 99202
   B. 99243
   C. 99203
   D. 99244

5. A pediatrician examines a newborn right after birth but is called away during the examination. The pediatrician returns later that day and completes the visit. The total time spent during that day is 25 minutes. Which code is reported?
   A. 99460
   B. 99221
   C. 99201
   D. 99462

6. A physician provides 75 minutes of inpatient critical care for a 30-day-old infant. Which code(s) will be reported?
   A. 99460
   B. 99468
   C. 99471
   D. 99291, +99292

7. An ED physician evaluates a patient in the ED. The patient's internist is called in to admit the patient to the hospital. What service does each physician report?
   A. ED physician reports ED code; internist reports initial hospital care for the admission.
   B. ED physician reports initial hospital care; no codes reported by internist.
   C. ED physician reports ED code and initial hospital care; no codes reported by internist.
   D. ED physician does not report any services; internist reports initial hospital care.

8. A 54-year-old established patient is seen for an annual examination. The physician provides a comprehensive physical and spends 15 minutes discussing the patient's anxiety. Which code is used?
   A. 99205
   B. 99386
   C. 99396
   D. 99401

9. A cardiologist asks a surgeon to stand by during a procedure. The surgeon sees patients in the hospital while on standby, but is available via beeper. The procedure takes 1.5 hours. Which code(s) are used?
   A. 99360
   B. 99360x3
   C. 99360, 99356
   D. This is not a reportable service.

10. A patient is in the hospital for a total hip replacement. The patient also has coronary artery disease and develops symptoms. The orthopedic surgeon puts a request in the patient's hospital chart for a cardiologist to see the patient and give his opinion on the severity of the problem. The cardiologist sees and evaluates the patient and puts his findings in the patient's chart. What code does the cardiologist report?
    A. Consultation code
    B. New patient code
    C. Subsequent hospital care code
    D. This is a professional courtesy; no codes are reported.

11. An internal medicine physician asks a local endocrinologist to evaluate a diabetic patient's ongoing bilateral lower extremity neuropathy. He needs an opinion on whether the patient's problem is related to the diabetes or if there is another problem. The endocrinologist performs a detailed history, a detailed exam, and moderate medical decision making (MDM). The endocrinologist writes a letter to the requesting physician indicating his findings. This is a Medicare patient who has never seen the endocrinologist before. Which code does the endocrinologist report?
    A. 99203
    B. 99243
    C. 99204
    D. 99254

12. An established patient is seen in his physician's office for a chief complaint of persistent cough. The physician performs a brief history and examines the respiratory system. MDM is straightforward. Which code does the physician use?
    A. 99211
    B. 99201
    C. 99213
    D. 99212

13. At an initial office visit by a patient with a 5-day history of right leg pain, swelling, and a hot spot on the right leg, the physician provides a detailed history and detailed exam, and MDM is moderate. The patient is concerned about thrombophlebitis because there is a family history of this problem. The physician counsels the patient for 40 minutes. The entire visit takes 65 minutes. Which code does the physician use?
    A. 99203
    B. 99204
    C. 99205
    D. 99202

14. A neonatologist is requested to attend a delivery due to concerns about the infant's possible respiratory problems. The pediatrician stabilizes the infant while still in the delivery room. What E/M code(s) does the pediatrician report?
    A. 99291
    B. 99460
    C. 99464, 99465
    D. 99464

15. A pediatrician stood by for 30 minutes during delivery by an obstetrician for a high-risk patient. The obstetrician delivered the baby and the pediatrician performed resuscitation. Which code(s) would be used for the pediatrician's services?
    A. 99464, 99460
    B. 99464
    C. 99465, 99360
    D. 99360

16. A 60-year-old patient recently moved to Phoenix and is seeing a new internist there. The patient has a long history of gouty arthropathy but presents today for his annual preventive medicine visit. The physician provides a comprehensive H&P, counsels the patient on diet, and orders exercise and blood work. Which code(s) would be used?
    A. 99205
    B. 99386
    C. 99396
    D. 99386, 99402

17. An ED physician sees a patient who was in a motor vehicle accident. The patient has scrapes, contusions, and two dislocations. The ED physician performs a comprehensive exam, a detailed history, and moderate MDM. Which code should be reported?
    A. 99243
    B. 99244
    C. 99284
    D. 99283

CHAPTER 14

CPT: Evaluation and Management Auditing

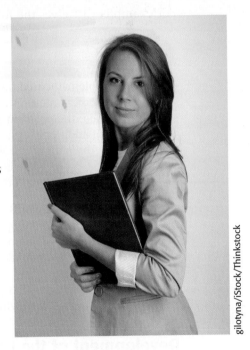

gilotyna/iStock/Thinkstock

CHAPTER OUTLINE

The Evaluation and Management Services Documentation Guidelines

Comparison of 1995 and 1997 Documentation Guidelines

Elements of Key Components

Working with the 1995/1997 History Guidelines

Working with the 1995 Examination Guidelines

Working with the 1995/1997 Medical Decision-Making Guidelines

Determining the E/M Level Based on the 1995 Documentation Guidelines

Applying the 1997 Documentation Guidelines to the Examination Key Component

Coding, Reimbursement, and Fraud

Auditing Tools

Auditing the Electronic Health Record System

LEARNING OUTCOMES

After studying this chapter, you should be able to:

1. State the origin of the documentation guidelines.
2. Understand the purpose of the documentation guidelines.
3. Understand how documentation translates into a level of E/M service.
4. Understand the differences between the 1995 and the 1997 documentation guidelines.
5. Code for E/M services from physician documentation, and use the 1995 documentation guidelines and the 1997 multispecialty and single-specialty documentation guidelines.
6. Understand the purpose of the audit process.
7. Understand E/M audit terminology.
8. Understand the tools used for auditing E/M services.
9. Successfully complete an audit form from documentation.
10. Be able to identify the audit pitfalls of an electronic health record system.

This chapter presents the concepts and practice coders need to assess the level of service (LOS) documented by a physician in order to assign appropriate CPT evaluation and management (E/M) codes. It explains the two sets of official documentation guidelines used to assign these codes based on the information in the physician documentation and to audit assigned codes to confirm their accuracy. It also provides an explanation of the potential problems in auditing the electronic health record (EHR) system.

Payers insist on objective verifiable assessments of E/M levels. For this reason, rules have been established to quantify these services. Following the rules permits coders, auditors, reviewers, and carriers to decide whether the E/M service a physician has reported is accurately supported by what he or she has documented. This validation in turn provides verification of the reimbursement level for the service. Physicians usually select the E/M level of service (LOS) for each patient encounter. It is the coders and/or the auditor's job to verify that the documentation meets the LOS chosen.

THE EVALUATION AND MANAGEMENT SERVICES DOCUMENTATION GUIDELINES

Recall from Chapter 13 that the coder must determine the level of each of the three key components:

- Is the history problem focused, expanded problem focused, detailed, or comprehensive?
- Is the examination problem focused, expanded problem focused, detailed, or comprehensive?
- Is the medical decision making straightforward, low, moderate, or high complexity?

For example, CPT gives the following guidance for determining the *level of history:*

- A *problem-focused history* requires a chief complaint and a brief history of present illness or problem.
- An *expanded problem-focused history* adds a problem-pertinent system review to the elements in the problem-focused history.
- A *detailed history* requires a chief complaint, and the history of present illness is required to be extended; the problem-pertinent system review is augmented by a review of a limited number of additional systems; and a pertinent past, family, and/or social history directly related to the patient's problem is added.
- A *comprehensive history* incorporates the same requirements as the detailed history and adds a review of all additional body systems and a complete past, family, and social history.

Study the underlined words. The coder is supposed to determine what is brief, extended, a limited number, and pertinent. The options are too vague to allow for accurate determination of the level of history, the first key component of the level of service. Likewise, the CPT definitions and terms used to describe the examination (such as limited and extended) and to discuss the MDM (such as minimal, low, moderate, and extensive) are all somewhat vague and qualitative. For this reason, documentation guidelines (DGs) have been written to create a specific set of points that can be analyzed and objectively scored when initially assigning or later verifying E/M code assignment.

Development of the Documentation Guidelines for E/M Services

The DGs grew out of a change in the way Medicare reimburses physicians. In 1992, based on a Harvard study initiated in December 1985 by Dr. William Hsiao and a multidisciplinary team of researchers, Medicare began to base payment on the resource-based relative value scale (RBRVS) methodology. Under this system, payment for services is determined by the costs needed to provide them rather than on the charges submitted. The costs of services were divided into three components: physician work, practice expense, and professional liability insurance.

As a result of this change, the American Medical Association (AMA) developed new E/M codes reflecting the RBRVS methodology. Physicians subsequently wanted a resource they could consult when determining the level of service to assign to their work. In 1994 the AMA and the Health Care Financing Administration (HCFA), now known as the Centers for Medicare and Medicaid Services (CMS), developed the *1995 Documentation Guidelines for Evaluation and Management Services*.

Medical specialty societies soon requested refinements to include guidelines for their own specialty E/M services. In 1997 the E/M guidelines were revised to include single-specialty and multisystem exams. The new version is referred to as the *1997 Documentation Guidelines for Evaluation and Management Services*.

Today physicians can use either the 1995 or the 1997 documentation guidelines to determine the LOS for E/M services, whichever is more advantageous to their practice. In other words, if using one or the other of the guidelines leads to a higher-level E/M code, that DG may be used.

Importance of Documentation Guidelines

When a physician provides services to a patient, the physician is required to record, or document, those services in the patient's medical record. The medical record chronologically documents the physician's care of the patient and verifies the services the physician reports on the patient's billing record. The documentation guidelines note that the medical record facilitates the physician's ability to evaluate and plan the patient's treatment and monitor care over time. It represents the communication and continuity of care and facilitates accurate and timely review of claims and payments, utilization reviews, and quality of care evaluations.

> **INTERNET RESOURCE: Documentation Guidelines for Evaluation and Management Services**
> **www.cms.hhs.gov**
> **Search for "documentation guidelines"**

The DGs emphasize a simple concept: "If it hasn't been documented, it hasn't been done." This phrase in effect underlies the entire concept of documentation of medical and surgical services. Medical students learn this concept in medical school, and when they become residents their commitment to documentation of services is apparent. However, after a period of time in practice, physicians are sometimes less attentive to documenting E/M services. When documentation is incomplete or inaccurate, third-party payers may downcode (reduce) the E/M service levels reported by physicians on claims. The 1995 and 1997 E/M documentation guidelines were put in place to ensure that documentation is complete and accurate and that it is correctly reported.

It is important to note that many physicians and health-care professionals are familiar with the SOAP method of documentation:

    S = subjective
    O = objective
    A = assessment
    P = plan

The three key components used to determine the LOS—history, examination, and medical decision making—can be matched to the SOAP method.

    S = subjective = history, what the patient indicates in his or her own words
    O = objective = examination, the physician's findings from examining the patient
    A = assessment = diagnosis
    P = plan = how to treat the diagnosis

The last two (A and P) equate to medical decision making, the third key component.

E/M services can supply up to 40% of the revenue of most physician practices, and carriers and the federal government auditing agencies are aware of the financial impact of E/M services. For that reason, E/M services are carefully monitored. (See the discussion of fraud in the Coding, Reimbursement, and Fraud section later in this chapter.)

> **INTERNET RESOURCE: Medicare learning network resources for E/M coding**
> **https://www.cms.gov/Outreach-and-Education/Medicare-Learning-Network**
> **-MLN/MLNProducts/index.html**

General Principles

Both the 1995 and the 1997 E/M documentation guidelines include the following general principles of documentation:

- The medical record should be complete and legible.
- Documentation for each patient encounter should include the following:
  - The reason for the encounter, the relevant history, physical examination findings, and prior diagnostic test results
  - Assessment, clinical impression, or diagnosis
  - Plan of care
  - Date and legible identity of the observer
- If not specifically documented, the rationale for ordering diagnostic and other services should be easily inferred.
- Past and present diagnoses should be accessible to the treating or consulting physician.
- Health risk factors should be documented.
- A patient's progress, response to, and changes in treatment and the physician's revisions of diagnoses should be noted.
- CPT and ICD-10-CM codes must be supported by the documentation.

CHECKPOINT 14.1

Answer the following questions.

1. What information must be documented for an expanded problem-focused history in addition to that documented in a problem-focused history? _____

2. The physician evaluated an established patient and documented an expanded problem-focused history and examination and straightforward MDM. The physician reported code 99213. Is the physician correct? What concept was used to correctly answer this question? _____

COMPARISON OF 1995 AND 1997 DOCUMENTATION GUIDELINES

The purpose of the DGs is to permit translation of physician documentation into levels of the three key components. History and medical decision making are assigned in the same way in both the 1995 and 1997 DGs; the guidelines differ only in the examination requirement.

The 1995 DGs have a single set of examination requirements with four levels: problem focused, expanded problem focused, detailed, and comprehensive:

- *Problem-focused (PF) exam:* A limited inspection of the affected body area or organ system
- *Expanded PF exam:* A limited look at any other symptomatic or related body areas or organ systems as well as the affected ones
- *Detailed exam:* Extended examination of affected body areas or organ systems and any other symptomatic or related body areas or organ systems
- *Comprehensive exam:* A general multisystem exam or a complete examination of a single organ system and other symptomatic or related body areas or organ systems

The 1997 DGs have two types of examination requirements: general multisystem examination requirements and specialty examination requirements. For both types of examinations, the guidelines specify body parts and organ systems and provide bulleted lists of the elements of examination—that is, the physician's actions in examining each of the parts or systems. For example, two bullets are listed for a multisystem examination of the skin:

- Inspection of skin and subcutaneous tissue (e.g., rashes, lesions, ulcers)
- Palpation of skin and subcutaneous tissue (e.g., by touch, pin, vibration, proprioception)

To work with the 1997 exam guidelines, the coder must consult the CMS document that shows the bulleted items.

The 1997 DGs define the multisystem examination levels as follows:

- *Problem focused:* One to five elements identified by bullets
- *Expanded PF:* At least six elements identified by bullets
- *Detailed:* At least two elements identified by bullets from each of six areas/systems, or at least 12 elements identified by bullets in two or more areas/systems
- *Comprehensive:* At least two elements identified by bullets from each of nine areas/systems

Specialty exam guidelines differ from general multisystem exam guidelines and can vary among the different specialties.

The 1997 documentation guidelines for specialty examinations provide specific rules for each of 11 different medical specialties. Besides showing bulleted elements, some of the listings appear in plain boxes, and others appear in boxes with shaded borders. For example, four of the systems in the musculoskeletal examination section—constitutional, musculoskeletal, skin, and neurological/psychiatric—appear inside shaded borders, while the remaining 11 areas, including cardiovascular and lymphatic, are in plain boxes.

The requirement for determining service levels for musculoskeletal examinations are:

- *Problem focused:* One to five elements identified by bullets.
- *Expanded PF:* At least six elements identified by bullets.
- *Detailed:* At least 12 elements identified by bullets.
- *Comprehensive:* All elements identified by bullets; document every element in each box with a <u>shaded</u> border and at least one element in each box with an <u>unshaded</u> border.

CHECKPOINT 14.2

Answer the following questions.

1. How has Medicare reimbursement been calculated since 1992? _____

2. What is the main difference between the 1995 and the 1997 documentation guidelines?

   _____

3. Are physicians allowed to use both the 1995 and 1997 documentation guidelines, or do they have to limit themselves to choosing one or the other? _____

ELEMENTS OF KEY COMPONENTS

Each key component has specific elements. The history key component comprises three elements:

1. History of present illness (HPI)
2. Review of systems (ROS)
3. Past, family, and/or social history (PFSH)

The examination key component has two elements:

1. Body areas
2. Organ systems

The MDM component has three elements:

1. Diagnoses and management options
2. Data review

Medicare's Incident-To Guidelines

When a licensed health-care professional other than a physician provides services to a Medicare patient, a special Medicare policy may apply. If the nonphysician provider (NPP) is working under the supervision of a physician, services can be billed and paid at the doctor's Medicare rate, rather than at the lower rate Medicare usually pays the NPP. This situation is stated as services provided incident to the physician. "Incident to" is a Medicare policy, and only Medicare defines the policy.

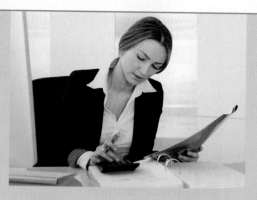

Under incident-to billing, the nonphysician provider is billing under the physician's name and provider number. This is different than billing as a credentialed provider under the NPP's own provider or billing number. Table 14.1 summarizes the rules for incident-to billing.

3. Overall risk, which comprises:
   a. Presenting problem
   b. Diagnostic procedures
   c. Management options

Remember that the goal of the DGs is to determine the level of service provided by the physician based on the information documented in the medical record. The history and examination key components use the same four levels:

1. Problem focused (PF)
2. Expanded problem focused (EPF)
3. Detailed (DET)
4. Comprehensive (COMP)

For the MDM key component, there is another set of four levels:

1. Straightforward (SF)
2. Low complexity (LOW)
3. Moderate complexity (MOD)
4. High complexity (HIGH)

The E/M services that require all three key components to assign the LOS are as follows:

- Office and other outpatient services: new patients (codes 99201–99205)
- Outpatient hospital observation services: initial care (codes 99218–99220)
- Hospital inpatient services: initial care (codes 99221–99223)
- Consultations (codes 99241–99255)
- Emergency department services (codes 99281–99285)
- Nursing facility services: initial care (codes 99304–99306)
- Domiciliary care services: new patients (codes 99324–99328)
- Home services: new patients (codes 99341–99345)

The E/M services that require two of the three key components to assign the LOS are as follows:

- Office and other outpatient services (codes 99212–99215)
- Hospital inpatient services: subsequent care (codes 99231–99233)
- Nursing facility services: subsequent care (codes 99307–99310)
- Domiciliary care services: established patients (codes 99334–99337)
- Home services: established patients (codes 99347–99350)

Table 14.1 Incident-To Versus Credentialed Billing

INCIDENT-TO BILLING	CREDENTIALED BILLING
NPP cannot see new patients.	NPP can see new patients.
Physician must be immediately available in the office suite.	Physician does not have to be present.
NPP bills E/M no higher than 99213.	NPP can bill all levels of E/M.
NPP cannot provide services in the hospital.	NPP is allowed to provide services in the hospital.
NPP bills under the physician's name and provider number.	NPP bills under own name and provider number.
NPP service is reimbursed same as provider.	NPP is reimbursed at 80% of the provider's amount.

Note: Services provided by NPPs must first meet the requirements of their state licensure.

Table 14.2 shows examples of this same information in another way. As it makes clear, new/initial codes require three key components, and established codes need two of the three key components.

Table 14.2 Number of Key Components Required for E/M Categories

E/M CATEGORY	CODES	NUMBER OF KEY COMPONENTS REQUIRED
New patients	99201–99205	3
Established patients	99212–99215	2
Initial hospital care	99221–99223	3
Subsequent hospital care	99231–99233	2
Office/outpatient consult	99241–99245	3
Inpatient consult	99251–99255	3

Note that only the MDM component differs for codes 99204 and 99205.

Determining which new patient code to assign requires identifying the level of service documented for each of the three key components and comparing the levels to those shown in Table 14.3, always remembering that the lowest key component controls the level of service.

Table 14.3 New Patient Codes and Level of Service

NEW PATIENT CODE	HISTORY	EXAM	MDM
99201	Problem focused	Problem focused	Straightforward
99202	Expanded problem focused	Expanded problem focused	Straightforward
99203	Detailed	Detailed	Low
99204	Comprehensive	Comprehensive	Moderate
99205	Comprehensive	Comprehensive	High

Assigning established patient codes requires matching the documented LOS to two of the three key components, as illustrated in Table 14.4.

Table 14.4 Established Patient Codes and Level of Service

ESTABLISHED PATIENT CODE	HISTORY	EXAM	MDM
99211	None	None	None
99212	Problem focused	Problem focused	Straightforward
99213	Expanded problem focused	Expanded problem focused	Low
99214	Detailed	Detailed	Moderate
99215	Comprehensive	Comprehensive	High

For initial hospital care, the levels of all three key components must be considered when assigning a code (Table 14.5).

Table 14.5 Initial Hospital Care Codes and Level of Service

INITIAL HOSPITAL CODE	HISTORY	EXAM	MDM
99221	Detailed or comprehensive	Detailed or comprehensive	Straightforward or low
99222	Comprehensive	Comprehensive	Moderate
99223	Comprehensive	Comprehensive	High

As shown in Table 14.6, two of the three key components are required for subsequent hospital care coding.

Table 14.6 Subsequent Hospital Care Codes and Level of Service

SUBSEQUENT HOSPITAL CODE	HISTORY	EXAM	MDM
99231	Problem focused	Problem focused	Straightforward or low
99232	Expanded problem focused	Expanded problem focused	Moderate
99233	Detailed	Detailed	High

WORKING WITH THE 1995/1997 HISTORY GUIDELINES

The first aspect of the history is the chief complaint (CC), defined in CPT as "a concise statement describing the symptom, problem, condition, diagnosis, or other factor that is the reason for the encounter, usually stated in the patient's words."

EXAMPLES
- This the first visit for a 45-year-old male patient with pain on urination.
- This a follow-up visit for an individual with type 2 diabetes.

The DGs indicate that the medical record must clearly reflect the CC. Statements such as "patient here for follow-up" and "new patient" do not identify a definitive presenting problem and thus do not qualify as appropriate descriptions of the chief complaint.

The History of Present Illness Element

Following determination of the chief complaint, the DGs cover the three elements of the history key component. Table 14.7 is a matrix of the DG requirements for the history key component.

Table 14.7 DG Requirements for the History Key Component

TYPE OF HISTORY	CHIEF COMPLAINT	HISTORY OF PRESENT ILLNESS	REVIEW OF SYSTEMS	PAST, FAMILY, AND/OR SOCIAL HISTORY
Problem focused	Required	Brief	Not required	Not required
Expanded problem focused	Required	Brief	Problem pertinent	Not required
Detailed	Required	Extended	Extended	Pertinent
Comprehensive	Required	Extended	Complete	Complete

The CMS documentation guidelines define the history of present illness (HPI) as "a chronological description of the development of the patient's present illness from the first sign and/or symptom or from the previous encounter to the present." The HPI includes these eight elements (Fig. 14.1):

1. *Location:* Where the pain, problem, or symptom is, such as chest, back, or abdomen
2. *Quality:* Description of the condition, such as dull, constant, sore, red
3. *Severity:* Most commonly a reference to the pain index, the patient's rating on a scale of 1 to 10
4. *Duration:* How long the patient has had the problem, such as 1 week, 1 day
5. *Timing:* When the problem occurs, such as after dinner, only in the morning, and so on
6. *Context:* The circumstances in which the problem has occurred, such as after a fall, while standing for a long time, and so on
7. *Modifying factors:* What the patient has done to make the problem better
8. *Associated signs and symptoms:* Other problems that occur with the primary problem, such as dizziness along with the pain

CHECKPOINT 14.3

Read the following scenarios and answer the questions.

1. The physician assistant (PA) sees an established patient who is covered by Medicare to review his blood pressure status and lipid profile since the last visit a month ago. This protocol was established by the physician on the patient's last visit. The physician was present in the office during the encounter. The billing for this visit went out under the physician's name and provider number to Medicare. This is an example of what type of billing? _____

2. If the above patient was new to the practice and was seen by the PA, could the service be reported under the physician's name and provider number? _____

3. In giving a history of her present illness, a patient states that she hurt her arm a week ago when she fell down a few stairs. Which elements of HPI are represented by that statement? _____

The documentation of the HPI can be brief, meaning a description of one to three of the eight elements, or it can be extended, a description of four or more of the elements or of the status of at least three chronic or inactive conditions. Although the 1995 DG does not explicitly state that documentation of three chronic or inactive conditions qualifies the HPI as extended, CMS has clarified that this criterion is applicable to the 1995 DGs as well as to the 1997 DGs, where it is stated.

EXAMPLE
The statement that "patient is here today for follow-up of his coronary artery disease, COPD, and peripheral vascular disease" qualifies as extended documentation of history.

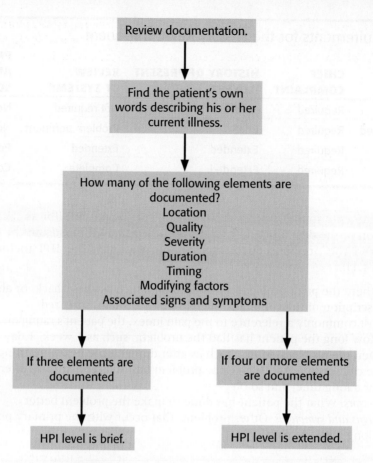

Figure 14.1 The steps for determining the level of history of present illness.

The documentation presented at the beginning of this chapter includes the following history of the patient's condition:

Patient is here today with left leg muscle pain for the past 6 months. It became worse 4 days ago, and the patient feels weak and tired. The patient has no shortness of breath, no stomach pain, no allergies; the patient feels distressed. There is nothing relevant in the patient's family history. The patient is 37 years of age, and is married with two children. The patient is not on any medications and has not had any surgeries.

From this documentation, the coder has to determine whether the history is problem focused, expanded problem focused, detailed, or comprehensive. To do so, the coder first determines the level of each of the three elements—history of present illness, review of systems, and past, family, and/or social history—documented by the physician.

The documentation provides information on the chief complaint (muscle pain) and the following four elements of HPI:

1. *Location:* Left leg
2. *Quality:* Worse
3. *Duration:* Six months; worse for 4 days
4. *Associated signs and symptoms:* Weak and tired

Thus, the documentation meets the criteria of the extended level.

The Review of Systems Element

According to CMS, the review of systems (ROS), "is an inventory of body systems obtained through a series of questions seeking to identify signs and/or symptoms which the patient may be experiencing or has experienced." The documentation of the ROS results from the physician's questions and the patient's answers or from the information the patient has provided on an intake form. If the information comes from an intake form, the relevant responses must be referenced in the physician's documentation. Figure 14.2 presents a decision tree on how to determine the level of review of systems.

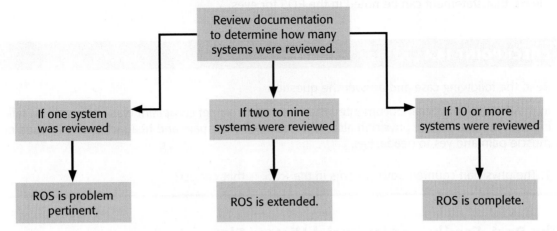

Figure 14.2 The steps for determining the level of review of systems.

The ROS inventories the following body systems:

- Constitutional (fever, weight loss)
- Eyes (pain, double vision, redness)
- Ears, nose, mouth, throat (pain, hearing difficulty)
- Cardiovascular (chest pain, edema, palpitations)
- Respiratory (wheezing, shortness of breath)
- Gastrointestinal (pain, bloating, constipation)
- Genitourinary (discharge, hematuria, burning sensation during urination)
- Musculoskeletal (pain, swelling, stiffness)
- Integumentary—skin and/or breast (rash, swelling, soreness)
- Neurological (headaches, trembling, lack of sensation)
- Psychiatric (feelings, depression, outbursts)
- Endocrine (excessive sweating or thirst)
- Hematologic/lymphatic (anemia, unusual bleeding or bruising)
- Allergy/immunologic (allergies, immune problems)

The three levels of ROS are problem pertinent, extended, and complete. At the problem-pertinent level, the physician documents the patient's positive and pertinent negative responses about the system directly related to the problems identified in the history of present illness. The documentation covers a single system.

At the extended level, the physician asks the patient about two to nine systems representing the system directly related to the problem plus additional systems. The documentation reports on both positive and pertinent negative responses from the patient.

> To report the higher levels of service, a comprehensive ROS is required. In many cases, physicians do not review 10 or more organ systems yet bill those higher LOS codes. As a result, the documentation does not meet the requirements for reporting the comprehensive level codes such as 99204, 99205, 99215, and 99255.

The complete ROS level covers all additional body systems directly related to the problems identified in the history of present illness. According to the DGs, "At least ten organ systems must be reviewed. Those systems with positive or pertinent negative responses must be individually documented. For the remaining systems, a notation indicating that all other systems are negative is permissible. In the absence of such a notation, at least ten systems must individually be documented."

Returning to the example presented earlier in this chapter, the documentation indicates that the patient is not experiencing shortness of breath, stomach pain, or allergies but does feel distressed. Four systems—respiratory, gastrointestinal, allergy/immunologic, and psychiatric—are identified in the documentation.

A body system can be documented in either the HPI or the ROS but not in both. However, if further questioning provides additional information about a body system, the system may be mentioned more than once.

A patient's statement that her eye has been red for 2 days is documented as location, quality, and duration under HPI. If the patient additionally states that she has no other visual problems, that statement can be noted in the ROS for eyes.

CHECKPOINT 14.4

Read the following case and answer the question.

In the ROS, the physician documented that the patient's chief complaint was chest pain. In talking with the patient, the physician also asked about muscle pain and headaches. She replied no to muscle pain and yes to headaches.

1. The physician counted both systems in the ROS. Is that correct? _____

The Past, Family, and/or Social History Element

The elements of PFSH are past history (the patient's past experiences with illnesses, operations, injuries, and treatments); family history (medical events in the patient's family, including diseases that may be hereditary or place the patient at risk); and social history (age-appropriate review of past and current activities such as marital status, alcohol or drug use, and employment). They are designated within the audit as none, pertinent, or complete. Figure 14.3 is a breakdown of how to determine the level of PFSH.

A pertinent PFSH involves one item from any one of the three types of history directly related to the problems identified in the HPI. A complete PFSH may require all three PFSH elements, or it may require only two of the three elements, depending on which E/M services are being provided.

For services that include a comprehensive assessment or reassessment of the patient, all three PFSH elements are required. These services are:

- Office/outpatient for new patients (codes 99201–99205)
- Initial observation care (codes 99218–99220)
- Initial hospital care (codes 99221–99223)
- Office/outpatient consultation (codes 99241–99245)
- Inpatient consultation (codes 99251–99255)
- Initial nursing facility care (codes 99304–99306)

> ● The key components for the subsequent hospital care codes 99231–99233 and subsequent nursing facility care codes 99307–99310 have an interval history requirement. Under the DGs it is not necessary to record information about PFSH for an interval history.

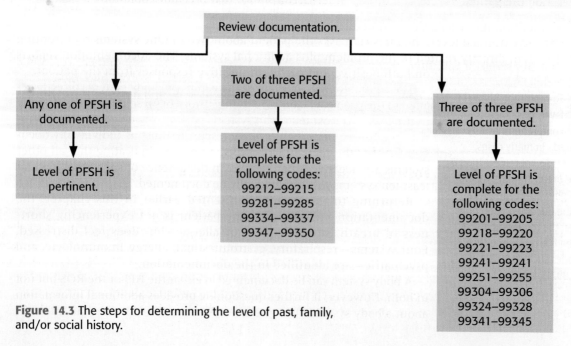

Figure 14.3 The steps for determining the level of past, family, and/or social history.

- Domiciliary care for new patients (codes 99324–99328)
- Home care for new patients (codes 99341–99345)

The services that require two of the three PFSH elements to meet the requirements for a complete PFSH are as follows:

- Office/outpatient for established patients (codes 99212–99215)
- Emergency department (codes 99281–99285)
- Domiciliary care for established patients (codes 99334–99337)
- Home care for established patients (codes 99347–99350)

CHECKPOINT 14.5

Read the following case and answer the question.

A patient was previously seen 2.5 years ago and is now seen for a worsening of her asthma. The physician did an extended HPI and ROS and documented that he asked if there had been any changes in the patient's medical history, or if she had changed jobs.

1. The physician notated that he had obtained a complete PFSH. Is the physician correct?

Additional Guidelines for ROS and PFSH

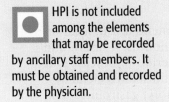

HPI is not included among the elements that may be recorded by ancillary staff members. It must be obtained and recorded by the physician.

ROS and PFSH obtained during an earlier encounter do not need to be recorded again if there is evidence that the physician reviewed and updated the information. A physician may update his or her own record, or may update a common record of other physicians in an institutional setting or group practice. The physician may document the review or the update by describing any new ROS and/or PFSH information or by noting the date and location of the earlier ROS and/or PFSH and indicating that there has been no change in the information.

The ROS and/or PFSH may be recorded by an ancillary staff member or may appear on a form completed by the patient. The physician must document that he or she reviewed the information in a note supplementing or confirming the information recorded by others.

If the physician is unable to obtain a history from the patient or other source, the record should describe the patient's condition or any other circumstance that precludes obtaining a history.

Putting the History Component Together

When the levels of the three elements of HPI, ROS, and PFSH have been determined, the coder can determine the level of the history key component, as shown in Figure 14.4 and Table 14.8. For example, the combination of a brief HPI, a problem-pertinent ROS, and no PFSH describes an expanded problem-focused level of service for the history component.

Table 14.8 History Key Component Example

ELEMENT	PROBLEM FOCUSED	EXPANDED PF	DETAILED	COMPREHENSIVE
HPI	Brief	Brief	Extended	Extended
ROS	None	Problem pertinent	Extended	Complete
PFSH	None	None	Pertinent	Complete

If, however, the levels of the elements fall into different columns in the chart, the coder determines the lowest level of service and assigns that level to the history component. For example, if the HPI is extended, the ROS is complete, and no PFSH is documented, the level of PFSH determines the history level, which in this case is expanded PF.

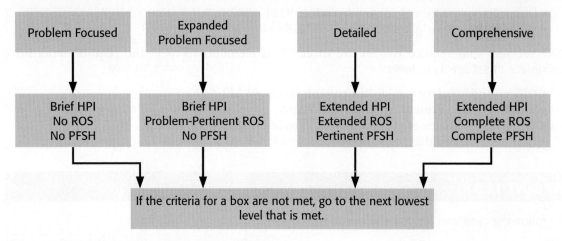

Problem Focused	Expanded Problem Focused	Detailed	Comprehensive
↓	↓	↓	↓
Brief HPI No ROS No PFSH	Brief HPI Problem-Pertinent ROS No PFSH	Extended HPI Extended ROS Pertinent PFSH	Extended HPI Complete ROS Complete PFSH

If the criteria for a box are not met, go to the next lowest level that is met.

Figure 14.4 The steps for determining the level of history.

Recall the example presented earlier in this chapter:

> Patient is here today with left leg (HPI–location) muscle pain (chief complaint; ROS–musculoskeletal) for the past 6 months (HPI–duration). It became worse (HPI–quality) 4 days ago, and the patient feels weak and tired (HPI–associated signs and symptoms). The patient has no shortness of breath (ROS–respiratory), no stomach pain (ROS–gastrointestinal), no allergies (ROS–allergies); the patient feels distressed (ROS–psychiatric). There is nothing relevant in the patient's family history (PFSH–family). The patient is 37 years of age, and is married with two children (PFSH–social). The patient is not on any medications and has not had any surgeries (PFSH–past).

Four of the eight elements of the history of present illness are documented: the location (muscle in left leg), the quality (pain, became worse), the duration (6 months, 4 days), and the associated signs and symptoms (weak and tired). This meets the criterion of at least four elements of extended HPI. The documentation includes review of the musculoskeletal system directly related to the problem plus four additional systems—respiratory, gastrointestinal, allergy, and psychiatric—placing the ROS at the extended level. Finally, past, family, and social history are all documented, meeting the criterion for the complete level.

Extended HPI and extended ROS both fall into the category of detailed history, while complete PFSH is part of comprehensive history (Table 14.9). Because at least one element (in this case, two elements) is at the lower level of detail, the documentation places history at the detailed level.

Table 14.9 History Key Component Example

	PROBLEM FOCUSED	EXPANDED PF	DETAILED	COMPREHENSIVE
HPI	Brief	Brief	Extended	Extended
ROS	0	Problem pertinent	Extended	Complete
PFSH	0	0	Pertinent	Complete

A detailed history complies with codes 99203 for new patients, 99214 for established patients, 99243 for office/outpatient consultations, and 99253 for hospital consultations.

WORKING WITH THE 1995 EXAMINATION GUIDELINES

As indicated previously, the guidelines for the examination key component differ in the 1995 and 1997 versions of the documentation guidelines. In the 1995 DGs, the examination key component is divided into two areas, the 12 organ systems and the seven body areas, as shown in Table 14.10.

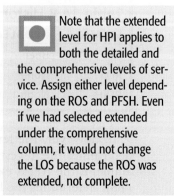

Note that the extended level for HPI applies to both the detailed and the comprehensive levels of service. Assign either level depending on the ROS and PFSH. Even if we had selected extended under the comprehensive column, it would not change the LOS because the ROS was extended, not complete.

Table 14.10 1995 DG Examination Key Component Division

ORGAN SYSTEM(S)	BODY AREA(S)
Constitutional (vital signs, general appearance)	Head, including the face
Eyes	Neck
Ears, nose, mouth, and throat	Chest, including the breasts and axillae
Cardiovascular	Abdomen
Respiratory	Genitalia, groin, buttocks
Gastrointestinal	Back, including spine
Genitourinary	Each extremity
Musculoskeletal	
Integumentary (skin)	
Neurological	
Psychiatric	
Hemic/lymphatic/immunological	

The 1995 DGs have four levels of examination:

1. *Problem focused:* A limited examination of the affected body area or organ system
2. *Expanded PF:* A limited examination of the affected body area or organ system and other symptomatic or related organ system(s)
3. *Detailed:* An extended examination of the affected body area(s) and other symptomatic or related organ system(s)
4. *Comprehensive:* A general multisystem examination or a complete examination of a single organ system

Because these criteria can make determining the level of examination from physician documentation difficult, an alternative methodology is generally accepted:

1. *Problem focused:* Examination of one body area/organ system
2. *Expanded PF:* Examination of two to four body areas/organ systems
3. *Detailed:* Examination of five to seven body areas/organ systems
4. *Comprehensive:* Examination of eight organ systems (not body areas) or a complete examination of a single organ system

According to the DGs, the physician should document abnormal and relevant negative findings of an affected or symptomatic body area or organ system. Simply indicating that there are abnormal findings without elaborating on what they are is insufficient. Furthermore, abnormal or unexpected findings of the unaffected or asymptomatic body area or organ system should be described. However, it is acceptable to report the presence of negative or normal findings related to unaffected/asymptomatic body areas or organ systems without elaboration. Finally, documentation of a general multisystem examination must include at least 8 of the 12 organ systems.

The documentation of the examination in the example presented earlier described the following:

The patient's blood pressure is 130/80; he weighs 180 lb; he is afebrile (constitutional—organ system); lungs are clear to auscultation (respiratory—organ system); no evidence of hepatosplenomegaly (gastrointestinal—organ system); neck is supple (neck—body area); cardiovascular is regular rhythm without murmur (cardiovascular—organ system); both legs appear normal; gait is normal, but the left leg is painful when manipulated; general muscle tone normal (musculoskeletal—organ system); no rash; skin texture and color are normal (skin—organ system).

Because nothing in the physician's documentation indicates whether the examination was limited or extended, the most useful methodology is based on the number of organ systems and body areas examined. (In fact, most auditors and reviewers prefer to use this methodology.) In the example, six organ systems and one body area were examined, for a total of seven. This complies with the detailed level of service for the examination.

WORKING WITH THE 1995/1997 MEDICAL DECISION-MAKING GUIDELINES

Medical decision making refers to the complexity of establishing a diagnosis and/or selecting a management option. Three factors go into measuring MDM. The first factor is the number of possible diagnoses and/or the number of management options that the physician must consider. Here the coder looks at the diagnoses the physician documents in assessing the patient. Second is the amount and/or complexity of medical records, diagnostic tests, and/or other information that must be obtained, reviewed, and analyzed. This includes documentation of the review and ordering of procedures to obtain data. Finally, the risks of significant complications, morbidity and/or mortality, comorbidities associated with the patient's presenting problems, the diagnostic procedures, and/or the possible management options are calculated. This is known as overall risk.

> Only conditions that affect the encounter being coded should be considered as relevant to MDM.

To determine the level of MDM, two of the three elements in Table 14.11 must be either met or exceeded.

Table 14.11 Medical Decision-Making Key Component

NUMBER OF DIAGNOSES OR MANAGEMENT OPTIONS	AMOUNT AND/OR COMPLEXITY OF DATA TO BE REVIEWED	RISK OF COMPLICATIONS AND/OR MORBIDITY OR MORTALITY	TYPE OF DECISION MAKING
Minimal	Minimal or none	Minimal	Straightforward
Limited	Limited	Low	Low complexity
Multiple	Moderate	Moderate	Moderate complexity
Extensive	Extensive	High	High complexity

Number of Diagnoses or Management Options

The DGs base determination of the level of the number of diagnoses on the following principles:

- Decision making is easier for a diagnosed problem than for an undiagnosed problem.
- The number and type of tests can be an indication of the number of diagnoses.
- Problems that are resolving or improving are less complex than those that are worsening or failing to change as expected.
- Seeking advice from others is an indication of complexity.
- For an established diagnosis, the documentation should indicate whether the problem is improved, well controlled, resolving, or resolved, or if it is instead inadequately controlled, worsening, or failing to change as expected.
- A problem that is not diagnosed can be stated as a "possible" or "rule out" diagnosis for purposes of determining the MDM level.
- Changes in treatment should be documented. Examples of such documentation are patient instructions, therapies ordered, and medications prescribed.
- Any consultations, referrals, or advice should be documented.

Amount and/or Complexity of Data

The DGs advise that three factors increase the amount and complexity of the data to be reviewed: (1) obtaining and reviewing old medical records and/or history from sources other than the patient, (2) discussing test results with the physician who performed or interpreted the test, and (3) the physician's personal review of an image, tracing, or interpretation.

Risk of Significant Complications, Morbidity, and/or Mortality

The DGs provide a table (Table 14.12) that shows common clinical examples in three categories—presenting problem, diagnostic procedures, and management options—to help the coder determine whether overall risk is minimal, low, moderate, or high. The documentation of one bullet in any box supports the level identified in the left column. The highest risk level in any one area establishes the overall risk. It is important to keep in mind that the examples in Table 14.12 are not absolute measures of risk.

Putting the Medical Decision-Making Component Together

The DGs do not have a point system methodology, but such a system is utilized by auditors and carriers to provide consistency in determining MDM. Table 14.13 indicates how points are assigned to the two elements of diagnoses/management options and data review to help provide a level of MDM. The third element, overall risk, is determined based on the table of risk presented below.

Table 14.12 Overall Risk

LEVEL OF RISK	PRESENTING PROBLEM(S)	DIAGNOSTIC PROCEDURES ORDERED	MANAGEMENT OPTIONS SELECTED
Minimal	• One self-limited or minor problem, e.g., cold, insect bite, tinea corporis	• Laboratory tests requiring venipuncture • Chest x-rays • EKG/EEG • Urinalysis • Ultrasound, e.g., echocardiography • KOH prep	• Rest • Gargles • Elastic bandages • Superficial dressings
Low	• Two or more self-limited or minor problems • One stable chronic illness, e.g., well-controlled hypertension, non–insulin-dependent diabetes, cataract, BPH • Acute uncomplicated illness or injury, e.g., cystitis, allergic rhinitis, simple sprain	• Physiological tests not under stress, e.g., pulmonary function tests • Non–cardiovascular imaging studies with contrast, e.g., barium enema • Superficial needle biopsies • Clinical laboratory tests requiring arterial puncture • Skin biopsies	• Over-the-counter drugs • Minor surgery with no identified risk factors • Physical therapy • Occupational therapy • IV fluids without additives
Moderate	• One or more chronic illnesses with mild exacerbation, progression, or side effects of treatment • Two or more stable chronic illnesses • Undiagnosed new problem with uncertain prognosis, e.g., lump in breast • Acute illness with systemic symptoms, e.g., pyelonephritis, pneumonitis, colitis • Acute complicated injury, e.g., head injury with brief loss of consciousness	• Physiological tests under stress, e.g., cardiac stress test, fetal contraction stress test • Diagnostic endoscopies with no identified risk factors • Deep needle or incisional biopsy • Cardiovascular imaging studies with contrast and no identified risk factors, e.g., arteriogram, cardiac catheterization • Obtain fluid from body cavity, e.g., lumbar puncture, thoracentesis, culdocentesis	• Minor surgery with identified risk factors • Elective major surgery (open, percutaneous, or endoscopic) with no identified risk factor • Prescription drug management • Therapeutic nuclear medicine • IV fluids with additives • Closed treatment of fracture or dislocation without manipulation

Continued

Table 14.12 *Continued*

LEVEL OF RISK	PRESENTING PROBLEM(S)	DIAGNOSTIC PROCEDURES ORDERED	MANAGEMENT OPTIONS SELECTED
High	• One or more chronic illnesses with severe exacerbation, progression, or side effects of treatment • Acute or chronic illnesses or injuries that pose a threat to life or bodily function, e.g., multiple trauma, acute myocardial infarction, pulmonary embolus, severe respiratory distress, progressive severe rheumatoid arthritis, psychiatric illness with potential threat to self or others, peritonitis, acute renal failure • An abrupt change in neurological, status, e.g., seizure, transient ischemic attack, weakness, sensory loss	• Cardiovascular imaging studies with contrast with identified risk factors • Cardiac electrophysiological tests • Diagnostic endoscopies with identified risk factors • Discography	• Elective major surgery (open, percutaneous, or endoscopic) with identified risk factors • Emergency major surgery (open, percutaneous, or endoscopic) • Parenteral controlled substances • Drug therapy requiring intensive monitoring for toxicity • Decision not to resuscitate or to de-escalate care because of poor prognosis

Table 14.13 Point and Level Assignment for MDM

DIAGNOSES/MANAGEMENT OPTIONS	POINTS	MAXIMUM POINTS
Self-limited (stable, improved, worsening)	1	2
Established problem (stable, improved)	1	
Established problem (worsening)	2	
New problem, no additional workup	3	1
New problem, additional workup planned	4	
DATA REVIEW		
Clinical lab tests—review and/or order	1	1
Radiology tests—review and/or order	1	1
Medicine section tests (ECG, EEG)	1	1
Discussions with physician who performs tests	1	
Independent review of x-rays, tracings, specimens	2	
Obtaining old records and/or history from other than patient	1	
Reviewing and summarizing old records	2	
OVERALL RISK		
Three factors:		
Presenting problem		
Diagnostic procedures ordered		
Management options		
Four levels:		
Minimal		
Low		
Moderate		
High		

The first element involves assigning a point value to the diagnoses and/or management options documented in the physician's assessment and plan.

EXAMPLE

Patient has a left swollen ankle. This is a new problem to this physician, and documentation indicates that no additional workup will be provided. The point value is 3.

The second element is for data review. Did the physician document laboratory tests, radiology tests, or medicine section testing? Was there discussion with the physician who performed the test? Did the physician document his or her own review of the tests performed? Were any old records requested or a history obtained from someone other than the patient, such as family members or caregivers? Any review or summarization by the physician of old records is also considered in the point system.

EXAMPLE

Continuing with the previous example: The physician orders an x-ray of the ankle. The point value is 1.

The third element, overall risk, involves using the Overall Risk portion in Table 14.13, which divides risk into three areas:

1. The risk associated with the presenting problem (chief complaint)
2. The risk associated with the diagnostic procedure the physician has ordered to provide additional information regarding the presenting problem
3. The risk associated with management options the physician has ordered or will perform to treat either the presenting problem or the diagnosis resulting from the patient encounter

Many times, MDM information is obtained by the physician but not recorded, particularly discussions with other physicians and/or review of old information.

EXAMPLE

Continuing with the previous example: A splint is applied to the ankle, and the patient is advised to take Tylenol or aspirin for pain and elevate the foot. In the presenting problem column of Table 14.12, a simple sprain appears in the low-risk area. Neither the diagnostic procedures nor management options column provides a higher level of risk, so the level of risk is low.

Determining the level of medical decision making involves combining the levels of the three elements of diagnoses and treatments, data, and risk, then matching those levels to the levels shown in Table 14.14. The MDM level is straightforward, low, moderate, or high, depending on which column of the table has two values that match or exceed the levels of the elements. In the example of the patient with the swollen ankle, the diagnoses and/or treatment options are at the multiple level (three diagnoses or treatment options), data are limited (two), and risk is moderate, making the MDM level moderate, because two of the three elements appear in that column. If no column contains two values, then the MDM level is at the level of the lowest element.

Table 14.14 Medical Decision-Making Level

FINAL MDM LEVEL	STRAIGHTFORWARD	LOW	MODERATE	HIGH
A. Number of diagnoses and treatment options	1 Minimal	2 Limited	3 Multiple	4 Extensive
B. Amount and/or complexity of data involved	0–1 Minimal	2 Limited	3 Moderate	4 Extensive
C. Risk of complications, morbidity, mortality	Minimal	Low	Moderate	High

Continuing the original documentation example from the beginning of the chapter:

The patient may have an underlying infection/virus or chronic fatigue syndrome (diagnoses—new problem, 4 points). He is being sent for x-rays, blood count, and metabolic panel. The ECG done here today is normal (data review—clinical lab, radiology, and medicine section tests, independent review, 5 points). I am prescribing Celebrex to help with the pain (overall risk—prescription drug management, moderate), and the patient is to return in 1 week.

Based on Table 14.14, diagnoses at four points are in the high category, as is data review at five points. Moderate risk falls into the moderate category. With two of the three elements in the high category column, the MDM key component is high.

DETERMINING THE E/M LEVEL BASED ON THE 1995 DOCUMENTATION GUIDELINES

The elements of the examination key component are shown in Table 14.15. The levels of the elements required for each code are discussed later in this chapter. In the example discussed earlier in this chapter, the key components were at the following levels:

- *History:* Detailed
- *Examination:* Detailed
- *Medical decision making:* High

> When a patient brings x-rays taken elsewhere to the treating physician and that physician reviews the x-rays during the E/M service, the review is part of data review (2 points) and should not be coded separately with a code from the Radiology section.

For a new patient, all three key components must be at the level reported, so the lowest key component controls the level of service. If the patient in the example is a new patient, based on the information on new patient codes, code 99203 is reported. If the patient is an established patient, code 99213 is reported because only two of the three key components must be at the level reported.

CHECKPOINT 14.6

Answer the following questions.

1. What is meant by a "modifying factor" in the HPI? _____

2. Can past problems and medications be counted in the ROS? _____

3. Which E/M services require all three key components? _____

Table 14.15 Examination Key Component

SYSTEM/BODY AREA(S)	ELEMENTS OF EXAMINATION
Constitutional	• Measurement of any three of the following seven vital signs: (1) sitting or standing blood pressure, (2) supine blood pressure, (3) pulse rate and regularity, (4) respiration, (5) temperature, (6) height, (7) weight (vital signs may be measured and recorded by ancillary staff) • General appearance of patient (e.g., development, nutrition, body habitus, deformities, attention to grooming)
Eyes	• Inspection of conjunctivae and lids • Examination of pupils and irises (e.g., reaction to light and accommodation, size, and symmetry) • Ophthalmoscopic examination of optic discs (e.g., size, C/D ratio, appearance) and posterior segments (e.g., vessel changes, exudates, hemorrhages)
Ears, nose, mouth, and throat	• External inspection of ears and nose (e.g., overall appearance, scars, lesions, masses) • Otoscopic examination of external auditory canals and tympanic membranes • Assessment of hearing (e.g., whispered voice, finger rub, tuning fork) • Inspection of nasal mucosa, septum, and turbinates • Inspection of lips, teeth, and gums • Examination of oropharynx: oral mucosa, salivary glands, hard and soft palates, tongue, tonsils and posterior pharynx

SYSTEM/BODY AREA(S)	ELEMENTS OF EXAMINATION
Neck	• Examination of neck (e.g., masses, overall appearance, symmetry, tracheal position, crepitus) • Examination of thyroid (e.g., enlargement, tenderness, mass)
Respiratory	• Assessment of respiratory effort (e.g., intercostal retractions, use of accessory muscles, diaphragmatic movement) • Percussion of chest (e.g., dullness, flatness, hyperresonance) • Palpation of chest (e.g., tactile fremitus) • Auscultation of lungs (e.g., breath sounds, adventitious sounds, rubs)
Cardiovascular	• Palpation of heart (e.g., location, size, thrills) • Auscultation of heart with notation of abnormal sounds and murmurs Examination of: • Carotid arteries (e.g., pulse amplitude, bruits) • Abdominal aorta (e.g., size, bruits) • Femoral arteries (e.g., pulse amplitude, bruits) • Pedal pulses (e.g., pulse amplitude) • Extremities for edema and/or varicosities
Chest (breasts)	• Inspection of breasts (e.g., symmetry, nipple discharge) • Palpation of breasts and axillae (e.g., masses or lumps, tenderness)
Gastrointestinal (abdomen)	• Examination of abdomen with notation of presence of masses or tenderness • Examination of liver and spleen • Examination for presence or absence of hernia • Examination (when indicated) of anus, perineum, and rectum, including sphincter tone, presence of hemorrhoids, rectal masses • Obtain stool sample for occult blood test when indicated
Genitourinary	Male: • Examination of the scrotal contents (e.g., hydrocele, spermatocele, tenderness of cord, testicular mass) • Examination of the penis • Digital rectal examination of prostate gland (e.g., size, symmetry, nodularity, tenderness) Female: • Pelvic examination (with or without specimen collection for smears and cultures), including: • Examination of external genitalia (e.g., general appearance, hair distribution, lesions) and vagina (e.g., general appearance, estrogen effect, discharge, lesions, pelvic support, cystocele, rectocele) • Examination of urethra (e.g., masses, tenderness, scarring) • Examination of bladder (e.g., fullness, masses, tenderness) • Cervix (e.g., general appearance, lesions, discharge) • Uterus (e.g., size, contour, position, mobility, tenderness, consistency, descent, or support) • Adnexa/parametria (e.g., masses, tenderness, organomegaly, nodularity)
Lymphatic	Palpation of lymph nodes in two or more areas: • Neck • Axillae • Groin • Other
Musculoskeletal	• Examination of gait and station • Inspection and/or palpation of digits and nails (e.g., clubbing, cyanosis, inflammatory conditions, petechiae, ischemia, infections, nodes) • Assessment of range of motion with notation of any pain, crepitation, or contracture

Continued

Table 14.15 *Continued*

SYSTEM/BODY AREA(S)	ELEMENTS OF EXAMINATION
	• Assessment of stability with notation of any dislocation (luxation), subluxation, or laxity
	• Assessment of muscle strength and tone (e.g., flaccid, cog wheel, spastic) with notation of any atrophy or abnormal movements
Skin	• Inspection of skin and subcutaneous tissue (e.g., rashes, lesions, ulcers)
	• Palpation of skin and subcutaneous tissue (e.g., induration, subcutaneous nodules, tightening)
Neurological	• Test cranial nerves with notation of any deficits
	• Examination of deep tendon reflexes with notation of pathological reflexes (e.g., Babinski)
	• Examination of sensation (e.g., by touch, pin, vibration, proprioception)
Psychiatric	• Description of patient's judgment and insight Brief assessment of mental status including:
	• Orientation to time, place, and person
	• Recent and remote memory
	• Mood and affect (e.g., depression, anxiety, agitation)

APPLYING THE 1997 DOCUMENTATION GUIDELINES TO THE EXAMINATION KEY COMPONENT

The coding workup to this point has been based on the 1995 E/M documentation guidelines. The difference between the 1995 and the 1997 DGs is in the examination criteria; history and MDM levels are the same in both versions. Using the same example of documentation presented earlier, this section examines the coding process for the examination key component using the 1997 DGs.

The General Multisystem Guidelines

With the 1997 DGs, the physician can choose to use either the general multisystem guidelines or the specialty-specific guidelines. Under the general multisystem guidelines, organ systems and body areas are combined, and the defining factor is the documentation of bulleted organ systems and body areas, as outlined in Table 14.15.

The 1997 general multisystem examination guidelines require the documentation described in Table 14.16.

Table 14.16 General Multisystem Guidelines

LEVEL OF EXAM	PERFORM AND DOCUMENT
Problem focused	One to five elements identified by a bullet
Expanded problem focused	At least six elements identified by a bullet
Detailed	At least two elements identified by a bullet from each of six areas/systems or at least 12 elements identified by a bullet in two or more areas/systems
Comprehensive	Perform all elements identified by a bullet in at least nine organ systems or body areas and document at least two elements identified by a bullet from each of nine areas/systems

Applying these guidelines to the original example presented earlier results in the following:

The patient's blood pressure is 130/80; he weighs 180 lb; he is afebrile (constitutional—1 bullet); lungs are clear to auscultation (respiratory—1 bullet); no evidence of hepatosplenomegaly (gastrointestinal—1 bullet); neck is supple (neck—1 bullet); the heart has regular rhythm without murmur (cardiovascular—1 bullet); both legs appear normal; gait is normal, but the left leg is painful when manipulated; general muscle tone normal (musculoskeletal—3 bullets); no rash; skin texture and color are normal (skin—1 bullet).

The total number of bullets comes to nine, which places this in the category of expanded problem focused. When put together with the history level of detailed and the MDM level of high and compared to the matrixes for new patients and existing patients, the resulting level of service is coded as 99202 for a new patient and 99213 for an established patient. By comparison, the codes using the 1995 guidelines were 99203 and 99214, respectively. Because results can vary depending on whether the 1995 or the 1997 guidelines are used, physicians must be careful in deciding which DG to use.

The Specialty-Specific Guidelines

Depending on the specifics of the case, the use of specialty-specific guidelines may be most appropriate. In some cases, however, they are not the best choice, and their use will lead to lower reimbursement. This section compares the use of the 1995 guidelines, the 1997 multisystem guidelines, and the specialty-specific guidelines in two different cases.

The Musculoskeletal Examination Guidelines

Because much of the patient's examination in this example is related to the musculoskeletal system, a physician can choose to use the single-specialty examination guidelines for the musculoskeletal system, which are listed in Table 14.17.

Table 14.17 1997 Musculoskeletal Guidelines

SYSTEM/BODY AREA(S)	ELEMENTS OF EXAMINATION
Constitutional	• Measurement of any three of the following seven vital signs: (1) sitting or standing blood pressure, (2) supine blood pressure, (3) pulse rate and regularity, (4) respiration, (5) temperature, (6) height, (7) weight (may be measured and recorded by ancillary staff.)
Head and face	
Eyes	
Ears, nose, mouth, and throat	
Neck	
Respiratory	
Cardiovascular	• Examination of peripheral vascular system by observation (e.g., swelling, varicosities) and palpation (e.g., pulses, temperature, edema, tenderness)
Chest (breasts)	
Gastrointestinal (abdomen)	
Genitourinary	
Lymphatic	• Palpation of lymph nodes in neck, axillae, groin, and/or other location
Musculoskeletal	• Examination of gait and station • Examination of joint(s), bone(s) and muscle(s)/tendon(s) of four of the following six areas: (1) head and neck; (2) spine, ribs, and pelvis; (3) right upper extremity; (4) left upper extremity; (5) right lower extremity; and (6) left lower extremity. The examination of a given area includes: • Inspection, percussion, and/or palpation with notation of any misalignment, asymmetry, crepitation, defects, tenderness, masses, or effusions • Assessment of range of motion with notation of any pain (e.g., straight leg raising), crepitation, or contracture • Assessment of stability with notation of a dislocation (luxation), subluxation, or laxity • Assessment of muscle strength and tone (e.g., flaccid, cog wheel, spastic) with notation of any atrophy or abnormal movements NOTE: For the comprehensive level of examination, all four of the elements identified by a bullet must be performed and documented for each of four anatomical areas. For the three lower levels of examination, each element is counted separately for each body area. For example, assessing range of motion in two extremities constitutes two elements.

Continued

Table 14.17 Continued

SYSTEM/BODY AREA(S)	ELEMENTS OF EXAMINATION
Extremities	[See musculoskeletal and skin]
Skin	• Inspection and/or palpation of skin and subcutaneous tissue (e.g., scars, rashes, lesions, cafe-au-lait spots, ulcers) in four of the following six areas: (1) head and neck, (2) trunk, (3) right upper extremity, (4) left upper extremity, (5) right lower extremity, and (6) left lower extremity. NOTE: For the comprehensive level, the examination of all four anatomical areas must be performed and documented. For the three lower levels of examination, each body area is counted separately. For example, inspection and/or palpation of the skin and subcutaneous tissue of two extremities constitutes two elements.
Neurological/psychiatric	• Test coordination (e.g., finger/nose, heel/knee/shin, rapid alternating movements in the upper and lower extremities, evaluation of fine motor coordination in young children) • Examination of deep tendon reflexes and/or nerve stretch test with notation of pathological reflexes (e.g., Babinski) • Examination of sensation (e.g., by touch, pin, vibration, proprioception) Brief assessment of mental status including: • Orientation to time, place, and person • Mood and affect (e.g., depression, anxiety, agitation)

The 1997 musculoskeletal guidelines require the levels of examination listed in Table 14.18.

Table 14.18 1997 Musculoskeletal Guidelines

LEVEL OF EXAM	PERFORM AND DOCUMENT
Problem focused	One to five elements identified by a bullet
Expanded problem focused	At least six elements identified by a bullet
Detailed	At least 12 elements identified by a bullet
Comprehensive	Perform all elements identified by a bullet; document every element in each box with a shaded border and at least one element in each box with an unshaded border

Application of these guidelines to the original example results in the following:

The patient's blood pressure is 130/80; he weighs 180 lb; he is afebrile (constitutional—1 bullet); lungs are clear to auscultation; no evidence of hepatosplenomegaly; neck is supple; the heart has regular rhythm without murmur; both legs appear normal; gait is normal, but the left leg is painful when manipulated; general muscle tone normal (musculoskeletal—3 bullets); no rash; skin texture and color are normal (skin—1 bullet).

Only the constitutional, musculoskeletal, and skin examination are relevant when these single-specialty documentation guidelines are applied, and the total number of bullets comes to five, making the examination key component problem focused. Comparing these results to the matrix produces an assignment of code 99201 for a new patient and 99213 for an established patient.

The reason the musculoskeletal-specific guidelines result in a lower new patient code and thus lower reimbursement is that several body areas that were examined—neck, cardiovascular, gastrointestinal, and respiratory—are not accounted for in the specialty-specific guidelines.

Coders must have knowledge of both the 1995 and 1997 guidelines in order to code for the most advantageous level of service for the physician's work. In this example, the 1995 guidelines provide the highest levels of reimbursement for both new and established patients and so are the most appropriate guidelines to use.

The Eye Examination Guidelines

Following is another case, this one involving an established patient, illustrating the use of the 1995 DGs, the 1997 multisystem DGs, and the 1997 eye DGs.

Established Patient

Patient is a 14-year-old female with a 3-day history of pinkeye. There has been no trauma or foreign body irritation. The patient also complains of itching and a purulent discharge in the left eye, visual changes negative.

BP 110/60, wt 105, respiration normal, both eyes examined.

Right eye: Within normal limits

Left eye: Erythema with a purulent exudate. Cobblestoning of left conjunctiva was noted, no hyphema noted bilaterally, and the extraocular muscles were intact bilaterally. Exam with ophthalmoscope was benign. No evidence of corneal abrasions.

Assessment: Acute bacterial conjunctivitis left eye

Plan: Sodium sulamyd ophthalmic solution twice a day in the left eye for 1 week. Use warm, moist compresses as needed.

> A negative statement is considered documentation in the HPI, just as a positive statement is considered documentation. For example, "No trauma or foreign body irritation" is documentation of context as is "There was trauma and foreign body irritation."

This established patient has presented to the physician with the chief complaint of pinkeye. The first key component to evaluate is the history key component, which breaks down into the three elements of history of present illness, review of systems, and past, family, and/or social history.

With regard to the history of present illness, five of the eight elements are documented, qualifying as extended documentation and meeting the requirement for the detailed level of history:

1. *Location:* Left eye
2. *Quality:* Red
3. *Duration:* Three days
4. *Context:* No trauma or foreign body
5. *Associated signs and symptoms:* Itching/discharge

Only one body system is identified in the documentation, the eyes, making the ROS problem pertinent, which falls under the expanded problem-focused level of history. There is no documentation of past, family, and/or social history, which also falls under the expanded problem-focused level. Because all three elements are not at the same level, the lowest level for the history key component—expanded problem focused—is selected.

For the second key component, the examination, information on blood pressure, weight, respiration, and both eyes are documented, qualifying as documentation of two organ systems: constitutional and eyes. According to the 1995 guidelines, the level of service is expanded problem focused (two to four body areas and/or organ systems).

Based on the documentation, the third component, medical decision making, is calculated as follows:

- *Diagnoses:* New problem, no additional workup = 3 points (moderate)
- *Data review:* Not documented = 0 points
- *Overall risk:* One bullet (management options selected: prescription drug management) = 3 (moderate)

With two values at the moderate level, the level of service of MDM is moderate.

Emergency Department E/M Billing: Physicians and Facilities

Evaluation and management services are a large aspect of emergency department (ED) work. Both the ED physicians and the facility code and bill these outpatient services.

ED Physician E/M Coding

CPT codes in the range 99281–99285 are used to report un-scheduled or episodic services for patients who are registered in the ED of a hospital-based facility and who present for immediate medical attention. The ED services codes are not appropriate for service in an office, an outpatient facility, or any setting other than the ED. These codes likewise are not reported for services provided in other areas of the hospital or for observation care.

ED services may be billed by physicians who are not assigned to the ED; any physician who provides services in the ED may use these codes. However, if a physician asks the patient to come to the ED as an alternative to the physician office, and the patient is not registered in the ED, that physician should report the appropriate office/outpatient visit codes. No distinction is made between new and established patients in the ED setting.

The physician level of service in the ED is similar to the LOS for an office visit. Providers must document and meet the history, examination, and MDM elements of the E/M code and report their services with place of service code 23 (hospital ED). Physicians reporting E/M services follow the standard documentation guidelines and may elect either the 1995 or the 1997 version. According to the American College of Emergency Physicians (www.acep.org), most use the 1995 guidelines.

> ■ Medicare Part B covers the physician services provided in the ED. The services of the facility—auxiliary personnel, drugs, and supplies—are considered Part A benefits.

A physician service includes obtaining the history; conducting the physical exam; ordering and interpreting the x-rays, ECG, cardiac monitoring, and laboratory tests; making an assessment; and ordering treatments. Additional services, such as suturing lacerations or applying a cast, are reported with the appropriate procedure codes.

When ED services are provided and reported for codes that may have a global period associated with them, specific exceptions apply to separate coverage by the ED physician. For example, when a patient presents to the ED with a fracture, typically the ED physician diagnoses and stabilizes the fracture and then refers the care to another physician (such as an orthopedic specialist). "Fracture care" has not been provided by the ED physician in this situation. Therefore, the ED physician bills for the ED services, and the specialist bills for the fracture care.

When a physician advises the patient to go to the ED for care and then subsequently is asked by the ED physician to come to the hospital to evaluate the patient and advise the ED physician about whether the patient should be admitted, the physician should bill as follows:

- If the patient is admitted to the hospital by the regular physician, the regular physician should bill only the appropriate level of the initial hospital care codes (99221–99223). All E/M services provided by that physician in conjunction with that admission are considered part of the initial hospital care when performed on the same date as the admission. The ED physician who saw the patient in the ED should bill the appropriate level of ED codes.
- If the ED physician—based on the advice of the regular physician who came to the ED to see the patient—sends the patient home, the ED physician should bill the appropriate level of ED service. The patient's regular physician may also bill the level of E/M code that the documentation supports.

ED Facility E/M Coding

CPT codes in the range 99281–99285 and 99288 are also used by the facility to bill for E/M services for patients in the ED. However, facilities do not follow the CMS documentation guidelines. Instead, each facility develops its own specific criteria for the five levels. For Medicare and Medicaid billing, according to CMS, the criteria the hospital develops must:

Critical care involves the direct delivery of medical care by a physician to a critically ill or critically injured patient. CPT code 99291 may be used in place of, or in addition to, a code for a medical visit or ED service. Critical care is one of the exceptions to the roll-up rule prohibiting two E/M services reported by a physician on the same day to the same patient.

- Follow the intent of the CPT code descriptor, relating the intensity of hospital resources to the different levels of effort represented by the CPT codes
- Use facility resources, not physician resources, as their basis
- Facilitate accurate payments and be useful for compliance and audits
- Meet HIPAA requirements
- Require only the documentation clinically necessary for patient care
- Discourage upcoding or gaming
- Be written or recorded and well documented, and provide the basis for selection of a specific code
- Be applied consistently across patients in the clinic or the ED
- Remain consistent with few changes
- Be readily available for fiscal intermediary (FI) or Medicare administrative contractor (MAC) review
- Result in coding decisions that can be verified by other hospital staff members or outside sources

The E/M levels for facilities may be very similar to physician E/M level assignments, but they should not rely on the three professional key components.

Because this was an established patient, only two of the three key components are required to be the same for code assignment. Both the history and the examination key components are at the expanded problem-focused level, so code 99213 is assigned.

The 1997 general multisystem guidelines base the level of service of the examination key component on the documentation of the number of elements examined. The physician examined one constitutional element and three elements related to the eyes, for a total of four elements, making the level of service of the examination problem focused.

For an established patient, the lowest level of service (in this case, problem focused) is dropped, and the lower of the two highest levels controls code assignment. The LOS is expanded problem focused, and the code is 99213, the same as when the 1995 guidelines were used.

Next, the 1997 eye examination guidelines are used. Four bullets in the section on eyes are documented—visual acuity, conjunctivae, pupil exam, and ophthalmoscope—making the examination LOS problem focused and the code 99213, as above.

CHECKPOINT 14.7

Answer the following question.

1. In what areas do the 1997 general multisystem exam requirements differ from the 1997 musculoskeletal exam requirements? _____

CODING, REIMBURSEMENT, AND FRAUD

Fraud occurs when a physician provides information (a claim for payment) that he or she knows is false and expects to result in a benefit (higher payment). It includes billing for services not provided and billing for services at a higher level than was provided.

When assigning an E/M code, a provider is required to be in compliance with the documentation guidelines provided by the AMA and CMS and to choose the code that most accurately represents the E/M service performed. Because E/M services make up more than 40% of physician services reported to Medicare Part B, the federal government and insurance carriers have a financial incentive to make sure they are not paying for services at higher levels than performed.

The Office of the Inspector General (OIG), a branch of the federal government's Department of Justice, audits agencies within the Department of Health and Human Services, which includes Medicare:

> The mission of the Office of Inspector General, as mandated by Public Law 95-452 (as amended), is to protect the integrity of Department of Health and Human Services (HHS) programs, as well as the health and welfare of the beneficiaries of those programs. The OIG has a responsibility to report both to the Secretary and to the Congress program and management problems and recommendations to correct them. The OIG's duties are carried out through a nationwide network of audits, investigations, inspections and other mission-related functions performed by OIG components.

The OIG has retrieved over $27 million dollars in overpayments from audits of E/M services, almost half the result of insufficient documentation by physicians. The OIG continues to monitor for intentional upcoding and/or downcoding. Upcoding—selecting a code that does not accurately represent the service provided in order to maximize reimbursement—is considered fraud. Downcoding—deliberately choosing a lower LOS—is seen as intent to encourage patients to return and utilize more physician services. For most physicians, however, downcoding is an attempt to play it safe and avoid carrier scrutiny. Both upcoding and downcoding are seen as intent to increase reimbursement and are under increased investigation by insurance carriers, CMS, and the OIG. Compliance with the documentation guidelines provides physicians with the necessary proof that they are coding correctly.

INTERNET RESOURCE: Office of Inspector General
http://oig.hhs.gov

Each year, the OIG develops a work plan related to investigation of physician services. In the work plan, the OIG describes the investigations it intends to conduct during that fiscal year. If new issues or priorities emerge, projects not included in the work plan may also be conducted. Nevertheless, E/M services are always prominent in work plans. The current OIG work plan, as well as previous years' plans, can be downloaded from the OIG website by selecting the publications link.

Auditing E/M Services

Monitoring the coding and billing process for compliance is the responsibility of the practice's compliance officer or of another staff member who is knowledgeable about coding and compliance regulations. The responsible person establishes a system for monitoring the process and performing regular compliance checks to ensure adherence to established policies and procedures.

An important compliance activity involves audits. An audit is a formal examination or review. An income tax audit is performed to find out whether a person's or a firm's income or expenses were misreported. Similarly, compliance audits judge whether the practice's physicians and coding and billing staff comply with regulations for correct coding and billing.

An audit does not involve reviewing every claim and document. Instead, a representative sample of the whole is studied to reveal whether erroneous or fraudulent behavior exists. For instance, an auditor might make a random selection, such as a percentage of the claims for a particular date, or a targeted selection, such as all claims in a period that have a certain procedure code. If the auditor finds indications of a problem in the sample, more documents and more details are usually reviewed.

External Audits

In an external audit, private payers or government agencies review selected records of a practice for compliance. Coding linkage, completeness of documentation, and adherence to documentation standards, such as the signing and dating of entries by the responsible health-care professional, may all be studied. The accounting records are often reviewed as well.

Payers use computer programs of code edits to review claims before they are processed. This process is referred to as a *prepayment audit*. For example, the Medicare program performs computer checks before processing claims. Some prepayment audits check only to verify that documentation of the visit is on file, rather than investigating the details of the coding.

Audits conducted after payment has been made are called *prepayment audit*. Most payers conduct routine postpayment audits of physicians' practices to ensure that claims correctly reflect performed services, that services are billed accurately, and that the physicians and other health-care providers who participate in the plan comply with the provisions of their contracts.

In a routine private-payer audit, the payer's auditor usually makes an appointment in advance with the practice to be audited and may conduct the review in the practice's office or by taking copies of documents back to the payer's office. Often, the auditor requests the complete medical records of selected plan members for a specified period. The claims information and documentation might include all office and progress notes, laboratory test results, referrals, x-rays, patient sign-in sheets, appointment books, and billing records. When problems are found, the investigation proceeds and may result in charges of fraud or abuse against the practice.

Internal Audits

To reduce the chance of an investigation or an external audit and to reduce potential liability when an audit occurs, the compliance plans of most practices require that internal audits be conducted regularly by the medical practice staff or by hired consultants. These audits are routine and are performed periodically without a reason to think that a compliance problem exists. They help the practice determine whether coding is being done appropriately and whether all performed services are being reported for maximum revenue. The goal is to uncover problems so that they can be corrected. Internal audits also help:

- Determine whether new procedures or treatments are correctly coded and documented;
- Analyze the skills and knowledge of the personnel assigned to handle medical coding in the practice;
- Find out whether training or additional review of practice guidelines is needed; and
- Improve communications among the staff members involved with claim processing: medical coders, medical insurance specialists, and physicians.

Internal audits are done either prospectively or retrospectively. A prospective audit (also called a *concurrent audit*), like a prepayment audit, is done before claims are sent to payers. Some practices audit a percentage of claims each day. Others audit claims for new or very complex procedures. These audits reduce the number of rejected or downcoded claims by verifying compliance before billing.

Retrospective audits are conducted after claims have been sent and the remittance advice (RA) has been received. Auditing at this point in the process has two advantages: (1) The complete record, including the RA, is available, so the auditor knows which codes have been rejected or downcoded, and (2) there are usually more claims to sample. Retrospective audits are helpful in analyzing the explanations of rejected or reduced charges and making changes to the coding approach if needed.

AUDITING TOOLS

Auditing involves answering some basic questions:

- Was the service a visit or a consultation?
- Should the service be based on the key components or on another factor, such as time spent?
- Was the service documented?
- Does the code reported require two or three key components?

The 1995 and 1997 DGs have reduced the amount of subjectivity involved in making judgments about E/M codes, such as one person's opinion of what makes an examination extended. They do this by describing the specific items that may be documented for each of the three key E/M components. They also explain how many items are needed to place the E/M service at the appropriate level.

> According to the CMS, E/M codes are the most frequently audited codes because of continual findings of poor documentation. When physicians use lower codes than warranted to avoid audits, their documentation often does not justify even the lower code levels, so their actions reduce legitimate revenue and still do not protect them from investigation.

The documentation guidelines have precise number counts of these items, and the counts can be used to audit as well as to initially code services. The audit double-checks selected codes based on the documentation in the patient medical record. The auditor looks at the record and, usually using an auditing tool such as that shown in Box 14.1, independently analyzes the services that are documented. The auditor then compares the codes that should be selected with the codes that have been reported. If these codes are not identical, the auditor has uncovered a possible problem in interpreting the documentation guidelines.

Many practices use this type of audit tool to help them conduct audits in a standard way. The tool is distributed to physicians and staff members to develop internal audits, not to make initial code selections. An experienced medical insurance specialist may be responsible for using the audit tool to monitor completed claims and to audit selected claims before they are released.

The audit tool that the practice uses should be easily understood and easy to use, especially by the staff members who will be using it. It should also clearly indicate whether it applies to the 1995 or the 1997 DGs or to both.

Using the Audit Form

An example follows of how to use the audit form to verify code selection for the history key component, focusing on the history of present illness element. After the coding has been done, the auditor examines the patient's medical record and analyzes the documentation. The HPI section at the top of Box 14.1, which reflects the documentation guidelines for HPI, is as follows:

HPI (HISTORY OF PRESENT ILLNESS)				BRIEF	EXTENDED
Location	Severity	Timing	Modifying factors	1–3 elements	4–8 elements
Quality	Duration	Context	Associated signs and symptoms		

Using this tool, the auditor checks off the appropriate items for HPI:

Patient's chief complaint: Right shoulder pain
History: The patient noted a sharp pain in the right shoulder about 3 days ago. The pain is worse when he lies on the arm.

BOX 14.1 E/M Code Assignment Audit Form

1995 DOCUMENTATION GUIDELINES

Patient: _____ MRN#: _____ Date of Service: _____

Provider: _____ Specialty: _____

HISTORY

CHIEF COMPLAINT: _____

History of Present Illness   **Review of Systems**   **PFSH**

Elements:

Location _____	Const	GU	Endocrine	Past
Quality _____	Eye	Integ (skin, breast)	Psych	Family
Severity _____	ENT	MS	Aller/Immuno	Social
Timing _____	Resp	Neuro	Hemato/Lymph	
Duration _____	Cardiovasc	Gastroint	All other Neg	

Context

Modifying Factors _____

Assoc. signs & sx _____

HPI   **ROS**   **PFSH**

1–3 = Brief   0 = None   0 = None

4+ = Extended   1 = Problem pertinent   1 = Pertinent

Or the status of at least 3   2–9 = Extended   2 = Complete (Est. Pt, ED)

chronic or inactive conditions   10+ = Complete   3 = Complete (New Pt, Consults)

To select Level of Service: HPI, ROS, PFSH selected must be in the same column below or select the column circled farthest to the left.

HISTORY	Problem Focused	Expanded PF	Detailed	Comprehensive
HPI	Brief	Brief	Extended	Extended
ROS	None	Problem Pertinent	Extended	Complete
PFSH	None	None	Pertinent	Complete

Est. Pt.	99212	99213	99214	99215
New Pt.	99201	99202	99203	99204, 99205
Off. Consult	99241	99242	99243	99244, 99245
Hosp. Consult	99251	99252	99253	99254, 99255
Hosp. Admit			99221	99221, 99222, 99223
Hosp. Follow up	99231	99232	99233	

Level of History: _____

EXAM-1995 Guidelines

Organ Systems   **Body Areas**

Constitutional	Musculoskeletal	Head, including the face
Cardiovascular	Neurologic	Neck
Eyes	Psychiatric	Chest, including breasts and axillae
ENT	Respiratory	Abdomen
GI	Skin	Genitalia, groin, buttocks
GU		Back, including spine
Hematologic/Lymphatic/Immunologic		Each extremity

Determine LEVEL OF EXAM:

Problem Focused Exam = 1 body area or organ system (limited exam of the affected body area/organ system) 99212, 99201, 99241, 99251, 99231

Expanded Problem Focused Exam = 2–4 body areas and/or organ systems (limited exam) 99213, 99202, 99242, 99252, 99232

Detailed Exam = 5–7 body areas and/or organ systems (extended exam) 99214, 99203, 99243, 99253, 99221, 99233

Comprehensive Exam = 8 or more ORGAN SYSTEMS
99215, 99204 and 99205, 99244 and 99245, 99254 and 99255, 99221 and 99222 and 99223,

Level of Exam: _____

MEDICAL DECISION MAKING

A. DIAGNOSIS OR MANAGEMENT OPTIONS

Number of Dx & Tx options	Points	# of Problems	Total
Self-limited or minor (stable, improved or worsening)	x1	Max #2	
Established problem (to examiner); stable, improved	x1		
Established problem (to examiner); worsening	x2		
New problem (to examiner) no additional workup planned	x3	Max #1	
New problem (to examiner) additional workup planned	x4		
TOTAL POINTS			

B. AMOUNT & COMPLEXITY OF DATA INVOLVED

		Total
Review and/or order of clinical lab tests	1	
Review and/or order of tests in Radiology Section (except Echo)	1	
Review and/or order of tests in Medicine Section (EEG, EKG, etc.)	1	
Discussion of test results with the performing physician	1	
Decision to obtain old records and/or additional history from other than patient	1	
Review and summarization of old records and/or obtained history from someone other than patient	2	
Independent visualization of image, tracing or specimen itself (not simply a review)	2	
TOTAL POINTS		

BOX 14.1 *Continued*

C. OVERALL RISK – USE TABLE OF RISK

OVERALL RISK	MINIMAL	LOW	MODERATE	HIGH
Presenting Problem	Minimal	Low	Moderate	High
Diagnostic Procedures	Minimal	Low	Moderate	High
Management Options	Minimal	Low	Moderate	High

DETERMINE MEDICAL DECISION-MAKING LEVEL

A. Number of Dx & Tx Options	1 Minimal	2 Limited	3 Multiple	4 Extensive
B. Amount and/or Complexity of Data Involved	0–1 Minimal	2 Limited	3 Moderate	4 Extensive
C. Risk of complications/morbidity/mortality	Minimal	Low	Moderate	High
FINAL MDM LEVEL Must have at least 2 in same column or select column 2nd from left	Straightforward	Low	Moderate	High

Established patient-office	**99212**	**99213**	**99214**	**99215**
New patient-office	**99201, 99202**	**99203**	**99204**	**99205**
Consult-office	**99241, 99242**	**99243**	**99244**	**99245**
Consult-hospital	**99251, 99252**	**99253**	**99254**	**99255**
Hosp. admit	**99221**	**99221**	**99222**	**99223**
Hosp. follow up	**99231**	**99231**	**99232**	**99233**

BILLED:
CPT code _____
    History _____
    Exam _____
    MDM _____
Was encounter based on counseling and/or
Coordination of care? Time _____
Modifiers _____
DX 1 _____
DX 2 _____

AUDIT:
CPT code _____
    History _____
    Exam _____
    MDM _____
Was encounter based on counseling and/or
Coordination of care? Time _____
Modifiers _____
DX 1 _____
DX 2 _____

Audit Findings: _____

Comments: _____

TABLE OF RISK	(1 bullet from any box supports level to left)		
Level of Risk	**Presenting Problem(s)**	**Diagnostic Procedure(s) Ordered**	**Management Options Selected**
Minimal	• One self-limited or minor problem, e.g., cold, insect bite, tinea corporis	• Laboratory tests requiring venipuncture • Chest x-rays • EKG/EEG • Urinalysis • KOH prep • Ultrasound, e.g., echocardiography	• Rest • Gargles • Elastic bandages • Superficial dressings
Low	• Two or more self-limited or minor problems • One stable chronic illness, e.g., well controlled hypertension, non-insulin dependent diabetes, cataract, BPH • Acute uncomplicated illness or injury, e.g., cystitis, allergic rhinitis, simple sprain	• Physiologic tests not under stress, e.g., pulmonary function tests • Non-cardiovascular imaging studies with contrast, e.g., barium enema • Superficial needle biopsies • Clinical laboratory tests requiring arterial puncture • Skin biopsies	• Over-the-counter drugs • Minor surgery with no identified risk factors • Physical therapy • Occupational therapy • IV fluids without additives
Moderate	• One or more chronic illnesses with mild exacerbation, progression, or side effects of treatment • Two or more stable chronic illnesses • Undiagnosed new problem with uncertain prognosis, e.g., lump in breast • Acute illness with systemic symptoms, e.g., pyelonephritis, pneumonitis, colitis • Acute complicated injury, e.g., head injury with brief loss of consciousness	• Physiologic tests under stress, e.g., cardiac stress test, fetal contraction stress test • Diagnostic endoscopies with no identified risk factors • Deep needle or incisional biopsy • Cardiovascular imaging studies with contrast and no identified risk factors, e.g., arteriogram, cardiac catheterization • Obtain fluid from body cavity, e.g. lumbar puncture, thoracentesis, culdocentesis	• Minor surgery with identified risk factors • Elective major surgery (open, percutaneous or endoscopic) with no identified risk factors • Prescription drug management • Therapeutic nuclear medicine • IV fluids with additives • Closed treatment of fracture or dislocation without manipulation
High	• One or more chronic illnesses with severe exacerbation, progression, or side effects of treatment • Acute or chronic illnesses or injuries that pose a threat to life or bodily function, e.g., multiple trauma, acute MI, pulmonary embolus, severe respiratory distress, progressive severe rheumatoid arthritis, psychiatric illness with potential threat to self or others, peritonitis, acute renal failure • An abrupt change in neurologic status, e.g., seizure, TIA, weakness, sensory loss	• Cardiovascular imaging studies with contrast with identified risk factors • Cardiac electrophysiological tests • Diagnostic endoscopies with identified risk factors • Discography	• Elective major surgery (open, percutaneous or endoscopic) with identified risk factors • Emergency major surgery (open, percutaneous or endoscopic) • Parenteral controlled substances • Drug therapy requiring intensive monitoring for toxicity • Decision not to resuscitate or to de-escalate care because of poor prognosis

Auditor's analysis: The HPI is extended; four elements are documented, as follows:
  Location: Right shoulder
  Quality: Sharp pain
  Duration: Three days ago
  Context: Worse when lies on arm

The auditor checks all the elements listed on the audit form to verify the overall selection of the E/M code.

Providing Feedback on Documentation Errors

Auditing E/M services gives the physician important feedback and helps identify errors about which the physician may be unaware. Some common errors include the following:

- The chief complaint is not documented or is too vague.
- The documentation does not support the level of service, and the service should be down-coded to a lower LOS.

EXAMPLE

The documented ROS does not support the comprehensive history level required for reported code 99204.

- The documentation supports a higher level of service, and the service should be upcoded.

EXAMPLE

The documentation identifies an expanded problem-focused LOS, but the physician reports a problem-focused LOS.

- Data review (tests ordered, discussion with other physicians) is performed but not documented.
- The documentation is illegible. If the auditor cannot read the documentation, it is disallowed.

Part of the audit process is to effectively present the audit findings to the physician and coding personnel. Presentation of audit results should be concise, relevant, and educational. A summary of the findings and detailed analysis, including statistics, should be provided. The statistics should include total number of records audited, the number of records that met the required LOS, the number of records that did not meet the required LOS, a listing of documentation errors, and the percentage of documentation errors.

Box 14.2 shows an example of a summary of the findings of an audit:

BOX 14.2 Audit Summary

Office Visits, Hospital Admissions, Hospital Visits, Consultations

Of the 189 E/M services audited:

- 55% of the E/M code levels were not supported.
- 14% were considered "not documented."
- 41% of documentation did not support the level of service billed.
- 15% were undercoded.
- 30% were coded correctly.

General Information

- Lack of understanding of documenting for consults vs. new patient services
  - Consults require all three key components to be documented
  - Requirement that "consultation" be specifically referred to in the documentation
  - Requirement that the request for a consultation and who requested the consultation must be stated in the record
- General lack of understanding of E/M requirements
  - When three of three key components vs. two of three key components are required
- Lack of physician signature on documentation will result in a finding of not documented.
- Illegible physician signature will result in finding of not documented.

Continued

BOX 14.2 *Continued*

- Many services were illegible.
- Laboratory services were billed but not documented.
- Ventilation management codes were billed, but documentation was for E/M services, not ventilation management.
- Critical care services were billed; documentation does not support critical care.
  - Time is not documented.
  - Patient is not critical.
  - Care is not critical.
  - Patient's location in critical care unit is not sufficient reason to report critical care codes.
  - Dates of service are incorrect.
- Psychiatry codes were used incorrectly.
  - Psychotherapy was billed, but documentation indicated that diagnostic interview service was provided.

Findings

E/M CODE BILLED BY PRACTICE	AUDITED CODE	HISTORY	EXAM	MDM	COMMENTS AND RECOMMENDATIONS
99213	99212	EPF	Illeg	Illeg	No signature
99214	99213	N/A	EPF	LOW	No signature
99215	99213	EPF	PF	LOW	No signature
99213	99212	PF	None	SF	No signature
99397	99397				No signature
99204	99203	EPF	EPF	LOW	
99204	99202	DET	EPF	MOD	
99215	99214	N/A	N/A	N/A	Code based on time—counseling and coordination of care.
99213	99213	EPF	EPF		
99213	99213	EPF	EPF	LOW	
99214	99214	DET	DET	MOD	
99214	99213	EPF	EPF		
99385	99213	EPF	NONE	LOW	Preventive medicine coding requires an exam.
99203	99202	EPF	DET	HIGH	
99243	99241	Brief	DET		Verify consultation request and report to surgeon. Documentation should indicate pre-op consultation—no HPI.
99397	99397				

Critical to the audit process is ensuring that the provider understands the audit results and that the person performing the audits is able to answer questions about the results. Basic facts and comments about the audit findings should be presented in a concise manner.

Office of the Inspector General and Compliance

The OIG does periodic studies related to medical coding. In one study, the OIG found that the billing of the higher level E/M codes was increasing. The time period studied was 2001 through 2010.

CMS was sent a list of 1,700 physicians who were consistently billing those high-level E/M codes in 2010 alone. In the outpatient setting the increase was 17%; for hospital visits the increase was between 6% and 9%. The ED codes showed the most pronounced increase at 21%.

It is important to understand, however, that reporting high-level codes does not mean fraud. The patient population may have increased in age, which can mean more complicated medical issues, or the physician practice may be seeing a more complex patient population. An example is patients requiring neonatology, oncology, and cardiothoracic surgery services.

What will matter when an auditor or the OIG examines the medical record is that the physician's documentation supports the level of service reported while meeting the medical necessity of providing the higher level of service. The OIG, in its report, recommends coding education as the number-one priority to ensure that claims are appropriate.

AUDITING THE ELECTRONIC HEALTH RECORD SYSTEM

EHRs are seen as tools for greater access to patient information and ease of documentation of patient encounters; however, they may also lead to noncompliance with documentation guidelines. There is a need to minimize the risk of liability when using EHRs.

- Many vendors of EHRs will state that their EHR can save coding staff expenses because their system will select the level of E/M based on the provider's documentation. While a system can calculate history and exam components, it cannot calculate medical necessity, which is the underlying concept of medical services.
- Studies have shown that cloning, which is a copy and paste process, was used when previous HPIs were cloned repeatedly and did not reflect the patient's current status.
  - Also, the ROS was cloned with a negative finding for one of the systems but there was contradictory evidence in the physician's note.
  - Cloning will also cause a problem when a problem-focused level of service is reported at a much higher level because the information from a previous high-level visit was populated or cloned into the lower-level visit.
  - Exams were identical from previous visits, or the exam contradicts what is in the HPI and/or ROS.
- Preventive medicine services have specific elements not based on medical necessity or on the key components of an E/M service. This allows for the use of a one-click option that populates the medical record with the standard preventive service elements, *but* the provider must take responsibility for performing all those elements and the system must allow for the provider to comment on any abnormal or unusual findings during the exam.

Is cloning ever correct? Yes, there are times when the physician can clone the previous HPI and ROS and then make changes where appropriate. Another issue is repeated information: This may suggest to the reviewer that the documentation does not reflect the current encounter. As a result of these issues, reviewers and auditors are changing how they do audits.

Prepopulated Fields

Some EHRs prepopulate fields with standard terminology and descriptions. Although this may expedite documentation for many physicians, some changes need to be made to reflect the specific findings for that visit.

EXAMPLE
The current encounter for flu shows an HPI for a sprained ankle.

Prompts

Some EHRs will prompt a provider to add documentation that would increase the level of service. While this is often seen as a positive element when the physician has forgotten to document something, it more often leads to inaccurate documentation and, more importantly, fraud.

Use of Templates

The EHR should mirror the handwritten documentation. The difference is that it is legible. EHR templates are generally customized to a specialty, so a spine surgeon's template would not look like a cardiologist's template. However, the use of templates can lead to a number of pitfalls.

Pitfall: In a hospital visit EHR system, the attending physician's documentation reads "d/w attending." The attending physician copied the resident's note into his own note, including the plan to "d/w attending." The reviewer would then suspect that the only documentation is the resident's, not the attending physician's documentation.

Pitfall: Rote notes are paragraph-upon-paragraph of facts not relevant to the current encounter with the patient. These facts appear to be "canned" EHR chart notes not associated with the current evaluation of the patient.

Pitfall: As mentioned earlier, cloning of notes can cause problems when, for example, the HPI from a previous visit is copied into the current visit, but those issues are not relevant because the patient is being seen for a different problem. Each record must stand on its own; cloning documentation from a previous encounter is not documentation of the current encounter.

Some EHR systems have the ability to copy and paste documentation from a previous patient encounter or from another patient's medical record. These functions can appear as "copy and paste," "copy note forward," and "save note as template" options. When the documentation is reviewed, all documentation in that EHR looks the same except for the name or the date or both.

EXAMPLES

- A patient is seen for three visits in one month and each visit documents a pap smear. The pap smear was done in the first visit and was not repeated in each subsequent visit. The error is a result of the copy and paste function.
- The patient's chief complaint is acute sinusitis and the ROS indicates no complaints of sinusitis.

Another problem related to the copy and paste function is referred to as a "pull forward." This feature is offered by the EHR companies as a positive quality that gives the provider the ability to identify information from a previous visit that can remind the provider to reconfirm or revise information related to the current visit. Studies of this pull-forward ability have shown that providers have signed off on duplicate information that was not applicable to the current visit and may also have misleading or erroneous information. Another risk can sometimes be the inability to identify the original source of the information.

Pitfall: "Exploding elements" occur when the EHR system automatically fills in information based on a selection made by the physician as indicated in the example below. An exploding element can also occur in systems where the EHR checks off elements as normal or negative automatically even though that element may not have been part of the current encounter.

EXAMPLES

- The provider selects a gastrointestinal exam and the system automatically fills in the description "abdomen soft and non-tender, normal bowel sounds, not distended, no organomegaly" when that is not the correct finding in the actual examination. It is now the responsibility of the provider to change that in the system. If the physician does not change it because of reliance on the EHR, then the physician is in danger of fraud and malpractice liability.
- Resolution: The EHR should require that the provider verify and click on each item within the exam elements as well as the history and medical decision making. This ensures that the medical record is patient specific.
- Resolution: Establish a committee to review and approve any EHR templates for accuracy and patient specificity. This committee should include the compliance director or compliance officer for that practice or facility.

Pitfall: "Negative defaults" are similar to exploding elements. Here, the system creates negative findings for all elements. This will also result in inaccuracies or incomplete information in the medical record.

Resolution: The provider must be required to specifically select and verify each element of the patient encounter.

Pitfall: The EHR must be able to reflect and trace any amendments and/or changes to the medical record. They must be dated and timed and easily identified for authentication during a review or audit. The tracing of those changes is essential to identify legitimate changes versus improper changes. The EHR would include the provider's credentials, signature (electronic), date, and time. There should be no opportunity to erase information already entered and authenticated.

Signatures

The health record requires the signature of the provider. In the case of EHR documentation, certain forms of the signature are accepted. A digitized signature that is an electronic image of the provider's handwritten signature is allowed. An electronic signature that includes a date and time stamp and a statement that the documentation was electronically signed by the provider is also allowed. Be cautious of "auto-authentication" or "auto-signature" systems, which may not allow the provider to review an entry prior to signing. Any documentation that states "signed but not read" is not acceptable.

An additional caution for EHR systems is the need for any personnel who document information to be identified. Systems with only a single authorization for a patient encounter may present a compliance problem. Ancillary personnel collect preliminary information related to vital signs and demographics and must be identified in the EHR.

1995 or 1997 Documentation Guidelines?

Organizations purchasing an EHR system for their physicians should select a system that allows for either set of documentation guidelines to be chosen by the provider at the time of the encounter. There are advantages to both sets. The 1997 DGs are generally found to be more advantageous to specific specialties such as ophthalmology and psychiatry, while other specialties and general practitioners will find the 1995 DGs more appropriate.

Chapter Summary

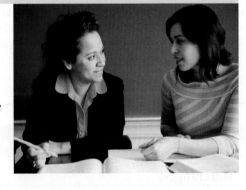

1. The documentation guidelines grew out of 1992 changes in the way Medicare reimbursed physicians, specifically the adoption of the RBRVS methodology. When the AMA developed new E/M codes reflecting the RBRVS methodology, physicians needed a resource on how to determine what level of service to assign to their work. The AMA and the HCFA developed the *1995 Documentation Guidelines for Evaluation and Management Services*. In 1997, the E/M guidelines were revised to include single-specialty and multisystem exams.

2. The purpose of the documentation guidelines is to translate physician documentation into the three key components of history, examination, and medical decision making so as to assign correct and appropriate codes to physician serves and obtain proper reimbursement. The guidelines support the need for thorough documentation that represents the communication and continuity of care and facilitates accurate and timely review of claims, payments, utilization reviews, and quality of care evaluations.

3. The documentation guidelines translate physician documentation into a chief complaint and the three key components of history, examination, and medical decision making. The chief complaint is always required to be documented. The history key component is made up of three elements: history of present illness, review of systems, and past, family, and/or social history. The examination key component rates the complexity of examination of body parts and organ systems. The medical decision-making key component comprises the number of diagnoses or management options, the amount and/or complexity of data reviewed, and the risk of significant complications, morbidity, and/or mortality. The levels of service of these key components are then translated into one of the four levels of E/M service: problem focused, expanded problem focused, detailed, and comprehensive.

4. The 1995 DGs have a single set of examination requirements. The 1997 DGs have two types of examination requirements: general multisystem examination requirements and single-specialty examination requirements. Providers can choose to use either the 1995 or the 1997 DGs. The main difference between the versions is in the way the examination key component level of service is determined; the history and medical decision-making components are determined the same way in both versions.

5. The result of studying the audit process and the documentation guidelines is to give providers and their coders the ability to determine whether the provider's documentation justifies the level of service reported. Using all the documentation guidelines—the 1995 and the 1997 multisystem and single-specialty versions—makes E/M compliance possible while ensuring appropriate reimbursement for the services reported.

6. The purpose of the audit process is to ensure accurate and compliant reporting of codes to payers so as to avoid accusations of fraud and to obtain the maximum appropriate reimbursement for services. Audits can be external, performed by payers or government agencies, or they can be internal, performed by a compliance officer or other skilled staff member to uncover possible problems so that they can be corrected.

7. To effectively audit E/M services, coders must know the terminology associated with auditing. The use of *brief* and *extended* in the HPI and the use of *pertinent* in both ROS and PFSH are examples. For MDM, coders must know what is associated with data review and overall risk. More generally, coders must understand upcoding and downcoding and their significance to the E/M audit process.

8. The tools used for auditing E/M services include audit forms and other tools that allow the individual reviewing coding to compare the documentation against the codes chosen and determine whether they are correct. The audit tool that the practice uses should be easily understood and easy to use and should clearly indicate whether it applies to the 1995 or 1997 DGs or to both.

9. It is virtually impossible to complete and present E/M audits without the use of an audit form. Coders should know what information belongs in HPI, ROS, and PFSH. They should know what information in the physician's documentation belongs in the examination section of the form and what belongs in the MDM section. The last element of the process is to put the pieces together to provide the appropriate E/M code based on the documentation reviewed.

10. The electronic health record brings its own set of audit concerns. Coders should be aware of the problematic issues associated with the use of EHRs. Specifically, watch for prompts, exploding elements, cloning (copy and paste functions), negative defaults, changes made to the record, and tracking of the signatures of anyone who documents in an EHR.

Review Questions

Matching

Match the key terms with their definitions.

A. audit
B. body areas
C. brief
D. constitutional
E. data review
F. documentation guidelines (DGs)
G. downcoding
H. extended
I. external audit
J. general multisystem examination requirements

K. history of present illness (HPI)
L. internal audit
M. organ systems
N. overall risk
O. past, family, and/or social history (PFSH)
P. prospective audit
Q. retrospective audit
R. review of systems (ROS)
S. specialty examination requirements
T. upcoding

1. _____ An element listed in both the ROS in history and in the examination key component

2. _____ An element of the 1995 and 1997 DG medical decision-making criteria

3. _____ Complications, morbidities, and mortalities associated with the patient's condition

4. _____ Determining whether the physician's documentation matches the level of service reported by an E/M code

5. _____ Reporting a level of service that is higher than the level documented

6. _____ A history element that identifies the chronology of the patient's illness or complaint

7. _____ A listing of four or more elements of HPI or two to nine elements of ROS

8. _____ Criteria established in 1992 as to how physicians can determine whether their documentation matches a level of service

9. _____ A listing of one to three elements of HPI

10. _____ An audit initiated by a medical practice to determine whether the codes selected are appropriate to the services documented

11. _____ An inventory of body systems presented by the patient in response to questions

12. _____ Reporting a level of service that is lower than the level documented

13. _____ An element of the history key component that relates to previous illnesses and family history

14. _____ Audits performed by payers or government agencies to determine whether a medical practice is adhering to documentation standards

15. _____ Part of the examination elements

16. _____ A refinement of the 1995 DGs

17. _____ An element of the 1995 and 1997 DG examination criteria that includes the neck

18. _____ An audit conducted prior to sending out claims to a payer

19. _____ One of the choices offered by the 1997 DGs at the request of specialty physicians

20. _____ An audit conducted after claims have been sent to the payer

True or False

Decide whether each statement is true or false.

1. _____ It is appropriate to use the 1995 DGs for the bullet method of determining the LOS for an E/M encounter.

2. _____ If the ROS has fewer than four elements documented, the ROS is considered brief.

3. _____ To qualify for a comprehensive exam, the physician must document an examination of eight organ systems.

4. _____ Question 3 relates to the 1995 documentation guidelines.

5. _____ As long as the chief complaint is documented, clarity about the presenting problem is not necessary.

6. _____ Past history includes a recitation of the relevant illnesses and surgeries of family members.

7. _____ The detailed levels of service under the 1997 general multisystem examination guidelines are the same as the 1997 single-organ system examination guidelines.

8. _____ Documentation of any key component at the highest level means that the patient encounter qualifies as the highest level E/M service.

9. _____ Historically speaking, the need for documentation guidelines resulted from the RBRVS program.

10. _____ Emergency department codes require only two elements of PFSH to qualify as the comprehensive LOS of the history key component.

11. _____ For the MDM key component, only two elements must be in the same column to select the level of MDM.

12. _____ All specialty physicians are required to use the specialty-specific 1997 documentation guidelines.

13. _____ Once the constitutional information is obtained for ROS, it can also be part of the constitutional requirement in the examination.

14. _____ In the physician's documentation, indicating an abnormal finding without elaboration is insufficient.

15. _____ The audit result will be affected by whether the E/M code requires three or two key components.

Multiple Choice

Select the letter that best completes the statement or answers the question.

1. Jane Robins, an established patient, presents with a chief complaint of a productive cough for 5 days after exposure to a friend who was ill with pneumonia. She has not had a fever. She is wheezing but has no muscle aches, dizziness, or headaches. What is the level of this patient's history using the 1995 documentation guidelines?
   A. 99203
   B. 99212
   C. 99213
   D. 99242

2. The physician examined Jane Robins's lungs and ears, nose, and throat (ENT). What is the level of this examination using the 1995 documentation guidelines?
   A. 99203
   B. 99212
   C. 99213
   D. 99242

3. After examining Jane Robins, the physician determined that she had bronchitis but sent her for a chest x-ray to rule out the possibility of pneumonia because of her previous exposure. What is the level of medical decision making using the 1995 documentation guidelines?
   A. Straightforward
   B. Low
   C. Moderate
   D. High

4. Using the three key components chosen for Questions 1–3, what E/M code should the physician report using the 1995 documentation guidelines?
   A. 99203
   B. 99212
   C. 99213
   D. 99242

5. Using the 1995 documentation guidelines, what E/M code would the physician report if Jane Robins was a new patient?
   A. 99202
   B. 99203
   C. 99204
   D. 99205

6. The physician examined new patient Jane Robins's lungs and ENT. What is the level of this examination using the 1997 general multisystem guidelines?
   A. 99201
   B. 99212
   C. 99213
   D. 99242

7. Using the findings in Question 6, what will be the result once all three key components for new patient Jane Robins are considered under the 1997 general multisystem guidelines versus the 1995 guidelines?
   A. The LOS does not change.
   B. The LOS is higher.
   C. The LOS is lower.
   D. The LOS is higher if Jane Robins is a new patient and lower if she is an established patient.

8. Arthur Martin, an established patient, has had difficulty walking due to pain in his right leg for the last 3 months. He has less pain when he stops walking. He denies pain while at rest; he has no other musculoskeletal pain and has no problems with impotence or urination. He denies any family history related to this problem that he knows of. Assess the level of history for this patient under the 1995 guidelines and select the correct E/M code.
   A. 99212
   B. 99213
   C. 99214
   D. 99215

9. The physical examination of Arthur Martin reveals a temperature of 98.1°F and BP of 135/76. The right leg is without any deformity and the skin on the right foot is cool and mottled. The neurological exam shows Arthur to be alert and oriented but with decreased sensation below the right knee. Both his cardiovascular and respiratory examinations are normal. Assess the level of examination under the 1995 guidelines and assign the correct E/M code.
   A. 99212
   B. 99213
   C. 99214
   D. 99215

10. Using Arthur Martin's details from Question 9, assess the level of examination for Arthur Martin under the 1997 general multisystem guidelines and assign the appropriate E/M code.
    A. 99212
    B. 99213
    C. 99214
    D. 99215

11. Arthur Martin has peripheral vascular disease, needs to begin a monitored walking program, and will need prescribed medication. He also has to stop smoking for his condition to resolve. A follow-up visit is to be scheduled for 1 month. Assess the level of medical decision making using the 1995 documentation guidelines and assign the appropriate E/M code.
    A. 99212
    B. 99213
    C. 99214
    D. 99215

12. Combining the three key component levels for Arthur Martin, what code will the physician report for this patient encounter using the 1995 documentation guidelines?
    A. 99212
    B. 99213
    C. 99214
    D. 99215

13. Sixteen-year-old Sandra Katz comes to the emergency department for right lower quadrant abdominal pain that started 4 hours ago. The pain was sudden onset and has remained steady. She is not nauseous and has not vomited. Her last menstrual period was normal, and she has not had any injury to account for this pain. Sandra has not had any surgeries, is not on any medications, and has no allergies. Her parents are in good health without any significant medical history. She does not drink or use drugs, and she denies sexual activity. What is the history level for this patient using the 1995 documentation guidelines?
    A. 99243
    B. 99253
    C. 99283
    D. 99284

14. The examination of Sandra Katz shows slightly hyperactive bowel sounds in the abdomen, no hepato-splenomegaly, no palpable masses, and some tenderness to deep palpation. The pelvic exam shows tenderness in the right adnexa but no adnexal masses; the cervix is not tender. Using the 1995 documentation guidelines, which code should be reported?

    A. 99243
    B. 99253
    C. 99283
    D. 99284

15. Continuing with Sandra Katz, urinalysis is done and is normal. The complete blood count (CBC) shows a low hematocrit level with mildly elevated white blood cell count. An independent review of the pelvic ultrasound shows no masses but some fluid in the deep pelvis. The onset of pain and the history are not typical for appendicitis. Possible options are a ruptured ovarian cyst or ovarian torsion. If pain persists, Sandra may need a laparoscopy. Her CBC is to be repeated. Using the 1995 documentation guidelines, which code should be reported?

    A. 99282
    B. 99283
    C. 99284
    D. 99285

16. Combining the three key component levels for Sandra Katz, what code will this physician report for this patient encounter using the 1995 documentation guidelines?

    A. 99243
    B. 99253
    C. 99283
    D. 99284

17. Helen Daniels, an established patient, sees her dermatologist due to recurrence of a rash on her forearm 4 days ago. The rash is itchy. The dermatologist's examination shows a 3- by 5-cm rash on the midforearm with scaly, erythematous, raised papules. He diagnoses the condition as recurrent eczematous dermatitis and prescribes 1% cortisone cream, an over-the-counter medication. What is the code for this patient encounter using the 1995 documentation guidelines?

    A. 99212
    B. 99213
    C. 99214
    D. 99215

18. If the MDM is straightforward, how does it affect the code selection for Helen Daniels's encounter?

    A. There is no impact because both the history and examination are at the same code level as straight-forward MDM.
    B. There is no impact because MDM is not required for an established patient encounter.
    C. It will impact the code selection because MDM controls the level of service.
    D. It will impact the code selection because straightforward MDM is the lowest-level MDM and will lower the level of service.

19. If the MDM for Helen Daniels's encounter is low, how does it affect the code selection?

    A. There is no impact because both the history and examination are at the same code level as low MDM.
    B. There is no impact because the lowest key component controls the level of service.
    C. It will impact the code selection because MDM controls the level of service.
    D. It will impact the code selection because low MDM is at a higher level than the history and examination key components.

20. HISTORY: Maxine Lee, a patient with unrelenting shoulder pain and decreased range of motion in the shoulder, is referred to a rheumatologist for an opinion about a diagnosis and about how to treat the condition once determined. In the rheumatologist's office, she tells the physician that the pain started 6 weeks ago after she lifted heavy suitcases during a family vacation. Motrin was used to alleviate the pain. There is no family history of rheumatoid arthritis, but Maxine is having increased difficulty with daily activities. She denies any respiratory or cardiovascular symptoms, has not been nauseous, and has no constipation problems or allergies. All other systems are negative as well. The patient had a knee arthroscopy 2 years ago, and she does smoke and drink occasionally. She is divorced with two children.

EXAMINATION: Musculoskeletal exam of the shoulders shows a very limited range of motion.

MEDICAL DECISION MAKING: X-rays of the shoulders were taken and reviewed. The patient has arthralgia of the shoulders and will need physical therapy and a stronger anti-inflammatory available only by prescription. If Maxine is not better in 2 weeks, her internist will consider cortisone injections and/or an MRI.

Which code should be reported for this patient encounter using the 1995 documentation guidelines?
A. 99241
B. 99242
C. 99243
D. 99244

CHAPTER 15

CPT: Anesthesia Codes

CHAPTER OUTLINE

Anesthesia Background

Types of Anesthesia

Anesthesia Organization

Anesthesia Services Package

Services Not Included in Routine Anesthesia Services

Anesthesia Modifiers

Qualifying Circumstances

Anesthesia Documentation

Anesthesia Time

Assigning Anesthesia Codes

Anesthesia Coding and Billing Resources

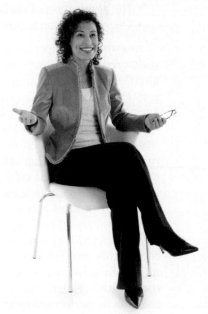

Tim Pannell/Fuse/Thinkstock

LEARNING OUTCOMES

After studying this chapter, you should be able to:

1. Describe the organization, guidelines, and key modifiers for the Anesthesia section in CPT.
2. Define the various anesthesia techniques: general, local, nerve block, regional, conscious sedation, and monitored anesthesia care.
3. Define the concept of a complete anesthesia service.
4. Explain when anesthesia modifiers and qualifying circumstances are reported.
5. Identify documentation necessary to code anesthesia services.
6. Calculate anesthesia time units and fees based on prescribed formulas.
7. Assign CPT anesthesia codes with appropriate HCPCS modifiers and physical status modifiers based on anesthesia procedural statements.
8. Discuss common coding mistakes and missed billing opportunities when reporting anesthesia services.

Anesthesiologists are active in many aspects of a patient's clinical treatment in addition to providing anesthesia during surgical procedures. They participate in acute and chronic pain management, critical care, ventilation assistance and management, anesthesia for deliveries, and intravascular catheterization procedures. Anesthesia services can be some of the most difficult to code, especially from a billing perspective. Anesthesiologists are not reimbursed according to the same payment methodology as other physicians, and individual payers have varying rules for coding and billing. Coding for anesthesia services is not routinely done by physician practices or health information management (HIM) coders; it is considered a coding specialty. However, it is important for all medical coders to have a basic understanding of this important topic.

ANESTHESIA BACKGROUND

The administration of anesthesia causes the loss of the ability to feel pain. The administered drug or other medical intervention causes partial or complete loss of sensation, with or without loss of consciousness. According to the American Society of Anesthesiologists (ASA), anesthesiology is essentially the practice of medicine that deals with the following:

- The management of procedures for rendering a patient insensible to pain and emotional stress during surgery and obstetrical procedures
- The evaluation and management of life functions under the stress of anesthetic and surgical manipulations
- The clinical management of a patient unconscious from any cause
- The evaluation and management of problems with pain relief
- The management of problems in cardiac and respiratory resuscitation
- The application of specific methods of respiratory therapy
- The clinical management of various fluids, electrolytes, and metabolic disturbances

Anesthesia services are provided by an anesthesiologist, anesthesiologist assistant, or a certified registered nurse anesthetist (CRNA). Anesthesiologists are physicians specializing in providing anesthesia and pain management services. Anesthesiologist assistants (AAs) are nonphysician master's-prepared allied health professionals who have successfully completed an accredited anesthesiologist assistant training program and who are certified by the National Commission for Certification of Anesthesiologist Assistants. AAs develop and implement anesthesia care plans and assist the anesthesiologist in monitoring the patient and carrying out specific tasks related to anesthesia, including delivery and maintenance of anesthesia. CNRAs are master's-prepared critical care nurses who have obtained additional training in providing anesthesia and who are certified by the Council on Certification of Nurse Anesthetists. These professionals specialize in anesthesiology and are regulated by the American Board of Anesthesiology, the ASA, and state laws. Most anesthesia groups are independent contractors and are not employed by hospitals. The anesthesiologist is ultimately responsible for the evaluation of the patient, development of the anesthesia plan, and provision of anesthesia services when services are directly performed by a CRNA or AA.

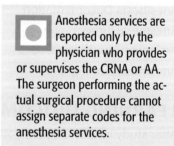 Anesthesia services are reported only by the physician who provides or supervises the CRNA or AA. The surgeon performing the actual surgical procedure cannot assign separate codes for the anesthesia services.

TYPES OF ANESTHESIA

The type of anesthesia the doctor chooses for a procedure depends on the type of procedure being performed plus the age and health of the patient. The choice is made after the anesthesiologist has interviewed and examined the patient and has obtained consent.

General Anesthesia

Under general anesthesia, the patient is rendered unconscious, pain free, and stable for the entire surgical procedure. Constant attendance of anesthesia personnel and monitoring are required. General anesthesia is performed when procedures are highly invasive, are long in duration, or do not permit patient movement. Some examples of procedures performed under general anesthesia are abdominal surgery such as hysterectomy and cholecystectomy, spine surgery, organ transplants, breast reconstruction, and sinus surgery. Examples of common medications used for general anesthesia are propofol, fentanyl, thiopental sodium (Pentothal), alfentanil, and succinylcholine.

The following steps are involved with administering general anesthesia:

1. *Preparation:* The anesthesiologist reviews the patient's history (allergies, previous anesthesia experiences, medications, treatments, etc.), performs a physical examination (including oral airway), and determines an anesthesia plan.
2. *Induction:* The anesthesiologist puts the patient to sleep (intubation).
3. *Maintenance:* While the surgeon operates, the anesthesiologist maintains the patient in an anesthetized state and monitors metabolic functions (temperature, pulse, respirations, and neuromuscular function).
4. *Emergence:* The anesthesiologist reverses the anesthetic agents and extubates the patient, who gradually regains consciousness and control of body functions such as breathing.
5. *Recovery:* After the surgeon has turned the patient over to the anesthesiologist, a postanesthesia care unit (PACU) monitors the patient for side effects of anesthesia. The anesthesia provider is responsible for the care of the patient until the patient is stable enough—breathing independently and able to answer questions appropriately—to be discharged to a room or from the facility. Postoperative pain management is started in the PACU.

Regional Anesthesia

Regional anesthesia numbs a part of the body without inducing unconsciousness. The patient is typically awake enough to respond to stimuli but is sedated and will not recall the procedure. This type of anesthesia is provided for procedures done below the diaphragm or on extremities and for patients for whom general anesthesia is a high risk. With this type of anesthesia, an IV is continuously instilling medication.

There are three types of regional anesthesia:

1. *Spinal anesthesia:* A single injection of the agent is made into the subarachnoid space between two lumbar vertebrae.
2. *Epidural anesthesia:* An agent is injected by inserting a catheter into the epidural space, numbing the chest and lower body. A catheter is left intact for continuous infusion of anesthetic. This is the approach commonly employed for labor and delivery.
3. *Intravenous regional block:* In this type, which is used for short-term procedures performed on extremities, a tourniquet is placed on the extremity. A common intravenous regional block is a Bier block, which is used for upper extremity procedures.

Peripheral Nerve Blocks

Nerve blocks involve injecting an anesthetic solution parallel to or surrounding a peripheral nerve or nerve plexuses such as the brachial plexus. The anesthetic solution diffuses from the outer surface (mantle) toward the center (core) of the nerve. The patient is awake throughout the procedure. This type of anesthesia is also used for controlling postoperative pain, often with trigger point or nerve injections.

Local Anesthesia

> According to the CPT, "local infiltration, metacarpal/metatarsal/digital block or topical anesthesia" is included in the surgical procedure code and cannot be billed separately.

Local anesthesia affects a specific, small area of the body and is common for procedures on the skin. Administration may be by injection, as a topical anesthesia, or by spray. The patient is not asleep. Procedures performed solely under local anesthesia are performed in a physician office or at the bedside and do not require an operating room (OR) or anesthesia staff. Local anesthesia is commonly used for mole removals, laceration repairs (suturing), catheter insertions, and pin removals. Examples of local anesthesia medications are lidocaine (Xylocaine), bupivacaine (Marcaine), chloroprocaine (Nesacaine), and procaine (Novocaine).

Monitored Anesthesia Care

Under monitored anesthesia care (MAC), the patient is not completely anesthetized and can respond to directions and questions. The administration of sedatives, hypnotics, and analgesics as well as anesthetic drugs commonly used for the induction and maintenance of general anesthesia is often a part of MAC. Patients are sedated with a tranquilizer preoperatively. The surgeon may or may not anesthetize the surgical incision site with a local anesthetic.

The patient is monitored throughout the procedure. In some cases, the surgeon may direct the patient to respond to areas of pain or to cough or breathe deeply. Examples of common procedures performed under MAC are podiatry procedures such as hammertoe repair, breast biopsy, carpal tunnel surgery, lesion removals, some hernia repairs, lymph node biopsy, and some gynecological procedures such as conization of the cervix.

Conscious Sedation: Not an Anesthesia Section Service

Conscious sedation (CS) is moderate anesthesia carried out by injecting a sedative and/or analgesic intravenously to relieve pain and anxiety during a medical procedure. Analgesics, unlike most anesthesia, relieve pain without the loss of consciousness, although they may have an amnesia effect after the procedure is completed. The patient remains awake and relaxed. Procedures performed under conscious sedation are typically done in an office or clinic setting, not in the OR.

Instead of an anesthesia provider, conscious sedation is done either by the surgeon or by a specially trained nurse who is supervised by the surgeon. The patient's consciousness and cardiac and respiratory function are monitored and documented throughout the procedure. The physician must be able to recognize deep sedation, manage the consequences, and adjust the level of sedation to a moderate or lesser level.

> Guidelines and codes for IV conscious sedation (99151–99157) are in the CPT's Medicine section, not the Anesthesia section. Moderate sedation codes are not used to report minimal or deep sedation, administration of pain medication, or MAC.

Differentiation of MAC and IV Sedation/Conscious Sedation

The difference between MAC and conscious sedation is under intense scrutiny by the medical and insurance communities. The scrutiny results from the lack of understanding between what is MAC and what is conscious sedation. There are some major differences. MAC allows a deeper sedation than does conscious sedation. MAC can easily be transitioned into general anesthesia for brief periods of time, permitting the performance of a wider range of invasive procedures. MAC requires a CRNA, AA, or anesthesiologist with the skill level to distinguish deep sedation from general anesthesia and to quickly return the patient to deep sedation. The provider must be prepared to convert to general anesthesia and maintain the patient's airway should the procedure require it or if the patient is uncooperative.

To pay for MAC, Medicare requires the following:

- A surgeon's request for MAC
- An anesthesia preoperative examination
- Continuous presence of anesthesia personnel
- Anesthesiologist presence for emergency treatment or diagnosis
- Continuous metabolic monitoring
- Oxygen administration, if indicated
- IV administration of scheduled pharmacological agents at the discretion of the anesthesia personnel

ANESTHESIA ORGANIZATION

Anesthesia codes are located in CPT in the Anesthesia section. The codes are also listed in the ASA's *Relative Value Guide,* which is published annually and contains anesthesia guidelines, modifiers, common procedures performed by anesthesiologists, and elements used in calculating anesthesia fees.

In CPT, anesthesia codes are grouped anatomically by body area, first from the head down to the feet, and then from the shoulder to the hand. The Anesthesia section is divided into 19 subsections, each covering general, regional, and local anesthesia (Table 15.1).

Table 15.1 Anesthesia Subsections

ANATOMICAL AREA(S)	CPT CODES
Head	00100–00222
Neck	00300–00352
Thorax (chest wall and shoulder girdle)	00400–00474
Intrathoracic	00500–00580
Spine and spinal cord	00600–00670
Upper abdomen	00700–00797
Lower abdomen	00800–00882
Perineum	00902–00952
Pelvis (except hip)	01112–01173
Upper leg (except knee)	01200–01274
Knee and popliteal area	01320–01444
Lower leg (below knee, includes ankle and foot)	01462–01522
Shoulder and axilla	01610–01680
Upper arm and elbow	01710–01782
Forearm, wrist, and hand	01810–01860
Radiological procedures	01916–01936
Burn excisions or debridement	01951–01953
Obstetrical	01958–01969
Other procedures	01990–01999

ANESTHESIA SERVICES PACKAGE

Anesthesia services for surgical procedures have one code that pays for the complete anesthesia service. The package includes the following:

Surgeons who render regional or general anesthesia report a code from the Surgery section (code range 10021–69990) with modifier –47. (Modifier –47 is never attached to an anesthesia code.) No additional payment is allowed; anesthesia services are considered part of the procedure.

- General, regional, and supplementation of local anesthesia
- Interpretation of lab values
- Placement of IVs for fluid and medication administration
- Arterial line insertion for blood pressure monitoring or other supportive services to provide the anesthesia care deemed optimal by the anesthesiologist during any procedure
- The usual preoperative and postoperative visits
- The administration of fluids and/or blood
- The usual monitoring services (temperature, blood pressure, oximetry, echocardiography (ECG), capnography, and mass spectrometry)

None of the following CPT codes can be billed in addition to a complete anesthesia service code, because these codes include anesthesia services: 31500 (intubation), 31505 (laryngoscopy, indirect), 31515 (laryngoscopy, direct), 31527 (laryngoscopy, with insertion of obturator), 31622 (bronchoscopy, diagnostic), 31645 (bronchoscopy), 36000 (introduction of needle or intracatheter, vein), 36010 (introduction of catheter, superior or inferior vena cava), 36400–36425 (venipuncture), and 62320–62327 (pain management).

SERVICES NOT INCLUDED IN ROUTINE ANESTHESIA SERVICES

Some services are not part of a complete anesthesia service package, and if provided they may be billed separately with the –59 modifier:

- Insertion of Swan-Ganz catheter (93503)
- Emergency intubation (31500)

- Central venous pressure line (36555 or 36556 for central venous catheter) through a separate stick
- Unusual forms of monitoring such as placement of central venous lines
- Pain management injections or placement of epidurals for postoperative pain management and not for anesthesia purposes (independent of the anesthesia service)
- Critical care visits (99291–99292)
- Arterial catheter (36620)
- Transesophageal echocardiography (TEE; 93312–93318) if performed for diagnostic purposes and not for monitoring the patient during surgery

■ **CASE SCENARIO**
A patient undergoes an anorectal procedure. Because of the patient's condition and chronic illnesses, the anesthesiologist places a Swan-Ganz catheter. Report codes 00902 and 93503–59.

Swan-Ganz Catheter Insertion

A Swan-Ganz catheter, also referred to as a *pulmonary catheter*, is a diagnostic tool used to monitor a patient's blood flow in the heart and lungs, measure blood pressure of the pulmonary artery and heart, monitor complications of a heart attack, and monitor effectiveness of medications. This procedure may also be referred to as a *right heart catheterization* and can be performed to diagnose heart failure, sepsis, and many other conditions. The catheter is inserted through a vein in the neck or groin and threaded up into the heart through the tricuspid and pulmonary valves and placed into the pulmonary (lung) artery for measuring and monitoring. An anesthesiologist or a surgeon may utilize this type of continuous monitoring in the critically ill patient who has the following:

- Abnormal pressures in the heart arteries
- Burns
- Congenital heart disease
- Heart failure
- Kidney disease
- Leaky heart valves (valvular regurgitation)
- Shock
- Acute respiratory distress
- Ventilator

The catheter has a port to allow for blood collection to measure oxygen consumption along with lumens to infuse solutions. The catheter may be left in place for several days to monitor a critically ill patient.

CPT code 93503, *Insertion and placement of flow directed catheter (e.g., Swan-Ganz) for monitoring purposes*, describes this service.

NOTE: Do not bill separately for a central venous pressure (CVP) port used to thread a Swan-Ganz catheter. It is appropriate, however, to bill both a CVP and a Swan-Ganz if they are two separate lines. An additional code from the cardiovascular section of CPT would be assigned for the CVP (i.e., 36555, 36556, 36620).

Transesophageal Echocardiography

Transesophageal echocardiography (TEE) is a diagnostic imaging test performed to view the heart, cardiac sac, and vessels in motion. The TEE is another method of performing ECG and is often performed by an anesthesiologist. Instead of having the ultrasound transducer pressing against the outside chest wall, an ultrasound transducer is inserted into the mouth and passed down the esophagus. This method of imaging is often chosen over the conventional method because the pictures are clearer for areas that are hard to view via the transthoracic method. In the traditional method, the ultrasound signal has to pass through skin, bone, and lungs before it reaches the heart, thus weakening the signal and producing a poor image. When the probe is inserted through the esophagus, it is closer to the internal structures and produces better imaging and Doppler quality. Structures commonly evaluated with TEE are the aorta, pulmonary artery, valves of the heart, both atria, atrial septum, left atrial appendage, and coronary arteries.

TEE is becoming the most powerful and relied-upon monitoring technique and diagnostic tool for the management of cardiac surgical patients for anesthesiologists. It can be used intraoperatively to provide information about the structure and function of the heart/great vessels in real time, enabling the anesthesiologist to manage a cardiac patient's physiology while providing updates and direction to the surgical team throughout the pre-, intra-, and postoperative period. TEE is usually considered diagnostic and performed by an anesthesiologist in the following situations:

- The surgical technique will be affected by the intraoperative TEE findings or the probe assists in surgical management decisions.
- Thoracic/cardiac structures and/or function were not adequately evaluated prior to surgery, making the TEE report necessary for a safe outcome of anesthesia and/or surgery.

TEE Coding

93312—Real-time with image documentation (2D); includes probe placement, image acquisition, interpretation, and report

93313—Probe only

93314—Image acquisition, interpretation, and report only

93315—For congenital cardiac anomalies; includes probe placement, image acquisition, interpretation, and report

93316—Probe only for congenital cardiac

93317—Interpretation and report only for congenital anomalies

93318—Monitoring purposes, includes probe placement, 2D image acquisition, and interpretation leading to ongoing (continuous) assessment of (dynamically changing) cardiac pumping function and therapeutic measures

NOTE: Modifiers affect physician and facility reimbursement. When a physician owns the equipment (e.g., TEE machine, ultrasound machine, lab equipment) used to perform a diagnostic service, he or she is entitled to payment for the use of the equipment. If a physician owns the equipment and is providing the interpretation of the study/test, bill the service globally with no modifier attached. This allows the physician to be reimbursed at 100% of the allowed amount for this procedure. If the physician is performing this procedure in a setting where he or she does not own the equipment, append the −26 modifier to reflect the professional component of the service instead.

Physicians should not report the TC (technical component) modifier with any code where there is a global component unless the physician performing the test owns the equipment but is sending the results out to another provider and not personally interpreting the results.

TEE Add-On Codes

Doppler echocardiography and color flow studies are not included in TEE codes 93312–93318; therefore, when these services are performed in conjunction with TEE, report add-on codes 93320, *Doppler echocardiography, pulsed wave and/or continuous wave with spectral display; complete*, 93321, *Follow-up or limited study*; or 93325, *Doppler echocardiography color flow velocity mapping*, in addition to the main procedure code.

NOTE: If the anesthesia provider performs the TEE, append the −26 modifier for the anesthesiologist's professional component of the service. If the anesthesiologist only provided anesthesia services for a TEE procedure, report anesthesia code 01922.

Obstetrical Anesthesia

Two questions must be answered before assigning codes for labor and delivery anesthesia:

1. Did the physician provide anesthesia for labor or only for delivery?
2. Was the delivery vaginal or cesarean?

For obstetrical anesthesia for vaginal delivery, two codes are available: 01960 and 01967. CPT code 01960 is used for anesthesia provided for a vaginal delivery only, regardless of type (epidural or general); and CPT code 01967 is used if the physician provided anesthesia for both labor and vaginal delivery. CPT code 01961 is assigned for a cesarean delivery only. Report 01967 when anesthesia is provided for both labor and C-section delivery but also report add-on code 01968 to represent the cesarean delivery if the patient labored and then required a C-section for delivery.

CHECKPOINT 15.1

Use Table 15.1 and the definition of a complete anesthesia service to determine the code(s) that can be reported for the following case.

A 43-year-old patient requires fusing of the lumbar spine due to traumatic injury. The surgeon asks the anesthesiologist to place an epidural for continuous infusion of pain medication for postoperative pain management. The possible codes are 22612 and 62326.

1. Which code(s) can be assigned? _____

2. Is a modifier needed to indicate that two distinct procedural services were performed?

   _____

ANESTHESIA MODIFIERS

All anesthesia services are reported using the five-digit CPT Anesthesia section codes 00100–01999 along with anesthesia modifiers. The modifiers are essential to identify who provided the anesthesia services, under what circumstances they were provided, and the status of the patient at the time of the anesthesia service. Three different categories of anesthesia modifiers can be appended to anesthesia codes: physical status modifiers, CPT professional services modifiers, and HCPCS Level II modifiers.

Physical Status Modifiers

Physical status modifiers are located on the inside cover of CPT (and in the Anesthesia guidelines) and are shown in Table 15.2. Based on the ranking system used by the American Society of Anesthesiologists, they depict the physical risk to the patient or the complexity of the anesthesia care. The ASA assigns reimbursement units to each modifier, which affects anesthesia fees.

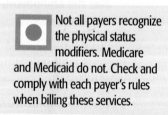 Not all payers recognize the physical status modifiers. Medicare and Medicaid do not. Check and comply with each payer's rules when billing these services.

Table 15.2 Physical Status Modifiers

MODIFIER	PHYSICAL STATUS
–P1	Normal, healthy patient
–P2	Patient with mild systemic disease
–P3	Patient with severe systemic disease
–P4	Patient with severe systemic disease that is a constant threat to life
–P5	Moribund patient who is not expected to survive without the operation
–P6	Declared brain-dead patient whose organs are being removed for donor purposes

CPT Modifiers

- Modifier –23 is appended only to anesthesia codes; it is never used with surgery codes or E/M codes.
- Modifier –47, anesthesia by surgeon, is never used by an anesthesiologist for anesthesia procedures.

Under certain circumstances, the CPT modifiers listed on the inside of CPT's front cover and shown in Table 15.3 may be used to explain circumstances that arise during surgery or in the OR. The modifiers (with the exception of modifier –23) can be assigned to diagnostic procedures anesthesiologists personally perform, not to anesthesia services.

Table 15.3 Applicable CPT Modifiers

MODIFIER	CIRCUMSTANCE
–22	Increased procedural services
–23	Unusual anesthesia reported when anesthesia is administered for a procedure that usually requires local anesthesia or none at all, but, because of unusual circumstances, must be done under general anesthesia. (For example, the physician requests general anesthesia to perform an examination of the ears and remove impacted cerumen in an autistic child. This procedure typically does not require general anesthesia and is normally performed in the office setting.)
–32	Mandated service
–50	Bilateral procedure
–51	Multiple procedures
–52	Reduced services
–53	Discontinued procedure, used when the physician elects to terminate or discontinue a procedure, usually due to the risk of the patient's well-being, after the surgical preparation of patient or induction of anesthesia (a copy of the operative report should be submitted with the claim)
–59	Distinct procedural service, used to indicate that a procedure or service was independent from other services provided that day only if no other modifier is appropriate
–74	Discontinued outpatient hospital/ambulatory surgery center procedure after the administration of anesthesia because of such circumstances as a threat to the patient's well-being. (For example, the physician encountered massive tumors and adhesions and could not complete the procedure because of extensive bleeding.)

HCPCS Level II Modifiers

HCPCS Level II modifiers, intended for use for Medicare patients and now widely accepted by all insurance carriers for reporting of anesthesia services, are located in the HCPCS code set (Table 15.4); they are not in CPT. Documentation to show medical necessity, such as an operative note, may be required for some payers. HCPCS coding is covered in Chapter 30 of this text.

Table 15.4 HCPCS Level II Anesthesia Modifiers

MODIFIER	DEFINITION	REPORTED BY	NOTES
–AA	Anesthesia personally performed by an anesthesiologist	Anesthesiologist	Anesthesiologist receives 100% of the allowed payment from the carrier. Services billed with the –AA modifier cannot be reported with any other anesthesia service billed with one of the supervising modifiers below.
MODIFIERS INDICATING THE ANESTHESIOLOGIST IS SUPERVISING/DIRECTING AN ANESTHESIA PROVIDER			
–AD	Medical supervision by a physician; more than four concurrent anesthesia procedures	Anesthesiologist	This is used to explain that the anesthesiologist is supervising or directing more than four anesthesia providers simultaneously.
–AQ	Physician providing service in an unlisted health professional shortage area (HPSA)	Anesthesiologist	
–QK	Medically directed two, three, or four concurrent anesthesia procedures involving qualified individuals	Anesthesiologist	Payment is 50% of the allowed amount from the carrier. This is used when the anesthesiologist supervised at least two but not more than four CRNAs.
–QS	MAC	Anesthesiologist or CRNA	If the physician personally performs the case, modifier –AA must also be submitted and payment is 100% of the allowed amount. If the physician directs four or fewer concurrent cases and two or more of these cases are MAC, modifier –QK must be reported with –QS and payment is 50% of the allowed amount. CRNA would report either –QZ or –QX in addition to –QS.
–QX	CRNA service with medical direction by a physician	CRNA	The physician is most often an anesthesiologist but may not always be. One CRNA to one physician.
–QY	Medical direction of one qualified nonphysician anesthetist by an anesthesiologist	Anesthesiologist	This modifier indicates to the carrier that the payment for the anesthesia service should be split 50/50 with the anesthesiologist and the CRNA the anesthesiologist is directing.
–QZ	CRNA not medically directed by a physician	CRNA	No payment reduction occurs when the CRNA is working independently of a physician.
–G8	MAC for deep complex, complicated, or markedly invasive surgical procedure	Anesthesiologist or CRNA	Used in lieu of –QS for Medicare patients with procedures of the face, neck, breast, male genitalia, or for procedures for access to central venous circulation, and appended to anesthesia codes 00100, 00300, 00400, 00160, 00532, and 00920.
–G9	MAC for patient who has history of severe cardiopulmonary condition	MAC	Used for at-risk Medicare patients with history of severe cardiopulmonary condition where MAC was chosen over general to avoid potential intraoperative complications.

■ CASE SCENARIO

A 69-year-old male Medicare patient has a hernia repair under MAC. The anesthesiologist is directing two CRNAs during the procedure. Report 00830–QS–QK for the anesthesiologist services and 00830–QS–QX for the CRNA services.

CHECKPOINT 15.2

Append all modifiers applicable to the anesthesia code in the following case.

A Medicare patient undergoes a radical hysterectomy for cervical cancer. The anesthesiologist is supervising two cases simultaneously. The CRNA provides the general anesthesia.

1. 00846–_____

QUALIFYING CIRCUMSTANCES

Qualifying circumstances (also called *modifying factors*) are particularly difficult situations under which anesthesia must be administered, such as extraordinary condition of the patient, notable operative conditions, and/or unusual risk factors. Four codes, as shown in Table 15.5, are used to report these circumstances. The codes increase the fee due to the complications with the administration of the anesthesia. The qualifying circumstances codes, found in the Medicine section of CPT, can be reported as additional procedure codes. They are also listed in the guidelines at the beginning of the Anesthesia section.

Qualifying circumstances codes are add-on codes (+), so they are always listed along with a code for the primary anesthesia procedure and are never used alone. If more than one qualifying circumstance applies, more than one code may be assigned.

Table 15.5 Qualifying Circumstances

MODIFIER	CIRCUMSTANCE
+99100	Anesthesia for patient of extreme age, under 1 year and over 70 years of age (list separately in addition to code for primary anesthesia procedure)
+99116	Anesthesia complicated by utilization of total body hypothermia (list separately in addition to code for primary anesthesia procedure)
+99135	Anesthesia complicated by utilization of controlled hypotension (list separately in addition to code for primary anesthesia procedure)
+99140	Anesthesia complicated by specified emergency condition (list separately in addition to code for primary anesthesia procedure), used when a delay in treatment would lead to a significant increase in the threat to life or body part

■ CASE SCENARIO

A patient is brought to the emergency department (ED) after a motor vehicle accident in which he was struck while riding his motorcycle. He sustained a near amputation of the right foot and has lost a considerable amount of blood. Report 99140 in addition to the anesthesia code for the surgical repair of the foot due to the nature of the circumstances.

ANESTHESIA DOCUMENTATION

Anesthesia coding is based on the services recorded in the anesthesia documentation. Each facility has a customized anesthesia record to capture anesthesia-specific clinical information. The record contains preoperative notes, intraoperative notes, and postanesthesia care unit documentation. Preoperative notes cover the patient's medical and surgical history, history of anesthetic complications, current medications, respiratory condition, and the chosen anesthesia. PACU documentation records the monitoring of the patient for immediate postoperative complications.

Intraoperative notes (Fig. 15.1) reflect the close monitoring of the patient during the procedure for any complications. Monitoring is done via a variety of mechanisms, such as heart monitoring, temperature probes, and pulse oximetry. Vital signs and ventilation are documented at 5-minute intervals during the procedure and are graphed using accepted standard symbols. Any medications or fluids provided during the procedure are also documented, as are anesthesia start and stop times and operation start and stop times. The coder must review this document to correctly ascertain anesthesia time.

In addition to the anesthesiologist's documentation, anesthesia coders have access to the operative report. All diagnoses and procedures are captured on this report, allowing the coder to sequence the highest-paying procedure first on the claim. If any intraoperative complications required CPR or other unusual anesthesia services, these would also be documented.

CHECKPOINT 15.3

Refer to Figure 15.1 to answer the following questions.

1. What type of anesthesia was provided? _____

2. What surgical procedure was performed? _____

3. What was the total anesthesia time? _____

4. Who provided the anesthesia care? _____

5. If a CRNA provided the care, did a physician supervise the work? _____

6. What is the anesthesia code for this procedure? _____

7. What physical status modifier should be appended? _____

REIMBURSEMENT REVIEW

Common Mistakes When Reporting Anesthesia Services

- Failing to use modifiers or using invalid modifiers
- Charging separately for services included in the anesthesia service
- Charging for procedures performed by the surgeon but billed under the anesthesiologist for payment
- Failing to code to the highest level of specificity and not combining all anesthesia units for services performed on a given day into one code
- Billing separately for verification of proper placement and localization of site by injecting a small amount of contrast. (This is not separately billable.)
- Failing to provide documentation that clearly states medical necessity for all additional procedures personally performed by either the anesthesiologist or anesthetist

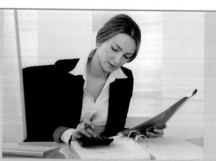

ANESTHESIA RECORD

		START	STOP
Anesthesia		0810	0951
Procedure		0814	0936
Room Time IN:	0800	OUT:	0950

Procedure(s) RT Hemicolectomy
Preop Diagnosis(es): Ulcerative Colitis
Surgeon: Walker

Date 10/14/04 **OR#** 3 **Page** of **PAM Check**

PRE-PROCEDURE

Pt Identified: ☑ ID Band ☐ Questioned ☐ Guardian
☑ Chart reviewed   ☑ Permit signed
☑ NPO since 10 PM   ☐ Full stomach
☑ Patient reassessed prior to anesthesia
☑ Surgical Site verified
☑ Peri-operative pain management discussed
☑ Oral airway examined
☐ Preop pain management injection site:
☑ Jewelry and nail polish removed
Pre-Anesthetic state: **Provider Time:**
☑ Awake   ☑ Anxious   ☐ Uncooperative
☐ Calm   ☐ Sedated   ☐ Reduced LOC

PATIENT SAFETY
☐ Anesthesia machine #   checked
☑ Critical clinical alarms checked & activated
☑ Secured with safety belt   ☐ Axillary roll
☑ Arm(s) secured on armboards   L   R☑
☑ Arm(s) tucked   L   R   ☐ Arms < 90°
☑ Pressure points checked, padded, monitored
☑ Eye Care: ☑ Taped closed   ☐ Ointment
      ☐ By surgeon ☐ Saline ☐ Goggles
Body Position: ☐ Lateral ☐ Dorsal ☐ Prone
      Supine   **TIME:**

MONITORS AND EQUIPMENT
Steth: ☑ Esophageal ☐ Precordial ☐ Suprasternal
☑ Non-Invasive B/P   ☐ V lead ECG
☑ Continuous ECG   ☐ ST / Dysrhy. analysis
☑ Pulse oximeter   ☑ Nerve stimulator:
☑ End tidal CO₂   ☐ Ulnar ☐ Tibial
☑ Oxygen / FiO₂ monitor   ☐ Facial ☐
☑ ET agent/analyzer   ☑ Fluid / Blood warmer
☑ Temp: Esoph(m)   ☐ Processed EEG
☑ Body warmer   ☐ Cell saver   ☐ ICP
☐ Airway humidifier: ☐ CPB   ☐ TEE
                                  ☐ Evoked potential:
☐ NG / OG tube
☐ Foley: ☑ OR   ☐ Ward   ☐ Doppler
☐ Arterial line
☐ C-line/CVP
☐ PA line
☑ IV(s) 18g IV (L) AC

Body Weight: 186   **Mucous Membranes:** Pink moist

ASA CLASS: 1 ② 3 4 5 E

ANESTHETIC TECHNIQUE
GA Induction: ☑ Intravenous ☐ Pre-O₂ ☐ RSI
☐ Cricoid pressure   ☐ Inhalation   ☐ IM   ☐ PR
GA Maintenance: ☐ Inhalation   ☑ Inhalation / IV
☐ GA / Regional combination   ☐ TIVA
☐ Sedation & Analgesia / Monitored Anesthesia Care
Regional: Epidural - ☐ Thoracic ☐ Lumbar ☐ Caudal
☐ SAB ☐ Ankle ☐ Femoral ☐ Interscalene
☐ CSE ☐ Bier ☐ Continuous Spinal ☐ Cervical Plexus
☐ Other:
Regional Technique: ☐ Position
☐ See remarks   ☐ Prep
☐ Local   ☐ Site
☐ Needle   ☐ Introducer
☐ LA
☐ Narcotic
☐ Additive
☐ Test dose Rx
☐ Attempts x   Level
☐ Catheter: ☐ Test dose response: +   —
L.O.R.   cm Skin   cm   ☐ Secured
☐ Difficult intubation
☐ Performed by: Vaughn

AIRWAY MANAGEMENT
☑ Oral ETT   ☐ RAE   ☐ L.T.A.   ☐ Magill forceps
☐ Nasal ETT   ☐ LMA #
☐ Stylet   ☐ Classic/Unique ☐ Fastrach ☐ ProSeal
☐ DL T   ☐ Flexible ☐ Other:
☑ Tube size: 7.0   ☐ FOI   ☐ Awake
☑ Blade: 3 Miller   ☐ Laser ETT ☐ LIS
☑ Attempts x   ☐ EMG ETT ☐ Bougie
☑ Grade: I ② III IV blind   ☐ Armored ETT ☐ TTJV
☐ Atraumatic intubation/LMA   ☐ DLT
☑ Secured at 21 cm   ☐ Bronchial blocker system
☑ ET CO₂ present
☑ Breath sounds = bilateral   ☐ Rigid FO laryngoscope
☑ Cuffed - min occ pressure
☐ Uncuffed ETT - leaks at   ☐ Nerve blocks / Topical
   cm H2O   Nebulizer - See Remarks
☐ Oral airway   ☐ Nasal airway   ☐ Bite block Two
Mask vent: ☑ Easy ☐ Head-tilt ☐ Max jaw-thrust ☐ handed/person
Circuit: ☑ Circle system   ☐ NRB ☐ Bain
☐ Mask case   ☐ Via tracheotomy / stoma
☐ Nasal cannula ☐ Simple O₂ mask ☐

TOURNIQUET	mmHg.	UP:	DOWN:

ANESTHETIC AGENTS		TIME:	800	820	900	930	1000										TOTALS
☑ Des ☐ Iso ☐ Sev ☐ Hal (ET%)			6	5	4.6	5.1	5-7										
☑ N₂O ☐ Air (L/min)				1	1	1	1	X									
Oxygen (L/min)			8	1	1	1	8	98									
Versed (mg)			2			1											
Fent (cc)			2		1	1/4											
( )																	
Lidocaine (mg)			65														
Propofol (mg)			160														
Zemuron (mg)			60														
( )																	
Zofran (mg)					4												
neostigmine/robinul (mg)					3/0.4 mg												

FLUIDS														
LR 1		LR1												
LR 2				LR2										

OUTPUT														
Urine (ml)		130/X		60/100	70/200									
EBL (ml)														
Gastric (ml)														

MONITORS														
ECG		ST	SR	SR	SR	SR	SR							
% Oxygen Inspired (FiO₂)		1.0	.50	.50	.50	.50	1.0							
O₂ Saturation (SaO₂)		98	98	97	98	98	98	99						
End Tidal CO₂		(+)	44	40	36	38	38	(+)						
Temp: ☑ C ☐ F			362	36	36	36.6	36.7							

PER-OP MEDS   TIME
reglan 10 mg IV 810
versed as above

Pre-procedure Vital Signs
Pulse 65   Resp 30
BP 127/90
Temp 102°   SaO₂ 97

VENT								
Tidal Volume (ml)		620	640	610				
Respiratory Rate (bpm)		30	10 (vent)	10	10-12			
Peak Pressure (cm H₂0)		20						
☐ PEEP ☐ CPAP (cm H₂0)	None	None						

SYMBOLS
V = ∧
∧ = BP CUFF PRESSURE
↕ = ARTERIAL LINE
X = MEAN ARTERIAL PRESSURE
● = PULSE
VENTILATION
O / SV SPONTANEOUS
Ø / AV ASSISTED
☒ / CV CONTROLLED
↑ = START ANESTH
↓ = START OPER.
◇ = END OPER.
□ = RESP
T = TOURNIQUET

Anesthesiologist: Morris
CRNA: Vaughn

Patient Identification (Addressograph Card)

Remarks: To OR 0800 - Routine monitors pre-O₂ → Smooth IV induction easy BMV and DLXT as above. uneventful GETA
① To RR c O₂ (98) VS stable in RR 136/78 92 R 22 T 36.8
① report care to RN @ 951

Figure 15.1 Anesthesia record.

ANESTHESIA TIME

Anesthesia time starts when the anesthesiologist begins to prepare the patient for the induction of anesthesia. The anesthesia staff must be continuously present in order for the time to be calculated. Anesthesia time ends when the anesthesiologist is no longer in personal attendance and the patient may be placed safely under postoperative supervision.

Generally, anesthesia time units are calculated in 15-minute intervals. That is, one time unit equals 15 minutes or a fraction thereof. However, this is determined by the payer's policy; a time unit can range from 10- to 30-minute intervals depending on the payer.

EXAMPLE

For one payer, 1 to 2 minutes would count as 0.1 unit, 3 minutes would be 0.2 unit, and so on.

Each preoperative encounter with the patient is added to the procedure time to compile total anesthesia time.

EXAMPLE

Surgery was 20 minutes in length. Preoperatively the anesthesia staff member spent 10 minutes starting the IV and interviewing the patient. Total anesthesia time was 30 minutes. Each 15-minute increment was equal to one time unit. Time in this case would be recorded as two time units.

> ● Time units are not recognized for code 01996.

> ● The formula for calculating anesthesia charges is (base units + time units + modifying factor units) × conversion factor = total anesthesia administration charge.

> ● Actual time units are paid. Do not round up to the next 15-minute increment. Instead, round to the 10th place. For example, anesthesia time is 85 minutes ÷ 15 minutes = 5.67. On the health-care claim, 5.7 time units are reported.

ASSIGNING ANESTHESIA CODES

The coder should follow these steps, which are also shown in Pinpoint the Code 15.1, for each anesthesia case:

1. Determine the payer (Medicare or other) to ascertain which codes and modifiers to assign. Remember that not all payers recognize qualifying circumstances and physical status modifiers.
2. Refer to the main term (anesthesia or analgesia) in the index for most patients, particularly for Medicare patients.
3. Look for the anatomical site of the procedure performed.
4. Locate the code(s) within the Anesthesia section of CPT.
5. Read and apply any notes or cross-references that may appear in the section.
6. For Medicare, determine who provided the anesthesia (CRNA or medical doctor). Was an MD in attendance or supervising the CRNA? The answer will determine which HCPCS Level II modifiers to apply for Medicare patients.
7. Assign the applicable physical status modifier (non-Medicare).
8. Determine the type of anesthesia that was administered (MAC or general).
9. Assign codes for any qualifying circumstances, if applicable (non-Medicare).
10. Assign any other applicable modifier(s).

EXAMPLE

An anesthesiologist provides general anesthesia services to a normal, healthy 56-year-old patient for transurethral resection of the prostate.

1. Patient is non-Medicare.

2. Under the main term anesthesia, locate the anatomical site.

3. Site is prostate.

4. There are three codes to choose from. Each must be referenced before selecting the most appropriate one: 00865 is not the correct choice, because it describes a radical prostatectomy; 00908 describes a perineal approach; 00914 accurately describes the procedure performed.

5. The anesthesiologist administered the anesthesia.

6. Patient is normal and healthy, so a –P1 modifier is appropriate.

7. There were no extenuating or qualifying circumstances. Report 00914–AA–P1.

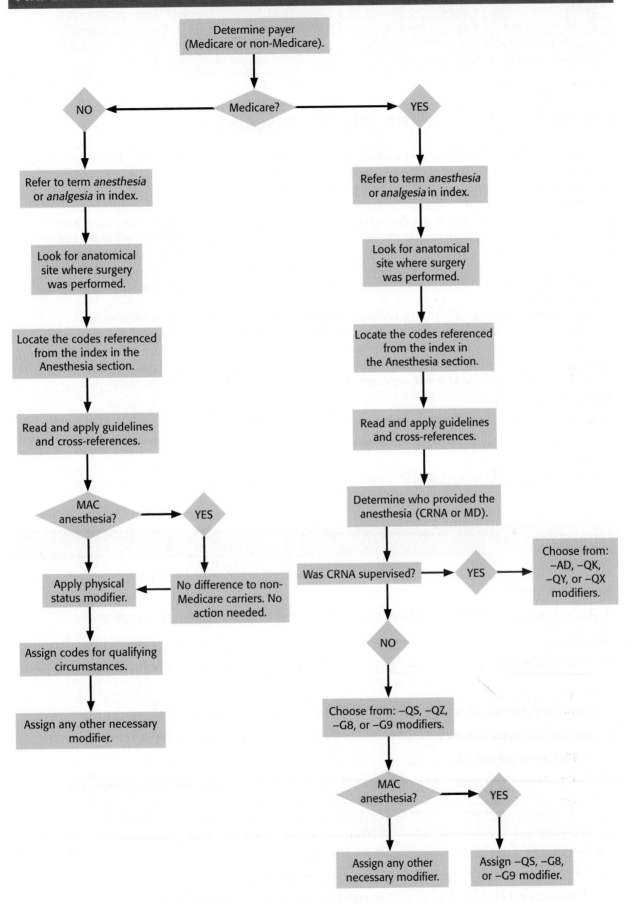

ANESTHESIA CODING AND BILLING RESOURCES

The most widely accepted sources for coding anesthesia services are (1) ASA's *Relative Value Guide,* (2) ASA's *CROSSWALK,* (3) the CPT codebook along with *CPT Assistant,* (4) the CMS's *Claims Processing Manual,* and (5) the CMS's *Conditions of Participation: Anesthesia Services.* The ASA publishes a monthly newsletter with helpful information for calculating anesthesia fees, practice management, and the like. Medicare has a dedicated webpage for anesthesia providers with billing and payment guidance along with educational resources specific to Medicare. Products and magazine articles are also available from commercial sources such as Decision Health's *Anesthesia & Pain Coder's Pink Sheet* and *Anesthesia & Pain Answer Book,* the American Academy of Professional Coders' (AAPC's) *Coding Edge,* and the American Health Information Management Association's (AHIMA's) *Journal of AHIMA.*

AAPC administers an anesthesia coding specialty examination for coders who work exclusively for anesthesia providers or anesthesia billing companies. Successful candidates will sit for the certification exam and be awarded the Certified Anesthesia and Pain Management Coder (CANPC™) credential. For more information about requirements for sitting for this exam, visit AAPC's website at www.aapc.com/certification/specialty/anesthesia-medical-coding-certification.aspx.

INTERNET RESOURCES: American Society of Anesthesiologists
www.asahq.org/

Medicare Anesthesia
www.cms.hhs.gov/center/anesth.asp

CHECKPOINT 15.4

Assign the anesthesia code and any applicable modifiers and qualifying circumstances for the following scenarios.

1. Radical prostatectomy for a Medicare patient. The anesthesiologist performs the anesthesia.

   _____

2. Correction of tetralogy of Fallot congenital heart defect with pump oxygenator in a 1-year-old girl.

   _____

3. Emergency appendectomy in a 28-year-old female who is otherwise healthy. _____

4. Hammertoe repair in a 66-year-old female with diabetes under MAC. The CRNA administered the anesthesia unsupervised. _____

5. A liver biopsy of a 42-year-old patient with cirrhosis of the liver under MAC in an ambulatory surgery center. _____

Chapter Summary

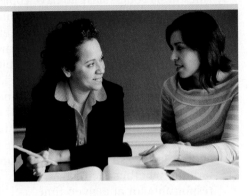

1. The complete anesthesia service includes the preoperative visit, anesthesia administration with intraoperative notes, and postanesthesia care. The preoperative care with the patient is provided to review the patient's medical and surgical history, including any previous anesthetic complications and respiratory issues. The intraoperative notes will reflect the monitoring of the patient during the procedure and his or her emergence from the anesthesia. Postoperative care consists of monitoring the patient for side effects from anesthesia and ensuring the patient is stable enough to breathe independently.

2. General anesthesia renders the patient unconscious and pain free, whereas regional anesthesia will numb only a part of the body without inducing unconsciousness. Nerve blocks are injected parallel to or surrounding a nerve or nerve plexus using various anesthetic solutions. Local anesthesia affects smaller areas of the body than does regional anesthesia and is usually administered by injection while keeping the patient awake. Conscious sedation is moderate anesthesia administered intravenously, and it relieves pains without the loss of consciousness. MAC allows the patient to respond to directions and questions and does not completely anesthetize the patient.

3. Anesthesia coding is a challenge because not all payers have the same requirements for reporting. Check with each payer or read the payer contract to determine how to report anesthesia codes. Most payers require the anesthesia code to be assigned with either a HCPCS modifier or a physical status modifier. Physical status modifiers are appended to anesthesia claims only and coincide with the anesthesia provider's ASA class. Some payers accept modifiers –P3 through –P5 and will reimburse these in addition to the procedure.

4. There can be many areas for error and missed billing in anesthesia coding. Many coders find the anesthesia modifiers an area of difficulty and this can affect reimbursement for the physician. Another area is in understanding what services are or are not included in the basic anesthesia service. Be sure to verify that time is accurately represented in both the anesthesia record and the billing system. Coders must understand that one anesthesia code can represent several surgical codes.

5. Anesthesia services are packaged into one payment. Complete anesthesia service includes the following:

   - General, regional, and supplementation of local anesthesia
   - Interpretation of lab values
   - Placement of IVs for fluid and medication administration
   - Arterial line insertion for blood pressure monitoring or other supportive services to afford the anesthesia care deemed optimal by the anesthesiologist during a procedure
   - The usual preoperative and postoperative visits
   - The administration of fluids and/or blood
   - Usual monitoring services (temperature, blood pressure, oximetry, ECG, capnography, and mass spectrometry)
   - Intubation
   - Laryngoscopy
   - Introduction or insertion of needle or catheter into vein
   - Venipuncture

6. Coders will use the anesthesia modifiers as needed based on the patient's physical status and under what circumstances the anesthesia is being provided. For physical status modifiers, almost any physical circumstances is captured by P1–P6, which range from "normal/healthy" to "brain dead." The qualifying circumstances modifiers indicate difficulty factors such as age, use of hypotension and hypothermia, and emergency conditions. The HCPCS modifiers generally relate to who provided the anesthesia service (anesthesiologist vs. CRNA) and whether or not the anesthesiologist was supervising or directing procedures involving qualified individuals.

7. Anesthesia coders have to have copies of insurance carrier contracts to determine how each carrier calculates anesthesia time, modifying factors, and base units. The formula for calculating anesthesia charges is (base units + time units + modifying factor units) × conversion factor = total anesthesia administration charge. Coders need a way to validate time and to determine discontinuous time if applicable.

8. If completed properly, the anesthesia record will contain all information necessary to assign anesthesia codes. It should include any preoperative interaction and services and postoperative services received in the recovery area. A copy of the operative report helps anesthesia coders ensure that they have captured all procedures and secondary diagnoses. It is important to determine the payer and the level of CRNA supervision in order to appropriately assign correct codes and modifiers. Coders must read documentation to determine whether the CRNA worked alone and how many rooms the anesthesiologist was responsible for at a given time.

Review Questions

Matching

Match the key terms with their definitions.

A. conscious sedation
B. postoperative anesthesia service
C. qualifying circumstances
D. monitored anesthesia care
E. physical status modifiers

F. general anesthesia
G. spinal anesthesia
H. preoperative anesthesia service
I. regional anesthesia
J. analgesic

1. _____ An anesthetic injection into the subarachnoid space

2. _____ The patient is rendered unconscious and is under constant attendance and monitoring

3. _____ Type of anesthesia that relieves pain without causing loss of consciousness

4. _____ Moderate anesthesia carried out by injecting a sedative and/or analgesic intravenously to relieve pain and anxiety during a medical procedure

5. _____ Add-on codes used to indicate operative conditions and/or unusual risk factors

6. _____ Part of the body is numbed without inducing unconsciousness

7. _____ Monitoring a patient for immediate postoperative complications

8. _____ The patient is not completely anesthetized and can respond to questions and directions

9. _____ Codes used with anesthesia codes to indicate patient's health condition

10. _____ Obtaining the patient's medical and surgical history and medications

True or False

Decide whether each statement is true or false.

1. __T__ Physical status modifiers are assigned with anesthesia codes.

2. __T__ An anesthesiologist's history and physical exam is separately reportable with an E/M code in addition to the anesthesia code for the same day of service.

3. __F__ Qualifying circumstances codes may be assigned for anesthesia services.

4. __F__ Use modifier –47 when the surgeon provides both the anesthesia and the surgical procedure.

5. __T__ Use qualifying circumstance modifier 99100 with code 00834 for patients younger than 1 year of age.

6. __F__ Once anesthesia has been provided, the anesthesiologist has no other responsibilities to the patient.

7. __T__ Use HCPCS modifier –QY for the anesthesiologist medically directing a CRNA.

8. ___T___ Modifier –P3 is appended to the surgery code whenever a patient has severe systemic disease.

9. ___F___ Anesthesia time begins when the patient is fully anesthetized.

10. ___F___ To find the anesthesia code in the CPT index, go to the anatomical site of the surgery.

Multiple Choice

Select the letter that best completes the statement or answers the question.

1. Which modifier is never used with anesthesia codes?
   A. –22
   B. –32
   C. –47
   D. –59

2. Surgeons who administer their own anesthesia use which modifier with the surgical code they submit?
   A. –23
   B. –47
   C. –32
   D. –22

3. Physical status modifiers are assigned for anesthesia services based on
   A. The payer
   B. The patient's age
   C. The patient's health
   D. Open versus closed procedure

4. Anesthesia was provided to a normal, healthy 75-year-old patient for a needle biopsy of the thyroid. What is the applicable code(s)?
   A. 00326–P2
   B. 00326–P1, 99100
   C. 00322–P1, 99100
   D. 00322–P2

5. A patient who has diabetes, controlled by diet and exercise, undergoes a transurethral resection of the prostate. What is the applicable code(s)?
   A. 00910–P2
   B. 00914–P2
   C. 00914–P3
   D. 00920–P3

6. An 82-year-old patient slipped on ice while crossing the street, sustaining a femoral neck fracture. Open treatment of the fracture with prosthetic replacement was performed. What is the applicable code?
   A. 01220
   B. 01230
   C. 01480
   D. 01462

7. A CRNA provides anesthesia on a patient during a radical mastectomy under the medical direction of an anesthesiologist. Code for the CRNA and the anesthesiologist:
   A. CRNA 00406–QY,   Anesth. 00404–QY
   B. CRNA 00406–QX,   Anesth. 00406–QX
   C. CRNA 00404–QX,   Anesth. 00406–QY
   D. CRNA 00404–QX,   Anesth. 00404–QY

8. An anesthesiologist provides anesthesia for an open lung biopsy on a patient with congestive heart failure. What is the applicable code(s)?
   A. 00540–P3
   B. 00540–P4
   C. 00560–P2
   D. 00560–P3

9. Anesthesia is provided for repair of a ruptured Achilles tendon without graft. What is the applicable code?
    A. 01462
    B. 01470
    C. 01472
    D. 01480

10. How do you report anesthesia services for multiple surgical procedures during the same session?
    A. Report the most complex procedure first, followed by the second procedure.
    B. Report the most complex procedure first, and report only half the time for the second procedure.
    C. Report the most complex procedure code, and also report the time for all the procedures combined.
    D. Report only the most complex procedure code.

CHAPTER 16

CPT: Surgery Codes

CHAPTER OUTLINE

IPGGutenbergUKLtd/iStock/Thinkstock

LEARNING OUTCOMES

After studying this chapter, you should be able to:

1. Describe the organization of the surgical section in CPT.
2. List components of a surgical package.
3. Define and cite examples of "separate procedure."
4. Distinguish between the CPT and Medicare definitions of a surgical package.
5. Discuss therapeutic versus diagnostic procedures and when to assign codes.
6. Identify whether a procedure is incidental or separately reported.

7. Utilize the following references to correctly report surgical services and modifiers: the National Correct Coding Initiative, the Medicare Physician Fee Schedule, the *Medicare Claims Processing Manual*, National Coverage Determination, Local Coverage Determination, third-party carrier medical policies, and specialty societies.

8. Differentiate between modifiers for physician use and hospital outpatient use.

9. Correctly assign modifiers for services performed during the global period.

10. Correctly assign CPT codes to basic procedural statements.

The Surgery section of CPT provides codes for surgical procedures performed in operating rooms (ORs), ambulatory surgery centers (ASCs) and hospital units, physician offices, and at the bedside. As a result, the Surgery section contains the greatest number of codes. To become successful in surgical coding, coders must be familiar with the format and organization of the surgical specialty subsections, have a fundamental understanding of anatomy and medical terminology, master the concepts of the surgical package, correctly apply modifiers, and adhere to payers' rules on billing surgery codes. These skills, along with communication with the provider and adequate documentation, are the formula to accurate surgical coding.

This chapter lays the groundwork for the surgical chapters that follow by discussing surgical concepts, terminology, and guidelines that are applied to all surgical coding, regardless of specialty. The chapter includes a basic introduction to each surgical subsection of CPT. For in-depth learning, this text dedicates a chapter to each surgical specialty focusing on common procedures performed and explaining the use of essential tools and resources to accomplish correct coding and reporting.

SURGICAL PROCEDURES: THERAPEUTIC AND DIAGNOSTIC

All significant procedures are assigned a CPT code for reporting and reimbursement. Significant procedures are incisions, excisions, biopsies, repairs, manipulation, amputation, endoscopies, destructions, suturing, and introductions. There are two categories of surgical procedures, diagnostic and therapeutic. It is very important to differentiate between the two. Surgery coding rules state that when a diagnostic and a therapeutic procedure are done at the same operative session on the same anatomical site, only the therapeutic procedure code is assigned.

EXAMPLE

Biopsy of a suspicious lesion followed by immediate excision of the entire lesion. The biopsy represents part of the overall excision or removal of the lesion and is not reported separately.

Diagnostic Procedures

Diagnostic procedures, like diagnostic tests, are performed to confirm a physician's "working diagnosis" or to assist in determining the physician's best course of treatment. Diagnostic procedures are means of assessing a patient's current state. The patient is experiencing signs or exhibiting symptoms, and these procedures are a way of evaluating and ruling out potential diagnoses. They involve examining a particular part of the body to identify the cause of the patient's pain, exploring the extent of an injury or disease, staging an illness such as cancer, and evaluating surrounding areas of question. Diagnostic procedures are typically invasive, whereby instruments are introduced into the body either through a natural orifice or by incising the skin, and are performed in the OR or in special treatment areas of the hospital such as the radiology department or the emergency department.

EXAMPLE

Examples of invasive diagnostic procedures are bronchoscopy, arthroscopy, endoscopy, laparoscopy, wound exploration, biopsy, and angiography.

Therapeutic Procedures

Therapeutic procedures involve treating or correcting a confirmed disease, condition, or injury (Box 16.1). They involve repairing or reconstructing defects or injuries, excising lesions or tumors, removing body parts or organs, transplanting organs, and so on. Diagnostic procedures may be converted to therapeutic procedures when circumstances warrant. In such a case, the

BOX 16.1 Surgical Terms Reflecting Therapeutic Procedures

Anastomosis	Manipulation
Arthrodesis	Reconstruction
Debridement	Reduction
Destruction	Release
Dilation	Removal
Excision	Repair
Extraction	Resection
Incision and drainage	Revision
Introduction	Suture
Lysis	Transplant

surgeon first performs a diagnostic procedure, then, upon confirming a condition, moves to a therapeutic procedure to treat it. As mentioned earlier, in the event that a surgeon performs a diagnostic procedure or evaluation of the surgical field and then proceeds with a therapeutic procedure at the same operative session, only the therapeutic procedure is reported. Examples of therapeutic procedures include hernia repair, appendectomy, polyp removal, hysterectomy, lesion removals, and vessel repairs.

Therapeutic procedures always include a diagnostic procedure on the same anatomical part when performed during the same session with limited exceptions. If the diagnostic procedure is performed prior to the surgical procedure and is the primary basis on which the decision to perform the surgical procedure is made, the two procedures may be reported with modifier –59 appended to the diagnostic service. However, if the diagnostic procedure is an inherent component of the surgical procedure, it cannot be reported separately.

Distinguishing Simple, Intermediate, and Complicated Procedures

Appending modifier –22 does not guarantee additional payment for surgical procedures. CPT states that the surgeon must perform and document the reason for the additional work and the amount performed, which must be substantially greater than typically required. The use of –22 is not justified based on time alone.

Code descriptors throughout CPT contain the words *simple, intermediate,* or *complicated.* CPT does not give clear directions on how to determine if a surgical procedure is simple, intermediate, complicated, or extensive. Many code descriptions require an interpretation of the level of the procedure. Of course, documentation is crucial in determining these factors. If a procedure is poorly described and details that support the procedure's complexity and the physician's level of skill are left out, the coder may have to assign a "simple" code that will not reimburse as much as an "intermediate" or " complicated" procedure. In this case, both the physician and the facility will not receive the maximum appropriate payment.

Well-run practices and facilities have clinical documentation improvement (CDI) programs in place to ensure that the medical records coders work with are an accurate depiction of what was done and, above all, are descriptive and complete.

At times, a coder may need to query the surgeon for clarifying or missing information before assigning a procedure code. Look for the presence of the following factors in the medical documentation when considering whether or not to query the surgeon for additional information. The presence of the details in the documentation will enable the coder to assign the most appropriate code when choosing among simple, intermediate, or complex codes. The following list can be used to guide physician documentation to ensure sufficient detail is provided for assigning the most specific code:

- *Length of the procedure.* If the procedure is documented as taking longer than usual, this may be an indication of a more extensive or complicated procedure.
- *Nature of wound closure.* The documentation must be specific about how the wound is closed.
- *Number of separate incisions.* More than the usual number or extent of incisions may be indicators of a more complex procedure.

- *Size of cyst or polyp.* If a cyst or polyp was abnormally large, this points toward a more extensive procedure. *The physician should always be queried if size is absent.*
- *Excessive bleeding.* If the patient suffered excessive bleeding, why this occurred and the amount of blood loss should be indicated, because it makes a difference when choosing simple versus complicated codes.
- *Presence of nerves, blood vessels, or tendons.* Each of these factors can complicate a procedure and should be documented.
- *Infection.* The presence of infection signifies a complicated procedure.
- *Treatment delay.* If treatment was not sought by the patient in a timely manner, the risk of complications increases and therefore constitutes a complex or complicated procedure.

ORGANIZATION

Surgery is the third designated section of the CPT book. The surgical section of CPT is the largest section of the book and is broken down into 17 subsections (Table 16.1). It provides codes for procedures performed by surgeons in any specialty—in essence, each organ system—and any place of service (POS). You can identify a surgical code by knowing what digit the code begins with. All "surgical" CPT codes begin with one of the following digits: 1, 2, 3, 4, 5, or 6. For example, the Integumentary System section is the first surgery subsection encountered. All the codes in this section begin with the numeral 1. The other subsections follow in the order shown in Table 16.1, with the corresponding number of the code range being the first digit of each code.

Most of these subsections are further subdivided into anatomical sites or organs within each respective body system. Each anatomical site is then further categorized by surgical method. See the outline in Box 16.2 for a visual explanation of this organization. The subsections within the Surgery section all mimic the same basic outline for consistency and ease of locating codes.

EXAMPLE
Subsection–Digestive

Anatomical site–Lip

Surgical Method–Excision

SURGERY CODING

The Surgery section guidelines must be read carefully. They provide directives on how to report codes for services within the section, define terms used within the section, and provide important information needed to correctly assign surgery codes. Instructional notes and definitions are also located throughout each subsection. Box 16.3 provides an example. They may be located at the beginning of each subsection, before or after a subheading, or in parentheses (parenthetical notes) below a specific code. Parenthetical notes offer quick reference to reporting a specific code, range of codes, or modifier usage. The importance of the

Table 16.1 Surgery Subsections

SUBSECTION	CODE RANGE
Integumentary System	10021–19499
Musculoskeletal System	20005–29999
Respiratory System	30000–32999
Cardiovascular System	33010–37799
Hemic and Lymphatic Systems	38100–38999
Mediastinum and Diaphragm	39000–39599
Digestive System	40490–49999
Urinary System	50010–53899
Male Genital System	54000–55899
Reproductive System Procedures	55920
Intersex Surgery	55970–55980
Female Genital System	56405–58999
Maternity Care and Delivery	59000–59899
Endocrine System	60000–60699
Nervous System	61000–64999
Eye and Ocular Adnexa	65091–68899
Auditory System	69000–69979
Operating Microscope	69990

BOX 16.2 Surgical Subsection Headings

Incision and Drainage
Biopsy
Excision
Introduction or Removal
Repair
Destruction
Endoscopy/Laparoscopy (if applicable)
Other Procedures

BOX 16.3 Example of a Subsection Note

SURGERY
INTEGUMENTARY SYSTEM
 DESTRUCTION
"Destruction means the ablation of benign, premalignant or malignant tissues by any method, with or without curettement, including local anesthesia, and not usually requiring closure."

CPT © 2017 American Medical Association, All Rights Reserved.

surgery subsection guidelines to correct coding cannot be stressed enough. Keep a close eye on the ▶◀ symbols for revised or new text within the notes because they may change from year to year.

NOTE: Make a habit of checking for notes at the beginning of the subsection or at the beginning of the surgical method in addition to above or below the code before assigning it.

Code Descriptors

In the Surgery section, code descriptors are very important. Coders sometimes highlight the semicolon and key words in the code descriptions such as *unilateral* or *bilateral* or words such as *each, lesions(s),* or *polyp(s)* to hone in on the specificity of the code. These key words indicate how many times a code should be listed and if modifiers are applicable. When the singular and the plural versions of words are present, it means that the code should only be listed once regardless of number. For example:

EXAMPLE
20550 *Injection(s); single tendon sheath, or ligament, aponeurosis (e.g., plantar "fascia").* This code would be listed only once even if several injections were performed in the same tendon sheath, ligament, or aponeurosis.

Other cautionary points:

- Be very careful when assigning the add-on code for a surgical microscope 69990. Some code descriptions include the use of a microscope; therefore, assigning this code in addition to the procedure code would be inappropriate. (This is further discussed in Chapter 27 of this text.)
- The term "complicated" appears in some code descriptions. If infection is present, if treatment is delayed, or if the surgery took longer than usual, then this code would be appropriate.
- Some codes do not permit the use of the −50 modifier, such as with 40843. The code description includes verbiage equivalent to this modifier, while other codes, such as 63030 or 69436, provide instructional notes to guide the coder to append the −50 modifier.

Add-On Codes

Add-on codes are seen throughout the Surgery section and other sections of CPT, and they are notoriously miscoded. Add-on codes are identified in the following ways:

1. In the CPT manual, an add-on code is designated by the "+" symbol. The code descriptor of an add-on code generally includes phrases such as "each additional" or "list separately in addition to primary procedure."
2. An add-on code can appear on the Medicare Physician Fee Schedule (MPFS) with a "ZZZ" in the Global Day Surgery column.
3. The code can be listed in Change Request (CR) 7501 Transmittal 2636 or subsequent ones as a Type I, Type II, or Type III add-on code.

The basic concept of add-on codes is that they are never coded independently—they are coded in addition to a primary procedure. They are always reported with the base code in their respective section. They are meant to be reported as a second or third procedure in addition to the primary procedure performed. Section guidelines and parenthetical instructions are helpful in guiding the coder to assign an add-on code. Appendix D of the CPT manual contains a master list of CPT-delineated add-on codes. However, this may not coincide with codes that are designated "ZZZ" on the MPFS or in Medicare transmittals.

For Medicare purposes, generally the add-on codes do have the "ZZZ" designation as the global surgery indicator but not always. Some codes depicted as add-on codes are not listed as "ZZZ" on the MPFS. Many of these codes are found in the Pathology and Laboratory and the Medicine sections of the CPT manual. For some codes, only the code descriptor indicates the add-on code classification.

EXAMPLE
Using Table 16.2 you can see that CPT add-on code 20936 is left off the MPFS status ZZZ list, but in the CPT manual the code is listed with the "+" preceding the code.

Most add-on codes have instructional notes indicating which code may be reported as a primary code; however, some do not.

EXAMPLE

For example, look at +49905 in the CPT manual. There is a parenthetical note that tells the coder not to report it with 44700. So, what do you report it with? If the procedure was done in conjunction with another intra-abdominal procedure, it may be reported in addition. However, third-party payers and local Medicare contractors may have policies specific to reporting this procedure, so it is best to check with the carrier for such conditions before reporting this code.

Table 16.2 Excerpt of MPFS Add-On Codes

CPT	DESCRIPTION	GLOB DAYS
19297	Place breast cath for rad	ZZZ
20931	Sp bone agrft struct add-on	ZZZ
20937	Sp bone agrft morsel add-on	ZZZ
20938	Sp bone agrft struct add-on	ZZZ
20985	Cptr-asst dir ms px	ZZZ
22103	Remove extra spine segment	ZZZ
49568	Hernia repair w/mesh	ZZZ
49905	Omental flap intra-abdom	ZZZ

REIMBURSEMENT REVIEW

CMS Add-On Codes

Coders need to be able to recognize add-on codes and know how to identify an appropriate primary code and when to append modifiers. The CPT manual is one source for identifying add-on codes. CMS CR 7501 Transmittal 2636 and the National Correct Coding Initiative (NCCI) are other sources.

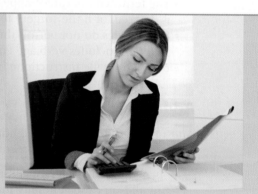

The CR 7501 Transmittal 2636 clarified that all add-on codes for Medicare are included whether they are "ZZZ" classified or not. Each update to the CR will include any new add-on codes or changes from the CPT manual, MPFS, or a designation by type of add-on code. For Types II and III, the Medicare contractors will create their own list of primary codes for each of those add-on codes.

CMS divides add-on codes into three categories, each for a designated reimbursement purpose. CR 7501 Transmittal 2636 publishes these codes for use by payers and contractors to properly reimburse claims containing add-on codes. This is a specific Medicare policy but may also be relevant to commercial claims, because many third-party payers mimic CMS policy or use the policy as a foundation in developing their own plan policies. All transmittals are posted on the CMS website at www.cms.gov/Regulations-and-Guidance/Guidance/Transmittals. Transmittal 2636 can be read in its entirety there by searching for the transmittal number.

Use of add-on codes as part of NCCI is discussed in the *Medicare Claims Processing Manual* (MCPM), Publication 100-04, Chapter 12 (Physicians/Non-Physician Practitioners), Section 30 (Correct Coding Policy), Section D.

As a general rule, add-on codes are eligible for payment as long as their listed primary procedure code is also eligible for payment (or reimbursable). Claims processing contractors are required to implement edits to ensure that Types I–III add-on codes are never paid unless a listed primary procedure code is also payable. Contractors are encouraged to develop primary codes for Type II and III add-ons listed in the transmittal. CMS annually updates the list of add-on codes with

Physician's Services

Physician's services are the first subsection of the Surgery Guidelines section. These services are applicable to physicians and their respective professional services performed in nonsurgical service areas, which should be reported using evaluation and management (E/M) codes. Codes from the Medicine section for noninvasive procedures, services, and reports are also often used in addition to surgical codes for surgeon reporting.

Separate Procedure

Seeing the words "separate procedure" in parentheses after a code description is a clue to ask the following question: Is this procedure an integral part of another procedure and more of an incidental procedure rather than the comprehensive procedure being performed?

EXAMPLE
31600 *Tracheostomy, planned (separate procedure).*

If a CPT code descriptor includes the term "separate procedure," the procedure is not to be reported separately with an associated procedure in an anatomically related region whether it be through the same skin incision, orifice, or surgical approach. It may be reported separately if it is performed

their primary procedure codes before January 1 based on changes to the CPT manual. Quarterly updates are issued, as necessary, via a change request.

The following are examples of each type of add-on code as defined by CMS:

- **Type I add-on codes** have a limited number of identifiable primary procedure codes. The CR lists the Type I add-on codes with their acceptable primary procedure codes.
- **Type II add-on codes** do not have a specific list of primary procedure codes. The CR lists the Type II add-on codes without any primary procedure codes. Claims processing contractors are encouraged to develop their own lists of primary procedure codes for this type of add-on code.
- **Type III add-on codes** have some, but not all, specific primary procedure codes identified in the CPT manual. The CR lists the Type III add-on codes with the primary procedure codes that are specifically identifiable. Contractors are encouraged to develop their own lists of additional primary procedure codes for this group of add-on codes.

ADD-ON	PRIMARY
Type I	
63048	63045–63047
96376 may be reported by facilities only	96365, 96374, 96409, 96413
Type II	
37186	As a Type II add-on code, CMS does not specify primary codes. The ACR/SIR (American College of Radiology/Society of Interventional Radiology) recommended the following primary codes, which may not be a listing of all possible primary codes: 37211–37214, 37215, 37216, 37220, 37221, 37222, 37223, 37224, 37225, 37226, 37227, 37228, 37229, 37230, 37231, 61630, 61635.
49905	List separately in addition to the code for the primary procedure.
Type III	
64727	37231, 61630, 61635

in an anatomically unrelated area through a separate skin incision, orifice, or surgical approach or at a different patient encounter on the same date of service. Modifier –59 or an anatomical modifier if appropriate may be appended to the "separate procedure" code to indicate that it qualifies as a separately reportable service.

An incidental procedure is performed at the same operative session as a more complex primary procedure. It is clinically related to the procedure being performed and would not usually be reported alone. It is a procedure that is commonly performed as part of the standards of medical treatment or is part of the package, including the services or supplies that are included in surgical procedures:

- Cleansing, shaving, and prepping the skin
- Draping and positioning of the patient
- Insertion of IV
- Sedative administration by the MD
- Surgical approach (evaluation of surgical field, simple debridement, simple lysis of adhesions, incising the skin or body part, isolation of nerves and tendons or bone limiting access to surgical field)
- Surgical cultures
- Wound irrigation
- Surgical closure of incision
- Application of dressings and removal of post-op dressings
- Surgical supplies, unless determined otherwise by payer policy (In this case, HCPCS codes are assigned for these.)
- Anesthesia administration

When a procedure is considered incidental to the primary procedure, *it is not separately reported*. Most of the procedures indicated as *separate procedures* are considered incidental. A separate procedure can sometimes be reported separately with a –59 modifier but is usually considered inclusive in a more comprehensive procedure.

EXAMPLES

31231 *Nasal endoscopy, diagnostic; unilateral or bilateral (separate procedure).*
31233 *Nasal/sinus endoscopy, diagnostic with maxillary sinusoscopy.*

Assignment of code 31231 would be accurate if the only procedure performed is looking in the nose with a scope. However, if this is done in addition to looking at the maxillary sinus as in 31233, it would be inappropriate to report 31231 in addition, because procedure code 31233 already includes what is being described in 31231.

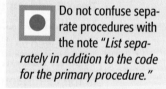 Do not confuse separate procedures with the note "*List separately in addition to the code for the primary procedure.*"

Unlisted Procedures

As noted in Chapter 12, unlisted procedure codes are used when a service that has no assignable CPT code is provided; that is, no specific code matches the documentation. Each subsection has unlisted procedure codes; the Surgery Guidelines section preceding the Surgery section of CPT lists them all in alphabetical order by their location within the Surgery section. Unlisted codes provide the means of reporting and tracking services and procedures until a more specific code is established in CPT to describe the procedure in question. Remember to first review HCPCS Level II codes (if the payer accepts them) and CPT Category III codes before assigning the unlisted code for that subsection and anatomical site. When performing two or more procedures that require the use of the same unlisted code, the unlisted code used should only be reported once to identify the services provided. Each time an unlisted procedure code is assigned, a special report or documentation supporting the service needs to be submitted for payment along with the claim. Refer to the guidelines at the beginning of each section to determine components of the special report. *CPT Assistant* also suggests providing the following:

1. The specific service performed (including any assistance necessary to carry out the service)
2. Whether the procedure performed was independent of other services provided, or if it was performed at the same surgical site or through the same surgical opening

3. The number of times the service was provided

4. Any extenuating circumstances that may have complicated the service(s) or procedure

> ⬛ Do not try to make an existing code "fit" what you are trying to describe! Instead, assign an unlisted procedure code for the appropriate subsection and anatomical site.

EXAMPLE

Arthroscopic metacarpophalangeal joint replacement with permanent prosthesis. Arthroscopic codes available for this joint are 29901 and 29902, but neither of these codes is accurate in this case. Code 26531 would be assigned if this procedure were performed "open." Therefore, an unlisted code 29999 is the appropriate code in this situation.

Modifiers are used to indicate that a service or procedure performed was altered by some specific circumstance, but not changed in its definition or code. Unlisted codes do not describe a specific procedure or service or component of a service; therefore, modifiers are not appended to these.

Surgical Package and the Global Period

In many cases the time, effort, and services of a physician when performing a surgical procedure are bundled together in a surgical package. CPT describes the surgical package as including local infiltration of anesthesia, the E/M visits either on the date of surgery or the day prior, immediate post-op care, writing of orders, evaluation of the patient in the recovery area, and any typical uncomplicated follow-up care. CPT also explains that follow-up care for complications, exacerbations, recurrence, and the presence of other diseases that require additional services is not included in the surgical package. The definition of the surgical package is also located in the Surgery Guidelines section of CPT. The exception to the global or surgical package is the E/M visit during which the decision for surgery was made. This type of E/M visit is not part of the surgical package even if provided on the day before or day of surgery. Modifier –57 is used to identify this scenario and is added to the E/M visit.

Coders need to know what is included in each payer's particular definition of a surgical package in order to correctly comply with payers' rules. For example, Medicare has its own definition of a surgical package. The Medicare-approved amount for the surgery or procedure includes payment for the same services related to the surgery as CPT, when provided by the physician who performs the surgery. It also includes the following items:

- *Preoperative visits, beginning with the day before a surgery for major procedures and the day of surgery for minor procedures.* Pre-op care includes the history and physical (H&P) and medical decision making (MDM) that occurs before surgery. It includes hospital admission or an office or outpatient visit that occurs before surgery, but it does not include the consultation or new patient office visit where the determination for surgery was made.
- *Preprocedure work such as obtaining a routine vascular and airway access.* If, however, a more invasive vascular access procedure, such as inserting a central line, is necessary, it is separately reportable.
- *Intraoperative services that are normally a usual and necessary part of a surgical procedure such as cardiopulmonary monitoring.* Exposure and exploration of the surgical field are integral to an operative procedure and are not separately reportable.
- *Complications following surgery that do not require additional trips to the operating room.* Control of postoperative hemorrhage is not separately reportable unless the patient must be returned to the OR for treatment. Modifier –78 in this case would be appended to the code for control of the hemorrhaging.
- *Routine postoperative visits (follow-up visits) during the postoperative period of the surgery that are related to recovery from the surgery.*
- *Postoperative pain management provided by the surgeon.*
- *Supplies, except for a few specific supplies provided in a physician's office.*
- *Miscellaneous services.* These include items such as dressing changes, local incisional care, removal of operative pack, removal of sutures and staples, line wires, tubes, drains, casts and splints, replacement lines, nasogastric and rectal tubes, and changes or removal of tracheostomy tubes.

The surgical package has a defined time frame for routine pre-op and post-op surgical care called the *global period*. The number of days in the global period is referred to as *global surgery days*. The global period is a payer concept under which a set amount is paid for all services furnished by the surgeon before, during, and after a particular procedure. This is important, because physicians can bill for work done *outside*—that is, before and after—the start and end dates of this global period.

Typical global periods are as follows:

- 0 days for simple procedures
- 0/10 (0 days pre-op/10 days post-op) for minor surgery
- 1/90 (1 day pre-op/90 days post-op) for major surgery

For example, with Medicare, a major procedure surgical package includes, in addition to the basic package mentioned earlier, a pre-op service day (1 day before or the day of surgery) and 89 days after, totaling 90 consecutive days. A minor procedure package includes everything in the basic package plus a pre-op service (1 day before or the day of surgery) and up to 10 days following surgery depending on whether the physician saw the patient the day before surgery or not. If so, 9 post-op days will be included in the global package. If the postoperative period is 0 days, post-operative visits are not included in the payment amount for the surgery. Payment is made in this instance if additional treatment is provided the same day or thereafter as long as it is a covered service. Services by other physicians are not included in the global fee for a minor procedure. Global periods can be calculated as follows:

- To determine the global period for major surgeries, count 1 day immediately before the day of surgery, the day of the surgery, and the 88 days immediately following the day of surgery. For example, if the date of surgery is April 5, the last day of the postoperative period would be July 2.
- To determine the global period for minor procedures, count the day of surgery and the appropriate number of days immediately following the date of surgery (either 0 or 10).

■ **CASE SCENARIO**

A patient has axillary hidradenitis and the physician performs code 11462, *Excision of skin and subcutaneous tissue for hidradenitis, axillary; with simple or intermediate repair*, on January 2. The patient comes back to the office for a post-op visit on January 12. Refer to Table 16.3 and find the code 11462. The visit on January 12 is not charged to the patient or the insurance carrier because this procedure carries 90 global days.

Bundling

Surgical packages are referred to as *bundled*, meaning that each package code contains all the related services. It is a coding error—and possibly fraudulent—to unbundle, or take apart and report codes that are included in a bundled code. For example, because a single code is available to describe removal of the uterus, ovaries, and fallopian tubes, physicians should not use separate codes to report the removal of the uterus, ovaries, and fallopian tubes individually.

The Medicare policy that explains what codes are part of the surgical package is called the *National Correct Coding Initiative*. Its purpose and format are explained in the following Reimbursement Review.

INTERNET RESOURCES: Correct Coding Initiative Updates
www.cms.gov/Medicare/Coding/NationalCorrectCodInitEd/index.html

Complete CCI Files: *Medicare Claims Processing Manual* (Publication 100-04), **Chapter 23, Section 20.9**
www.cms.hhs.gov/manuals/104_claims/clm104index.asp

CPT Modifiers

Under certain circumstances, the CPT modifiers listed inside the CPT manual's front cover may be used to explain circumstances that arise during surgery or in the operating room. Refer to Table 16.4 for a list of applicable surgery modifiers. The modifiers listed can be appended to all surgical codes. The CPT modifiers are also known as *HCPCS Level I modifiers*.

Table 16.3 Excerpt From MPFS Showing the Global Days (GLOB DAYS) Column

CPT/ HCPCS	DESCRIPTION	WORK RVU	NON-FACILITY PE RVU	FACILITY PE RVU	MP RVU	NON-FACILITY TOTAL	FACILITY TOTAL	GLOB DAYS
11444	Exc face-mm benign lesion + marg 3.1–4 cm	3.14	3.48	2.19	0.3	6.92	5.63	10
11446	Exc face-mm benign lesion + marg > 4 cm	4.48	4.05	2.78	0.43	8.96	7.69	10
11450	Exc skin and subcutaneous tissue for hidradenitis	2.73	5.04	2.03	0.34	8.11	5.1	90
11451	Exc skin and subcutaneous tissue for hidradenitis	3.94	6.62	2.55	0.53	11.09	7.02	90
11462	Exc skin and subcutaneous tissue for hidradenitis	2.51	5.12	2.02	0.32	7.95	4.85	90
11463	Exc skin and subcutaneous tissue for hidradenitis	3.94	6.84	2.69	0.54	11.32	7.17	90
11470	Exc skin and subcutaneous tissue for hidradenitis	3.25	5.07	2.27	0.4	8.72	5.92	90
11471	Exc skin and subcutaneous tissue for hidradenitis	4.4	6.72	2.77	0.58	11.7	7.75	90
11600	Exc tr-ext mlg + marg < 0.5 cm	1.31	2.64	0.97	0.1	4.05	2.38	10
11601	Exc tr-ext mlg + marg 0.6–1 cm	1.8	2.71	1.22	0.12	4.63	3.14	10

Note: PE = physician expense; RVU = relative value unit.

When reporting more than one procedure or service at the same operative session or during the post-op or global period, modifiers are required to "paint a clearer picture" of the circumstances surrounding the episode of care. There are modifiers applicable to the Surgery section, which are detailed later in this chapter. Remember that not all of these modifiers are reportable by outpatient facilities; only those on the approved list of modifiers for facilities, located on the front cover of the CPT manual, are reportable.

Services Not Included in the Global Surgery Package

The following services are not included in the payment amount for a global surgery package and may be paid separately. In many instances, coders need to use appropriate modifier(s) when submitting claims for these services:

- The initial consultation or evaluation of the problem by the surgeon to determine the need for surgery. A –57 modifier would apply in this circumstance.
- Visits unrelated to the diagnosis for which the surgical procedure is performed, unless the visits occur due to complications of the surgery.
- Treatment for the underlying condition or an added course of treatment that is not part of the normal recovery from surgery.
- Diagnostic tests and procedures, including diagnostic radiological procedures.
- Distinctly unrelated surgical procedures during the postoperative period. (A new postoperative period begins with the subsequent procedure.)
- Treatment for postoperative complications that requires a return trip to the operating room or procedure room. An OR is a place of service specifically equipped and staffed for the sole purpose of performing procedures. It does not include a patient's room, a minor treatment

National Correct Coding Initiative: Compliant Coding for Medicare Beneficiaries

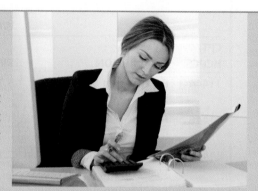

Compliant coding for Medicare beneficiaries follows Medicare's national policy on correct coding, the National Correct Coding Initiative (NCCI). NCCI controls improper coding that would lead to inappropriate payment for Medicare claims. It has coding policies that are based on the following:

- Coding conventions in CPT
- Medicare's national coverage and payment policies
- National medical societies' coding guidelines
- Medicare's analysis of standard medical and surgical practice

CMS updates correct coding combinations each quarter in the MCPM (Publication 100-04), Chapter 12 (Physicians/Non-Physician Practitioners), Section 30 (Correct Coding Policy), Section D. NCCI has many thousands of CPT code combinations called *NCCI edits* that are used by computers in the Medicare system to check claims. Edits are code combinations that are screened against each other to determine if both codes in the combination can be reported at the same time. The NCCI edits are available on the CMS website. There are two groups of edits: one for physicians and the other for institutions or facilities. NCCI edits apply to claims that bill for more than one procedure performed on the same patient (Medicare beneficiary), on the same date of service, by the same performing *provider*. Claims are denied when codes reported together do not "pass" an edit.

NCCI prevents billing two procedures that, according to Medicare, could not possibly have been performed together. Here are examples:

- Reporting the removal of an organ both through an open incision and with laparoscopy
- Reporting female- and male-specific codes for the same patient

Organization of the NCCI Edits

NCCI edits are organized into the following categories:

- Column 1/column 2 code pair edits
- Mutually exclusive code edits
- Modifier indicators

Column 1/Column 2 Code Pairs

In the NCCI column 1/column 2 code pair edits, two columns of codes are listed. Most often, the edit is based on one code being a component of the other. This means that the column 1 code includes all the services described by the column 2 code(s), so the column 2 code(s) cannot be billed together with the column 1 code for the same patient on the same day of service. Medicare pays for the column 1 code only; the column 2 code(s) are considered bundled into the column 1 code.

EXAMPLE

Column 1	Column 2
27370	20606, 64530, 76000

If 27370 is billed, neither 20606, 64530, nor 76000 should be billed with it, because the payment for each of these codes is already included in the column 1 code.

Mutually Exclusive Code Edits

NCCI mutually exclusive code (MEC) edits are included with the column 1/column 2 pairs and no longer listed separately. According to CMS regulations, both services represented by these codes could not have reasonably been done during a single patient encounter, so they cannot be billed together (e.g., laparoscopic and open appendectomy). If the provider reports both codes from both columns for a patient on the same day, Medicare pays only the lower valued code.

EXAMPLE

Column 1   *Column 2*
11444   11100

This means that a coder/biller cannot report 11100 when reporting 11444. They would be mutually exclusive of each other because a biopsy is a diagnostic procedure usually performed at a session previous to the therapeutic excision. The excision is the more invasive procedure and both procedures would not be performed on the same lesion at the same time.

Modifier Indicators

In CPT coding, modifiers show particular circumstances related to a code on a claim. The NCCI modifier indicators control modifier use to "break," or avoid, NCCI edits. NCCI modifier indicators appear next to items in both the NCCI column 1/column 2 code pair list and the MEC list. An NCCI modifier indicator of 1 means that a CPT modifier *may* be used to bypass an edit (if the circumstances are appropriate). An NCCI modifier indicator of 0 means that use of a CPT modifier will not change the edit, so the column 2 codes or mutually exclusive code edits will not be bypassed.

Resubmit claims with a modifier indicator of "9" if the NCCI modifier indicator "9" appears on a claim denial. This means that the original edit was a mistake and is being withdrawn, or the edit was deleted.

EXAMPLE

Flu vaccine code 90656 includes bundled flu vaccine codes 90655 and 90657–90660. It has an NCCI indicator of 0. No modifier will be effective in bypassing these edits, so in every case only CPT 90656 will be paid.

■ CASE SCENARIO

A patient undergoes biopsy of a salivary gland under general anesthesia. The anesthesia code would be 00100. The information listed below is an excerpt from the Medicare NCCI edits for physicians with respect to code 00100. Any code listed in column 2 is considered part of the anesthesia code 00100 and should not be billed separately unless one of the elements above applies. In this case, 36010 can never be coded at the same time as 00100.

COLUMN 1	COLUMN 2	MODIFIER 0 = NOT ALLOWED 1 = ALLOWED 9 = NOT APPLICABLE	COLUMN 1	COLUMN 2	MODIFIER 0 = NOT ALLOWED 1 = ALLOWED 9 = NOT APPLICABLE
00100	31500	9	00100	36405	1
00100	31505	1	00100	36406	1
00100	31515	1	00100	36410	1
00100	31527	1	00100	36420	1
00100	31622	1	00100	36425	1
00100	31645	1	00100	36430	1
00100	36000	1	00100	36440	1
00100	36005	1	00100	36600	1
00100	36010	0	00100	36620	9
00100	36011	1	00100	36625	9
00100	36012	1	00100	36640	1
00100	36013	1	00100	43752	1
00100	36014	1	00100	61026	1
00100	36015	1	00100	61055	1

NCCI Code Pair Edits

Table 16.4 Surgery Modifiers and CMS Acceptance

MODIFIER	SURGERY MODIFIER	GLOBAL SURGERY DAYS MODIFIER	GLOBAL SURGICAL PACKAGE MODIFIER	MEDICARE ACCEPT	PREFERRED REPLACEMENT	MEDICAID ACCEPT	PREFERRED REPLACEMENT
−22	Y	N	N	Y		N	
−23	N	N	N	Y		Y	
−24	N	Y	N	Y		Y	
−25	N	N	N	Y		Y	
−26	Y	N	Y	Y		Y	
−32	N	N	N	N		N	
−33	N	N	N	Y		Y	
−47	N	N	N	N		N	
−50	Y	N	N	Y		Y	
−51	Y	N	N	Y		Y	
−52	Y	N	N	Y		Y	
−53	Y	N	N	Y		Y	
−54	Y	N	Y	Y		Y	
−55	Y	N	Y	Y		Y	
−56	Y	N	Y	Y		N	
−57	N	Y	Y	Y		Y	
−58	Y	Y	N	Y		N	
−59	Y	N	Y	N	XE, XS, XP, XU	Y	
−62	Y	N	N	Y		Y	
−63	Y	N	N	N		Y	
−66	Y	N	N	Y		Y	
−73	Y	N	N	Y		Y	
−74	Y	N	N	Y		Y	
−76	Y	Y	N	Y		Y	
−77	Y	Y	N	Y		N	
−78	Y	Y	N	Y		Y	
−79	Y	Y	N	Y		Y	
−80	Y	N	N	Y, for MDs only	AS for RNs or PAs	Many state plans do not	No known replacement
−81	Y	N	N	N		N	
−82	Y	N	N	Y		Y	
−99	N	N	N	N		Y	
−TC	N	N	Y	Y		Y	

room, a recovery room, or an intensive care unit (unless the patient's condition was so critical there would be insufficient time for transportation to the OR).

- If a less extensive procedure fails and a more extensive procedure is required, the second procedure is separately payable.
- For certain services performed in a physician office, separate payment may be made for a surgical tray. In addition, drugs, splints, and casting supplies are separately payable under the reasonable charge payment methodology.
- Immunosuppressive therapy for organ transplants.

Patient follow-up care related to a surgical diagnostic service—an endoscopy, for example—only includes the care related to the recovery from the diagnostic procedure. Any treatment for a condition that was diagnosed as a result of this diagnostic procedure is not included and should be reported separately.

Special Documentation

Any procedure or service that is new, unusual, or coded to an unlisted procedure code requires documentation such as a special report to be submitted to support the procedure performed and substantiate medical necessity of that treatment method. Also, procedure codes with modifiers –22, –23, –59, –62, –66 –80, –81, –82, and –99 routinely require additional documentation to substantiate the services. Insurance companies typically have edits built into their adjudication systems to automatically place a claim on hold or deny it and to request medical record documentation for review. Typically, the history and physical and operative report will suffice. Essentially, what the modifier indicates is that payment is affected either positively or negatively and the report is going to justify why. The following must be included in a special report:

- Description of the nature, extent, and need for the procedure
- Time and effort
- Equipment necessary
- Complexity of symptoms
- Final diagnosis
- Pertinent physical findings
- Diagnostic and therapeutic procedures
- Concurrent problems
- Follow-up care necessary

CHECKPOINT 16.1

Using Table 16.3 and the Reimbursement Review, answer the following questions.

1. Is code 11471 a major or minor procedure? _____

2. Is 11446 a major or minor procedure? _____

3. Can 36640 be reported separately from 00100? _____

INTERNET RESOURCE: Medicare Global Surgery Days
Medicare determines the global surgery days for each procedure code in CPT.
This information is located at
www.cms.gov/Medicare/Medicare-Fee-for-Service-Payment/PhysicianFeeSched/
PFS-Relative-Value-Files.html

OPERATIVE REPORT

An operative report is generated each time a health-care provider performs a significant procedure, regardless of the complexity of the procedure performed or the place of service in which it is provided. It is a regulatory requirement by various organizations, such as the Department of Health and Environmental Control, and the Medicare Conditions of Participation that this report be generated immediately upon completion of the procedure to describe in detail, at a minimum, the procedure performed and by whom, observations and findings, preoperative and postoperative diagnoses, any implants placed within the body, specimens removed, and the condition of the patient at the completion of the procedure. This report is used by both facility and physician coders to assign ICD-10, CPT, and HCPCS codes for services rendered.

Box 16.4 illustrates a sample operative report with an explanation of the components that can help a coder to identify and abstract important information needed to assign codes. Notice that the surgeon did not describe procedure #1 within the body of the report. Just because something is listed at the top of the report under "Operation" or "Procedure Performed," that does not mean it actually was performed. If the procedure is not described within the body of the report, a code cannot be assigned because there is no "proof" that the procedure was actually performed. Furthermore, it cannot be billed or reported to the insurance carrier.

NAME: Jack Russell   DATE: 3/31/xx

SURGEON: Marc Barfield, MD   ASSISTANTS: None

ANESTHESIA: General with endotracheal intubation, left scalene block

ANESTHESIOLOGIST: Felix Munger

PREOPERATIVE and POSTOPERATIVE DIAGNOSIS:
1. Impingement left shoulder with partial rotator cuff tear.
2. Residual adhesive capsulitis left shoulder.

OPERATION:
1. Manipulation left shoulder under general anesthesia.
2. Arthroscopy left glenohumeral joint-diagnostic.
3. Arthroscopic assisted subacromial decompression left shoulder, bursectomy, acromioplasty with resection of coracoacromial ligament.

The top portion of the report is somewhat standardized by regulatory agencies to list patient name, date of service, surgeon, assistant surgeons, anesthesiologist, pre-op and post-op diagnoses, and procedures performed. Read the entire report. Never assign codes just from this section alone. All the procedures listed here should be described below in the body of the report.

PROCEDURE: The patient was brought to the operating room with the scalene block intact and carefully transferred to the operating table. After adequate general anesthesia with endotracheal intubation had been obtained, he was placed in the right lateral decubitus position. Axillary roll was inserted. Subsequently, the left upper extremity was placed in 12 pounds of counter traction. The left shoulder was prepped and draped in a routine sterile box fashion.

This is a standard introduction paragraph discussing induction of anesthesia, positioning the patient, and cleansing and prepping the site of operation.

The bony landmarks were outlined. The portals were established and infiltrated with 0.25% Marcaine with epinephrine. Subsequently, through the posterior portal, the glenohumeral joint was distended with sterile saline and then arthroscopy was carried out. In the glenohumeral joint, the patient had residual of adhesive capsulitis. Scarring was appreciated more so than active synovitis. Actually, his motion prior to arthroscopy was significantly improved with only slightly or mildly limited motion at extremes. Biceps tendon was intact with no indication of significant synovitis. No profound degenerative changes.

This paragraph describes procedure #2 above.

Going into the subacromial space, redirection was then carried out. Lateral portal was established. The patient had profound chronic bursitis. The bursa was resected to allow better visualization. Hemostasis was checked and obtained by means of the SERFAS ablator. Going anteriorly, he had a large hook on the anterior aspect of the acromion. This was resected with a 5.5 incisor followed by resection of coracoacromial ligament. All these findings were documented.

Going medially, he was decompressed over to the (acromioclavicular) AC joint. Hemostasis was checked and maintained by means of Bovie coagulator. After adequate decompression and adequate resection of coracoacromial ligament with the muscle bundles of the deltoid musculature being exposed, the bursectomy was completed. No significant bleeding was encountered. The shoulder joint was then generously irrigated.

These paragraphs describe procedure #3 above.

Arthroscopic sites were approximated with the approximating clips. Sterile dressing was applied. The patient was then awakened and taken to the recovery room in satisfactory condition. The patient tolerated the procedure well with no known intraoperative complications.

This is a standard conclusion paragraph discussing wound closure, dressings, waking the patient, and transferring to the recovery room. In this section, the surgeon may indicate that he or the anesthesiologist administered a pain block to help with post-op pain control. If this is done, it can be coded separately.

Use Box 16.4 to answer the following questions.

1. Was there an assistant surgeon in this case? _____

2. Was the procedure performed via an open or endoscopic approach? _____

3. What type of anesthesia was provided? _____

4. Did the patient have any synovitis? _____

5. Which shoulder was operated on? _____

6. Would the arthroscopy of the glenohumeral joint be coded separately from the procedures described for procedure #3? _____

SURGERY MODIFIERS

CPT/HCPCS Level I modifiers along with anatomical HCPCS Level II modifiers and modifiers approved for hospital outpatient use are located on the inside front cover of CPT. Surgery modifiers are used to indicate the following:

1. A procedure was performed bilaterally.
2. More than one procedure was performed at the same time.
3. An assistant surgeon participated.
4. A service or procedure was increased or decreased.
5. Part of a service was performed.
6. Unusual events occurred during a procedure or service.
7. Anatomical location is indicated.
8. A service has two parts or components, a technical component and a professional component.
9. More than one procedure or service was performed on the same day or within the global period (described in the Surgery section guidelines).

Proper Use

Coders must become familiar with the modifiers that affect their work environment (physician office, surgical practice, facility-based outpatient, etc.). For example, a coder employed by a hospital or facility can use the modifiers approved for hospital outpatient use. A coder employed by a physician private practice or a billing company hired by a physician is coding for physician professional services and can use any of the modifiers listed. HCPCS Level II anatomical modifiers may be assigned by all providers and facilities. The contracts between physicians and payers specify which modifiers are recognized by the payer.

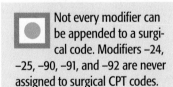 Not every modifier can be appended to a surgical code. Modifiers –24, –25, –90, –91, and –92 are never assigned to surgical CPT codes.

Modifiers are not appended to Category III codes, HCPCS supply codes, or unlisted procedure codes. Modifier –51 is never appended to add-on codes. The –51 modifier-exempt codes do not allow the use of the –51 modifier, but in some cases an anatomical modifier may be permitted.

INTERNET RESOURCE: Medicare Modifiers:
MCPM, Chapter 12, Sections 20, 40, and 140.3.3,
explain modifier use and effect on payment.
http://www.cms.gov/Regulations-and-Guidance/
Guidance/Manuals/Internet-Only-Manuals-IOMs.html

Periodically, Medicare issues its own guidelines or clarifications about modifier use and coding issues. Whenever CMS sees the need to do this, it will issue a program memorandum.

Modifier Descriptions

The Level I/CPT modifiers in Table 16.4 and HCPCS Level II anatomical modifiers listed in Box 16.5 are used for reporting procedures. The Level II anatomical modifiers specify laterality in terms of digits, extremities, coronary arteries, and the eyes. This specificity is not available in the Level I/CPT modifiers.

Modifier –22, Unusual Procedure or Service

The services provided are different from what is included in the code description. Usually, this is extra time spent or prolonged cleansing or some other added complexity. For some reason, the procedure was more complex than usual (e.g., increased risk, difficulty, hemorrhage [blood loss over 600 mL], unusual findings). There may have been a complication that cannot be identified by using another CPT code. The procedure may have taken longer than usual. To justify the use of this modifier, work and effort would be increased by about 30% to 50%. Additional time alone will not constitute use of the –22 modifier.

This modifier triggers the payer to review the claim carefully, so most practices send an operative note or letter explaining the circumstances with the claim. When the claim is paid as submitted, reimbursement is typically 20% to 30% higher, but often payers reject the –22. The most important issue for use of this modifier is that the complicating factor be carefully documented.

EXAMPLE

Excision of a lesion on an obese patient in the crease of the neck. The obesity makes it more difficult to reach the lesion so it warrants a modifier. The surgeon would report 11422–22.

BOX 16.5 HCPCS Level II Surgery Modifiers

Code	Description	Code	Description
LT	Left side	RC	Right coronary artery
RT	Right side	TA	Left foot, great toe
E1	Upper left, eyelid	T1	Left foot, second digit
E2	Lower left, eyelid	T2	Left foot, third digit
E3	Upper right, eyelid	T3	Left foot, fourth digit
E4	Lower right, eyelid	T4	Left foot, fifth digit
FA	Left hand, thumb	T5	Right foot, great toe
F1	Left hand, second digit	T6	Right foot, second digit
F2	Left hand, third digit	T7	Right foot, third digit
F3	Left hand, fourth digit	T8	Right foot, fourth digit
F4	Left hand, fifth digit	T9	Right foot, fifth digit
F5	Right hand, thumb		
F6	Right hand, second digit		
F7	Right hand, third digit		
F8	Right hand, fourth digit		
F9	Right hand, fifth digit		
GA	Waiver of liability on file		
LC	Left circumflex, coronary artery		
LD	Left anterior descending coronary artery	CA	Procedure payable only in the inpatient setting performed emergently on an outpatient who expires prior to admission
		SG	ASC facility service
		TC	Technical component

Modifer –23 Unusual Anesthesia

Report modifier –23 when general anesthesia is administered for a procedure that usually requires local anesthesia or none at all. Modifier –23 is assigned to the basic anesthesia service to identify why an anesthesia code is being reported for a service that does not usually require anesthesia. Modifier –23 is only appended to anesthesia codes. It is never used with surgery codes or E/M codes.

EXAMPLE

Diagnostic bronchoscopy for mentally ill patient who becomes combative when treated. Report 00520–23

Modifier –32 Mandated Service

Modifier –32 denotes that a procedure is performed at the request of the patient's insurance carrier or an outside organization such as a governmental agency or worker's compensation organization. Payers may request services be performed for second opinions or for disability determinations.

EXAMPLE

Nerve conduction study requested by insurance carrier prior to surgical intervention. Report 95907–32.

Modifier –47, Anesthesia by Surgeon

Modifier –47 is used when regional nerve block or general anesthesia is administered by the surgeon without a certified registered nurse anesthetist (CRNA) or anesthesiologist. It is not used in conjunction with anesthesia codes but simply appended to the CPT code for the procedure. This modifier is not accepted by Medicare.

EXAMPLE

Physician performed a paracervical nerve block for a cervical conization procedure. The physician would report 57520–47.

Modifier –50, Bilateral Procedures

Modifier –50 is used when the exact same procedure is performed on both the left and right side of a paired body part or organ. Paired body parts are as follows: eyes, ears, sinuses, nostrils, breasts, lungs, ovaries, kidneys, ureters, arms, legs, feet, hands, testicles, vas deferens, and fallopian tubes. If a procedure was only carried out on one of the parts of the pair, it would be considered unilateral and the HCPCS Level II RT or LT modifiers would be more applicable.

Unless otherwise stated in the code description, surgical procedures are unilateral. Before using this code, be sure the code description does not state "one or both or bilateral." This is used to indicate bilateral procedures performed at the *same* operative session. Do not use RT and LT when modifier –50 applies. Payers typically pay 1½ times the unilateral allowed amount for a bilateral procedure.

> List the most complex or major procedure first because it will receive full reimbursement. The second procedure code with the –51 modifier will receive 50% of the allowed amount.

EXAMPLE

For bilateral turbinate reduction, the surgeon would report 30130–50.

Modifier –51, Multiple Procedures

Modifier –51 is used when more than one *surgical* procedure is performed on the *same* day or at the *same operating session by the same provider*. The procedures can be performed on the same body part or different body part through the same incision or a different incision. Medicare will only pay for up to five procedures before a review is conducted by the medical director to determine if the procedures were properly coded and the documentation supports the claim. Medicare does not require that physicians use the –51 modifier because the approved procedures are paid on the physician's fee schedule and are ranked automatically by Medicare. It is, however, in the best interest of the practice to rank the procedure codes with the highest RVU code first and any other codes second with the –51 modifier to ensure the code with the highest reimbursement is listed first. This modifier is not used with add-on codes, Category III codes, or –51 modifier-exempt or unlisted procedure codes.

EXAMPLE

EXAMPLE

For probing of the right nasolacrimal duct and a nasal septoplasty, the surgeon would report 68811–RT, 30520–51.

CPT Appendix E lists all codes that are exempt from the –51 modifier use. The code descriptions for these exempt codes should alert the coder that a –51 modifier is not necessary with phrases such as "each additional" or "list separately in addition to code for." These procedures also may be staged procedures, and thus additional procedures are expected.

EXAMPLE

⊙31500 *Intubation, endotracheal, emergency procedure.*

Modifier –52, Reduced Services

When a procedure is partially reduced, modifier –52 is used. This alerts the payer that the service was not completed to its full extent. Each payer has its own policy regarding this modifier. Documentation should accompany the claim. Typically, payers pay 50% of the allowed amount.

EXAMPLE

The doctor performed a procedure unilaterally but the code description indicates bilateral. Modifier –52 should be reported only when no other procedure code that describes the partially reduced services exists. If a more appropriate procedure code is available, it should be reported in place of using modifier –52.

■ **CASE SCENARIO**
A patient had a left extremity arterial study. A –52 modifier would be appropriate here because the code specifies bilateral. The surgeon would report 93923–52.

Modifier –53, Discontinued Procedure

Modifier –53 is used by the physician to indicate that a procedure that had been started was terminated for some reason such as threat to patient, instrument failure, power outage, fire, arrhythmia, or hypotension. This is not used to report elective cancellations prior to a procedure being started. It is the equivalent of the facility modifiers –73 and –74. This modifier, however, is not specific to whether or not anesthesia is indicated. Typically, insurance carriers will reimburse the physician 25% of the allowed amount with this modifier.

■ **CASE SCENARIO**
A planned colonoscopy with polyp removal was terminated halfway through the procedure because the patient developed an arrhythmia. The surgeon would report 45378–53.

Modifier –54, Surgical Care Only

Modifier –54 is used by the surgeon who actually performed the surgery and did not/will not provide the pre-op or post-op care. This is a "split-care modifier," indicating that more than one provider is involved. There must be a written agreement for the transfer of care or a note in the medical record.

■ **CASE SCENARIO**
A patient is on vacation and is involved in a car accident. The patient undergoes an open reduction of the fourth left finger. The patient is to follow up with a physician in her hometown for post-op care. The surgeon would report 26615–F3–54.

Modifier –55, Postoperative Management Only

Modifier –55 is used by a physician who performed only post-op management and neither evaluated the patient prior to the procedure nor performed the actual procedure. Payment for the post operative, post discharge care is split between two or more physicians when the physicians agree on the transfer of care. The physician providing postoperative care would add modifier –55 to the surgical procedure code.

Modifier –56, Preoperative Management Only

Modifier –56 is appended to the code submitted by a physician who only examined a patient preoperatively. For example, the physician may have intended to perform the planned procedure, but circumstances changed. If a physician other than the surgeon provides preoperative care, modifier –56 should be billed with the surgery code.

Modifier –58, Staged or Related Procedure by the Same Physician During the Postoperative Period

To use modifier –58, the surgeon should have documented in the medical record that a staged procedure was planned. Do not use this modifier with codes that already have language in their code definition indicating multiple sessions. This modifier is used when a procedure was planned prospectively, was more extensive than the original procedure, or is for therapy following a diagnostic surgical procedure and each of the stages of the procedure is performed by the original surgeon. A new postoperative period begins with each subsequent procedure. Multiple-session services, as defined in CPT, may not be billed with this modifier, as in code 67145, *Prophylaxis of retinal detachment without drainage, one or more sessions; photocoagulation,* because this code is meant to include all sessions for the predefined treatment.

Modifier –58 is not used to report a problem or complication resulting from the original surgery that required a return to the OR. The key is to know what the post-op period or allowed global surgery days are for each code.

Modifier –59, Distinct Procedural Service

Modifier –59 is used to report two codes that normally are packaged but were performed as two distinct procedures. One procedure is performed independent of the other or is unrelated to the other. Use the –59 modifier if the procedures are done at different sites or organs, a separate incision was made, a separate excision was done, or when the physician is treating a separate injury.

EXAMPLES

• Arthrocentesis of the elbow is done (20605), and also of the ankle (20605–59). Because they are two distinct and different sites, use the code twice, appending the –59 to the second code.

• Excision of a lesion on the right breast is done, and an incision and drainage is done on a different and separate lesion of the right breast. The second procedure is reported with a –59.

Modifier –62, Two Surgeons

Modifier –62 is applicable when the procedure requires 50% of each surgeon's skill/time. This applies when the two surgeons are participating in the same procedure. However, if two surgeons are operating at the same time but performing two different procedures, then this modifier does not apply.

EXAMPLES
- A neurosurgeon will perform a spinal arthrodesis
- A thoracic surgeon is requested by the neurosurgeon to create an anterior approach through the thoracic cavity for an anterior lumbar arthrodesis with instrumentation. The thoracic surgeon would report 22558–62. The neurosurgeon would report 22558–62, and 22845.

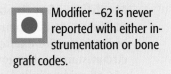 Modifier –62 is never reported with either instrumentation or bone graft codes.

Modifier –63, Procedure Performed on Infants Less Than 4 Kg

Modifier –63 is used to capture services on neonates and infants weighing less than 4 kg. Procedures on neonates and infants may involve increased complexity and physician work associated with this type of patient. The concept of this modifier is similar to that of modifier –22 in that the circumstances are much riskier or more complex, thus warranting extra physician work. CPT Appendix D states that this modifier is not used with the E/M, Anesthesia, Radiology, Pathology and Laboratory, or Medicine sections.

> ### ■ CASE SCENARIO
> A premature infant undergoes procedure to close a patent ductus arteriosus by ligation. The surgeon would report 33820–63.

Modifier –66, Surgical Team

Modifier –66 is used mainly in transplant procedures or multiple-trauma cases when the skill of several different surgeons is required. This is appended to the procedure code to report professional fees.

Modifier –73, Discontinued Outpatient Procedure Prior to Anesthesia Administration

At times, an intended procedure may be discontinued before anesthesia induction, requiring the –73 modifier. A patient could be prepped preoperatively and taken to the OR where the procedure is then canceled. This modifier is reported by the facility.

> ### ■ CASE SCENARIO
> A patient is prepped preoperatively and taken to the OR. The anesthesiologist cancels the procedure due to an abnormal heart rate. The facility would report the procedure code for the scheduled procedure with a –73 modifier.

Modifier –74, Discontinued Outpatient Procedure After Anesthesia Administration

Modifier –74 is used only in facilities to indicate that a procedure was terminated after local or general anesthesia was given. This includes situations when the patient is actually in the OR and anesthesia has been started *or* when sedation was given in the holding area.

> ### ■ CASE SCENARIO
> A planned colonoscopy with polyp removal was terminated halfway through the procedure because the facility was required to evacuate due to a fire on the second floor. Code 45378–74 would be reported.

Modifier –76, Repeat Procedure or Service by Same Physician

Modifier –76 is used to report a second procedure that was previously performed that same day. This is usually used to report radiology, lab, and minor procedures such as repeat blood sugars, EKGs, and chest x-rays. By appending this modifier, it alerts the payers that it is not a duplicate charge. Some payers recognize this and some do not. The exact same procedure or service must be repeated in order to use this modifier.

> ### EXAMPLE
> Repeat CAT scan of the head following trauma to monitor intracranial hemorrhaging. Code 70460–76 would be reported.

Modifier –77, Repeat Procedure or Service by Another Physician

Another physician of the same group to which the original physician performing the procedure belongs would qualify to use modifier –77 in addition to any physician outside the practice.

> ### ■ CASE SCENARIO
> An adult patient had a tonsillectomy and adenoidectomy earlier in the day. The surgeon was called back to the hospital 2 hours later for post-op bleeding that required a return trip to the OR to cauterize the area for bleeding control. The physician on call for the group practice was called 6 hours later due to additional post-op bleeding and had to cauterize the area again. The on-call physician would report 42971–77.

Modifier –78, Unplanned Return to OR for a Related Procedure During the Postoperative Period

Modifier –78 is used when the surgeon must perform additional surgery for a reason related to the original surgery during the global period. This is usually done because of hemorrhage or a failed flap or graft. Most payers recognize this as a secondary procedure for a related complication. To use this modifier, the patient must be taken back to the OR. The global days do not "reset" for the original procedure, and procedures reported with modifier –78 do not have a global period. The physician is only paid for the intraoperative service part of the payment allowed for the procedure. Payment is based on the intraoperative value of the code that describes the treatment of the complication. Procedures with a zero-day global period have no intraoperative value; thus, payment is made at the full fee schedule amount (less other reductions, such as the facility fee).

The physician and facility must bill the code that best describes the procedures performed in that second session. If one does not exist, an unlisted procedure is filed. The original surgery code should not be used unless the exact same procedure was carried out a second time, in which case the –76 or –77 modifier would instead apply.

> ### ■ CASE SCENARIO
> An adult patient had a tonsillectomy and adenoidectomy earlier in the day. The surgeon was called back to the hospital 2 hours later for post-op bleeding that required a return trip to the OR for bleeding control. The surgeon would report 42971–78.

Modifier –80, Assistant Surgeon

Medicare requires the use of HCPCS modifier –AS for assistant surgeons who are not physicians, such as nurse practitioners.

Modifier –80 is used to indicate that an assistant was required to perform the surgery. Modifier –80 (assistant surgeon) is widely used for complex spine, cardiac, or abdominal procedures. The assistant surgeon would submit the same CPT code as the surgeon with the –80 modifier appended. The assistant surgeon will be paid at 20% of what is allowed for the procedure. The head surgeon will be paid at 80% of the allowed reimbursement.

Modifier –81, Minimum Assistant Surgeon

Minimum assistants provide no hands-on care. Medicare does not pay for a minimum assistant surgeon on many procedures.

Modifier –82, Assistant Surgeon (When Qualified Resident Surgeon Is Not Available)

Modifier –82 is used in teaching hospitals (or rural hospitals) when a surgical resident is not available or there is no adequate training program locally for the medical specialty needed to perform the procedure. The physician who assists the primary surgeon would append this modifier.

Modifier –91, Repeat Clinical Diagnostic Laboratory Test

Modifier 91 is used when the same laboratory test is repeated on the same day to obtain multiple test results. Do not use this modifier when tests are rerun for confirmation of the original result or tests are rerun due to problems with specimens or equipment. This modifier is also not used when the standard one-time result is all that is required. Note that there are codes that already describe a series of test results, such as glucose tolerance tests or evocative suppression tests.

Modifier –95, Synchronous Telemedicine Service Rendered Via a Real-Time interactive Audio and Video Telecommunications System

Modifier 95 is used when a patient is provided with a key component oriented E/M service from a physician or other QHP who is located at a distant site. The services provided must meet the E/M requirements as if rendered during a face-to-face service.

Modifier –96, Habilitative Services

Habilitative services help individuals to learn skills and functions for daily living that have not been developed already. Append modifier –96 when a service or procedure may be either habilitative or rehabilitative but is provided for habilitative purposes. The modifier is appropriate for physicians or QHPs providing the service or procedure.

Modifier –97, Rehabilitative Services

Rehabilitative services help the patient to keep, get back, or improve skills and functioning that were lost or impaired because of sickness, injury, or disability. The modifier is appropriate for physicians or QHPs providing the service or procedure.

Modifier –TC (Technical Component)

Charges may be submitted by facilities for use of equipment. The total allowed payment for a procedure requiring the use of special equipment is split between the physician, who submits a –26 modifier, and the facility. TC is not used by a physician. If a physician is submitting charges for use of special equipment and he owns the equipment and is performing the interpretation of the results obtained by using the equipment, no modifier is necessary.

Modifier Methodology

The coder must determine if a modifier is required. Keep in mind that no matter how automated coding or electronic records become, modifier assignment is a learned skill in which an educated decision must be made that takes into consideration all circumstances. Remember, not all circumstances or codes warrant a modifier. Answer the questions and follow the steps provided in Pinpoint the Code 16.1 to determine the need for a modifier.

Procedure Sequencing

The primary or principal procedure should also be linked to or referenced to the primary or principal diagnosis. List the most extensive/heaviest weighted/highest grouped procedure code first, which is always going to be a therapeutic procedure. All procedures other than the principal procedure should have a –51 modifier, with the exception of add-on, unlisted, Category III, and –51 modifier-exempt codes, and codes reported by facilities.

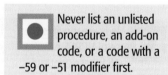

Never list an unlisted procedure, an add-on code, or a code with a –59 or –51 modifier first.

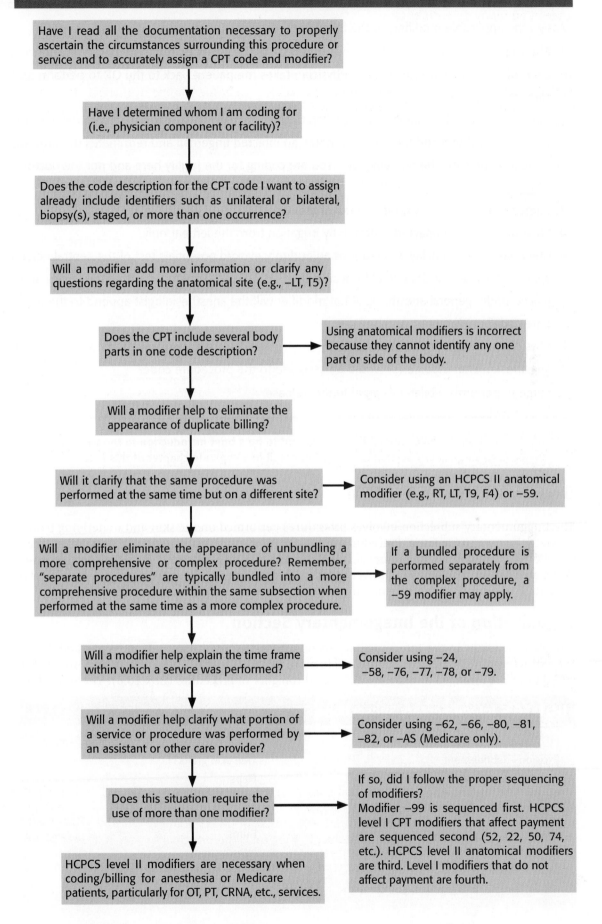

Have I read all the documentation necessary to properly ascertain the circumstances surrounding this procedure or service and to accurately assign a CPT code and modifier?

Have I determined whom I am coding for (i.e., physician component or facility)?

Does the code description for the CPT code I want to assign already include identifiers such as unilateral or bilateral, biopsy(s), staged, or more than one occurrence?

Will a modifier add more information or clarify any questions regarding the anatomical site (e.g., –LT, T5)?

Does the CPT include several body parts in one code description? → Using anatomical modifiers is incorrect because they cannot identify any one part or side of the body.

Will a modifier help to eliminate the appearance of duplicate billing?

Will it clarify that the same procedure was performed at the same time but on a different site? → Consider using an HCPCS II anatomical modifier (e.g., RT, LT, T9, F4) or –59.

Will a modifier eliminate the appearance of unbundling a more comprehensive or complex procedure? Remember, "separate procedures" are typically bundled into a more comprehensive procedure within the same subsection when performed at the same time as a more complex procedure. → If a bundled procedure is performed separately from the complex procedure, a –59 modifier may apply.

Will a modifier help explain the time frame within which a service was performed? → Consider using –24, –58, –76, –77, –78, or –79.

Will a modifier help clarify what portion of a service or procedure was performed by an assistant or other care provider? → Consider using –62, –66, –80, –81, –82, or –AS (Medicare only).

Does this situation require the use of more than one modifier? → If so, did I follow the proper sequencing of modifiers? Modifier –99 is sequenced first. HCPCS level I CPT modifiers that affect payment are sequenced second (52, 22, 50, 74, etc.). HCPCS level II anatomical modifiers are third. Level I modifiers that do not affect payment are fourth.

HCPCS level II modifiers are necessary when coding/billing for anesthesia or Medicare patients, particularly for OT, PT, CRNA, etc., services.

Assign the applicable modifiers to the following scenarios.

1. Physician performs cautery of the nose for epistaxis. Patient goes home and 6 hours later comes back with the nose bleeding again. Physician takes the patient back to the OR to perform further cautery and packing. _____

2. Patient is prepped for surgery and is taken to the OR. Anesthesia is administered. Patient's extremity is scrubbed and the physician notes an infected fingernail and terminates the procedure for fear of infecting the operative site. You are coding for the facility here and not the doctor.

   _____

3. Surgeon performs an ectropion repair of the left lower lid. _____

4. Surgeon removes impacted cerumen by irrigation from the left ear only. _____

5. Child has a speech delay and requires an auditory evoked potentials test of the central nervous system. Because the child would not sit still, the child was taken to an outpatient facility and placed under general anesthesia. What modifier will the anesthesiologist append to the procedure code? _____

6. Physician performs tendon procedure on the left hand. He also performs both local and regional anesthesia. What modifier(s) would be assigned to the procedure code? _____

7. Surgeon performs a bilateral carpal tunnel release. _____

NOTE: Remember, the following sections are meant to be a brief introduction to the various body systems. Each surgical CPT section is covered in detail in a separate chapter of this text.

INTEGUMENTARY SYSTEM

The Integumentary subsection involves procedures performed on the skin and underlying tissues down to the nonmuscle fascia. Procedures in this section include lesion removals, skin grafts, breast procedures, skin biopsies, nail removal, and debridement of wounds and burns. This section is not designated for dermatologists exclusively. Many different types of physician specialties report codes from this subsection, such as plastic surgeons, family practitioners, and general surgeons.

Organization of the Integumentary Section

The main headings in the Integumentary section are as follows: Skin, Subcutaneous and Accessory Structures; Nails; Pilonidal Cyst; Introduction; Repair (Closure); Destruction; and Breast. The subsections are arranged by anatomical site and category of procedure (Box 16.6). These sections,

BOX 16.6 Integumentary Subsections

Incision and drainage	Adjacent tissue transfer or rearrangement
Excision—debridement	Free skin grafts
Paring or curettement	Flaps
Biopsy	Other procedures
Removal of skin tags	Pressure ulcers
Shaving	Burns
Excision—benign lesions	Introduction
Excision—malignant lesions	Mohs micrographic surgery
Repair—simple, intermediate, and complex	Repair and/or reconstruction

which are further broken down into subsections or categories by surgical method or body part, are used as main terms to locate codes in the Index.

Specific coding guidelines are found throughout this chapter that pertain to differentiating between simple, intermediate, and complex skin repairs; skin grafting with various materials; and determining the size of lesions removed and square surface area of skin repaired or grafted. These must be read along with instructional notes/parenthetical notes before assigning a code from these sections. Procedures in each of these categories are discussed in great detail in Chapter 17.

Code Assignment

To locate the surgical code, remember to look for the action words such as "biopsy," "excision," "repair," procedure names, and specific body parts such as "breast." Thoroughly review the code descriptions and instructional notes. Pay close attention to the approach to the procedure and technique utilized.

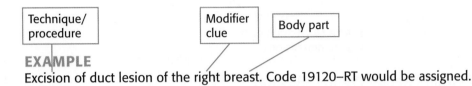

EXAMPLE
Excision of duct lesion of the right breast. Code 19120–RT would be assigned.

Incision and Drainage

When incision and drainage (I&D) and foreign body removals are referenced in the Integumentary subsection, they are referring to superficial procedures. The coder should check the Musculo-skeletal section for a more specific code for the depth of the procedure and anatomical site if it goes beyond the subcutaneous tissue.

Excision and Destruction

The size and type of skin lesion will determine the mode of treatment. Modalities of treatment include paring, shaving, excision, and destruction. To properly code procedures involving skin lesions, you must first differentiate between these treatment modalities.

Methods of Lesion Removal

1. *Excision* is surgically removing or cutting out part or all of a tumor, lesion, organ, or structure with a scalpel, sharp instrument, laser, loop electrode, or hot knife.
2. *Paring* is trimming or gradual reduction in size by slicing.
3. *Shaving* is slicing a raised lesion or mole off at skin level by using a razor or surgical blade.
4. *Destruction* is eradicating or exterminating all or a portion of a lesion, growth, or structure. Tissue is destroyed by force, chemicals, heat, or freezing. Key words used include *destruction, ablation, desiccation, fulguration,* and *cauterization*.

Assigning Codes for Lesion Removals

To properly code lesion removal procedures, you must know the following:

- Site
- Number of lesions
- Depth of the lesion
- Size of the lesion
- Behavior of the lesion (malignant or benign) (Lesion removal codes are designated by this.)

Excision codes already include the direct, primary, and simple repair or closure of the defect. Any closure other than a *simple closure* is coded separately.

The codes are assigned based on the greatest diameter (width) of the lesion being excised or destroyed, not according to the size of the incision necessary to access the lesion. The size of the lesion is taken from the physician's operative report or office procedure note. If there is no documentation in the physician's operative note or chart, it is permissible to use the excision code with the *smallest size* for that anatomical area, but it is not recommended. It is better to query the physician for this information. Never guess or assume the size of the specimen or lesion.

Repair (Closure)

When coding wound repair, three factors must be considered:

1. Size of wound in centimeters (cm). If the size is reported in millimeters (mm), it must be converted to centimeters (cm) by moving the decimal point. For example, if the lesion is 11 mm it is 1.1 cm. (Do not confuse the size of the lesion with the size of the specimen or size of the defect. See Fig. 16.1.)
2. Complexity of repair
3. Site of wound repair

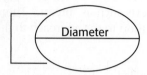

Figure 16.1 Lesion or wound dimensions.

Three Types of Wound Repair (Suture Closure)

Guidelines are located under the Repair heading in the Integumentary section with definitions for repair types:

1. *Simple*—superficial wound repair involving epidermis, dermis, and a minimal amount of subcutaneous tissue requiring one-layer suturing. Dermabond is a skin adhesive, or "skin glue," that when used to close a minor laceration is considered a simple repair. If the closure was done with tape or adhesive strips, this is included in the E/M code and not billed separately. This is done for superficial wounds and is an inherent component of all surgical procedures; it is not coded separately.
2. *Intermediate*—closure of one or more of the subcutaneous layers and superficial fascia, in addition to the skin. You can also use this code when the wound has to be extensively cleaned due to contamination or removal of small pieces of foreign material before suturing.
3. *Complex*—complicated closure including scar revision, debridement, extensive undermining, stents, or retention sutures, and more than layered closure. Repair of traumatic avulsions or lacerations may fall into this category. Repair of extensive nerve, blood vessel, or tendon damage may also be reported when the wound is complex.

> Pay attention to the type of suture used to close a wound or surgical site. Typically, if two different types of suture are used (one being absorbable such as Vicryl, chromic, catgut, or Dexon), an intermediate repair is likely.

CHECKPOINT 16.4

Assign CPT codes for the following statements.

1. Excision of malignant lesions, 1.1 cm, upper arm; 0.1 cm, foot _____

2. Needle core biopsy of both breasts (not using imaging guidance) _____

3. Simple incision and removal of foreign body, subcutaneous tissue _____

MUSCULOSKELETAL SYSTEM

The Musculoskeletal System subsection is the largest subsection of the Surgery section. Many different procedures can be performed on the bones, tendons, soft tissue, and muscles of the body. Common procedures include reduction of fractures and dislocations. It is important to have a good knowledge of all the bones of the body and their locations, tendons, and muscles. This section of the book is arranged starting from a general section that applies to the entire body and then from the head down to toes. Box 16.7 lists the sections contained in this part of the CPT manual.

BOX 16.7 Musculoskeletal Section Headings

General	Forearm and Wrist
Head	Hand and Fingers
Neck (Soft Tissues) and Thorax	Pelvis and Hip Joint
Back and Flank	Femur (Thigh Region) and Knee Joint
Spine (Vertebral Column)	Leg (Tibia and Fibula) and Ankle Joint
Abdomen	Foot and Toes
Shoulder	Application of Casts and Strapping
Humerus (Upper Arm) and Elbow	Endoscopy/Arthroscopy

Within each section is a consistent arrangement of subsections that makes finding codes easier. You will see this breakdown throughout the entire section. Each body site is identified and then the following terms appear:

- Incision
- Excision
- Introduction or Removal
- Repair
- Revision and/or Reconstruction
- Fracture and/or Dislocation
- Manipulation
- Arthrodesis
- Amputation
- Other Procedures

Chapter 18 of this text discusses musculoskeletal procedures in further detail.

Accurately Coding Orthopedic Procedures

The coder should pay close attention to the type of service provided and the extent of services by carefully reading the medical record and then reading the code description in its entirety to catch such phrases as *closed, open, with or without manipulation, with traction, with or without internal or external fixator*, or *with grafting*. There are many "separate procedures" located in this section, particularly in the arthroscopic procedure sections. Orthopedic procedures are coded by the surgical approach to the procedure. Note that many of these procedures can be done using either a traditional open method or an arthroscopic method.

Open Treatment

An open procedure involves making an incision and surgically opening the body at the site of the injury or ailment. Uncomplicated soft tissue closure may be involved. This approach is considered major surgery because of the large, deep incisions made, and it poses more risk and most often requires general anesthesia. Clues to look for are words ending in "-otomy."

> **EXAMPLE**
> 23105 *Arthrotomy, glenohumeral joint, with synovectomy, with or without biopsy.*

Closed Treatment

A closed procedure does not involve making a large incision and surgically opening the site of injury or area in need of repair or treatment. Closed procedures are primarily performed endoscopically (through a scope) through small incisions. Clues to look for are words that end in "-oscopy."

EXAMPLE

29820 *Arthroscopy, surgical, shoulder; synovectomy, partial.*

Coders should make a special effort to code by type of treatment. Coders must also determine if the treatment is for a traumatic injury (accident) or medical condition (ongoing condition). When it comes to excision, biopsies, and I&D, do not immediately turn to the Integumentary section. In the Musculoskeletal section, several codes exist that are more specific to the anatomical part than the Integumentary section codes are and should be used in place of the Integumentary section codes. As in all subsections of the Surgery section, a biopsy of a structure is not billed separately when an excision, destruction, removal, repair, or fixation procedure is also performed at the same operative session unless it is of a different site.

> ■ The term "specify" following a code description in this section is a cue to send an operative note or special report with the claim.

Wound Exploration

The wound exploration codes are for traumatic wounds that result from *acute* or *penetrating trauma* (e.g., gunshot, stabbing). These codes include basic exploration and repair of the area. They also include dissection to determine depth of penetration of the wound, debridement, removal of foreign body, and ligation or coagulation of minor subcutaneous and/or muscular blood vessels or the subcutaneous tissues, muscle fascia, and muscle. These codes are used when the repair requires enlargement of the existing wound for cleaning, determination of the extent of the wound, and repair. If the wound did not require enlarging or if deeper structures of the muscle fascia and beyond were not explored, you would use a repair code from the Integumentary section. If the wound is more severe than the wound exploration would encompass or if the repair was done to major structures or major blood vessels, the repair code would come from the specific area of the musculoskeletal section. The following rules apply when coding wound explorations:

- These are coded in addition to the E/M service with modifier –25 on the E/M code if the E/M services meet the requirement for modifier –25.
- Codes are used for acute and penetrating injuries only.
- Surgical exploration is through the current wound with possible enlargement.
- Muscle fascia and beyond are explored.
- Skin and subcutaneous exploration is coded to the Integumentary section when no enlargement of the wound, extension, dissection, or the like is required.
- Layered closure is expected.
- Drains may or may not be placed.
- Debridement and removal of foreign body are included.
- Ligation of minor subcutaneous and/or muscle blood vessels is included.
- If a thoracotomy or laparotomy was performed, the wound exploration is bundled into the more extensive procedures.

> ■ **CASE SCENARIO**
>
> A man is stabbed in the thigh and goes to the emergency department (ED). The surgeon removes the knife and explores the extent of the penetration. He finds that the femoral artery has been nicked. He proceeds to repair the femoral artery; therefore, he would not code for the wound exploration but would instead code for the artery repair.

Injection of Sinus Tracts, Joints, Tendons, and Trigger Points

Arthrocentesis describes the procedure to aspirate the joint, remove fluid, *or* insert a therapeutic substance. Pay attention to the size of the joint being injected. They are broken down into three groups: small, intermediate, and major (20600–20611). If a more extensive procedure is being done to the same joint that is being injected, the injection would be bundled into the more complex procedure. Tendon injections are coded to 20550–20551. Trigger point codes 20552–20553 are based on the number of muscle groups injected, not on the number of times the needle is inserted. Trigger point injections are typically done for pain management purposes.

Fixation Devices

Fixation device codes can only be coded when not included in the original code description for the procedure performed. When coding the application of an external fixation device, you need to know how many planes the appliance will cross (20690–20692). It is not uncommon to have an external fixation device adjusted and then subsequently removed. (See codes 20693–20694. Examples of external fixators are Orthofix, Ace-Fischer, Ace Unifix, Hoffmann, Ilizarov, and Monticelli-Spinelli.) When removing an internal fixation device, it is normally coded to 20670–20680. Be sure to check the Index to see if there is a more specific code for the particular body site from which the implant is being removed. If removal of an internal fixation device is done in conjunction with another procedure at the same site, do not code it separately.

Foreign Body Removal

Two factors affect coding for removal of a foreign body: the site and whether the foreign body is superficial or deep. Some of the code sections have a specific code for foreign body removal and some do not. They are usually found under the subheading in each body section, "Introduction or Removal." For those that do not have a specific code, the coder should refer back to the "general" section of the musculoskeletal subsection using the parenthetical notes. Foreign bodies can be anything that is "foreign" to the body (e.g., metal, gravel, bullet, or an orthopedic device) and embedded in tissue, bone, or a joint, or it could be a "loose" body of natural tissue or bone that "broke off" (e.g., a bone chip or cartilage).

Fractures

The following questions must be answered in order to assign the appropriate code for fracture repair:

1. Where is the fracture or dislocation?
2. Is the treatment open or closed?
3. Was a reduction/manipulation of the fracture performed?
4. Was an internal or external fixation device applied?
5. Was percutaneous or skeletal fixation applied?
6. Was infection present, was treatment delayed, or did the surgery take longer than usual?

Fracture care is coded by the type of treatment (open, closed, percutaneous fixation), *not the type of fracture* (this is for ICD-10 diagnosis coding). There is no correlation between the type of fracture sustained and the type of treatment received (i.e., closed fracture and closed treatment). A closed fracture could require open treatment for adequate repair.

Open Treatment

An open treatment procedure involves making an incision and surgically opening the site of the fracture for repair and treatment. Uncomplicated soft tissue closure may be involved. Most often, internal fixation is applied (screws, plate, wire, rod) but not always. Additionally, if the fracture is opened at a site remote from the fractured bone to insert an intramedullary nail, it is considered an open treatment.

Closed Treatment

A closed treatment procedure does not involve making an incision and surgically opening the site of the fracture in order to repair it. It includes manipulating the fracture (reducing it); application of the cast, splint, or bandage; and application of a traction/immobilization/stabilization device.

Percutaneous Skeletal Fixation

A fixation device or appliance is placed across the fracture site with C-arm x-ray imaging assistance.

Guidelines

Application and removal of the *first* cast or traction device are considered bundled for all orthopedic procedures. If a cast, splint, or strapping is applied as a result of or during a surgical procedure, do not assign a code for this. It is considered part of the overall comprehensive surgical code. When coding for replacement of the first cast or traction device or when the cast or strapping is an initial service performed without a restorative treatment or procedure, use the 29000–29799 code series during the period of follow-up care. These codes can be used if the physician applying a temporary cast is not the physician performing the fracture reduction. Application of temporary casts, splints, or strapping is not considered part of the preoperative care. This should be billed accordingly, not as part of the surgical procedure, with a –56 modifier. Assign the code for cast removal only for casts applied by another physician for professional component coding. Otherwise, the removal of a cast, strapping, or splinting is included in the application.

According to Medicare rules and regulations, splints, casting supplies, and surgical dressings are separately payable under the reasonable charge payment methodology. In this case, an HCPCS code is also assigned (physician office only) for the actual splint or casting materials.

> ● If a cast is placed on a patient and no surgery was performed, CPT guidelines state to code using the appropriate level E/M code (outpatient or ED service) plus the codes for any supplies.

Arthroscopy

Many procedures on joints are done arthroscopically or endoscopically. Terms such as *portals, trocars, cannula,* and *scope* indicate an arthroscopic procedure. Arthroscopy codes are located at the end of the Musculoskeletal section.

> ● Diagnostic arthroscopies should not be coded when a surgical arthroscopy is performed.

Look up the word *arthroscopy* in the Index and find the appropriate site. If there is no code in that body section for arthroscopy, then the codes listed are "open" and cannot be used in lieu of a more specific arthroscopy code. If this happens, you will need to use an unlisted code. Synovectomy of the joint is always included in a more extensive arthroscopic or open procedure unless it is an extensive synovectomy performed in more than two compartments.

CHECKPOINT 16.5

Use the CPT book to assign codes to the following statements. Do not forget to append modifiers if needed.

1. Humeral osteotomy _____

2. Closed treatment of sesamoid fracture _____

3. Open treatment of right talus fracture _____

4. I&D of left foot bursa _____

5. Right elbow joint arthrodesis _____

RESPIRATORY SYSTEM

The Respiratory System subsection includes many procedures on the sinuses, nose, larynx, trachea, bronchi, lungs, and pleura. Box 16.8 lists the headings within the respiratory section.

Many of the procedures in this body system are performed via a scope and will be located in the Index or under the words *endoscopy, laryngoscopy,* or *bronchoscopy.* It is very important to thoroughly read the operative note to determine if the procedures were carried out unilaterally or bilaterally and if they were open, closed, or endoscopically performed. Codes in the nasal and sinus endoscopy section are unilateral procedures and if done bilaterally would require a –50 modifier. Keep in mind that most of

BOX 16.8 Respiratory Section Headings

Nose

Accessory Sinuses

Larynx

Trachea and Bronchi

Lungs and Pleura

the procedures on the sinuses are done endoscopically but at times may be done by making an incision in the mouth through the gum. Chapter 19 of this text discusses the respiratory system and associated procedures in further detail.

Nasal Procedures

Procedures done on the nose can be done with or without an endoscope. Be sure to determine which approach was used—internal or external and with or without a scope. Common procedures on the nose are septoplasty, removal of polyps, turbinate excisions, and treatment of epistaxis (nosebleeds). Other nasal procedures, if not performed alone, such as control of nasal hemorrhage, ligation of arteries, and fractures of turbinates, are usually components of the major procedure being performed.

Excision of Nasal Polyps

Nasal polyps described as simple are limited to one polyp or one polyp per side of the nose. These are usually pedunculated (hanging from a stalk) and are easy to remove. Simple excisions are typically performed in the physician office. Excision of multiple polyps or more than one per side is extensive. Extensive polyp removal usually involves sessile polyps (with a thick base) whose removal requires more effort, skill, and time. Extensive excisions are typically performed in an ASC. If you cannot determine whether the excision is simple or extensive, query the physician. If a polyp is removed from both sides of the nose, a −50 modifier is required.

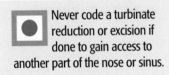
Never code a turbinate reduction or excision if done to gain access to another part of the nose or sinus.

Excision of Turbinates or Turbinate Reduction

A turbinate excision or reduction procedure is performed for turbinate hypertrophy from chronic inflammation or infection. This can lead to persistent sinus infections. Turbinates can be reduced by removing part of the lining and/or part of the bone itself with cautery, laser, or excision. Submucosal resection means that the surgeon performs submucosal removal of the lining of the turbinate, not actually removing part of the bone itself (30140). At times, when turbinates are enlarged and obstructing the nasal airway, they may be "fractured" to reposition them (30930).

Rhinoplasty

Rhinoplasty is performed for both cosmetic and therapeutic purposes. This procedure reshapes the external portions of the nose and may or may not involve the cartilage and bone. The extent of this procedure varies. There are two conditional phrases to keep in mind, *primary* and *secondary*. Primary refers to the first rhinoplasty procedure done and secondary refers to follow-up or a second rhinoplasty procedure.

There are three types of revision:

- *Minor revision (30400)* involves only the nasal cartilage for external parts of the nose.
- *Intermediate revision (30410)* involves an osteotomy for the external cartilage of the nose (removal of a hump or elevation of the tip).
- *Major revision (30420), or primary septorhinoplasty,* includes repair done on the internal and external parts of the nose and cartilage (elevation of nasal tip), grafts, osteotomy, and reshaping of a deviated septum. Code 30520 would not be coded separately. If grafts are obtained, musculoskeletal codes 20900–20926 and 21210 may be used for obtaining the tissue.

Nasal Septal Deviation

When the nasal septum is not midline, or straight, it may obstruct air movement. Septoplasty is a procedure that "straightens" the septum. Septoplasty with cartilage graft is included in code 30520. Surgeons refer to septoplasty as *submucous resection*. Modifier −50 does not apply to septoplasty procedures.

Nasal Hemorrhage

If bleeding occurs as a late complication and requires a significant separately identifiable service after the patient has been released from an endoscopic procedure, the cautery and packing can be billed with a –78 modifier. To code control of nasal hemorrhage, the coder must decide if this was an anterior or posterior control:

- *Anterior (30901–30903):* Key phrases to look for are *insertion of gauze packing, anterior packing,* or *cauterization.*
- *Posterior (30905–30906):* Key phrases to look for are *insertion of nasal stents, balloons, tampons, catheters,* or *posterior nasal packing.*

Procedures on the Larynx

Procedures on the larynx include laryngoscopies for biopsy, removal of foreign bodies, dilation of the larynx, and diagnostic examination of the pharynx and larynx. These can be performed for diagnostic or surgical purposes depending on the procedure's goal. There are two kinds of laryngoscopies, direct and indirect. Indirect laryngoscopy is performed with the use of mirrors to view the larynx, pharyngeal walls, oropharynx, and posterior third of the tongue. People with strong gag reflexes and small children have difficulty with this procedure. Direct laryngoscopy requires a scope to be passed through the mouth and pharynx to the larynx. This would be done in a facility under general anesthesia. A microscope may be used to magnify the image of the larynx. If the word *microlaryngoscopy* is mentioned in the operative note, then it would be appropriate to assign either 31526 or 31531.

> As with all scope procedures, a diagnostic laryngoscopy is always included in a surgical laryngoscopy.

> Many codes in this section include the use of an operating microscope, so do not code 69990 separately in this instance.

Procedures on the Lungs, Trachea, and Bronchi

Bronchoscopies are performed for dilation of the trachea; biopsies of the lung, bronchus, and trachea; bronchial lavage; removal of foreign bodies; tumor removal; lung brachytherapy; and aspiration. Bronchoscopies are automatically considered a bilateral procedure. Do not assign a –50 modifier if performed on both lungs. Bronchoscopies can be performed either by using a flexible fiber-optic or rigid bronchoscope (also known as an *open-tube bronchoscope*). Fluoroscopy is an inherent component of some of the bronchoscopy codes. The rigid scope would be used to remove foreign bodies or to remove a large biopsy sample. The flexible bronchoscopy is more commonly performed and utilizes fiber-optic light to better view the bronchioles, etc.

> When a bronchoscopy with brushings or washings is performed, this is considered a diagnostic bronchoscopy and not a biopsy.

CHECKPOINT 16.6

Use the CPT book to assign codes to the following statements. Do not forget to append modifiers if needed. Some of the following procedures require two codes. (*Hint:* For endoscopic procedures, read the notes before the endoscopic code group carefully.)

1. Surgical thoracoscopy with excisions of pericardial and mediastinal cysts _____

2. Surgical nasal/sinus endoscopy with left maxillary antrostomy _____

3. Planned tracheostomy on infant _____

4. Hematoma drainage from nasal septum _____

5. Laser destruction of two intranasal lesions, internal approach _____

CARDIOVASCULAR SYSTEM

The Cardiovascular System subsection covers procedures on the heart, veins, and arteries. Thousands of procedures are done each year on blood vessels, ranging from heart bypasses to creating access to vessels for chemotherapy and dialysis to varicose vein and hemangioma treatments. Box 16.9 lists the two cardiovascular section headings. This section of CPT is one of the most complex of all and contains numerous subsections.

The most difficult part of coding cardiovascular cases is determining how many codes are needed. Some of the services provided to treat or evaluate cardiology patients are actually located in the Medicine section of CPT. Codes from three different sections of the manual could potentially be assigned. The Cardiovascular System subsection of CPT houses the surgical codes (33010–37799). The Medicine section contains codes (92950–93799) for the cardiac-related nonsurgical services. Radiology codes (75557–75774) may also be assigned when imaging is used to perform a service on the heart such as nuclear studies involving angiography (e.g., catheterizations and angioplasties).

In coding cardiovascular services, the coder must determine if the procedure was invasive or noninvasive. Invasive procedures involve entering the body (cutting through the skin) to correct a problem, examine the internal part of the body, or remove a mass or foreign body. Noninvasive procedures do not require cutting the skin and are performed on the outside of the body. They are diagnostic in nature rather than therapeutic. The cardiovascular area of coding is extensive and complex and is covered in the detail necessary to understand this coding in Chapter 20 of this text.

Pacemaker and Pacing Cardioverter Defibrillator

The purpose of a pacemaker is to electrically stimulate the myocardium of one or more chambers of the heart to contract when the heart fails to do so on its own. A pocket is created and a generator and leads are placed inside the chest. A pacemaker may either be permanent or temporary. A pacemaker has two components: the pulse generator and leads (electrodes). The pulse generator contains four elements: the battery, the electronic circuit, the connector, and the sealed encasement. The electrodes are either inserted via a vein (transvenous) or placed on the surface of the heart (epicardium). A temporary pacemaker does not include an internally placed pulse generator because the device is temporary. The term *battery* is used interchangeably for the pulse generator. The battery alone is never replaced. The leads are always left in place unless they are defective. When a battery replacement is necessary, two codes are required to capture each step of the procedure. One describes the removal of the pulse generator and the second describes the reinsertion of the pulse generator. Other codes capture both the removal and replacement. Electrophysiological evaluation of the cardioverter-defibrillators can be done at the time of initial implantation or replacement or at any time subsequent to the initial placement. Codes from the Medicine section are assigned to capture this.

■ Cardioverter-defibrillators use multiple leads even if placed in a single chamber.

To correctly code pacemaker and cardioverter-defibrillator services, the coder must know the following:

1. Where were the electrodes (leads) placed: atrium, ventricle, or both?
2. Is this the initial placement, replacement, or repair of all of the components of a pacemaker or some of the components?
3. Was the approach transvenous or epicardial?

Codes for pacemaker services are reported based on what is inserted, replaced, or revised. Codes in this section are grouped this way but not clearly labeled this way or divided into subsections. The code groupings are shown in Box 16.10.

BOX 16.10 Pacemaker Code Groupings

Insertion of pacemaker	Insertion of transvenous electrodes, permanent pacemaker, or cardioverter-defibrillator
Insertion or replacement of temporary transvenous pacemaker or electrode	Transvenous electrode repair
Insertion of new or replacement electrodes (leads)	Revision or relocation of pulse-generator pocket
Insertion and replacement of pulse generator	Insertion or repositioning of cardiac venous system pacing electrode
Device replacement	Removal procedures
Repositioning of pacemaker or cardioverter-defibrillator	Insertion, replacement, or removal of pacing cardioverter-defibrillator pulse generator or electrodes

Heart and Great Vessels

Heart and great vessel codes describe electrophysiological procedures for arrhythmias and major cardiac procedures to repair or replace the aortic, mitral, tricuspid, and pulmonary valves. Coronary artery bypass grafts (CABGs) are also in this section and codes are based on the type of material used to perform the bypass. There are vein-only codes (33510–33516) to represent that only vein(s) are used as the bypass graft material. Codes 33517–33530 represent bypass grafts that combine both veins and arteries to accomplish the graft procedure, but these codes represent the vein portion only and they are all add-on codes. They must be reported in addition to the artery-only codes (33533–33536). Note that the artery-only codes can be reported on their own when the bypass graft material is from an artery.

Open and endovascular repairs of the thoracic aorta are represented by codes 33860–33891. It is important for coders to understand the different approaches available for these types of repairs. The open method is a far riskier procedure and requires a longer recuperative period, while the endovascular repair is less invasive, less risky, and has a shorter recuperation time. The coding structure, however, is more detailed for endovascular repairs, and the guidelines must be carefully reviewed.

The heart and lung transplant codes break down into whether or not the patient is receiving both heart and lung(s) or just the heart. The standard breakdown of codes is the same in this section as it is in all CPT sections related to transplants. Three procedures need to be considered in transplant coding: the removal of the organ from the donor, the backbench work, and the actual transplant into the recipient.

Procedures on Veins and Arteries

Carefully review the introductory notes and guidelines that precede procedures on veins and arteries. Instructions for reporting are contained within those paragraphs. Embolectomy and thrombectomy procedures are covered in this section, as are endovascular repairs of abdominal aortic aneurysms and iliac aneurysms. The section then goes into the open repairs of aneurysms in various locations. Bypass grafts (other than coronary) are covered here based on the type of material used for the graft, similar to the CABG section. The three types of bypass grafts are vein only, in situ vein, and other than vein.

Vascular injections require extensive knowledge of the vascular systems, and CPT has provided some assistance with this in Appendix L of the CPT book. Coders need to understand the order of each vessel within each vascular family to select the right code(s). This coding is further broken down into the type of catheterization: nonselective or selective. A nonselective catheterization is included in a select catheterization, and each time the surgeon views the injection of dye through the catheter an additional service is coded to reflect the radiological supervision and interpretation.

Central venous access devices provide access for chemotherapy infusions, for administration of medications or fluids, and to obtain blood and cardiovascular measurements. These procedures are represented by codes 36555–36598 and are divided into five types of services: insertion, repair, partial replacement, complete replacement, and removal. The guidelines that precede these codes define what qualifies as a central venous access device in terms of where the catheter/device terminates and whether it is centrally inserted or peripherally inserted. The Central Venous Access table at the beginning of the central venous access codes section is used to locate appropriate codes based on the "who, what, where, why, and how" concept: the intent (why) of the procedure, what is inserted, how it is inserted, and where it is inserted.

The Cardiovascular System subsection continues with transcatheter procedures (37184–37217) for thrombectomies, stent placements, thrombolysis infusions, and vena cava filters as examples. Coding for dialysis access and endovascular revascularization of the lower extremity blood vessels is also provided.

Varicose Veins

Codes in this section describe treatment for varicose veins. Treatment for severe varicose veins involves ligating, dividing, and ultimately stripping the diseased veins. Other treatments for less severe varicosities include:

- *Sclerotherapy*—chemical injection producing scarring of the vein to close off blood flow
- *Electrodessication*—applying electrical current to close off veins
- *Laser therapy*—use of laser beams to close off veins

The VNUS closure is a new technique for the treatment of superficial varicose veins. It is minimally invasive. A thin catheter is inserted into the vein, and the catheter delivers radio-frequency energy to the vein wall, causing it to heat, collapse, and seal shut. This procedure should be coded 36475–36476. Many payers consider this procedure to be experimental, so it should be preauthorized before performing it to ensure coverage.

> INTERNET RESOURCE: To view varicose and spider
> veins and read about common treatments, go to
> www.veinclinics.com

Hemangiomas and Arteriovenous Malformations

There are two prominent vascular anomalies that often require surgical intervention: hemangioma and venous malformations. Hemangiomas (often called *birthmarks* or *port-wine stains*) are benign neoplasms comprised of capillaries and venules in superficial and/or deep dermis, most often of the head and neck. In some cases, hemangiomas can be life threatening or severely problematic (interfering with eating, breathing, seeing, hearing, speaking, etc.) and require immediate aggressive intervention. Venous malformations are abnormal collections of dilated blood vessels (arteries, veins, capillaries) and lymphatic vessels that are present at birth. These anomalies, hemangiomas and venous malformations, can be treated in many ways: laser therapy (17106–17108), embolization (36475–36479, 37241–37244), or sclerotherapy (36468–36471). Treatment depends on the type of anomaly. Laser therapy is the method of choice for capillary malformations because they tend to be flat. Embolization is a way of occluding (closing) one or more blood vessels with various substances (e.g., alcohol, glue, oil) and it is also used to treat arterial malformations. Sclerotherapy is often used to treat venous malformations by injecting clotting material.

CHECKPOINT 16.7

Use the CPT book to assign codes to the following statements. Do not forget to append modifiers if needed. Some of the following procedures require two codes. (*Hint:* For endoscopic procedures, read the notes before the endoscopic code group carefully.)

1. Ligation of secondary varicose veins, left and right legs _____

2. Excision of infected abdominal graft, surgical care only _____

3. Patient is placed on heart/lung bypass and the main pulmonary artery is opened in order to remove the blockage and interior lining of the artery. The artery was then sutured closed and the pulmonary endarterectomy was accomplished. _____

4. Insertion of transvenous electrodes for dual-chamber pacing cardioverter-defibrillator

_____

HEMIC AND LYMPHATIC SYSTEMS; MEDIASTINUM AND DIAPHRAGM

Codes in these subsections encompass procedures on the spleen, bone marrow, lymph nodes, mediastinum, and diaphragm. Common procedures are splenectomy, lymph node biopsy, lymph node excision, and bone marrow transplants. Procedures performed on the hemic and lymphatic system are further discussed in Chapter 20 of this text.

Lymph Node Biopsy

Lymph node biopsy is removal of part of a lymph node for examination as opposed to complete removal of the entire node. Biopsies may be performed open (38500–38530) or laparoscopically (38570–38589). About 30% of the body's lymph nodes are located in the head and neck; however, keep in mind that lymph nodes are located throughout the body. Coders must pay attention to the site of the biopsy/excision and the depth (superficial or deep). Coders then must determine if the biopsy was performed via needle aspiration, skin incision, or laparoscopically. Lymphadenectomy refers to removal of one or more lymph nodes. The term "complete" when describing neck dissection is synonymous with "radical." When a radical dissection is carried out, all lymph nodes in that area are removed. If a complete cervical lymphadenectomy was performed, all lymph nodes in the five lymphatic regions of the neck would be removed. Lymphadenectomy is different from excision of lymph nodes in the code range 38500–38555.

DIGESTIVE SYSTEM

The Digestive System subsection encompasses many parts of the body, beginning with the lips and mouth and ending with the anus. Box 16.11 lists the headings located in this section. Procedures performed on the digestive system are further discussed in Chapter 21 of this text.

BOX 16.11 Digestive Section Headings	
Lips	Intestines (Except Rectum)
Vestibule of Mouth	Meckel's Diverticulum and the Mesentery
Tongue and Floor of Mouth	Appendix
Dentoalveolar Structures	Rectum
Palate and Uvula	Anus
Salivary Gland and Ducts	Liver
Pharynx, Adenoids, and Tonsils	Biliary Tract
Esophagus	Pancreas
Stomach	Abdomen, Peritoneum, and Omentum

Also included are procedures on internal organs that aid in digestion such as the pancreas, appendix, gallbladder, and liver. Many of the procedures performed on the digestive system are done endoscopically such as colonoscopy, cholecystectomy, appendectomy, hernia repair, and esophagogastroduodenoscopy (EGD). The open procedure codes for a site cannot be assigned to describe a closed procedure of the same site (i.e., percutaneously performed or done by endoscope), and open procedure codes cannot be used if the procedure was done laparoscopically.

■ **CASE SCENARIO**
A patient is seen for an open gastric Roux-en-Y bypass (43846) for morbid obesity. The patient previously had an adjustable gastric band placed with subpar weight-loss results. The surgeon must remove the gastric band before proceeding to the gastric bypass. The band is

CPT © 2017 American Medical Association, All Rights Reserved.

Tonsils and Adenoids

Tonsillectomy and adenoidectomy codes are considered bilateral, so do not use a −50 modifier. Pay close attention to the age of the patient because codes for this procedure are age specific. There are codes for removing tonsils and adenoids together and codes for removing them separately. Make sure you know which was removed and verify that with the pathology report. After codes 42830–42836, the word *primary* or *secondary* appears. A primary procedure is when the designated procedure has not been performed prior to the current episode of care. Secondary means that this procedure has been performed in the past and the tissue has regrown.

Lips

Be careful when coding procedures involving lips. If the incision or repair crosses the vermilion border, this falls into the digestive category. If it does not cross this border, it would be classified in the Integumentary section.

Esophagogastroduodenoscopy

EGD codes are chosen based on whether the procedure was a diagnostic or surgical procedure. The coder must read the procedure to verify that the scope passed through the stomach into the duodenum. If not, the procedure is not an EGD and is coded as an upper endoscopy. Fluoroscopy may be used to verify positioning of devices introduced into the esophagus. See code series 43200–43273 for notations to code radiological supervision/interpretation.

Appendectomy

This can be done open (44950–44960) or laparoscopic (44970–44979). Incidental appendectomies are not coded separately with other open abdominal procedures. If the appendix is removed for an indicated purpose, it can be coded separately using 44955 in addition to another major surgery.

Colonoscopy

To code colonoscopies correctly, coders must first read the endoscopy report and determine how much of the bowel was visualized and where and how the scope was inserted. The scope can be inserted through the rectum or through a colostomy or colotomy. Second, the coder must determine if the procedure was diagnostic or surgical in nature. A diagnostic colonoscopy does not entail obtaining any biopsies or removal of polyps. A biopsy involves obtaining a sample of tissue, not removing the entire lesion or polyp. Various methods are used to obtain biopsies and remove polyps, each of which has a respective code assignment.

Check with the patient's insurance carrier for colonoscopy medical policies. Some carriers require a −52 modifier instead of the −53 modifier.

EXAMPLE

45380, *Colonoscopy, flexible, proximal to splenic flexure with biopsy,* should be reported for the removal of a portion of a polyp. Code 45385 is used when the entire polyp is removed by the snare technique.

A colonoscopy is coded if the scope is passed beyond the splenic flexure or beyond more than 60 cm of colon. If a patient is scheduled for and fully prepped for a colonoscopy and the scope is not passed beyond the splenic flexure due to unforeseen circumstances, report code 45378 with a −53 modifier per the endoscopy instructions located in this section.

Colonoscopy With Polyp Removal

Polyp removal is reported when the entire polyp is removed. More than one method of removal may be used. When different polyps are removed by *different* techniques/methods, report each technique but watch for different techniques incorporated into one code.

EXAMPLE

If a polyp is completely removed from the ascending colon using the snare technique and a second polyp is removed using hot biopsy forceps, both codes (45384 and 45385) are reported.

If several polyps are removed by the *same* technique, the appropriate code is only reported once because the CPT code descriptions indicate more than one tumor, polyp, or lesion. If one polyp, tumor, or lesion is removed with both snare and hot biopsy techniques, report only the code for the snare technique.

Hemorrhoidectomy

A hemorrhoidectomy can be achieved by surgically excising the hemorrhoid, attaching rubber bands, or using a laser. Complex hemorrhoids are bleeding, prolapsed, or thrombosed or require plastic skin closure (e.g., anoplasty). An important note is located beneath code 46262 referring the reader to various codes according to the procedure performed.

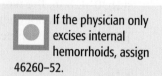 If the physician only excises internal hemorrhoids, assign 46260–52.

Cholecystectomy

This procedure involves removing the gallbladder. This can be performed as an open (47600–47620) or laparoscopic (47562–47570) procedure. Removal includes destruction by morcellation coagulation, a laser technique.

Hernia Repairs

There are several types of hernias, including inguinal, umbilical, and incisional. Each has its own code assignment. Pay close attention to whether the hernia is an initial hernia or a recurrent one and whether it is incarcerated or reducible. Inguinal hernias can be repaired with an open or laparoscopic procedure. Be careful not to code insertion of mesh for any hernia repair other than the incisional or ventral hernia. A separate code for the mesh (49568) is used in addition to the code for incisional and ventral hernia repairs *only*. Many terms are used to describe the types and locations of hernias:

- Inguinal—common hernia of the inguinal canal in the groin
- Lumbar—a very rare hernia occurring in the lumbar region of the torso
- Incisional—hernia occurring at the site of a previous incision
- Femoral—common hernia occurring in the femoral canal in the groin
- Epigastric (umbilical)—hernia located above the navel or inside of the belly button indentation
- Spigelian hernia—usually located above the inferior epigastric vessel along the outer border of the rectus muscle
- Hiatal hernia—occurs when a part of the stomach slides above the diaphragm
- Reducible—hernia in which the organs can be returned to normal position by the surgeon manipulating the viscera

---

CHECKPOINT 16.8

Use the CPT book to assign codes to the following statements. Do not forget to append modifiers if needed. Some of the following procedures require two codes. (*Hint:* For endoscopic procedures, read the notes before the endoscopic code group carefully.)

1. Secondary adenoidectomy, 10-year-old patient _____

2. Endoscopic placement of gastrostomy tube with radiological S&I _____

3. Simple ileostomy revision _____

URINARY SYSTEM

The urinary system is responsible for maintaining a steady balance in the fluid and chemical composition of the blood and for disposing of waste products from the blood. This system consists of the kidneys, ureters, bladder, and urethra. A common acronym used in this specialty is *KUB* for kidneys, ureters, and bladder. Box 16.12 lists the headings in this section. Procedures on the urinary system are further discussed in Chapter 22 of this text.

This section's subheadings are further subdivided following the consistent theme of incision, excision, introduction, repair, and laparoscopy. Many diagnostic procedure codes located in this section evaluate the functionality of the urinary system, such as flow of urine, volume, pressure, and muscle function. The body has two kidneys and two ureters, so the –50 modifier is appended if procedures are performed on both sides. Pay close attention to the site where the procedure is being performed. It is easy to confuse urethra and ureter.

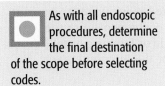 As with all endoscopic procedures, determine the final destination of the scope before selecting codes.

Procedures in this section range from minor procedures such as treatment of ureter and urethral strictures, dilation of the bladder, and biopsy of the bladder to more complex operations including removal of kidney stones, tumor removals, suspension procedures for urinary incontinence, and kidney transplants. Many of the procedures involve inserting a cystoscope in which the procedure is carried out through the scope.

Endoscopy

Codes for cystoscopy and urethroscopy are combined under the term *cystourethroscopy*. Many procedures can be done via the cystourethroscope, so the coder must choose carefully among the many codes available and the site of the cystourethroscopy (e.g., bladder, urethra, ureter). The terms *cystoscopy, urethroscopy,* and *cystourethroscopy* are used interchangeably. Be sure to identify how the scope is inserted. Was it inserted transurethrally or through an existing stoma?

Foreign Body Removal

Code range 52310–52315 includes any substance not native or natural to the urethra or bladder such as a stone, catheter tip, or stent. A simple procedure usually lasts less than 15 minutes in duration. Wording to look for to determine whether to assign a simple or complicated code includes large, numerous calculus, condition of the foreign body, and location of the stent.

Prostate Procedures

Prostate surgery is commonly performed cystoscopically. Codes are designated by treatment method. The prostate may be treated by various methods such as microwave thermotherapy or laser vaporization. Some of the prostate procedures are carried out endoscopically while others are performed open.

MALE GENITAL SYSTEM

The male reproductive system consists of the penis, testicles (epididymis, scrotum, vas deferens, spermatic cord, seminal vesicles), and prostate. Box 16.13 provides a listing of the male genital system section headings.

Procedures located in this section encompass treatment for undescended testicles, orchiectomy, vasectomy, hydrocele, spermatocele, circumcision, and lesions of the penis. Some of the procedures in this section are differentiated by age. Many procedures on the male anatomy are found in the urinary section of the CPT manual. When coding procedures involving the male genitourinary system, combination coding may occur, with codes being assigned from both the Urology and the Male Genital System sections. Procedures on the male genital system are discussed further in Chapter 23 of this text.

Orchiopexy

Sometimes the testicle does not descend into the scrotum and remains in the pelvis. Surgery is performed to pull the testicle down and secure it in the scrotum. Pay close attention to which testicle is being repaired (left, right, or both) and how the surgery is performed because more than one technique can be used to perform an orchiopexy. Laparoscopic orchiopexy is reported with 54692.

Destruction of Lesions

Lesions are typically destroyed by laser. These codes are designated as simple or extensive. If there are more than just a few lesions, if more time than usual was required, if the lesions were large, if different methods of destruction are used, or if they are on different parts of the penis, use the extensive code. As a stated rule, when assigning destruction of lesions on male or female genitals, always assign a code from the male or female genital system section and not the integumentary section, because they are more specific to the body system.

Orchiectomy

There are times when a testis must be removed for treatment of testicular cancer or prophylactically due to cancer of other parts of the male reproductive system (prostate). Sometimes only a partial orchiectomy is required for other problems associated with the testicle. Orchiectomy can also be done laparoscopically using 54690.

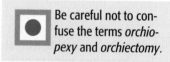 Be careful not to confuse the terms *orchiopexy* and *orchiectomy*.

Circumcision

The surgeon removes the foreskin by excising the skin. When assigning a code, read the operative note to determine the method used. There are two methods: excision or use of clamps. The age of the patient also plays a role in correct code choice. A newborn is a baby who is up to 28 days old.

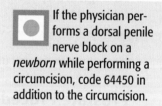 If the physician performs a dorsal penile nerve block on a *newborn* while performing a circumcision, code 64450 in addition to the circumcision.

Sterilization (Vasectomy)

The vas deferens are cut to permanently sterilize the male. In some cases, men change their mind and want to be able to procreate again. A vasovasostomy or vasovasorrhaphy is performed to reconnect the vas deferens (55400). This code is inherently bilateral so no –50 modifier is necessary.

CHECKPOINT 16.9

Use the CPT book to assign codes to the following statements. Do not forget to append modifiers if needed.

1. Discontinued contact laser vaporization of prostate _____

2. Incisional biopsy of testis followed by radical orchiectomy for tumor, inguinal approach

   _____

3. Simple electrodesiccation of four lesions on penis _____

4. Radical perineal prostatectomy _____

FEMALE GENITAL SYSTEM; MATERNITY CARE AND DELIVERY

When a pelvic exam is performed in conjunction with a gynecological procedure, the pelvic exam is not billed separately.

The female genital/reproductive system is much more complex than the male system and consists of the following: uterus, ovary, fallopian tubes, vagina, vulva, clitoris, vestibule (urethral meatus, Bartholin's and Skene's glands, and the vaginal orifice). The Female Genital System section is subdivided into seven sections (Box 16.14). There are two ovaries and two fallopian tubes so when procedures are performed on both sides, a –50 modifier is appended. There is one exception to this—sterilization, the code for which is inherently bilateral. Some of the procedures located in this section include ovarian cystectomy, lysis of pelvic adhesions, hysterectomy, dilation and curettage (D&C), removal of genital lesions, and sterilization. Many of the procedures performed on the female abdomen can be done laparoscopically, hysteroscopically, or by colposcopy, instead of the traditional open method. Laparoscopic procedures are performed using trocars and cannulas inserted into the abdomen, allowing for use of a scope to repair, excise, and evaluate abdominal and pelvic contents. A hysteroscope is used to visualize the uterine contents and perform diagnostic and therapeutic procedures such as D&C and removal of uterine fibroids. Pay close attention to the approach in the operative note. To code from this section, the coder should have a good foundation of anatomy and know the differences between the vulva, labia, vagina, and other organs. Female genital and obstetrical coding is discussed in greater detail in Chapter 24 of this text.

BOX 16.14 Female Genital Section Headings

Vulva, Perineum, and Introitus	Oviduct/Ovary
Vagina	Ovary
Cervix Uteri	In Vitro Fertilization
Corpus Uteri	

Laser Ablation of the Cervix

This procedure is performed to destroy precancerous changes in cervical tissue. At times, the dysplasia converts to carcinoma in situ of the cervix. Treatment typically is laser ablation of the cervix (LAC) 57513 or cold knife conization (CKC) 57520. If conization was done via a loop electrosurgical excision of the cervix (LEEP), use code 57522.

Sterilization

The sterilization procedure is often referred to as "tying tubes." Pay attention to the method used, because it can be either laparoscopic or open. Varying methods exist to achieve this. Sometimes the fallopian tubes are clamped with Hulka clamps or they are cut and fulgurated (cauterized). Material may be placed inside the fallopian tube to provide a mechanical occlusion.

Lesion Removal From Vulva

Lesions can be biopsied and/or removed. There are times when destruction of a lesion is appropriate, as in condyloma (56501–56515). See the definitions at the beginning of the lesion removal section to help you determine the extent of the vulvectomy.

Maternity Care and Delivery

Uncomplicated maternity care includes routine antepartum, delivery, and postpartum care. This is called the *maternity* or *OB package*. The concept of this package is that the physician will be paid for the approximate 10 months of care in one payment. It is very important to understand the definitions of each of the following:

- *Antepartum care/period* includes initial and subsequent H&P; measurement of weight, BP, and fetal heart tones; routine chemical urinalysis; monthly visits up to 28 weeks and biweekly visits up to 36 weeks; and weekly visits until delivery. All E/M services pertaining to these services are included. Any visits during this period other than those listed would be reported separately.

- *Delivery services* include admission to the hospital; admission H&P; and management of uncomplicated labor, vaginal delivery, or C-section. Delivery of placenta, induction of labor with Pitocin, artificial rupture of membranes (AROM), and vacuum extraction are all considered part of the delivery package and are not coded separately.
- *Postpartum care/period* includes hospital and office visits following delivery.

Before assigning any delivery codes, verify if the patient had a previous C-section or not. If so, very specific codes in the 59610–59622 range must be used indicating this. These may indicate a vaginal delivery after a previous C-section (VBAC) or an attempted vaginal delivery after C-section completed by C-section, and so on.

There are instances when a physician may only provide one or two of the three phases of obstetrical care (antepartum, delivery, postpartum). In such a case, assign the code as appropriate for the extent of the care provided.

> ▢ Episiotomy or vaginal repair performed by a consulting physician is reported with 59300. If performed by the attending physician, it is included in the OB package for the vaginal delivery.

■ **CASE SCENARIO**

Suzie Q saw Dr. Lee for 7 months of her pregnancy but then her husband got transferred out of state. She resumed her care with Dr. Shaw for the remaining 2 months and subsequent delivery and postpartum visit. Dr. Lee would bill 59426 and Dr. Shaw would bill 59425 and 59410.

NOTE: Maternity is discussed further in Chapter 24.

Abortion

Codes exist for the treatment of blighted ovum, incomplete abortion (spontaneous miscarriages), and elective abortions. Pay attention to the stage of the pregnancy (first or second trimester, etc.) and whether the abortion was missed or incomplete. A *missed abortion* is the retention of the products of conception after fetal death prior to 22 weeks of gestation. A blighted ovum would be considered a missed abortion because the mother did not begin to expel any products of conception. An *incomplete abortion* is where the woman begins to miscarry but does not expel all the products of conception. *Induced abortion* is the elective termination of pregnancy prior to 22 weeks' gestation via D&C, dilation and evacuation (D&E), intra-amniotic injections, or vaginal suppositories. Codes 59840–59841 should not be used for the completion of a spontaneous abortion. Use 59812 for this service.

CHECKPOINT 16.10

Use the CPT book to assign codes to the following statements. Do not forget to append modifiers if needed.

1. Routine obstetric care/vaginal delivery, previous cesarean delivery _____

2. Missed abortion surgically completed in first trimester _____

3. Cesarean delivery, including postpartum care, and total hysterectomy following attempted vaginal delivery; patient had previous cesarean delivery _____

4. D&C, postpartum hemorrhage _____

5. Simple destruction of four lesions, vulva _____

CPT © 2017 American Medical Association, All Rights Reserved.

NERVOUS SYSTEM

This section is subdivided into three main sections, as listed in Box 16.15. It is further subdivided into sections specific to skull-based surgery, neurostimulator insertions, aneurysm repair, shunt insertions, laminectomies, and nerve injections and repairs.

BOX 16.15 Nervous System Section Headings

Skull, Meninges, and Brain

Spine and Spinal Cord

Extracranial Nerves, Peripheral Nerves, and Autonomic Nervous System

---

This section is truly dedicated to the subspecialty of neurosurgery; therefore, codes from this section would be reported by neurosurgeons with the exception of nerve injections, epidural injections, and nerve repairs. It is very common for neurosurgeons to utilize an assistant surgeon because of the tedious nature of procedures involving the brain and spine, allowing for modifier –80 usage. At times, orthopedic surgeons and neurosurgeons will perform complex spinal column procedures where each physician will carry out very specific procedures independently of the other and utilize the –62 modifier. The majority of procedures located here would be very difficult for an entry-level coder to assign.

Pain management is a growing subspecialty of neurology, and anesthesia and is widely accepted as treatment for disk herniations, radiculopathy, and intractable pain. Pain management codes encompass epidural steroid injections, nerve injections and destructions, neurostimulator insertion, pain pump insertions, and intricate epidural catheter insertions involving heating the intervertebral disk. As with the Cardiovascular section, additional codes may be located in the Medicine section for services performed, such as neurostimulator programming and electromyography. Many of the procedures performed in this section require the use of a surgical microscope to visualize nerves and intricate anatomy. Pay close attention to the code descriptions in this area because some include the use of the microscope whereas others do not. CPT code 69990 is assigned when microsurgical dissection or microsurgical repair of a nerve is done unless the code description already includes this.

An anatomy book is very helpful in this section when determining which nerves are peripheral, cranial, and spinal. It is also invaluable when visualizing the spine and its vertebrae.

Spinal Injections and Pain Management

Spinal injections are commonly performed for diagnostic and therapeutic purposes for patients with chronic back pain. Injections are performed typically after all conservative measures have been taken and the pain persists. Types of injections include trigger point injections, hypertonic saline injections for epidural lysis of adhesions, epidural steroid injections, spinal nerve blocks, and facet joint injections.

To correctly code spine injections or pain blocks, the coder must determine at least the following three things: what was injected (steroid or anesthetic), where the needle was inserted (cervical, thoracic, or lumbar), and if it was a single injection or a continuous infusion or regional injection. A list of common steroids and anesthetics is provided in Box 16.16. The documentation needs to support the codes. See codes 62320 and 62324 for an example.

BOX 16.16 Examples of Anesthetic Agents and Steroids

Anesthetics

Lidocaine, bupivacaine (Marcaine, Sensorcaine), ropivacaine (Naropin), morphine (Duramorph)

Steroids

methylprednisolone (Solu-Medro), triamcinolone (Aristocort, Kenalog, Aristospan), Depo-Medrol

---

Nerve Blocks

Peripheral nerves are injected for pain management purposes. For example, the greater occipital nerve is injected for chronic or ongoing headaches. Surgeons commonly inject nerves as a post-op pain control method. Injections are also performed in the sympathetic nerves (stellate ganglions) for analgesia.

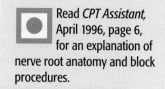
Read *CPT Assistant*, April 1996, page 6, for an explanation of nerve root anatomy and block procedures.

Transcutaneous Electrical Nerve Stimulator

In a transcutaneous electrical nerve stimulation (TENS) procedure, electrodes attached to a battery pack are placed on the skin to stimulate the muscles and nerves. This is used routinely for sprains and strains of the back and neck and may be used in physical therapy or performed during chiropractic treatment. Do not forget to capture the HCPCS code for the actual unit provided—E0720, E0730, or A4595.

Blood Patch

This is carried out for treatment of spinal fluid leakage following a lumbar puncture or epidural injection. Blood is drawn from the patient's arm and injected into the epidural space. It is very common to develop a postdural puncture headache after having a myelogram done or after having an epidural placed for labor and delivery.

Lumbar Puncture

This is also known as a *spinal tap*. This procedure is performed for diagnostic purposes when spinal fluid is needed for analysis. A needle is inserted into the subarachnoid space in the lumbar region. The color of the fluid can indicate hemorrhage, infection, or other complication. Sometimes, a therapeutic spinal puncture to drain excess fluid off the spine is required for a condition known as *pseudotumor cerebri*. This is not done for the same reasons a diagnostic lumbar puncture is performed. Assign 62272 for this service.

Chemodenervation

Chemodenervation involves injecting a chemical substance to interrupt nerve function. This type of injection is not being performed for cosmetic purpose but rather for treatment of neurological disorders such as tics. It does not matter how many injections are performed or how many muscles are injected, the code is only assigned once per session. You must also assign the HCPCS code for the drug injected.

Neurosurgery

Neurolysis

This involves injecting a nerve with a neurolytic agent (alcohol, phenol, iced saline, ethanol) to destroy the nerve. This is provided to patients with chronic pain and those with cerebral palsy who have muscle spasms. You must determine the targeted nerve and whether a single nerve or multilevel injection was done. Pay attention to the code descriptions to determine if they are unilateral or bilateral.

Nerve Decompression

Nerve decompression, transposition, or neuroplasty is the freeing of an intact nerve from scar tissue or entrapment. It can also be called *neurolysis*, so be careful. You must read the operative note to determine if the nerve was moved or if it was injected.

EYE AND OCULAR ADNEXA; AUDITORY SYSTEM; OPERATING MICROSCOPE

Codes in this section include procedures on the eyeball, anterior and posterior segment, ocular adnexa, and conjunctiva and procedures on the inner and outer ear. The codes are arranged by anatomical part and then by procedure on that part. Box 16.17 lists the headings for this section.

For the most part, the outline of this section follows the template used in other sections, grouping procedures by incision, excision, repair, and other procedures. Typical procedures performed on the eye are foreign body removal, cataract removal, glaucoma surgery, laser surgery for vision correction, strabismus surgery on the muscles of the eye, and retinal procedures. Codes for examinations of the eye are captured in the Medicine section.

Codes for the auditory system include procedures on the external ear, middle ear, inner ear, and temporal bone. Common procedures performed on the ear are foreign body removal, insertion of ventilation tubes, tympanoplasty, and cochlear implants. The microscope code 69990 may be assigned in addition to the procedure codes in some circumstances. Notes located prior to code 69990 explain that this code should not be assigned in addition to procedures where use of the microscope is an inclusive component. Procedures on the eye and ear are discussed further in Chapter 26 of this text.

Eye

Procedures and services in this section are performed by an ophthalmologist and never by an optometrist. When coding procedures for eyes and eyelids, be sure to remember to use modifiers. HCPCS Level II modifiers are required for use when billing eyelid procedures (E1, E2, etc.). Remember to use the −50 modifier when coding procedures on both eyes. Some procedure code descriptions in this section are specific to whether a patient has had prior surgery on the eye. Be sure to read the parenthetical notes following codes. These are your instructions for going to other sections of the CPT if necessary to capture all services provided and to select the most appropriate anatomical code.

Foreign Body Removal

For foreign body removal from the eye, codes are differentiated by compartment of the eye and whether a corneal slit lamp is used. Numerous notes related to this that provide instructions on code assignment are located prior to code 65205.

Cataract

When coding cataracts, the coder must determine what type of procedure was performed. Three different methods of cataract extraction are used: intracapsular (ICCE), extracapsular (ECCE), and extracapsular complex requiring devices not routinely used in cataract surgery. Routine cataract surgery involves removing the cataract and replacing the old lens with a new lens. There are times, however, when a new lens is not placed immediately after the cataract extraction. In this case, assign code 66985 when the patient returns for the lens placement. It is not uncommon for patients to come in and have the newly implanted lens exchanged (66986) due to failure of the implant or to have it repositioned (66825).

Lesion Removals

If the excision involves only skin of the eyelid, use a code from the Integumentary section. If it involves lid margin, tarsus, or otherwise, use codes 67840–67850, 67961–67966. Chalazion excision has its own code assignment (67800–67808).

Glaucoma Surgery

Glaucoma is a condition in which the aqueous humour cannot drain from the anterior segment of the eye. There are two types of glaucoma surgery: laser and incisional. Trabeculoplasty, iridotomy, and iridoplasty are laser treatments. Trabeculectomy is an incisional procedure that basically creates a drain for the aqueous humour. This procedure is usually performed ab externo—from the outside of the eye. At times when a trabeculectomy is not indicated, an aqueous humour shunt may be placed. This tube is placed into the anterior chamber between the cornea and the iris.

Vision Correction Surgery

Many people are taking advantage of the availability of technological advances to eliminate the need for glasses. Two procedures are done frequently to correct vision by altering the surface of the cornea: photorefractive keratectomy (PRK) and laser-assisted in situ keratomileusis (LASIK).

Ear

The ear is a paired body part and would require the use of the LT or RT modifiers with code assignment.

Foreign Body Removal

It is very common for children to place objects (peas, crayons, beads, etc.) in their ears that become lodged there. More often than not, this requires surgical removal under anesthesia (69200–69205).

Ventilation Tube Insertion

One treatment for otitis media is insertion of tubes in the tympanic membrane to promote drainage (69436). These tubes are often called *PET tubes* or *ventilation tubes*. A myringotomy alone may be done for infection where an incision is made and fluid is suctioned out and/or the eustachian tube is inflated. *This does not involve inserting tubes*. Codes from 69420–69421 are assigned instead.

Tympanoplasty

Perforation of the tympanic membrane can occur from trauma, infection, tube placement, or from foreign objects being pushed too far into the ear canal. It is not uncommon when tubes are removed for a tympanic membrane repair to be required to patch the "hole" left from the tubes. These codes are differentiated by whether the tympanic membrane was simply repaired or whether the eardrum was repaired or reconstructed.

Operating Microscope

The microscope is utilized for intricate procedures involving the eyes, ears, nerves, and vertebrae. Some carriers may consider the microscope to be an inherent portion of the surgical procedure, meaning it is routinely used and in many cases must be used to carry out the surgery. Instructional notes located prior to the 69990 code explicitly list codes where it is inappropriate to also report the use of a microscope. Read the surgical codes carefully to verify whether or not the code description includes language such as "microsurgical" or "microvascular." The prefix "micro" indicates that the use of the surgical microscope is already built into the payment for the surgical procedure and would not be reported separately. Code 69990 is reported without appending any modifier.

> ■ Do not assign 69990 unless the operative note specifies the use of a microscope. Loupes or magnifying lenses are not the same thing as a microscope.

CHECKPOINT 16.11

Assign the CPT code and applicable modifier to the following statements.

1. Extracapsular cataract removal with insertion of intraocular lens prosthesis, mechanical technique, left _____

2. Excision of scleral right lesion _____

3. Chalazion excision, right eye, during the global period of a strabismus surgery _____

4. Impacted cerumen removed from both ears _____

Chapter Summary

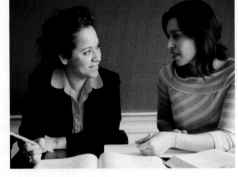

1. In general, the organization of the surgical sections in CPT follows the same format. Each section is subdivided by body areas, working from the head to the feet and then further subdivided as follows: Incision and Drainage, Biopsy, Excision, Introduction or Removal, Repair, Destruction, Endoscopy/Laparoscopy (if applicable), Other Procedures.

2. The surgical package includes local infiltration of anesthesia, any E/M visits either on the date of surgery or the day prior unless the decision for surgery was made at the time of the E/M service, immediate post-op care, writing orders, evaluating the patient in the recovery area, and any typical uncomplicated follow-up care. Follow-up care for complications, exacerbations, recurrence, and the presence of other diseases that require additional services are not included in the surgical package.

3. The major difference between the American Medical Association definition and Medicare's definition of surgical package from what is in the guidelines is the number of days pre-op and post-op that are included in the global surgery days. The national global policy for surgical procedures is a concept under which a "single fee" is billed and paid for all services furnished by the surgeon before, during, and after the procedure. This can range from 0 to 10 days for minor surgery and up to 90 days for major surgery.

4. Coders can identify whether a procedure is surgical or diagnostic by recognizing suffixes of medical terms and looking for key words discussed within the chapter that indicate the service is diagnostic or therapeutic.

5. "Separate procedure" codes are located throughout the codebook and should not be assigned if they are performed as part of a more comprehensive procedure.

6. Throughout the chapter the coder was introduced to references commonly used in assigning surgical codes; this is reinforced throughout the text. Recognizing references needed and how to use them to correctly report surgical services and modifiers is an important skill to attain. Common sources include the National Correct Coding Initiative, the Medicare Physician Fee Schedule, the *Medicare Claims Processing Manual*, National Coverage Determination, Local Coverage Determination, third-party carrier medical policies, and specialty societies.

7. Coders must pay attention to modifiers designated for physician use and those for facility use. Most of these modifiers are identical. The modifiers are located on the inside cover of the CPT codebook and labeled as such.

Review Questions

True or False

Decide whether each statement is true or false.

1. __F__ Being aware of payer coding and reporting requirements is unnecessary because it does not influence correct coding.

2. __F__ CPT modifiers are the same for both physician and outpatient facilities.

3. __F__ The modifier –51 for multiple procedures can be used in the Radiology section.

4. __T__ The modifier –50 for bilateral procedures is used to describe bilateral views (x-rays) taken of both knees (see code 73565).

5. __T__ All HCPCS Level I and II modifiers are appropriate to use for coding in all settings.

6. __F__ CPT does not have a way to capture the charges for the technical component of a procedure or service.

7. ___T___ A special report is only required when submitting a claim with an unlisted procedure code.

8. ___T___ The Neurology section of CPT is dedicated solely to neurologists and neurosurgeons, and codes from this section should not be reported by physicians of other specialties.

9. ___T___ If the procedure note indicates that the physician utilized magnifying loupes to visualize blood vessels, 69990 is reported in addition to the procedure code.

Multiple Choice

Select the letter that best completes the statement or answers the question.

1. CMS provides a Change Request transmittal that lists types of add-on codes without any primary procedure codes. Which type is correct?
   A. Type I
   B. Type II
   C. Type III
   D. Type IV

2. A designated separate procedure may be reported when (choose two answers)
   A. It is the only procedure performed
   B. It is reported with modifier 59
   C. It is performed in a separate site during the associated procedure
   D. It is an incidental procedure performed during the associated procedure

3. The Medicare Physician Fee Schedule is a tool to help the coder do the following (select all that apply):
   A. Look up codes without having to use the CPT book
   B. Determine if a code has a physician or technical component
   C. Determine if a code can be billed bilaterally
   D. Obtain the global days for a procedure
   E. Sequence codes in highest value code order

4. Select the correct code for removal of both tonsils and adenoids in a 12-year-old patient.
   A. 42836
   B. 42826
   C. 42825
   D. 42821

5. Select the correct code for biopsy of a lesion of the earlobe.
   A. 11440
   B. 11100
   C. 69100
   D. 69105

6. Select the correct code for removal of a foreign body of the left deep calf muscle.
   A. 20525
   B. 20103
   C. 20520
   D. 11043

7. Select the correct code(s) for excision of two nasal polyps in the physician's office.
   A. 30300
   B. 30110
   C. 30115
   D. 30110, 30110–51

8. Select the correct code for drainage of a cervical lymph node abscess.
   A. 38308
   B. 38505
   C. 38300
   D. 38510

9. Select the correct code for cystotomy with excision of ureterocele, bilateral.
   A. 51530
   B. 51535–50
   C. 51065
   D. 51535

CHAPTER 17

CPT: Integumentary System

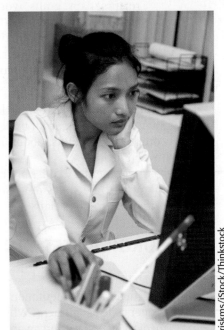

riskms/iStock/Thinkstock

CHAPTER OUTLINE

LEARNING OBJECTIVES

After studying this chapter, you should be able to:

1. Define the surgical procedures common to the integumentary system: incision and drainage, biopsy, destruction, debridement, excision, repair, and Mohs micrographic surgery.
2. Differentiate among simple, intermediate, and complex wound repairs.
3. Explain guidelines for coding excision of lesions.
4. Accurately calculate measurements for lesion excisions.
5. Differentiate among the various types of skin grafts.
6. Describe the difference between a flap and a graft.

7. Determine when it is appropriate to assign lesion excisions with flap and graft closure.
8. Use the Rule of Nines to assign codes for burn treatment.
9. Describe the four types of debridement codes.
10. Describe the difference between selective and nonselective wound debridement.
11. Understand both the therapeutic and cosmetic breast procedures and the methods for treatment of the breasts.

This chapter focuses on the procedural coding and terminology of surgical cases involving problems of the integumentary system. It covers anatomical structures, common conditions that are surgically treated, and surgical procedures performed on the skin and subcutaneous tissue as well as the breasts and nails. Chapter 16 introduced key CPT surgical concepts such as the surgical package, separate procedures, modifiers, global period, and recognizing when a procedure is a diagnostic or therapeutic service. This chapter introduces additional terminology that is used throughout CPT and encountered when reading surgical documentation.

Two main specialties treat diseases, disorders, and injuries of the skin and underlying tissue: dermatology, and plastic and reconstructive surgery. Dermatology is a branch of medicine that specializes in diagnosing and treating diseases and disorders of the skin, its structure, and its function; it includes nails, hair, and sweat glands. The plastic and reconstructive surgery specialty concentrates on the repair and reconstruction of defects of the integument and its underlying musculoskeletal system to restore function and appearance. Plastic surgeons perform procedures on the following body parts:

- Skin, subcutaneous tissue, and musculature (e.g., scar revisions, lesion removals, complex repairs, flaps, grafts, wound care, and tattoo removal)
- Craniofacial structures (from trauma or birth defects)
- Breast (e.g., reconstruction, reduction, and augmentation)
- Hand (e.g., injury repairs and replantation)
- Lips, palate, and oropharynx
- Microvasculature

Plastic surgeons are most known for their aesthetic or cosmetic surgery to reconstruct, smooth, augment, tighten, or lift undesirable features of one's body by performing procedures such as body contouring, facelifts, abdominoplasty (tummy tuck), rhinoplasty (nose job), and blepharoplasty (eyelid lift).

Integumentary codes are not reserved exclusively for use by dermatologists or plastic surgeons. Many of these codes are also routinely assigned by emergency department (ED) physicians and primary care physicians.

SURGICAL TERMINOLOGY

Coders are expected to have a broad knowledge of medical terminology in order to read and interpret medical documentation. Differentiating between surgical terms and techniques is paramount to proper code assignment. When assigning codes from the Surgery section, it is advantageous to have a medical dictionary and an anatomy atlas available for reference. A foundation in anatomy and medical terminology is essential when coding in general but particularly for surgical services. A coder who masters the terminology can visualize and mentally follow along with what is taking place during the surgery as documented in the medical record. This enables the coder to identify all procedures that should be coded and to recognize when a procedure is a component of a more comprehensive procedure. Knowledge of these terms also promotes efficiency in locating codes in CPT, because many of these terms are main headings or subheadings.

> Do not assign codes for documentation that contains technical words and procedures you do not understand. Take the time to look them up in references.

The terminology can seem overwhelming. When reading medical documents, coders are bound to come across words they do not recognize. Coders must at a minimum memorize basic prefixes, suffixes, and root words to be able to break complicated words into smaller parts to decipher their meaning. Some of these common terms are located near the front of the CPT manual and should be reviewed. Also review the suffixes noted in Table 17.1.

Table 17.1 Common Surgical Suffixes

SUFFIX	DEFINITION	EXAMPLE
-centesis	Puncturing a cavity to remove or inject fluid	arthrocentesis
-desis	Fixation or fusing permanently	arthrodesis
-ectomy	Partial or total removal of a body part, bone, or tissue	colectomy
-graphy	Use of x-ray or fluoroscopy for viewing anatomy during a procedure	radiography
-lysis	Destruction, breaking down, or freeing	enterolysis
-ostomy	Creating a hole or opening from the inside to the outside of the body or creating an opening within the body	colostomy
-otomy	Making an incision or opening into	laparotomy
-pexy	Surgical fixation of an organ	mastopexy
-plasty	Repair or reconstruct	mammaplasty
-rrhaphy	Use of sutures to repair or reduce	herniorrhaphy
-scopy	Surgical intervention using an endoscope to visualize internal structures	laparoscopy
-tripsy	Crushing, pulverizing, destroying	lithotripsy

Table 17.2 Directional Terms

TERM	DESCRIPTION
Anterior	Toward the front or in front of
Distal	Farthest from where that point attaches to the trunk of the body
Dorsal (dorsum)	Toward the backside of the body
Inferior	Below
Lateral	Toward the outer edges of the body or away from the middle
Medial	Toward the middle of the body
Posterior	Toward the back of or the back surface
Proximal	Closest to where that point attaches to the trunk of the body
Superior	Above
Ventral	Toward the front side of the body

Directional Terms

When coders read medical documentation, they must master medical terms describing location and direction, as shown in Table 17.2 and Figure 17.1. Directional terms are widely used in operative reports and x-rays to indicate the precise location of a body part. CPT codes also contain these terms.

EXAMPLES

- 11755 *Biopsy of nail unit (e.g., plate, bed, matrix, hyponychium, proximal and lateral nail folds) (separate procedure).*
- 11750 *Excision of nail and nail matrix, partial or complete (e.g., ingrown or deformed nail), for permanent removal; with amputation of tuft of distal phalanx.*
- 12020 *Treatment of superficial wound dehiscence; simple closure.*
- 19020 *Mastotomy with exploration or drainage of abscess, deep.*
- 49560 *Repair initial incisional or ventral hernia; reducible.*
- 54160 *Circumcision, surgical excision other than clamp, device, or dorsal slit; neonate.*
- 21282 *Lateral canthopexy.*

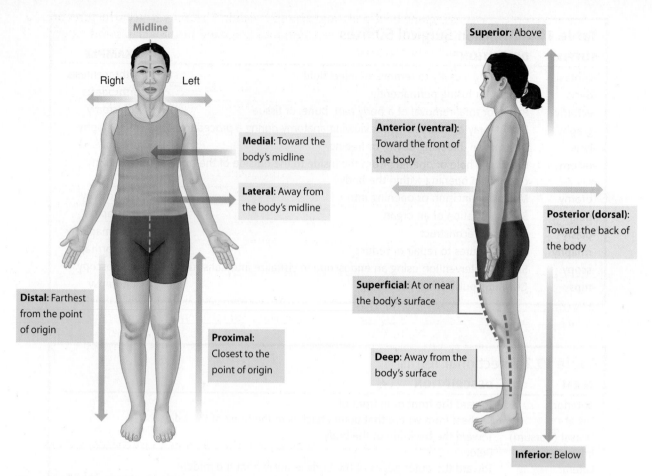

Figure 17.1 Directional terms in anatomy.

Midline

Right | Left

Medial: Toward the body's midline

Lateral: Away from the body's midline

Distal: Farthest from the point of origin

Proximal: Closest to the point of origin

Superior: Above

Anterior (ventral): Toward the front of the body

Posterior (dorsal): Toward the back of the body

Superficial: At or near the body's surface

Deep: Away from the body's surface

Inferior: Below

INTEGUMENTARY ANATOMY

When reading an operative note, the coder must be able to recognize what type of repair was performed or how deep a debridement was based on the anatomical landmarks and descriptions. Recognition begins with the basic anatomy of the skin, as shown in Figure 17.2.

The integument is made up of two parts: the cutaneous membrane, or skin, and the accessory structures. The cutaneous membrane is made up of two layers: epidermis or superficial epithelium (epithelial tissues) and the dermis, which is composed of connective tissues. The epidermis is the outside layer of skin. The dermis, or dermal layer, is the second layer of skin containing blood vessels (capillaries), hair follicles, nerves, and glands. The dermal layer is dense with connective tissue and is woven to this subcutaneous layer to secure the skin in place, stabilizing the position of the skin but allowing separate movement. It is strong from the collagen fibers and elastic, with water aiding in flexibility. Bruises visible in the skin are the result of damage to the tiny capillaries. Below the dermis is a subcutaneous layer of loose connective tissue, also known as the *superficial fascia* or *hypodermis*. The subcutaneous layer contains mostly fat cells and superficial fascia. The hypodermis is not technically part of the integumentary system, despite its name.

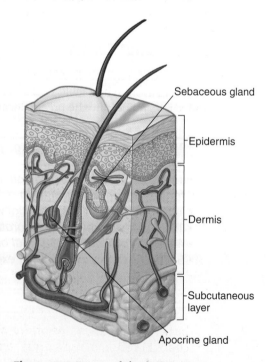

Sebaceous gland

Epidermis

Dermis

Subcutaneous layer

Apocrine gland

Figure 17.2 Layers of the integument.

The accessory structures include hair, nails, and exocrine glands. These accessory structures are considered part of the integumentary system, because they originate in the dermis and extend through the epidermis to the skin's surface.

The skin is the largest organ of the body and performs these functions:

- Protects the body as a barrier against the environment, fluid loss, abrasion, and shock
- Maintains body temperature by keeping in heat and allowing sweat out to cool the body
  - Produces vitamin D_3
  - Stores lipids

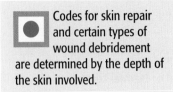
Codes for skin repair and certain types of wound debridement are determined by the depth of the skin involved.

The skin repairs minor abrasions and injuries itself. Cells from the epidermis break away and form a sheet across the wound. For deeper wounds, a clot forms in the wound bed, and blood flow increases, bringing cells into the wound to form a scab. Granulation tissue fills the wound and there is intense growth of epithelial cells beneath the scab.

INTEGUMENTARY ORGANIZATION

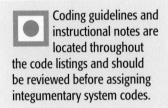
Coding guidelines and instructional notes are located throughout the code listings and should be reviewed before assigning integumentary system codes.

Integumentary codes are arranged by anatomical site and category of procedure. The main headings are Skin, Subcutaneous and Accessory Structures; Nails; Pilonidal Cyst; Introduction; Repair (Closure); Destruction; and Breast. These sections are further broken down into subheadings, as shown in Box 17.1.

MODIFIERS

Table 17.3 outlines the CPT modifiers most commonly used in the Integumentary System section and why. Documentation must support the use of the modifiers.

Note that modifier –50 is commonly misused in the Integumentary System section when reporting lesion removals or skin repairs when performed on both arms and/or both legs. The code descriptors for lesion removals and skin repairs include several body parts that are not paired body organs, so it is inappropriate to use LT or RT or –50 in these situations. You may recall that these modifiers are used when performing procedures on paired body parts or organ systems. The skin is one organ system. The code descriptions do not accommodate these modifiers because many body parts are grouped under one code and would not describe in any further detail to which one it applies.

EXAMPLE

Excision of 2.5-cm benign lesion of the right shoulder. **The correct code assignment is 11403** *Excision, benign lesion including margins, except skin tag (unless listed elsewhere), trunk, arms or legs, excised diameter 2.1 to 3.0 cm.* **Here, the RT modifier would not differentiate arms from legs. Without the operative report, the insurance carrier or other third party would not glean any clarification by appending this modifier.**

Modifier –59 is used with skin lesion excisions to identify lesions removed from separate incisions in the same body category, as in code 11403 in the previous paragraph that describes several anatomical sites. By appending modifier –59, the provider is alerting the payer that additional work was involved because each lesion was removed individually through separate incisions from a different area on the body but incorporated within the one CPT code.

Modifier –51 is also used to identify multiple procedures. For physician coders, the –51 modifier goes on any code not listed as the primary procedure, with the exception of those not permitting –51 modifier assignments such as add-on codes and those that are –51 modifier exempt.

EXAMPLE

The physician excises a 1.5-cm lesion from the left arm, a 2.0-cm lesion from the upper back, and a 1.0-cm lesion from the right leg. According to the code description in base code 11400, the back, arms, and legs are grouped into one category. A code should be submitted for each of these excisions because they were separate lesions on parts of the body requiring removal through separate incisions; they just so happen to fall into the same body category according to CPT and must be distinguished by appending the –59 modifier to the second and third codes. Codes: 11402, 11402–59, –51, 11401–59, –51.

Codes in this section would not typically be reported with global surgery modifiers –54, –55, and –56 because of the nature of the specialty and procedures performed.

COMMON DISEASES AND DISORDERS OF THE INTEGUMENT

A wide variety of conditions affect the skin, including skin injuries. The most common of these conditions are presented here. Treatments for these conditions are discussed immediately following this section. Burns, wound care, breast procedures, and cosmetic surgery are discussed separately in this chapter.

Skin Neoplasms

Benign lesions, or neoplasms, are abnormal noncancerous growths on the skin that tend not to spread to surrounding tissue. These lesions are removed because of their cosmetic appearance, suspicion of malignancy, or inconvenience of location on the skin. These include seborrheic keratosis, pigmented nevus (mole; plural *nevi*), dermatofibroma, and keratoacanthoma.

Lipomas (tumor) also fall into this category. These are benign tumors composed of fatty tissue. Code assignment is based on the location and depth of the tumor.

Malignant lesions or neoplasms are cancerous lesions and are dangerous because of their unregulated growth and invasion of nearby tissues (e.g., basal cell carcinoma, melanoma, squamous cell carcinoma) and must be removed.

Other Nonneoplastic Lesions and Growths

BOX 17.1 Integumentary System Sections and Subsections
Skin, Subcutaneous, and Accessory Structures
Introduction and Removal
Incision and Drainage
Debridement
Paring or Cutting
Biopsy
Removal of Skin Tags
Shaving of Epidermal or Dermal Lesions
Excision—Benign Lesions
Excision—Malignant Lesions
Nails
Pilonidal Cyst
Introduction
Repair (closure)
Repair—Simple
Repair—Intermediate
Repair—Complex
Adjacent Tissue Transfer or Rearrangement
Skin Replacement Surgery
Surgical Preparation
Autografts/Tissue Cultured Autograft
Skin Substitute Grafts
Flaps (Skin and/or Deep Tissues)
Other Flaps and Grafts
Other Procedures
Pressure Ulcers (Decubitus Ulcers)
Burns, Local Treatment
Destruction
Destruction, Benign or Premalignant Lesions
Destruction, Malignant Lesions, Any Method
Mohs Micrographic Surgery
Other Procedures
Breast
Incision
Excision
Introduction
Mastectomy Procedures
Repair and/or Reconstruction
Other Procedures

Lesion is a "catchall" word for many things removed from the body. This is a universal term to look up in CPT in lieu of the following words: macule, papule, nodule, plaque, wheal, vesicle, bulla, scales, fissure, crust, erosion, ulcer, atrophy, scars, and warts. The term *lesion* is used to locate procedure codes in the CPT Index because entries for individual skin ailments are not usually indexed. Scars are revised surgically to reduce disfigurement or to improve function when a scar limits

Table 17.3 Integumentary System Modifiers

MODIFIER	DESCRIPTION	USAGE
–25	Significant, separately identifiable evaluation and management (E/M) service by the same physician on the same day of the procedure or other service	Typically used to differentiate a lesion removal, biopsy, and wound care from the E/M service
–50	Bilateral procedure	Used to report procedures of the breast
–51	Multiple procedures	Used to report subsequent procedures excluding add-on or modifier –51 exempt codes
–52	Reduced services	Used to report any service that was not carried out to the fullest extent of the code. A portion of a procedure may have been eliminated or partially completed.
–58	Staged or related procedure or service by the same physician during the postoperative period	Used to report staged breast reconstruction or skin grafting (particularly the cultured skin grafts)
–59	Distinct procedural service	Commonly used to report skin lesion removals, repairs, or grafts when removing and repairing body areas that are combined in one code descriptor
–78	Unplanned return to the operating room by the same physician for a related procedure during the postoperative period	May be required for postoperative complications such as hematoma, graft failure, or infection
–79	Unrelated procedure or service by the same physician during the postoperative period	Used to report tissue transfers following Mohs procedures and different sites of treatment from the original procedure done in the global period of the original procedure
–80	Assistant surgeon	Some surgeries allow for reporting of an assistant surgeon. Double check the Medicare Physician Fee Schedule (MPFS) to confirm if the procedure allows for an assistant first.
E1, E2, E3, E4	Upper and lower right and left eyelids	Blepharoplasties. Do not use for eyelid lesion removals or repair.

Medicare has national and local medical necessity policies that regulate surgical removal of skin lesions with restrictions on the size and diagnosis and method of removal. Removal of certain benign skin lesions that do not pose a threat to health or function are considered cosmetic and are not covered by Medicare.

the flexibility of the skin. Warts are products of viral infection. Growths include verruca vulgaris (common wart), condyloma acuminatum (genital wart), and molluscum contagiosum. Molluscum contagiosum is a highly contagious skin condition that presents as discrete pimple-like skin eruptions or a small, flat rash with tiny flesh-colored bumps. It hides from the immune system and spreads by physical contact with the waxy core, which is located inside the lesion.

Abscesses

An abscess is a circumscribed collection of pus of any size in any location, and represents an infection. Abscesses usually have one or more of these symptoms: redness, warmth, tenderness, fluctuance, edema, or lymphangitis. Various types of abscesses are carbuncles, suppurative hidradenitis, cysts, furuncles, postoperative wound infections, or paronychia. Treatment for an abscess(es) is (are) to incise and drain it, as discussed later in this chapter.

Cysts

Cysts are soft, raised cavities usually filled with a liquid or semisolid material. These are usually caused by infection, the presence of a foreign body, or blockage of a gland. Cysts can either be excised or incised and drained. Common types of cysts are sebaceous and epidermoid cysts.

Hidradenitis

Hidradenitis is a chronic abscessing and subsequent infection of the sweat gland in the axilla, groin, or abdomen. Codes for this are provided at the end of the skin, subcutaneous, and accessory structures section.

Pilonidal Cyst or Sinus

A pilonidal cyst is an abscess, a pocket of pus below the skin. It consists of entrapped epidermal tissue. A sinus cavity is usually present and may have fluid or tracts. These types of cysts are usually located at the base of the tail bone in the area where the buttocks begin. In some cases, these cysts have accompanying sinus tracts. These sinuses are not at all associated with the sinuses in your head! A sinus is a cavity or a passageway that links the abscess with the outer skin, which allows it to drain. Not everyone who has a pilonidal abscess has a pilonidal sinus. In differentiating which codes to assign, there are three from which to choose. For a small or simple sinus, the physician uses a scalpel to completely excise the cyst and sinus and any inflamed tissue. The wound is sutured in a single layer, and the procedure is reported with code 11770. Code 11771 would be assigned if a sinus is superficial to the underlying fascia but has subcutaneous extensions. The physician uses a scalpel to completely excise the tract and affected tissue. The wound may be sutured in several layers or packed and left open to heal from the inside out. Code 11772 is used when sinuses are present with subcutaneous extensions and/or if tissue re-arrangement was necessary to close the wound. This procedure would result in a larger defect that would require a flap or complex closure. The surgeon may elect to pack the wound and allow the deeper tissue to heal from the inside out with a staged closure once all drainage has stopped and granulation tissue has formed. If the cyst is only incised and none of it is removed, use codes 10080–10081.

Ulcers

Skin ulcers can be caused by a variety of factors, such as trauma, exposure to heat or cold, problems with blood circulation, constant pressure, and neuropathy. Three common types are pressure ulcers, venous stasis ulcers, and nonhealing wounds.

Skin Tags

Skin tags are small, usually benign, painless flesh-colored growths of tissue on the skin's surface that are usually located on the neck, face, and axilla.

> **INTERNET RESOURCES: Descriptions of Skin Diseases**
> *Electronic Textbook of Dermatology*
> www.telemedicine.org/stamford.htm
> *Atlas of Dermatology*
> http://atlases.muni.cz/atl_en/sect_main.html

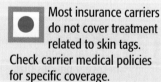
Most insurance carriers do not cover treatment related to skin tags. Check carrier medical policies for specific coverage.

Skin Wounds

There are six types or classifications of skin injuries. Each differs according to depth, entry into the skin, and whether there are clean or jagged edges of skin. The type and extent of injury are the basis for accurately assigning codes for level of treatment provided.

1. *Laceration*—an open wound caused by blunt trauma to the body or by cutting or tearing of the skin and subcutaneous layers with a saw or other sharp object, leaving jagged edges
2. *Puncture*—an injury sustained from a needle, pipe, nails, or objects that penetrate the skin and create a hole but do not tear the skin

3. *Abrasion*—superficial damage to the epidermis that may bleed slightly but does not scar, such as carpet burns
4. *Avulsion*—a sudden, traumatic tearing away of tissue
5. *Incision*—an open wound caused by cutting into the skin by a sharp object such as a knife, glass, or razor blade, leaving clean skin edges
6. *Burn*—an injury or destruction to layers of skin from intense heat as a result of exposure to a fire or too much sun or contact with hot objects or corrosive chemicals. Burns are classified based on the depth of damage to integument and total body surface area injured.

Nails

- HCPCS Level II anatomical modifiers (TA–T9 and FA–F9) should be used to indicate which fingers and toes are biopsied or repaired to avoid claim denials.
- Medicare generally excludes routine nail care, but certain conditions are covered.
- Medicare requires G0127 to be reported for trimming of dystrophic nails.

The nail consists of structures such as the nailbed, matrix, and nail plate. Nail care is a very important aspect of care for people with diabetes. Trimming of nondystrophic nails or debridement of nails using an electrical sander or grinder is performed every 3 months. The nail codes are assigned based on how the nails are trimmed and the number of nails. Common procedures carried out on nails include evacuation of subungual hematoma (11740), matrixectomy (11750), and avulsion of the nail plate for chronic ingrown nails or for severe onychomycosis (11730–11732). Evacuation of a hematoma is carried out by using a needle, drill, or other instrument such as a cautery probe to puncture a hole into the nail to remove the trapped blood under the nail. Avulsion here involves using a nail elevator to tear the nail from the nail plate. Code descriptions state specific numbers of nails or "each."

The *CPT Professional Edition* provides two illustrations of the nail for reference when reading medical documentation pertaining to the nail.

> ■ **CASE SCENARIO**
> A patient presents complaining of chronic ingrown toenail of the right great toe. After digital anesthesia is administered, a nail splitter is used to cut proximally and create a smooth, straight edge. The free lateral nail now is grasped with a hemostat and removed. The lateral nailbed and matrix are now exposed for ablation. Code 11730–T5 is assigned.

COMMON PROCEDURES PERFORMED ON THE INTEGUMENT

Incision and Drainage and Foreign Body Removal

The surgical technique of drainage involves removal of liquid, pus, or blood from an area by inserting a needle or catheter and sucking or aspirating the material. Key words to look for are *stabbing, suction, needle puncture, evacuation, aspiration, arthrocentesis,* or *creation of a window.* When the surgeon performs an incision, a cut is made into the body with a sharp instrument such as a scalpel or scissors for purposes of gaining access to a site or to drain a site. Words ending in *-otomy* depict incision.

Incision and drainage (I&D) is a minor procedure commonly performed under local anesthesia in an office setting, although in some cases general anesthesia and an operating room (OR) are required. Conditions treated by I&D include abscess, cyst, boil, hematoma, acne, carbuncle, and wounds. I&D codes require that an incision has been done, as compared to puncture aspiration, another form of drainage carried out by inserting a needle into the site and drawing out fluid.

It is easy to confuse I&D of a site with aspiration. These are not the same technique. Aspiration does not involve incising the skin. Read the documentation carefully.

The code descriptions for I&D and foreign body (FB) removal refer to a superficial procedure. If the procedure involves a deep incision, the coder should check the Musculoskeletal System section for a more specific code depending on the depth of the procedure and anatomical site. A foreign body removal usually includes I&D, which is then not reported unless the documentation states that more than a single incision was made for the procedure. CPT considers removing joint prostheses and implants as retained FB removals.

EXAMPLES
- 10120 *Incision and removal of foreign body, subcutaneous tissues; simple.*
- 11450 *Excision of skin and subcutaneous tissue for hidradenitis, axillary; with simple or intermediate repair.*

■ **CASE SCENARIO**
A patient is experiencing pain and complaining of a growth that weeps fluid at the base of his tail bone. Upon examination, it is determined that he has a pilonidal cyst. The physician shaves this area and incises the skin to allow drainage of the cystic fluid. Curettage is also performed and the skin is closed primarily. Code: 10081.

Biopsy

A biopsy—the process of obtaining living tissue samples for analysis—is a very common procedure. A biopsy may be done independently to make a diagnosis or as a related part of another surgical procedure, often to confirm a suspected diagnosis. A biopsy does not treat or repair a problem. The sample of tissue removed is sent to a pathologist for examination under a microscope and interpretation. Many surgical procedures routinely involve removing tissue that may be submitted for pathological examination. This is a component of the procedure and routinely carried out, so a biopsy code would not be appropriate to assign in addition to the procedure code. Biopsy coding requires the coder to read and interpret the documentation to determine what type of biopsy occurred. There are five types of biopsy techniques:

> ● Report code 10030 if a catheter is used for percutaneous image guidance to drain an abscess, hematoma, seroma, cyst, or lymphocele of the soft tissue. This code is reported for each separate catheter collection. This is not reported for needle drainage or fine needle aspiration.

1. Incisional biopsy—In an incisional biopsy, performed by an incision, a portion or a sample of the lesion or tumor is removed and sent for pathological examination. Key words to look for include *sample, portion, piece,* and *partial.*

EXAMPLE
11100 *Biopsy of skin, subcutaneous tissue, and/or mucous membrane (including simple closure), unless otherwise listed; single lesion.*

2. Excisional biopsy—In contrast, in an excisional biopsy, the entire lesion, tumor, or other tissue is removed as one specimen and sent to pathology. Key words to look for include *removed in toto* (meaning the whole thing), *entirely dissected free, excised en-block, margins are clear,* and words that end in *-ectomy.*

EXAMPLE
11600 *Excision, malignant lesion including margins, trunk, arms, or legs; excised diameter 0.5 cm or less.*

3. Aspiration—Fluid or tissue is aspirated with a needle and cells are sent to pathology to be examined under a microscope (Fig. 17.3). This may be done with or without x-ray imaging guidance. Key words to look for include *needle, syringe, fluid withdrawal,* and *cytopathology.*

EXAMPLE
10021 *Fine needle aspiration; without imaging guidance.*

4. Percutaneous needle core biopsy—A large-bore needle is inserted into a suspicious site and a core of tissue is removed (see Fig. 17.3). A small nick or incision is made to place the needle through to retrieve tissue, not fluid. A radiologist typically performs this procedure. Key words to look for include *stereotactic x-ray, ultrasound,* and *probe.*

EXAMPLE

19100 *Biopsy of breast; percutaneous, needle core, not using image guidance.*

> If a code exists that specifically describes a biopsy of a particular site, it should be assigned rather than a code from the biopsy range.

5. Punch biopsy—This is used to biopsy small areas where a 3- to 4-mm cylindrical core of tissue is removed. It can be used to remove an entire lesion if it is small enough. This technique differs from needle core biopsies because it does not go deeper than the subcutaneous fat. Key words to look for include *trephine, biopsy punch,* and *stretching of skin perpendicular to skin tension lines.*

EXAMPLE

There is no code assigned just for punch biopsies. These fall under

11100 *Biopsy of skin, subcutaneous tissue and/or mucous membrane (including simple closure), unless otherwise listed; single lesion.*

> Simple repair or closure is always included in the biopsy service and is not coded separately.

In many cases, biopsies are initially performed in an office setting, perhaps with the punch and aspiration techniques. Once pathology results are received, the physician will then determine if further surgery is required such as an excision of the entire lesion. Physicians routinely will remove an entire lesion or mass and refer to this as an "excisional biopsy." This is somewhat of a misnomer, because, by definition, a biopsy is removing a sample from the suspicious site, not the entire thing. However, it is a biopsy in the sense that the physician is removing something that requires pathological examination before a diagnosis can be confirmed.

> A biopsy and excision performed on the same site are not both coded; only the excision code is assigned. Excision procedures include biopsies.

Pay close attention to the details in the operative report. A biopsy code is not assigned separately if an excision code description includes "with or without biopsy." In using the wording "unless otherwise listed" in the code descriptions, CPT is suggesting that the coder should reference a specific anatomical site for a more specific biopsy code before assigning codes 11100–11101.

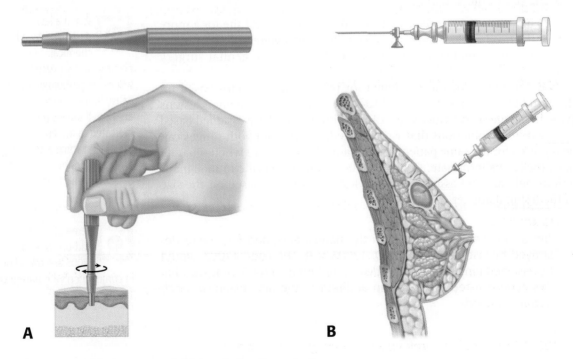

A

B

Figure 17.3 Biopsies. A. Punch biopsy. B. Needle aspiration.

EXAMPLE

Biopsy of skin, outer ear, would be assigned 69100 instead of 11100 because it is exclusive to that anatomical site and better describes "where" the biopsy was taken.

Some biopsy sites, particularly incisional and excisional, require closure or repair. If more than simple repair or closure is needed, then the repair would be coded separately. (The levels of repair are discussed later.) A biopsy code can be assigned separately from an excision *if* the excision is performed on a different site from the biopsy. A –59 modifier is required on the second code to identify the separate and distinct site.

EXAMPLE

Biopsy of the neck performed followed by excision of a 0.4-cm lesion of the scalp. Codes: 11420, 11100–59.

> Although actinic keratoses (AKs) may be considered either precancers or early cancers, they are categorized as premalignant growths and are medically necessary to treat before they become invasive. Seborrheic keratoses (SKs), on the other hand, are benign tumors (warts), so destruction may not be covered if they are not inflamed or irritated.

Destruction

Destruction involves eradicating or obliterating all or a portion of a lesion, growth, or structure. Destruction of lesions uses various methods, such as ablation, obliteration, vaporization, cryosurgery, laser or chemical procedures, and electrosurgical annihilation. Tissue is destroyed by force, chemicals, heat, or freezing. Key words are *destruction, ablation, desiccation, fulguration,* and *cauterization* (to cauterize is to use heat or chemicals to burn or cut). Ablation uses energy such as radio frequency or heat to remove tissue on the surface of the body or organ while not harming the surrounding tissue. Cryosurgery uses liquid nitrogen to freeze a lesion or growth by applying it to the skin with a cotton swab, sprayer, or cryoprobe.

Destruction procedures can be performed in an office setting with local anesthesia, but, depending on the area treated and the number of lesions, general anesthesia may be required. In most cases, closure or repair is not required after destruction.

To correctly code these procedures, the coder must know the following:

- Whether the lesion(s) is premalignant, benign, or malignant
- Lesion site
- The number of lesion(s)
- The depth of the lesion(s)
- The size of the lesion(s)

CPT instructions refer the coder to a specific anatomical site for a more appropriate code before assigning a code from this general lesion range. For example, genital condylomata are coded from the genital surgery codes.

Codes 17000–17004 are assigned for premalignant lesions based on the number of lesions. Codes 17110–17111 are used for benign lesions (which include scars, which are cicatricial lesions) and are assigned based on the number of lesions that were treated. Codes from both ranges can be reported for the same patient on the same day of service when separate diagnoses are appropriate. Codes 17260–17286 are specific to malignant lesions only and are assigned for *each* lesion destroyed based on the size of the lesion diameter.

> When a lesion is destroyed by a laser, chemical, freezing, or electrocautery procedure, there will be no pathology report because there is no specimen to analyze. If the lesion size is not indicated in the operative note, the best practice is to query the physician on the size, number of lesions, and type of lesion.

EXAMPLES

- Ten actinic keratosis lesions on the hands, ears, and face were destroyed by laser. Codes: 17000, 17003 × 9. The code 17003 would be assigned nine times. The code description for 17003 indicates that this code is listed separately in addition to the first lesion *for each lesion removed.*

> Remember that add-on codes such as 17003 are coded only in conjunction with parent code 17000.

Introduction

In surgical terminology, introduction means insertion of an instrument, substance, or appliance into the body that performs a function, assists in treatment, monitors body functions, or marks a site. Key words: *insertion, injection, percutaneous placement, intubation,* and *catheterization.*

EXAMPLE
11900 *Injection, intralesional; up to and including 7 lesions.*

Paring

Paring means trimming or gradual reduction in size by slicing. Picture a potato or carrot peeler and how a thin layer is trimmed off with each stroke.

EXAMPLE
11055 *Paring or cutting of benign hyperkeratotic lesion (e.g., corn or callus); single lesion.*

Be careful! CPT directs the coder out of the Integumentary System section to other surgery sections for destruction of lesions of specific anatomical sites for a more appropriate code.

Shaving

Shaving involves slicing a raised lesion or mole entirely off at skin level (i.e., flush with the skin) by using a razor or surgical blade; this is in contrast to paring, where layers are sliced off gradually. Shaving is also carried out in orthopedic procedures of the joints where cartilage is removed with a shaver.

EXAMPLE
11300 *Shaving of epidermal or dermal lesion, single lesion, trunk, arms, or legs; lesion diameter 0.5 cm or less.*

CHECKPOINT 17.1

Assign codes to the following procedures. Include any necessary modifiers.

1. A patient has been complaining of a nonhealing surgical wound. The patient underwent an arthroplasty of the left index finger proximal interphalangeal (PIP) joint. The skin over the joint has been chronically infected. The physician debrides the skin surface. _____

2. A patient presents to the office with a tender 2.0-cm cyst located in the right axilla. The patient says she has had this for 2 weeks and thinks it is from an ingrown hair. The physician uses a scalpel to puncture the cyst and proceeds to drain the pustule. _____

3. A patient was hit in the left upper arm with an 85-mph fastball while playing baseball. Over the course of the day, the arm became bruised and began to swell. Two days later, he went to the physician who diagnosed him with a hematoma and recommended draining the pooled blood. The patient tolerated the procedure well. _____

4. A women is seen in the dermatologist's office for a chronic rash with raised lesions on her stomach. The physician examines the rash under magnification and decides to biopsy two lesions. He stretches the skin perpendicular to the tension lines and inserts the trephine to sample the skin to rule out lupus. _____

5. A patient presents to the office with two dermatofibroma on her right leg and one on her left. The nurse practitioner uses liquid nitrogen to destroy them. _____

6. Laser destruction of four premalignant lesions. _____

Excision

An excision involves surgically removing or cutting out part or all of a tumor, lesion, organ, or tissue with a scalpel, sharp instrument, laser, loop electrode, or hot knife. Key words to look for are *debulking, trimming, wedging, removing, excising, dissecting,* and *biopsy.*

Three common surgical techniques are used for excising lesions of the integument. Two methods are located in the Integumentary System section, and both methods are represented by the same group of codes:

- Simple
- Wide

Simple excision removes a full-thickness lesion (through the dermis) and includes direct closure of the skin. Wide excision removes a lesion or tumor, its capsule, and a margin of normal tissue.

EXAMPLE

11401 Excision, benign lesion including margins, except skin tag (unless listed elsewhere) trunk, arms or legs: excised diameter 0.6cm or to 1.0cm.

Radical excision is the third method. As the name indicates, radical excision involves the removal of the growth, its capsule, and the entire area of tissue or bone encompassing the growth. A radical excision is located within the Musculoskeletal System section of CPT.

To properly code excisions, the coder must have the following data:

- Morphology (type) of lesion: malignant or benign
- Anatomical site of lesion
- Number of lesions
- Depth of the lesion
- Size of the lesion
- Surgical technique (shaving, excision, destruction, etc.)
- Type of closure or repair to site

The operative report or procedure note along with the pathology report will provide this necessary information. Note that all excision codes include simple closure. Repair by intermediate or complex closure is separately reportable.

Two distinctly separate code ranges are available for excisions: benign lesions and malignant lesions. After this division, codes are grouped by body part and then by size of lesion. The codes are assigned based on the *diameter* of the lesion being excised, including any margins, not according to the size of the incision necessary to access the lesion. Asymmetrical or irregular-shaped lesions are assigned codes based on the *longest* dimension. The *margin* of skin is the additional skin excised beyond or bordering the actual lesion. This is done to ensure that the entire lesion is removed. Surgeons typically make the excision slightly larger than the actual lesion, creating a larger defect. The resulting defect is called an *ellipse*. The ellipse is drawn so that the resulting scar runs parallel with existing skin creases. This ensures that the scar is as narrow and short as possible. A visual example of this is shown in Figure 17.4. This is also illustrated in the *CPT Professional Edition,* Example B, located adjacent to the guidelines for excising benign lesions. The ellipse also allows for the surgeon to sew a straight line when closing the wound. If this technique is applied, the size of the repair for other than a simple repair would be the length of one end of the ellipse to the other.

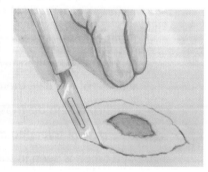

Figure 17.4 Ellipse.

Other forms of lesion removal that do not involve a full-thickness excision of the skin, such as shaving, paring, and removal of skin tags, are located under those respective headings prior to the Excision heading. Codes for excision should be assigned to *each* lesion excised, regardless of the number of lesions removed.

CPT codes 11400–11446 should be used when the excision is a full-thickness (through the dermis) removal of a lesion, including margins, and includes simple (nonlayered) closure and is specific to benign lesions only.

> Pay particular attention to how the size of a lesion is stated. Physicians may report the size as inches, centimeters, or millimeters.

If a mix of benign and malignant excisions is performed, each lesion excision is reported individually.

Following an excision, any closure other than a simple closure is billed separately.

BOX 17.2 Converting to Metric Units

1 mm	=	0.1 cm
10 mm	=	1 cm
1 in.	=	2.54 cm
1 sq. in.	=	6.452 sq cm

Measurement of Lesions

Many of the codes in the Integumentary System section involve measurements. All integumentary codes are based on centimeters excised, repaired, or otherwise treated. If the measurements are in millimeters, they must be converted to centimeters to accurately code the service (Box 17.2). For the most part, it is a matter of moving the decimal point to the left.

EXAMPLES

A physician excises a 1.5-cm (width) × 2.0-cm (length) benign lesion from the top of the hand. The largest dimension is 2.0 cm; therefore, the code is 11422.

2-in × 3-in lesion = 6 sq in

6 sq in × 6.452 = 38.71 sq cm

If the diameter of a lesion is 5 mm, then it would be 0.5 cm

Converting a 5-in laceration would look like this: 5 in × 2.54 cm = 12.7 cm

The following points should be observed:

- The size of the lesion should be taken from the physician's op note or office notes. If there is no documentation, query the physician for this information.
- Never guess or assume the size of the specimen or lesion; instead, query the surgeon.
- The pathology report is also a source for measurements.
- If both sources have a size listed and they are not the same, use the physician's measurement. The formalin preservative may shrink the size of the tissue sample, so always report the pre-excision size if it is available.

Study the illustration shown in Figure 17.5 and review the following example. The *CPT Professional Edition* also provides an illustration of this within the Excision-Benign Lesions section, Example A.

EXAMPLE

Removal of a benign lesion of the back with an actual diameter of 2.0 cm × 1.0 cm. The physician determines that the appropriate margin required for this excision is 0.2 cm. The greatest clinical diameter of the lesion is 2.0 cm. An additional 0.2-cm margin is excised around the entire lesion. The excised diameter is then equal to the greatest clinical diameter (2.0 cm) and an additional margin of 0.4 cm (0.2 cm added on either side of the lesion). The total excised diameter is 2.4 cm, which codes to CPT code 11403.

There is one exception to how measurements are described in Integumentary System codes. Codes for flaps and grafts are reported in square centimeters (cm²), not by the diameter of the lesion or length of repair.

It is important for facility and surgeon claims to match. It is not uncommon for the surgeon not to wait for the pathology report to report a final diagnosis for a biopsy or lesion excision; therefore, the diagnosis that the facility bills might not match the surgeon's bill, which would cause claim denials to either entity. Ideally, the diagnoses and CPT codes that both parties submit should match for the same service performed on the same day.

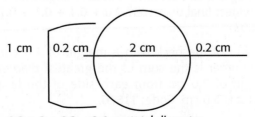

0.2 + 2 + 0.2 = 2.4 cm total diameter

Figure 17.5 Diameter of a lesion.

When multiple lesions are treated, report the most complex (largest lesion) procedure first and the others with a –51 or –59 modifier depending on the code description and the location of the lesions.

> **EXAMPLE**
>
> If two lesions of the hand (0.5 cm each) and two lesions of the neck are removed (0.7 cm each), assign a –59 modifier for each separate lesion and site because the code description includes several body sites. Codes: 11420, 11420–59, 11421–59, 11421–59.

If two lesions are removed through one incision, only one code is assigned. The size of the two lesions and the space between the lesions are added together.

> **EXAMPLE**
>
> Two 0.3-cm hand lesions located 0.5 cm apart are removed through one incision. 0.3 cm + 0.3 cm + 0.5 cm = 1.10 cm. Code: 11422.

In most cases, modifiers –RT and –LT do not apply to lesion removals or repairs in the integumentary section. Because many different anatomical sites are "grouped" or classified into codes for removal and repair, assigning one of these modifiers would not be describing a paired body part.

> **EXAMPLE**
>
> Excision of a 0.5-cm nevus from the right ear is coded as 11440. The code description for 11440 includes lesion removal from the face, ears, eyelids, nose, lips, and mucous membrane. Applying the RT modifier does not differentiate the right ear from the right eyelid.

Lipomas (tumors) are tricky to code. Pay very close attention to the code description. If the description says, "unless listed elsewhere," refer to the most specific code in the most specific body category. Code to the most appropriate anatomical site regardless of the depth of the lipoma (tumor) even if the term *skin* is mentioned. Use the Integumentary System code only when there is no specific code in the Musculoskeletal System section.

> **EXAMPLE**
>
> 11406 *Excision, benign lesion including margins, except skin tag (unless listed elsewhere), trunk, arms, or legs*; excised diameter over 4.0 cm.

A Note on Malignant Lesions

If a physician excises a malignant lesion and sends the specimen to pathology intraoperatively (during the procedure) to determine if the margins are "clear," and further excision is done until the pathologist confirms for the surgeon that the margins are "clear," only one excision code is assigned. This code is for the final greatest width of the lesion.

> **EXAMPLES**
>
> The surgeon excises a 2.0-cm × 1.0-cm lesion of the shoulder with a 0.1-cm margin on both sides and sends it to pathology. The pathologist says the margins are not clear. Surgeon excises an additional 0.1-cm margin all around. Pathologist finally confirms that the margins are free of disease. What is the widest final diameter? 2.0 + 0.1 + 0.1 + 0.1 + 0.1 = 2.4 cm. Code: 11603.
>
> A 1.0-cm malignant lesion of the neck with a margin of 2.0 cm is excised. The excised diameter is the sum of the greatest diameter (1.0 cm) plus the margin of 2.0 cm from each side of the lesion (2.0 + 2.0). Total diameter is 5.0 cm. Code: 11626.

What happens if a physician removes a lesion and the pathology report states that the lesion is of unknown neoplastic behavior? This

If lesion size is not indicated in the op note, the best thing to do is query the physician on the size and type of lesion. If this is not done, you are forced to use a code for the smallest size lesion (0.5 cm), which in most cases is not reimbursable in the outpatient setting.

Note that when a lesion is removed from a previous mastectomy site, the site is considered the "trunk" and not the "breast" because the breast is no longer there, *unless* a partial mastectomy or lumpectomy was performed and the woman still has breast tissue remaining.

Remember to add the margins (M) for both ends of the lesion to the diameter (D) of the lesion itself. Think times two! Total diameter × D + (M × 2).

If a malignant lesion is excised on one visit and a re-excision is performed on a separate visit (could be weeks or months later) to verify that all the cancer is gone, code to the excision of a malignant lesion, even if the second re-excision pathology report states that margins are benign or clear.

CPT © 2017 American Medical Association, All Rights Reserved.

documentation means it is uncertain as to whether it is benign or malignant, which has a direct impact on CPT code assignment. In this case, the surgeon's documentation should reflect the surgical approach. The CPT code that best describes the extent of the procedure performed should be reported. A lesion that is judged probably benign might be excised with minimal surrounding tissue removal, but one judged more suspicious might be excised with greater tissue margins.

Wound Repair (Closure)

A repair surgically closes a defect, restores shape or functionality, or reconnects to an anatomical body part, which usually involves suturing and possibly replacement of tissue. Key words to look for include *stitching, closure, correction, anastomosis, restoration, suturing, reduction,* and words ending in *–rrhaphy.*

Codes for repair are not based on whether the lesion removed is malignant or benign. Instead, code assignment is based on depth of skin, technique, and materials used. As mentioned earlier, CPT defines three levels of wound repair complexity:

- Simple
- Intermediate
- Complex

 "Bring together, sew together, add together."

Codes are grouped within each level by anatomical sites and size of wound. The size of the wound is determined by adding the length of all wounds in the same classification or anatomical group. With wound repairs, the lengths of multiple wounds are added together by repair group or classification and by complexity.

EXAMPLE
13160 *Secondary closure of surgical wound or dehiscence, extensive or complicated.*

Medicare requires code G0168 to be submitted when a repair is performed with tissue adhesive only. However, G0168 is bundled to all wound repair codes and cannot be reported separately if also assigning a code in the 12001–13160 range. For non-Medicare patients, if the repair is performed solely with tissue adhesive, only the E/M code for the visit is assigned.

Simple Repair
A simple repair is made for a superficial wound repair involving the epidermis, dermis, and a minimal amount of subcutaneous tissue requiring one-layer suturing. This type of repair is referred to as "direct" or "primary" closure. If the closure was done with tape, staples, Dermabond, glue, or adhesive strips, this service is included in the E/M code and not billed separately. Likewise, when lesions were removed and only simple repair was necessary to close the wound, the simple repair is not coded separately. A simple repair is included in the lesion removal "package" and payment. Running subcuticular suture involves the epidermis and part of the dermis.

EXAMPLE
Excision of a 3.0-cm nevus from the left shoulder. Only the epidermal and part of the dermal layers were repaired. Code: 11403. The simple repair is included in the code for the lesion removal.

Intermediate Repair
An intermediate repair involves closure of one or more of the subcutaneous layers and superficial fascia, in addition to the skin. Often, two different types of suture are used to close the wound. There are several names or types that serve varying purposes. Some are used for closing deep tissue and dissolve internally, while others are used for the superficial layers of skin and require removal. Common suture brands include Chromic, Vicryl, Monocryl, Prolene, and Ethilon. An intermediate repair indicates that a layered closure took place. One layer is closed with one type of suture and the second layer is closed with a different suture type. Reference to buried suture indicates a layered closure took place. The buried sutures provide support to the wound and prevent tension on the skin wound edges. An intermediate repair code can also be reported when the wound has to be extensively cleaned due to contamination or removal of small pieces of foreign material before suturing, even if the suturing is simple. This is an important exception that is often overlooked in the coding process. Running subcutaneous suture is used to close the deep portion of incisions created during surgery. Sizes 3-0 and 4-0 suture materials are typically used for subcutaneous suturing.

Look at code 12031 in CPT. It includes intermediate repair of wounds of the scalp, axillae, trunk, and/or extremities (excluding hands and feet). As you can see, many significantly different sites are "grouped" or "classified" into this code. For example, a 2.5-cm wound of the right leg and a 3.1-cm wound of the back were both repaired with intermediate repair. The coder should add the lengths of both of these wounds together and use the sum to base code assignment. In this case 2.5 + 3.1 = 5.6 cm. Code: 12032.

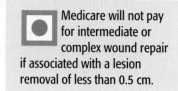 Medicare will not pay for intermediate or complex wound repair if associated with a lesion removal of less than 0.5 cm.

Complex Repair

A complex repair or closure includes scar revision, debridement, extensive undermining, stents, or retention sutures, and more than layered closure. Repair of traumatic avulsions or lacerations may be in this category. When the wound is complex, repair of extensive nerve, blood vessel, or tendon damage may also be reported. Irregular or jagged wounds often require complex repairs.

EXAMPLE

The physician repairs a 7.6-cm knife laceration of the right forearm. The physician had to repair all layers of the skin and debride foreign material from the wound. Because the length of the repair is 7.6 cm, two codes are required: 13121 and 13122. Note that add-on code 13122 specifies "each additional 5cm or less."

Wound repairs include simple ligation of vessels; simple exploration of surrounding tissue, nerves, vessels, and tendons; and simple debridement (cleaning or removing of tissue until normal-appearing, healthy tissue is exposed). If gross contamination is encountered and requires extensive debridement, the wound requires extensive cleansing, or significant amounts of tissue are removed, this is coded separately.

Lengths of wounds or defects caused by lesion removal are only added together if the repair is the same complexity and from the same body category or group depicted in the code description.

Repair sites and types must match to be added. Lengths cannot be added together if the type of repair is not the same or if the repairs were done on different sites.

EXAMPLE

A 2.5-cm simple repair of the arm and 3.1-cm intermediate repair of the leg. These procedures cannot be added together because they are two different complexities of repair even though they are in the same anatomical group.

If multiple types of repair are performed, the most complex type is coded as the primary procedure. Report modifier −59 for any additional repairs. Although modifier −51 is the multiple procedure modifier, CPT specifies the use of modifier −59 for multiple repair codes.

Debridement is coded separately from wound repairs if gross contamination is encountered and requires extensive debridement, the wound requires extensive cleansing, significant amounts of tissue are removed, or the wound is packed and closed at a later encounter.

EXAMPLE

Simple repair of the lower leg and intermediate repair of the foot are performed. The intermediate repair of the foot is coded and listed first followed by the simple repair of the leg.

Assigning Codes for Wound Repair

To properly assign codes for wound repair, the following factors (Pinpoint the Code 17.1) must be considered:

1. What is the length of wound in centimeters (cm)? If the size is reported in millimeters (mm), it must be converted to cm by moving the decimal point. For example, if the lesion is 11 mm, it is 1.1 cm. (Do not confuse the size of the lesion with the size of the specimen or size of the defect left.)
2. What type of wound (wound dehiscence, burn, laceration) is it?
3. Where is the site of the wound repair?
4. How many wounds were repaired?

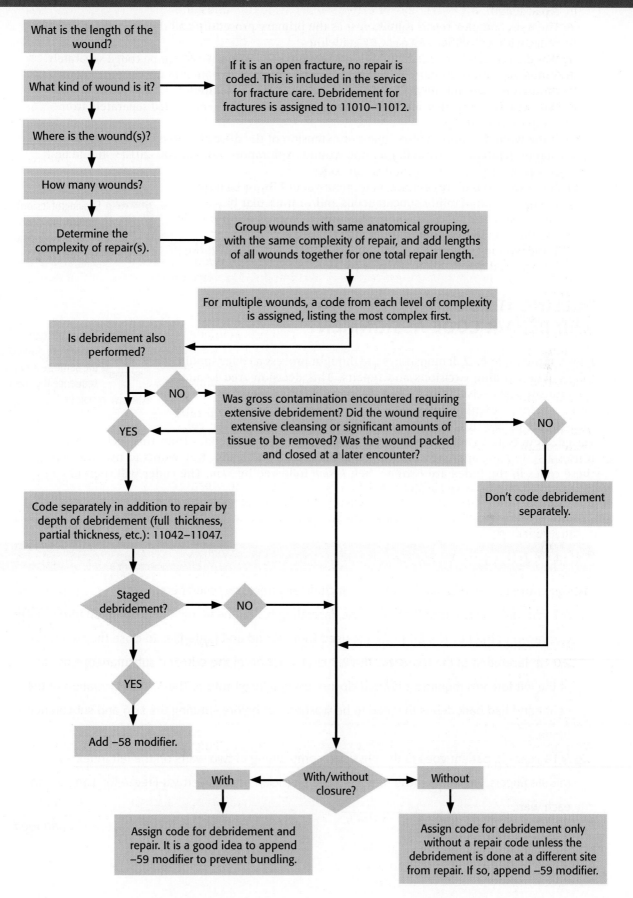

What is the length of the wound?

What kind of wound is it? → If it is an open fracture, no repair is coded. This is included in the service for fracture care. Debridement for fractures is assigned to 11010–11012.

Where is the wound(s)?

How many wounds?

Determine the complexity of repair(s). → Group wounds with same anatomical grouping, with the same complexity of repair, and add lengths of all wounds together for one total repair length.

For multiple wounds, a code from each level of complexity is assigned, listing the most complex first.

Is debridement also performed?

NO

YES ← Was gross contamination encountered requiring extensive debridement? Did the wound require extensive cleansing or significant amounts of tissue to be removed? Was the wound packed and closed at a later encounter? → NO → Don't code debridement separately.

Code separately in addition to repair by depth of debridement (full thickness, partial thickness, etc.): 11042–11047.

Staged debridement? → NO

YES

Add –58 modifier.

With/without closure?

With → Assign code for debridement and repair. It is a good idea to append –59 modifier to prevent bundling.

Without → Assign code for debridement only without a repair code unless the debridement is done at a different site from repair. If so, append –59 modifier.

5. What was the complexity of repair for all wounds? Group the same anatomical groups, with the same complexity of repair, and add lengths of all wounds together for one total repair length.

6. The most complex repair is listed first as the primary procedure and then the lesser repair codes with a modifier –59 per CPT guidelines.

7. Was debridement provided? If this is documented and extensive, it can be coded separately.

8. Simple ligation or cautery of blood vessels and simple exploration of nerves or tendons through the wound site are routine and are not coded separately.

9. If nerves, blood vessels, and tendons are repaired, then these are coded separately from complex wound repairs.

10. If the wound requires enlargement or extension of the dissection to determine penetration or depth of the wound, then the wound exploration codes 20100–20103 should be reported instead of the wound repair codes.

11. If the wound requires debridement, removal of FBs, or ligation or coagulation of minor subcutaneous and/or muscular blood vessels(s) of the subcutaneous tissue, muscle fascia, and/or muscle, use the wound exploration codes 20100–20103.

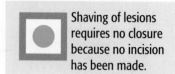

Shaving of lesions requires no closure because no incision has been made.

12. If the wound requires a thoracotomy or laparotomy, report those services and not the wound repair codes.

PULLING IT TOGETHER: EXCISION AND REPAIR CODE ASSIGNMENT

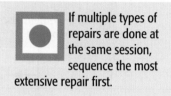

If multiple types of repairs are done at the same session, sequence the most extensive repair first.

Pinpoint the Code 17.2 demonstrates the thought process a coder should follow when coding excisions and repairs. This decision tree is only used for surgical excisions and is not meant for shaving, destruction, or paring. Before assigning any codes for excisions or repairs, make sure measurements are in centimeters; if they are not, they must be converted. New coders can use this decision tree when assigning codes from this section because it uses a systematic approach that can be applied time and again. Key words to use in locating these codes in the Index are *Excision* then *Lesion* followed by *Skin*. The coder will then have to choose from *Benign* or *Malignant*.

CHECKPOINT 17.2

Assign codes to the following procedures. Include any necessary modifiers.

1. A 7-year-old boy fell from his tree house, lacerating his forehead, right hand, and left forearm. He was taken to the ED. The ED physician used Dermabond and butterflies to close the superficial 2.0-cm laceration of the forehead. The 2.5-cm laceration of the skin and subcutaneous tissue of the left forearm required a layered closure using a Vicryl suture. The 3.0-cm laceration of the right hand had bark debris that had to be washed out before suturing the skin and subcutaneous tissue. _____

2. A 19-year-old patient goes to the physician complaining of two warts on the left index and middle fingers. He wants these removed. The physician applies Verruca-Freeze for 1 minute to each wart. _____

Continued

CPT © 2017 American Medical Association, All Rights Reserved.

3. A 63-year-old female noticed a purplish irregular lesion on her lower leg. She has already had a basal cell carcinoma removed from her left shoulder. The 1.7-cm lesion was removed with a 0.2-cm margin. Simple repair was performed. Pathology confirmed basal cell carcinoma.

   _____

4. A patient has been complaining of a nonhealing surgical wound. The patient underwent an arthroplasty of the left index finger PIP joint. The skin over the joint has been chronically infected. The doctor debrides 10 sq cm of skin and subcutaneous tissue and performs a complex layered closure. _____

5. A 3.0-cm, full-thickness benign lesion is removed from the patient's upper back. A second benign lesion is also removed from the midback measuring 2.2 cm. The physician uses Vicryl to repair the subcutaneous layer and Monocryl to close the skin in both sites. _____

SKIN GRAFTS AND FLAPS

The skin is the body's first defense against injury and infection by microorganisms. When skin is damaged, the body can regenerate only the epidermal layer. At times, skin injuries and defects from lesion removal destroy deeper structures such as the dermal and subcutaneous tissues. This damage requires more than simple, intermediate, or complex closure. Alternative methods of repair are adjacent tissue transfer or tissue rearrangement and skin grafting with either the patient's own skin or skin substitutes. The success of the skin graft will depend upon the location and size of the injury, along with the patient's healing abilities and blood supply.

> Be sure that the measurements used are square centimeters and not just centimeters. Finding square centimeters is like measuring a room for carpet in your house. Multiply length (L) times width (W) to get the square area. L x W = square centimeters. For example, if a 2 x 3 cm defect was closed, the code assigned is based on 6 sq cm (2 x 3 = 6).

Codes for tissue transfers/arrangements (flaps) are assigned based on location of the defect and surface area to cover (size of defect). To assign codes for skin grafts, the type of graft is located first (i.e., split-thickness, full-thickness, xenograft) followed by the location of the defect, and surface area (size of defect). It is critical to read the operative report in its entirety to determine the type of graft, flap, or tissue rearrangement carried out, where the tissue is coming from (donor site), the recipient site, the size of the defect where the graft is placed, and if any additional repair to the donor site is required. It is also important to ascertain if a skin substitute is used in the repair. The area is measured in square centimeters (cm² or sq cm). The coder is often required to calculate the square centimeters to derive the correct flap or graft size before assigning the code. If the operative report describes deeper structures such as muscle, fat or fascia, or microvascular anastomosis of other than skin and vessels, other CPT codes may be more appropriate from the Musculoskeletal section of CPT.

Skin flap and graft codes are not located centrally in one subsection of the Integumentary chapter. Instead, they are located in different areas under codes 14000–15777, 15840–15845, 15922, 15934, 15944, 15952, 19364, 19637, and 19369 so the coder needs to have a good understanding of this and not skip the Index and go right to the graft section of the chapter.

Skin grafts are obtained by using an instrument called a *dermatome* to slice the skin away from the donor site at very precise thicknesses. It is similar to a hand-held cheese slicer or vegetable peeler that is dragged across the skin. The surgeon may *mesh* the graft by running it through a special processor that places holes in the tissue to allow it to expand to cover more area.

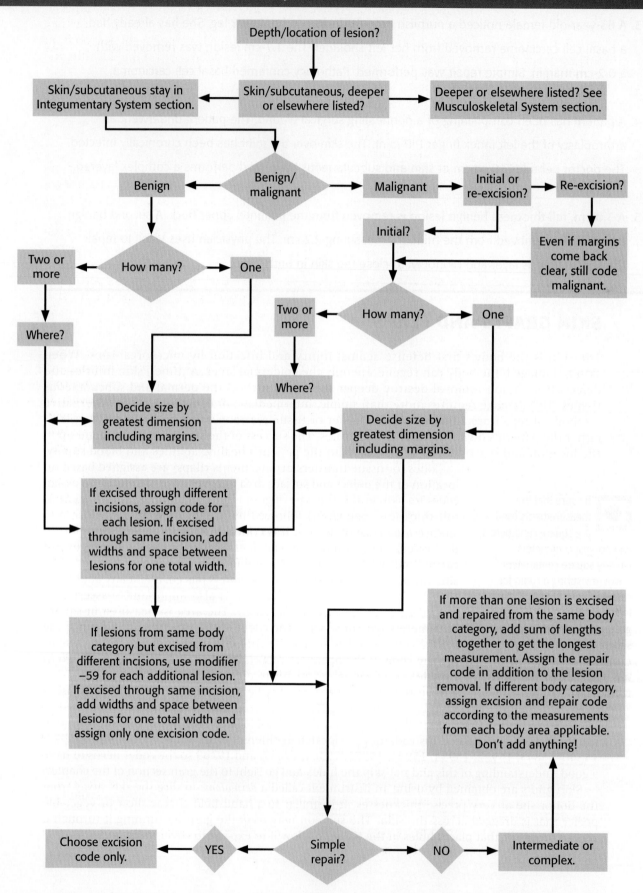

Depth/location of lesion?

Skin/subcutaneous stay in Integumentary System section. ← Skin/subcutaneous, deeper or elsewhere listed? → Deeper or elsewhere listed? See Musculoskeletal System section.

Benign ← Benign/malignant → Malignant → Initial or re-excision? → Re-excision?

Initial? ← Even if margins come back clear, still code malignant.

Two or more ← How many? → One

Where?

Two or more ← How many? → One

Where?

Decide size by greatest dimension including margins.

Decide size by greatest dimension including margins.

If excised through different incisions, assign code for each lesion. If excised through same incision, add widths and space between lesions for one total width.

If lesions from same body category but excised from different incisions, use modifier –59 for each additional lesion. If excised through same incision, add widths and space between lesions for one total width and assign only one excision code.

If more than one lesion is excised and repaired from the same body category, add sum of lengths together to get the longest measurement. Assign the repair code in addition to the lesion removal. If different body category, assign excision and repair code according to the measurements from each body area applicable. Don't add anything!

Choose excision code only. ← YES ← Simple repair? → NO → Intermediate or complex.

Free Skin Grafts

Skin grafting procedures are assigned from code range 15040–15278. There are many types of grafting procedures and types discussed in this section. *Free skin grafts* get their name because they are completely freed from the donor site and placed at a recipient site. No vascular connection from the donor site is left intact with these grafts. Free skin grafts are sections of skin that fall into one of these four categories:

1. Autograft/Tissue Cultured Autograft
2. Acellular Dermal Replacement
3. Allograft/Tissue Cultured Allogeneic Skin Substitute
4. Xenograft

An autograft is a piece of skin taken from the patient's own body to cover a defect so the donor and recipient site is the same individual. The patient's own skin is used whenever possible to reduce the risk of rejection. The term *allograft* refers to a graft obtained from a source other than the patient's body. It is either a donation from a cadaver or is a manmade synthetic material.

To understand free skin grafting, the coder must be able to distinguish between the recipient site (site receiving the graft) and the donor site (site where graft was harvested from). If the donor site requires more than simple repair after harvesting the tissue, an additional repair code is required. Sometimes, a graft is necessary to close the defect at the donor site. If so, this is coded separately in addition to the original skin graft. If a lesion is excised and immediately closed with a free skin graft, code the excision of the lesion in addition to the graft.

Surgical Preparation

Codes 15002–15005 are used to report the initial preparation of the graft recipient site, which needs healthy bleeding tissues to receive the graft. The initial preparation includes cleansing, removing any nonviable tissue, or excision of tissue or incisional or excisional release of scar contracture resulting in an open wound. Surgical preparation maximizes the chances of survival of the graft to be placed. Usually, the recipient site contains uneven layers or multiple layers that could pose a problem with connecting the surfaces of the donor graft to the recipient site. The layers may also cause the graft site to be very visible with a less than adequate cosmetic effect.

> Do not assign codes 15002–15005 for non-incisional or excisional debridement (VERSAJET™ or manual removal) of tissue reported with a code from the Medicine section because these are not considered to meet the definition of surgical preparation.

As stated in the CPT Surgical Preparation section, 15002, "Surgical preparation or creation of recipient site by excision of open wounds, burn eschar, or scar (including subcutaneous tissues); first 100 sq cm or 1% of body area of infants and children" and 15004, "Surgical preparation or creation of recipient site by excision of open wounds, burn eschar, or scar (including subcutaneous tissues, or incisional release of scar contracture, face, scalp, eyelids, mouth, neck, ears, orbits, genitalia, hands, feet and/or multiple digits); first 100 sq cm or 1% of body area of infants and children." The operative words here are *excision of tissue or incisional or excisional release.* This type of preparation requires the use of a scalpel.

CPT provides parenthetical instruction to report 15002–15005 in conjunction with the codes for skin graft or replacement when preparation of the recipient site is performed.

> Report codes 15002–15005 in addition to the code for the respective skin grafts or replacement codes 15050–15261, 15271–15278 if the skin is intact.

Debridement of skin that is *nonintact* to prepare the site to receive a skin graft is generally included in the skin graft service and not coded separately. However, if the recipient site requires debridement of *intact* skin to prepare for a free skin graft, use code 15002–15005 in addition to the code for the graft when the site is prepared prior to receiving the graft (i.e., removing scar tissue or eschar).

Codes 15002–15005 are not used to report debridement of nonintact necrotic skin lesion removals, or for chronic wounds that are intentionally allowed to heal secondarily from the inside out. These services are reported with codes from the Medicine section.

Table 17.4 provides a short list of graft categories and descriptions to assist coders in determining the uses and respective CPT code ranges.

Autografts

The autograft can be of various thicknesses, shapes, and sizes. The purpose of the autograft is to actually replace the skin that was damaged or removed. There are four categories of autograft indicative of the source of tissue: split thickness, full thickness, epidermal, and dermal. Each category of autograft has its respective CPT code range.

Split-Thickness Grafts (STGs or STSGs). Split-thickness skin grafts get their name because they contain only part of the dermal layer in some areas of the graft. It is used for areas that do not require a complete dermal covering but do require a complete epidermal layer. Split-thickness grafts are most typically used for non-weight-bearing parts of the body or for infected or large wounds resulting from burns. The code range is 15100–15101, 15120–15121. This code range is also assigned for thin grafts (0.010–0.015 inches), moderately thick grafts (up to 0.015 inch, which includes more of the dermis), and thick grafts (greater than 0.015 inches but does not include all of the dermis) because these all contain varying percentages of epidermis and dermis.

Full-Thickness Grafts. Full-thickness grafts (FTGs or FTSGs) are used to replace areas that are missing epidermal and dermal layers of skin. The code range is 15200–15261. They include an equal and continuous section of both layers of the skin and all of the skin elements including blood vessels but none of the underlying fat. The blood vessels will begin to grow from the recipient area into the transplanted skin within 36 hours of grafting. Full-thickness grafts are used for weight-bearing portions of the body and friction-prone areas, such as feet and joints. Donor sites are typically the thigh, abdomen, postauricular skin, and inguinal folds.

Full-thickness grafts are also located in the Eye and Ocular Adnexa section of CPT and reported with codes 67961 or 67966.

Table 17.4 Free Skin Grafts and Skin Substitutes

GRAFT CATEGORY	DESCRIPTION	CPT CODE(S)
Pinch	Small (typically 2 cm or smaller) pieces of tissue that are used to repair tips of digits or other small areas	15050
Epidermal	Grafts composed of the epidermis, the outermost layer of skin	15110–15116
Dermal	Grafts composed of the dermis the second layer of skin immediately below the epidermis	15130–15136
Split thickness	Grafts composed of the full layer of epidermis and part of the dermis	15100–15101, 15120–15121
Full thickness	Grafts composed of the full layer of both the epidermis and dermis	15200–15261
Tissue-cultured epidermal autograft	Cultured skin with only an epidermal layer (e.g., CEA, Epicel®, EpiDex®). For treatment of deep dermal or full-thickness wounds where adequate donor sites not unavailable.	15150–15157
Acellular dermal replacement	A tissue-derived or manufactured device that provides immediate temporary wound closure. It incorporates into the wound and promotes generation of new skin that can support epidermal tissue (e.g., Integra®).	15271–15278
Allograft	Cadaveric human skin (from skin banks)	15271–15278
Skin substitute grafts	Non-autologous human skin, non-human skin substitute grafts (xenograft), and biological products that form a sheet scaffolding for skin growth.	15271–15278

DIAGNOSIS: Full-thickness skin injury, right elbow.
OPERATION: Skin graft.

This 33-year-old male was pushed through a glass storm door window and sliced skin off his right medial elbow area. He was seen in the ED and sent home using saline moistened dressings and referred to a plastic surgeon. The patient is seen today in the outpatient surgery center. The wound was full thickness, partially granulating, and covered with fibrinous debris with uneven skin margins and required a 60 sq cm. full thickness skin graft. The wound was painted with ethylene blue as a marker and then the VERSAJET was used to remove the outer layer of granulation tissue. There are no gouges or exposed fat in the wound bed. Using a dermatome, a full-thickness skin graft was harvested from the right left shoulder and passed through the mesher. It was then placed over the wound. Fibrin glue was used to adhere the graft to the wound bed. A foam bolster was applied.

Answer: 15220, 15221 x 2 for the skin graft. Documentation notes a 60 sq cm. full-thickness autograft from the patient's own shoulder. Do not assign 15002 because surgical preparation was performed by using the VERSAJET and it is not considered to be surgical preparation. With skin grafts, codes are assigned based on the recipient site and the depth or thickness of the graft.

Epidermal Graft. Epidermal grafts (15110–15116) are composed of the epidermis, the outermost layer of skin. This type of closure is used when direct suture closure or adjacent tissue transfer is not feasible. The graft is used in many cases to perform the final stage of wound closure. Frequently, it is used in conjunction with dermal allografts in treating ulcers of the lower extremities.

Dermal Graft. Dermal grafts (15130–15136) are composed of the dermis, the second layer of skin immediately below the epidermis. The epidermis and subcutaneous fat are removed. This type of graft is used instead of fascia in various plastic procedures. It serves as a filler and provides a localized correction to an area, such as the border of the lip, forehead lines, depressed scars, or the deep hollow beneath the eyes.

Pinch Graft. Pinch grafts are very small (typically 2 cm or smaller) pieces of tissue that are used to repair tips of digits or other small areas. They heal quickly and resist infection. Refer to CPT code 15050 to report pinch graft services. As indicated in the code descriptor, this code would be used only once, regardless of the number of pinch grafts performed to cover a defect 2 cm or less.

Other Grafts. There are other autografts located in this chapter but these grafts have different compositions of tissue and are not just skin or subcutaneous tissue. These particular grafts, similar to the previously mentioned autografts, serve a specific purpose of replacing tissue and are chosen based on their size, location of defect, and physical composition.

Composite grafts (15760–15770) include more than one tissue type, such as the cartilaginous skin found in the ear or nose. This graft type is used to fill in a defect and to provide skin and structural support (cartilage) in the recipient site; therefore, it minimizes scar contraction and distortion because it imitates the tissue and function of the tissue in the recipient area.

Derma-fascia-fat grafts (code 15770) are composed of the dermal layer, fascia, and subcutaneous fat. Indications for this graft are primarily the same as the composite graft in that the purpose is to blend-in or fill-in defects left behind by surgical excisions, atrophy, and so on. The tissue may be grafted in three ways: complete portion (containing all three of the layered components), individual parts (grafted layer by layer), or inserted in combination (such as a fascia-fat layer, later covered by a dermal layer). The technique used to attach the graft is not relevant to code assignment.

Tissue-Cultured Autograft

An autograft as described earlier is harvested from the patient's own body and applied to another area requiring coverage. A tissue-cultured autograft is one that has been first cultured in the laboratory from skin cells harvested from the patient and under controlled conditions grown into sheets of graft material to produce "new skin." The autograft is then applied to the patient's wound.

When the surgeon harvests skin—or more specifically, keratinocytes—and dermal tissue for the cultured autograft, CPT code 15040 *Harvest of skin for tissue cultured skin autograft, 100 sq cm or less* is reported. The skin is removed by using a dermatome to obtain a split-thickness graft. The tissue is sent to a lab and the layers of skin are separated and placed in a special solution that stimulates the skin cells to divide and generate tissue.

Surface area and location matter when assigning codes for the placement of the cultured autograft. The code range is 15150–15157. Codes are reported according to the number of square centimeters used. Either code 15150 or 15155 is reported for the first 25 sq cm. If more than 25 sq cm is used, add-on codes are required for reporting additional square centimeters from 1 *up to* 75 (15151 or 15156). The measurements of the two codes—base code (25 sq cm) plus the add-on code (additional 1 to 75 sq cm)—can add up to 100 sq cm. If the graft tissue required is larger than 100 sq cm (total sq cm of base code plus add-on), then either 15152 or 15157 is also reported to capture each 100 sq cm beyond the first 100 sq cm and/or each additional 1% of body surface or fraction thereof of each. Laboratories can only culture a limited amount of autograft; therefore, for large surface areas this procedure is often performed in stages. Modifier –58 is required to indicate that the procedure is being conducted in stages.

■ **CASE SCENARIO**

A patient suffered extensive road rash to the back when she crashed her motorcycle. The surgeon provided temporary wound closure until the patient's cultured skin was ready to be permanently placed. He placed 150 sq cm of cultured epidermal autograft to the upper and mid-back. This requires reporting three codes: 15150, 15151, 15152. Note that add-on code 15152 states "or part thereof" indicating that the additional sq. cm. autograft does not have to be 100 sq. cm. to use code 15152

The FDA as well as CMS state that skin substitutes are a one-time use item because they have a finite shelf life. Even if the surgeon does not use all of the material to cover the ulcer, wound, or burn, the entire piece of material is billed regardless of the size of the piece applied.

Skin Substitute Grafts

Skin substitutes (15271–15278) are successful in improving wound healing, controlling pain, and improving function and cosmetic appearance. Skin and dermal substitutes refer to nonpermanent grafts. A bilaminate skin substitute is a manufactured product composed of human cells in a bovine (cow) collagen matrix. Skin substitutes are favored for some wound coverage because they are flexible, pliable, and biodegradable. They also resist the stress of stretching and pulling, and allow fibroblast in-growth. Skin substitutes have less risk of disease transmission than traditional cadaver allografts. The substitute has two layers: an outer epidermal layer of silicon rubber and an inner layer of flexible nylon fabric. The inner fabric contains porcine collagen, which promotes fibroblast in-growth and patient acceptance. The artificial skin product TransCyte is made by culturing human neonatal fibroblasts on a synthetic nylon mesh dressing. Once optimal growth is achieved, it is then transplanted or grafted to the patient's wound. When applying a tissue-cultured allogenic skin substitute, report 15002–10005 for preparation of the graft site prior to applying a tissue-cultured allogenic skin substitute—do not report an excisional debridement code.

Acellular dermal replacements are bioengineered artificial skin substitutes. They may go by the names *neodermis, skin substitute, AlloDerm, Integra, Oasis, Surgisis,* or *Dermagraft.* These are temporary skin substitutes used to cover wounds until skin autografts can be harvested and placed. CPT defines acellular dermal replacements as "A tissue-derived or manufactured device that provides immediate, temporary wound closure and that incorporates into the wound and promotes the generation of a neodermis that can support epidermal tissue." These products usually consist

HCPCS codes Q4100–Q4114 should be reported per sq cm for the graft material in addition to the CPT code for the grafting procedure *if* the physician is performing the procedure in his office or is bringing the material with him to the facility. Facility codes will be assigned based on charges entered via the charge master for OR supplies and services. Reporting the HCPCS code for the supply is challenging; it requires the coder to know the brand name of the material and the amount of material applied or the entire size of the material. Because these codes are reported by sq cm, the quantity in the unit's column of the claim form must reflect the correct amount applied.

of a silicone outer epidermis and an inner layer of porous lattice fibers made from a collagen/glycosamine or bovine cartilage mix. They are used to provide full-thickness skin coverage in burn victims when autografting is not an option. The products are also FDA approved for treatment of noninfected partial and full-thickness skin ulcers due to venous insufficiency and neuropathic diabetic foot ulcers. The dermal replacement is applied and in time the patient's dermal cells travel into the graft area. Once new dermal growth has appeared, an epidermal graft may be applied. Wound care centers see many patients receiving this type of graft. Codes are assigned based on anatomic site and upon documentation of the size of the total defect treated. These codes are reported for the total body surface area treated, not per wound site.

> **◉** Unlike the adjacent tissue transfer coding guidelines, when lesions are excised and then repaired with a free skin graft (split thickness or full thickness), the excision of the lesion(s) may be reported separately with codes from the 11400–11471 and 11600–11646 code ranges.

Allografts are used to temporarily cover wounds from burns, traumatic skin injuries, and areas of soft tissue infection or necrosis. An allograft (homograft or allogeneic graft) is a graft transplanted between genetically nonidentical individuals of the same species (i.e., cadaver). The graft protects the exposed recipient site from infection and maintains the overall viability of the underlying tissue until a more suitable autograft can be obtained or cultured later.

A xenograft is a graft transferred from an animal of one species to one of another species, typically porcine (pig) or bovine (cow). Acellular xenografts actually incorporate into the skin during the healing process are not removed but rather become a permanent *implant* of the skin. This is not the case with regular xenografts. Allograft and xenograft tissue, once placed, only lasts a few days, at which time the material is either replaced with more xeno- or allograft material or the autograft procedure can be performed.

Flaps and Adjacent Tissue Transfer or Rearrangement

Flaps and tissue transfers or arrangements differ from skin grafts because they carry their own blood supply. The procedures are carried out when the donor site and the recipient site are in close proximity. The flaps or tissue transfers are not completely severed from the donor site, so the vascular bed is still attached to feed the tissue with adequate blood supply. The *CPT Professional Edition* provides illustrations and descriptions of adjacent tissue repairs.

Skin flaps are used for wound coverage when inadequate vascularity of the wound bed prevents free skin graft survival. Usually, surgeons use tissue transfer to minimize scarring when repairing wounds that are too large or deep for a complex repair. This procedure is most likely to be used for the hand, face, or neck areas, but can be placed anywhere on the body. Each flap is different in the way the skin is incised, undermined, and moved to cover the defect area, leaving the base or connected portion intact. Tissue rearrangement involves freeing skin and subcutaneous tissue and reconfiguring a flap. Flaps are categorized into two major categories: local and distant. *Local* is what the name implies because the wound or defect is adjacent to, in close proximity to, or in the local area of the donor tissue. Local flaps remain attached to their blood supply. Distant flaps are used to cover wounds that are not adjacent to the defect. These may be transferred directly, tubed, or transferred by the microvascular technique.

Adjacent Tissue Transfer or Rearrangement

An adjacent tissue transfer (ATT) or rearrangement includes excising the lesion; therefore, an excision code is not reported in addition to codes 14000–14032. The defect size includes both the original defect being repaired and the secondary defect created by the ATT or rearrangement.

> **EXAMPLE**
> A lesion was excised from the trunk leaving a 7 sq cm defect requiring a rotation flap. After placing the rotation flap, a second defect of 12 sq cm required closure. The ATT code to be reported will be 14001 to include the size of both defects (19 sq cm).

- Codes are reported based both on the anatomical site and the size of the defect repaired, not the size of the tissue flap used.
- The defect size is measured in square centimeters. The code descriptors allow for adjacent tissue transfer for rearrangement of a defect measuring 10 square cm or less, and also for defects measuring 10.1 square cm to 30.0 square cm.

- Adjacent tissue transfer or rearrangement, more than 30 sq cm, unusual or complicated, any area, as stated in the code descriptor, should be reported when the size of the defect is greater than 30 sq cm.
- Additionally, this code may be reported when the physician performs an unusual or complex tissue transfer or rearrangement. CPT does not define unusual or complicated; instead, this determination is made by the physician.
- Code 14300 may be reported for any anatomical area.

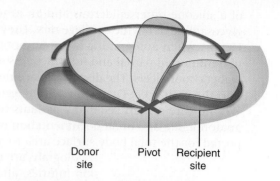

Figure 17.6 Flaps and pivot point.

Adjacent Tissue Transfer/Flaps. To perform an adjacent tissue transfer (e.g., rotation flap, advancement flap and double pedicle flap), a tissue flap is created by surgically freeing the skin and underlying subcutaneous tissue and/or fascia.

- The base of the tissue flap remains connected to one or more borders of the donor site, thus maintaining the blood supply to the surgically created flap.
- Once the flap has been freed from the donor site, it is moved to cover the site of the defect, where it is sutured into place.
- The recipient site may be a laceration or a defect created by removal of a lesion.
- Transfer of the tissue flap may create an exposed area, or secondary defect, at the donor site.
- This may be closed by primary suturing of the wound edges. In some cases, however, a separate graft or flap may be required to close the tissue flap donor site.
- When another graft or flap is required for closure of the donor site, this is considered an additional procedure, and should be reported with a separate CPT code.

Surgeons may use one of four major types of local flaps:

1. Advancement flap
2. Rotation flap
3. Transposition flap
4. Interpolation flap

The rotation, transposition, and interpolation flaps are very similar. Each has a pivot point where the flap is still attached to the vascular bed and rotated (Fig. 17.6). The difference between these flaps is the degree of rotation or arch.

Adjacent tissue transfer involves freeing tissue from around the wound and literally rearranging/transferring it to an adjacent area to cover the defect. Look for all elements of the procedure: lesion removal, development of the flap, and transfer or rearrangement of the surrounding tissue to accomplish final closure. Look for key words such as the following:

- A-T flap
- Z-plasty
- W-plasty
- V-Y plasty
- O-Z plasty
- Rotation flaps
- Advancement flaps (single or double)
- Rhomboid flaps
- Bilobed flaps
- Double pedicle flap

Any excision of lesion that is repaired by an adjacent tissue transfer or flap is included in the transfer code and is not coded separately. The NCCI includes a modifier indicator of "1" for the edits bundling 11400–11646 to 14000–14350. This means that you may use modifier –59 (Distinct procedural service) to override the edits "when the lesion excision and adjacent tissue transfer occur at different anatomical locations or during separate operative sessions."

If two lesions from the same site category are removed and each defect requires an adjacent tissue transfer, each transfer is reported with a –59 modifier on the second code as long as each defect has distinct margins and is not contiguous.

Advancement Flap. An advancement flap moves directly forward without lateral movement. It requires undermining and advancing or moving a flap of tissue forward in the direction of the wound. These flaps are used to repair relatively square wounds. The defect is located at the tip of the flap. Two skin incisions are made in the donor skin parallel to the wound edges. One edge of the wound is thus used as the leading edge of the flap. Pedicle flaps cannot be performed in areas with movement or variable tension such as hands and neck or over joints. An example is the Kutler flap, which is a form of the V-Y advancement flap. An incision is made in the shape of "V" and sutured in the shape of "Y" to lengthen an area. Kutler flaps are used for repairs on the fingers where flaps are created on each side of the finger and then moved toward the tip of the finger to create a normally shaped fingertip.

Rotation Flap. A rotation flap is a semicircular flap of skin that is freed by incising the skin on three sides to create flap and rotated into position over the wound site. In Figure 17.6, the flap with the largest arch would represent a rotation flap.

EXAMPLE
A surgeon removes a lesion measuring 2.5 cm x 2 cm from a patient's left forearm. To repair this primary defect, the surgeon creates a rotation flap measuring 4 cm x 2.5 cm. To determine the total square area of the primary defect, multiply 2.5 x 2 for a total of 5 sq cm. To determine the size of the secondary defect multiply 2.5 x 4 for a total of 10 sq cm. Code 14021 is assigned representing 15 sq cm.

Transposition Flap. A transposition flap is a rectangular skin flap that is rotated into the defect around its pivot point, most commonly at a 90-degree angle. A transposition flap moves sideways about a pivot point into an adjacent defect. Usually, it is designed as a rectangle. Examples of this type of flap are the bilobed flap (Fig. 17.7), the Z-plasty, melolabial flap (nasolabial flap), and the rhomboid flap (actually shaped like the geometric shape with 60-degree and 120-degree angles). The Z-plasty is commonly used to treat scars by lengthening, straightening, or realigning the scar to help reduce tension on the wound. A "Z" type of incision is made and two triangular flaps are interposed to exchange width and length. The bilobed flap has two lobes or pedicles. The primary lobe is transposed to cover the defect and the secondary lobe is used to close the defect left from the donor site.

Interpolation Flap. The interpolation flap rotates about a pivot point into a nearby but not adjacent defect, with the pedicle passing above or below a skin bridge. In this type of flap, the flap does not border the defect and has to cover intact skin between the donor and recipient site. An example is an island pedicle flap where the pedicle consists solely of the supplying artery and veins and possibly a nerve.

Distant and Other Flaps
CPT codes 15570–15776 are used for flap grafts. The pedicle is created anywhere on the body, stretching the skin to a nearby site, and suturing it in place. The flap is actually staged whereby the pedicle is severed once the recipient site begins to create its own blood supply to the flap. Codes 15733–15738 and 15756 refer specifically to muscle, myocutaneous, or fasciocutaneous flaps. In order to assign these codes, these tissues must be specified in the documentation of the donor tissue flap development being used to graft.

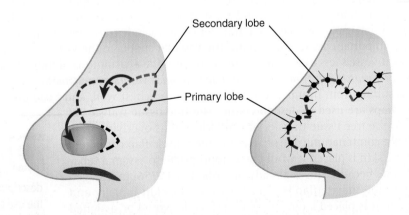

Figure 17.7 The bilobed flap.

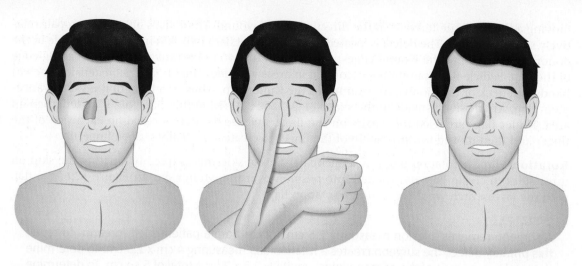

Figure 17.8 The tubed pedicle flap.

Distant flaps require two or more operations. The first operation consists of creating the flap and transferring it to the recipient site. The second operation is required to then detach the flap at the donor end once the blood vessels have developed at the other end and the surgeon feels the flap will be viable once severed from the base of the flap. There are three major categories of distant flaps: direct flap, tubed flap, and microvascular flap.

Direct Flap. A direct flap is transferred to a distant site directly so that the donor and recipient sites are attached. The flap is divided or separated 1–3 weeks after the first stage.

Tubed Flap. The tubed flap is a flap of skin elevated from a distant site from the defect and then sewn down its long edges forming a tube or stalk, leaving one end attached to the site of origin (donor site) and the other is attached to the site to be grafted (recipient site) (Fig. 17.8). The pedicle maintains the blood supply into that flap, keeping it viable. The new blood supply from the donor site is incorporated from the distant end of the flap. The procedure begins with the lifting of a large flap of skin by making a U-shaped incision. The long (lateral) edges of the skin flap are stitched together to form a tube to prevent the underside of the skin flap from drying out. The free end of the tube is then attached to the recipient site while the other end of the tube remains attached. For tubed flaps, tissue must be taken from distant parts of the body in stages. After a number of weeks, the tube is cut near the recipient area leaving enough skin on the graft to shape and model as needed to fully cover the defect. The remaining tube can be repositioned back to its original donor site by opening the tube and suturing it back into place. Report codes 15570–15576 for creation of the direct or tubed pedicle flap. 15600–15630 are reported for the delay or sectioning of the pedicle. 15650 is used to describe the final transfer or separation of the pedicle flap.

Microvascular Flaps. A microvascular flap is a type of distant flap in which the tissue is transferred from one area of the body to another using microsurgical techniques. As the name implies, microsurgical procedures require the use of an operating microscope. The free flap, with its vascular pedicle, is divided completely from its donor vessels and anastomosed to the recipient vessels at the recipient site. It should be noted that all of the free tissue transfer codes include transferring a portion of the fascia. The fascia is very important because it contains the vascular supply to the skin. Microsurgery includes the anastomosis of vessels less than 2 mm in diameter and the anastomosis of individual nerve fibers.

Code 15756 *Free muscle flap or myocutaneous flap with microvascular anastomosis* is used to cover soft tissue defects resulting from trauma, reconstruction of the chest wall, and head and neck surgery. Myocutaneous flaps are used to describe either the free tissue transfer of a muscle only or the free tissue transfer of a muscle and its overlying skin. 15756 is used as a combination code so when a free muscle flap combined with its overlying skin is placed it would be inappropriate to assign a separate skin graft code because this is already described in 15756. In a staged procedure where the muscle flap is placed without the skin initially and a separate skin graft is placed later, the skin graft code would be assigned separately on a subsequent claim with a –58 modifier. The preparation and debridement of the recipient site (prior to the actual creation and transfer

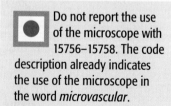

Do not report the use of the microscope with 15756–15758. The code description already indicates the use of the microscope in the word *microvascular*.

of the flap) including the microdissection of arteries, veins, and nerves of the recipient site is not included in the free flap graft code, and should be reported separately. Examples of free muscle flaps are latissimus dorsi flap, serratus anterior flap, gracilis flap, rectus abdominis flap, tensor fascia lata flap, and extensor digitorum brevis. As with other flap and graft procedures, if a skin graft is needed to close the donor muscle flap site, a separate graft code is assigned to close the secondary defect. The donor site is always closed at the time of the initial free flap, either directly or with a skin graft.

Code15757 is used to report free skin flaps with microvascular anastomosis. Examples of free skin flaps are: free scapula, parascapula, groin flap, lateral arm, gluteal flap, and medial thigh flap.

Free fascial flaps (15758) involve only the elevation and transfer of the fascia. They are used when soft tissue coverage is needed without the bulk of muscle. Free fascial flaps are limited in use compared to other types of free flap grafts. The fascial flaps are usually covered with a skin graft, which would be coded separately. These could be used to cover joints and the dorsum of the hand. Examples of fascial flaps are: lateral and radial forearm flap and temporalis flap.

Skin Graft and Tissue Transfer Coding Steps

Successful graft and tissue transfer code assignment requires that you follow the steps below. See Pinpoint the Code 17.3.

1. **Determine if there was a lesion removal also performed.** If lesion removal is performed simultaneously with a flap or tissue transfer, do not assign a separate code for the lesion removal. It is included in the flap procedure. It is, however, separately reportable with the free skin graft. There are three exceptions to this rule. The first exception is if the flap or transfer is staged, which means the surgeon removed the lesion at a previous operative session. In this case, both the lesion removal and the repair can be separately reported; however, the flap code must have a –58 modifier if the tissue transfer occurs during the excision's 10-day global period. The second exception pertains to lesion removals and adjacent tissue transfers performed on the same day during the same operative session but on separate sites. For example, if a lesion is removed from the shoulder as well as from the forearm and the forearm defect requires an adjacent tissue transfer, both can be reported but the lesion removal code must be appended by the –59 modifier to indicate that these are separate lesions and sites. The third exception applies to lesion removal with complex repair. Both codes may be reported if it is performed at the same session.
2. **Determine what type of graft or tissue transfer/flap is performed.** Differentiate transfers from repairs/grafts and flaps.
3. **Determine the anatomic area and the size of the defect in square centimeters.** Consider each repair separately if more than one repair type is performed at different sites. These should each be calculated separately by type and not added together. If the surgeon uses more than one type of flap to close a defect, a code for each flap or graft is separately assigned based on the defect's size.
4. **Report surgical preparation for skin grafts separately if the surgeon removed intact tissue.**
5. **Assign the HCPCS code for the allograft if supplied by the physician.** Facility coders should check the charges in the facility computer system to see if this was captured in the chargemaster. If not, assign the HCPCS code for the supply.
6. Append modifiers if necessary for staged procedures (–58) or separate sites (–59).

CHECKPOINT 17.3

Assign codes to the following procedures:

1. A patient is treated for a chronic venous stasis ulcer of the lower calf. The patient has been managed in the wound care clinic for 8 weeks with debridement, whirlpool therapy, and compression dressings and is now ready today for graft closure. An acellular graft is applied to the 5 cm x 12 cm ulcer site. _____

2. Split-thickness autograft, 80 sq cm., lower leg, staged procedure. _____

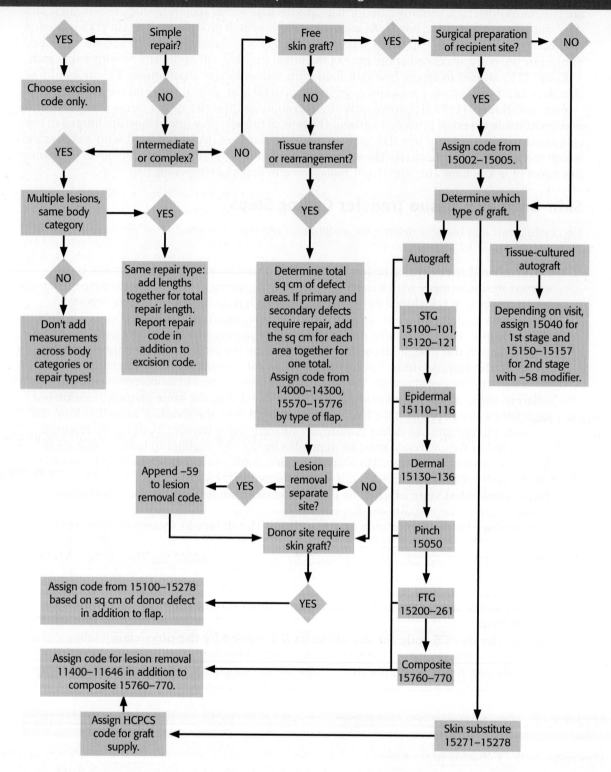

BURNS

Burns are a type of injury caused by heat, cold, electricity, chemicals, light, radiation, or friction. Two million people in the United States each year are treated for burn injuries. According to WebMD, burn injuries account for an estimated 700,000 annual ED visits per year, with 45,000 requiring hospitalization. It is important to learn about burn types and treatments because it is likely coders will encounter these when coding ED visits and inpatient records. Table 17.5 and Figure 17.9 illustrate the type of burns.

It is important for the ICD-10 diagnosis codes specifying the percentage of body area burned to be linked to the respective dressing or debridement code for demonstration of medical necessity.

Burn acuity is judged by the amount of skin surface affected, the severity, the depth of the burn, and resultant complications. Burns that extend deep may cause permanent injury and scarring and not allow the skin in that area to return to normal function. First-degree burns are minor in nature and only involve the epidermis and can be treated at home with basic first aid and over-the-counter pain relievers. Second-degree burns involve the epidermis and part of the dermis. These can also be treated at home unless the skin becomes infected. Third-degree burns involve the epidermis, dermis, and subcutaneous layers of skin. These layers are destroyed and precipitate complications such as dehydration, infection, and loss of limb. Muscle, bone, blood vessel, and epidermal tissue can all be damaged, with subsequent pain due to profound injury to nerves. The more body surface area (BSA) involved in a burn, the greater the morbidity and mortality rates and the greater the management challenge.

CPT contains a section that includes local treatment of burns, but this section does not include skin grafting and medical management services. CPT codes 16000–16030 describe burn dressing

Table 17.5 Types of Burns

BURN TYPE	SKIN LAYER(S)	FEATURE
First-degree	Epidermis	Superficial reddened area of skin. Redness, swelling, pain to touch. Similar to a sunburn.
Second-degree	Epidermis, superficial dermis, and/or partial deep reticular dermis. Partial-thickness superficial or partial-thickness deep	Redness, blistering, pallor. Skin blanches with pressure and is still moist. Extremely painful.
Third-degree	Complete dermis, full thickness	Grayish white ash or black char with necrosis. Leather appearance. Loss of feeling. The epidermis is lost with damage to the subcutaneous tissue, which requires surgical intervention for wound healing such as debridement and grafting. Dermis and underlying tissue and possibly fascia, bone, or muscles are damaged.
Fourth-degree	Complete dermis, fat, and muscle; may include bone and joints	Dry, crispy, black charred tissue. Loss of feeling because nerves are destroyed. Function of area is lost or severely limited. Amputation or extensive surgical intervention is required. Death may result.
Scald	Epidermis, superficial dermis	Caused by hot liquids or gases such as hot water, grease, or radiator fluid.
Chemical	Epidermis, dermis	Direct skin exposure to strong acid or base solutions causing redness, pain, blistering, and in some cases necrosis of skin. Some agents cause deep-tissue burns.
Electrical	Can damage all layers of skin	Occur to the skin when directly exposed to an electrical current from, for example, a live wire or electrical outlet.
Contact	Epidermis	Deep burns that are contained where the skin comes in direct contact with hot objects such as curling irons, muffler tail pipes, hot irons, cigarettes, and stoves.

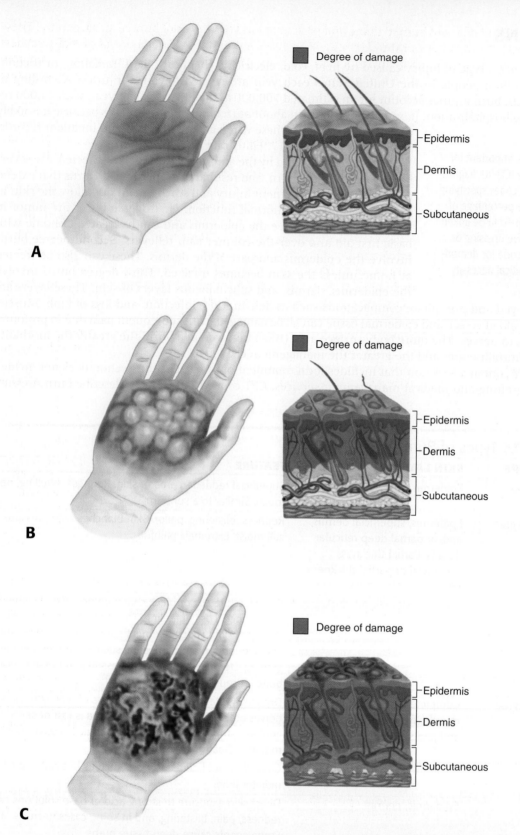

Figure 17.9 Burn. A. First-degree burn. B. Second-degree burn. C. Third-degree burn.

and/or debridement of burned tissue and pertain to local treatment of burned surfaces only. These codes refer to treatment of the skin surface or dressings and/or debridement of partial-thickness burns. Full-thickness debridement of skin is not located in this subsection of CPT. It is reported separately, however, if the surgeon must debride deeper layers of tissue; use CPT codes 11042–11047.

The codes are differentiated by size: small, medium, or large. Code 16000 is the only code in this series that refers to the "specific type of burn; first degree." Dressing and debridement codes 16020–16030 are used for either initial or subsequent treatments and are assigned based on what percentage of body surface was involved. Body surfaces are divided into small (less than 5%), medium (5%–10%), and large (over 10%). The coder should be familiar with the Rule of Nines, which is used to calculate the percentage of a body burned by dividing the total BSA into 9% or multiples of 9% segments. Refer to your codebook for the Rule of Nines used to estimate body surface. In an infant or child, the "rule" deviates because of the large surface area of a child's head. *CPT Professional Edition* includes a table in this section titled the "Lund-Browder Diagram and Classification Method Table for Burn Estimations." The coder can locate the body part affected and the age of the patient to assist in selecting the appropriate code based on percentage of body surface burned.

Small burns or minor burns are treated with a silver sulfadiazine (Silvadene) dressing in the ED or the physician office. In this case, CPT code 16020, *Dressings and/or debridement of partial-thickness burns, initial or subsequent; small,* would be reported.

> **E/M codes reported with burn codes 16000–16036 will be denied unless the E/M code is reported with a –25 modifier. As always, the E/M service must be documented and be separately identifiable from the burn care.**

> **When 16035 is billed, the ICD-10 code reported should indicate the burn was full thickness or deeper; otherwise, carriers will deny 16035 and 16036.**

■ CASE SCENARIO

A patient was camping and poured lighter fluid on to a charcoal grill, causing the flame to flare up and burn his hands, arms, neck, and face. He was taken to the local ED and determined to have 25% total body surface area (TBSA) first-degree burns and 4% second-degree burns on the hands. First-degree burn treatment was provided to his face, arms, and neck and second-degree treatment with Silvadene and gauze was provided to the hands. Codes: 16000, 16020.

Burn patients commonly undergo an escharotomy to relieve pain and pressure at the burn site when eschar is prominent. Escharotomy (16035) is an incision made through the eschar (dead tissue or scab) into the fat layer below. The aim of the escharotomy is to release the pressure over the involved deeper tissues and to restore circulation to this tissue. Escharotomy is indicated for circumferential full-thickness burns. Escharotomy may be reported for each anatomical area in which it is performed. Use modifier –59 to identify each area treated.

As described earlier, codes 15002–15005 describe burn and wound preparation or incisional or excisional release of scar contracture, resulting in an open wound requiring a skin graft. Such wound preparation is required when the site has uneven layers or multiple layers. Uneven or multiple layers could cause the graft not to adhere or connect to the wound surface and thus fail or "die." Report this procedure in addition to the code for the actual graft. This excisional preparation is coded *once per recipient area* by the size of the excision.

CHECKPOINT 17.4

Assign codes to the following procedure. Include any necessary modifiers.

1. The patient was burned on his upper arm and now suffers pain from the burn scar (eschar) in that area. The surgeon makes three incisions around the scar to release the constriction and pain caused by the scar. _____

WOUND CARE AND DEBRIDEMENT

The primary goals of active wound care are to debride the wound of devitalized tissue, cleanse the wound, promote coverage of the skin defect, and restore function to the tissue and surrounding area. Wound care services include assessment of the wound, debridement (selective or nonselective), cleansing of the wound, and dressing of the wound (including application of topical ointments, wound bed protection, and bulk dressing).

Debridement is the removal of dead, necrotic, devitalized, or damaged tissue (including cartilage) and/or foreign material from a wound. This can be accomplished surgically by using a sharp instrument such as a scalpel or scissors, or nonsurgically by using wet-to-dry dressings, whirlpool baths, or application of medications that contain enzymes to dissolve dead tissue. A debridement is done to leave behind viable tissue and promote healing. Phrases to indicate this procedure include "tissue was removed until healthy-appearing tissue was encountered" or "tissue was sharply debrided until bleeding tissue was visualized."

The objective is to preserve granulation tissue (pink) in the wound and remove fibrin tissue (white, yellow, or green tissue) or necrotic (black) tissue. Debridement is indicated when a wound is erythematous, shows fluctuance, or has discolored discharge. Debridement is performed at the bedside, in the OR, or in a wound care clinic. Anesthesia is necessary when debriding deep wounds or when bone biopsies are obtained.

EXAMPLE
11000 *Debridement of extensive eczematous or infected skin; up to 10% of body surface.*

Several codes in the Integumentary System section of CPT and in the Medicine section encompass some level of surgical debridement. The coder must make an educated decision about which code to assign based on the following:

- Why the debridement is being performed
- Where it is being performed
- Who performed the procedure
- The depth of the debridement
- The type of wound dressing applied

Debridement is commonly performed on soft tissues of the body. This tissue connects, supports, or surrounds other structures and organs of the body. Partial-thickness debridement includes the epidermis and part *but not all* of the dermal layer of skin. Full-thickness debridement involves epidermis and dermis layers. Debridement of a wound may be any type of debridement, such as mechanical, surgical, autolytic, or chemical. Refer to Table 17.6 for a list of common surgical and excisional debridement methods and their respective CPT codes (see Chapter 29 for a discussion of nonexcisional methods). Selective debridement refers to controlled debridement of a targeted area of skin where tissue is removed leaving behind healthy, undamaged tissue. Instruments such as scissors and forceps are used to cut the tissue along the margin of viable and nonviable tissue, which requires a greater set of skills by a qualified health-care provider. In contrast, nonselective debridement methods are not as controlled; therefore, they do not have the ability to target certain tissues and run the risk of damaging healthy tissue. Debridement is also carried out on joints and nerves to remove scar tissue or other material.

Debridement Codes

Surgical debridement codes are divided into four sections:

1. Codes 11000 and +11001
   - Based on body surface percentage
2. Codes 11004 through +11008
   - Specific to necrotizing soft tissue infections
   - Specific to anatomical locations
3. Codes 11010–11012
   - Specific to debridement associated with open fractures and/or dislocations
   - Based on depth

Table 17.6 Surgical/Excisional Methods

Code(s)	Description	Code(s)
97602	Debridement of extensive eczematous or infected skin	11000–11001
97602	Debridement of skin, subcutaneous muscle, and fascia for necrotizing tissue	11004–11006
97602	Debridement of skin by depth including removal of foreign material for open fracture and/or dislocation	11010–11012
97602	Debridement of skin by depth	11042–11047
97602	Excision of pressure ulcers	15920–15999

4. Codes 11042–11047
   - For all other types of debridement (ulcers, injuries, infections, etc.)
   - Based on depth, not on location.
     - If reporting a single wound/ulcer, and so on, base the code on the depth of the wound. Examples: Subcutaneous, muscle, bone
     - If reporting multiple wounds/ulcers, and so on, combine (sum) the surface area of the wounds that are at the same depth.

■ CASE SCENARIO

A patient has two ulcers, one on the heel and one on the hip; both ulcers go down to the bone. The heel ulcer is 4 sq cm. The hip ulcer is 10 sq cm. The coder will report code 11044, *Debridement, bone (includes epidermis, dermis, subcutaneous tissue, muscle, and/or fascia, if performed); first 20 sq cm or less*. This code was selected based on the total square centimeters of the two debridement (14 cm). Note that code 11044 is an out-of-sequence code.

■ CASE SCENARIO

A patient has two wounds, one on the abdomen and one on the thigh. The abdominal wound is 16 sq cm. The thigh wound is 10 sq cm. The coder will report code 11042 for the first 20 sq cm and add-on code +11045 to represent the additional 6 sq cm. If the physician treated all four wounds during the same session, the coder would report 11042, 11042-59, +11045-59.

Wounds are classified into stages developed by the Agency for Health Care Research and Quality (AHRQ) Clinical Practice Guidelines (Table 17.7).

Clinical studies show that as deep ulcers heal, the lost muscle, fat, and dermis are *not* replaced. Per the *National Pressure Ulcer Advisory Panel (NPUAP) Report*, Vol. 4, No. 2, September 1995, granulation tissue fills the defect before re-epithelialization. Knowing this, it is not appropriate to reverse-stage a healing ulcer when documenting wound status. In other words, a stage III pressure ulcer does not become a stage II or stage I pressure ulcer during healing. The provider must methodically record the wound's healing progress by noting an improvement in the characteristics (size, depth, amount of necrotic tissue, amount of exudate, etc.). Invariably, stage III and IV wounds require skin grafting, skin flaps, musculocutaneous flaps, or free flaps for final closure.

Codes 11000–11001 refer to debridement of extensive eczematous or infected skin and are assigned according to the percentage of body surface affected. Codes 11004–11006 are assigned for debridement of necrotizing soft tissue of the genitalia or abdominal wall only. Codes 11010–11012

Table 17.7 Wound Stages

Stage	Description
I	Nonblanchable erythema of intact skin, the heralding lesion of skin ulceration. In individuals with darker skin, discoloration of the skin, warmth, edema, induration, or hardness may also be indicators.
II	Partial-thickness skin loss involving epidermis, dermis, or both. The ulcer is superficial and presents clinically as an abrasion, blister, or shallow crater.
III	Full-thickness skin loss involving damage to or necrosis of subcutaneous tissue that may extend down to, but not through, underlying fascia. The ulcer presents clinically as a deep crater with or without undermining of adjacent tissue.
IV	Full-thickness skin loss with extensive destruction, tissue necrosis, or damage to muscle, bone, or supporting structures (e.g., tendon, joint capsule). Undermining and sinus tracts also may be associated with Stage IV pressure ulcers.

involve debridement associated only with open fractures or dislocations. This type of debridement can be performed at any stage of the fracture care—before, during, or after the surgical treatment of the fracture. Codes 11042–11047 are based on thickness of the debridement. These codes are assigned for debridement of gangrene, ulcers, and nonhealing wounds. According to many carriers, this type of surgical debridement is only medically necessary if infected, necrotic, devitalized, or nonviable tissue is present. Do not report these codes for washing bacterial or fungal debris from lesions, paring or cutting of corns or calluses, incision and drainage of abscess including paronychia, trimming or debridement of nails, avulsion of nail plates, acne surgery, destruction of warts, or burn debridement. Providers instead should report these procedures when reasonable and necessary using the appropriate CPT or HCPCS codes that accurately describe the service such as those located in the Medicine section.

● Debridement performed as part of a primary procedure is included in that procedure unless the debridement is extensive.

● It is very common to provide multiple debridement in a span of several days or weeks, as in the case of open fracture and non-healing wounds. In these cases, the –58 modifier would be applied during the global period. Debridement of superficial tissue is not coded separately in this case.

■ CASE SCENARIO
A physician sees a patient in the office and debrides 15 sq cm of skin and subcutaneous tissue from a nonhealing surgical wound. Code: 11042.

Code range 15920–15999 is used specifically to code debridement or excision of pressure ulcers. Note, however, that these codes are only for pressure ulcers of the coccyx, sacrum, ischium, or trochanter. What about the other sites of the body previously mentioned that are prone to pressure ulcers? Debridement codes from the 11042–11047 range would apply as well as additional codes from the flap or graft subsection if repair was also done. Codes are specific to the site of the ulcer. Pay close attention to the wording of these code descriptors. These codes are combination codes in that the code description includes excision and repair (e.g., flap closure, ostectomy) all in one code. It is incorrect to assign codes for tissue flaps, grafts, or repairs in addition to these codes. CPT does direct the coder to assign codes for muscle or myocutaneous flap closure in addition to these services. Many of these codes also depict excision with ostectomy. In the case of ischial ulcer excision *without* ostectomy, report code 15946 with a –52 modifier to reflect that the ostectomy was not performed because this code does not have a companion code for *without* ostectomy.

● Debridement codes are reported for each site treated. The additional sites would be coded and appended with the –59 modifier.

● Codes 97597–97606 cannot be reported in conjunction with 11040–11044.

● 97602 has a status indicator "B" on the MPFS database, meaning that it is not separately payable under Medicare.

Medicare does not consider the following services to be debridement services:

- Removal of necrotic tissue by cleansing, scraping (other than with a scalpel or a curette), chemical application, and/or wet-to-dry dressing technique
- Trimming of callous or fibrinous material from ulcer margins
- Cleaning and dressing of small or superficial lesions
- Removing coagulation serum from normal skin surrounding an ulcer

Local infiltration, metacarpal/digital block, and topical anesthesia are included in the reimbursement for debridement services and are not separately payable.

Medical necessity must be documented in the patient's medical record based on the following criteria:

1. Treatment will significantly improve the wound in a reasonable period of time.
2. The expectation is that the dressing will significantly improve healing and tissue viability, reduce or control tissue infection, and allow tissue preparation for surgical grafting.
3. Additional precautions, such as appropriate bedding, padding, and patient turning, have been taken to prevent the formation of new or perpetuation of existing ulcers or wounds.
4. A treatment plan is established at the beginning of any debridement therapy outlining specific goals, duration, frequency of dressing, number/amount of dressings to be used at one time (if more than one), size of dressing, modalities, expected duration of need, and other pertinent factors as they may apply. An explanation should be provided for any deviation from this plan.

Wound Dressing

Surgical dressings must be ordered by a physician or an NP, clinical nurse specialist, certified nurse-midwife, or PA who is acting within the scope of his or her legal authority as defined by state law or regulation. Alloplastic dressings are man-made coverings used to aid healing of ulcers or wounds. As discussed earlier, these are not skin grafts but rather temporary wound coverings. Composite dressings such as Tegaderm, Telfa, and Viasorb are used for wounds with minimal to heavy drainage, healthy granulation tissue, or necrotic tissue. Most composite dressings have three layers: (1) a semiadherent or nonadherent layer that touches the wound and protects the wound from adhering to other material—drainage passes through it into the next layer, which is absorptive; (2) an absorptive layer that wicks drainage and debris away from the wound's surface and helps liquefy eschar and necrotic debris, facilitating autolytic debridement; and (3) an outer bacterial barrier layer, which may have an adhesive border, that allows moisture vapor to pass from the wound to the air and keeps bacteria and particles out of the wound.

A signed order for the dressing must be present along with a treatment plan for the wound care. The order should include type of dressing, size of dressing, and frequency of changes. Both primary and secondary dressings are covered when either of the following criteria is met: (1) They are medically necessary for the treatment of a wound caused by, or treated by, a surgical procedure; or (2) they are medically necessary when debridement of a wound is medically necessary.

A new order is required for wound dressing in the following circumstances:

1. When a new dressing is added
2. When the quantity of an existing dressing increases
3. Every 3 months for each dressing being used, even if the quantity remains unchanged

Dressings may be used as long as necessary until the wound is healed or a permanent skin graft is performed.

Many wound care items are not covered. Review the list below and make sure that the physician is aware. An advance beneficiary notice (ABN) may be required.

1. Dressings for cutaneous fistula drainage that has not been caused by or treated by a surgical procedure
2. Dressings for stage I pressure ulcers
3. Dressings for first-degree burns
4. Dressings for traumatic wounds that do not require surgical closure or debridement
5. Skin sealants or barriers, wound cleansers or irrigating solutions, solutions used to moisten gauze (e.g., saline), topical antiseptics, and topical antibiotics

6. Enzymatic debriding agents
7. Surgical tray items such as gauze or other dressings used to debride a wound, but not left on the wound

According to CMS policy, the use of skin substitutes (15271–15278), or skin substitute material (Q4100–Q4111) is considered not reasonable and necessary when used for or with the presence of cellulitis, osteomyelitis, necrotic ulcer, draining wound, or bone-exposed wound bed. Q4100–Q4111 are payable by contractor discretion. Dressings used for mechanical debridement are typically covered. Check your local CMS contractor for specific Local Coverage Determinations (LCDs).

Hyperbaric Oxygen Therapy (HBO²)

Hyperbaric oxygen therapy utilizes a pressure chamber to administer oxygen under pressure. It boosts wound healing by hyperoxygenation of tissue, which promotes vasoconstriction and has antibacterial effects. These chambers provide tissue oxygen levels of greater than 11 times normal, quickly feeding tissue that is hypoxic, or oxygen deprived, with much needed oxygen to stimulate wound healing. Hypoxic or ischemic wounds such as diabetic wounds, venous stasis ulcers, failing grafts and flaps, necrotizing soft tissue infections, and refractory osteomyelitis can all benefit from this therapy. It is primarily used to aid in healing of diabetic ulcers, venous stasis ulcers, and arterial insufficiency ulcers.

> CMS has very strict coverage policies for HBO² therapy, requiring specific diagnoses. Check for LCDs in your state.

To report this service, 99183 is submitted for each session during which the physician is in personal attendance. Per CPT, any E/M service provided in a hyperbaric oxygen facility in conjunction with this service should be reported with the appropriate E/M code.

States have specific rules for if and when a physician must be present during this service. These rules vary from requiring the physician to check in with the patient at least every 30 minutes during each patient treatment and at the end with an expected response time of 1 minute for an emergency to requiring the physician to be in continuous attendance within the immediate hyperbaric oxygen area. Coverage is also limited to place of service and diagnosis.

MOHS MICROGRAPHIC SURGERY

Mohs micrographic surgery is a surgical technique used to remove the three most common types of skin cancer: basal cell carcinoma (BCC), squamous cell carcinoma (SCC), and melanoma. It offers a strong cure rate of approximately 98% and spares healthy tissue. Mohs is the standard of care when a tumor is either in a critical location (either cosmetic or functional), recurrent, has ill-defined margins, or is large (over 2 cm) or aggressive in its growth. The surgery is unique in that the surgeon acts as both the surgeon and the pathologist.

Procedure

The surgery is typically performed in stages in the outpatient office under local anesthetic by a dermatologist. A thin layer of the tumor is removed, marked, and frozen and stained so that it can be examined under the microscope. A two-dimensional diagram is drawn of the specimen. The saucer-shaped specimen is further divided, numbered, and colored into units called *tissue blocks*. All of these steps are mapped on the Mohs operative map. This map precisely outlines the residual tumor and allows for examination of 100% of the surgical margin, thus sparing normal surrounding tissue. If malignant cells are still found at the margins, the surgeon will repeat the process. Each layer that is removed and examined is called a "stage," and it may take any number of stages to remove an aggressive tumor.

Code Assignment

Each stage of the Mohs procedure is coded separately. Code descriptions for the number of specimens and the stage should be read carefully. When additional layers are removed, add-on codes 17312 or 17314 are used. Should any stages require more than five tissue blocks, use code 17315 and indicate the number of units over five taken in each layer.

EXAMPLE

Cancers of the neck and right upper back are treated by Mohs micrographic surgery in one stage each. Codes: 17311, 17313.

EXAMPLE

A cancer of the nose requires a first and second stage of Mohs micrographic surgery. Codes: 17311, 17312.

Repairs and grafts/flaps may be done to close the defect created by the removal of the tumor. In this case, these are coded separately. Any such reconstructions are not routine or expected work in conjunction with Mohs micrographic surgery.

If a definitive diagnosis of a tumor is not available, the Mohs surgeon may obtain a biopsy to confirm the diagnosis of skin cancer before initiating the surgery. The biopsy and the frozen section surgical pathology code 88331 may be additionally reported with a modifier –59. Code 11100–59 is reported for the biopsy procedure, and 88331–59 for the pathology interpretation of the skin biopsy specimen. Any other pathology service associated with MOHS surgery is included in the MOHS codes.

INTERNET RESOURCE: Visit the Mohs College website for a patient education video explaining Mohs surgery.
www.mohscollege.org/about/video_patient_education.php

CHECKPOINT 17.5

Assign codes to the following procedures. Include any necessary modifiers.

1. A patient is being treated for injuries sustained in a motor vehicle accident earlier in the day. Debridement is necessary on his right foot down to the muscle and on his right hand down to the subcutaneous tissue. _____

2. The surgeon performed Mohs surgery on an upper extremity malignancy. He performed a first-stage excision with seven tissue blocks. The frozen section examined by the surgeon revealed that the tumor was still present. A second-stage excision was performed with four tissue blocks and the tumor was still present. A third-stage excision with four tissue blocks revealed no tumor present in the margins. _____

BREAST PROCEDURES

Procedures performed on the breast may be for therapeutic or cosmetic purposes. Mammaplasty refers to various surgical techniques used to change the size or shape of a patient's breast(s). Cosmetic procedures on the breast are most often performed by plastic surgeons but may also be performed by dermatologists. Breast mastectomies are primarily performed by general surgeons but may also be performed by plastic surgeons. Breast reconstruction procedures are performed by plastic surgeons.

The diagnostic and therapeutic procedures used to diagnose, stage, and treat breast disease are rapidly becoming less drastic and less invasive. Breast imaging procedures such as mammography, ultrasonography, magnetic resonance imaging (MRI), fine needle aspiration (FNA), core biopsy, and surgical excisional biopsy are routinely performed in diagnosis and management of breast disease. Many surgical physician practices can perform breast ultrasonography and ultrasound-guided biopsy in the office setting. Trends now show that excisional breast biopsy is being superseded by FNA biopsy for palpable breast lesions and by percutaneous biopsy for nonpalpable breast lesions. Stereotactic and ultrasound-guided needle core biopsies are less-invasive alternatives to open surgical biopsies for most patients with nonpalpable breast lesions whereby tissue must be sampled to achieve a diagnosis.

Breast biopsies are performed using the following methods:

- FNA
- Needle core biopsy
- Open biopsy (excisional or incisional)

Fine-Needle Aspiration

Fine-needle aspiration (FNA) biopsy samples cells from lesions for cytological analysis rather than removing the lesion itself. FNA is not a biopsy where tissue is taken and examined. CPT codes 10021–10022 include preparation of smears, if prepared. These codes do not specify an anatomical part and are used if FNA is performed anywhere on the body. FNA is typically the first step in the evaluation of breast masses. A local anesthetic is usually not needed. The tip of the needle is advanced into the lesion before any suction is performed to avoid collection of tissue outside the lesion. Once the tip is in place, strong suction is applied, and the needle is moved back and forth within the lesion repeatedly along a 5- to 10-mm long track to loosen and collect cells. The needle is then withdrawn from the breast and the sample expelled onto prepared glass slides, spread into a thin smear, and fixed according to the preferences of the cytology laboratory. Assign codes 10021–10022 depending on whether imaging guidance was utilized.

INTERNET RESOURCE: Visit *MedlinePlus* to view illustrations of FNA. http://nlm.nih.gov/medlineplus/ency/imagepages/17016.htm

Needle Core Biopsy

Needle core biopsy removes a narrow cylinder of tissue that is submitted for standard pathological rather than cytological analysis. Needle core biopsy is ideal for sampling large lesions and not ideal for small, nonpalpable lesions. If the mass is palpable, the surgeon can perform the biopsy in the office. Injection of a local anesthetic is required. A large needle is placed either by hand or with a biopsy gun device into the mass. A small "nick" is made in the skin with a scalpel to create an entry point for the biopsy needle into breast tissue and then into the lesion.

If the lesion is nonpalpable but detected on mammography, stereotactic image-guided biopsy is the preferred approach. When possible, needle core biopsy is performed with ultrasound guidance, which confirms needle position within the lesion as the procedure is done. Stereotactic mammography-guided needle core biopsy is performed if the lesion is not visualized on ultrasound.

Biopsy code 19100 is assigned for each lesion or site biopsied. The code description is specific to a biopsy not using imaging guidance and is a designated separate procedure.

Open Biopsy

Open biopsy can be either incisional or excisional. The difference is based on the amount of breast tissue or lesion removed.

Incisional Breast Biopsy

Incisional biopsy (19101) is cutting of breast tissue where a small portion or slice of a lesion is removed. Incisional biopsies are typically performed on large lesions.

Cytological analysis is conducted on specimens obtained through FNA. This involves spreading a fluid specimen on a glass slide for examination at the cellular level under a microscope. Pathological analysis is conducted on tissue obtained from core biopsies, excisional biopsies, and surgical resections. It is performed by a combination of macroscopic and histological examination of the tissue and at times may involve other chemistry and other laboratory tests.

Do not assign 19100 to report FNA. 19100 is for reporting needle core biopsies only.

When coding breast biopsies requiring imaging assistance, be sure to note that the codes now include the imaging portion of the biopsy, if performed. Coders will no longer report the radiology imaging codes 76942, 77002, 77012, or 77021. CPT codes 19081–19086 now include the imaging services when performed.

Remember that add-on codes such as 19291 and 19295 are coded only in conjunction with a parent code.

Excisional Breast Biopsy

Excisional biopsy (19120) involves removing an entire lesion (male or female). This type of biopsy is carried out when the mass is larger than 4 cm or so in diameter, is deeper and harder to reach, or contains microcalcifications.

Excisional Biopsy With Needle Localization

Needle localization is the placement of a guide wire. Insertion of a localization device (e.g., guide wire) is most often done preoperatively in the radiology department, and if that is the case, would not be coded separately by the surgeon. This procedure is coded separately if done in a different location. Codes for insertion of the guide wire (19281–19288) vary based on the method of guidance used: mammogram, stereotactic, ultrasound, or MRI. All specimens excised with a previously placed marker are immediately radiographed (76098) to confirm that the lesion has been excised in its entirety. In rare circumstances, the surgeon may place the localization device and surgically excise the lesion, in which case he would report both services with 19125/19126 for the excision and a code from 19281–19288 for the localization. Device placement and surgical excision is also discussed in Chapter 27.

When coding for this procedure, it is important to differentiate whose work is being coded (i.e., radiologist, surgeon, or facility). Each entity codes for its portion of the service and uses modifiers to indicate such.

■ CASE SCENARIO

A female patient undergoes an excisional breast biopsy of the right breast with placement of a preoperative needle guide wire in the radiology department via stereotactic guidance. The radiologist places the guide wire before the patient is taken to the OR. The surgeon removes the suspicious lesion that is indicated by the guide wire and confirms via x-ray that the lesion has indeed been removed. The radiologist would bill for the guide wire insertion: code 19283–26–RT. The surgeon would bill for the excisional biopsy: code 19125–RT. The facility would report codes 19125–RT–TC, 19283–RT–TC, and 76098.

Image-Guided Placement of Metallic Marker

After needle core biopsy, areas where lesions were biopsied can be difficult to re-identify, particularly after needle core biopsy, because the lesions may be altered and be made even less conspicuous. Placement of a marker (clip, pellet, wire) to aid in relocating the lesion is reported separately from the biopsy code for each site marked. Code selection depends on the type of imaging used to place the marker: mammography (19281–19282), stereotactic (19283–19284), ultrasound (19285–19286), or magnetic resonance (19287–19288). In some cases, once the mass is excised from the breast, the surgeon will place a clip in the area where the mass was removed for future reference or marking when additional surgery or follow-up is likely.

Be sure to read the pathology report before finalizing an incisional biopsy code. If the report indicates the lesion was removed entirely or *in toto*, an excisional biopsy code must be assigned instead.

INTERNET RESOURCE: Read the *American Journal of Roentgenology* article at the following website for information and illustrations of metallic clip insertions. www.ajronline.org/cgi/content/full/175/5/1353

Breast Reduction

Reduction mammaplasty, more commonly referred to as *breast reduction*, is the reduction of large breasts by excising excessive tissue and fat, thereby reducing overall cup size. Most women who have the surgery have very large, sagging breasts referred to as *pendulous breasts* that restrict their activities and cause back, neck, and shoulder ailments. Basically four different techniques are used in reduction mammaplasty:

- Pedicle method (and all its variations)
- Free nipple graft
- Stevens Laser Bra
- Liposuction only

There are surgical and scar pattern differences with these methods and not everyone is a candidate for all of the different types of reductions. Size of the breast and the patient's medical history are considered when determining the best approach. Regardless of technique (with the exception of the free nipple graft), CPT code 19318 is assigned for this procedure. The breasts are a paired body part, so if the reduction is performed on both breasts, append the –50 modifier.

Pedicle Method

The pedicle method of breast reduction reduces breast appearance, volume, and contour, while maintaining breast function and nipple sensation. The pedicle method refers to the location of the blood and nerve supply—not where the incisions are placed and subsequent scars will result. This is the method that the majority of surgeons choose.

Pedicle methods vary by the way the blood and nerves are maintained from different areas of the breast and where the incisions are made in relation to this (Box 17.3).

Free Nipple Graft

In the case of very large breasts, however, women are sometimes faced with the free nipple graft (FNG) procedure. The pedicle, along with its blood and nerve supply, must be severed, and the nipple-areola complex detached and grafted back on as a skin graft after the reduction is completed. Function and sensation are lost with this method.

Stevens Laser Bra

The Stevens Laser Bra is a new technique that uses a laser and the skin that would normally be discarded during breast reduction surgery. This technique creates an "internal bra" to provide a permanent support system and a more natural effect in the long term for patients. The incision patterns are the same as with most of the anchor-style pedicle methods, as is the preservation of the pedicle. The Laser Bra is attached internally to the chest wall.

Liposuction-Only Breast Reduction

Liposuction can be used to remove excess breast tissue. It is sometimes referred to as the "scar-less" breast reduction procedure. Two small incisions large enough for the cannulas to be inserted are all that is visible compared to the large incisions under the breast and around the nipple in other methods. Cannulas are inserted and tumescent fluid is injected, which separates the tissue from the fat. Liposuction is then performed on each breast. This procedure takes less time than traditional breast reduction methods; however, it does not include the benefit of a breast lift.

Nipple Reconstruction

Nipple reconstruction is performed for two purposes: as the last phase of breast reconstruction postmastectomy or to correct inverted nipples. Reconstruction is accomplished by harvesting a skin graft from various donor sites on the body. A thin circular layer of skin is removed from the recipient breast and the graft is placed onto the reconstructed breast to resemble the areola or it is molded into a representative nipple. Code 19350 includes repair of the donor site with suture. Code 19355 is reported for correction of inverted nipples. These codes are unilateral so modifiers LT, RT, or –50, if performed bilaterally, are applicable. The surgeon may elect to insert a biological implant to support the nipple; this is reported with +15777. Surgical tattooing may also be used during reconstruction to tint the areolar grafted skin to the pigment that most resembles that of the areola. Report codes 11920–11922 for the tattooing based on the area (in square centimeters) of skin treated. Notice that these codes are not specific to breasts or a site other than skin so anatomical modifiers do

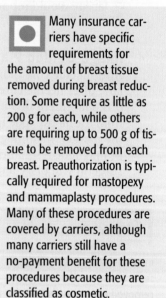

If breast reduction is done with areolar reconstruction, code both 19318 and 19350.

Many insurance carriers have specific requirements for the amount of breast tissue removed during breast reduction. Some require as little as 200 g for each, while others are requiring up to 500 g of tissue to be removed from each breast. Preauthorization is typically required for mastopexy and mammaplasty procedures. Many of these procedures are covered by carriers, although many carriers still have a no-payment benefit for these procedures because they are classified as cosmetic.

not apply. Tattooing is also used in reconstruction following trauma or removal of cancer from an eyelid, eyebrow, or lip.

Mastectomy

Breast cancer continues to be a top national health concern. It ranks number one in occurrence and number two in death among women. Mastectomies are performed for carcinoma of the breast, severe fibrocystic disease, or as preventative therapy in women who have a very strong family history of breast cancer. Each code differs in the amount of tissue removed and if lymph nodes and underlying muscle were taken. Mastectomy procedures are categorized by CPT into four areas:

1. Gynecomastia
2. Partial (lumpectomy)
3. Simple, Complete
4. Subcutaneous
5. Radical

Do not assign code 19300 to female patients.

Physicians need to specifically state that they paid attention to the surgical margins to help the coder differentiate between an excisional biopsy and a lumpectomy. Excision is a removal of the lesion without specific attention to adequate surgical margins. During excision, the visible mass is removed but unless frozen section was performed, there is no guarantee that the margins are clear before the case is ended. Additionally, the intraoperative placement of a clip (or clips) is not separately reported with partial mastectomy procedures.

Mastectomy for Gynecomastia

Gynecomastia is a condition that affects enlarged breasts in males. Surgical treatment involves performing a mastectomy (19300), otherwise known as breast reduction, whereby the excess breast tissue is removed. This can be done through a periaereolar incision. The surgeon cuts away the excess glandular tissue, fat and skin from around the areola and from the sides and bottom of the breast. Major reductions that involve the removal of a significant amount of tissue and skin usually require larger incisions placed under the breast.

Partial Mastectomy

Partial mastectomy (19301–19302) is also referred to as wide local excision lumpectomy, segmental mastectomy, or quadrantectomy. Lumpectomy involves excision of all cancerous tissue and a margin of normal tissue around the tumor to ensure microscopically clean margins. It involves removal of the breast tumor and a small amount of surrounding tissue that may include the underarm lymph nodes. An incision is made in the skin over the site of malignancy. This procedure may be performed with the patient under local anesthesia, but sedation or general anesthesia is usually advisable if a significant amount of tissue is to be excised.

19302 is assigned if the surgeon also performs axillary lymphadenectomy. The documentation may state partial mastectomy with sentinel node biopsy. Lymph nodes are connected as a chain with the sentinel node being the first of the axillary lymph node chain. Even after the lymph nodes are located, it is difficult to determine where the lymph node chain starts. Dye is injected to assist the surgeon in identifying the sentinel node. The surgeon can observe the flow of dye through the lymph nodes to locate the first node. The surgeon can then remove the first few nodes sequentially to test for metastasis. If the first few lymph nodes are benign then that means the cancer has not spread. The injection is coded separately with 38792. A separate incision is made and lymph nodes between the pectoralis major and minor muscles and nodes in the axilla are removed. Not all axillary lymph nodes have to be removed in order to assign this code.

Simple, Complete Mastectomy

A simple, complete mastectomy (19303) procedure entails removing the entire breast tissue, but axillary tissue is not removed. At times, the surgeon may remove the sentinel lymph node. This node is the first axillary node into which the breast drains.

Subcutaneous Mastectomy

Subcutaneous mastectomy (19304) (also called a skin-sparing mastectomy) is a procedure in which the surgeon dissects the breast tissue from the pectoral fascia and from the skin preserving the nipple and areolar

If the surgeon performed and documented extra work to spare the nipple—which can be difficult because of the need for an adequate blood supply—report the -22 modifier and send the operative report.

tissue but removing the rest of the breast. Breast tissue is removed but the skin and pectoral fascia are not removed. In a male subQ mastectomy, only about 200 grams of tissue are removed versus moderate to extensive amounts of tissue or anterior chest wall in a mastectomy in this range. This procedure is routinely performed for women who have a high risk for breast cancer or those with benign disease when the physician is concerned about increased risk cancer development in the breast tissue.

Radical Mastectomy

Radical mastectomy (19305–19306) involves removing the entire breast, the axillary lymph nodes, and the pectoral tissue behind the breast. It is a procedure of last resort for recurrent breast cancer that has spread to the chest wall or for those with tumors of the pectoralis muscle. This procedure is the most disfiguring of all mastectomies. In 19305, the breast tissue including pectoral muscles, axillary pectoral major and minor and axillary lymph node is removed. In 19306, breast tissue is dissected from the pectoral fascia and pectoral muscles and axillary pectoral muscles are removed. All tissue within the vicinity of the internal mammary lymph nodes, sternum, rectus fascia, latissimus dorsi muscle and the clavicle are removed.

Modified radical mastectomy requires that the entire breast tissue is removed along with the axillary contents (fatty tissue and lymph nodes) and may involve the pectoralis minor muscle but does not resect the pectoralis major muscle. This saves the patient from having a more extensive procedure but is more difficult for the surgeon to accomplish.

Additionally, intraoperative placement of clips is not separately reported with total mastectomy procedures.

> INTERNET RESOURCES: Visit the breastcancer.org website to view illustrations of the radical and modified radical mastecomy procedure.
> http://www.breastcancer.org/radical_mastectomy.html
> http://www.breastcancer.org/modified_radical_mastectomy.html

> If a breast biopsy is performed at the same session as a mastectomy, it is not coded separately unless the biopsy is performed to decide whether the mastectomy is to be done and if a previous biopsy had not been obtained. If a mastectomy is performed as a result of a positive breast biopsy performed at the same session, append a –58 modifier to the mastectomy code to show a staged procedure. Breast biopsy 19101 (Biopsy of breast; incisional) will always be denied when billed with 19316 (Mastopexy), 19318 (Reduction mammaplasty), 19324 (Mammaplasty; without implant), 19325 (Mammaplasty; with implants) or 19355–19369 (Breast reconstruction codes).

 Excisions of breast lesions are not coded separately from a mastectomy.

Breast Reconstructions

Mastectomy patients are offered the opportunity to reconstruct the absent breast either immediately after the mastectomy or at some time after the procedure once the patient has recovered or completed adjuvant therapy. According to the New York Times, "66,000 women in the U.S. had mastectomies in 2006 and 57,000 had reconstructive breast surgery." These procedures are quite complex and vary in technique. Implant surgery is the most popular reconstruction and often performed immediately after the mastectomy by first placing a tissue expander to stretch the tissue ad prepare it for subsequent prosthetic implant insertion. Other techniques require transferring abdominal tissue to the breast or latissimus tissue with flap reconstruction. Patients may elect to have a mold of their breast made prior to mastectomy to be used to create a custom breast implant. Report 19396 for the preparation of the moulage. The actual insertion of the custom implant will be reported at a separate session using 19340 or 19342.

When assigning codes for breast reconstruction, the coder needs to read the documentation and determine which breast was treated, what type of reconstruction technique was applied, and whether or not an implant was inserted.

Tissue Expanders

A tissue expander is a plastic balloon that is placed under the skin and filled with saline. Through a small injection port under the skin, saline is injected incrementally into the expander over a period of weeks or months, gradually filling it to the desired size while stretching the overlying skin. Tissue expanders may be inserted under the skin anywhere on the body. The purpose is to stretch or expand the skin in preparation of a staged reconstruction or to receive an implant. 11960 is used to report insertion of tissue expanders in other parts of the body aside from the breast. 19357 is used to report insertion of a tissue expander in preparation for later breast reconstruction with permanent mammary implant. It also includes subsequent expansion of the balloon. If for some reason a tissue expander is removed without immediate insertion of a permanent implant as in the case of an infection in the breast capsule, assign code 11971.

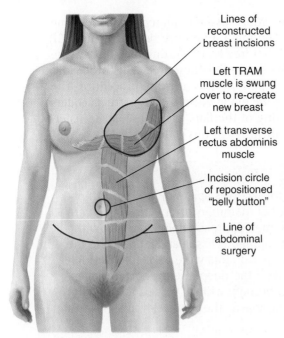

Figure 17.10 TRAM flap. From Gylys, B. *Medical Terminology Systems*, 8E. F.A. Davis, 2017.

Most local CMS carriers cover the TRAM flap but they don't cover a revision to the abdomen when the TRAM flap creates dog ears. Dog ears are triangular shaped ends of poorly healed incisions that stick up on each end of the incision resembling a dog's ears. CMS as well as many commercial carriers view this as cosmetic and not medically necessary.

Do not report the use of the microscope (69990) separately because it is included in breast reconstruction surgeries 19367–19369.

Insertion of Prosthetic Implant

Implant insertion post-mastectomy is performed the same way as a cosmetic breast augmentation. When the physician has determined that the tissue has been stretched adequately enough to allow for insertion of a permanent implant, report 11970 for removal of the temporary tissue expander and exchanging it with a permanent implant. For cases when a tissue expander is removed at a prior visit, the surgeon will place the permanent implant at a separate visit. In this case, when the patient does come back later for insertion of a breast implant, 19342 *Delayed insertion of breast prosthesis following mastopexy, mastectomy, or in reconstruction* is reported.

Implants come with the risk of complications and likelihood of future operations. According to studies, within five years of implant placement, more than one third of patients have undergone a second operation for ruptured implants or infections.

Tranverse Rectus Abdominis Myocutaneous (TRAM) Flap

The TRAM flap is a form of a pedicle flap where the rectus abdominis muscle along with soft tissue and blood vessels is rotated and used to reconstruct a new breast (Fig. 17.10). An oval section of skin, fat, and muscle is taken from the lower half of the abdomen and slid up through a tunnel created under the skin of the abdomen to the breast area. Blood vessels remain attached to the base of the flap an anywhere else along the pedicle when possible. The tissue is pulled out through the mastectomy site and shaped into a natural-looking breast and sewn into place. The procedure takes 3-4 hours to complete. 19367 is assigned for this procedure. All TRAM procedures include the following components:

- Creation of the breast pocket (capsule)
- Elevation of the abdominal flap
- Muscle dissection
- Flap transfer
- Fascial closure (donor site) with or without mesh
- Abdominal closure including umbilical repair or reconstruction
- Breast contouring

Blood vessels that are cut during the elevation of the flap and transfer are reanastomosed in the chest area using a microscope. The term *supercharging* appears in the code descriptor for 19368. This means that an additional artery is included with the flap when it is harvested from the abdomen to provide more blood supply to the flap. To report the microvascular anastomosis use code 19368.

Code 19369, *Breast reconstruction with transverse rectus abdominis myocutaneous flap (TRAM), double pedicle, including closure of donor site*, is reported for a unilateral breast reconstruction when both rectus muscles are used instead of one or the other as in the above TRAM procedure.

Deep Inferior Epigastric Perforator (DIEP) Free Flap

The DIEP flap (19364) utilizes the epigastric perforator, which is the main blood vessel that runs through the deep abdominal tissue used to reconstruct the breast. In DIEP flap reconstruction, only skin, fat, and blood vessels are removed from the lower abdomen below the belly button to the mons pubis. Muscle is spared in this technique. Because no abdominal muscle is removed, most women recover more quickly from DIEP compared to TRAM reconstruction.

The TRAM and DIEP have the same goal in mind and utilize tissue obtained from the same area but are very different in technique and execution. The main difference between the DIEP and TRAM procedures is the TRAM is a flap and the DIEP is a free graft. During the DIEP, tissue is completely detached from the abdomen and reanastomosed to the chest area. This procedure requires a highly skilled plastic surgeon specially trained to perform this intricate procedure. The surgeon must use the microscope to microsurgically repair the blood vessels. CPT instructs coders to not assign 69990 in addition to 19364 because harvesting of the flap, microvascular transfer, closure of the donor site, and shaping of the breast are all inclusive in this code.

> **■ CASE SCENARIO**
> Under high-power magnification, the pectoralis major muscle was split along the fourth rib. The deep perichondrium was then incised and the internal mammary artery and veins were identified. An oval incision was made in the lower abdomen approximately 2 cm below the umbilicus. Dissection was carried down through the subcutaneous tissue and fat down to the rectus abdominis fascia. The fascia was incised and the perforators were dissected through the rectus abdominis muscle. The flap was harvested with the deep inferior epigastric vessels visualized as they entered the muscle. The flap was brought with its vessels through the rectus abdominus muscle leaving all muscle behind and intact. The flap was transferred to the chest with microvascular anastomosis and secured.

Latissimus Dorsi Flap

The latissimus dorsi muscle located on the side of trunk just adjacent to the breast tissue can be used to reconstruct the breast (19361). A section of skin, fat, and latissimus dorsi muscle is detached and slid around through a tunnel under the skin to the breast area. The muscle-skin flap remains attached to the blood vessels and is then rotated to the front of the chest through a tunnel under the patient's armpit and is then pulled out through the mastectomy incision. As with all flaps, blood vessels remain attached and preserved as much as possible. The tissue is shaped into a natural-looking breast and sewn into place. If blood vessels were severed during the elevation of the flap and transfer, they can be reanastomosed to the vessels in the chest area; however, 69990 cannot be reported in addition. In most cases, when using this type of flap reconstruction, patients also require insertion of an implant because there isn't an abundance of fatty tissue on this part of the back to create a sizable breast. If an implant is also placed, assign 19340 in addition.

Revision of Reconstructed Breast

It is not uncommon in patients that have had breast reconstruction for them to have subsequent surgery or staged surgery where the breast is revised. Tissue may be rearranged to correct asymmetry. Tissue may be revised or scars may be excised because of contracture or wound breakdown. Implants may be removed and replaced with a different kind or size to improve the appearance or fit. Common diagnoses submitted with this procedure are scar or fibrosis of skin, mechanical complication of breast implant, and late effect of surgical care.

Mastopexy

Mastopexy (19316) is a breast lift usually done for cosmetic purposes. Various factors play a role in the sagging of a woman's breast(s): pregnancy, nursing, and the forces of gravity and aging. As the skin loses its elasticity, the breasts often lose their shape and firmness and begin to sag. Mastopexy raises and reshapes sagging breasts. At times, this procedure may be done in an effort to make breasts symmetrical after a woman has had a mastectomy—surgical removal of the breast—with reconstruction on the opposite side.

> Some states require every health policy to provide coverage for reconstructive surgery on each breast on which a mastectomy has been performed and reconstructive surgery on a nondiseased breast to produce a symmetrical appearance. Surgery on the nondiseased breast should be preauthorized, because carrier and state rules differ.

Augmentation

Breast augmentation is a cosmetic procedure to enhance the existing breast. A pocket is created between the breast and the pectoral muscles, and an implant is inserted with the end result being a larger breast. Augmentation can also be performed by rearranging the fat and mammary tissue, which does not require the insertion of an implant. This procedure is reported using codes 19324 and 19325. This procedure is most commonly performed in women; however, with the explosion of the cosmetic industry, men are also undergoing this procedure to obtain more defined "pecs" (pectoralis major muscles). Medicare covers implants inserted in a postmastectomy reconstruction for breast cancer patients.

Breast Capsulotomy

Capsule formation and contracture are common complications of breast augmentation. Formation of a capsule can cause distortion of the breast. A capsulotomy is usually performed in this case: An incision is made in the capsule to relieve tightness around the implant, but no capsule tissue is removed. The implant may be temporarily removed and replaced or not replaced at all. Manual capsulotomy can also be performed by applying pressure to the breast without using anesthesia. To report this service, use code 19370 with the respective LT or RT modifier.

> HCPCS codes for the implant supply should also be reported. Code L8600 is used to describe breast silicone or saline implants.

Breast Capsulectomy

Periprosthetic capsulation is the most common complication resulting from breast implantation. Fibrous sacs of scar tissue that encapsulate the implant become contracted, causing pain and distortion of the breast, and, depending on the degree of contracture, may require removal. Capsulectomy (19371) is the surgical removal of the capsular contracture or adhesive scar tissue. The implant is temporarily removed and the surgeon removes this tissue and revises the pocket and then places the implant back into the breast. This code does not include the reinsertion of the breast implant. The code assigned for reinsertion of the breast implant depends on whether the patient had the initial breast procedure done for reconstruction postmastectomy or post–cosmetic breast augmentation.

> It is considered incorrect to bill a periprosthetic capsulectomy (19371) with delayed insertion of breast prosthesis (19342) when the procedures are accomplished during the same operative session. The reason the breast implant was placed originally will determine the correct code. Choose from either 19325 or 19340.

■ CASE SCENARIOS
- A patient has a unilateral breast capsulectomy postaugmentation with removal of the implant and reinsertion of the breast implant. Codes: 19371, 19325–51.

- A patient has a unilateral breast capsulectomy with removal of the implant postreconstruction and a new implant is replaced. Codes: 19371, 19340–51.

Implant Removal or Exchange
Unfortunately, breast augmentation surgeries run the risk of complications with the mammary implant rippling, rupturing, or becoming dislodged from the breast capsule. If the implant was silicone and the material leaks beyond the capsule, infiltrating surrounding tissue into the breast capsule, assign 19330, *Removal of mammary implant material,* to account for the work entailed in retrieving all of the silicone material. Do not assign this code when a saline implant ruptures. Saline implants may leak or develop ripples and can be removed and exchanged/replaced with a new implant. To report this service, use code 19325 for cosmetic augmentation patients and 19340 for postmastectomy patients.

SKIN RESURFACING

Dermatologists and plastic surgeons are performing these procedures more often now for a couple of reasons. Some individuals who want to appear younger are looking for noninvasive ways to turn back the clock. Once thought of as cosmetic procedures, insurance carriers are now paying for many of these procedures to treat surface skin conditions such as actinic keratosis before they progress to more serious conditions requiring invasive surgery.

Dermabrasion

Dermabrasion is a surgical procedure that scrapes away the outermost layer of skin with a motorized instrument that uses a wire brush or a burr. The instrument sands down the skin and penetrates the dermis layer of skin to reach smoother, wrinkle-free skin. This technique is very similar to sanding and stripping wood to reveal the smooth untainted wood beneath the rough or painted outer surface. Dermabrasion is most often used to improve the look of scars on the face or to smooth out fine facial wrinkles, especially around the mouth. This procedure lowers raised lesions or thins tissue to regenerate skin with a smoother appearance.

It can also be utilized to remove the precancerous growths called *keratoses* that reside on the superficial layers of the skin. CO_2 laser dermabrasion to treat a basal cell carcinoma is also assigned with codes 15780–15783. Segmental dermabrasion may be covered as treatment for conditions such as rhinophyma.

Coding for dermabrasion is based on the location and the size of the area. Use code 15780, *Dermabrasion; total face* (e.g., for acne scarring, fine wrinkling, rhytids, general keratosis), for the total face, 15781 for a segment of the face, and 15782 for regional dermabrasion of an area other than the face. Use 15783, *Dermabrasion; superficial, any site* (e.g., tattoo removal), for a superficial site. This code indicates that it should be used to remove a tattoo; however, codes 15780–15782 are more suitable for tattoo removal because these procedures penetrate into the dermal layer of skin where the tattoo resides. Code 15783 only affects the superficial layer of skin.

Dermaplaning

Dermaplaning is used to treat deep acne scars. Dermaplaning utilizes a handheld instrument called a *dermatome* to slice off layers of skin with an oscillating blade. The area of skin is "skimmed" off evenly, making the skin flush with the deepest point of the scar or skin defect. This provides a smoother appearance of the entire area. It is not uncommon for the procedure to be performed more than once, or in stages, especially when scarring is deep or a large area of skin is involved.

Both dermabrasion and dermaplaning can be performed on small areas of skin or on the entire face. They can be used alone or in conjunction with other procedures, such as a facelift, scar removal or revision, or chemical peel.

COSMETIC PROCEDURES

Abdominoplasty

Abdominoplasty is considered to be, in most cases, a cosmetic procedure performed on the abdomen to remove excess skin and fat, in addition to plicating, or tightening, the stomach muscles to obtain a flatter, tighter abdomen. Many women have historically undergone this procedure after having multiple children such that the abdominal wall is stretched so much it no longer retains its elasticity or if they developed rectus diastasis during pregnancy. Rectus diastasis is separation between the left and right sides of the rectus abdominis muscle, leaving a ridge-like appearance down the front of the abdomen from the breastbone to the belly button. Abdominoplasty repairs weakened or separated muscles, creating an abdominal profile that is smoother and firmer. Report code 17999

> Most carriers consider dermabrasion procedures to be cosmetic and will only reimburse for them under certain medical circumstances. For example, Aetna states that it considers dermabrasion—whether by dermaplaning or CO_2 laser—medically necessary "for removal of superficial basal cell carcinomas and precancerous actinic keratoses" only when the patient meets two criteria: (1) Conventional methods of removal such as cryotherapy, curettage, and excision are impractical due to the number and distribution of the lesions, and (2) the patient has failed a trial of 5-fluorouracil (5-FU; Efudex). Check with individual carriers for specific policies.

> CPT codes 15780, 15782, and 15783 have an assistant surgeon indicator of 0, which means an assistant surgeon fee is payable for 15780 but requires documentation to substantiate medical necessity. These codes include 90 days of follow-up care.

> Check carrier websites and LCDs for payer policies specific to this procedure.

Table 17.8 Abdomen Panniculus/ Apron Grading Scale

GRADE	DESCRIPTION
1	Covers only the hairline to the mons pubis but does not cover the genitalia
2	Covers genitalia in line with upper thigh crease
3	Covers upper thigh
4	Covers midthigh
5	Covers knees or beyond

for abdominoplasty. Abdominoplasty is never covered by insurance.

Panniculectomy

A panniculectomy is a lipectomy or removal of excess skin that can be performed on the abdomen, thighs, legs, upper arms, buttocks, and other areas. Panniculectomy, on the other hand, is not primarily a cosmetic procedure. This procedure differs from abdominoplasty in that it is performed to reduce the health risk of the patient. More and more patients are undergoing bariatric surgeries, resulting in drastic weight reduction and leaving behind an apron of redundant skin around the abdomen called *abdominal panniculus*. These skinfolds become problematic because they retain moisture and become irritated or inflamed when they rub against the underlying skin. The skinfolds can harbor bacteria, resulting in chronic infections. Abdominoplasty tightens the muscle and removes excess skin and fat, but a panniculectomy only removes excess skin and fat. Aprons are graded on a scale of 1 to 5—the higher the grade, the higher the health risk associated with the condition. The larger the apron or panniculus, the more difficult it is for the patient to walk, dress, exercise, bathe, or perform other activities. See Table 17.8 for further details. This procedure is usually considered to be medically necessary for the patient who has had significant weight loss following the treatment of morbid obesity and when there are medical complications such as candidiasis, intertrigo, or tissue necrosis that is unresponsive to oral or topical medication. CPT instructs the coder to report codes 15830, +15847 for panniculectomy with abdominoplasty.

Liposuction

Liposuction, or suction-assisted lipectomy, refers to the removal of unwanted fatty tissue, using suction by inserting a cannula under the skin. Tumescent fluid is injected to break up the fatty tissue and liquefy it, making it easy to suction out. It also has some anesthetic properties. Liposuction is commonly performed on the abdomen, the breasts during reduction mammaplasty, the thighs, the buttocks, and under the chin. Liposuction is primarily a cosmetic procedure, but it is also used to enhance or contour during therapeutic procedures. Liposuction differs from lipectomy in that it uses suction to remove the tissue instead of using a scalpel or electrosurgery (Bovie) to excise the tissue surgically. Liposuction is reported by using codes 15876–15879, depending on which area of the body is treated.

Rhytidectomy

A facelift, or rhytidectomy, is a cosmetic surgical procedure performed on the face to improve the appearance of the skin, giving it a more youthful look. This is accomplished by removing excess facial skin, with or without the tightening of underlying tissues of the face and neck, resulting in tighter-looking skin. During the procedure, the surgeon makes incisions at the temples above the hairline continuing down in front of the ear, around the earlobe, and to the lower scalp. If the patient has sagging of the neck tissue and the neck is also lifted, another incision is made under the chin. The surgeon then separates the skin from the underlying fat and muscle and any excess fat is trimmed or suctioned away around the neck and chin to contour the area. Tissue is repositioned and the muscles are tightened. Excess skin is removed. Codes used to report rhytidectomies are located in the 15824–15829 series. Codes are assigned based on where on the face and/or neck the procedure was performed. If the surgeon frees the superficial musculoaponeurotic system (SMAS) from the skin and creates a flap, assign 15829. What is interesting is that CPT considers facelift procedure codes to be unilateral, so if the lift is done on both sides of the face, the –50 modifier is appended.

When liposuction is performed as part of a facelift repair, it is not reported separately. It is considered an integral component of the facelift procedure.

For a very few conditions, rhytidectomy is considered medically necessary to correct a functional impairment as a result of a disease such as facial paralysis. Often, this procedure is performed in conjunction with other procedures to correct the impairment.

CHECKPOINT 17.6

Assign codes to the following procedures. Include any necessary modifiers. In some cases, more than one code is required.

1. A 47-year-old female patient underwent a routine mammogram. The patient has had chronic fibrocystic disease, but this mammogram showed a small calcification not palpable to the touch. The radiologist performed an ultrasound-guided percutaneous needle core biopsy of this lesion of the right breast. _____

2. A patient undergoes a lumpectomy of the right breast for biopsy suspicious for malignancy. The 4.0-cm lesion with 0.2-cm margins was sent for frozen section. The pathologist confirmed the specimen to be malignant and that the margins were clear. _____

3. Surgical removal of excess skin and tissue, upper arm and hand. _____

4. Rhytidectomy of glabellar frown lines. _____

Chapter Summary

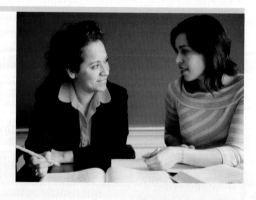

1. I&D procedures require an incision to open the affected site and allow for drainage. Biopsy is a diagnostic procedure that allows a sample of tissue to be removed and sent for pathology testing and interpretation. Destruction uses various methods to eradicate a lesion but is not considered to be a full-thickness excision. Excisions are the removal of full-thickness (i.e., through the dermis) lesions. This method is used for both benign and malignant lesions, and understanding the guidelines for lesion measurement is essential to correct coding. Debridement is the removal of devitalized tissue to promote repair and healing as well as function to the affected area. Mohs micrographic surgery is a technique where the surgeon acts as surgeon *and* pathologist. If either the surgery or the pathology review is performed by different physicians, Mohs codes cannot be reported. Mohs is specific to basal cell carcinomas, squamous cell carcinomas, and melanomas.

2. There are basically three types of wound repairs: simple, intermediate, and complex. Simple repairs are for superficial wound repair involving the epidermis, dermis, and a minimal amount of subcutaneous tissue requiring one-layer suturing. The simple repair is included in the lesion removal "package" and payment. Intermediate repair is closure of one or more of the subcutaneous layers and superficial fascia, in addition to the skin. This type of repair can also be assigned when the wound has to be extensively cleaned due to contamination or removal of small pieces of foreign material before suturing, even if the suturing is simple. A complex repair is associated with complicated closure including scar revision, debridement, extensive undermining, stents, or retention sutures, and is more than layered closure.

3. Code to the most appropriate anatomical site regardless of the depth of lesion, which may require making a decision between using codes in the Integumentary System or Musculo-skeletal System sections. With excisions, a specimen is removed from the body using varying techniques, whether it is a partial or complete removal, and sent to pathology for examination. Lesion excision codes are based on the following seven basic factors:

   a. Where the lesion is located
   b. Type of lesion
   c. Morphology of the lesion (benign or malignant)
   d. Number of lesions
   e. Diameter

4. Measuring a lesion requires that you determine the greatest clinical diameter of the lesion plus that margin required for complete excision. In CPT, this is defined as the lesion diameter plus the *narrowest* margins required. The measurement is made prior to excision.

5. Skin graft coding differentiates between the autografts from the patient's own skin, such as split thickness skin grafts, full thickness skin grafts, epidermal only grafts, dermal only grafts, and adjacent tissue transfers. The non autografts are skin substitute grafts.

6. Flaps and tissue transfers or arrangements differ from skin grafts because they carry their own blood supply. They are most commonly used when the donor site and the recipient site are in close proximity. The flaps or tissue transfers are not completely severed from the donor site, so the vascular bed is still attached to feed the tissue with adequate blood supply. The *CPT Professional Edition* provides illustrations and descriptions of adjacent tissue repairs. Skin grafts are completely freed from the donor site and placed onto the recipient site, no connection remains.

7. When an excision is performed and the method of closure is an adjacent tissue transfer, the excision procedure is included in the adjacent tissue transfer procedure. When the method of closure is a graft or other type of flap, the excision is reported in addition to the closure procedure.

8. The Rule of Nines is used to calculate the percentage of a body burned by dividing the total body surface area into multiples of 9% segments. For example, if both an arm and a leg are burned, this represents 27% of the body surface area. The arm is 9% and each leg is 18%.

9. The debridement codes are divided into four sections. The first is based on the body surface percentage debrided, the second is based on debridement of necrotizing soft tissue infections, the third is specific to open fractures and dislocations, and the fourth is for all other types of debridement such as ulcers, injuries, and infections.

10. Selective debridement refers to controlled debridement of a targeted area of skin where tissue is removed leaving behind healthy, undamaged tissue. Instruments such as scissors and forceps are used to cut the tissue along the margin of viable and nonviable tissue, which requires a greater set of skills by a qualified health-care provider. In contrast, nonselective debridement methods are not as controlled; therefore, they do not have the ability to target certain tissues and run the risk of damaging healthy tissue. Whirlpool therapy and maggot therapy are some examples of this type of debridement.

11. The diagnostic and therapeutic procedures used to diagnose, stage, and treat breast disease are rapidly becoming less drastic and less invasive. Breast procedures are inherently unilateral; therefore, if the same procedures are done on both breasts, a −50 modifier is needed. Some of the breast procedures are fine needle aspiration, needle core biopsy, open biopsy, placement of metallic marker(s), breast reduction and mastectomy. Understanding the difference between these procedures and their coding requirements is essential to the coder.

Matching

Match the key terms with their definitions.

A. paring
B. dermabrasion
C. dorsal
D. shaving
E. incisional biopsy

F. excision
G. proximal
H. excisional biopsy
I. debridement
J. intermediate repair

1. _____ Slicing a raised lesion or mole entirely off at skin level

2. _____ Trimming or gradual reduction in size by slicing

3. _____ Surgically removing or cutting out part or all from the body

4. _____ Removal of dead, necrotic tissue

5. _____ Closest to where that point attaches to the trunk of the body

6. _____ Toward the backside of the body

7. _____ Entire lesion, tumor, and so on, is removed

8. _____ Layered closure/repair of a wound

9. _____ Portion or a sample of the lesion or tumor is removed through an incision

10. _____ Scraping away the outermost layer of skin with a motorized instrument

True or False

Decide whether each statement is true or false.

1. __F__ I&D of abscess of the left thigh would always be coded as 27301; the code is specific to the thigh region.

2. __T__ Excision of a 3.0-cm hyperkeratosis of the scalp is coded as 11423.

3. __T__ Needle cauterization of a subungual hematoma is coded as 11740.

4. __F__ Suture repair of a 12.0-cm laceration of the right lower leg in which fascia, subcutaneous layer, and skin are closed is coded 13121 and 13122.

5. __F__ The dermis is the thick, outer layer of the skin.

6. __T__ Layered closure is an example of an intermediate wound repair.

7. __T__ Debridement is never coded as a separate procedure.

8. __T__ A shallow wound in the epidermis that could be repaired with a simple repair required extensive cleansing due to contamination. An intermediate wound repair code should be assigned.

9. __T__ Before you can assign a code for shaving a lesion, you must know if the lesion was benign or malignant.

10. __F__ One 0.5-cm benign lesion of the hand was removed and another 0.5-cm benign lesion of the foot was removed. Multiple lesions were excised and both anatomical areas are grouped into the same code descriptor, so the diameters of the lesions are added together.

11. __T__ When coding for skin grafts, simple closure of the donor site is included in the service for the graft and is not coded separately.

12. __T__ Simple closure is not included in the excision of a lesion.

Multiple Choice

Select the letter that best completes the statement or answers the question.

1. In which of these cases would the coder add the lengths of the defects?
   A. Removal of benign lesions from neck
   B. Simple closure of lacerations on the trunk
   C. Intermediate closures of lacerations on arm and face
   D. Excision of lesion on left leg with simple repair and excision of lesion on back with intermediate repair

2. Wound exploration does not include which of the following?
   A. Laparotomy
   B. Debridement
   C. Foreign body removal
   D. Wound enlargement

3. The physician excised a benign lesion on the face measuring 2.0 cm × 0.6 cm × 3.0 cm. The correct code would be
   A. 17000
   B. 11444
   C. 11643
   D. 11443

4. When coding wound repairs with varying complexity, which of the following is true?
   A. The codes are listed with the largest repair size listed first.
   B. Only the most complex repair code is listed.
   C. The most complex repair code is listed first followed by the other repairs.
   D. The order in which the codes are listed does not matter.

5. Per CPT guidelines, if a lesion is biopsied and the remainder of the lesion is removed, what code(s) is (are) assigned?
   A. Code for the biopsy and the lesion excision with a –59 modifier on the excision code.
   B. Code for the lesion excision only.
   C. Code for the biopsy only.
   D. Code for the biopsy and the lesion excision with a –59 modifier on the biopsy code.

6. Which of the following procedures describes destruction of a lesion?
   A. Paring
   B. Shaving
   C. Removal
   D. Laser removal

7. A patient is seen in the ED after cutting his hand with a band saw. The ED physician indicates that the wound required extensive cleansing and multiple-layer closure. What kind of wound repair was done?
   A. Intermediate
   B. Simple
   C. Tissue rearrangement
   D. Complex

8. For a superficial incision and drainage of the shoulder, the code would be assigned from which range?
   A. 21501–21510
   B. 23030–23031
   C. 10040–10180
   D. None of the above

9. In an excision of a 3.0- x 2.5-cm lipoma of the back, the incision was carried down to and through the subfacial fascia. A layered closure was performed with 2-0 Vicryl and 1-0 Monocryl. Which codes apply to this procedure?
   A. 11403, 12032
   B. 21932, 12032
   C. 21925, 12031
   D. 21930, 12031

10. In a suture repair of a 9.0-cm laceration of the left lower leg, fascia, subcutaneous layer, and skin were closed. Which code(s) apply(ies) to this procedure?
    A. 12034
    B. 13121, 13122
    C. 12004
    D. 13120, 13121

11. A patient has two benign lesions on the left leg: one is 2 cm, the other is 2.5 cm. The surgeon will use chemosurgery to perform destruction of the lesions. Which code(s) apply to this procedure?
    A. 17263, 17262–51
    B. 17000 x 2
    C. 17000, +17003
    D. 17110

12. A patient was treated at the ambulatory surgery center for a 3.3-cm lesion on his cheek. A previous biopsy indicated the lesion was a malignant melanoma and the patient is now seen for Mohs surgery. The lesion required three stages of excision with four blocks in the first stage, three blocks in the second stage, and two blocks in the third stage. Which codes apply to this procedure?
    A. 17311, +17312 x 2, +17315 x 9
    B. 17311, +17312 x 2
    C. 17313, +17314 x 2, +17315 x 9
    D. 17313, +17314 x 2

13. A layered closure is an example of which type of repair?
    A. Skin graft
    B. Intermediate closure
    C. Rotation flap
    D. Adjacent tissue transfer

14. What is the code or codes for suction lipectomy of the right and left thighs?
    A. 15877, 15878
    B. 15878, 15877
    C. 15879–50
    D. 15879

15. What is the code for mastectomy with removal of the right axillary lymph nodes including the pectoralis minor muscle but not the pectoralis major?
    A. 19305
    B. 19307
    C. 19303
    D. 19306

16. A surgeon performs three percutaneous needle core biopsies on the right breast and two percutaneous needle core biopsies on the left breast. One incision was made on each breast. The surgeon supervised and interpreted the ultrasound imaging. The biopsies were performed in the outpatient surgery setting. Which codes apply to this procedure?
    A. 19100, 19100–59
    B. 19081, +19082
    C. 19083, +19084
    D. 19085, +19086

17. Mohs surgery was provided to a patient with a malignancy on his head. The surgeon provided both the surgery and the pathology services. There was a first-stage excision with 10 tissue blocks and a second-stage excision with 6 tissue blocks. Which codes apply to this procedure?
    A. 17311, 17312, 17315 x 6
    B. 17311 x 2, 17315 x 6
    C. 17313, 17314, 17315
    D. 17313, 17314, 17315 x 6

18. A patient has a squamous cell carcinoma on his left thigh. The 2.1-cm lesion is excised and a simple repair is performed to repair the resulting defect. The total defect size for both defects is 10.1 cm². Which code(s) apply(ies) to this procedure?

    A. 14021
    B. 11603
    C. 14001
    D. 11603, 14001

19. A patient with insulin-dependent diabetes has a 4- x 4-cm (16-cm²) ulcer involving the skin and subcutaneous tissue of the left foot. The surgeon debrides the area. Which code(s) apply(ies) to this procedure?

    A. 11042
    B. 11043
    C. 11044
    D. 11042, 11045

20. A patient suffered burns on the arm, torso, and leg. The surface size of the area to be excised involves 20 sq cm of the arm, 80 sq cm on the torso, and 30 sq cm on the leg. The total area to be excised is 130 sq cm. Treatment included excision of burn eschar and then placement of a split-thickness skin graft to each of the three areas. Which codes apply to this procedure?

    A. 15002, 15003, 15100, 15101
    B. 15002, 15003, 15100, 15100, 15100
    C. 15001, 15101
    D. 15002, 15002, 15002, 15100, 15100, 15100

21. A male patient was treated at the ambulatory surgery center for a 3.3-cm lesion on his cheek. It was excised, found to be basal cell carcinoma, and a full-thickness skin graft is excised from his shoulder and placed on the 10-sq cm defect. Which codes apply to this procedure?

    A. 15240, 11646
    B. 15240, 15000
    C. 15350, 15000, 11644
    D. 15240, 11644

CHAPTER 18

CPT: Musculoskeletal System

CHAPTER OUTLINE

Organization
Modifiers
Intraoperative Services and Image Guidance
Surgical Techniques
General Musculoskeletal Procedures
Spine
Fracture and Dislocation Treatment
Arthroscopy/Endoscopy
Shoulder, Elbow, and Wrist
Hand
Hip
Knee
Foot

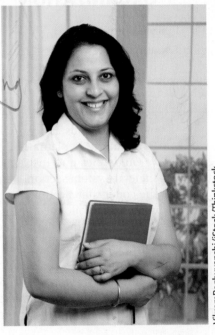

*Ch. 18 T&F
19 T&F
20 Matching*

VikramRaghuvanshi/iStock/Thinkstock

LEARNING OUTCOMES

After studying this chapter, you should be able to:

1. Assign codes for procedures commonly performed on the muscles, bones, and joints.
2. Recognize when to use modifiers when coding orthopedic services.
3. Determine intraoperative services and imaging guidance work for orthopedic procedures and know when they are separately reportable.
4. Define common musculoskeletal system surgical techniques.
5. Understand the physical structure of the spine and its coding guidelines.
6. Describe the guidelines for coding fractures and explain the correct assignment of casting/strapping codes.
7. Describe the guidelines for the use of codes in the endoscopy/arthroscopy section of the musculoskeletal surgery codes in CPT.
8. Assign codes for common shoulder, elbow, and wrist procedures.
9. Discriminate between flexor and extensor tendons of the hand, describing common tendon repair procedures.

635

10. Assign codes for hip arthroplasty based on the components used.
11. Identify the compartments of the knee and assign arthroscopic procedure codes based on these structures.
12. Describe the differences between common bunionectomy techniques.

Musculoskeletal codes make up the largest subsection of the CPT Surgery section, because many different procedures can be performed on the bones, tendons, soft tissue, and muscles of the body. These codes are primarily used by orthopedic surgeons, emergency department (ED) physicians, and urgent care centers. Orthopedics (alternate spelling is orthopaedics) is the subspecialty of medicine that deals with prevention and treatment of injuries and diseases of bones, muscles, joints, and ligaments. Correct code assignment in this section is dependent on the coder being able to determine if the treatment provided is for a traumatic injury (accident) or a medical condition (ongoing condition).

In an orthopedic practice, HCPCS codes are routinely assigned for drugs, splints, casting material, etc. When a practice dispenses durable medical equipment (DME) such as splints or crutches in the office, a separate claim is filed to the DME MAC. HCPCS coding is discussed in Chapter 30 of this text.

This chapter focuses on the procedural coding of surgical cases involving problems of the musculoskeletal system. It covers anatomical structures, terminology, common conditions surgically treated, and surgical techniques.

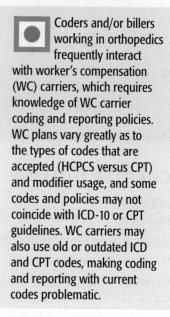

Coders and/or billers working in orthopedics frequently interact with worker's compensation (WC) carriers, which requires knowledge of WC carrier coding and reporting policies. WC plans vary greatly as to the types of codes that are accepted (HCPCS versus CPT) and modifier usage, and some codes and policies may not coincide with ICD-10 or CPT guidelines. WC carriers may also use old or outdated ICD and CPT codes, making coding and reporting with current codes problematic.

ORGANIZATION

The CPT's Musculoskeletal System section begins with definitions, such as open versus closed treatment. The General section then covers instructions for coding non–site-specific procedures. After that, the codes are organized by body part from the head down to the toes. Each anatomical site consistently groups its procedures under the same subheadings, as appropriate, which makes finding codes easier (see Box 18.1). Three of the subheads appear only under the General main heading: Wound Exploration, Replantation, and Grafts.

Guidelines and instructional notes appear throughout the Musculoskeletal System section. Also note that the word *specify* appears in some code descriptions, alerting the coder that a claim attachment (such as an operative note) may need to be submitted with the claim to provide specifics. CPT also uses terms and phrases such as *each, each additional, single,* and so on, indicating that it is necessary to indicate the number of bones, muscles, tendons, joints, or fingers/toes treated.

EXAMPLES
28308 Osteotomy, with or without lengthening, shortening or angular correction, metatarsal; *other than first metatarsal, each.*
28220 *Tenolysis, flexor, foot; single tendon.*

MODIFIERS

Modifiers are frequently used with orthopedic services. Box 18.2 outlines the modifiers most commonly used in the Musculoskeletal System section and explains how and why they are used. With numerous procedures performed on the extremities, hands, and feet, many codes in this section are also commonly subject to global surgery modifiers –54, –55, and –56 because of the nature of the specialty and procedures performed.

BOX 18.1 Musculoskeletal Subheadings

Incision

Excision

Introduction or Removal

Repair, Revision, and/or Reconstruction

Fracture and/or Dislocation

Arthrodesis

Amputation

Other Procedures

BOX 18.2 Orthopedic Modifiers

MODIFIER	DESCRIPTION	EXAMPLE OF USAGE
−25	Significant, separately identifiable evaluation and management (E/M) service by the same physician on the same day of the procedure or other service	Typically used to differentiate an injection or wound care from the E/M service.
−50	Bilateral procedure	Used to report procedures of the arms, legs, hands, and feet and both sides of spine.
−51	Multiple procedures	Used to report subsequent procedures excluding add-on or modifier −51 exempt codes.
−52	Reduced services	Used to report any service that was not carried out to the fullest extent of the code. A portion of a procedure may have been eliminated or partially completed.
−54	Surgical care only	Used frequently in fracture treatment but may apply to other trauma care.
−55	Postoperative management only	Used frequently in fracture treatment but may apply to other trauma care.
−56	Preoperative management only	Used frequently in fracture treatment when family practice MD diagnoses and refers to orthopedist.
−57	Decision for surgery	Appended to the E/M service when surgeon determines surgery is required (a major surgery with a 90-day global period).
−58	Staged or related procedure or service by the same physician during the postoperative period	Used to report a planned hardware removal within the global period.
−59	Distinct procedural service	Commonly used to report procedures on different compartments of the knee.
−62	Two surgeons	Used to report two surgeons who are not usually of the same specialty working as primary surgeons to perform a complex procedure. Commonly used to report spine procedures where a general surgeon opens the neck or abdomen to access the spine and the orthopedic surgeon performs the bone work.
−76	Repeat procedure or service by the same physician or other qualified health-care professional	Reported when physician performs an identical procedure on a patient within the postoperative period of the first surgery.
−77	Repeat procedure or service by another physician or other qualified health-care professional	Reported when a different physician performs an identical procedure on a patient within the postoperative period of the first surgery.
−78	Unplanned return to OR by the same physician for a related procedure during the postoperative period	May be required for postoperative complications such as hematoma, graft failure, or infection.
−79	Unrelated procedure or service by the same physician during the postoperative period	Used to report a procedure in the global period of an original procedure that is not staged and is seemingly unrelated to a previous one. For example, fracture care for a broken wrist in the postoperative period of an ACL repair.

Continued

BOX 18.2 Continued

MODIFIER	DESCRIPTION	EXAMPLE OF USAGE
–80	Assistant surgeon	Some surgeries allow for reporting of an assistant surgeon. Double-check the Medicare Physician Fee Schedule to determine whether the procedure allows for an assistant before coding.
AS	Physician assistant, nurse practitioner, or clinical nurse specialist services for assistant at surgery	Used in place of modifier –80 for Medicare recipients.
RT/LT	Right or left	Used to distinguish which arm, leg, hand, etc.
F1–F9	Finger modifiers	Used when performing procedures on fingers such as fracture repair, tendon reconstruction, or amputation.
TA–T9	Toe modifiers	Used when performing procedures on toes such as bunion or hammertoe correction or amputation.

■ CASE SCENARIOS

• A 65-year-old woman with obesity and end-stage degenerative arthritis endured as much pain and loss of mobility in her knees as she could tolerate. Despite the difficulty she would have during rehabilitation because of her weight, she and her orthopedic surgeon agreed during an office visit that she should have a total knee replacement (TKR) in each knee. The surgeon would report 9921x–57 for the office visit because the decision to perform surgery took place at this visit, and the surgery would take place the next day.

• An orthopedist in Florida sees a winter visitor who had a fracture repair of the humerus in Michigan 1 week before traveling. The surgeon in Michigan would report 27447–54 and the surgeon in Florida would report 27447–55.

Misadventure

Patients may develop complications while still under the global care period for a surgery. These can be the result of additional injury, accident, infection, or an unforeseen problem with a surgically implanted device. Some complications are clearly related to the original procedure, such as infection or implant malfunction, whereas others are due to injuries or procedures that seem to have nothing to do with the original surgery or operative site, such as a car accident. Carriers are not consistent with what they consider to be a postoperative complication and when and how to report modifiers –78 and –79. Orthopedic coders have to seek assistance from insurance companies regarding their position and requirement for what they consider a postoperative complication and how they want them reported.

Medicare states all postoperative complications are covered under the surgery code, while most commercial carriers consider all post-op complications reimbursable with either a –78 or –79 as unrelated to the surgery.

REIMBURSEMENT REVIEW

Furnace bid code

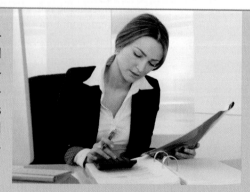

Medicare's rules for reporting postoperative complications differ from those of commercial carriers. Under Medicare's global surgery policy, all postoperative complications that do not require a return trip to the operating room are considered components of the global surgical package. But commercial carriers will often pay for the treatment of post-op complications and the associated supplies regardless of whether there was a return to the OR.

INTRAOPERATIVE SERVICES AND IMAGE GUIDANCE

Included Services

The National Correct Coding Initiative (NCCI) policy manual and the American Academy of Orthopaedic Surgeons (AAOS) each provide guidance on what is always included in a surgical procedure. Services integral to a defined procedure are included in the procedure based on the standards of medical/surgical practice. It is inappropriate to separately report services that are integral to another procedure with that procedure.

Many NCCI edits are based on the standards of medical/surgical practice. Services that are integral to another service are component parts of the more comprehensive service. The AAOS has developed a list of 11 generic intraoperative services that are common to most orthopedic procedures. When these services are billed with an orthopedic procedure, these services will be included in the global surgical fee.

1. Local infiltration of medications, anesthetic, or contrast agent before, during, or at the conclusion of the operation
2. Suture removal by operating or designee
3. Surgical approach, with necessary identification, isolation, and protection of anatomical structures, including hemostasis and nerve stimulation, or skin scar revision
4. Wound culture
5. Wound irrigation
6. Intraoperative photos and/or video recording, excluding ionizing radiation
7. Intraoperative supervision and positioning of imaging and/or monitoring equipment by operating surgeon or assistant
8. Insertion, placement, and removal of surgical drain, re-infusion devices, irrigation tube, catheter, or suction device
9. Closure of wound and repair of tissues divided for the initial surgical exposure, partial or complete
10. Application of initial dressing, wound vacuum device, orthosis, continuous passive motion, splint or cast, including traction, except where specifically excluded from the global package
11. Preparation and insertion of synthetic bone substitutes

This list mirrors that of the NCCI global surgery package but with these additional services:

- Cleansing, shaving, and prepping of skin
- Insertion of intravenous access for medication administration
- Insertion of urinary catheter (general anesthesia cases only)
- Sedative administration by the physician performing a procedure
- Application, management, and removal of postoperative dressings and analgesic devices (peri-incisional)
- Application of TENS unit
- Institution of patient-controlled analgesia (PCA)
- Preoperative, intraoperative, and postoperative documentation
- Surgical supplies, except for specific situations where Centers for Medicare and Medicaid Services (CMS) policy permits separate payment

Surgeons may elect during some orthopedic procedures (particularly those of the spine and at times the hand) to utilize intraoperative neurophysiology testing to ensure proper functioning of nerves. Intraoperative neurophysiology testing (95940–95941) should not be reported by the surgeon performing the operative procedure. This testing is considered to be part of the global package. It is felt that the surgeon cannot monitor the patient and perform the surgery at the same time. However, if a second physician performs the testing, it is separately reportable using codes located in the Medicine section of CPT (i.e., 95822, 95940–95941, 95925).

Image Guidance

If a physician requires image guidance during a surgical procedure, the coder should determine if the service is separately reportable by first checking the code description and any parenthetical notes in CPT as well as the NCCI edits. Aside from straight x-ray codes, the following common imaging codes are reported with codes in the Musculoskeletal System section of CPT:

- 76000 Fluoroscopy (separate procedure), up to 1 hour physician time or other qualified health-care professional time, other than 71023 or 71034
- 77002 Fluoroscopic guidance for needle placement
- 20696 Application of multiplane, unilateral, external fixation with stereotactic computer-assisted adjustment including imaging; initial and subsequent alignment(s), assessment(s), and computation(s) of adjustment schedule(s)
- 20697 Exchange of strut, each
- +20985 Computer-assisted surgical navigation procedure for musculoskeletal procedures, image-less (list separately in addition to code for primary procedure)
- 0054T Computer-assisted musculoskeletal surgical navigational orthopedic procedure, with image-guidance based on fluoroscopic images (look for instruments such as VectorVision and the OEC FluoroTrak)
- 0055T Computer-assisted musculoskeletal surgical navigational orthopedic procedure, with image-guidance based on CT/MRI images

REIMBURSEMENT REVIEW

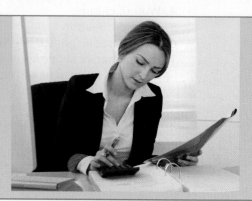

Check with insurance carriers to determine if they recognize and reimburse Category III codes for computer-assisted navigational devices for orthopedic procedures (most Medicare payers do not), because many carriers consider their use to be investigational and nonpayable.

Codes 76000, 77002, and 0054T–0055T indicate the use of fluoroscopic C-arm imaging. Codes 0054T and 0055T indicate the use of a computer with an optical or electromagnetic sensor to track surgical instruments. The computer uses stored images to display the position of the surgical instruments and the devices' predicted path. If the surgeon is using the imaging to simply view the anatomy, evaluate a joint in motion, or confirm placement of a wire or screw, report 76000.

EXAMPLE

Physician performs a computer-assisted total knee replacement using fluoroscopic imaging techniques. Adequacy of the arthroplasty is confirmed with intraoperative C-arm fluoroscopy. A reference frame (tracker) is attached to the femur. The C-arm fluoroscope, retrofitted with a calibration target for image-guided surgery, is brought in to obtain images of the joint. The patient and C-arm are tracked by an optical camera interfaced with the image-guided surgery (IGS) system. Multiple stored images are simultaneously displayed on the IGS monitor. The system then tracks the surgical instruments (drill guide or probe) and displays their position relative to the stored images. Small stab incisions allow precise insertion of the drill guide in predetermined safe zones, and large-diameter cannulated screws are placed percutaneously into the femur and tibia to stabilize the implant. Code 0054T would be submitted in addition to the code for the TKR.

SURGICAL TECHNIQUES

Coders learning how to code procedures often ask, "How can I determine what is 'significant' to code?" The answer is that you must first know the meaning of the surgical root procedures. Think about the definition of a significant procedure and look for those key words. Pay close attention to

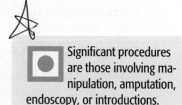

Significant procedures are those involving manipulation, amputation, endoscopy, or introductions.

BOX 18.3 Musculoskeletal System Acronyms

AC	acromioclavicular
ACL	anterior cruciate ligament
AKA	above-knee amputation
BKA	below-knee amputation
CMC	carpometacarpal (joint)
CTR	carpal tunnel release
DDD	degenerative disk disease
DIP	distal interphalangeal joint
DJD	degenerative joint disease
FB	foreign body
Fx	fracture
LCL	lateral collateral ligament
MCL	medial cruciate ligament
MCP	metacarpophalangeal (joint)
MPJ	metatarsal phalangeal joint
MTP	metatarsophalangeal (joint)
NSAID	nonsteroidal anti-inflammatory drug
OATS	osteochondral autograft transfer system
ORIF	open reduction with internal fixation
PCL	posterior cruciate ligament
PIPJ	proximal interphalangeal joint
ROM	range of motion
SLAP	superior labrum anterior and posterior
Sx	surgery
TENS	transcutaneous electrical nerve stimulation
TKR	total knee replacement
TPI	trigger point injection
UCL	ulnar collateral ligament
UE	upper extremity

the type of service provided and the extent of services by carefully reading the medical record and then reading the code description in its entirety to catch phrases such as *closed, open, with or without manipulation, with traction, with or without internal or external fixator, with grafting,* and so on. Key acronyms are listed in Box 18.3.

Amputation

Amputation means detachment by surgical or traumatic means of a limb, body part, or appendage. Disarticulation is amputation of a limb by cutting through a joint rather than cutting through bone at any point of the limb. Key words: *amputation, exarticulation, complete removal.*

EXAMPLE

27590 *Amputation, thigh, through femur, any level.*

Arthrodesis

Arthrodesis or fusion is the permanent joining together of bones by mechanical implant such as screws or wire or by graft to make them immobile. Key word: *arthrodesis.*

EXAMPLE

28750 *Arthrodesis, great toe; metatarsophalangeal joint.*

Arthrotomy

An arthrotomy is a surgical incision into a joint as an approach to a therapeutic surgery, to explore the joint, provide drainage, or possibly remove a foreign body.

EXAMPLE

23040 *Arthrotomy, glenohumeral joint, including exploration, drainage, or removal of foreign body.*

Arthroscopy

In the procedure called *arthroscopy,* the surgeon makes two small incisions in the skin and inserts pencil-sized instruments that contain a lens and lighting system to magnify and visualize the structures inside the joint. By attaching the arthroscope to a miniature camera, the surgeon is able to see the interior of the joint.

EXAMPLE

29888 *Arthroscopically aided anterior cruciate ligament repair/augmentation or reconstruction.*

Arthroplasty

An arthroplasty is a procedure to restore range of motion by realigning or reconstructing a dysfunctional joint. This includes reconstruction of a joint, which may involve replacement of the joint with a prosthesis.

25441 *Arthroplasty with prosthetic replacement; distal radius.*

Endoscopy

Endoscopy is a surgical approach or technique that uses an endoscope (a lighted tubular instrument) to visualize the internal body. It is proven to reduce surgical risks and postoperative recovery time. Endoscopic procedures are performed by making small incisions into the skin and inserting an endoscope to view the surfaces of organs, joints, and the digestive tract, allowing the physician to take pictures, obtain biopsies, remove foreign bodies, and remove and repair organs. The scope can also be inserted into a natural orifice such as the mouth or rectum. Key words: *arthroscope, arthroscopy, endoscope, endoscopy, laryngoscopy, laryngoscope, bronchoscopy, bronchoscope, scope, trocar, sleeve.*

EXAMPLE

29804 *Arthroscopy, temporomandibular joint, surgical.*

Exostectomy

An exostectomy is removal of a benign tumor or calcification of bone called "exostosis" from one of the bones of the feet.

EXAMPLE

28288 *Ostectomy, partial, exostectomy or condylectomy, metatarsal head, each metatarsal head.*

Lysis

Lysis means to cut loose or through, or to free something from another. This may be performed with an instrument such as a scalpel, by Bovie cautery, or by manually freeing with hands. Key words: *release, divide, destroy*; words ending in *-lysis.*

EXAMPLE

29825 *Arthroscopy, shoulder, surgical; with lysis and resection of adhesions, with or without manipulation.*

Manipulation

Manipulation is a very important term in musculoskeletal system coding. It refers to the maneuvering or movement of a joint or body part by the surgeon's hands so that fragments of fractured bone or displaced joints are brought into normal anatomical alignment. Key words: *adjustment, manipulation.*

EXAMPLE

27860 *Manipulation of ankle under general anesthesia (includes application of traction or other fixation apparatus).*

Reduction

Reduction is another key term; it means that the physician aligns the fracture bones back into their original anatomical alignment, either manually or surgically. Nonsurgical reduction may involve the use of traction, for example, to pull the bones back into position. Key words: *open reduction, closed reduction.*

EXAMPLE

23505 *Closed treatment of clavicular fracture; with manipulation.*

Release

Release refers to the decompressing or loosening of a tendon, muscle, or nerve from surrounding tissue that is binding or impeding movement. Key words: *freeing, decompression, relaxing, relieving, lysing.*

28035 *Release, tarsal tunnel (posterior tibial nerve decompression).*

Replantation

Replantation indicates reattachment of a body part that was traumatically removed in its entirety from the body. Key words: *reattachment, replantation, reconstruction.*

20838 *Replantation, foot, complete amputation.*

Revision

Revision means surgery on a joint or body part previously repaired to again make minor repairs or repeat any portion of the original surgery.

> Most of the mus-culoskeletal NCCI edits have the modifier indicator of "1," so the use of an appropriate modifier (usually –59) can override them.

27134 *Revision of total hip arthroplasty; both components, with or without autograft or allograft.*

Sequestrectomy

Sequestrectomy involves removal of dead bone that is fragmented away from healthy bone.

23170 *Sequestrectomy (e.g., for osteomyelitis or bone abscess), clavicle.*

Traction

Traction is force applied by weights or other devices to treat bone injuries or muscle disorders. It is most often used as a temporary measure when operative fixation is not available for a period of time. Traction is usually applied to the extremities, neck, back, or pelvis. There are two types of traction: skeletal and skin. Skin traction imposes a force on the limb through the use of a strapping or adhesive tape that is applied directly to the skin. The straps are then attached to a traction cord and pulley system that uses 5 to 7 pounds of weight on the end to provide a continuous pulling force. Skeletal traction is invasive and requires inserting a pin, wire, or screw into the bone most distal from the fracture site. Skeletal traction is applied when heavier weight is necessary or needed for an extended period of time. The pin is placed through the skin and subcutaneous tissue through the bone and exits the opposite side. A clamp is attached to the pin to connect it to the continuous traction cord. Skeletal traction is used to treat fractures of the femur and humerus and dislocations of the hip (Fig. 18.1).

20661 *Application of halo, including removal; cranial.*

GENERAL MUSCULOSKELETAL PROCEDURES

Diagnostic and Therapeutic Procedures

Some procedure codes include the word *diagnostic* in the code description. But a therapeutic procedure always includes the diagnostic portion; therefore, only the therapeutic portion is coded. Diagnostic procedures are just that: They do not treat or repair a problem. Diagnostic procedures are carried out to determine the extent of a problem and "diagnose" it. They are a "look and see" type of procedure. Therapeutic procedures often result after a diagnostic procedure identified a problem. Therapeutic procedures involve repairing an injury or defect, excising a lesion or body part, destroying tissue, etc. When the procedure extends beyond just looking, it is no longer a diagnostic procedure.

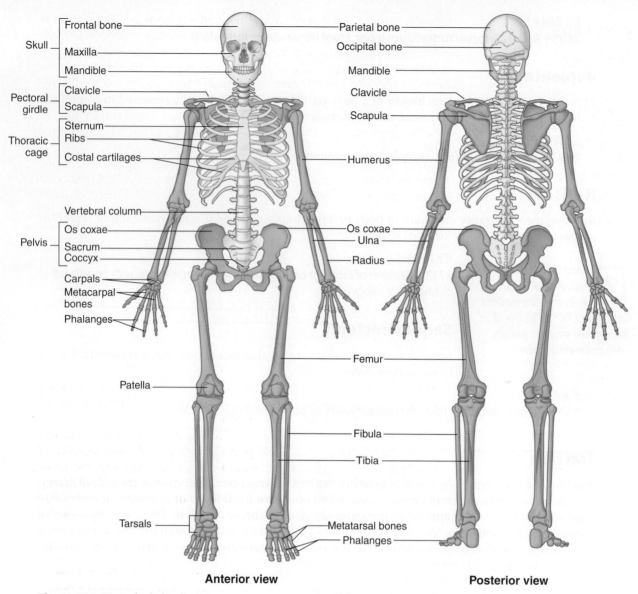

Figure 18.1 Musculoskeletal system.

Labels (Anterior view):
Skull — Frontal bone, Maxilla, Mandible
Pectoral girdle — Clavicle, Scapula
Thoracic cage — Sternum, Ribs, Costal cartilages
Vertebral column
Pelvis — Os coxae, Sacrum, Coccyx
Carpals
Metacarpal bones
Phalanges
Patella
Tarsals
Metatarsal bones
Phalanges

Labels (Posterior view):
Parietal bone
Occipital bone
Mandible
Clavicle
Scapula
Humerus
Os coxae
Ulna
Radius
Femur
Fibula
Tibia

Anterior view   **Posterior view**

Injection of Joints, Tendons, Trigger Points, and Sinuses

Arthrocentesis is the procedure to aspirate the joint and remove fluid, and/or inject a therapeutic substance. Codes from the range 20600–20610 are selected according to the size of the joint: small, intermediate, or major. If a more extensive procedure is done to a joint that is also being injected, the injection would be bundled into the more complex procedure. Tendon injections are coded to 20550–20551.

> ■ **CASE SCENARIO**
> A patient complains of shoulder pain when raising the right arm or when trying to lift, push, or pull objects. Physician diagnosed tendonitis and injected the shoulder with corticosteroids. Code: 20610–RT.

Trigger point injections (TPIs) are used to treat pain. TPI injections are used to treat painful areas of muscle that contain trigger points, which are knots of muscle that form when muscles do not relax. Trigger points are coded by the number of muscle groups

> For a number of codes in this section, per CPT notes, code the appropriate radiology codes if imaging guidance is used.

The patient's medical record must also include the reason for the injection and the injection site. If you are coding for a physician office visit, don't forget to include the appropriate J code that represents the medication. When injections, whether to joints or skin, are performed in the physician's office, the HCPCS code for the medication administered is coded separately with a J code.

Medicare requires HCPCS G codes for injections of the sacroiliac joint instead of codes from the CPT Musculoskeletal System section.

A biopsy of a musculoskeletal structure is not billed separately when an excision, destruction, removal, repair, or fixation procedure is also performed unless it is of a different site.

Remember: If lipomas are excised from skin or subcutaneous tissue, it is appropriate to assign a code from the Integumentary System section only if there is no specific code in the Musculoskeletal System section. If a lesion is deeper than the superficial fascia, assign a code from the Musculoskeletal section.

injected, not the number of times the needle is inserted. The needle is inserted into the muscle and then slightly withdrawn and re-angled, and medication is injected in a fan distribution. The needle may be withdrawn and reinserted in different locations of the same muscle, so the coder must be sure to determine which muscles were injected. Trigger point injections (20552–20553) have no laterality because they are based on the number of muscles treated, so left versus right side of body is not important; therefore, –LT, –RT, and –50 modifiers will not apply.

Codes 20500–20501 refer to injecting sinus tracts. These cavities or abscesses are not located in the nasal sinuses. These are abscesses or pockets of infection that can develop as a result of puncture wounds or skin abscesses that burrow or create tracts in the soft tissue and muscle. Use these codes for injection of dye prior to some diagnostic radiology procedures as well.

EXAMPLE

In the office, an orthopedic physician injects the right wrist with a mixture of lidocaine and Depo-Medrol with the use of a C-arm to confirm needle placement in the joint. Codes: 20605–RT, 77002, and J1030.

Excisions

Codes from the Excision sections cover primarily removal of tumors or cysts from the soft tissue or bone, synovectomy and bursectomy of tendons and joints, and partial or complete removal of bone. Codes 20150–20251 are organized by the structure being biopsied, the depth of the biopsy, and the biopsy technique. When it comes to excisions and biopsies, coders often make the mistake of immediately turning to the Integumentary System section. Depth of excision and the most specific anatomical site should be considered. If the incision goes beyond the superficial fascia, the Musculoskeletal System section is the most appropriate section from which to code. The excision includes the administration of anesthesia, the incision into the area, removal of the tissue, and suturing the site.

EXAMPLE

25065 *Biopsy, soft tissue of forearm and/or wrist; superficial.* Even though the descriptor in this procedure codes says "superficial," this code would be more appropriate to assign than an Integumentary System code because it is specific to the forearm and indicates "soft tissue."

Specific CPT guidelines address the excision of soft tissue tumors. The codes break down into subcutaneous, fascial/subfascial, and radical resection of bone. The depth of the excision and the level of work determine what is included and/or excluded in the excision services.

Subcutaneous soft tissue tumors. These tumors are usually benign and are resected without removing a significant amount of normal tissue. Tumor measurement follows lesion excision measurement guidelines in the Integumentary System section. Excision includes the following:

- Perform a simple or intermediate repair.
- Perform a simple or marginal resection of tumors confined to subcutaneous tissue below the skin but above the deep fascia.
- Dissect or elevate tissue planes to allow for resection of tumor.
- Appreciable vessel exploration and/or neuroplasty are separately reportable.

Fascial/subfascial soft tissue tumors. Codes are based on size and location of tumor. Tumor measurement follows lesion excision measurement guidelines in the Integumentary System section. Excision includes the following:

- Perform a simple or intermediate repair.
- Resect tumors confined to subcutaneous tissue within or below the deep fascia but not involving bone.
- Dissect or elevate tissue planes to allow for resection of tumor.
- Resect usually benign, often intramuscular tumors, without removing a significant amount of normal tissue.
- Appreciable vessel exploration and/or neuroplasty are separately reportable.

Radical resection of soft tissue tumors. Radical resection is commonly used for malignant or very aggressive benign tumors. Codes are based on size and location of tumor. Tumor measurement follows lesion excision measurement guidelines in the Integumentary System section. Resection includes the following:

- Perform a simple or intermediate repair.
- Resect tumors with wide margins of normal tissue.
- Dissect or elevate tissue planes to allow for resection of tumor.
- Tumors may be confined to a specific layer but radical resection may involve removal of tissue from one or more layers.
- Appreciable vessel exploration and/or neuroplasty repair or reconstruction are separately reportable.

Radical resection of bone tumors. Radical resection is commonly used for malignant or very aggressive benign bone tumors. Codes are based on size and location of tumor. Tumor measurement follows lesion excision measurement guidelines in the Integumentary System section. Resection tumors includes the following:

- Perform a simple or intermediate repair.
- Resect tumors with wide margins of normal tissue.
- Dissect or elevate tissue planes to allow for resection of tumor.
- Removal of entire bone may be required.
- Tumors may be confined to a specific layer but radical resection may involve removal of tissue from one or more layers.
- If surrounding soft tissue is removed, do not report radical resection of soft tissue tumor codes.
- Appreciable vessel exploration and/or neuroplasty repair or reconstructions are separately reportable.

Foreign Body Removal

Two factors affect coding for removal of a foreign body (FB): the site and whether the foreign body is superficial or deep. Some of the code sections have a specific code for FB removal and some do not. This is usually found under the "Introduction or Removal" subheading in each body section. Foreign bodies can be anything that is "foreign" to the body (such as metal, gravel, bullet, or an orthopedic device) and embedded in tissue, bone, or a joint or it could be a "loose" body of natural tissue or bone that "broke off" (such as bone chip or cartilage) and is blocking movement or blood flow or is floating in a joint causing pain.

EXAMPLE
24200 *Removal of foreign body, upper arm or elbow area; subcutaneous.*

Assign codes to the following procedures for the physician. Include any necessary modifiers.

1. A 6-year-old child was helping his father clear out brush and small trees from their yard and got a large splinter embedded in his right hand that required removal. The splinter was located deep in the palm of the hand. _____

2. A data entry operator has been suffering from chronic tendonitis in the right index finger. The physician injects the finger with 0.5 mL lidocaine and 0.25 mL Celestone Soluspan.

   _____

3. A patient suffers a nasty fall from the top flight of the stairs. The patient is complaining of neck and left shoulder pain. The physician identifies three trigger points: the right trapezius, the right deltoid, and the right levator scapulae muscles and injects these with a mixture of lidocaine and Marcaine. _____

4. Diagnosis: Soft tissue tumor of the back. Procedure: Excision of soft tissue tumor. Patient presents with tumor on the upper right back. Skin is incised down through the deep dermal layers to the deep subcutaneous tissue. The cyst was removed en bloc. The cyst measured 5.5 x 2.7 x 1.2 cm.

   _____

SPINE

Understanding the spinal anatomy is the first step in the process of accurately assigning CPT codes for procedures on the spine (Fig. 18.2).

The spine, also known as the vertebral column or spinal column, consists of 26 bones: 24 separate vertebrae separated by impact absorbing cartilage, the sacrum, and the coccyx. The spine has five major regions:

1. **Cervical:** There are seven vertebrae in the neck or cervical region of the spine identified as C1–C7. The first cervical vertebra, C1, is referred to as the "atlas" and supports the skull. The skull pivots on the atlas when moving up and down.

2. **Thoracic:** There are 12 vertebrae in the chest or thoracic region identified as T1–T12. These vertebrae are larger and stronger than cervical vertebrae. The spinous processes of the thoracic vertebrae point inferiorly to help lock the vertebrae together, each one forming a joint with ribs on either side of the spine to form the rib cage that protects the vital organs of the chest.

3. **Lumbar:** There are five vertebrae in the lower back or lumbar region of the spine identified at L1–L5. Lumbar vertebrae are the largest and strongest of the vertebrae. The lumbar vertebrae support all weight from the upper body, which is why this area of the spine is prone to disease and injury.

4. **Sacral:** The sacrum is formed by the fusing of vertebrae S1–S5. The sacrum is a flat, triangular bone found in the lower back and wedged between the two hip bones.

5. **Coccygeal:** The coccyx is the only bone located in the coccygeal region. The coccyx is also known as the tailbone. The coccyx sustains our body weight while sitting.

Each vertebra has six structural components: the vertebral body, pedicle, lamina, spinous process, transverse process, and vertebral foramen (see Fig. 18.2). The body of the vertebra (the round, solid portion of the vertebra) bears the weight of the body and is the largest of the six components. Projecting from the back of each vertebral body are two short stalks of bone called

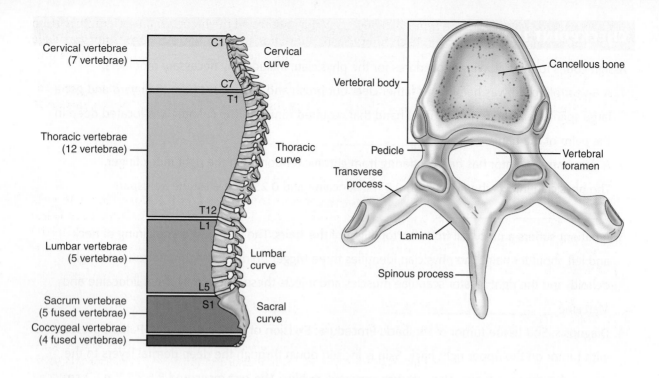

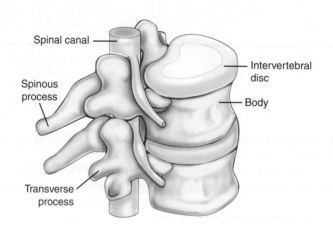

Figure 18.2 Spine Anatomy (a) The vertebral column (b) Vertebral body (c) Intervertebral disc. From Hoffman, G. and N. Sullivan, *Medical-Surgical Nursing: Making Connections to Practice*, F.A. Davis Company, 2017.

pedicles. They form the sides of the vertebral foramen. The lamina are flat plate-like bones that connect the pedicles on either side of the vertebral body forming the back wall or roof of what is called the vertebral arch. The transverse processes are thin bones that project out from the left and right sides of the vertebral body. These bony projections are an attachment site for muscles and ligaments of the spine. The spinous process extends posteriorly from the end of each transverse process. (These are the knobs that you see in a person's back when they bend over.) Between the body, transverse processes and spinous process is the vertebral foramen, a hollow space or spinal canal that contains the spinal cord and meninges.

When reading medical documentation, vertebrae are referred to by their location (spine section or region) and number sequence. Figure 18.2 illustrates this numbering methodology. For example, patient is diagnosed with a pathological fracture of the T4 vertebrae. This tells us the affected vertebra is the fourth one located in the thoracic section of the spine.

Between each vertebra is an intervertebral disc that is attached to the vertebral body above and below it. The discs are meant to cushion the spinal column and absorb some of the force caused by movement—walking, jogging, dancing, jumping, etc. Without these cushions, the vertebrae would fracture from "banging" into each other and the brain would suffer injury from the jarring it would sustain. Each intervertebral disc has an outer band of fibrous fibrocartilage called the annulus fibrosus that encapsulates the disc's gelatinous core called the nucleus pulposus.

Procedures on the spine may be performed by orthopedic surgeons or neurosurgeons. Additional spinal procedures, such as those involving the disc, facet, or nerve roots are discussed in Chapter 26 of this text.

INTERNET RESOURCE:
Visit http://www.spineuniverse.com/anatomy to view
animations and learn more about the anatomy and physiology of the spine.

When reading medical documentation and assigning spinal procedure codes, the coder must understand the difference between the terms *vertebral segment* and *vertebral interspace.*

A vertebral segment refers to a single vertebral bone complete with its bony articular processes and laminae. A vertebral interspace is the non-bony compartment between two vertebral bodies that contains the intervertebral disc which is made up of the nucleaus pulposus and annulus fibrosus.

Common Spinal Problems and Procedures

Back pain is a symptom of all back ailments and injuries. Weight, age, diet, exercise, and occupation all affect spine health. The following list includes the most common spinal disorders. Some of these disorders occur over time as part of a degenerative process as we age while others are acquired from overuse or occupational hazards that lead to injuries.

Disc Prolapse or Disc Bulge—The disc is attached to the vertebral bodies above and below it. These discs cushion and soften the forces created by walking and jumping, which might otherwise fracture the vertebrae or jar the brain. Prolapse occurs when the intervertebral disc shifts or slips out of the interspace. When the disc's position changes, nerve impingement often occurs.

Disc Herniation—As explained above, each intervertebral disc is composed of a band of fibrous fibrocartilage (annulus fibrosus) that surrounds a gelatinous core, called the nucleus pulposus. When the disc's outer band weakens or breaks open, the nucleus will extrude through the wall of this capsule but stay within the disc itself. Herniation (or herniated nucleus pulposus [HNP]) occurs when the nucleus extrudes through the disc wall and the nucleus sac ruptures causing fluid inside the nucleus to leak out. The disc's gelatinous material then places pressure on nearby nerve roots or the spinal cord causing pain and/or numbness. Once fluid leaks out of the disc, the intervertebral disc space height "shrinks" placing tension on surrounding ligaments and narrowing the opening where the nerve roots exit.

Degenerative Disc Disease (intervertebral disc degeneration)—The discs located between each vertebra lose their cushioning and begin to break down with age (shrink and lose height). As they deteriorate, the vertebral bones begin to rub causing back pain.

Spondylolisthesis—Referred to as "slipped vertebrae," spondylolisthesis most commonly occurs in the lumbar spine (L4–L5) when one vertebra slips forward over the vertebra below. Physicians classify the severity of this condition into five grades based on the percentage of the vertebral body that slipped over the bottom vertebra. Grade 1 being up to 24% and the most severe Grade 5 with 100% or complete slip.

Fractured Vertebrae—Fractures commonly occur due to the osteoporosis disease process that weakens the bone making it brittle. The bones fracture under the stress of supporting the body's weight. Some fractures are a result from traumatic injury such as falls or vehicular accidents.

Diseases and disorders involving the disc, spinal cord, or nerves are further discussed in Chapter 26 of this text. Some spinal surgeries require the use of codes from both the Musculoskeletal and Nervous System sections such as when a decompression is performed along with a spinal fusion. This chapter only discusses procedures that fall within the reporting of the Musculoskeletal section.

In the past, invasive spinal procedures were performed in the hospital requiring inpatient hospitalization and long recuperation periods. Today, with advanced spinal fusion techniques and decreased scarring these procedures are performed on an outpatient basis.

Arthrodesis

Arthrodesis, or fusion, is indicated to treat the conditions mentioned above when conservative measures have failed. Fusion of the vertebra is achieved by removing the disc between two vertebrae and using a bone graft to fuse two vertebral segments together into one long bone, which permanently immobilizes an interspace. The transverse processes are fused to stabilize the vertebral segments. The grafts may be autogenous (taken from the patient's hip) or allogenic (received from a bone bank harvested from cadavers). Bone grafts are often paired with metal implants referred to as "instrumentation" to maintain the spinal stability and correct any spinal deformity such as loss of disc space. Report all structural allografts using code 20931.

Surgeons can use various approaches when performing a spinal fusion. Documentation should be carefully read to determine which approach is applied.

> When an interbody spinal fusion device (IFD) is placed and bone grafting is packed into the IFD, CPT codes are reported for each procedure.

The posterior approach is the conventional approach. It uses an incision made over the vertebra posteriorly, or on the patient's back, where muscle is stripped off the vertebrae to gain access. Conversely, the anterior approach with the patient lying supine accesses the affected vertebra by making an incision anteriorly on the body either in the front or the side of the neck (anterior interbody) or transorally (through the mouth) for cervical fusions or through the abdomen to access thoracic or lumbar vertebrae by pushing organs and structures aside. The CPT Professional Edition contains illustrations throughout the spine section of various approaches, segmentation, and instrumentation.

Detailed documentation is essential considering that the following approaches are coded with a different series of codes:

- Transforaminal interbody fusion (TLIF)—incision is made posteriorly but more to the side.
- Lateral extracavitary (codes 22532–22534)
- Anterior or anterolateral or anterior interbody fusion (ALIF) use codes 22548–22586, and codes 22808–22812
    - Note that code 22551 includes the services of both arthrodesis and discectomy, therefore you would not report code 63075 with code 22551. If only arthrodesis is performed report code 22554. See the note below code 22554.
    - Be aware of the phrase "including minimal discectomy to prepare interspace other than for decompression" in codes 22554–22558. This not the same as the discectomy indicated in code 22551. If the discectomy is performed to prepare the interspace report code 22554. If a discectomy is performed for any other purpose during an arthrodesis report code 22551.

EXAMPLES

- During an anterior spinal fusion to stabilize the spine, a discectomy was performed to provide access to the surgical site C5–C6. Report code 22554.

- During an anterior spinal fusion to treat a herniated disc, the surgeon also performed a discectomy, osteophytectomy, and decompression of spinal cord. Report code 22551.

- Transoral approach or anterior interbody—incision is made in the front of the body (side of neck through the sternocleidomastoid and platymal muscles for cervical fusion) or through the abdomen using a retroperitoneal approach to access the lumbar spine (22548).
- Posterior or posterolateral or lateral transverse process use codes 22590–22632, and codes 22800–22804 for spinal deformity. The incision is made through the posterior body or patient's back. Posterior fixation is accomplished by placement of graft between the vertebra and/or applying segmental or non-segmental fixation. Posterolateral fixation is obtained by fixation of the transverse processes. The term posterolateral gutter fusion may be used during a posterolateral spinal fusion when the bone graft is placed between the transverse processes of the affected vertebrae.

When coding a spinal fusion, consider the reason for the procedure. Review the documentation to determine why the fusion is necessary. If the surgeon is performing the fusion for pain or instability, coders should reference one of the following code series:

> When it comes to choosing the correct CPT code for a spinal fusion, count vertebral interspaces instead of vertebrae to choose the correct code.

22532–22534 (lateral extracavitary)
22548–22585 (anterior or anterolateral)

CPT © 2017 American Medical Association, All Rights Reserved.

22590–22632 (posterior)
22633–22634 (combined posterior or posterolateral)

If the surgeon performed the fusion for a spinal deformity (e.g., scoliosis or kyphosis), look to CPT codes 22800–22819. This code series was created for, and intended to be used for, fusion procedures performed on patients with congenital spinal deformities, not for degenerative scoliosis.

Instrumentation

Spinal instrumentation consists of two types: segmental and non-segmental. At the beginning of the Spinal Instrumentation section of the Musculoskeletal section, definitions are provided for these as well as instructions for reporting insertion of spinal instrumentation separately. CPT specifies that modifier –62 may not be reported for instrumentation procedures.

Non-segmental instrumentation is fixated at each end of the implant and may span several vertebral segments without attachment to any additional segments. The Harrington rod is an example of this type of instrumentation. The rod is attached to the spine by hooks on the top and bottom. This device can be adjusted to ratchet and stretch the spine if needed.

Segmental instrumentation is described as fixation at each end of the implant (construct or rod) in addition to at least one bony attachment or spinal segment. Typical segmental instrumentation would be plates attached by screws or placement of pedicle screws in the lumbar spine. The anterior instrumentation codes +22845 to +22847 are used for both segmental and non-segmental instrumentation. Only the posterior instrumentation codes break down into segmental and non-segmental.

Codes for instrumentation are reported in addition to the arthrodesis procedure codes and in addition to bone graft procedures. Minimal wiring using devices such as a Songer cable are not separately reported. Report the appropriate add-on CPT code based on approach and instrumentation:

+22840 to +22844 (posterior instrumentation, with separate codes for segmental and non-segmental)
+22845 to +22847 (anterior instrumentation, representing both segmental and non-segmental)
+22848 (pelvic fixation)
+22853 to +22859 (insertion of interbody or intervertebral biomechanical devices)

Instrumentation removal is reported with codes 22850, 22852, 22855. If the surgeon removes instrumentation and inserts new instrumentation at different levels, only the codes for insertion are reported. For example, if a surgeon removes instrumentation at L2–L3 and inserts new instrumentation from L3–L5, only the new instrumentation codes should be reported, not codes for both the removal of the old instrumentation and the insertion of new instrumentation. If the surgeon removes old instrumentation at L1–L24 and reinserts new instrumentation at the same level, the reinsertion code 22849 should be used.

EXAMPLE
During an anterior spinal fusion to stabilize the spine, a discectomy was performed to prepare the interspace C5-C6. Anterior instrumentation and structural allograft were also performed. Report code 22554, +22845 and +20931.

Spinal Prosthetic Devices

When the intervertebral disc is removed, an interbody spinal fusion device (IFD) is placed. In addition to instrumentation, surgeons may use this prosthetic device also known as a biomechanical device to fill the void left from removing the disc. A device commonly used is referred to as a "cage" because of its wire structure. The device bridges the gap created when a disc is removed or when a vertebra is fractured or diseased. Bone grafting is packed into the cage and grows through the holes and fuses the vertebrae. Methylmethacrylate (i.e., bone cement) is one of the more common IFDs. Report the application of the biomechanical device(s) using add-on code +22851. Coders should report this code per interspace, not per segment or per device. Append modifier –59 (distinct procedural service) for each code that indicates an additional interspace.

EXAMPLE
Arthrodesis is performed and a cage is placed at L1 and L3. Report +22851 × 2 in addition to the arthrodesis procedure.

When performing an interbody fusion, it may be necessary at times to apply posterior instrumentation. You would not report an interbody arthrodesis and a posterior or posterolateral arthrodesis at the same level. In this scenario, report the interbody fusion and posterior instrumentation codes. These procedures are considered mutually exclusive if performed at the same level.

Type of Graft

When assigning codes for grafts, first consider the type of bone graft used. Allograft is bone obtained from a donor—not from the patient. The allograft is purchased from a bone bank and comes in a bottle or a package. Autografts are obtained from the patient's body, usually the hip. Report bone graft codes once per operative session. CPT specifies that modifier 62 is never used with bone graft codes 20900–20938.

The spinal bone graft codes include:

+20930 (allograft or osteopromotive material for spine surgery, morselized)

+ 20931 (allograft for spine surgery, structural)

+20936 (autograft, local, obtained from same incision)

+20937 (harvest of graft through separate skin incision, commonly iliac crest)

+20938 (autograft, structural, bicortical, or tricortical through separate skin or fascial incision.)

Note: CPT has several examples of arthrodesis coding with bone grafts and instrumentation to assist coders. These examples are under the Spine (Vertebral Column) section header in the CPT book.

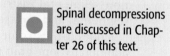 Spinal decompressions are discussed in Chapter 26 of this text.

CPT instructs the coder to report 38220 for bone marrow aspiration, if bone marrow is aspirated from the body and then mixed with the bone graft material.

FRACTURE AND DISLOCATION TREATMENT

A fracture is a break, crack, or disruption of a hard surface such as bone or cartilage. *Closed* fractures (such as greenstick, linear, spiral, or comminuted) do not break through the skin, whereas *open* fractures (such as compound, puncture, missile, or infected) create a wound on the outside of the skin caused by bone puncturing out through skin and/or blood vessels. Open wounds often involve debris such as dirt, gravel, and glass and run the risk of contamination.

Dislocation is a condition in which bones that meet at a joint are separated. X-rays are obtained to rule out additional fractures. A dislocation may cause ligament or nerve damage and take 2 to 3 months to heal. The obvious treatment for this type of injury is to put the "joint back in place" or put the bones back into anatomical alignment.

If a closed reduction is attempted, fails, and is followed by an open reduction, no code is assigned for the closed reduction.

CPT code assignment for fractures depends on whether the fracture being treated requires open or closed treatment. Fracture care is coded by the *type of treatment,* not by the *type of fracture,* which determines the ICD-10 diagnostic code. There is no correlation between the type of fracture the patient has and the type of treatment the surgeon performs. For example, a closed fracture could require open treatment for adequate repair.

Closed Treatment of Fractures

Codes indicating "manipulation" can be assigned even if the fracture reduction is not accomplished or successful.

Closed treatment means that no incision is made in the procedure. Instead, the fracture is repaired by reducing it and applying the cast, splint, bandage, or other stabilization device (Box 18.4).

In closed treatment, codes are assigned based on whether or not manipulation was performed. Closed treatment without manipulation indicates that no attempt was made to align the fracture and that a cast,

BOX 18.4 Stabilization Devices

Splints (static splint and dynamic splint)	MindSet toe splint (for broken toes)
Charnley's traction unit	Dynamic hip screw/plate
Baron's tongs	Lag screw
Crutchfield tongs, and halo skull traction	Tapes
Hamilton-Russell's traction	Kirschner wire and Steinmann pin
Balanced suspension and fixed skeletal traction	Dunlap's skin traction

splint, or traction device was applied. Review the following codes and notice the presence or absence of manipulation:

> **Assign debridement codes 11010–11012 with the open fracture treatment if the wound required *extensive* cleansing.**

EXAMPLES

22310 *Closed treatment of vertebral body fracture(s), without manipulation, requiring and including casting or bracing.*
22315 *Closed treatment of vertebral fracture(s) . . . , with and including casting and/or bracing by manipulation or traction.*

Open Treatment of Fractures

Open treatment involves making an incision to surgically access the fracture for repair and treatment. (Open treatment is also referred to as ORIF or open reduction with internal fixation.) It is only performed in the operating room. Open treatments are necessary when muscles, ligaments, or skin are disrupted; the fracture cannot be manipulated manually; or fractures have not healed after closed treatment.

> **If bone graft harvesting is required, it may be billed separately ONLY when it is not listed as part of the treatment code description.**

Typically, internal fixation is applied during open treatment. Internal fixation is a means of securing bones together with surgical hardware such as nails, screws, plates, rods, or wire. Fixation devices are often left inside the body permanently or for an extended period of time. If a device is later removed, this procedure is normally coded to 20670–20680, but the coder should check for a more specific code for the particular body site.

Application of Casts, Strapping, and Traction

> **Fracture re-reduction during the global period must be coded using the modifier –76 or –77, depending on whether the physician who performed the initial fracture reduction also did the re-reduction.**

Casts, straps, or splints (see Box 18.4) are usually applied following fracture treatment. Codes for these procedures are located in CPT near the end of the Musculoskeletal System section in the code range 29000–29799. Casting involves immobilization of a bone or joint with a plaster or fiberglass molded support that remains on for 4 to 6 weeks. Strapping entails wrapping a joint with bandages to restrict movement and is commonly used to treat sprains, strains, and dislocations. Splinting requires the application of a support made of wood, metal, plastic, or plaster to prevent movement of a joint or protect an injured part of the body. A static splint does not allow any movement; a dynamic splint allows limited movement. (Note that slings, Ace bandages, and air casts are considered supplies and are not part of casting or strapping services.)

> **Application of the first cast or strapping is incidental to fracture or dislocation treatment and is not separately reported at the time of fracture treatment; however, physicians may report the supply of the cast or strapping material with HCPCS codes.**

Coders must be clear about when this service can be billed. Application and removal of the *first* cast or other traction device are considered bundled for all global procedures. If a cast, splint, or strapping is applied by the treating physician as a result of or during a surgical procedure, it is not coded, because it is part of the overall comprehensive surgical code. But if the cast requires replacement because it is loose, broken, or cracked or if the physician must remove the cast to assess the healing process, a code from the 29000–29450 range can be assigned.

Application of a temporary cast, splints, or strapping is not considered part of preoperative care for a physician who *does not then treat the fracture*. This service should be billed with the appropriate casting or strapping code and an E/M code if appropriate. (Does the E/M service meet the criteria of significant and separately identifiable from the cast application? If it does, report modifier –25 with the E/M code.) Do not report a surgical procedure code with modifier –56.

Traction performed at the time of fracture or dislocation treatment is not coded separately if the fracture code descriptor includes traction, for example, 27502, *Closed treatment of femoral shaft fracture, with manipulation, with or without skin or skeletal traction.*

Pinpoint the Code 18.1 provides a decision tree for deciding when to assign codes for these services in the physician office or hospital.

Percutaneous Skeletal Fixation

Another type of fracture treatment is percutaneous skeletal fixation, in which a fixation device or appliance is placed through the skin across the fracture site utilizing imaging assistance. This type of fixation does not require making incisions into the skin and typically accompanies a closed reduction to keep bone fragments together in proper alignment. During fracture treatment by percutaneous skeletal fixation, the fracture fragments are not viewed directly but rather via fluoroscope or x-ray in order to place the fixation across the fracture site; therefore, fluoroscopy is considered integral to this service and is not coded separately.

External Fixation Devices

External fixation is any means of securing or fixing bone ends or fragments in proper anatomical alignment from outside the body without nailing, wiring, rodding, screwing, or plating the bones together on the inside. The coder will immediately know such a device was placed by recognizing the names of the devices. Common types of external fixation devices are as follows:

- Orthofix
- Ace-Fischer
- Ace Unifix
- Hoffman
- Ilizarov (ring) (multiplane system)
- Hybrid (multiplane system)
- Monticelli-Spinelli

It is common to have an external fixation device adjusted as the fracture is healing and then subsequently removed. External fixation may be billed separately *only* when it is not listed in the description for the procedure performed. When coding the application of an external fixation device, the coder needs to know how many planes the appliance will cross to determine whether to use a uniplane or multiplane code.

Assign codes for cast removal only for casts applied by another physician for professional component coding. Otherwise, the removal is included in the application.

Assign 99070 or a HCPCS level II code to bill for cast or strapping supplies in addition to the treatment code. The HCPCS codes are more specific; CPT 99070 is not specific.

Remember that if a physician other than the surgeon provides follow-up care, that physician reports that care with the same surgery code and the modifier –55. This code/modifier can be billed only once to cover all routine follow-up care during the procedure's global period. In this case, the surgeon should report the surgery code and the modifier –54.

The AAOS states in the *Complete Global Service Data for Orthopedic Surgery* that intraoperative photos, video imaging, and other imaging or monitoring equipment used by operating surgeon or assistants as a generic intraoperative service are bundled into the global service package.

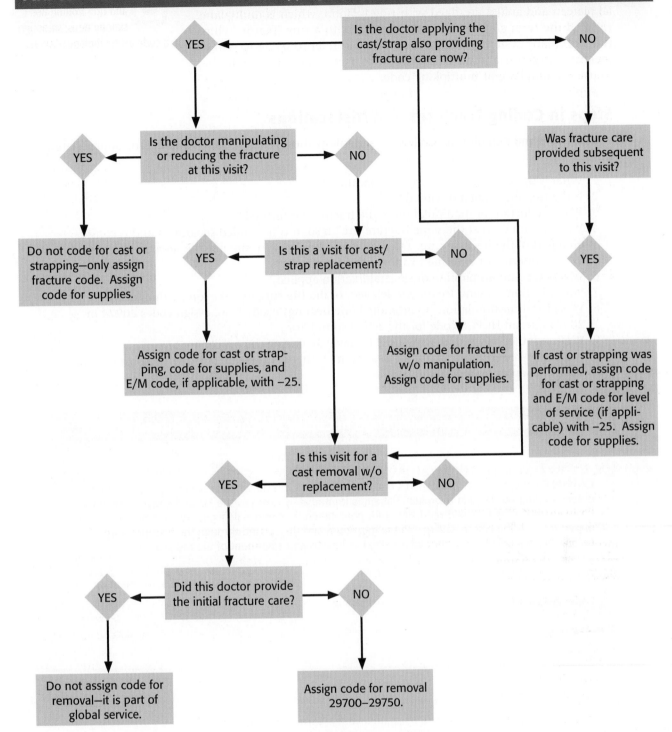

Is the doctor applying the cast/strap also providing fracture care now?

YES → Is the doctor manipulating or reducing the fracture at this visit?

NO → Was fracture care provided subsequent to this visit?

Is the doctor manipulating or reducing the fracture at this visit?

YES → Do not code for cast or strapping—only assign fracture code. Assign code for supplies.

NO → Is this a visit for cast/strap replacement?

Is this a visit for cast/strap replacement?

YES → Assign code for cast or strapping, code for supplies, and E/M code, if applicable, with –25.

NO → Assign code for fracture w/o manipulation. Assign code for supplies.

Was fracture care provided subsequent to this visit?

YES → If cast or strapping was performed, assign code for cast or strapping and E/M code for level of service (if applicable) with –25. Assign code for supplies.

Is this visit for a cast removal w/o replacement?

YES → Did this doctor provide the initial fracture care?

NO

Did this doctor provide the initial fracture care?

YES → Do not assign code for removal—it is part of global service.

NO → Assign code for removal 29700–29750.

Surgeons use uniplane fixators almost exclusively for shaft fractures, especially midshaft tibia fractures. Most intra-articular fractures (e.g., tibial plateau and ankle) are fixed with ring fixation, which is multiplane. (*Hint:* If the term *olive wire* is used, this refers to a ring fixator, which is a multiplane system.) Operative reports will refer to *spanning,* which means to go across a joint. This term is not used to determine whether to use the uniplane or multiplane code.

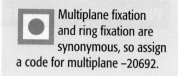

Multiplane fixation and ring fixation are synonymous, so assign a code for multiplane –20692.

Steps in Coding Fractures and Dislocations

Use Box 18.5 and Pinpoint the Code 18.2 and follow these decision steps to assign the appropriate fracture care code:

1. What is the site of the fracture or dislocation?
2. Is the treatment open or closed?
3. Was a reduction or manipulation of the fracture performed?
4. Was traction used at the same fracture site? If so, it is not coded separately and is considered part of the fracture care. Traction of another fracture site may be separately reported.
5. Was an internal or external fixation device applied?
6. Was percutaneous pinning or skeletal fixation applied?
7. Was infection present, treatment delayed, or did the surgery take longer than usual?
8. Was electrical stimulation (to promote bone healing) used? If so, assign codes 20974 or 20975 plus an HCPCS code for the actual stimulator.
9. Was computer-assisted imaging used to navigate during the procedure?
10. Is this a re-reduction or an initial treatment? If this is a re-reduction in the global period, assign the appropriate modifiers.

BOX 18.5 Example of Following Steps In Coding Fractures and Dislocations

1. Where

7. No delay
10. Initial

EXAMPLE Patient sustains a Bennett's fracture of the right thumb while at basketball camp. The thumb is very swollen but no skin is broken. Patient is immediately taken to the ED and x-rays were obtained. Physician performs a closed reduction with percutaneous pinning. Two pins were used: The first was placed through the first metacarpal to the trapezium and the second through the first metacarpal to the second metacarpal. X-ray confirmed excellent reduction and alignment of the metacarpal.

2. Closed

3. Reduction

4. No
5. Internal
6. Pinning

8 & 9. No mention

Code: 26650–RT

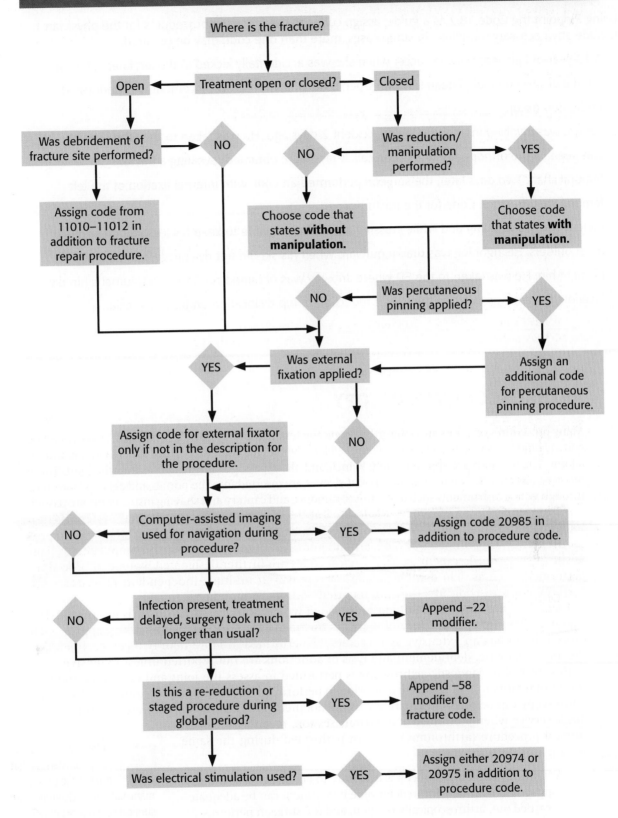

Using Pinpoint the Code 18.2 as a guide, assign codes to the following procedures for the physician. Include any necessary modifiers. In some cases, more than one code may be required.

1. A 19-year-old girl was playing soccer when she was accidentally kicked in the left knee. She suffered a displaced tibial plateau fracture. Open reduction with screw placement was performed under fluoroscopy. _____

2. Patient was involved in a four-wheeler accident 2 days ago. He was taken to the ED where he was seen by the orthopedic surgeon on call. X-rays were obtained revealing a fracture of the left femoral shaft. Two days later, the surgeon performed an ORIF with internal fixation of the left femoral shaft fracture. Code for the fracture repair. _____

3. Patient was water skiing and while crossing a wake was unable to keep his legs square beneath his shoulders. His right leg was drawn outward when his ski did not disengage. He felt a pop in his right hip. He was taken to the ED where an x-ray was obtained confirming a traumatic hip dislocation. Patient was taken to the OR for reduction of hip dislocation under anesthesia.

_____

ARTHROSCOPY/ENDOSCOPY

Many procedures on joints are done arthroscopically (endoscopically). The terms *portals*, *trocars*, *cannula*, and *scope* indicate an arthroscopic procedure, which involves making two or three small incisions around a joint. The incisions are approximately ¼ inch and allow passage of instruments into the joint. These incision sites are referred to as *portals*. Trocar sleeves are inserted into the portals and act as a "pipeline" through which instruments such as cannulas, cameras, and cautery and shaving instruments are passed.

Arthroscopy/endoscopy codes are located at the end of the Musculoskeletal System section under codes 29800–29999. Codes in this section describe both diagnostic and therapeutic procedures. They are grouped by body part and joint and then by type of arthroscopy, either diagnostic or surgical (therapeutic). The surgical codes are further designated by type of procedure performed, such as debridement, repair, or removal. If multiple independent procedures are performed arthroscopically, they are reported with a –51 modifier.

Diagnostic arthroscopies should not be coded when a surgical arthroscopy is performed. For example, synovectomy of the joint is always included in a more extensive arthroscopic or open procedure, unless an extensive synovectomy is performed in more than two compartments of the joint. Likewise, debridement and lysis of adhesions are not reported unless extensive.

However, if a diagnostic arthroscopy is performed to assess the joint and determine the best course of treatment and results in a decision to perform an open surgical procedure, the diagnostic arthroscopy can be reported separately using modifier –59. The modifier indicates a distinct diagnostic service when performed at a separate session, meaning the open surgical procedure (arthrotomy) was not performed during the same session as the arthroscopy.

- At times, a surgeon may feel it is necessary to do a diagnostic arthroscopy to visualize the joint to determine if treatment can be adequately carried out, arthroscopically or open, and the surgeon performs an arthrotomy during the same session, in which case the diagnostic arthroscopy can be reported separately with a –51 modifier.
- Conversely, if the procedure was started as an arthroscopic procedure and it could not be completed arthroscopically, resulting in an open procedure, only the open procedure is reported.

> Coders need to assess the circumstances that result in the performance of both a diagnostic and surgical scope procedure to know whether both or only one is reportable. In general, surgical endoscopy or arthroscopy includes diagnostic endoscopy/arthroscopy, but not always.

- There may be situations when a surgeon performs one procedure arthroscopically and for whatever reason may need to perform a second procedure at the same session via open arthrotomy approach. If this occurs, code the diagnostic arthroscopy separately with a –51 modifier. Refer to the note in CPT that precedes the Endoscopy/Arthroscopy section codes (29800–29999).

Codes for arthroscopic procedures are located by looking up the word *arthroscopy* in the Index and finding the appropriate site. Codes may also be located by searching for the site and then the term *arthroscopy*. If an arthroscopic code for the body part necessary is not indicated as such, then the codes listed are "open" and cannot be used in lieu of an arthroscopic code. If this happens, an unlisted arthroscopic procedure code must be assigned.

> The arthroscopic code section makes several cross-references to codes for "open procedures" for quick locating. Be careful not to assign an open procedure code if the surgery was done arthroscopically.

EXAMPLE

Arthroscopic removal of a loose body from the right hip. The word *arthroscopic* is not located in the Index, but the word *arthroscopy* is. There are two main terms located here—Diagnostic and Surgical. Now the coder must determine if the procedure performed was a diagnostic or a surgical arthroscopy. If the physician does not just explore the joint but removes a loose body, it is a surgical procedure. By finding the subterm hip, the coder is directed to the range 29861–29916. Each code within this range should be read before assigning code 29861.

CHECKPOINT 18.3

Assign codes to the following procedures for the physician. Include any necessary modifiers. In some cases, more than one code may be required.

1. What modifier is needed when a diagnostic scope was performed and results in the decision to do an open procedure? _____

2. Can you use a –59 modifier when an attempted arthroscopic procedure cannot be accomplished and an open procedure is done instead? _____

3. The standard medial and inferior lateral portals were established and diagnostic arthroscopy was carried out. The meniscus was then contoured back medially and laterally. _____

4. Code for a synovial biopsy and diagnostic arthroscopy of the left hip. _____

5. Code for a surgical arthroscopy of the left ankle with removal of foreign body. _____

SHOULDER, ELBOW, AND WRIST

A working knowledge of the shoulder anatomy is required to properly assign codes for shoulder arthroscopies. This knowledge enables the coder to understand when additional codes are required to fully describe the complete service provided.

The bones of the shoulder are the clavicle, scapula, and humerus. The scapula (shoulder blade) has several facets on the anterior and posterior sides, as seen in Figure 18.3. The acromion is the bony end of the scapula and clavicle. These bones meet to form the acromioclavicular joint. The coracoid process and the spine are attachment sites for muscles and ligaments. The glenoid fossa (cavity) is the shoulder socket. The head of the humerus fits in the glenoid fossa, thus creating the glenohumeral joint (Fig. 18.4). The glenoid labrum is a strong rim of cartilage that forms around the glenoid fossa, securing the humerus in the socket.

The shoulder section of codes in the Musculoskeletal System section covers procedures on the scapula, humeral head and neck, sternoclavicular joint, clavicle, acromioclavicular joint, and shoulder joint.

> **INTERNET RESOURCES: The shoulder joint can be further explored at**
> **Shoulderdoc.co.uk or Innerbody.com**
> **www.shoulderdoc.co.uk/article.asp?article=1177**
> **www.innerbody.com/image/skel17.html**

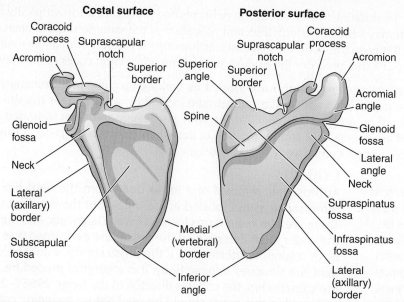

Costal surface

- Coracoid process
- Suprascapular notch
- Acromion
- Superior border
- Superior angle
- Glenoid fossa
- Neck
- Lateral (axillary) border
- Subscapular fossa
- Medial (vertebral) border
- Inferior angle

Posterior surface

- Suprascapular notch
- Coracoid process
- Superior border
- Superior angle
- Spine
- Acromion
- Acromial angle
- Glenoid fossa
- Lateral angle
- Neck
- Supraspinatus fossa
- Infraspinatus fossa
- Lateral (axillary) border

Figure 18.3 Scapula: Anterior and posterior views. From Roy, S, et al. *The Rehabilitation Specialist's Handbook, 4E,* F.A. Davis Company, 2013.

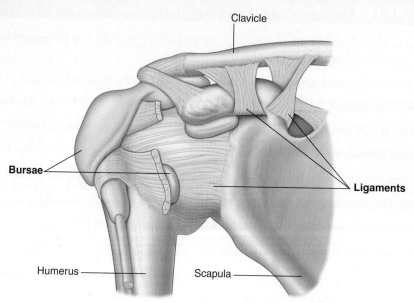

- Clavicle
- Bursae
- Ligaments
- Humerus
- Scapula

Figure 18.4 Shoulder joint. From Thompson, G. *Understanding Anatomy & Physiology: A Visual, Auditory, Interactive Approach,* F.A. Davis Company, 2013.

Shoulder Procedures

Rotator Cuff Syndrome Treatment

The rotator cuff is the group of four tendons and muscles that surround the shoulder joint: supraspinatus, infraspinatus, subscapularis, and teres minor. These muscles and tendons connect the humerus with the shoulder blade and hold the ball of the humerus firmly in the shoulder socket. When the rotator cuff is injured, it is the tendons of the rotator cuff connecting the rotator cuff muscles to the bone that are injured. Rotator cuff injuries are acquired from repeated overuse, for example, from doing things above the head or swimming or pitching a baseball. Rotator cuff syndrome involves diseases of the tendons of the rotator cuff and usually refers to a partial or complete tear in one or more of these tendons. A partial tear involves damage to the soft tissue, but the tendon is not completely frayed or severed. A complete tear is a full-thickness tear that splits the soft tissue into two pieces, most commonly tearing where it attaches to the head of the humerus. Tears can be treated either open (23410–23420) or arthroscopically (29827). Acromioplasty (23130), in which the acromioclavicular ligament is divided and part of the acromion removed, is often performed as part of a rotator cuff repair and is not coded separately.

Note that it is not uncommon to use an open code for the mini-open rotator cuff repair for large partial-thickness tears and an arthroscopic code for the debridement or subacromial decompression. According to AAOS, excision of the distal clavicle (23120, 29824), partial acromioplasty (23130, 29826), coracoacromial ligament release (23415), and biceps tenodesis (23430, 29828) are *not* included in the rotator cuff repair. This philosophy conflicts with the NCCI policy manual and NCCI edits, which state, "CMS considers the shoulder joint to be a single anatomic structure. A CCI procedure to procedure edit code pair consisting of two codes describing two shoulder joint procedures should never be bypassed with a CCI-associated modifier when performed on the ipsilateral shoulder joint."

> According to the American Medical Association, the following three major tendons must be torn in order to report code 23420: (1) supraspinatus, (2) subscapularis, and (3) infraspinatus.

Small partial-thickness tears of the rotator cuff are usually debrided using code 29823. A chronic rotator cuff repair is carried out for ruptures that occur over a long period of time with repeated use, such as in pitching a baseball (23412). An acute repair (reconstruction) would be done on a traumatic injury (all four tendons attached to the four muscles are torn) (23410).

According to AAOS, CPT code 29826, arthroscopic decompression, is an add-on code and cannot be reported as a stand-alone code. If an arthroscopic decompression is the only procedure performed, the most appropriate codes to use are 29822 (limited debridement) or 29823 (extensive debridement), depending on the extent of the work involved.

Impingement Syndrome Treatment

Impingement syndrome involves compression of the rotator cuff tendons and/or subacromial bursa by the acromion and the overlying coracoacromial ligament. This is treated with a coracoacromial ligament release (23130 or 23415) or included in the subacromial decompression (29826) if done arthroscopically. Sometimes, an open acromioplasty or acromionectomy is performed (23130). If a complete acromioclavicular joint resection including excision of the distal 1 cm of the clavicle is done (Mumford procedure) in conjunction with subacromial decompression, this is coded separately.

EXAMPLE

PREOPERATIVE DIAGNOSIS: Right shoulder impingement and right rotator cuff strain.

POSTOPERATIVE DIAGNOSIS: Same.

OPERATIVE PROCEDURE: Right shoulder arthroscopy and partial acromioplasty, coracoacromial ligament excision, bursa excision, and distal clavicle excision.

INDICATIONS: Patient is a 54-year-old woman who injured her right shoulder while at work and has persistent signs and symptoms of shoulder strain and impingement. Despite cortisone injection and conservative treatment with anti-inflammatory and physical therapy, she had persistent pain, worse with abduction, internal rotation, and adduction.

DESCRIPTION OF PROCEDURE: She was brought to the operating room following adequate general endotracheal anesthesia and was placed in a beach chair position upright. The right upper extremity and shoulder were prepped and draped in the usual fashion and injected with 15 cc of the 50% of 0.5% Marcaine and 1% lidocaine, both with epinephrine. Following this, a lateral portal site was created via a #11 blade, then the scope was placed. The underside of the acromion was identified as well as the distal tip of the clavicle. Using a shaver, the bone was exposed and then Vulcan electrocautery was used to remove all soft tissue and electrocauterize any bleeders, followed by the aggressive debridement of the underside of the acromion removing sharp points. There was a notable spike at the end of the distal clavicle and at the articulation with the medial aspect of the acromion; these were also debrided.

Thorough irrigation was performed followed by closure of the wound with monofilament Nylon suture #4-0 and subcutaneous section of portal sites as well as the remaining joint with the remaining 15 cc of 50% 0.5% Marcaine and 1% lidocaine both with epinephrine.

CODES: 29824–RT, +29826–RT.

Adhesive Capsulitis Treatment

Usually a manipulation under anesthesia is performed (23700) to treat adhesive capsulitis (a *frozen shoulder*), during which the shoulder is forced through various ranges of motion to break up scar tissue in the joint. Sometimes an arthroscopic procedure, lysis of adhesions, is required (code 29825). Manipulation in addition to the arthroscopy is not coded separately; it is bundled into the more extensive procedure.

Shoulder Instability Treatment

Instability of the shoulder (*subluxation*) usually requires a *thermal* capsulorrhaphy using a heated probe to shrink the joint capsule, making it tighter or more stable. If this is done, use code 29999.

SLAP Lesion Repair

A SLAP (superior labrum anterior and posterior) lesion is a tear or detachment of the superior glenoid labrum and runs from front to back or from anterior to posterior. The glenoid labrum is the ring of fibrocartilage that surrounds the glenoid, creating a deep shoulder socket that stabilizes the joint. This tear involves the rim above the middle of the socket, causing separation of the labrum from the upper rim of the shoulder cavity and may also involve the biceps tendon.

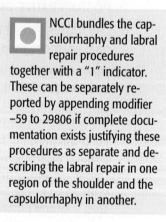

Before assigning any unlisted code, check the CPT Category III codes. In the case of Medicare, be sure to reference HCPCS for a more specific code.

Arthroscopic repair of the SLAP lesion and shoulder stabilization is coded 29807. If a tear occurs, joint instability or dislocation may be imminent.

Bankart Lesion Repair

A Bankart lesion is a tear of the anterior glenoid labrum with a detached inferior glenohumeral ligament. More specifically, it is a tear of the glenoid rim below the middle of the glenoid socket that also involves the inferior glenohumeral ligament. Assign CPT code 29806 as well as a code for repair of any labral lesion. Similar to the rotator cuff, surgeons often perform arthroscopic procedures to reconstruct unstable shoulders. The Bankart repair involves repairing a tear of the antero-inferior labrum (the fibrocartilaginous lining of the glenoid fossa) while also tightening the anterior capsule (capsulorrhaphy). This is typically done arthroscopically and involves imbrication of the inferior glenohumeral ligament and/or rotator interval closure. The anterior capsule is a separate anatomical structure from the labrum. When coding for arthroscopic stabilization, the coder needs to determine from the documentation whether a capsulorrhaphy was performed as part of the procedure. A true arthroscopic Bankart procedure should contain both a labral repair (29807) and a capsulorrhaphy (29806).

Elbow Procedures

The elbow joint consists of the head of the radius and olecranon of the ulna and the medial and lateral epicondyles of the humerus. The primary stability of the elbow is provided by the ulnar collateral ligament, on the medial (inner) side of the elbow. The medial epicondyle is the attachment point for the tendons of the muscles that flex the elbow. The lateral epicondyle is where the muscles that extend the elbow are attached. The olecranon is the "pointed" part of the elbow. The capitulum is located on the lateral side of the distal humerus and articulates, or connects with, the cup-shaped depression on the head of the radius. It is only located on the front and lower part of the humerus.

NCCI bundles the capsulorrhaphy and labral repair procedures together with a "1" indicator. These can be separately reported by appending modifier −59 to 29806 if complete documentation exists justifying these procedures as separate and describing the labral repair in one region of the shoulder and the capsulorrhaphy in another.

Bursectomy

The bursa is located between the ulna and the skin at the posterior tip of the elbow. The olecranon bursa allows for the skin to glide easily over the bone. Normally, the bursa is a flat sac, and it is hard to tell it is even there. If the bursa becomes irritated or inflamed, a condition known as *bursitis* develops. Typically this problem is treated by injecting the elbow with steroids or by aspirating the fluid from the bursal sac. In severe cases, an excision of the olecranon bursa (a bursectomy; code 24105) may be performed.

Tennis (Golfer's) Elbow Repair

One of the most common injuries to the elbow occurs on the lateral, or outer, side of the elbow—it is called *lateral epicondylitis*, or *tennis elbow*. A tear may also be medial. Three surgical procedures in the code range 24357–24359 are used to treat this condition.

Wrist Procedures

The wrist is a very complex joint. It comprises 6 muscles, 8 carpal bones along with the distal radius and distal ulna, 18 joints, 4 ligaments, and 10 tendons. The tendons that flex or bend the wrist and fingers are located on the palmar side of the wrist. Extensor tendons are located on the back of the hand and straighten the fingers and thumb.

Arthroscopy

An arthroscopic procedure is usually done for synovectomy for arthritis or synovitis (29844). Code 29846 is also done for debridement of arthritis.

Carpal Tunnel Release

Carpal tunnel is a term used to describe compression of the median nerve as it passes through the tunnel, or flexor retinaculum. Code 64721 is reported for open carpal tunnel release (CTR); code 29848 if it is done arthroscopically. Tenolysis or tenosynovectomy of flexor tendons, release or exploration of the ulnar nerve, and excision of subcutaneous tumor of wrist are included in this procedure.

> **INTERNET RESOURCE:** More information is available from AAOS on carpal tunnel syndrome. http://orthoinfo.aaos.org/topic.cfm?topic=a00005

DeQuervain's Release

DeQuervain's tendinitis occurs when tendons on the thumb side of the wrist become swollen or irritated from overuse. The irritation causes the lining (synovium) around the tendon to swell. Code 25000 reports an incision to treat inflammation of the tendon sheaths of the thumb muscles causing pain at the wrist.

Colles Fracture

Code 25600 reports closed treatment of a Colles fracture, which involves the distal radius and is usually caused by falling on an outstretched hand in trying to brace or break the fall, for example, as can occur when skating.

Ganglion Cyst

A ganglion is a benign, fluid-filled tumor of a tendon sheath, ligament, or joint capsule. They commonly grow from a stalk between two of the wrist bones. Codes 25111–25112 report excision.

> **INTERNET RESOURCE:** More information on ganglion surgery can be found on the AAOS website at http://orthoinfo.aaos.org/topic.cfm?topic=a00006

CHECKPOINT 18.4

Assign codes to the following procedures for the physician. Include any necessary modifiers. In some cases, more than one code is required.

1. The patient is a 20-year-old minor league baseball player with chronic left elbow pain. Patient throws side-arm and after MRI of the left elbow is diagnosed with medial collateral ligament tear. He undergoes a repair of the ligament with local tissue. _____

2. The patient is diagnosed with a rotator cuff tear. MRI confirms the diagnosis and patient undergoes a left arthroscopic repair of the rotator cuff. _____

3. A patient has chronic right lateral epicondylitis. He is taken to the OR and an incision is made over the lateral epicondyle. The underlying bone is noted to have a very sharp ridge. An osteotome is used to remove this ridge down to healthy smooth bone. _____

4. Procedure: Excision of right volar ganglion cyst, radial side. Keith is a 34-year-old man with a work-related injury to the left wrist. He had a painful right volar ganglion cyst, which continued to increase in size, giving him pain and some numbness and tingling in the thumb and index finger. The ganglion cyst was excised. _____

5. Nine months after a right humeral fracture repair a patient returns to his physician with pain in the fracture area. The patient had not returned before this time for fracture care follow-up and now has a nonunion of the humeral fracture. The surgeon does an iliac graft to repair the nonunion. _____

HAND

The anatomy of the hand is extremely complex. Coders need to take time to study this anatomy because proper code assignment is dependent on this knowledge. The bones that form the hand are the carpals, metacarpals, and phalanges. The carpal bones are small bones that form the wrist and are arranged in two rows, proximal and distal. Each of the eight carpal bones is given a specific name: scaphoid, lunate, triquetrum, pisiform, trapezium, trapezoid, capitate, and hamate. The bones in the palm of the hand are the metacarpals. These five bones make up the base of each finger. Each finger is referred to as a *digit*. Four of the digits are made up of three phalanges: proximal, middle, and distal. The thumb, also known as the *pollex*, has two phalanges: proximal and distal.

The hand has 27 bones (including the 8 from the wrist), 13 muscles, 14 joints, and many tendons on the palmar and dorsal sides. The metacarpals and phalanges all have a base, a shaft, and a head. The base of the bone is closest to the wrist. The head of the bone is the farthest from the wrist, with the shaft connecting these ends. The movements of the hand are controlled by two sets of muscles and tendons: the flexors, for bending the fingers and thumb, and the extensors, for straightening out the digits. The flexor muscles are located on the underside of the forearm and are attached by tendons to the phalanges of the fingers. The extensor muscles are on the back of the forearm and are similarly connected. The human thumb has two separate flexor muscles that move the thumb in opposition and make grasping possible. Flexor muscles contract to bend a joint (palmar flexion is bending fingers toward the palm), while dorsal flexion turns the hand posterior to the palm.

Extensor tendons are located on the dorsum (or back) of the hand. These tendons attach to muscles that allow the hand or fingers to extend (open). Flexor tendons are located on the palm of the hand. Flexor tendons attach to muscles that cause the hand or fingers to bend.

Fascia deep in the forearm partitions the muscles into two compartments: anterior and posterior. At the wrist, the deep fascia forms fibrous bands called *retinacula*. The retinacula function much like wide rubber bands that keep the tendons close to the bones but allow movement. The flexor retinaculum covers the surface of the carpal bones on the palmar side of the wrist. Flexor tendons and the median nerve pass through this tight space between the carpal bones and the retinaculum. The extensor retinaculum of the wrist is located on the dorsum (back) of the wrist. It runs transversely across the back of the wrist and connects to the radius and ulnar bones with fibrous branches of connective tissue that extend down into the wrist bones, creating a series of sheath-like compartments or tunnels through which the tendons of the extensor muscles pass to reach the fingers. The extensor retinaculum has six compartments, and these six compartments contain nine tendons. Each tendon is encased in a tendon sheath (synovium).

- Compartment 1—abductor pollicis longus and extensor pollicis brevis (This is the compartment commonly released for deQuervain's syndrome.)
- Compartment 2—extensor carpi radialis longus and extensor carpi radialis brevis
- Compartment 3—extensor pollicis longus
- Compartment 4—extensor digitorum and extensor indicis
- Compartment 5—extensor digiti minimi
- Compartment 6—extensor carpi ulnaris

Common Disorders and Procedures on the Hand

Dupuytren's Contracture Repair

Dupuytren's contractures occur when the palmar fascia thickens and shortens (contracts), causing a permanent flexion. This results in the fourth or fifth fingers being drawn in toward the palm in a flexed position. The repair, a fasciotomy, is coded either 26040 or 26045. Sometimes repair involves more fascia from the palm and requires extensive fasciectomy; codes range from 26121 to 26125. The key to coding Dupuytren's contracture surgery is to determine the number of fingers involved and/or whether or not just the palm is affected. If fingers are also involved, use the add-on code +26125 for each additional digit released.

Ganglion Cyst

Ganglion cysts also appear on or near the tendons and joints of the dorsum and palm of the hand and wrist. They are treated by excision (code 26160).

Amputation

Amputation, or removal of the hand or finger, typically results from accidental trauma with cutting instruments. In partial amputation, some soft tissue is still connected to the rest of the hand. By definition, a complete amputation occurs when an entire limb or appendage is detached from the body. In this case, it would be complete severing of the hand or finger. Do not code an amputation when it may be an avulsion—not actually involving bone work. Avulsion is the tearing away of skin and muscle and may include a portion of bone. Avulsion may also be referred to as a *partial* or *incomplete amputation*.

There are two types of amputation procedures: primary and secondary. Primary amputations are for the definitive surgical treatment. Secondary amputations are performed at a later date, usually following previous vascular reconstructive procedures. Surgeons use two amputation-repair techniques: open and flap. With the open technique, used when infection is present, the surgeon does not close the stump wound with skin flaps immediately upon removing the limb, but rather leaves it open, allowing the wound to drain freely. Once the infection is gone, another surgery is performed for stump closure. The flap amputation technique is used when no infection is present. The limb is removed and anterior and posterior flaps are created to close the wound.

> ● Don't code an amputation when what actually was done was an avulsion that did not involve bone work. Avulsion is skin and tissue only. Coders have to read the op note closely to capture the work that was actually performed in cases where a surgeon partially amputates a patient's finger but not the entire digit.

> ■ **CASE SCENARIO**
>
> A 29-year-old male patient accidentally injured the fourth finger of his right hand with the drive chain on his motorcycle. The chain amputated the tip of the patient's fourth finger at the mid-nail level and left an additional 4 centimeters of mangled finger and bone below the amputation. The surgeon amputated the mangled portion of the finger and sharply debrided the injury at the amputation site, including the bone, with a rongeur. The surgeon carried out sterile Betadine and saline irrigation, then created a V-Y flap to cover the remainder of the finger and sutured it with 5-0 Nylon. The surgeon then cleaned the fourth finger with saline and Betadine and used single 5-0 Nylon to repair the less-than-half-centimeter laceration. By removing the bone with the rongeur and closing the injury with a V-Y flap closure, the surgeon should report code 26952–F8, *Amputation, finger or thumb, primary or secondary, any joint or phalanx, single, including neurectomies; with local advancement flaps (V-Y, hood)*, to represent the surgeon's work amputating the finger and dissecting the tissues to the bone.

Replantation of Finger

At times, a finger may be salvaged and reattached instead of finalizing a partial amputation or closing the wound site from where the finger was traumatically amputated. Replantation codes 20816–20827 involve cleansing the amputation site; debridement of devitalized tissue; shortening of the bone; internal fixation; repair of tendons, arteries, veins, and nerves; and skin closure including skin flaps and grafts.

CPT instructions direct the coder to code replantation of *incomplete* digit amputation excluding thumb with codes for repair of bones, ligaments, tendons, nerves, or blood vessels with modifier –52.

INTERNET RESOURCE: Visit the American Society for Surgery on the Hand for more information and illustrations of hand procedures. www.assh.org

Tendon Repairs

Tendon repairs are performed to treat traumatic injury (lacerations) or congenital deformities of the hand. These are usually very complex procedures. They include the following integral components: tenosynovectomy, tenolysis (freeing of tendon from adhesions), tendon retrieval and preparation of ends, suture and repair of tendon, and application of traction. The type of tendon repair is selected based on which digit was affected, whether a flexor or extensor tendon is repaired, and the amount of physical therapy the patient undergoes. Tendon repair, or tenorrhaphy, is when torn ends of a tendon are sutured together. Tendon advancement is the moving forward of the end of the tendon from its original location and then making it secure. The surgeon will choose a repair based on the proximity from the tendon insertion site to the laceration.

Codes for tendon repair have the qualifying terms in their code descriptions: primary or secondary. The primary repair is considered to be the first time the tendon is repaired, which is immediately after the injury. Secondary repair is a repair that is done after the primary repair or occurs at a date much later than the injury where the tendon sheath has healed. These repairs are typically harder to perform because of scar tissue at the end of the tendon and in the bed where the tendon lies. Delayed primary repair is the late initial repair and is considered "secondary repair" from a CPT standpoint.

Flexor tendon repair is more technical and difficult than extensor repairs because flexor muscles are stronger and require more secure suturing for initial attachment. A longer follow-up period is also required. The type of tendon repair is selected based on the digit that was injured, whether it was a flexor or extensor, the anatomical zone where injury occurred, the proximity from the insertion site to the laceration, and the amount of preoperative and postoperative physical therapy the patient undergoes. A code is used for *each* tendon repaired. These anatomical zones are defined as "in no man's land" or "not in no man's land." These references are indicated in the CPT code descriptions for 26350–26358. No man's land is located between the A1 pulley and the insertion of the superficialis tendon. "A pulleys" are the annular part of the fibrous sheaths of the fingers. The A1 pulley is the first annular pulley near the head of the metacarpal bone and lies in the flexor groove in the deep transverse metacarpal ligament.

Flexor Tendon Zones. These six compartments or zones contain nine tendons. Each tendon is encased in a tendon sheath (synovium). A *compartment release* involves an incision into the tendon sheath to decompress the tendon(s) found within that compartment. Use CPT codes 25000–25025 to report decompressions.

Extensor Tendon Zones. The extensor tendons of the hand are superficial and highly susceptible to injury from lacerations, bites, burns, or blunt trauma. Extensor tendon injuries are commonly diagnosed in the ED. Some of them can be repaired in the ED, whereas others require the skill of a hand surgeon. The dorsum of the hand, wrist, and forearm are divided into eight anatomical zones to facilitate classification and treatment of extensor tendon injuries.

Tendon Grafts

Tendons may not be able to be repaired directly by suture if a loss of tendon length occurs due to, for example, contracture or trauma. Primary tendon grafting may be performed when the annular pulley system is intact and there is adequate skin coverage and an intact digital nerve.

The procedure for an autogenous tendon graft itself is coded separately only when it is not included in the description for the basic procedure. If it is not, see codes 20900–20926. To report these codes in addition to the primary procedure, harvesting of the graft should be made through a *separate incision* from the primary procedure. *One-stage-grafting* procedures involve the replacement of a damaged tendon sheath with a graft after the reaction to the injury has subsided and the tendon has retracted. This includes excision of tendon remnants and release of joint contractures. The A2 and A4 pulleys are reconstructed by harvesting the graft using either a flexor tendon or a strip of the wrist extensor retinaculum. See code 26358, *Repair or advancement, flexor tendon, in zone 2 digital flexor tendon sheath; secondary, with free graft, each tendon*, as an example.

Two-stage-grafting procedures involve an initial procedure in which a silicone or plastic tube or rod is inserted to create a tendon sheath. The second stage of the procedure involves removing the plastic tube, harvesting a tendon graft, and grafting the tendon. See codes 26390 and 26392 for two stages of grafting of flexor tendons and 26415 and 26416 for extensor tendons.

If a procedure is planned beforehand to be performed in stages or if a second procedure is performed during the global period that is more extensive than the primary procedure was, think about appending the –58 modifier, indicating a planned staged procedure, to avoid reduction in payment or denial for procedures performed during the global period.

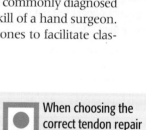

When choosing the correct tendon repair code, the coder needs to answer these questions:

1. Which digit and/or hand is affected?
2. Is the tendon a flexor or extensor?
3. Which anatomical zone is involved?
4. Is the procedure a repair, advancement, or graft?
5. Is it a primary or secondary repair?
6. Was a microscope used? Check the code description to be sure the word "microvascular" is not already included in the code description.

Tendon Pulley

The tendon sheath consists of *annular* pulleys that provide mechanical stability and *cruciate* pulleys that provide flexibility. The A1, A2, and A3 pulleys are located over the metacarpophalangeal, proximal, and interphalangeal and distal interphalangeal joints. The A2 and A4 pulleys are located over the middle portion of the proximal and middle palm at the proximal edge of the A1 pulley. If the patient has tenosynovitis and requires tenosynovectomy and excision of one slip of the flexor digitorum superficialis (FDS), code 26145 would be assigned. Tendon pulley reconstruction is an integral part of tendon repair. Trigger finger is a chronic inflammation of the tendon sheaths of the finger flexors that forms a nodule on the tendon sheath. The tendon can no longer glide smoothly and requires incision into the tendon sheath also referred to as *A1 pulley release* (code 26055). Reconstruction is assigned to codes 26356 for primary tendon repair, 26390 or 26415 for first-stage reconstruction, and 26392 or 26416 for second-stage reconstruction.

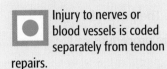 Injury to nerves or blood vessels is coded separately from tendon repairs.

INTERNET RESOURCE: Visit handsurgery.com to read more about trigger fingers. www.handsurgery.com/trigger.html

■ **CASE SCENARIO**

A patient suffers from right thumb stenosing tenosynovitis. Physician performs a right thumb A1 pulley release. Local anesthesia was given to the volar aspect of the thumb. Through a transverse incision in the MP crease, full-thickness skin flaps were raised with gentle spreading dissection. The radial and ulnar neurovascular bundles were then carefully swept to their respective sides. The pulley was divided longitudinally along its mid portion, exposing the underlying undamaged flexor pollicis tendon. There was no tenosynovial hypertrophy and no tenosynovectomy was required. Following visualization of the full release, the tendon was placed through a passive/active range of motion and no further impingement was noted. Report code 26055.

Hand Joint Arthroplasty

The carpal bones of the hand are subject to wear and tear from age and degeneration from arthritis. They can be replaced with artificial joints as a last resort in the treatment of pain and disfigurement of the hands and fingers. Hand arthroplasty codes are located in the 25441–25449 code range.

Codes 25441–25446 describe procedures that include excision of the bone(s) named in the code descriptor and their replacement with a prosthetic device. For wrist arthroplasty without replacement with an artificial device, refer to code 25332, *Arthroplasty, wrist, with or without interposition, with or without external or internal fixation.*

Facility coders, do not forget to assign a HCPCS code for the implant: L8630–L8631, L8658–L8659.

Arthroplasty does not always have to include placing an artificial joint in the affected area. It also can pertain to an operation that as much as possible restores the integrity and functionality of a joint. In hand surgery, arthroplasty most commonly is used to repair or correct cartilage damage and joint dislocations caused by various forms of arthritis.

INTERNET RESOURCES: Visit Hand University.com and read more about hand surgery and see anatomical illustrations of many common hand procedures. http://ww2.handuniversity.com/handschool.asp

Visit the American Society of Surgery of the Hand (ASSH) to learn more about disorders of the hand and hand anatomy. www.assh.org/Public/HandAnatomy/Pages/default.aspx

Assign codes to the following procedure for the physician. Include any necessary modifiers. More than one code may be required.

1. The patient is a 65-year-old female with a firm lump over the volar aspect of her right hand. The mass is consistent with Dupuytren's contracture. The right extremity is prepped and an incision is made over the fifth ray. Dissection was carried down through the subcutaneous layers. The pretendinous fascia was excised over the fifth ray approximately 3 cm in length. The same procedure was repeated and fascia was also removed from the fourth ray. _____

HIP

The hip is also called the *coxal joint* and is the ball-and-socket joint where the head of the femur fits deep into the acetabulum (Fig. 18.5). It is held there by the acetabular labrum and the articular capsule made of ligamentous fibers called the *retinacular*.

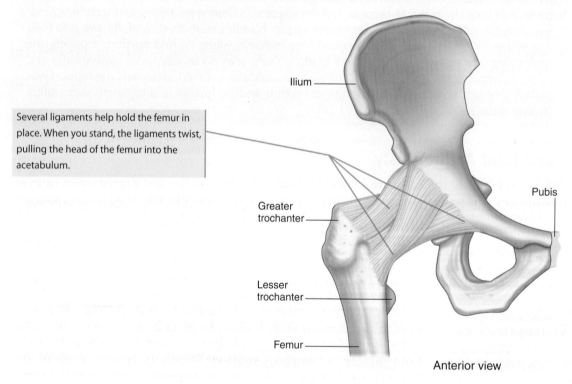

Several ligaments help hold the femur in place. When you stand, the ligaments twist, pulling the head of the femur into the acetabulum.

Ilium

Greater trochanter

Lesser trochanter

Femur

Pubis

Anterior view

Figure 18.5 Hip joint. From Thompson, *G. Understanding Anatomy & Physiology: A Visual, Auditory, Interactive Approach*, F.A. Davis Company, 2013.

Common Disorders and Procedures on the Hip

Arthroplasty

When conservative treatments fail to address a patient's pain or loss of function, orthopedists can choose from a number of surgical options to repair damage done by hip arthritis, including hemiarthroplasty (27125, *Hemiarthroplasty, hip, partial [e.g., femoral stem prosthesis, bipolar arthroplasty]*); total hip replacement (27130, *Arthroplasty, acetabular and proximal femoral prosthetic replacement [total hip arthroplasty (THA)], with or without autograft or allograft*; and 27132, *Conversion of previous hip surgery to total hip arthroplasty, with or without autograft or allograft*). CPT Professional Edition includes illustrations of codes 27125 and 27130 to assist the coder in assigning the correct arthroplasty code based on the components used. Code 27132 is reported when a patient has had a prior procedure, such as a hemiarthroplasty or hip fracture reduction, and subsequently undergoes a total hip replacement. If the surgeon is performing a staged revision, 27132 is also reported. During the first stage, the physician removes the implant and places a spacer (27091, *Removal of hip prosthesis; complicated, including total hip prosthesis, methylmethacrylate with or without insertion of spacer*). The second stage is when the spacer is removed and the total hip prosthesis is reimplanted (27132).

Hip arthroplasty codes include the following component procedures and should not be coded separately: capsulotomy/capsulectomy, bone grafting, bone biopsy, injection of the joint, tenotomy, arthrotomy, acetabuloplasty, osteotomy, percutaneous skeletal fixation, fracture care, manipulation of the joint, and use of the microscope.

Arthroplasty Revisions

Hip revisions are performed in the acetabulum, liner, and femur (stem) because of infection or implant malfunction. Revision codes are assigned based on which components are replaced:

27134, *Revision of THA, both components*
27137, *Revision of THA, acetabular component only*
27138, *Revision of THA, femoral component only*

Girdlestone Salvage Procedure

The Girdlestone procedure (27122, *Acetabuloplasty; resection, femoral head [e.g., Girdlestone procedure]*) is only rarely performed and usually only for long-standing infection. The physician incises the hip capsule and removes the femoral head and neck, creating a resection arthroplasty, in which no true hip joint remains. A curette is used to remove any necrotic bone or infected material.

Code Assignment

Before assigning a code to hip arthroplasty, the coder should obtain answers to the following questions first:

1. Was this procedure an initial or revision arthroplasty?
2. Was this a total or partial replacement?
3. What components were replaced?
4. Was this a conversion of a previous hip fracture reduction to a prosthetic joint?

EXAMPLE

DIAGNOSIS: DJD, left hip.

OPERATION: Total hip arthroplasty, left hip. Implantation of #4, 28-mm porous ceramic femoral component and 54-mm acetabulum component.

Physicians may elect to inject their arthroplasty patients who are anemic with erythropoietin (trade names: Epogen and Procrit) to prepare them for upcoming joint replacement surgery. During joint replacement surgery, patients can lose two or more units of blood. When reporting these injections, use J0885 for Epogen/non-ESRD. In the "units" field of the claim form, report one unit of J0885 for every 1,000 units of erythropoietin that the surgeon administers to the patient.

PROCEDURE: Incision was made and carried down to the deep fascia. The short external rotator tendons were taken down from their insertion into the femur to gain access to the hip capsule. A capsulotomy followed by capsulectomy was carried out. The femoral neck osteotomy was performed with a sagittal saw. A bone chisel was used to open the superolateral neck. A canal finder was placed into the femur to incrementally ream the canal and allowed for a good fit of the rasp component. Next, attention was turned to the acetabulum where a capsulectomy was done. The acetabulum was exposed and reamed with the hemispherical reamers to 52 mm, 2 mm smaller than the component to be inserted. Morselized bone was grafted to the acetabulum. The acetabulum shell was inserted into a press-fit mode and fixed with screws. The trial acetabular liner and the trial femoral component were placed in the hip along with the trial ball head. The hip was reduced and taken through range of motion and was found to have excellent stability. The hip was dislocated and the trial components were removed and the permanent components placed. The site was irrigated and the tendon was reattached to the deep fascia. The wound was then closed in layers with a drain in place.

CODE: 27130–LT. The bone graft, tenotomy, capsulotomy/capsulectomy, and tenorrhaphy are all components of the comprehensive code 27130.

INTERNET RESOURCE: Visit the University of Wisconsin Health Orthopedics and Rehabilitation site where you can take on the role of the surgeon and perform hip and knee replacement surgery. www.edheads.org/activities/hip

---

CHECKPOINT 18.6

Assign codes to the following procedure for the physician. Include any necessary modifiers.

1. A patient was running and felt a sharp pain in his hip and his right leg collapsed. He was taken to the ED, where an x-ray confirmed a traumatic tear to the labrum of his right hip. Patient was taken to the OR for an arthroscopic labral repair under anesthesia. _____

KNEE

The knee is considered to be the largest, most complicated joint in the human body. Because the knee supports nearly the entire weight of the body, it is the joint most vulnerable both to acute injury and the development of osteoarthritis.

The knee consists of the tibiofemoral joint, patellofemoral joint, meniscus (medial and lateral), patellar ligament, lateral fibular collateral ligament, medical tibial collateral ligament, and the anterior cruciate and posterior cruciate ligaments (ACL and PCL, respectively) (Fig. 18.6). The knee joint has two articulations, or places of contact between bones or between bones and cartilage: one between the femur and tibia (tibiofemoral joint), and one between the femur and patella (patellofemoral joint). The tibiofemoral joint is between the condyles of the femur and tibia. The patellofemoral joint is located between the patella and the surface of the femur. The patellar ligament connects the quadriceps femoris muscle tendon over the patella and attaches it to the tibia. The medial and lateral collateral ligaments (MCL and LCL, respectively) connect the femur to the tibia on the left and right side of the knee. The meniscus acts as a cushion between the surfaces of the bones. The ACL and PCL limit movement of the knee anteriorly and posteriorly. The ACL runs from the posterior femur to the anterior side of the tibia and prevents hyperextension. The PCL runs from the anteroinferior femur to the posterior side of the tibia and prevents hyperflexion.

There are three compartments to the knee: medial, lateral, and patellar. The *medial compartment* is separated from the lateral compartment by the ACL and PCL. It is bordered by the medial tibial plateau on the bottom and the medial femoral condyle on the top. This is the side closest to the opposite knee. The *lateral compartment* is bordered by the lateral tibial plateau on the bottom and the lateral femoral condyle on the top. The popliteus tendon and the fibular collateral ligament surround the compartment. This is the side farthest from the opposite knee. The *patellar compartment* is located in front of the knee joint and behind the kneecap over the edge of the femur.

> Code assignment for knee arthroscopy is based on procedures performed in each compartment, so coders must be able to identify and differentiate among these compartments.

Common Knee Injuries and Procedures

Repair/Removal of Meniscus

The meniscus is made of a very strong substance called *fibrocartilage*. The meniscus covers the cartilage and prevents it from wearing out from vigorous activities and the natural aging process.

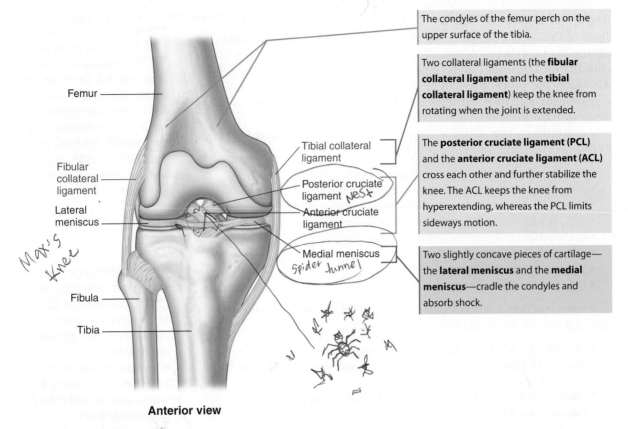

Femur

Fibular collateral ligament

Lateral meniscus

Max's Knee

Fibula

Tibia

Tibial collateral ligament

Posterior cruciate ligament *Nest*

Anterior cruciate ligament

Medial meniscus
spider tunnel

The condyles of the femur perch on the upper surface of the tibia.

Two collateral ligaments (the **fibular collateral ligament** and the **tibial collateral ligament**) keep the knee from rotating when the joint is extended.

The **posterior cruciate ligament (PCL)** and the **anterior cruciate ligament (ACL)** cross each other and further stabilize the knee. The ACL keeps the knee from hyperextending, whereas the PCL limits sideways motion.

Two slightly concave pieces of cartilage—the **lateral meniscus** and the **medial meniscus**—cradle the condyles and absorb shock.

Anterior view

Figure 18.6 Knee joint.

⬤ *Chondroplasty* is incorrectly used synonymously with the term *notchplasty*. A chondroplasty debrides articular cartilage and not bone. A notchplasty is not a full chondroplasty. During a notchplasty, the surgeon debrides bone to enlarge the U-shaped notch that the ACL and PCL pass through so they will fit properly. According to AAOS, notchplasty is reported with unlisted procedure code 27599 or 29999.

Traumatic meniscal injury commonly happens when a bent knee is suddenly twisted during, for example, athletic events. Degenerative tears occur gradually over a long period of time. There are several types of meniscal tears—medial, lateral, radial, and bucket-handle tears. These are classified by the actual location of the tear.

The meniscus can be repaired or removed depending on how much is torn or where the tear is located. Tears that occur in the outer edge of the meniscus tend to respond to meniscal repair because this area of the meniscus has blood flow to aid in healing. The inner part of the meniscus does not have blood supply and would not heal if repaired and must be removed.

If a repair was done (code 29882 or 29883), the operative note will describe where sutures were placed into the meniscus. If the meniscus could not be repaired, it will have been removed via meniscectomy by trimming or debriding part of it or by removing the meniscus (code 29880 or 29881). (Documentation may mention the use of basket forceps, which indicates that a meniscectomy was performed.)

Chondroplasty

At times, as a result of a meniscal tear, the articular cartilage may also become torn or irregular, necessitating treatment. A chondroplasty (29877) is performed to shave or debride the articular cartilage. Chondroplasty includes synovectomy, loose body removal, articular shaving or curettement, and removal of chondral bodies. This code is only used once regardless of how many areas are debrided. This procedure may be performed at the same time as a notchplasty. A notchplasty is carried out with the intent to widen the anterior portion and recess of the roof of the intercondylar notch by removing 3 to 5 mm of bone from the lateral femoral condyle.

Repair of Ligament Tears

Tears of the ACL, PCL, LCL, and MCL are usually sports-related injuries or results of accidents. Repair of the ACL involves using sutures to anchor the torn ligament to its original point of attachment on the femur. Although the procedure can be done by open repair, it is most often accomplished arthroscopically using 29888 or 29889. Terms used are *repair* or *reconstruction*.

According to the AAOS's *Complete Global Service Data* guide, code 29888 includes the following procedures:

- Minor synovial resection for visualization
- Articular shaving, debridement, chondroplasty
- Notchplasty (debridement of the intercondylar notch of the femur)
- ACL stump removal (replacement of ligament)
- Intra-articular ligament reconstruction
- Harvesting of graft
- Diagnostic arthroscopy
- Internal fixation of graft

Reconstruction involves grafting of a tendon and is accomplished through one of three methods:

- The patellar tendon is harvested (autograft) to create the new ACL.
- Two small portions of hamstring tendon are harvested (autograft) to create the new ACL.
- Donor tendon, or allograft, is used instead of the patient's own tendon to rebuild the new ACL.

In all three methods, the new tendon is inserted through holes drilled in the tibia and femur, pulled through, and secured in position with bioabsorbable or metal screws. When the tendon is harvested from the patient, harvesting takes place at the same time as the reconstructive surgery.

Even though reconstruction of a torn ACL is significantly more complicated than a repair, it is still assigned the same procedure code. If a separate incision is made to harvest the patellar tendon, hamstring, or other graft, 20926 may be applicable.

It is very common after an ACL repair to develop localized anterior arthrofibrosis where fibrous scar tissue develops at the base of the tibial insertion (this is also called a *cyclops lesion*). Treatment for this is arthroscopic debridement.

INTERNET RESOURCE: Visit Andreas C. Staehelin's website for an ACL repair. www.staehelin.ch/ait/aitacl.html

Synovectomy

Synovitis is the inflammation and/or overgrowth of the synovial (joint-lining) membrane. This is particularly painful, mainly during motion, due to the swelling from fluid collection in the synovial sac. It is treated by synovectomy (29875 or 29876), in which the synovial membrane is removed. The only time a synovectomy is reported in addition to any other arthroscopy code is if an extensive synovectomy in two or more compartments of the knee is performed; otherwise, it is included in the surgical arthroscopy.

Plica Syndrome

In utero, the fetal knee is divided into three separate compartments that eventually evolve into one synovial membrane. Plica syndrome is caused by bands or folds in the synovium that are fused during joint development. The synovial membrane aids in reducing friction in the joint. Normal smooth movement of the knee can be affected by damage to these bands because of chronic overuse or as a result of injury. Synovectomy is performed to remove these bands (29875).

Read the operative note thoroughly to determine what has been debrided. The meniscus encases the articular cartilage and is commonly referred to as *cartilage*. If the meniscus is arthroscopically debrided, assign code 29881 or 29880. If the articular cartilage is debrided, assign 29877.

If Medicare is the primary insurance, you must use code G0289 for chondroplasty when the surgeon performs both chondroplasty and meniscectomy in separate compartments on a Medicare patient during the same session, instead of the CPT surgical code 29877.

If meniscectomy and chondroplasty are done in the same compartment, the chondroplasty is considered bundled and cannot be coded separately, per the AAOS's *Complete Global Service Data* guide and the Medicare NCCI. If however, a chondroplasty and meniscectomy are performed at the same operative session but in *different* compartments, assign a –59 modifier to the second procedure.

Osteochondritis Dissecans Treatment

Osteochondritis dissecans results from a loss of blood supply to an area of bone beneath the surface of a joint from injury to the bone under the articular cartilage. The joint surface above the affected bone may deteriorate or detach, resulting in a loose body. The lateral aspect of the medial femoral condyle and the weight-bearing surface of the medial and lateral femoral condyle are most likely affected. The condition is treated using the procedures described in code range 29885–29887.

Treatment of Arthritis

Osteoarthritis is a pathological progressive disease that attacks the joint cartilage and results in exposure of the underlying bone and reduction of the joint space, forcing bones to rub together. Abrasion arthroplasty (29879), typically performed to relieve this condition, involves use of a motorized shaver to smooth down articular cartilage to expose bleeding subchondral bone or drilling holes to create microfractures to enhance blood flow to promote healing and regeneration of cartilage. This procedure is different from the chondroplasty described in 29877 where cartilage is simply debrided to smooth the edges.

An OATS procedure (or *osteochondral autograft transfer system*) (29866) may also be indicated for people with arthritis. During an OATS arthroscopic procedure, articular cartilage is removed from a healthy site and "plugged" into defects in the cartilage where the cartilage is worn through. Joint replacement and fusion of the joint are also modes of treatment.

> Before assigning 29879, confirm that the operative report describes debriding of the cartilage down to bleeding bone or that microfracture was performed.

INTERNET RESOURCE: Walk through an OATS procedure.
www.isakos.com/innovations/oats2.aspx

Harvesting of Chondrocytes

Harvesting of chondrocytes may be a last-resort option for patients with arthritis or those with severe cartilage injuries. The procedure is done in two stages. The first stage entails arthroscopically harvesting the patient's own cartilage cells (chondrocytes) and sending them to a processing facility for cultivation. Essentially it is like "cloning" your own cartilage. In the second stage, these cells (or Carticel) are then implanted back into the patient's knee. The cells will, over time, integrate with surrounding tissue to produce new articular cartilage. The second stage of this procedure is similar to the OATS procedure described above. This procedure may also be called *Genzyme biosurgery* or *Carticel repair*, named after their respective manufacturers. For payers that accept HCPCS codes, S2112 would be appropriate for the first stage; otherwise, 29999 is assigned. Codes 29866 or 27416 are used for the second stage.

> At the second-stage visit, 20926, *Tissue grafts, other,* can also be reported with 27416 or 29866 as long as the –58 modifier is appended to 27416 or 29866. The surgeon harvests the chondrocytes weeks ahead of time and plans in advance to perform this second procedure.

INTERNET RESOURCE: Visit the Doe Report website to see animations of the surgeries discussed above.
www.doereport.com/categories.php?CatID=000&TL=1

Knee Arthroplasty

Similar to the hip arthroplasty, a knee replacement can involve the total knee or a single component. The components are medial and lateral. It is important to read the operative report to determine the extent of the arthroplasty. Codes are assigned based on whether the medial or lateral compartment or both compartments are replaced.

Total Knee Replacement (TKR)

In a TKR, the surgeon makes a midline incision over the knee and dissects down to expose the knee joint. Ligaments and soft tissues are released. The surgeon uses a cutting-alignment tool called a *jig* to remove both femoral condyles and the medial and lateral compartments of the tibial joint surface. Damaged cartilage on the joint surface of the patella is removed and a prosthesis is placed. The tibial and femoral components are secured with glue and/or bone screws and the incision is closed. The procedure includes synovectomy, removal of loose bodies, debridement of the knee, meniscectomy, lateral retinacular release, ligament or capsular release or reconstruction, manipulation of the knee, and arthrotomy. Code 27447 is used to report a TKR with the appropriate –RT or –LT modifier. In unusual circumstances, a surgeon may perform bilateral knee replacements and this would be indicated with the –50 modifier. Code 27446, *Arthroplasty, knee, condyle and plateau; medial or lateral compartment,* is assigned for hemiarthroplasty.

Arthroplasty Revisions

Revision may be performed because of infection, inflammatory reaction, or failure of the implant. If a knee replacement surgery fails, codes for revision surgery are reported. CPT directs the coder to use 27486 or 27487. If the failure of the TKR requires a revision to only one component, use 27486, *Revision of total knee arthroplasty, with or without allograft; one component.* For the entire knee, assign 27487, *Femoral and entire tibial component.* If the knee fails during the global period of the initial placement, use modifier –78 with these codes. An osteotome or saw is used to loosen the cement or bone and the prosthesis is forced out with a mallet. The surgeon then makes bone cuts to accommodate the new component. Donor bone or allograft may or may not be packed into the defect from the original compartment. The component is then placed into the new compartment and cemented.

EXAMPLE

Code 27488, *Removal of prosthesis, including total knee prosthesis, methylmethacrylate with or without insertion of spacer, knee,* is used to report removal of the prosthesis and placement of a spacer in the open space where the prosthesis used to be. The spacer prevents the soft tissues from compressing the joint space. According to AAOS's *Complete Global Service Data for Orthopaedic Surgery,* code 27488 includes a synovectomy (29876), removal of foreign body (29874), capsulotomy (27435), knee ligament reconstruction (27427 and 27429), partial excision of the bone (27360), chondroplasty (29877), and arthrotomy with biopsy (27330). Therefore, these services should not be billed separately.

Patients who undergo knee replacement surgery are often placed in a continuous passive motion (CPM) machine to force the knee joint into flexion in a very slow, gradual motion designed to prevent scarring and stiffness of the joint. CPM following knee replacement surgery lessens the likelihood of a patient requiring knee manipulation. CMS policy limits CPM (E0935) to a 21-day period of time following knee replacement surgery.

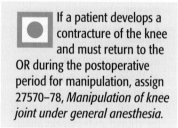 If a patient develops a contracture of the knee and must return to the OR during the postoperative period for manipulation, assign 27570–78, *Manipulation of knee joint under general anesthesia.*

EXAMPLE

DIAGNOSIS: Advanced osteoarthritis, left knee.

OPERATION: Knee replacement.

PROCEDURE: The patient was placed in a supine position, with the draped leg set on a thigh support or in a leg holder so the knee was free to flex to at least 120°. A sandbag or other bump was affixed to the table to help maintain flexion of the knee. A small incision was made in the medial compartment, leaving the patella and the suprapatellar synovial pouch intact. The meniscus was removed. A jig was used to make cuts into the medial femoral condyle and tibial plateau. Peg holes were made into the bone and the components were secured into position.

CODE: 27446–LT.

Knee Arthroplasty Coding Steps. Before assigning a code to knee arthroplasty, the coder should obtain answers to the following questions:

1. Is this procedure an initial or revision arthroplasty?
2. Is this a total or partial replacement?
3. If partial, which compartment is replaced?
4. For revisions, is it one component or all components?

Use the steps outlined in Pinpoint the Code 18.3 to assist in assigning codes for arthroplasties and revisions.

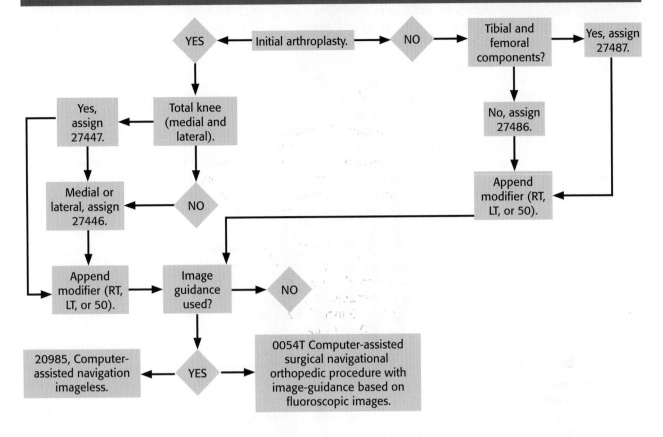

CHECKPOINT 18.7

Assign codes to the following procedures for the physician. Include any necessary modifiers. In some cases, more than one code is required.

1. A patient sustained a twisting injury to the left knee after getting the heel of her shoe caught in a sidewalk crack. MRI confirmed an anterior horn medial meniscus tear. Surgeon performs arthroscopic meniscal repair and synovectomy of the medial compartment. _____

2. A patient with long-standing osteoarthritis undergoes chondroplasty on the right knee to repair damage to the articular cartilage. Cartilage is debrided using a microdebrider device until bright red bleeding bone is encountered. _____

FOOT

The foot has 26 bones, 33 joints, 107 ligaments, and 20 muscles. A network of muscles, tendons, and ligaments supports the bones and joints in the foot. The foot has three main parts: the forefoot, the midfoot, and the hindfoot (Fig. 18.7). The *forefoot* is composed of the five toes (called *phalanges*) and long metatarsal bones. The big toe (hallux) has two phalanges, two joints (interphalangeal

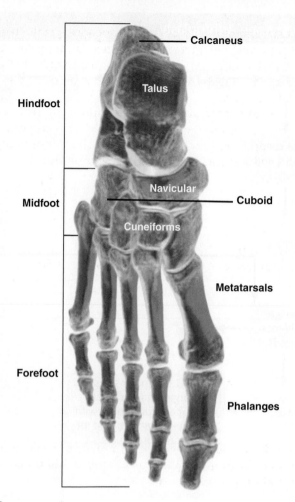

Calcaneus

Talus

Hindfoot

Midfoot

Navicular — Cuboid

Cuneiforms

Metatarsals

Forefoot

Phalanges

Figure 18.7 Joints of the foot. From Thompson, G. *Understanding Anatomy & Physiology: A Visual, Auditory, Interactive Approach,* F.A. Davis Company, 2013.

joints), and two tiny, round *sesamoid bones* that enable it to move up and down. The other four toes each have three bones and two joints. The forefoot bears half the body's weight and balances pressure on the ball of the foot. The *midfoot* has five tarsal bones forming the arch, and serves as a shock absorber. The bones of the midfoot are connected to the forefoot and the hindfoot by muscles and the plantar fascia (arch ligament). The *hindfoot* is composed of three joints and links the midfoot to the ankle (talus).

A doctor of podiatric medicine (DPM), a physician who specializes in podiatry, is the only health-care professional whose total training focuses on the foot and ankle. As a specialist in foot care, a DPM, or *podiatrist,* receives extensive training in the diagnosis, treatment, and prevention of foot and ankle disorders by medical and surgical means. More than 70% of all people in the United States will have painful foot problems at some time during their lifetime due to sports injuries, arthritis, poor shoe fit and selection, ingrown toenails, warts, and plain old genetics. Because of this, orthopedic practices are now incorporating orthopedic physicians who are subspecialists in foot and ankle injuries.

> T-modifiers must be applied for procedures on the phalanges of the toes because many procedures can be done on different toes at the same time. If only metatarsal work was performed, the T– modifiers will not apply; instead, use –LT or –RT.

Common Podiatric Surgeries and Conditions

The common disorders of the foot include bunions, heel pain/spurs, hammertoes, neuromas, ingrown toenails, warts, corns, and calluses. A podiatrist provides care for sprains, fractures, infections, and injuries of the foot, ankle, and heel. Refer to the anatomical drawings in the professional edition of the CPT manual for illustrations of the following bunion correction surgeries.

Bunion Correction

A bunion refers to the enlargement of a joint where bone forms at the base and side of the joint. The correct term for the abnormal enlargement of the metatarsal phalangeal joint (MPJ) is *hallux valgus,* the angulation or deviation of the big toe out of place where the enlargement forces the the great toe toward the other toes. Bunions can also occur on other toes. A bunion of the fifth metatarsal is referred to as a *bunionette*.

Several procedures are available for treating bunions of the great toe, (code range 28289–28299). Coding for bunion surgery is very challenging because not all bunion deformities are the same. To complicate this task further, there are numerous techniques for each procedure. All bunion procedures include the following procedures:

- Arthrotomy
- Capsular release and reconstruction
- Synovectomy
- Synovial biopsy
- Extensor tenotomy (release)
- Removal of medial eminence and osteophyte excision when done on the first MPJ
- Articular shaving
- Internal fixation
- Removal of bursal tissue
- Capsular arthroplasty
- Excision of synovial cysts or bone
- Splinting/casting
- Revision of scar
- Tenolysis
- Capsulotomy
- Sesamoidectomy

The metatarsal osteotomy is the most common bunion procedure performed. The professional edition of CPT has an illustration of this technique in addition to illustrations of various other bunionectomy techniques.

CPT code 28292 is a radical bunionectomy requiring more bony work for subluxed joint.

CPT code 28299 is a *double osteotomy* done for people who have severe hallux valgus that cannot be repaired by osteotomy of the first metatarsal. This procedure represents the performance of more than one type of osteotomy.

CPT code 28899, unlisted procedure, is now used for bunionectomy including tendon transfer release. The tendon transplant is the major part of this procedure.

> When performing procedures on phalanges and metatarsals, physicians will use the words *proximal* and *base* when referring to the same anatomical site. These words are synonymous.

> Hammertoe arthroplasty includes tenotomy, capsulotomy, internal fixation, implant insertion, excision of exostosis, hemiphalangectomy, local bone graft, phalangectomy, synovectomy of PIP joint, extensor tenotomy, and tenolysis.

Ostectomy, Partial Excision (Bunionette)

A separate procedure is reported with code 28110, *Ostectomy, partial excision, fifth metatarsal head (bunionette)*. Arthrotomy is performed to expose the MPJ, and resection of the exostosis or lateral eminence is performed. The procedure includes excision of bursa, exostosis, repair of capsule, capsulorrhaphy, repositioning of the tendon, tenolysis, and release of joint contracture.

Hallux Varus

Hallux varus results when the MPJ bulges inward, causing the great toe to turn outward away from the other toes. The big toe begins to deviate away from the midline of the foot and looks as if it is separating from the foot. Treatment involves extensor hallucis brevis tendon transfer to pull the toe back to midline. Another technique used is called a *reverse Austin bunionectomy.*

Hammertoe Repair

Hammertoe is a deformity of the toe in which the PIP joint cannot be straightened. *Rigid* hammertoes are fixed in one position and require removal of bone to return the toe to the normal position. *Flexible* hammertoes can be manually straightened or may require tenotomy because the joint is not "frozen" in place. Hammertoe correction (28285) may be called an arthroplasty because the joint may require bone remodeling. Hammertoes on the fifth digit have their own associated CPT code (28296) because the technique used to repair the foot is slightly different. Incision is made under the toe (plantar side) rather than the dorsal approach and usually involves plastic surgery skin repair. The procedure involves proximal phalangectomy of the fifth toe and includes skin graft closure, arthrodesis, excision of neuroma, as well as the components of code 28285.

Hallux Rigidus Repair

Hallux rigidus is arthritis of the MPJ restricting the motion of the great toe; it can result from trauma, previous surgery, or a congenital condition. Mild cases can be corrected with cheilectomy (28289), where excess bone around the joint is removed. Severe cases may require fusing of the joint (28750) or osteotomies to decompress the joint.

Plantar Fasciitis Treatment

Plantar fasciitis is inflammation of the sole of the foot (plantar fascia). To treat this, the plantar fascia is incised or excised depending on the extent of the fasciitis (28008 or 28060, 28062, 28250, 29893). Radical fasciotomy incorporates an additional transverse incision through the fascia at the midsection. Code 28890 is used for plantar fascia shock wave treatment done before the surgical incision or excision is performed.

Treatment of Morton's Neuroma

Morton's neuroma is a benign nerve tumor usually occurring between the third and fourth interdigital metatarsal interspace. A conservative treatment option is injection of the neuroma with steroids. Surgical treatment involves excision of the neuroma (28080). This does not include excision of neuroma between metatarsal bones.

Heel Spur Surgery

A heel spur is a small projection or bony exostosis that develops where the plantar fascia meets the calcaneus and is caused from straining the attachment. Surgical treatment includes osteotomy of the calcaneus (28119), which may include plantar fascia and tarsal tunnel release.

Exostosis

Exostosis is a benign tumor or cyst of a bone. New growth of bone forms on top of existing bone and may sometimes be covered in cartilage. It is important to read the operative report to clearly determine if the exostosis was actually removed without removing the underlying bone. Exostectomies (28288) can be carried out where the mass is simply excised or with the assistance of saucerization. Saucerization includes removing the subperiosteal new bone with the attached cyst contents and curettaging the remaining cortical bone to leave a shallow dip, like a saucer.

> **EXAMPLE**
> 28120 *Partial excision (craterization, saucerization, sequestrectomy, or diaphysectomy) bone; talus or calcaneus.*

Repair of Tarsal Tunnel Syndrome

Tarsal tunnel syndrome is similar to carpal tunnel in the wrist in that the posterior tibial nerve that runs along the inside of the ankle into the foot is compressed in the flexor retinaculum, causing pain in the foot. An incision is made on the medial side of the ankle and the nerve is traced and freed from any constricting tissue (28035).

> **INTERNET RESOURCE:** Visit surgery.com to view videos and images of podiatric surgeries and pictures of foot deformities.
> www.surgery.com/guide/podiatry-surgery

Assign codes to the following procedures for the physician. Include any necessary modifiers. In some cases, more than one code is required.

1. An avid runner has been experiencing chronic plantar fasciitis. She has already tried conservative methods including anti-inflammatories, injections, and rest. She is also experiencing numbness of the fourth toe on the left foot. Physician performs a partial fasciectomy and removal of Morton's neuroma on the left foot. _____

2. A patient has been suffering from large bony bunion prominence of the right great toe for 2 years. She has changed footwear and still has pain with activity. She wants to have this bunion removed. Her great toe has severely deviated toward her other toes. Physician performs a first metatarsal osteotomy and fixation with screw. _____

3. A patient contracted osteomyelitis of the fourth left toe. A skin incision was made along the lateral border of the fourth metatarsal and carried down to the subcutaneous tissue. Dissection was carried down to the base of the metatarsal where an osteotomy was made. The bone was delivered from the wound and sent to pathology. There was erosion of the head consistent with osteomyelitis. The toe was amputated. _____

INTERNET RESOURCES: Visit the Florida Podiatric Medical Association for useful links to resources at
http://fpma.com/cms/index.php?option=com_content&view=article&id=11

The American Podiatric Medical Association (APMA) maintains an online podiatry coding resource center that offers a brief free trial for new users.
www.apmacodingrc.org

The American Academy of Orthopaedic Surgeons is a specialty organization that serves as an authoritative body for orthopedic practitioners. They publish the *Complete Global Service Data for Orthopaedic Surgery.*
www.aaos.org

State podiatric medical associations provide resources and links on their association websites, as well.

Chapter Summary

1. Assigning codes for procedures commonly performed on the muscles, bones, and joints requires familiarity with the organizational format of this subsection and a thorough understanding of anatomy and terminology. Procedures are located in the Index by looking up the anatomical site, and then the surgical root word such as *arthroscopy,* eponym, or the procedure performed.

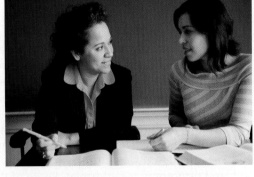

2. Modifiers are a very important component of coding and should be used when necessary to describe the circumstances of the service as well as who performed them.

3. AAOS has identified 11 intraoperative services that should not be coded separately when performing orthopedic procedures. Reporting imaging guidance requires a review of CPT and NCCI guidelines.

4. Common surgical techniques used with the musculoskeletal system include (a) amputation, detachment of a limb; (b) arthrotomy, a surgical incision into a joint; (c) arthroscopy/endoscopy, using an arthroscope to view the interior of a joint; (d) fusion (also called *arthrodesis*), joining bones; (e) lysis/release, cutting loose, or decompressing; (f) manipulation, aligning body parts manually; (g) reduction, aligning body parts either surgically or manually; and (h) revision, surgically correcting a previous repair.

5. The spine is divided into the cervical, thoracic, lumbar, and sacral sections. There are seven cervical vertebrae, twelve thoracic, five lumbar and five sacral vertebrae. The five sacral vertebrae are fused into one solid bone. Arthrodesis is one of the most common procedures on the spine and the coder must know the various approaches such as anterior, anterolateral, posterior, posterolateral. The coder must also know the difference between the vertebral disc versus the vertebral disc space. Co-surgery is common in the anterior approach to arthrodesis but know when you can apply the co-surgery modifier and to which codes that modifier can be appended.

6. Fracture guidelines are located in the beginning of the CPT's Musculoskeletal System section. Codes are assigned based on the type of fracture treatment, not the fracture type. There are three types of fracture treatment: closed, open, and percutaneous skeletal fixation. Choose codes based on whether a fracture or dislocation is being treated. If a fracture is reduced or manipulated, assign the code with those terms in the description. If an external fixation device is used along with the fracture treatment, assign this separately if the code description for the fracture treatment does not already include external fixation. Application and removal procedures for the *first* cast or traction device are considered bundled for all procedures when a cast, splint, or strapping is applied during a surgical procedure.

7. Arthroscopy/endoscopy codes are located at the end of the musculoskeletal section under codes 29800–29999. Codes in this section describe both diagnostic and therapeutic procedures. They are grouped by body part and joint and then by type of arthroscopy, either diagnostic or surgical (therapeutic). Diagnostic arthroscopies should not be coded when a surgical arthroscopy is performed.

8. Procedures on the shoulder, elbow, and wrist are used to treat various common injuries and conditions. Knowledge of anatomy and pathology is required to select correct codes.

9. Extensor tendons are located on the dorsum (or back) of the hand. These tendons attach to muscles that allow the hand or fingers to extend out/open. Flexor tendons are located on the palm of the hand. Flexor tendons attach to muscles that cause the hand or fingers to bend. They are both grouped into zones on the hand for identification.

10. Tendon repair, or tenorrhaphy, is a procedure for suturing together the torn ends of tendons. Tendon advancement is used to advance or move forward the end of a tendon from its original location. The tendon is then made secure. Codes for tendon repair are assigned based on technique used and whether the repair is a primary or secondary repair. A primary repair is considered to be the first time the tendon is repaired, which is immediately after the injury. A secondary repair is a repair that is done after the primary repair or occurs at a date much later than the injury, after the tendon sheath has healed.

11. Hip arthroplasty codes are assigned based on whether it is an initial or revision arthroplasty and whether it is a total or partial replacement (based on components used). The codes must reflect the component(s) replaced and whether it is a conversion of a previous hip fracture reduction to a prosthetic joint.

12. Recognizing anatomical landmarks for arthroscopic knee surgery is critical for adhering to coding guidelines. Knee arthroplasty codes are assigned based on whether the procedure is an initial or revision arthroplasty, and whether it is a total or partial replacement. If the arthroplasty is a revision, codes are chosen based on which components are replaced.

13. Assigning codes for bunion procedures is based on the technique used, whether an osteotomy was performed, and if so where it was performed. All bunionectomy procedures include the same basic components: synovectomy, extensor tenotomy, removal of exostosis, tenolysis, capsulotomy, and articular shaving. The coder must focus on exactly where the incision and osteotomy is performed. Some of the procedures are carried out for deformities in the interphalangeal joint and some for deformities in the metatarsal phalangeal joint.

Matching

Match the key terms with their definitions.

A. external fixation
B. lysis
C. fusion
D. arthrotomy
E. casting

F. arthroplasty
G. replantation
H. trigger point injection
I. chondroplasty
J. traction

1. _____ A procedure involving injections used to treat painful knots of muscle that form when muscles do not relax

2. _____ Immobilization of a bone or joint with a plaster or fiberglass molded support that remains on (usually) for 4 to 6 weeks

3. _____ Reattachment of a body part that was traumatically removed in its entirety from the body

4. _____ Realigning or reconstructing a dysfunctional joint

5. _____ Force applied by weights or other devices to treat bone injuries or muscle disorders

6. _____ Any means of securing or fixing bone ends or fragments in proper anatomical alignment from outside the body without nailing, wiring, rodding, screwing, or plating the bones together on the inside

7. _____ The decompression or loosening of a tendon, muscle, or nerve from surrounding tissue that is binding or impeding movement

8. _____ Surgical incision into a joint as an approach to a therapeutic surgery

9. _____ The permanent joining together of bones by mechanical implant such as screws or wire or by graft to make them immobile

10. _____ Debridement of articular cartilage

True or False

Decide whether each statement is true or false.

1. __T__ Debridement is never coded as a separate procedure.

2. __F__ The removal of a biplane external fixator from the humerus under general anesthesia is assigned 20693.

3. __F__ A synovectomy is always included in a surgical arthroscopy and is never coded separately.

4. __T__ An ED physician examines a boy's arm and determines that the radial shaft is broken. She places a cast on the arm and refers him to the orthopedic surgeon for fracture reduction. The correct code for the ED physician's service is 25500.

5. __F__ The arthroscopic thermal capsulorrhaphy of the left shoulder and manipulation under anesthesia is coded 23700–RT, 29999.

6. __T__ A labrum is a piece of bone that encircles the glenohumeral joint.

7. __T__ A shoulder manipulation and a shoulder arthroscopy should both be coded when performed at the same time.

8. __F__ The correct code for the excision of a recurrent ganglion cyst of the wrist is 25112.

9. __T__ Fluoroscopy is included in fracture treatment and is not coded separately.

10. __T__ The patient sustained a fracture of the radial shaft. Six weeks after the fracture reduction, x-rays demonstrate a nonunion requiring a fracture re-reduction. The same surgeon performed both procedures within 6 weeks of each other. The doctor should append the –76 modifier to the re-reduction code.

Multiple Choice

Select the letter that best completes the statement or answers the question.

1. Select the correct code(s) for closed treatment of a distal radial fracture with manipulation and external fixator application.
   A. 25605, 20690
   B. 25600, 25611–51
   C. 25607
   D. 25600, 20690

2. Select the correct code(s) for injection of lidocaine and Depo-Medrol to the left knee and right great toe.
   A. 20550
   B. 20600, 20610
   C. 20526, 20600–51
   D. 20612, 20612–59

3. Select the correct code(s) for arthroscopy of the right knee with synovectomy of the medial compartment and meniscectomy of the medial and lateral compartments.
   A. 29876–RT, 29880–RT–51
   B. 29875–RT, 29880–RT–51
   C. 29876–RT, 27333–RT–51
   D. 29880–RT

4. Select the correct code(s) for when a patient has two hammertoes repaired, one on the left third toe and the second on the left fourth toe.
   A. 28285–50
   B. 28285–LT, 28285–59
   C. 28285–LT, 28285–LT-51
   D. 28285–T2, 28285–T3

5. An excision of bone is an
   A. Exostectomy
   B. Ostectomy
   C. Osteotomy
   D. Arthrodesis

6. Select the correct code for wound exploration of the shoulder.
   A. 20120
   B. 20610
   C. 20103
   D. 21501

7. Select the correct codes for excision of a 3.0- x 2.5-cm lipoma of the back, where the incision was carried down to and through the superficial fascia and a layered closure was performed with 2-0 Vicryl and 1-0 Monocryl.
   A. 11403, 12032
   B. 21931, 12032
   C. 21925, 12031
   D. 21931, 12031

8. Cast codes are not coded when
   A. An ED physician applies the cast for support and refers the patient to an orthopedist
   B. A physician is reapplying a cast at a follow-up appointment
   C. A doctor performs fracture care
   D. A doctor applies a splint in the office after performing a detailed exam, reviewing a CT scan of the wrist, and coordinating rehab services

9. Select the correct code(s) for a percutaneous repair of a ruptured Achilles tendon on the patient's left foot, with application of a short leg cast.
   A. 27650–LT
   B. 27652–RT
   C. 27654–RT
   D. 27650–RT, 29405–RT

10. If an arthroscopic rotator cuff repair is performed, but it cannot be completed under this technique and is converted to an open procedure
   A. Only the open procedure is reportable
   B. Both the open and arthroscopic procedures are reported
   C. Both the open and arthroscopic procedures are reported with the –59 modifier appended to the open procedure code
   D. Both the open and arthroscopic procedures are reported with the –52 modifier appended to the open procedure code

11. Casting/splinting/strapping should not be reported separately if a _____ is also performed.
   A. Restorative treatment
   B. E/M service
   C. Treatment to afford comfort to the patient
   D. All of the above

12. If a physician treats a fracture, dislocation, or injury with a cast, splint, or strap as an initial service without any other definitive procedure or treatment and only expects to perform the initial care, the physician may report
   A. An E/M service
   B. A casting/splinting/strapping CPT code, an E/M code, and a casting supply code
   C. A cast/splint/strap HCPCS supply code
   D. A fracture reduction care code with a –54 modifier

13. When it is necessary to perform skeletal/joint manipulation under anesthesia to assess range of motion, reduce a fracture, or for any other purpose during another more major procedure in an anatomically related area, the corresponding manipulation code (e.g., CPT codes 22505, 23700, 27275, 27570, 27860) is
   A. Separately reportable
   B. Reported with a –59 modifier
   C. Not reported separately
   D. Reported separately with 23700 for a shoulder dislocation

14. Select the correct code(s) for a left shoulder arthroscopy, arthroscopic subacromial decompression, open rotator cuff repair, and repair of a SLAP lesion.
   A. 23412, 29826, 29807
   B. 23412
   C. 29807, 29826, 29827–51
   D. 23412, 29826–51, 29807–51

15. Select the correct code(s) for a right knee arthroscopy with medial and lateral meniscectomies and chondroplasty of the patellofemoral joint.
   A. 29877–RT
   B. 29880–RT
   C. 29881–RT, 29877–RT
   D. 29880–RT, 29877–RT–59

16. Select the correct code(s) for a posterior lumbar arthrodesis at L3–L5.
    A. 22614 × 3
    B. 22612
    C. 22600
    D. 22612, 22614

17. Arthrodesis is performed using a metal cage; a hole is drilled in the interspace and a metal cage is place in the hole. Another metal cage is placed in the same interspace and filled with autogenous, morselized bone graft from a separate incision. Code for the application of the metal cages and the bone graft.
    A. 22851, 20937–51
    B. 22851 × 2, 20937–51
    C. 22851
    D. 22851, 20937

CHAPTER 19

CPT: Respiratory System

CHAPTER OUTLINE

Organization

Respiratory Anatomy

Common Procedures of the Nose

Common Procedures of the Sinuses

Common Procedures of the Larynx

Common Procedures of the Pharynx

Common Procedures of the Lungs and Bronchi

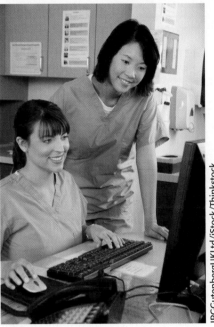

IPGutenbergUKLtd/iStock/Thinkstock

LEARNING OUTCOMES

After studying this chapter, you should be able to:

1. Understand the coding structure and its relationship to the anatomy of the respiratory system in order to code this system's procedures correctly.
2. Describe the purpose of the common procedures on the lower respiratory system: laryngoscopy, tracheostomy, bronchoscopy, thoracoscopy, and thoracentesis.
3. Assign codes to nasal and septal fracture repairs depending on technique, type of fracture, and age of fracture.
4. Explain the difference between turbinate excision, reduction, and submucous resection and when these are appropriate to report.
5. Understand the differences between various endoscopic sinus procedure codes and how to report multiple surgeries at the same session.
6. Determine when it is appropriate to separately report image guidance when performed with sinus endoscopies.
7. Recognize when to assign laryngectomy codes when performed with pharyngectomy and/or radical or modified neck dissection.
8. Distinguish between the various pharyngectomy codes and assign the correct code based on the technique applied.

9. Differentiate between lung wedge resection, lobectomy, segmentectomy, and pneumonectomy procedures.
10. Identify the three components of work for lung transplantation and appropriate codes to assign for each.

This chapter covers the anatomical features of the respiratory system and its common conditions and surgical procedures. Because many of these procedures are done endoscopically, this approach is emphasized for mastery of the associated coding. This chapter discusses from the simplest to the highest level of procedure for most complex otorhinolaryngological and pulmonology surgical services.

Otorhinolaryngology is a surgical subspecialty that concentrates on the medical and surgical treatments of diseases related to the nose, sinuses, ears, and throat (pharynx and larynx). Pulmonology is a medical subspecialty that concentrates solely on the medical and minor surgical treatment of the trachea and lungs. Diagnostic and some therapeutic endoscopic procedures on the lungs are performed by pulmonologists.

Pulmonologists and thoracic and general surgeons obtain additional training in performing video-assisted thoracic surgery (VATS), which is an important development in performing thoracic and lung surgery. VATS follows the same concept as laparoscopic procedures but instead of making the small incisions in the abdomen, they are instead made in the thoracic chest wall. The trocars are inserted and a small video camera is used to view the cavity and all the instruments required to carry out the procedures. Open surgical procedures on the lungs are performed by general surgeons, not pulmonologists.

Surgical procedures on the sinuses, nose, and throat are commonly performed endoscopically under general anesthesia by otorhinolaryngologists, physicians who specialize in otorhinolaryngology. These physicians are commonly referred to as *ENT* (ear, nose, and throat) *specialists*.

> Procedures on the nasal septum and nasal bones are performed by ENT specialists even though codes for nasal fracture repair are located in the Musculoskeletal System section of CPT and not the Respiratory System section.

INTERNET RESOURCES: The American Academy of Otolaryngology—Head and Neck Surgery is a specialty organization that serves as an authoritative body for ENT practitioners. www.entnet.org

The American Thoracic Society is another physician specialty organization that provides clinical practice guidance, clinical resources, patient educational material, etc., in addition to coding and reimbursement guidance. www.thoracic.org

ORGANIZATION

The CPT respiratory surgical codes cover procedures on the sinuses, nose, larynx, trachea, bronchi, lungs, and pleura. Code assignment requires careful review of the procedural/operative note to determine the following:

1. The extent of the procedure
2. The technique or approach (open or closed) used by the surgeon
3. The type of procedure—whether it is diagnostic or surgical in nature
4. Whether the procedure was unilateral or bilateral
5. Whether the procedure is considered a component of another major procedure (Many nasal procedures, such as control of nasal hemorrhage, ligation of arteries, and repair of fractures of turbinates, are components of a more major procedure.)

The Respiratory System subsection is arranged by body area from the top down—the nose to the lungs. It includes the following headings:

- Nose
- Accessory Sinuses
- Larynx

> The National Correct Coding Initiative (NCCI) edits bundle many respiratory procedures into more comprehensive procedures. Most edits have the modifier indicator of "1," so the use of an appropriate modifier (usually –59) can override them.

- Trachea and Bronchi
- Lungs and Pleura

Within each heading is one or more of these subheadings:

- Incision
- Excision
- Introduction (and Removal)
- Removal of Foreign Body
- Repair
- Destruction
- Endoscopy
- Other Procedures

RESPIRATORY ANATOMY

The respiratory system is responsible for conducting air, exchanging gases (oxygen is inhaled and diffused into the blood while carbon dioxide is diffused from the blood into the lungs and exhaled), producing sound, smell, and protecting the body from airborne infection.

**INTERNET RESOURCE: Visit
www.innerbody.com/image_card06/card13.html
to view images of the respiratory anatomy.**

Upper Respiratory Tract

The upper respiratory tract consists of the nose, nasal cavity, paranasal sinuses, and pharynx. The primary function of these structures is to conduct air into the lungs (Fig. 19.1).

Nose and Nasal Cavity

The nasal bone projects from the skull to form the bridge of the nose. The lateral nasal cartilage shapes each side of the nose. The alar cartilages shape the nasal alae. The nasal septum lies in the middle of the nasal cavity and so is called the *medial wall*. The two outer lateral walls of the nasal cavity have three very thin, curved, projecting bones called *turbinates* (Fig. 19.2).

Three sets of paired turbinates—inferior, middle, and superior—secrete mucus and can swell or shrink, affecting the size of the nasal passages. These are also called *nasal conchae*. They are called conchae because of the way they curve up and around similar to a conch shell. They consist of a thin, spongy bony plate and a thick mucoperiosteum that contains a cavernous vascular bed. The paired nasal conchae create air turbulence.

Reporting of turbinate procedures is tricky. The inferior turbinate is the most important of the three and the largest. It is located on the lateral wall of the nasal cavity and separates the middle from the inferior meatus. A meatus is a natural opening within the body. The inferior meatus communicates via vibration with the ethmoid, palate, and maxilla bones. It is very large and extends from the front to the rear of the nose. The middle turbinate is part of the ethmoid labyrinth and separates the superior and middle meatus. The superior turbinate is also part of the ethmoid labyrinth that projects from the lateral wall of the nose. Each of the spaces above or below the turbinates has its own name. The space above the superior turbinate is the sphenoethmoidal recess. The remaining spaces are considered to be below each of the other turbinates.

Sinuses

The sinuses are responsible for humidifying the air, filtering it for particles, and warming it before it enters the lungs (Fig. 19.3). They cleanse air with their mucous-lined walls. The paranasal sinuses are air pockets within the frontal, ethmoid, sphenoid, and maxillary bones. The two frontal sinuses are located within the frontal bone in the area of the forehead just over the eyes. The ethmoid sinus is a collection of small cavities contained within the ethmoid labyrinth of bone. These cavities are located behind the bridge of the nose just between the eyes. The two maxillary sinuses are located within the maxillary bone. These are found on either side of the nose just below the eyes. The antrum refers to the paranasal cavities or sinuses lined with mucous membrane located under

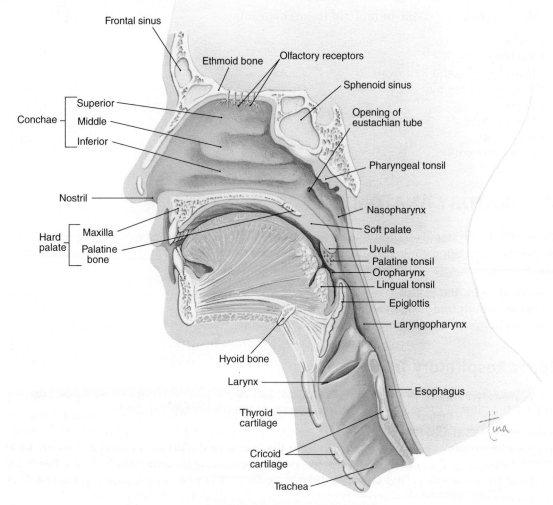

Figure 19.1 Anatomy of the upper respiratory tract.

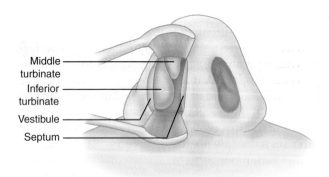

Figure 19.2 Basic anatomy of the nose.

the eye in the maxillary bone. For example, the maxillary sinus is also referred to as the *maxillary antrum*.

The two sphenoid sinuses are deeply seated in the skull behind the nose and eyes. The sinuses drain into the nasal cavity via the meatuses and the sphenoethmoidal recess. The middle meatus is particularly important because that is where the frontal, maxillary, and part of the ethmoid sinuses open into the nasal cavity. This area is called the *osteomeatal complex*. Any inflammation or infection that causes blockage in this sensitive area can occlude the other sinuses that drain into the osteomeatal complex. When obstruction occurs, the mucus is retained in the sinus cavity. These stagnant secretions thicken and provide a medium for bacterial growth. These changes lead to damage and dysfunction of the cilia (microhairs) that line the sinuses. The retained secretions and infection lead to further tissue inflammation, which in turn leads to further blockage. This repetitive cycle typically leads to chronic sinusitis. Removal of this diseased tissue and obstruction is necessary to im-

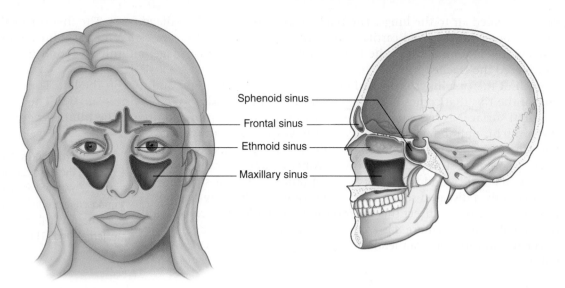

Figure 19.3 Sinuses.

prove sinus drainage. The uncinate process is a mound of bone after the infundibulum that is present as the ethmoid bullae is entered.

The sinuses are in distinct and separate anatomical locations, so procedures in each sinus cavity require separate and significant amounts of work and skill to maneuver within such an area so close to the brain. A procedure code is therefore assigned for each sinus cavity examined.

Pharynx

The pharynx, or throat, is where the oral cavity and the nasal cavity meet. (The oral cavity or mouth contains the hard palate, soft palate, tongue, and uvula.) The pharynx is divided into regions: nasopharynx, oropharynx, and laryngopharynx. The *nasopharynx* is posterior to the nasal cavity and is where the eustachian tube opens into the throat. This area also contains the pharyngeal tonsil on the posterior wall. The pharyngeal tonsil (adenoid) is located where the nasal cavity joins the pharynx. Tonsils are arranged in a ring around the pharynx and are named according to their location. The *oropharynx* extends posterior to the oral cavity from the soft palate to the level of the hyoid bone. Lingual tonsils are found here at the very back of the tongue. Palatine tonsils are found on each side of the pharynx on the lateral walls. The *laryngopharynx* extends from the hyoid bone to the top of the esophagus.

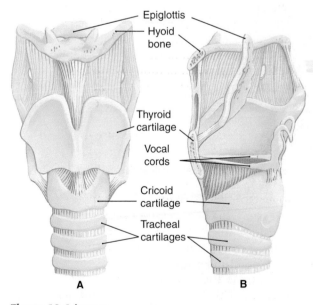

Figure 19.4 Larynx.

Lower Respiratory Tract

The lower respiratory tract consists of the larynx, trachea, lungs, bronchi, bronchioles, and alveoli. The larynx is the passage from the pharynx to the lungs and where we produce speech. The larynx is supported by the thyroid cartilage and the cricoid cartilage, which serves as the base of the larynx (Fig. 19.4). The epiglottis is attached to the thyroid cartilage and closes off the larynx during swallowing to prevent food from entering the lungs. The larynx connects to the pharynx and trachea. It serves two functions: to prevent food from entering the trachea and to produce sound. Through the larynx (voice box) are the vestibular folds (ligaments) referred to as the *false vocal cords*. Just beyond the false vocal cords are the true vocal cords that produce sound. Beneath the true vocal cords is the infraglottic space that connects the larynx to the trachea. The trachea carries inhaled air to the lungs. The trachea consists of 18–22 cartilage rings. The first tracheal ring resides under thyroid cartilage and cricoid cartilage and serves as a landmark during laryngoscopy. Examination of the larynx ends at the cricoid cartilage; anything beyond this is considered the trachea.

Each of the two lungs is divided into lobes: three on the right and two on the left. The surface of the ribs that comes in contact with the thoracic wall is called the *costal surface*. The mediastinal surface, as the name suggests, faces the mediastinum and houses the hilum whereby the bronchi, pulmonary vessels, lymphatic vessels, and nerves pass. Each lung is subdivided into bronchopulmonary segments (Fig. 19.5). Each segment is supplied by its own bronchus and a branch of the pulmonary artery and vein. This segmentation allows a surgeon to remove only a diseased segment while leaving healthy lung segments untouched. Bronchi direct the air into the bronchioles, which contain the alveoli. This is where gas exchange occurs. Any blockage in the lower respiratory tract can lead to respiratory distress or, even worse, failure.

> ◉ Procedures done on the nose can be done with or without an endoscope. Code by (1) the approach, whether internal or external, and (2) the use of a scope.

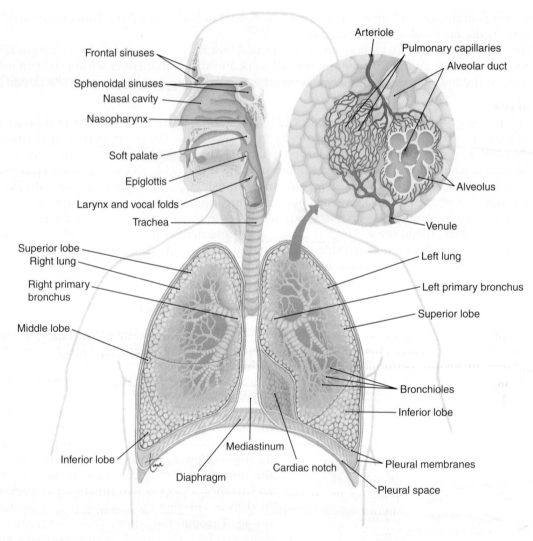

Figure 19.5 Respiratory tract.

COMMON PROCEDURES OF THE NOSE

Removal of Nasal Polyps

Codes in the nasal and sinus endoscopy section are classified unilateral procedures and if done bilaterally require a –50 modifier. If a polyp is removed from both sides of the nose, report a –50 modifier.

Nasal polyps can emanate from the lining of the nose or paranasal sinuses. Most polyps are benign, pedunculated (hanging from a stalk) growths that are easy to remove. A nasal polyp described as *simple* is limited to one polyp or one polyp per side of the nose. Simple excisions are typically performed in the physician's office (30110). Excision of multiple polyps—more than one per side—is considered *extensive*. Extensive polyp excision usually involves *sessile* polyps (with a thick base) whose removal requires more effort, skill, and time; this procedure is typically performed in an outpatient clinic (30115). If the coder cannot determine if the excision is simple or extensive, the physician must be queried for accurate coding.

> **INTERNET RESOURCE:** More about nasal polyps and endoscopic images can be found at: www.emedicine.com/ped/topic1550.htm#target1

Removal of Foreign Body

Children are famous for inserting things in to their noses. Some common items (referred to as *foreign bodies*) are beans, crayon tips, beads, eraser tips, paper wads, and pebbles. Packing from previous nasal surgery is also referred to as a *foreign body* for CPT coding; thus, packing removal post-surgery is coded as a foreign body removal (but only if packing is removed by a different provider than the one who did the previous surgery). Codes are available for an office procedure, for one requiring general anesthesia, and for a procedure done via lateral rhinotomy (surgical incision into the nose). The code range is 30300–30320.

Resection of Turbinates

Turbinates are removed (resected) or reduced because of turbinate hypertrophy from chronic inflammation or infection, which if left untreated can lead to persistent sinus infections. The usual procedure involves repair of an anatomically deviated, obstructing *inferior* turbinate.

The inferior turbinates can be reduced or removed with or without endoscopy. The procedure involves removing part of the lining and/or part of the bone itself with cautery, laser, debridement, cryotherapy, radio-frequency ablation, or excision (all coded to 30130). Submucosal resection of the inferior turbinate means that the submucosal lining of the turbinate is removed, but not part of the bone itself (30140). If turbinates are cauterized but not excised, either code 30801 or 30802 is assigned. Turbinates are also called *nasal conchae*, so concha bullosa resection is coded as a turbinectomy. Turbinates can also be injected to reduce their size (30200).

At times, turbinates may be "fractured" to reposition them when they are enlarged and obstructing the nasal airway (30930). Fracturing a turbinate is never coded separately unless this is the only procedure performed. Do not report this if the surgeon fractures the middle turbinates medially to provide access for sinus procedures. This is considered part of the sinus surgery. CPT considers the fracture (30930) inclusive of 30140, *Submucous resection inferior turbinate, partial or complete, any method.* A parenthetical note instructs coders to not report 30130 or 30140 in conjunction with 30801, 30802, or 30930. If, however, the turbinate fracture was performed on the opposite side from the submucous turbinectomy, it may be reported by appending the –59 modifier.

Assign only one turbinate procedure code per turbinate. Never code middle turbinate reduction, fracture, or excision if done to gain access to another part of the nose or the ethmoid sinus. However, middle turbinate surgery is not considered access to the frontal or sphenoids and may be reported separately.

CPT codes 30130 and 30140 are used to report procedures of the inferior turbinate. There are two other turbinates in the nose (middle and superior), but there isn't a specific code for these like there is the inferior turbinates. To report submucous resection of the turbinate (SRT), code 30140, the operative report should describe the surgeon making an incision in the mucosa and preserving it versus removing it by creating a flap that is raised to access the inferior turbinate. The incision is carried deeper through the submucosal tissue until the inferior turbinate mucoperiosteum bone is reached. The mucoperiosteum is then elevated (with an instrument called a *Freer elevator*) to expose the bony turbinate. The elevator is shaped for use in blunt dissection and tissue manipulation in small spaces. A chisel or forceps is used to resect portions of the bone. The flap is then returned to its normal position. A statement such as "I excised the turbinate" is not adequate documentation to support this technique.

EXAMPLE
The inferior turbinates were injected bilaterally. A flap 2.5 cm wide and 2 cm high was elevated. Vasomotor tissue was then removed from each inferior turbinate and the flaps returned to their normal position. Code: 30140–50.

CPT code 30130 describes the removal of all or part of a turbinate. However, it does not extend down into the submucosal layer of nasal tissue. An incision is made around the base of the turbinate and it is chiseled or drilled away from the lateral wall of the nose. The surgeon does not make an incision into the mucosa to resect the turbinate but rather excises mucosa and bone at the same time, cutting out the mucosa and the bone completely. This is commonly referred to as *outfracturing* the bony turbinate. Most insurance carriers will bundle turbinate excision procedures into the ethmoidectomy procedure codes if these two procedures are performed at the same time because the middle and superior turbinates are part of the ethmoid labyrinth. Therefore, if the middle turbinate is removed while performing an ethmoidectomy or polypectomy, it is not reported separately.

> ● Do not report turbinate excision codes when performed simply to access the ethmoid.

EXAMPLE
The turbinates were injected with 0.05% Xylocaine with 1:100,000 epinephrine. The Takahashi forceps were then utilized to infracture and excise the protruding ends of the inferior turbinates on both sides. Code: 30130–50.

CPT codes 30130 and 30140 should be reported separately when performed on the inferior turbinates on opposite sides of the nose. Turbinate excision codes are not problematic when reported with maxillary, frontal, or sphenoid procedures because anatomically they are not connected. For excision of superior or middle turbinates, use CPT code 30999 and not 30130.

> ● Modifier –50 should be appended to any turbinate procedure code when performed bilaterally because these codes are intended to be unilateral. Likewise, if a procedure is performed unilaterally, append the appropriate RT or LT modifier to designate which side is treated.

Turbinate Reduction

Turbinate reduction can be accomplished in different ways. The goal of turbinate reduction procedures is to make the turbinates smaller, thus allowing more room for flow through the nasal cavity. Read the operative report carefully to determine the method of turbinate reduction. One method of reducing the turbinates is with radio-frequency ablation (RFA). The term *coblation*—which is a method of surgically removing, destroying, or shrinking tissue via radio-frequency waves using low-heat electrosurgical equipment—may be used to indicate RFA as well. CPT does not contain the term *radio-frequency*. The Index to CPT does, however, include the word *ablation*. The codes for turbinate ablation are located under 30801–30802. CPT code 30802 is for intramural ablation or cauterization of the deeper mucosa, whereas 30801 is for superficial ablation that involves only the outer layer of the mucosa.

EXAMPLE
The inferior nasal turbinate was infiltrated with 0.75% Marcaine with epinephrine. Four submucosal tunnels were then made beginning at the caudal aspect of the turbinate. The tunnels were made with a Coblator setting of 4 and a coagulation setting of 6. The turbinate was then crushed and fractured laterally. Code: 30802.

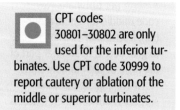

> ● CPT codes 30801–30802 are only used for the inferior turbinates. Use CPT code 30999 to report cautery or ablation of the middle or superior turbinates.

The second method of turbinate reduction is accomplished by making two parallel incisions on the turbinate's medial surface from the anterior tip to the turbinate's mid one-third posterior aspect followed by dissection and removal of the mucosa. If the operative report states *incision of the mucosa along with outfracturing or incision with partial resection (partial removal of the turbinate without resecting the whole turbinate) and fracture,* you should report 30140–52.

EXAMPLE

Physician injected both the right and left inferior turbinates with local and made an incision on the front of the turbinates with a #15 blade. He inserted a Xomed XPS shaver turbinate blade through the incision and evacuated submucosal tissue down to the periosteum and then fractured the turbinates. Code: 30140–52–50.

Concha Bullosa Excision

The term *bullosa* refers to a bubble-like or balloon-like structure. A middle turbinate that has an air cell in it or has become filled with air is called a *concha bullosa*. A concha bullosa is considered to be an extension of the ethmoid sinus because the middle and superior turbinates are part of the ethmoid labyrinth. There is a common misconception that a concha bullosa is another term for turbinate. It is true that each turbinate has a concha. A concha bullosa, however, is an enlargement or ballooning of the concha of the middle or superior nasal turbinate. It can become very large and contribute to sinus obstruction requiring reduction.

There is a strong association between the presence of a concha bullosa and septal deviation toward the opposite side from the concha bullosa. Concha bullosa are routinely treated via endoscopic resection. The scope is inserted and a scalpel is placed parallel to the endoscope to incise and resect the concha bullosa. The surgery's intent is to resect the concha bullosa, while preserving the middle turbinate's integrity and mucosa on both sides of the preserved lamella. Resection of areas of exposed bone is also performed. The procedure is reported with CPT code 31240. If procedures are performed on the other turbinates at the same operative session, these can be reported together because they are not bundled, according to the NCCI. The documentation must be very detailed to support reporting these procedure codes separately. There are three turbinates on each side of the nose, so it makes sense to use modifier –59 to designate that this procedure was performed on a different and separate turbinate from the inferior or superior.

If the surgeon performs CPT code 31240 with 30130 or CPT 30140 on the same side, both are billable as long as the two procedures were performed on separate turbinates. The same is true if these procedures are performed on opposite sides.

EXAMPLE

If the surgeon performs a right middle turbinate excision (30130) and an endoscopic resection of a concha bullosa (31240) of the middle turbinate on the left side, 30130 and 31240–59 may be reported.

INTERNET RESOURCE: Visit the YouTube website and watch the video of Resection of a Large Concha Bullosa by Michael Hawk, MD. He does an excellent job of describing endoscopic resection of concha bullosa and pointing out anatomical landmarks.
www.youtube.com/watch?v=2t4JrHSUW7Q

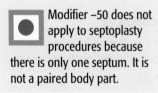

Modifier –50 does not apply to septoplasty procedures because there is only one septum. It is not a paired body part.

Septoplasty

A deviated septum is one that is not midline and obstructs air movement. Surgeons refer to septoplasty as *submucous resection* (30520). The surgeon straightens or reshapes the septum by removing a portion of the septum or excess cartilage and/or supporting the deviated area with a graft. Septoplasty with cartilage graft obtained from the septum itself or local area is included in this code. If the graft is from another source—a bone graft, a cartilage graft—the grafting is separately reportable from the graft code range. Use code 20912 if the graft is obtained from outside of the septal area and transferred to the septum. Assign code 21235 if cartilage is obtained from the ear. If bone is transferred from a second site outside the septum, use 20900.

Rhinoplasty

Nasal deformities can result from a congenital anomaly or trauma. Rhinoplasty reshapes (revises) the external portions of the nose. Its code range is 30400–30462. There are two conditional phrases to keep in mind, primary and secondary. A primary procedure refers to the first or initial rhinoplasty procedure, and secondary refers to follow-up or a second rhinoplasty procedure. The extent of this procedure varies, and it can be done for cosmetic or therapeutic purposes:

- Minor revision involves only the nasal cartilage for external parts of the nose.
- Intermediate revision involves an osteotomy for the external cartilage of the nose (removal of a hump or elevation of the tip).
- Major revision (primary septorhinoplasty) includes repair done on the internal and external parts of the nose as well as cartilage (elevation of nasal tip), grafts, osteotomy, and reshaping of a deviated septum.
- If grafts are obtained, musculoskeletal codes 20900–20926, 21210 may be used for obtaining the tissue.

Rhinoplasty is often cosmetic. Linking a diagnosis that demonstrates medical necessity—along with supporting documentation—is usually needed if insurance coverage is sought, such as in congenital deformity or traumatic injury.

> Except for rhinoplasty and excision of a dermoid cyst, procedures on the skin of the nose are located in the Integumentary System section.

Repair of Nasal Vestibular Stenosis

Nasal vestibular stenosis (30465) is the narrowing of the nasal inlet resulting in airway obstruction caused by nasal trauma, infection, or disease process. It commonly involves nasal valve collapse, which is caused by the narrowness and weakness at the nasal valve, the narrowest part of the nasal airway.

Alar batten grafts are used to treat nasal valve collapse caused by a weak nasal sidewall. In this procedure, grafts are obtained and placed in the nasal valve area to support the nasal walls and keep the openings patent. Parenthetical notes are present providing direction to the coder stating that 30465 does not include obtaining a graft. Codes 20900–20926 and 21210 are separately reportable. Coders should also note that 30465 describes a bilateral procedure. If only one side is repaired, modifier –52 (reduced services) should be appended.

Control of Nasal Hemorrhage

Nose bleeds or nasal hemorrhages, see Table 19.1, also referred to as *epistaxis*, can occur spontaneously due to blood vessels residing close to the surface of the lining of the nose or from trauma. To code control of nasal hemorrhage, the coder must decide if this was an anterior or posterior control and whether it is simple or complex. Nasal hemorrhage may also be treated endoscopically (31238).

> *Initial* in the description for 30905 refers to the initial bleed of that current episode—not that this is the very first nosebleed the patient has had. Likewise, *subsequent* for 30906 refers to the current episode of care.

Table 19.1 Anterior and Posterior Nasal Hemorrhage Control

LOCATION	CONTROL	SIMPLE	COMPLEX
Anterior (30901–30903)	Cautery performed or packing placed through the front of nose.	Limited cautery with gauze packing	Extensive packing or medical use of drugs such as cocaine
Posterior (30905–30906)	Packing placed or cautery performed via the mouth up the back side of the nasopharynx. Nasal stents, balloons, catheters, or tampons may be used.	N/A	N/A

• Cautery and control of bleeding during a nasal or sinus procedure is considered incidental or integral to the primary procedure being performed and is not reported. Do not assign codes 30901–30905 separately.

• If bleeding occurs as a late complication and requires a significant separately identifiable service after the patient has been released from an endoscopic procedure, the cautery and packing can be billed with a –78 modifier.

Treatment of Blockage of Nasolacrimal Duct

Have you ever wondered why your nose runs when you cry? The nasolacrimal duct carries excess tears from the eyes to the nose. When it becomes blocked—usually at the far end just before it enters the nose—the eye cannot properly drain and bacteria and debris may collect. Dacryocystorhinostomy can be performed to unblock the duct. A probe is inserted transnasally through an endoscope and the blocked nasolacrimal duct is enlarged by the surgeon.

Other approaches for nasolacrimal duct procedures including dilation, probing, and stent insertion are located in the Eye and Ocular Adnexa chapter of CPT.

Nasal Fracture Procedures

Nasal fracture is a vague term. Before assigning a code for repair, the coder has to have more information, such as answers to the following questions:

• Where is the fracture—nasal bone or septum?
• What type of repair was performed—closed with or without manipulation or stabilization or open with or without stabilization?
• Was the nasal fracture complicated?
• Is the fracture acute or old? Is this an acute injury or a nonunion or malunion?

Treatment of nasal fractures is aimed at restoring nasal airway patency and optimal airflow and reestablishing the cosmetic appearance of the nose. Treatment within the first hours of injury is optimal for nasal fractures. If this window of time is not feasible, treatment should be sought within 3 to 7 days maximum. Delay in treatment beyond 7 to 10 days poses significant risk of the bones healing incorrectly. Manipulation of the bones is difficult because the fracture fragments are not mobile. Many surgeons recommend delaying fracture correction for several months to allow for complete healing and have the patient return for a corrective rhinoplasty with osteotomy.

Repair Methods

Nasal and septal fracture repairs are reported using codes 21310–21337. The treatment options depend on the extent of the injury. Codes differ if the fracture was of the nasal bone and/or septum, and by whether the approach was open or closed, without manipulation, and with or without stabilization.

Closed Treatment. If the surgeon does not surgically open the fracture site, assign a closed repair code. This type of reduction is performed for unilateral or bilateral fractures of the nasal bones, or if the fracture of the nasal–septal complex is insignificant. If the fracture of the nasal–septal complex is less than one-half of the width of the nasal bridge, then closed reduction is indicated. If there is a resultant deformity following treatment, an open reduction may be needed.

Three methods are used for closed nasal fracture repair and each method corresponds to a specific code:

1. Without manipulation
2. With stabilization
3. Manipulation without stabilization

Code 21310, *Closed treatment of nasal bone fracture without manipulation,* is assigned when the fracture is nondisplaced and no manipulation is needed. Code 21315, *Closed treatment of nasal bone fracture; without stabilization,* is performed by placing nasal elevators into the nostrils and physically moving the bones back into alignment. If the surgeon places a splint on the nose after realigning the fracture, assign 21320. The splints can either be internal or externally taped to the nose. Facility coders would also assign an HCPCS code for the supply of the splint.

Open Treatment. Open reductions are performed for more complex nasal fractures. This entails manipulating the bones back to their original location by making an incision in the skin. This procedure is indicated for fractures involving dislocation of the nasal bones and the septum. It is also indicated for a septal hematoma or for open fractures where the nasal bone has perforated the skin.

Open fracture treatment is rarely performed on acute fractures unless one of the complex fractures above is present. They are more commonly performed when a closed reduction has failed and/or the fracture is displaced or when the patient is experiencing fracture sequelae. Incisions are made inside the nose to reach the nasal bone and septum. Skin incisions may also be required to adequately align the fracture with nasal elevators. Fracture fragments may be removed in order to achieve proper alignment. Report 21325 for open repair without stabilization. If the reduction must be held in place with wires, screws, or plates, report 21330. If the nasal dorsum and nasal septum are both fractured and repaired via open treatment, 21335, *Open treatment of nasal fracture, with concomitant open treatment of fractured septum,* should be used.

If the nasal septum was previously reduced by closed manipulation and it fails to heal properly or produces unsatisfactory results, open incisional repair is indicated. According to the American Academy of Otolaryngology–Head and Neck Surgery, the diagnosis of nasal fracture must have been billed within the last 6 months in order to report 21325, 21330, or 21335.

Documentation

Determining the status of a fracture and whether or not the fracture is beyond the healing stage is critical to choosing the correct repair code. Unfortunately, this is not a simple thing to assess, and documentation is key. The AAFPRS does not specify exactly how many days after a fracture occurs that the fracture diagnosis can be considered acute. Their coding guidelines clearly state that nasal fracture codes should be used to describe the treatment of acute fractures only. They, along with the American Society of Plastic Surgeons, do state that if the fracture no longer moves, it is not acute and cannot be reported with nasal fracture repair codes. If the bones are not mobile or the time period since fracture is greater than 6 weeks, then report the nasal bone or septal repair as a rhinoplasty. If the fracture is no longer acute, it would be considered a late effect of the fracture.

There is debate in the medical community on whether to report nasal fracture or rhinoplasty codes. According to the recommendation from the American Academy of Facial Plastic and Reconstructive Surgery (AAFPRS), treatment of healed fractures and the sequelae of trauma, such as malunion and nasal airway obstruction, are coded using the rhinoplasty series (30400–30420).

The caveat to assigning an accurate code for nasal fracture treatment is that there isn't a specific nasal fracture care code in CPT to capture the work, skill, and time involved in treating an old fracture where the nasal bone has already healed. This is harder to repair because the surgeon has to do more bony work to refracture the bone and then manipulate and stabilize the fracture site. The extra work is not reflected in the relative value unit (RVU) for the nasal fracture repair codes. This is why some ENT surgeons are reporting the rhinoplasty codes because the RVU is higher and captures some of the components of the repair; however, it does not completely capture all of the bony work.

CPT codes 30400–30420 are typically set up to be denied automatically by carriers because the codes describe cosmetic procedures of the nose and septum. Be prepared to appeal and fully describe the service. Send the operative report with the claim and a letter explaining the circumstances surrounding the patient's injury and sequelae.

The procedure and the circumstances surrounding the fracture must be well documented as well as the type of repair performed. The documentation should state that injury to the nasal dorsum and/or septum was from a traumatic injury and describe details of how the fracture was reduced. Nasal fractures often are accompanied by fractures of the septum.

INTERNET RESOURCE: The American Academy of Family Practitioners (AAFP) discusses nasal fracture management and treatment options and provides illustrations. www.aafp.org/afp/2004/1001/p1315.html

COMMON PROCEDURES OF THE SINUSES

Three types of access for sinus procedures are common:

- Intranasal—using a surgical instrument other than a scope placed in the nostrils to perform a procedure
- Extranasal—making an incision in the facial area to access the nasal sinuses
- Endoscopic—inserting an endoscope through the nostrils to perform the procedure

The most frequently performed access is via an endoscope. A diagnostic sinus endoscopy involves inspecting the nasal cavity, middle and superior meatus, the turbinates collectively, and the sphenoethmoid recess. For treatment, endoscopic surgery is typically performed as an outpatient procedure under general anesthesia lasting from 1 to 3 hours. After surgery, the sinus is packed with temporary sponges or sterile packing at the surgical site; the packing is removed days later in the office at a postoperative visit.

Sinus Endoscopy Procedures

Sinus endoscopy is used to perform diagnostic and therapeutic procedures in the nose and sinuses. Sinus endoscopy is indicated when a patient acquires nasal polyps, mucoceles or tumors of the sinus cavities, or experiences recurrent acute or chronic sinusitis and associated chronic sinus headaches. It is also medically necessary for cerebrospinal fluid leaks, juvenile angiofibroma, nasolacrimal duct obstruction, and choanal atresia. Typically, patients should have undergone accepted medical therapies such as nasal sprays, antibiotics, nasal lavages, and allergy immunotherapy with no significant signs of improvement before sinus surgery is performed.

Endoscopic sinus surgery is also referred to as *functional endoscopic sinus surgery (FESS)*. A separate code is assigned for each sinus entered. These codes are unilateral, so if the procedure is performed on both sides of a pair of sinuses, a –50 modifier is needed. Many times, the surgeon will enter all four pairs of sinuses to remove diseased tissue, take cultures, or open up blocked entrances to promote proper drainage, so assigning more than one code is very common. FESS involves the insertion of the endoscope into the nose for a direct visual examination of the openings into the sinuses. With the thin fiber-optic scope and microtelescopes and instruments, abnormal and obstructive tissues are removed without making any external incisions and is all accomplished through the nostrils. The advantage of this procedure is that the surgery is less extensive than performing these procedures by open incision, there is often less removal of normal tissues, and it can frequently be performed on an outpatient basis. The code range for sinus endoscopic surgeries is 31231–31298. Nasal/sinus endoscopy codes include the word *with* rather than the word *for*. *With* means that the procedures included in the code description are performed in addition to the surgical endoscopy, allowing for the assignment of only one code that includes two procedures. For example, 31267, *Nasal/sinus endoscopy, surgical; with maxillary antrostomy; with removal of tissue from maxillary sinus.* The goals of FESS are to open the ostium, the small openings that connect the paranasal cavities to the nasal cavity; to promote drainage of mucus; to reduce the incidence of infection; and to remove any diseased tissue from the sinus cavity. If the ostia get blocked by infection, scarring, trauma from nasal septal deviation, or polyps, then the mucus cannot flow from the sinus cavities and becomes a breeding ground for bacteria.

Each sinus endoscopy procedure encompasses the same basic preparation and components. Once the patient is asleep, cotton patties (pledgets) with decongestant liquid are placed in specific locations in the nasal cavity. Many surgeons use cocaine-soaked cotton to provide the vasoconstriction (decongestion). After a few minutes, the nasal endoscopes are brought into the field. The nasal passages are examined by passing the endoscope into the meatuses of the nasal anatomy. In most cases, the initial access to the sinuses is achieved under the middle turbinate. It is usually pushed toward the midline, but some patients may require partial removal to provide access to the sinuses or to create a wider drainage path. The area under the middle turbinate (middle meatus) is where most of the sinuses drain. The uncinate process is the first structure that is then encountered. This small crescent of bone and membrane is the main drain or channel for the sinuses. Many people require removal of the uncinate process because it can become narrowed by mucus clinging to the sides, making drainage slower. If the uncinate is removed, there is nothing in the way to direct or slow the drainage and the drainage pathway for the maxillary sinus, anterior ethmoid sinuses, and frontal recess is opened. The uncinate process is partially removed in most endoscopic procedures, with the exception of procedures on the sphenoid sinus.

Once the uncinate process is removed, the surgeon can see the natural opening to the maxillary sinus and can see the anterior ethmoid sinuses using the endoscope. From here, each sinus procedure is a bit different and is explained below. Sometimes, sinus surgery may require simultaneous repair of the nasal septum. After surgery, the sinus is packed with temporary sponges or sterile packing at the surgical site and removed days later in the office at a post-op visit. The use of packing will depend on the extent of surgery and physician preference.

> ■ Many of the codes in the 31238–31298 range have a "Do not report" note indicating that there are other nasal/sinus endoscopy codes that cannot be reported together if performed on the same or ipsilateral side.

Parenthetical notes located in the sinus endoscopy code section are instrumental in guiding the coder to proper code assignment when multiple sinus endoscopy procedures are performed at the same operative session. The *CPT Professional Edition* of CPT has an anatomical and procedural illustration located at the beginning of the sinus endoscopy section demonstrating the locations of each sinus and how the endoscope is introduced in the nasal cavity.

Suctioning of Material From Sinuses. When a surgeon suctions purulent mucoid material from any of the sinuses, this is not to be considered as tissue removal. If a sinus endoscopy is performed and no tissue is excised or the ostia is not enlarged for the sinus, then it is inappropriate to report codes 31238–31294. It is, however, appropriate to report 31231, *Nasal endoscopy, diagnostic, unilateral or bilateral (separate procedure)*. If there is endoscopic nasal/sinus debridement and not just suctioning of mucus or pus (i.e., removal of infectious or necrotic material or tissue or polyp), 31237, *Nasal/sinus endoscopy, surgical; with biopsy, polypectomy or debridement (separate procedure)*, may be reported. The concept of debridement applies to the sinuses as well: Tissue is removed until healthy tissue is seen. Do not report 31254, 31255, 31267, or 31288 because these procedures require a sinusotomy or ethmoidectomy to be performed. Code 31237 is commonly performed in a period some time after a patient has undergone a FESS to remove blood clotting or scar tissue, and so on. Suctioning of purulent material from sinuses during the performance of codes 31254/31255, 31267, or 31288 is part of the procedure itself and not assigned separately. Code 31237 is not reported for each sinus debrided on the same side. For example, if the ethmoid and maxillary sinuses are debrided on the left side of the nose, then 31237 is only reported once. If one sinus on the right is debrided and another sinus on the left is debrided, then 31237–50 should be reported.

EXAMPLE

The maxillary trocar was introduced and the maxillary sinus was inspected using a 0° and 30° telescope. The middle meatus was found to be obstructed completely by soft tissue. The sinus was irrigated and there was good exit of the irrigating fluid. Code: 31231. Do not confuse this procedure with 31000, *Lavage by cannulation; maxillary sinus (antrum puncture or natural ostium)*. The cannula or trocar is inserted into the sinus through an opening in the middle meatus, antral puncture beneath the inferior turbinate, or through natural ostium. It does not, however, require the use of an endoscope.

Maxillary Sinusoscopy

Codes for maxillary sinusoscopy are reported with codes 31233, 31256, and 31267. Code 31233 is a diagnostic maxillary sinusoscopy via the inferior meatus or canine fossa puncture. The surgeon punctures the inferior meatus with an instrument such as a trocar or makes an incision of the mucosa into the canine fossa of the maxilla to examine the maxillary cavity. The scope is inserted and the area is examined. No biopsy is done or tissue removed during this diagnostic procedure. In 31256 the scope is inserted into the maxillary sinus as in 31233 and the surgeon performs an antrostomy, which creates an opening for mucus to drain freely from the maxillary sinus by enlarging the maxillary ostium that has been covered by scarring or disease. Key words or anatomical landmarks to look for are *antrostomy, enlarging of the natural opening or ostium*. In addition to the antrostomy, if tissue is removed such as a thickened, infected mucous membrane lining the sinus cavity, or if maxillary cells, a mucocele, or a polyp is removed from the maxillary sinus, 31267 is assigned.

> ● Do not report both 31256 and 31267 if they are performed on the same side in the same sinus cavity.

Frontal Sinusoscopy

The frontal sinus has veins that penetrate the posterior sinus wall and on the opposite side go directly to the dura of the brain. These veins can transfer organisms to the brain via an infection in the frontal sinus cavity. Patients who have contracted acute frontal sinusitis are typically admitted to the hospital for aggressive antibiotic and steroid therapy. If within 24 hours of treatment the sinusitis isn't improving, the sinus should be surgically debrided and drained.

The frontal sinus anatomy and its drainage path are somewhat complex. The frontal sinus is a direct extension of the frontal recess. Frontal ethmoidal cells do not reach above the frontal beak and do not penetrate into the floor of the frontal sinus. The passageways are very narrow and before the scope can enter the frontal sinus, the anterior ethmoid sinuses have to be removed. What makes the procedure difficult is that several of the anterior-most ethmoid cells are in the frontal recess. This area is hard to reach and very narrow and is very close to the eye and brain. Special instruments and techniques are needed to safely remove the last of these ethmoid sinuses. Once all of the ethmoid cells in the frontal recess have been removed, the surgeon can see into the frontal sinus. If the opening to the frontal sinus is especially small, silicone stents may be placed and remain for 2 or 3 weeks to prevent the sinus from trying to heal closed.

A frontal sinusoscopy procedure is reported with code 31276. Unlike the maxillary and sphenoid sinuses, there is no distinct code for a diagnostic frontal sinusoscopy. Code 31276, *Nasal/sinus endoscopy, surgical with frontal sinus exploration, including removal of tissue from frontal sinus when performed,* is accomplished by inserting the endoscope into the frontal sinus and removing diseased or polypoid tissue using a scalpel or forceps, if indicated. A diagnostic frontal sinusoscopy is not reported with 31276 just because the code description says *exploration, including removal of tissue*. To meet the criteria for reporting 31276, the surgeon must at least perform a sinusotomy. If the ENT opens up the ostium to allow the patient to breathe better, the physician is performing a frontal sinusotomy, which is part of 31276. Code 31276 includes exploration of the sinus anatomy, subluxing the agger nasi cells, and removal of obstructing frontal recess cells, polyps, or scar tissue. Sometimes, if necessary, the surgeon may remove intersinus septi from the dome of the ethmoid and skull base. The physician may also remove ostetic bone between the frontal sinus and a supraorbital ethmoid cell. Just looking into the frontal sinus does not fulfill the requirements for reporting code 31276. If the surgeon does not open the ostium of the frontal sinus—if he or she simply just looks—the coder should instead report 31231.

> ● Before assigning 31276, make sure the surgeon has documented the dissection and removal of obstructing frontal recess cells, polyps or scar tissue, and intersinus septi from the ethmoid dome and skull base.

With a microdebrider using a straight 40° blade and a 60° blade, the frontal ethmoid recess was cleared and the frontal sinuses cannulated bilaterally. Code: 31276–50.

Sphenoid Sinusoscopy

The sphenoid is located at the base of the skull in a wedge-shaped bone between the back of the nasal space and the brain. The sphenoid sinus is the farthest back of all the sinuses. Codes for sphenoid sinusoscopy include 31235, 31287, and 31288. Code 31235 is a diagnostic sphenoid sinusoscopy via the inferior meatus or canine fossa puncture. The surgeon punctures the sphenoid sinus after maneuvering through the ethmoids or by cannulation of the sphenoid drainage system that enters the sphenoethmoidal recess. The scope is inserted and the area is examined. No biopsy is performed nor tissue removed during this diagnostic procedure. For code 31287, the scope is inserted into the sphenoid sinus (as for code 31235) through the ethmoid sinus. The surgeon uses forceps and punches a hole through the ostium into the sphenoid sinus. The middle turbinate may be resected and/or fractured to allow better access. If the surgeon removes any polyps or diseased tissue, 31288 is assigned.

EXAMPLE

The physician completed the ethmoidectomy posteriorly on the left side and entered the sphenoid sinus. Care was taken to inspect the eyes and ballot the eyes repeatedly. Code: 31287.

REIMBURSEMENT REVIEW

Nasal/sinus endoscopy procedures are paid via multiple endoscopy rules. When multiple endoscopies that share the same base endoscopy are performed on the same date of service, they are termed *related*. Typically, these endoscopies are performed through the same orifice (i.e., nose, throat). When listing these procedure codes on the claim, the coder should determine which endoscopy has the highest value based on the RVU price, which is usually paid at 100% of the fee schedule allowed amount. Payment for any subsequent endoscopies will be reimbursed at the difference between the subsequent 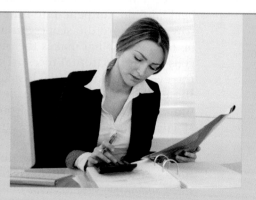 endoscopy RVU price and the base endoscopy RVU price. The secondary endoscopies are reduced by the percentage that is representative of the value of the base endoscopy.

Procedures that are included in the multiple endoscopy edits are those procedures on the National Physician Fee Schedule Relative Value File, published by the Centers for Medicare and Medicaid Services (CMS), that have an indicator of "3" in the Multiple Procedure ("Mult Proc") field. The base endoscopy for these procedures is indicated in the "Endo Base" field. The majority of the procedures affected by this reduction methodology are shoulder and knee arthroscopies, laryngoscopies, bronchoscopies, and colonoscopies. Note that sinus endoscopies are not included in this methodology because they do not have the indicator of "3" in the Multiple Procedure field.

EXAMPLE

A patient is seen in the physician office and has an indirect laryngoscopy with biopsy (31510 with an RVU 5.28) and an indirect laryngoscopy with injection of the vocal cords (31513 with an RVU 3.41). Code 31510 will be reimbursed at 100% of the allowed amount and 31513 will be reimbursed at an RVU of 1.87, which is 54.8% of the secondary endoscopy code's RVU.

Sinus Endoscopy With Balloon Catheter

When sinus endoscopy (with or without video) is used with a balloon catheter to open the ostia to the frontal, maxillary, or sphenoid sinuses, the work is similar to when a surgeon is using forceps, a microdebrider, or a laser because the end result is displacement of bone and mucosa. The balloon is placed by using the assistance of a sinus endoscope to position the balloon prior to and during the cannulation of the ostia. The scope is also used to confirm that the ostia was successfully dilated. During this sinusotomy procedure, bone and mucosa are moved by inflating the balloon (similar to the technique used in vessel angioplasty), which forces the mucosa and bone to shift and packs the mucosa against the ostia wall, significantly enlarging the ostia of the affected sinus. No tissue removal is involved in this procedure. Surgical sinus endoscopy code 31256, 31276, or 31287 is assigned based on the sinus ostia treated.

Ethmoid Sinusoscopy

Resection of the uncinate process and infundibulum is part of an ethmoidectomy procedure.

Ethmoid sinusoscopies are reported with codes 31254 and 31255. Unlike with the maxillary codes, there is no code for a diagnostic ethmoid sinusoscopy. Recognizing anatomical landmarks can assist in assigning the correct codes. The uncinate process is a mound of bone after the infundibulum that is present as the ethmoid bullae is entered. Once you see the terms *infundibulum* or *uncinate process*, you know that the ethmoid sinus has been entered. The basal lamella of the middle turbinate divides the ethmoid air cells into anterior and posterior groups. The agger nasi air cell is classified as an extramural ethmoid air cell,

CPT	DESCRIPTION	MULT PROC	RVU FACILITY	RVU NON-FACILITY	ENDO BASE
31510	Laryngoscopy with biopsy	3	3.13	5.28	31505
31511	Remove foreign body, larynx	3	3.42	5.29	31505
31512	Removal of larynx lesion	3	3.36	5.2	31505
31513	Injection into vocal cord	3	3.41	3.41	31505
31527	Laryngoscopy for treatment	3	5.02	5.02	31525
31528	Laryngoscopy and dilation	3	3.75	3.75	31525
31529	Laryngoscopy and dilation	3	4.21	4.21	31525
31530	Laryngoscopy w/fb removal	3	5.16	5.16	31525
31628	Bronchoscopy/lung bx, each	3	5.10	10.71	31622
31629	Bronchoscopy/needle bx, each	3	5.45	15.81	31622
31630	Bronchoscopy dilate/fx repr	3	5.45	5.45	31622
31631	Bronchoscopy, dilate w/stent	3	6.17	6.17	31622

Current Procedural Terminology © 2016 American Medical Association, All Rights Reserved.

According to CMS's fee schedule, the four FESS procedures have zero global days. Therefore, any services performed after the day of surgery should be separately payable by carriers that follow CMS payment guidelines.

If a patient visits the ENT office the next day to be evaluated postoperatively or to have packing removed and replaced, the office visit would be coded as an established patient visit 9921x. No modifier is needed because the examination is not being performed during the global period of another procedure.

because it projects anterior to the ethmoid bone. In 31254, the scope is inserted into the anterior ethmoid sinus and the surgeon debrides the cavity by taking down air cells. If the physician takes down the ethmoid air cells anterior to the "grand lamellae," it is an anterior ethmoidectomy. If he goes beyond the grand lamellae, it is a posterior or "total" ethmoidectomy and reported with 31255. This procedure is also referred to as an *anterior posterior ethmoidectomy (APE)*.

> When listing sinus endoscopy codes on the claim, be sure to properly link the diagnosis code for the sinus disease to the respective CPT code for the sinus treated.

EXAMPLE

The left middle turbinate was retracted to the midline and the uncinate process was exposed. A left anterior ethmoidectomy was performed removing polypoid tissue and mucoid material. The stenotic middle meatus was enlarged using up-biting and side-biting forceps. Code: 31254.

Image Guidance

Many ENT surgeons are using CT image guided technology when performing intricate sinus endoscopies. Stereotactic computer-assisted navigation (SCAN), for example, provides the surgeon with a clear view of intracranial and extracranial structures such as areas near the eyes, brain, major veins, arteries, and nerves that may be encountered during FESS. A computer is used to correlate the scope's orientation to the CT image viewed on a monitor to assist the surgeon in navigating the sinus cavities. It provides image enhancement when scarring may be present and usual anatomical landmarks are no longer in place, or on complex sinus cases where the anatomy may be distorted. The idea behind using this technology is to avoid complications and reduce the risk of puncturing the cerebral spinal fluid or injuring the eye because the sinus cavities share a thin common wall with the eye cavity and/or the brain.

SCAN is reported by ENT physicians during sinus endoscopy surgery using CPT code +61782. This is an add-on code and is not bundled into the codes for sinus endoscopy procedures. Documentation should be present in the operative report indicating the use of this technology. Some key terms to look for are *3D visualization, 3D stereotactic visualization, image guided technique,* and *InstaTrak system.* Some Medicare carriers may have Local Coverage Determinations with restrictions on reporting these codes and their medical necessity, so coders should check their state's CMS carrier website for policies pertaining to this.

Sinusotomy or Sinus Endoscopy With Sinusotomy? Do not confuse the two approaches to sinus surgery. When a sinusotomy is performed in conjunction with a sinus endoscopy, only one service may be reported. CPT manual instructions indicate that surgical sinus endoscopy includes a sinusotomy (if appropriate) and a diagnostic sinus endoscopy. However, it may be medically necessary in extreme cases when a sinusotomy and a sinus endoscopy are performed to evaluate adequacy of the sinusotomy and visualize the sinus cavity for disease. If this in fact occurs, it is appropriate to report the sinus endoscopy CPT code rather than the sinusotomy CPT code. Here is why: The sinus endoscopy codes have a higher RVU and require greater work, and surgical sinus endoscopies include a sinusotomy and diagnostic sinus endoscopy. If, however, a procedure is planned as a sinus endoscopy and the surgeon cannot fully complete the surgery endoscopically due to scarring or an intricate anatomy, for example, and the procedure is converted to an open sinusotomy technique, then only the open procedure code can be reported. Keep in mind that certain types of sinusoscopies require an incision (sinusotomy) into the sinus cavity to accomplish the sinusoscopy. In those cases the sinusotomy is included in the sinusoscopy procedures.

> Sinus endoscopy codes are unilateral so if the procedure is performed on both sides, a –50 modifier is needed. If all four sinuses were examined bilaterally, four CPT codes would be listed, each with a –50 modifier.

Assigning Sinus Endoscopy Codes

You can use the following steps and Pinpoint the Code 19.1 as guides in assigning codes for sinus endoscopy procedures.

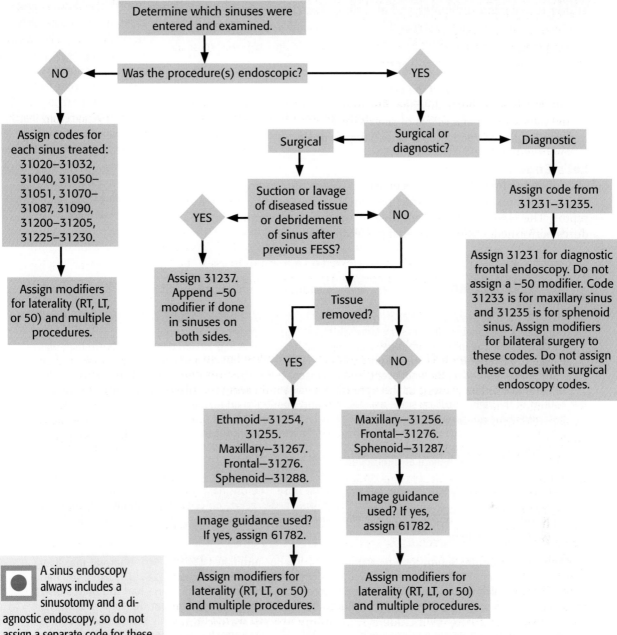

Determine which sinuses were entered and examined.

Was the procedure(s) endoscopic?

NO → Assign codes for each sinus treated: 31020–31032, 31040, 31050–31051, 31070–31087, 31090, 31200–31205, 31225–31230.

Assign modifiers for laterality (RT, LT, or 50) and multiple procedures.

YES → Surgical or diagnostic?

Surgical → Suction or lavage of diseased tissue or debridement of sinus after previous FESS?

YES → Assign 31237. Append –50 modifier if done in sinuses on both sides.

NO → Tissue removed?

YES → Ethmoid—31254, 31255. Maxillary—31267. Frontal—31276. Sphenoid—31288.

Image guidance used? If yes, assign 61782.

Assign modifiers for laterality (RT, LT, or 50) and multiple procedures.

NO → Maxillary—31256. Frontal—31276. Sphenoid—31287.

Image guidance used? If yes, assign 61782.

Assign modifiers for laterality (RT, LT, or 50) and multiple procedures.

Diagnostic → Assign code from 31231–31235.

Assign 31231 for diagnostic frontal endoscopy. Do not assign a –50 modifier. Code 31233 is for maxillary sinus and 31235 is for sphenoid sinus. Assign modifiers for bilateral surgery to these codes. Do not assign these codes with surgical endoscopy codes.

A sinus endoscopy always includes a sinusotomy and a diagnostic endoscopy, so do not assign a separate code for these procedures. All diagnostic nasal and sinus endoscopies include interior nasal cavity, middle and superior meatus, turbinates, and sphenoethmoid recess procedures. Do not code these separately from 31231–31235. If all of these elements are not fully examined append modifier –52 (reduced services) if a repeat examination is not planned. If a repeat examination is planned, append modifier –53 (discontinued procedure).

1. What sinuses were examined?
2. Was the entire procedure performed endoscopically?
3. Was this procedure diagnostic or surgical? Code only the surgical endoscopy.
4. If surgical, was tissue removed or polyps excised?
5. Was the exact same procedure done bilaterally or unilaterally? There are many times when different procedures are performed on the same sinuses but on different sides. This would not be considered bilateral unless the exact procedure was performed on the same sinuses on both sides.
6. Was image guidance used?

■ CASE SCENARIO

A patient has chronic sinusitis of the ethmoid and frontal sinuses due to enlarged turbinates and allergies. Physician performs anterior surgical ethmoidectomy and frontal sinus exploration bilaterally. Codes: 31254–50, 31276–50.

INTERNET RESOURCE: Visit the ENT USA website and read more about endoscopic sinus surgery and view pictures and videos of sinus surgery. www.entusa.com/endoscopic_sinus_surgery.htm

Let's Code It

The following operative report is dissected using color coding to help you understand and apply the abstracting concept when reading an operative report. The colors are representative of separate and significant procedures performed. Code the following operative report.

Control of bleeding is an integral component of endoscopic procedures and is not separately reportable. If bleeding occurs in the postoperative period requiring a return to the operating room, a code for bleeding control may be reported with modifier 78 indicating that the procedure was a complication of a recent procedure. If the bleeding is not severe enough to warrant the need for the operating room, it is not separately reportable.

PREOPERATIVE DIAGNOSIS: Chronic airway obstruction, chronic rhinosinusitis, mass lesion, left maxillary sinus.

OPERATION: Submucous resection of the inferior turbinates. Bilateral maxillary FESS antrostomy wtih removal of mucocele right maxillary sinus. Bilateral endoscopic ethmoidectomy.

PROCEDURE: The inferior turbinates were injected bilaterally. A flap 2.0 cm wide and 2.5 cm high was elevated. Vasomotor tissue was removed from each inferior turbinate and the flaps returned to their normal position. Using the endoscope and microscope, the right sinus area was then examined. The right middle turbinate was gently elevated. The uncinate process was reflected anteriorly. The natural ostium of the right maxillary sinus was located and opened in an inferior posterior direction, creating an antrostomy approximately 2.2 cm in size. A large mucocele was found filling the maxillary sinus. Extremely viscid mucus was located in this area. This was all removed. The right anterior ethmoid air cells were taken down. Mucosal edema was noted in this area. The edema was traced into the posterior ethmoid air cells which were also removed.

Attention was then directed to the left side of the nose. The uncinate process was removed and the maxillary sinus ostium located. The ostium was enlarged creating an opening in an inferior posterior direction. The anterior and posterior air cells were also opened in similar manner to the right side. Packs were placed bilaterally.

Answer Rationale: Submucous resection of the inferior turbinates (30140–50). Bilateral maxillary FESS antrostomy (31256–LT) with removal of mucocele right maxillary sinus (31267–RT). Here you had to discern which maxillary sinus had the antrostomy performed and which one had the antrostomy with mucocele or tissue removed. CPT instructs that both cannot be reported for the same side. It is a common trap to assign either 31267–50 or 31256–50 if you do not thoroughly review the operative report. Bilateral endoscopic ethmoidectomy (31255–50): We know this was done bilaterally because the procedure is explained for both left and right sides. This was a complete ethmoidectomy because both the anterior and posterior ethmoids were entered and tissue removed.

Assign codes to the following procedures. Include any necessary modifiers.

1. Bilateral inferior turbinate reduction _____

2. Nasal sinus endoscopy with maxillary antrostomy, anterior ethmoidectomy, bilateral

    _____

3. Removal of a Lego from a child's nose under anesthesia _____

4. Diagnosis: right nasal polyp. Procedure: excision of nasal mass. An incision was made along the dome-like polyp just posterior to the nasal sill. This continued laterally underneath the right inferior turbinate. The lesion was bluntly dissected. It was removed in its entirety. _____

5. Diagnosis: deviated septum with hypertrophic turbinates. Procedure: septoplasty and submucous resection of inferior turbinates. The deviated parts of the quadrilateral cartilage were resected. A nasal speculum was then used to expose the inferior turbinate on the right. The soft tissues were elevated off the inferior turbinate bone, which was then resected. A Bovie suction was placed in the resected cavity to shrink it. The same procedure was carried out on the opposite side. The mucoperichondrium of the septum was reapproximated with 4-0 catgut. _____

6. Diagnosis: intranasal tumor. Procedure: removal of nasal tumor. A right intercartilaginous incision was made and the entire nasal dorsum was exteriorized. There was a tumor on the lateral nasal bone measuring 1–2 cm. A retractor was placed in the nose. The tumor was removed down to the underlying bone. A Denver splint was applied to the nose. _____

7. Diagnosis: persistent epistaxis. Procedure: nasal endoscopy with cauterization. During the past few days patient has had persistent brisk bleeding. The scope was inserted into the nose and the nasal passages were suctioned of blood clots. A very brisk bleeding arteriole was located on the left floor of the nose. It was cauterized. A similar arteriole was encountered on the right side and was also cauterized. _____

8. Diagnosis: pansinusitis; nasal polyposis. Procedure: shaver-assisted intranasal polypectomy with ethmoidectomies. The patient had huge polyps present exuding from the middle meati bilaterally. The bulk of the polyps were snared. The remaining polyps were debrided. Anterior–posterior ethmoidectomies were accomplished. _____

COMMON PROCEDURES OF THE LARYNX

Laryngoscopy can be performed for diagnostic or surgical purposes, depending on the goal for the procedure. Laryngoscopies are performed for biopsy, removal of foreign body (FB), dilation of the larynx, diagnostic examination of the pharynx/larynx up to the first tracheal ring, injection of vocal cords, and excision of lesions of the larynx/pharynx. Laryngoscopies are indicated when a patient complains of persistent sore throat, difficulty swallowing, or persistent hoarseness. As with all scope procedures, a diagnostic laryngoscopy is always included in a surgical laryngoscopy. Examination can be of the pharyngeal region, larynx, and vocal cords, arytenoid, cricoid cartilage, epiglottis, and first tracheal ring.

Laryngoscopy is either direct or indirect. Indirect laryngoscopy is performed with the use of mirrors to view the larynx, pharyngeal walls, oropharynx, and posterior third of the tongue. A mirror is placed in the back of the throat and another is held outside the mouth. This procedure can be difficult to perform on patients who have strong gag reflexes. Direct laryngoscopy requires a scope to be passed through the mouth and pharynx to the larynx to directly view the larynx and surrounding area without the use of mirrors. This would be done in a facility under general anesthesia. A microscope may be used during the direct procedure to magnify the image of the larynx. If the word *microlaryngoscopy* is mentioned in the operative note, then it would be appropriate to assign either 31526 or 31531. A parenthetical note is present that informs the coder not to separately assign 69990 for the operating microscope because it is part of the following procedures: 31526, 31531, 31536, 31541, 31561, and 31571.

> ● If general anesthesia is not administered, a surgical (operative) laryngoscopy code cannot be assigned. Instead use the flexible fiber-optic or direct laryngoscopy codes.

> ● If the physician indicates that a microscope was used to perform the laryngoscopy, assign a code that states "with operating microscope or telescope" in lieu of also assigning 69990. Such codes include 31526, 31531, 31536, 31541, 31545, 31546, 31561, and 31571.

Flexible Fiber-Optic Laryngoscopy

Flexible fiber-optic laryngoscopy is a method of direct visualization of the larynx using a flexible scope that permits the attachment of instruments at the end. Examination is of the same areas as the laryngoscopy procedures but instead of inducing general anesthesia, a topical anesthesia with a vasoconstrictor is applied and the scope is advanced through the nasal cavity into the larynx and pharynx.

The following must be considered when assigning a laryngoscopy code:

- Was the laryngoscopy diagnostic or surgical? Think about what the purpose is. Remember that as soon as a biopsy is done or tissue is removed, it is no longer a diagnostic study.
- Was the laryngoscopy direct or indirect or flexible fiber-optic?
- If it was direct, did it require a microscope or flexible fiber-optic scope?
- Was a lesion removed and a biopsy taken of a separate area? If so, the biopsy can be coded separately if the site of the biopsy is different than the site of removal or ablation.
- Was stroboscopy used; that is, did the physician insert a strobe light to better visualize the movement of the vocal cords?

EXAMPLE

Patient is placed under general anesthesia. Laryngoscope is inserted and the vocal cords are examined. Leukoplakia is identified and the physician utilizes a microscope to obtain a small biopsy.

Code: 31536   Hint that this is a direct operative procedure.   Look for a code that states operative microscope.   Hint that this is a direct operative procedure.

Laryngectomy

Laryngectomy is the surgical removal of the larynx because of malignancy of the larynx or the immediate area such as the thyroid. The malignancies may be primary or secondary or of uncertain behavior. Laryngectomy may also be incident to trauma to the throat area. The code range for laryngectomy procedures is 31360–31395. These codes include qualifiers such as "with" or "without," "partial," "subtotal," and "radical neck dissection." The coder needs to read the operative report carefully to seek the information necessary to make decisions in code assignment based on these qualifiers.

Cervical Neck Dissection

The lymph nodes of the neck are divided into seven regions or levels. These levels correspond to anatomical landmarks of the nodes of the neck, musculature, and vasculature. These levels are used in reading and reporting imaging of the neck and in cervical neck dissections. Some lymph nodes are not part of any of these levels, and are described by their anatomical location. The number of lymph node levels removed does not correlate to whether the dissection was radical or modified.

Radical neck dissection consists of:

- Cervical lymphadenectomy (all nodes of the lateral neck, under the chin and mandible, supraclavicular nodes) (Level I)
- Dissection of the submandibular and posterior triangles (Levels III and V)
- Sternocleidomastoid (SCM) muscle
- Spinal accessory nerve
- Internal jugular vein

Radical neck dissection does not include removal of the suboccipital nodes, periparotid nodes (except infraparotid nodes located in the posterior aspect of the submandibular triangle), buccinator nodes, retropharyngeal nodes, and midline visceral (anterior compartment) nodes. Modified radical neck dissection is a scaled-down version of a radical neck dissection in an effort to improve a patient's quality of life. One or more nonlymphatic structures are preserved: spinal accessory nerve, internal jugular vein, or SCM muscle. The structure(s) preserved should be specifically named in the operative report similar to the following: "modified radical neck dissection with preservation of the internal jugular vein." The term *selective* neck dissection is an indicator that a modified radical neck dissection was performed.

INTERNET RESOURCE: Visit www.cancernetwork.com/oncology-journal/current-concepts-surgical -management-neck-metastases-head-and-neck-cancer/ to learn more about radical neck dissections.

Laryngectomy Procedure

The skin incision for a laryngectomy may be made with a scalpel or electrocautery inferior to the mastoid tip with a straight line to the trapezius. Incisions may be extended vertically overlying the anterior border of the trapezius to the mastoid tip or toward the clavicle. A flap is elevated in the subplatysmal plane, immediately above anterior and external jugular veins. Strap muscles are transected with a hemostat or cautery. The thyroid isthmus is divided and the thyroid gland is dissected away from the trachea (may remove ipsilateral lobe along with larynx). Two to four centimeters of the inferior skin flap is trimmed and the subcutaneous fat is removed in preparation for the lower border of the tracheostomy site to mature (tracheostoma). Soft tissue is cleaned off the anterior tracheal wall and an incision is made between the second and third rings. The incision is continued superolaterally into the trachea. The endotracheal tube is pushed into the stoma. A scalpel is used to cut the anterior tracheal wall. After the anterior wall of the tracheostoma is created, the endotracheal tube is removed and a flexible tube is placed into the stoma and sutured to the chest. A radical or modified radical neck dissection may also be performed. Constrictor muscles from the thyroid ala are detached with a cautery or scalpel blade. The suprahyoid musculature is dissected off the superior border of the hyoid bone with monopolar dissection. The larynx is entered from above. Most often, it is entered from the vallecula. The surgeon will palpate the vallecula with his finger while inserting a retractor through the mouth and will confirm the end of the retractor immediately above the hyoid. The surgeon will cut into the neck until he sees the retractor appear into the neck wound. The neck is then dissected laterally from the point of entry to expose the supraglottis. The diseased side of the larynx is separated from posterolateral wall mucosa with scissor cuts. Final separation of the larynx is performed from below with scalpel incision of the posterior tracheal wall. The larynx is removed from the patient with upward traction on the larynx to permit inspection of the surgical margin, esophageal introitus, and trachea as the final cuts are made.

A nasogastric feeding tube is placed and the pharynx is closed with sutures. The tracheostoma is completed by suturing the undersurface of the upper and lower flaps to the cartilage of the

Laryngectomy codes with bilateral neck dissection cannot be appended with a −50 modifier when neck dissection is carried out bilaterally. We only have one larynx. According to the CMS physician fee schedule, these codes have a bilateral indicator of "0." When a total laryngectomy with bilateral radical neck dissection is performed, the −50 modifier should not be appended. Instead, report code 31365, *Laryngectomy; total, with radical neck dissection,* to identify the total laryngectomy and radical neck dissection on one side of the neck and use code 38720–59, *Cervical lymphadenectomy (complete),* to identify the radical neck dissection on the opposite side of the neck.

Use Table 19.2 to help guide you as to when it is appropriate to report cervical node dissection in addition to the laryngectomy or pharyngectomy procedure. Cervical node dissection can be reported when it is performed with another procedure that does not include neck dissections in the description.

Table 19.2 Laryngectomy or Pharyngectomy

PROCEDURE CODE	CERVICAL DISSECTION CODE	SEPARATELY REPORTABLE?	MODIFIER FOR DISSECTION
31360	38724	Y	−58 or −59 or −51
31365	38724	Y, if performed on opposite side from radical	−58 or −59 or LT/RT
31367	38724	Y	−51
31368	38724	Y, if performed on opposite side from radical	−58 or −59 or LT/RT
31390	38724	Y, if performed on opposite side from radical	−58 or −59 or LT/RT

trachea. The platysma is sutured closed and the skin is stapled. In 31360 and 31365, the surgeon may also remove a portion of the base of the tongue and upper esophagus.

Subtotal supraglottic laryngectomies are performed through the thyroid cartilage without radical neck dissection (31367). The epiglottis, false vocal cords, part or all of the hyoid bone, and superior part of the laryngeal cartilage are removed. A horizontal neck incision is made when performing a subtotal supraglottic laryngectomy with radical neck dissection (31368). Code 31370 is an operation to remove the epiglottis, false vocal cords, and superior half of the thyroid cartilage. It is performed with only partial removal of the supraglottic structures. A supracricoid laryngectomy is also reported with 31367. It differs from the code described below because this procedure removes the entire larynx. This technique is similar to a supraglottic laryngectomy in which the surgeon contains the resection to the laryngeal structures above the vocal cord/arytenoid areas only. The laryngectomy code includes all related laryngeal tissue/cartilage procedures and a tracheotomy. If the surgeon also removes lymph nodes, you should separately report this surgery using 38720–38724.

Partial Laryngectomy

The intended goal of a partial laryngectomy is to avoid a permanent tracheostomy, maintain laryngeal speech, and preserve the swallowing function. Partial laryngectomy codes are assigned based on the approach: horizontal (31370), laterovertical (31375), anterovertical (31380), or antero-latero-vertical (31382). A supracricoid partial laryngectomy is a horizontal partial laryngectomy technique. A supracricoid laryngectomy includes removal of the entire supraglottis, the false and true vocal cords, and the thyroid cartilage, including the paraglottic and preepiglottic spaces. In some cases, one arytenoid may be resected. The cricoid cartilage, hyoid bone, and at least one arytenoid are saved. This technique spares speaking and swallowing functions.

Vertical partial laryngectomies are performed for early glottic carcinoma. A low collar incision is made and the tracheostomy is placed through a separate horizontal incision below the collar incision. The surgeon develops subplatysmal flaps, exposing the larynx by separating the strap muscles vertically and incising the external perichondrium and along the superior and inferior borders of the thyroid cartilage. Laryngofissure is performed with an oscillating saw and may be referred to as a *midline thyrotomy*. This step is performed for all vertical partial laryngectomy procedures unless the anterior commissure is involved. Once the laryngofissure is completed and the incision in the cricothyroid membrane is made, the vocal cords are inspected from below. If the anterior commissure is disease free, the internal mucoperichondrium is divided at or near the anterior commissure. The entire vocal cord is then resected. In the laterovertical approach (31375), the vocal cord and adjacent cartilage are resected.

The anterovertical approach (31380) is performed by making incisions in both halves of the thyroid cartilage. The affected areas of the vocal cords are resected. The antero-latero-vertical (31382) procedure also removes part and sometimes all of the arytenoid.

> If the coder reads that hypopharyngeal and oropharyngeal wall excisions were carried out during a laryngectomy, this is a clear indication that a pharyngolaryngectomy was performed because these excisions are not part of a laryngectomy.

Pharyngolaryngectomy

A pharyngolaryngectomy is performed to remove malignant tumors from the larynx that have also spread into the pharynx. A pharyngolaryngectomy may also be indicated when both the larynx and pharynx have been severely damaged by disease or injury. A pharyngolaryngectomy includes the removal of the larynx and the pharynx. This procedure always includes

In a laryngotomy, an incision is made over the larynx to bring the larynx into open view. The surgeon can remove a tumor, laryngocele, or vocal cord without removing the larynx itself. Read the documentation carefully before assigning a code to be sure the larynx was partially or totally removed before assigning a laryngectomy code.

a radical neck dissection. The discerning factor in code assignment here is whether reconstruction with a myocutaneous flap using the pectoris major muscle was performed. Assign 31390 when the procedure has no reconstruction and 31395 when neck reconstruction is done at the same operative session.

The procedure is performed by turning the patient's head to one side and making two curved incisions, one from just behind the ear to the chin, and the other low down on the neck. Another small incision is made below this in the trachea (i.e., a tracheostomy) to create the permanent stoma. After the larynx has been removed, the areas of the pharynx affected by the tumor are cut out and the slit in the esophagus is sutured closed. A nasogastric tube is then inserted through the nose and down the esophagus to the stomach. The esophagus connection to the mouth is reconstructed by a skin graft, complete with blood supply and muscular support, taken from the chest, back, or forearm. A skin graft from the thigh is used to repair the area from which the main graft is taken. A more radical version of this procedure involves the removal of part of the esophagus, and sometimes, the thyroid and parathyroid glands as well. In this case more extensive grafting is needed, and often a section of small intestine is used to replace the esophageal section removed. Some cases require a two-stage operation. Final plastic reconstruction is performed about 3 weeks after the initial operation.

Let's Code It

PREOPERATIVE DIAGNOSIS: Squamous cell carcinoma left oropharynx, hypopharynx, and larynx.
PROCEDURES: Pharyngolaryngectomy, left modified neck dissection, right neck dissection, left pectoralis major flap, resection of pharyngeal wall, pharyngoplasty.

Apron incision was made through the skin and subcutaneous tissue through the platysmal muscle. Flaps were elevated superiorly with preservation of the fascia of the submandibular glands. Flaps were elevated inferiorly and posteriorly on the left side to the anterior border of the trapezius. The sternocleidomastoid muscle was divided anteriorly and superiorly on the left side sparing the spinal accessory nerve. The posterior triangle soft tissue contents from the trapezius up to the level of the digastric were dissected free. The external jugular and the internal jugular veins were ligated. The level IV nodal contents were brought from posterior to anterior along the deep cervical fascia. The tissue was divided high to preserve the phrenic nerve. The jugular vein and Level II–III nodes were brought anteriorly and the jugular vein was ligated. Level I nodes were then removed from the submandibular and submental region.

On the right, a level I–IV neck dissection was performed. A deep plane of dissection was carried out along the deep cervical fascia. Over the carotid sheath, nerves along with the carotid and jugular vein were spared. The strap musculature was divided and the left upper thyroid gland was divided from the lower half and reflected free from the trachea. The right thyroid lobes were divided similarly. The trachea was divided below the second tracheal ring and the tracheostomy was created. The dissection was carried along the line between the trachea and the esophagus to the inferior aspect of the cricoid cartilage.

A forcep was inserted into the oral cavity and used to demarcate the left piriform sinus that was subsequently incised. Scissors were used to extend the cut along the aspect of the left piriform sinus from inferior to superior. The tumor was visualized and then resected with 10-mm margins along the posterior hypopharyngeal and oropharyngeal wall. The dissection was advanced around the vallecula and into the left tongue base. The tumor was resected completely. Attention was moved to creating and harvesting the pectoralis major flap.

The pectoralis major flap was elevated and transferred through a subcutaneous tunnel from the chest to the neck. The chest donor site did not need complex closure and was closed with 3-0 Vicryl in an interrupted fashion. The flap along with the soft tissue of the neck was used to perform pharyngoplasty.

Answer Rationale: 31360. Neck dissection was not radical because it spared the spinal accessory nerve on the left. Code 31395 is not assigned here because laryngectomy or pharyngolaryngectomy codes do not include the hypopharyngeal or oropharyngeal wall excisions. The following codes are represented within the operative report but all are included in code 31360: 42894, 15733, 38724, 42950.

Steps in Assigning Laryngectomy Codes

To ensure consistency in the approach to code assignment, coders should use the following steps and the decision tree shown in Pinpoint the Code 19.2 to walk through the logic.

1. Determine if the laryngectomy included a pharyngectomy. If so, discern if it was done with or without reconstruction.
2. Determine if the laryngectomy was a partial or total laryngectomy.
3. Determine if the procedure was performed with or without radical neck dissection.
4. For a partial laryngectomy, determine if it was horizontal, laterovertical, anterovertical, or antero-lateral vertical.

PINPOINT THE CODE 19.2: Laryngectomy

COMMON PROCEDURES OF THE PHARYNX

A pharyngectomy is the partial or total removal of the pharynx. The code range for a pharyngectomy is 42890–42894. A pharyngectomy procedure is performed to treat cancers of the pharynx such as throat cancer and hypopharyngeal carcinoma. A total or partial pharyngectomy is usually performed for cancers of the hypopharynx in which all or part of the hypopharynx is removed. Whether a pharyngectomy is performed in total or with only partial removal depends on the localized amount of cancer found. This procedure can be performed alone or in conjunction with partial laryngectomy, complete laryngectomy, or esophagectomy. When the procedure involves removal of the larynx it is called a *pharyngolaryngectomy*,

CPT code 42894 does not include the work of developing the flaps; therefore, it would be appropriate to report it separately by using 15733. Additionally, if a free flap is performed for reconstruction, it should also be reported separately.

which is discussed in the next section. Well-localized, early-stage hypopharyngeal tumors can be treated by a partial pharyngectomy. Following a total or partial pharyngectomy, the surgeon may also need to reconstruct the throat so that the patient can swallow. Code 42890 is assigned for limited pharyngectomy. If radical neck dissection is also performed, CPT instructs physicians to bill 38720 separately. If a modified radical neck dissection is performed, assign 38724 instead of 38720. Code 42892 is reported if the lateral pharyngeal wall is resected and closed with advancement of the lateral and posterior pharyngeal walls. If the pharyngeal walls are resected and require closure with a myocutaneous or fasciocutaneous flap, or a free muscle, skin, or fascial flap with microvascular anastomosis, assign 42984.

Pharyngectomy Procedure

A vertical neck incision is made in the form of a half "H" or "T" on the side of the patient's neck from the vertical limb of the anterior border of the trapezius to the horizontal limb at the level of the thyrohyoidal membrane. The incision is deepened and the strap muscles are retracted. Flaps are elevated until the larynx is exposed. The anterior jugular veins and strap muscles are left undisturbed. The SCM muscle is then identified. The layer of cervical fibrous tissue is incised longitudinally from the hyoid above to the clavicle below. Part of the hyoid is then divided, which allows the surgeon to enter a loose compartment bound by the sternomastoid muscle and the pharynx and larynx. Using scissors, the surgeon performs bilateral, direct cuts, separating the pharynx from the larynx. The larynx is retracted. The incisions are made and the pharynx is removed. The wound is thoroughly irrigated; all clots are removed; and the wound is closed. The pharyngeal wall is closed in two layers. In code 42892, the surgeon removes the diseased pharyngeal wall or piriform sinus. In code 42894, in addition to the previous procedures, the surgeon also creates a myocutaneous flap and reconstructs the pharyngeal area using muscle from the chest (pectoralis major). This is called a *tubed pectoralis major myocutaneous flap*. The flap is rotated and pulled through a tunnel created and sutured at the pharynx. Microvascular free flaps are increasingly being used for reconstruction of pharyngoesophageal defects including the jejunal flap, the tubed radial forearm flap, and the anterolateral thigh flap. Other methods include colon interposition and gastric pull-up and are reported separately.

Coders should use the decision tree shown in Pinpoint the Code 19.3 to aid in correct pharyngectomy code assignment.

PINPOINT THE CODE 19.3: Pharyngectomy

Tracheostomy

A tracheostomy is a surgical procedure performed in the front of the neck. An incision is made through the neck and into the trachea to provide access to the windpipe. A tracheostomy tube is then placed into the windpipe below the larynx. This artificial opening is used to assist people with breathing who otherwise cannot breathe on their own. It can be performed either emergently as in the case of trauma or foreign body in the proximal windpipe, or it can be planned as part of managing patients with cancer of the neck and other illnesses. At times, stroke victims may suffer from paralysis of the muscles that affect swallowing, which necessitates assistance in breathing. The word *tracheostomy* is used synonymously with tracheotomy, which is somewhat inaccurate. Tracheotomy is the actual act of making a horizontal incision in the neck, dissecting through muscle and tissue and entering the trachea. The tracheostomy or "stoma" is what is created once the incision is made and the tube is inserted by sewing the skin and the tissue layers around the tube to maintain the opening. Tracheostomy can be either temporary or permanent. Codes are selected based on age, circumstance (planned or emergent), and approach—transtracheal or cricothyroid. The transtracheal approach is the most common, where the incision is made just above the sternal notch at the second or third tracheal ring. The cricothyroid is higher up the neck.

> ### ■ CASE SCENARIO
> A 35-year-old patient sustained severe head trauma in a motorcycle accident. A transtracheal tracheostomy was performed in the ED and he was placed on 28% oxygen. The tracheostomy stayed in place for a month while he was in rehabilitation. Code: 31603.

COMMON PROCEDURES OF THE LUNGS AND BRONCHI

Bronchoscopy and Tracheobronchoscopy

A bronchoscopy involves inserting a scope either through the mouth or nose to view the airway and lungs to diagnose disease. Bronchoscopies are performed for dilation of the trachea; biopsies of the lung, bronchus; and trachea; bronchial lavage; removal of FB; tumor removal; lung brachytherapy; and aspiration. Bronchoscopy codes include fluoroscopic guidance when performed; therefore, the fluoroscopy would not be reported separately.

Bronchoscopies can be performed either by using a flexible fiber-optic or rigid bronchoscope (also known as an *open-tube bronchoscope*). Fluoroscopy is an inherent component. Use of the rigid scope requires anesthesia and would be used to remove FBs or a large biopsy sample. The flexible bronchoscopy is more commonly performed and utilizes fiber-optic light to better view the bronchioles, and so on. Fiber-optic bronchoscopy typically includes viewing the nasal cavity, pharynx, larynx, and trachea, so when coding a bronchoscopy with nasal endoscopy and laryngoscopy, only report the bronchoscopy code. Code selection can be verified by consulting the NCCI edits. See Table 19.3 for an example. The highlighted areas show that these procedures are bundled into the bronchoscopy procedure.

When reviewing bronchoscopy reports, it is essential that the coder note the definitions of "brushings, washings, bronchial alveolar lavage, and total lung lavage" as defined by CPT. Cell washing or lavage involves the aspiration of small amounts of instilled sterile saline or secretions from the larger airways that are then sent for culture and/or cytology examination. Tissue is sampled by irrigating with saline and then suctioning the fluid. See CPT code 31622 for this code description. Brushings or protected brushings involve passing a catheter through the bronchoscope into an area of diseased lung tissue.

Rigid bronchoscopy is performed for FB removal from the lung, and flexible scopes are used in screening procedures for suspected cases of aspiration, for obtaining small tissue samples, and other procedures.

As with all endoscopic procedures, a diagnostic bronchoscopy is part of a surgical bronchoscopy and not reported separately.

Table 19.3 Bronchoscopy NCCI Edits Excerpt

COLUMN 1	COLUMN 2	EFFECTIVE DATE	DELETION DATE	MODIFIER
31622	31231	20030701	*	1
31622	31500	19960101	19960101	9
31622	31525	19960101	*	1
31622	31526	19960101	19960101	9
31622	31535	19960101	*	1
31622	31536	19960101	19960101	9
31622	31540	19960101	19960101	9
31622	31541	19960101	19960101	9
31622	31575	19960101	*	0
31622	31717	19960101	*	1
31622	31720	19970101	*	1
31622	31725	19970101	*	1

* Indicates deletion date is blank.

For brushings, use code 31623 one time regardless of the number of times the brush is passed.

The seal on the catheter is broken and the uncontaminated brush is used to obtain a culture by combing or brushing the mucous lining. This may include several passes of the brush. This brush is called a *protected specimen brush (PSB)*. Code 31623 describes this procedure. When a bronchoscopy with brushings or washings is performed, this is considered a diagnostic bronchoscopy and not a biopsy.

If a physician performs a percutaneous needle biopsy of the lung and a fine needle aspiration of the lung, codes 32405 and 10022 are reported together. Code 32405 describes the percutaneous needle biopsy in which a small piece of tissue is taken through the needle and examined. Code 10021 describes the fine needle aspiration where fluid or tissue is aspirated with a long needle and the cells are examined cytologically.

If the code description includes the word *lungs* the code is considered bilateral.

If both bronchial or endobronchial biopsy(s) and transbronchial biopsy(s) are performed during the same session, CPT allows you to report both 31625 and 31628. The NCCI, however, does not permit coding this combination (31625 and 31628) unless the biopsies occur on different sites of the lung or different lesions, in which case the −59 modifier is appended to the second code.

Transbronchial Lung Biopsy

Transbronchial lung biopsy involves inserting a bronchoscope into the bronchus using forceps to puncture the bronchus and through the bronchial wall to then take samples of lung tissue. Here, the pulmonologist obtains tissue from the lung's periphery using fluoroscopic guidance or blindly. The coder must review the operative note to determine the exact site of biopsy and review the path report for the presence of lung tissue if the physician only documents transbronchial lung biopsy. Confirm with the surgeon if the intent of the procedure was a lung biopsy or bronchial biopsy. This code assignment should be based on the intent to obtain *lung* tissue, not bronchial tissue. Code 31628 is used for this procedure regardless of the number of biopsies obtained from a single lobe. If more than one lobe is biopsied, also assign the add-on code 31632.

Physician performs a transbronchial lung biopsy of the left lung. Path report reflects epithelial cells and macrophages of the lung indicating inflammation. Code: 31628–LT.

Thoracoscopy

Diagnostic thoracoscopy is the direct examination of the pleural cavity using a scope. The *pleura* is the space between the lining of the outside of the lungs and the wall of the chest. Thoracoscopy is a less invasive means of treating pleural disorders because it allows the physician to view and surgically treat the pleura without having to open up the chest to access the lung. This procedure is done to

- Assess lung disease such as cancer
- Biopsy lung tissue for analysis
- Determine the cause of fluid in the chest cavity
- Introduce medications or other treatments directly into the lungs
- Treat collected fluid, pus, or blood in the pleural space

A thoracoscopy can be performed under general or local anesthesia. An incision is made between two ribs and the scope is inserted to view the chest cavity. Surgical thoracoscopies (32650–32674) are not bundled and can therefore be reported separately for each procedure.

Thoracentesis

A thoracentesis is a procedure to remove fluid from the pleura, which is the chest cavity outside of the lung. The fluid is collected and then sent off for analysis. The test is performed to determine the cause of the fluid accumulation or to relieve the symptoms associated with the fluid accumulation. Thoracentesis is indicated when a patient has pleural effusion, which is the accumulation of excess fluid between the layers of the pleura. This procedure may also be carried out to diagnose or assist in treating the following:

- Pneumonia
- Hemothorax
- Pulmonary occlusive disease
- Pulmonary embolism
- Asbestos-related pleural effusion

When performing this procedure, the physician may simply puncture the skin and advance the needle into the pleural cavity to remove fluid (32554) without imaging guidance or she may elect to place a catheter (32556) without imaging guidance. Codes 32555 and 32557 represent these services with imaging guidance. These thoracentesis codes do not reflect any type of indwelling procedure. For an indwelling tunneled pleural catheter with cuff, use code 32550. These procedures differ from pneumocentesis, which is the actual puncturing of the lung to remove fluid.

Thoracotomy

A thoracotomy is an incision into the chest wall and into the deeper structures of the thoracic cavity. It is performed to gain access to the thoracic organs such as the heart, lungs, esophagus, or thoracic aorta and for approaches to the anterior spine when performing diskectomy or spinal fusions.

Performing a thoracotomy is the first step in many lung surgeries including lobectomy or pneumonectomy and would therefore not be coded separately. Codes 32100–32160 describe thoracotomy procedures where incisions are made into the chest, but do not go as far as the

---

Review the pathology report and confirm site of biopsy to determine if a code for bronchus or lung biopsy is warranted. Both the bronchus and lung have upper, middle, and lower lobes.

Bronchoscopies are automatically considered a bilateral procedure. Do not assign a –50 modifier if performed on both lungs.

A diagnostic thoracoscopy is always included in a surgical thoracoscopy. If a surgical thoracoscopy was scheduled and attempted but the procedure could not successfully be completed endoscopically, the open procedure code should be submitted in lieu of the endoscopic code.

Instructional notes direct the coder not to report the radiology imaging guidance codes 76942, 77002, and 77012, 77021, and 75989.

lung itself. CPT has instructional notes within this section that direct the coder to other codes for resections of lung or for lung volume reduction. If any portion of the lung is removed, an excision code should be used. Thoracotomies are bundled with more extensive procedures such as lobectomies and open heart surgery.

Various approaches are used for a thoracotomy: medial, posterolateral, and anterolateral. The only difference in these procedures is where on the thorax the incision is made. The medial approach includes a sternotomy, which provides wide access to the mediastinum. A posterolateral thoracotomy is made over the fifth intercostal space and allows access to the pulmonary hilum (pulmonary artery and pulmonary vein). It is carried out as the approach for a pneumonectomy and lobectomy. An anterolateral thoracotomy is performed on the anterior chest wall and would be done when the physician needs access to the heart to perform open chest massage during trauma cases. This approach requires a rib spreader to open the cavity protected by the rib cage.

Pneumonectomy

If a surgeon takes a wedge biopsy of the lung and sends it to pathology for a frozen section and the results are positive for malignancy and the surgeon subsequently performs a more extensive procedure such as a lobectomy, both procedure codes can be reported. Code for both the subsequent lobectomy (32480–32486) and the diagnostic wedge biopsy (+32507).

If a portion of the bronchus next to a preserved segment of lung must be removed for closure to preserve function of the lung and requires plastic closure, assign code +32501, *Resection and repair of portion of bronchus [bronchoplasty] when performed at time of lobectomy or segmentectomy.* According to CPT, this code can only be reported with 32480, 32482, and 32484. CPT also instructs physicians not to use 32501 to report closure of the proximal end of a resected bronchus.

Surgeons recommend pneumonectomy if the position of a lung tumor is central within the lung and involves either the two lobes on the left or the three lobes on the right. A total pneumonectomy (32440) is removal of the entire lung. A sleeve pneumonectomy (32442) also includes resection of the tracheal carina with end-to-end anastomosis of the trachea and contralateral main stem bronchus. Extrapleural pneumonectomy (32445) additionally consists of resection of the parietal pleura, which is the thoracic lining of the ribs, diaphragm, and mediastinum.

A wedge resection (32505) is the removal of a portion of lung, less than an anatomical segment, and can be performed in any portion of a diseased lung. It may also be referred to as a limited resection or a wedge biopsy in that the lesion is excised as well as a margin of the surrounding normal lung. Code 32505 is specifically *therapeutic*. Although the surgeon typically reserves wedge resections for lesions that he expects to be benign, the specimen may turn out to be cancerous. The add-on code 32506 is reported when additional wedge resections are performed during the same session on the same side (ipsilateral) as the initial wedge resection. Code 32506 is reported in addition to code 32505. The add-on code 32507 is reported when a *diagnostic* wedge resection is followed by anatomical lung resection and it is reportable with codes 32440, 32442, 32445, 32480–32488, 32503, and 32504.

■ **CASE SCENARIO**
A patient was admitted to the hospital for malaise and irregular heart rate. Chest x-ray showed a nodule in the left upper quadrant. CT scan showed a 2.0-cm noncalcified soft tissue nodule in the apical posterior left upper lobe and nonspecific soft tissue density in the right lower lobe. Diagnosis was (1) emphysema and (2) well-marginated nodule in LLL. On day 4 of her admission, the patient underwent a left lateral thoracotomy with wedge resection of the left upper lobe. Pathology came back as benign, hemithorax lymph node sampling. On day 7 her chest tube was removed and on day 8 she was discharged home. Code: 32505.

Lobectomy and Bilobectomy

The surgeon will elect this type of operation if she thinks the cancer is isolated in one or two lobes of the lung. It is the most common type of operation for lung cancer. A lobectomy (32480) is the removal of a single lobe of the lung. This code describes either the removal of one of the three lobes in the right lung or removal of one of the two lobes in the left lung.

A bilobectomy (32482) is removal of two lobes of the right lung (i.e., right upper and right middle). A bilobectomy is not removal of one lobe from each lung, but rather the right lung exclusively.

The surgeon can make an incision in the patient's side between two of the ribs and around to the back or the incision can be made vertically through the sternum. The incision is carried deep through all the soft tissue and muscle layers and the ribs are spread open using a rib spreader. In the vertical approach, the sternum is split with a saw and rib spreaders are used to pull the rib cage open. The affected lobe(s) are removed and blood vessels and bronchial tubes are clamped off. Once the operation is complete, the incision is closed and a chest tube is placed. For the vertical incision, the sternum is wired back together and skin is then sutured closed.

Segmentectomy

Each lobe of the lung is divided up into multiple segments (Fig. 19.6). A segmentectomy (32484) is removal of one of the divisions of a lobe. The approach and operation are essentially the same as a lobectomy. CPT code 32501 describes a resection of anything other than a total lung that requires a bronchoplastic repair. A sleeve lobectomy (32486) is similar to a lobectomy but also includes removal of a portion of the bronchus going to the remaining lung. Most commonly, sleeve lobectomies are upper lobectomies. Surgeons may elect this route to avoid removing the entire lung if the cancer is central and affecting one of the bronchi. In this scenario a simple lobectomy cannot be done. The operation involves removing the affected section of the bronchus and any surrounding cancer in the lobe plus a section of the bronchus going to the lower lobe.

Completion pneumonectomy (32488) is a secondary operation in which the lung tissue remaining after previous lung excision surgery is entirely removed. For example, a portion of a lung (i.e., lobe) has been removed previously for a cancerous tumor. The cancer recurs and it is necessary to remove all of the remaining lung tissue. This subsequent removal of the remaining lung tissue on that lung is termed a *completion pneumonectomy*.

Lung Volume Reduction

Lung volume reduction surgery (LVRS) is performed on patients who typically have emphysema or some other type of pulmonary disease such as chronic obstructive pulmonary disease

> According to the CMS's physician fee schedule, this procedure is not a bilateral procedure. Do you know why? Bilobectomy is not performed on the left lung because there are only two lobes in total on that side. If both lobes of the left lung are removed, this would be considered a pneumonectomy, not a lobectomy.

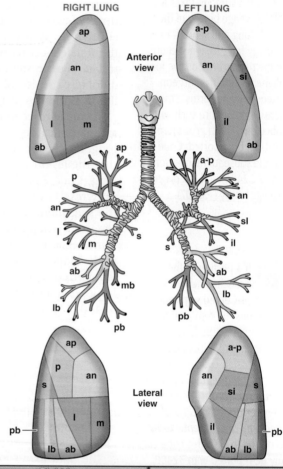

Right Lung			Left Lung	
Right upper lobe	**Right middle lobe**	**Right lower lobe**	**Left upper lobe**	**Left lower lobe**
ap - apical	**l** - lateral	**s** - superior	**a-p** - apical-posterior	**s** - superior
an - anterior	**m** - medial	**ab** - anterior basal	**an** - anterior	**ab** - anterior medial basal
P - posterior		**lb** - lateral basal	**sl** - superior lingula	**lb** - lateral basal
		pb - posterior basal	**il** - inferior lingula	**pb** - posterior basal
		mb - medial basal		

Figure 19.6 Segments of the lung.

Many of the lung lobectomies, seg-mentectomies, and wedge resections can also be performed via thoracoscope. Refer to codes 32650–32674 to assign codes using this technique.

Lung volume reduction reflects both unilateral and bilateral proce-dures as represented by the parenthetic "s" after the word "lung." It is generally a bilateral procedure.

If any additional procedures must be carried out on the donor lung such as repair or resection, assign codes 32491, 32505–32507, 35216, or 35276. For example, if a direct repair of an intrathoracic blood vessel of the donor lung is required, this is separately reported us-ing 35216, *Repair blood vessel, direct; intrathoracic, without bypass,* with a –51 modifier.

(COPD) where the most damaged areas of lung tissue are removed. It is also referred to as *reduction pneumoplasty, lung saving,* or *lung contouring.* By removing this diseased tissue, the healthy lung tissue is decompressed allowing it room to expand. Twenty to thirty-five percent of diseased lung tissue is removed to provide adequate room for the healthy lung tissue to expand and contract when inhaling and exhaling to carry out gas exchange in the blood. LVRS is performed to improve the patient's quality of life until a lung transplant is achieved. Assign code 32491 for this procedure.

Lung Transplants

Lung transplantation is complex surgery performed to remove a diseased lung(s) and replace with lung or lungs from a donor. Transplants may be indicated in patients with COPD, cystic fibrosis, pulmonary fibrosis, or pulmonary hypertension. Transplant services are reported using codes 32850–32856.

Transplant services consist of three components. The first component is the harvesting of the lung from a cadaver or living donor. Preparation of the organ includes harvesting and preservation of the organ as well as dissection of the organ from surrounding soft tissues. Organs must be perfused with a cold preservation solution and be kept cold until it is implanted. This process is reported using code 32850.

The second component of physician work is what is termed "backbench work"; work done on a separate table from the operating table where the patient is laying. Backbench work includes standard preparation of a donor organ (allograft), such as dissecting and removing unneeded soft tissue and tailoring or reconstructing the organ by altering or revising the pulmonary venous/atrial cuff, pulmonary artery, and bronchus in order to render the organ (allograft) ready to be transplanted. Backbench work is reported using a CPT code from 32855–32856.

The third component of physician work is the actual transplant (allotransplantation), which includes removal of the diseased lung, transplantation of the new lung (allograft), and the usual and customary care of the patient included in the surgical package. This last step is reported using CPT codes 32851–32854 depending on whether the transplant was a single lung with or without cardiopulmonary bypass or if the transplant was a double lung transplant with or without cardiopulmonary bypass.

Postoperative Spirometry

A post-transplant service such as spirometry analysis is conducted by the pulmonologist. Once the patient is discharged from the hospital post-transplant, the patient will be required to perform daily spirometry tests so the pulmonologist can monitor lung function. Patient-initiated spirometric recording requires the patient to perform the spirometry at specific times each day. The results are stored in a small computer that is part of the spirometer and at various scheduled times, the patient is contacted and the data are downloaded via modem from the spirometer's computer to a computer located at the hospital or provider's office. The physician analyzes the data at least once a week (and more often if necessary) and makes an interpretation so that complications such as organ rejection, infection, or bronchiolitis obliterans are recognized early. CPT codes 94014–94016 in the medicine section are reported for spirometric recording and physician review and interpretation. These codes are reported every 30 days and no sooner. These codes are intended to describe transtelephonic spirometry and should be reported with diagnosis code Z94.2.

EXAMPLES
- Code 94014, *Patient-initiated spirometric recording per 30-day period of time; includes reinforced education, transmission of spirometric tracing, data capture, analysis of transmitted data, periodic recalibration and interpretation by a physician or other qualified health-care professional,* is used to report the global service.

- Code 94015, *Patient-initiated spirometric recording per 30-day period of time; recording (includes hook-up, reinforced education, data transmission, data capture, trend analysis, and periodic recalibration),* is used to report the technical component.
- Code 94016, *Patient-initiated spirometric recording per 30-day period of time; physician review and interpretation only by a physician or other qualified health-care professional,* is used to report the professional component.

CHECKPOINT 19.2

Assign codes to the following procedures. Include any necessary modifiers.

1. Direct diagnostic laryngoscopy and tracheoscopy with operating microscope

   _____

2. Bronchoscopy with biopsy of bronchus and transbronchial biopsy of lung _____

3. Insertion of tube for tube thoracostomy for drainage of hemothorax _____

4. Planned tracheostomy on infant _____

5. Microlaryngoscopy with biopsy of posterior larynx _____

6. Patient developed a cough with thick sputum production along with dyspnea on exertion. Bronchoscopy was ordered. The flexible bronchoscope was inserted. Forceps were advanced through the suction channel of the scope into the left lower lobe bronchus and bronchioles. Significant infiltrate was encountered in the tracheobronchial tree and aspirated. The fluoroscope was utilized and the biopsy forceps were advanced into the bronchiole. Six biopsies were obtained from the bronchus and bronchioles and the forceps and scope were removed. _____

7. A 73-year-old man with a history of asbestos exposure was admitted for increasing dyspnea and dry cough. He denied fever, chills, sweats, or hemoptysis. X-rays showed large effusion. Thoracentesis with removal of 2 L of fluid was performed. The next day under ultrasound guidance, a French pigtail drainage catheter was placed, and 7 L of fluid was removed. Fluid continued to drain and 2 days later he had a thoracoscopy with pleurodesis and decortication. Code for the last procedure(s). _____

Chapter Summary

1. Proper code assignment is largely dependent on knowing the anatomy of the organ system being treated and looking for anatomical landmarks to recognize when the surgeon is leaving one area and entering another. Surgeries are commonly reported with several CPT codes for each procedure performed such as in endoscopic sinus surgery. The coder must be able to discriminate when the surgeon has moved to another sinus cavity to capture all services rendered.

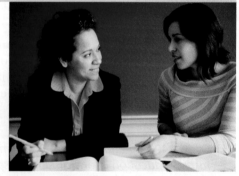

2. Laryngoscopies can be either diagnostic or therapeutic and are commonly provided for biopsies, removal of FBs, dilation of the larynx, and examination of the pharynx/larynx. Tracheostomies are provided either emergently or as

CPT © 2017 American Medical Association, All Rights Reserved.

planned procedures to provide access to the windpipe. Patients need tracheostomies because they cannot breathe on their own. Bronchoscopies provide dilation, biopsies, removal of FBs, or lung brachytherapy and aspiration. Thoracoscopies are performed to assess cancer, to biopsy lung tissue, to find the cause of fluid

in the chest cavity, to introduce medications or other treatments directly into the lungs, and to treat collected fluid, pus, or blood in the pleural space. Thoracentesis procedures are done to remove fluid from the pleura in order to determine the cause of the fluid accumulation or to relieve the symptoms. Thoracentesis can also provide information on possible cases of pneumonia, hemothorax, occlusive disease, embolism, and pleural effusion.

3. Codes assigned to nasal and septal fracture repairs require the coder to determine where the fracture is (nasal bone or septum), what type of repair was performed (closed with or without manipulation or stabilization or open with or without stabilization), and if the fracture is acute or old (malunion, nonunion, or sequelae). Closed fracture repairs are performed on acute injuries and open repairs on old fractures. Rhinoplasty codes may be indicated to report the complexity of the open fracture repair for old fractures.

4. Turbinate excision can be performed by removing part of the turbinate or all of it. Code 30130 describes the removal of all or part of an inferior turbinate when the incision does not extend down into the submucosal layer of nasal tissue. The surgeon does not make an incision into the mucosa to resect the turbinate but rather excises mucosa and bone at the same time, cutting out the mucosa and the bone completely. Submucosal excision means excising the turbinate by making an incision in the mucosa and preserving it versus removing it by creating a flap that is raised to access the inferior turbinate. Turbinate reduction is not removing the turbinate but rather making it smaller by shrinking it with radio-frequency ablation or incising it to reduce the air cells and fracture it. Procedures on the middle turbinate cannot be reported if performed at the same session and same side as an ethmoidectomy.

5. For an endoscopic diagnostic evaluation of the nasal sinuses, the following services are included: inspection of the interior of the nasal cavity, the middle and superior meatus, the turbinates, and the sphenoethmoid recess. When coding for a surgical sinus endoscopy, the diagnostic endoscopy is included and any sinusotomy required to perform the surgical endoscopy is included.

6. Endoscopic sinus surgery codes are assigned based on which sinuses were entered, what was done within each sinus cavity, and if tissue was removed. The code with the highest RVU is listed first on the claim form. All other procedures in separate sinuses are reported with the −51 modifier. Bilateral procedures are reported with the −50 modifier unless the carrier requires reporting on two lines. Some procedure codes, such as turbinate excisions and ethmoidectomies, will require the −59 modifier if performed at the same time.

7. Image guidance is used during surgical sinus endoscopies when the anatomy is hard to navigate due to extensive disease, scarring from previous surgery, and when previous surgery has changed the sinus anatomy because anatomical landmarks were removed.

8. Laryngectomy procedures can be performed with or without pharyngectomy and with or without neck dissection. Tracheostomy is always performed. The type and location of the neck incision gives the coder an idea of what procedure is being performed. A low collar or midline cervical incision is made for a total laryngectomy without neck dissection and a horizontal neck incision is made for total laryngectomy with neck dissection. Incisions made through the thyroid cartilage are for supraglottic subtotal laryngectomies. Pharyngectomy incisions are made on the side of the neck in a half "H" or "T" on the side. The coder must thoroughly read the operative report to capture the approach and to determine if the larynx and/or pharynx were partially or totally removed, if neck dissection was performed, and whether or not reconstruction was required.

9. Code 42890 is assigned for limited pharyngectomy. If radical neck dissection is also performed, CPT instructs physicians to bill 38720 separately. If a modified radical neck dissection is performed, assign 38724 instead of 38720. Pharyngectomies differ from laryngectomies for the obvious reason that they are different anatomical parts of the throat. Hypopharyngeal and oropharyngeal wall excisions are not part of a laryngectomy. Code 42892 is reported if lateral pharyngeal wall is resected and closed with advancement of the lateral and posterior pharyngeal walls. If the pharyngeal walls are resected and require closure with myocutaneous flap, assign 42894.

10. Lung tissue is removed for diagnostic and therapeutic purposes. Each of the following procedures removes tissue but in varying amounts and locations: Lung wedge resection is considered to be a biopsy where a small wedge of tissue is removed from any part of the lung. It is performed for diagnostic purposes. Lobectomy requires removing one of the five lung lobes in its entirety. Segmentectomy is the removal of a segment or segments of any of the lobes of the lung. Pneumonectomy is the complete removal of one of the two lungs.

11. Transplant services consist of three components: harvesting and preservation (32850); back-bench work, which consists of preparing the organ for transplant (32855–32856); and transplantation (allotransplantation), which includes removal of the diseased lung, transplantation of the new lung (allograft), and the usual and customary care of the patient included in the surgical package (32851–32854).

Review Questions

Matching

Match the key terms with their definitions.

A. antrum
B. concha bullosa
C. lobectomy
D. osteomeatal complex
E. ostium
F. pneumonectomy
G. radio-frequency ablation
H. segmentectomy
I. thoracotomy
J. turbinates

1. _____ method of surgically removing turbinates

2. _____ the paranasal cavities

3. _____ removal of one of the divisions of a lobe

4. _____ a nasal bone that has become filled with air

5. _____ removal of a single lobe of the lung

6. _____ middle meatus

7. _____ removal of the entire lung

8. _____ performed to gain access to the thoracic organs

9. _____ bones located inside the nose shaped like a shell

10. _____ openings that connect the paranasal cavities to the nasal cavity

True or False

Decide whether each statement is true or false.

1. __T__ The sphenoid sinus opens into the osteomeatal complex.

2. __T__ Middle turbinate procedures can never be reported at the same time as an ethmoidectomy on the same side.

3. __F__ A sleeve pneumonectomy is reported with 32486.

4. __T__ Arytenoid cartilage is part of the larynx.

5. __F__ Separate codes are used for harvesting a lung from a live versus a cadaver donor.

6. __T__ Lobectomies and wedge resections can be performed endoscopically.

7. _____ The uncinate process is part of the ethmoid.

8. __T__ An endoscopic segmentectomy can be performed by a pulmonologist.

9. __T__ There are three different kinds of turbinates: inferior, anterior, and superior.

10. __T__ There are five sinus cavities: maxillary, sphenoid, ethmoid, paranasal, and frontal.

11. ___F___ Each lung has three lobes: superior, middle, and inferior.

12. ___T___ Codes 31020 and 31256 can be reported together when both are performed.

13. ___F___ A flexible fiber-optic laryngoscopy is routinely performed under topical anesthesia.

14. ___F___ All nasal endoscopies are unilateral.

Multiple Choice

Select the letter that best completes the statement or answers the question.

1. A patient undergoes nasal endoscopy with bilateral partial ethmoidectomies. What procedure does this describe?
   A. 31255–50
   B. 31237–50
   C. 31231
   D. 31254–50

2. A patient had an endoscopic exam of the left nasal cavity and left ethmoid sinus with removal of polyp. On the right side, the physician examined the nasal cavity and performed a partial anterior ethmoidectomy. What procedure does this describe?
   A. 31254–RT, 31237–59
   B. 31254–RT, 31237–LT
   C. 31254–50
   D. Both A and B

3. A patient with liver carcinoma with bilateral pulmonary metastasis is seen for surgical excision. Incision was made between the fourth and fifth ribs and carried through the deeper tissues. The fifth rib was transected and a rib spreader was placed. Exploratory thoracotomy was conducted locating a mass in the apical segment of the left upper lobe (LUL). An apical segmentectomy was performed. What procedure does this describe?
   A. 32503
   B. 32484
   C. 32505
   D. 32442

4. The natural ossea was enlarged to create an opening for draining of the maxillary sinus. What procedure does this describe?
   A. 31256
   B. 31237
   C. 31267
   D. 31231

5. A perpendicular plate of the anterior ethmoid was found to be causing severe septal deviation. It was elevated off the mucoperiosteum and the bone was removed in pieces with forceps. What procedure does this describe?
   A. 31237
   B. 31255
   C. 31254
   D. 31020

6. A patient has adenocarcinoma of the upper lobe of left lung. Two intercostal incisions were made in the chest wall and advanced into the chest cavity. A trocar was inserted into the first incision. The chest cavity was examined through direct visualization. Images were obtained of the lesion. Blood vessels and bronchial tubes were clamped at the segments of the lung containing the mass. The mass was removed by dividing the vessel and bronchial tubes and removing the segment. Trocars were removed. What code describes this procedure?
   A. 32669
   B. 32484
   C. 32480
   D. 32663

7. A patient was in an altercation 3 months ago where his nose was broken. It was reduced in the ED. He is seen for major repair of the septum because of chronic sinusitis and a feeling of fullness in the nose. The physician performs reconstruction rhinoplasty with major repair of the septum. What procedure does this describe?

   A. 21335
   B. 21336
   C. 30420
   D. 30450

8. A patient with hemoptysis is treated with bronchoscopy. The bronchoscope is inserted, noting any abnormalities. The vocal cords are visualized with structure and function noted. The bronchoscope is then inserted through the upper airway and into the tracheobronchial tree. The patient has mild erythema throughout. In the right lower lobe, blood is seen coming from the right posterior basilar segment. Sterile saline washings of this bronchus are obtained and sent for culture and cytological examination. What procedure does this describe?

   A. 31623
   B. 31623–50
   C. 31622
   D. 31622–50

9. A patient was seen in the ED because of a stab wound to the chest creating a lung laceration. He was taken to the OR after an emergency thoracotomy was performed in the ED with insertion of a chest tube. The chest was entered through the thoracotomy incision and the pleura was dissected off the area of bleeding. The arterial intercostal space artery was bleeding. This was repaired with 3-0 Prolene. The laceration was identified in the lower-most portion of the upper left lobe posteriorly. The stapling device was placed over this laceration and repaired. What procedure does this describe?

   A. 32110
   B. 32503, 32110
   C. 32480
   D. 32480, 32110

10. A 33-year-old male who worked as a chemical operator, presented for evaluation of sinus problems and nasal congestion that had plagued him for many years. Clinical examination was significant for a severely deviated anterior septum, and bilateral inferior turbinate hypertrophy. The patient underwent a nasal septoplasty combined with partial resection of the inferior turbinates. What procedure does this describe?

    A. 30520, 30140–50
    B. 30520, 30130–50–51
    C. 30520, 30140–52–50
    D. 30520–22

11. A patient had a CT scan 1 week ago due to increasing shortness of breath and persistent cough. Lesions were noted and surgery was scheduled. The right upper and lower lobes were removed through an intercostal incision between the fourth and fifth ribs. A wedge resection was performed on the middle lobe and frozen section pathology revealed it was positive for malignancy. The patient is diagnosed with non–small-cell carcinoma of the right lung. What procedure does this describe?

    A. 32480 x 2
    B. 32482
    C. 32482, 32505
    D. 32480, +32507

12. What code(s) would be assigned for diagnostic bronchoscopy with bronchial biopsy?

    A. 31622, 31625
    B. 31625
    C. 31662
    D. 31622, 31625–59

13. A patient has laryngeal cancer and has had a tracheostomy for over a year. The patient requires a revision of the stoma with reconstruction with local flap because of irritation and breakdown from the artificial larynx device. What procedure does this describe?
    A. 31613
    B. 31750
    C. 31614
    D. 31611

14. A patient is diagnosed with three lesions on the right lung. Bronchoscopy was performed and two transbronchial lung biopsies were done on one lobe and another transbronchial lung biopsy was done on the second lobe. What procedure does this describe?
    A. 31628, +31632
    B. 31628 x 3
    C. 31628
    D. 31625

15. A surgical thoracoscopy with excisions of pericardial and mediastinal cysts was performed. What procedure does this describe?
    A. 32661–22
    B. 32661, 32662–51
    C. 32662–22
    D. 32659

CHAPTER 20

CPT: Cardiovascular, Hemic, and Lymphatic Systems

CHAPTER OUTLINE

Cardiovascular Anatomy

Cardiovascular System Coding Issues

Hemic and Lymphatic Systems Organization

Hemic and Lymphatic Anatomy

Common Conditions of the Hemic and Lymphatic Systems Requiring Treatment

Mediastinum and Diaphragm Anatomy

Common Conditions of the Mediastinum and Diaphragm Requiring Treatment

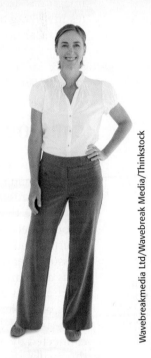

LEARNING OBJECTIVES

After studying this chapter, you should be able to:

1. Identify the anatomical structures of the cardiovascular system.
2. Describe the most common conditions that require treatment in the cardiovascular system.
3. Describe the difference between a pacemaker and cardioverter defibrillator.
4. Understand the most common abbreviations and acronyms used in cardiovascular coding.
5. Define the three types of coronary artery bypass procedures.
6. Understand endovascular versus open cardiovascular procedures.
7. Define the three types of services in heart transplants.
8. Define the five vascular systems and the concept of vascular families.
9. Describe central venous access devices.
10. Identify the anatomical structures of the hemic and lymphatic anatomy and their purpose.
11. Describe the most common conditions that require treatment in the hemic and lymphatic systems and the mediastinum and diaphragm systems.

In this chapter, procedures on the arterial and venous systems (cardiovascular) and the lymphatic system are discussed. This chapter also covers the major heart procedures, such as coronary artery bypass grafts and the interventional cardiovascular procedures. Cardiac catheterizations are discussed in Chapter 29.

Three types of physicians report codes from the cardiovascular section: cardiologists, cardiovascular surgeons, and vascular surgeons. Cardiologists are internal medicine physicians who specialize in the diagnosis and treatment of heart diseases and disorders; for example, they would perform pacemaker and cardioverter procedures. Cardiologists are not surgeons; therefore, they do not perform invasive surgery such as open-heart surgery. The invasive treatments are performed by a cardiovascular surgeon. A cardiovascular surgeon performs therapeutic procedures on the heart and the great vessels of the chest such as coronary artery bypass grafts and valve procedures. Vascular surgeons perform the extremity vascular procedures and aortic aneurysm repairs in the abdominal aorta.

Tasks that commonly prevent beginning coders from properly assigning codes from the cardiovascular section successfully include understanding the terminology, keeping separate in their minds "where" in the cardiovascular system the procedure is being performed, and determining how many codes are needed. Potentially, codes from three different sections of the CPT book could be assigned. The Cardiovascular System section of CPT (33010–37799) houses the surgical codes. The Cardiovascular block within the Medicine section (92920–93799) contains codes for the cardiac-related nonsurgical services. Diagnostic tests on the cardiovascular system are located in the Medicine section of CPT. Radiology codes would be assigned when imaging is used to perform a service on the heart, such as nuclear studies involving angiography.

> Remember that some of the services provided to treat or evaluate cardiovascular patients are located in the Medicine section of CPT. Examples are cardiac catheterizations and electrophysiology studies.

The Cardiovascular System section in CPT is arranged by anatomical part and then by procedures performed on that part. There are only two subsection headings in this section. The first is Heart and Pericardium and the second is Arteries and Veins.

CARDIOVASCULAR ANATOMY

The cardiovascular system consists of the heart, arteries, capillaries, and veins of the body. The heart is made up of three layers: the endocardium, which is the innermost layer of muscle; the myocardium (middle layer), and the epicardium, the outermost layer. The pericardium is the membrane that surrounds or encases the heart. The circulatory system consists of two types of blood vessels—arteries and veins. Arteries carry blood from the heart to the rest of the body. Veins return blood from the body to the heart. Arteries have thick walls to withstand the tremendous pressure created by the heart pumping blood through the body at great velocity. Veins have thin walls and can be superficial (close to the surface of the skin) or deep. Veins return blood to the heart against gravity and therefore have valves inside to prevent backflow of blood. Superficial veins of the legs are connected to the deeper veins by a network of communicating veins. These veins are also called *perforating veins* because they pass through the fascia. Arteries and veins are connected by a network of vessels called *capillaries*. Capillaries carry materials from the blood to the tissues.

Heart

The location and basic structure of the heart can be described as follows:

- The heart is located in the mediastinum.
- The mediastinum is the middle of the chest cavity between the lungs (side to side) and the sternum and vertebrae (front to back).
- The heart is behind the sternum, between the lungs, and in front of the esophagus.
- The right and left atria are the upper chambers (Fig. 20.1).
- The right and left ventricles are the lower chambers.

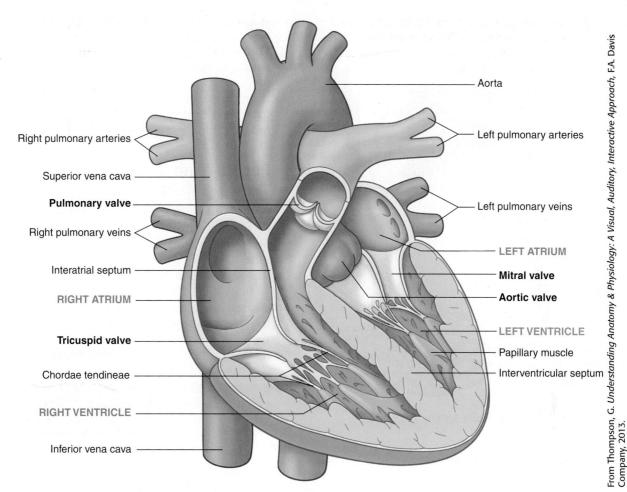

Right pulmonary arteries

Superior vena cava

Pulmonary valve

Right pulmonary veins

Interatrial septum

RIGHT ATRIUM

Tricuspid valve

Chordae tendineae

RIGHT VENTRICLE

Inferior vena cava

Aorta

Left pulmonary arteries

Left pulmonary veins

LEFT ATRIUM

Mitral valve

Aortic valve

LEFT VENTRICLE

Papillary muscle

Interventricular septum

Figure 20.1 The heart.

Heart Function

The following are the functions of the heart and related anatomy:

- The right atrium receives deoxygenated blood from the superior and inferior venae cavae.
- Blood passes through the tricuspid valve to the right ventricle.
- Blood then passes from the right ventricle through the pulmonic valves to the main pulmonary artery and then branches into the right and left pulmonary arteries into the lungs.
- The lungs release carbon dioxide and absorb oxygen.
- Oxygenated blood leaves the lungs via four pulmonary veins and moves into the left atrium.
- The left atrium sends the blood through the mitral valve into the left ventricle.
- The left ventricle contracts and sends blood through the aortic valve into the aorta.
- The aorta sends blood to the body—the blood gives off oxygen and picks up carbon dioxide via the capillaries.
- Capillaries become veins, the veins take the blood back to the heart, and the cycle begins again.

The heart itself gets blood from the right and left coronary arteries, which branch off the aorta. This is done immediately after the blood leaves the left ventricle (Fig. 20.2).

Valves

The valves of the heart include the following (Fig. 20.3):

- *Tricuspid*: located between the right atrium and right ventricle
- *Mitral*: located between the left atrium and left ventricle
- *Aortic*: located between the left ventricle and aorta
- *Pulmonic*: located between the right ventricle and pulmonary artery

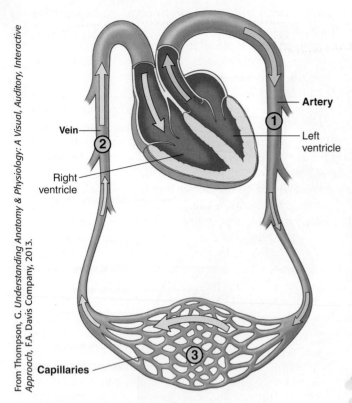

From Thompson, G. *Understanding Anatomy & Physiology: A Visual, Auditory, Interactive Approach*, F.A. Davis Company, 2013.

Figure 20.2 The vascular system.

Aorta

The aorta exits the heart from the left ventricle, rises up and arches to the left (aortic arch) and down behind the heart, through the chest cavity into the abdominal cavity, branching into the two iliac arteries in the lower abdomen.

Pericardium

The pericardium is the sac around the heart, and pericarditis is inflammation of the pericardium. The layers of the pericardium contain a small amount of lubricating fluid between them. When the pericardium becomes inflamed, the amount of fluid between the two layers increases, squeezing the heart and restricting its pumping. Depending on the severity of the fluid accumulation or the elasticity of the pericardium, either a pericardiocentesis or pericardiectomy will be performed. Pericardiocentesis (33010–33011) involves using local anesthesia and inserting a needle into the pericardial space, then

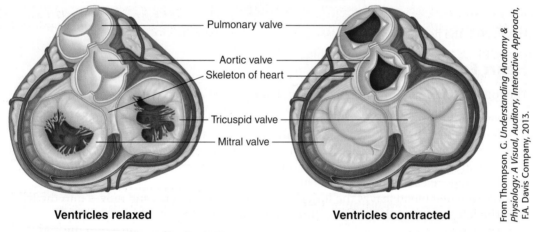

Figure 20.3 The heart valves.

From Thompson, G. *Understanding Anatomy & Physiology: A Visual, Auditory, Interactive Approach*, F.A. Davis Company, 2013.

inserting a catheter to allow the fluid to drain. This can be done by using anatomical landmarks, ultrasound, or echocardiogram guidance. Pericardiectomy is a much more involved procedure performed under general anesthesia. An incision is made in the sternum and the pericardium is cut away while the heart is beating. If cardiopulmonary bypass is required, 33031 is assigned.

CARDIOVASCULAR SYSTEM CODING ISSUES

Pacemakers and Implantable Defibrillator Systems

Pacemakers "pace" the heart into a regular rhythm and provide electrical stimulation to all chambers of the heart. The purpose of a pacemaker is to electrically stimulate the myocardium of one

CPT © 2017 American Medical Association, All Rights Reserved.

or more chambers of the heart to contract when the heart fails to do it on its own. An implantable defibrillator system is similar to a pacemaker and serves the same purpose, but the technology is somewhat different. It is implanted in patients who are at risk of sudden cardiac death due to ventricular fibrillation. Its advanced technology has the ability to detect and treat atrial and ventricular arrhythmias as well as the ability to perform biventricular pacing.

A pacemaker has two components: a pulse generator and leads (electrodes). The pulse generator contains four elements: the battery, the electronic circuit, the connector, and the sealed encasement. The term *battery* is used interchangeably for the pulse generator.

A pacemaker may either be temporary or permanent. Temporary pulse generators (33210–33211) are attached *externally*. Temporary pacemakers are designated separate procedures and therefore not reported separately when a more intensive procedure is performed at the same time and/or in the same site. For example, when a coronary artery bypass graft (CABG) is performed, the surgeon will place two transvenous leads after the CABG so that if the patient suffers any kind of arrhythmia, the leads can quickly be attached to an external generator to correct the problem. The temporary pacemaker is included in the CABG code and is not reported separately. The pulse generator of a temporary pacemaker is located outside the body and may be taped to the skin or attached to a belt. The leads for a temporary pacemaker can be positioned in a number of ways: inserted through a vein (transvenously) and positioned on the inside of the heart (endocardially), attached to the outside surface of the heart (epicardially), or inserted through the skin (transcutaneously), such as via a needle placed directly through the chest wall.

> ◉ Arrhythmia is a condition in which the heart does not beat regularly in a steady rhythm. Atrial fibrillation and bradycardia are the most common forms of arrhythmia and are treated with implantation of a pacemaker.

A permanent pacemaker is a surgically implanted device about the size of a pager. One method of insertion is to create a pocket below the collarbone so that the generator and leads can be placed inside the chest. The electrodes are either inserted transvenously to the heart and are connected to the pacemaker or placed epicardially.

CHECKPOINT 20.1

Assign the CPT code(s) for the following situation.

1. A 70-year-old male patient with a history of coronary artery disease presents with chest pain and indications of myocardial infarction. A pacing catheter is passed into the right ventricle with attachment to an external pulse generator. _____

> ◉ Before attempting to code pacemaker procedures, coders should read the instructional notes and guidelines preceding code 33202.

Epicardial pacemakers are permanent pacemakers placed through an open incision in the sternum called a *thoracotomy*. They can also be placed through an epigastric xiphoid incision or via an endoscopic approach. The open approach is reported with code 33202, while the endoscopic approach is reported with code 33203.

Transvenous pacemakers are the most commonly placed permanent pacemakers (33206–33208). The codes for this type of pacemaker include the insertion of the entire system, including the generator. Occasionally, a surgeon will implant an additional electrode to achieve pacing of the left ventricle. This is called *biventricular pacing*. If this occurs, placement of the extra electrode is reported separately using 33224 or 33225. Biventricular pacing is also called *resynchronization therapy*.

EXAMPLE

Code 33224 represents insertion of a biventricular electrode into a pacemaker or implantable defibrillator system previously placed in the patient. Code 33225 and an add-on code are reported when the biventricular electrode is inserted at the same session as the pacemaker/implantable defibrillator system.

Codes 33212–33221 are reported when only the pulse generator is inserted and the existing electrodes remain in place. Do not report the removal of pulse generator codes with 33212–33221. If the old pulse generator is removed and replaced, report codes 33227–33229 to represent the removal and replacement of the pulse generator and to indicate that the existing electrodes remain in place. If the pulse generator and the transvenous electrodes are removed and replaced, report 33233 for the generator removal, 33234 or 33235 for the electrode removal, *and* one code from the 33206–33208 series based on the type of pacemaker system being inserted.

Pacemakers can be upgraded from a single-chamber to a dual-chamber system. Report code 33214 to represent this service, being careful to note the inclusions: removing the previously placed generator, testing the new electrode, and inserting the new generator.

> Repositioning of pacemaker electrodes is reported with either 33215 or 33226. Code 33226 includes the removal and insertion/replacement of the existing generator.

CHECKPOINT 20.2

Assign the CPT code(s) for the following situations.

1. A patient's original pulse generator has reached the end of its life and needs to be replaced. The physician will remove the old generator and put in a new one. The existing two electrodes will remain in place. _____

2. Subcutaneous removal of pacing cardioverter-defibrillator pulse generator, electrodes removed by thoracotomy. _____

The skin pocket where the pulse generator for a pacemaker or implantable defibrillator system is located may need to be revised or relocated due to infection or injury to that area. Revision of the skin pocket is included in codes 33206–33249 and codes 33262–33264. If the revision involves an incision and drainage or debridement procedure, CPT allows for coding those procedures with codes 10140, 10180, 11042, 11043, 11044, 11045, 11046, and 11047 from the Integumentary System section of CPT.

Electrophysiological evaluation of the implantable defibrillator system can be done at the time of initial implantation or replacement or at any time subsequent to the initial placement. The codes from the Medicine section that are assigned to capture these services are 93640–93642.

Pinpoint the Code 20.1 illustrates a decision tree to correctly code pacemaker services. You must know the following:

> For relocation of the skin pocket, report code 33222 for the pacemaker or 33223 for the implantable defibrillator system. Do not report the relocation codes with incision and drainage or debridement codes. The relocation codes also should not be reported with complex wound repair codes 13100, 13101, or 13102.

1. Is the pacemaker temporary or permanent?
2. Is it single chamber or dual chamber? To determine this, determine where the electrodes (leads) were placed: atrium, ventricle, or both? A single-chamber system has one electrode in the right atrium or right ventricle. A dual-chamber system has one electrode in the right atrium and one in the right ventricle.
3. What was the approach: transvenous (endocardial) or epicardial?
4. Is this the initial placement, replacement, or repair of a pacemaker? If this is a repair or re-placement, is it of all of the components of a pacemaker or just an electrode or generator?
5. Was a single-chamber pacemaker converted to a dual-chamber system?
6. Was more than one physician involved in placing the pacemaker? What portions did each physician complete?

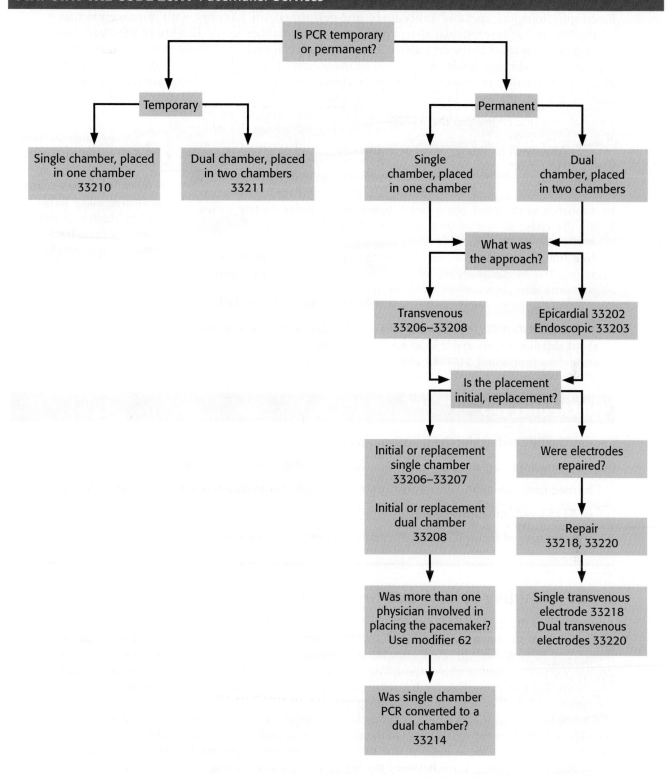

EXAMPLE

Cardiologist performs surgical creation of a pocket for a pulse generator and inserts a permanent pacemaker with transvenous insertion of atrial and ventricular electrodes. Report code 33208.

Electrophysiological Operative Procedures

Electrophysiological *operative* procedures are performed on patients with supraventricular dysrhythmias. Supraventricular dysrhythmias are abnormalities in the rhythm of the heart and are specifically located in the area above the atrioventricular node, not in the ventricle itself. Most commonly the abnormality is tachycardia, an irregular and rapid heart rate. Ablation is a form of destruction of abnormal heart tissue. It can be cryotherapy, the use of cold to destroy the tissue, or radio-frequency, the use of heat to destroy the tissue.

Codes 33250 and 33251 are ablation procedures and differ by whether or not cardiopulmonary bypass is performed during the procedure. Codes 33254–33256 represent ablation and reconstruction of the atria, limited or extensive, and are not reported with other open-heart procedures; however, CPT provides add-on codes +33257 through +33259, representing the same services, and these codes can be reported with other open-heart procedures. Refer to the notes below the codes in the section where CPT specifically states "Do not report 33254–33256 with" for clarification.

> Always carefully review the parenthetical notes under these and any CPT codes. They provide coding instruction regarding "do not report" or "report in conjunction with" guidance. This is essential coding information.

Note that the procedures described in this section are emphasized as operative. The Medicine section of CPT has other codes for electrophysiological procedures that are less invasive. These procedures are done via the insertion of catheters. The codes for these procedures are 93600–93662.

> INTERNET RESOURCE: The following website provides additional information about ablation surgery and is in an easy-to-read format:
> www.ehow.com/about_5147793_ablation-surgery.html

CHECKPOINT 20.3

Assign the CPT code(s) for the following situations.

1. Coronary artery bypass graft ×3 was performed, and during the same session the surgeon performed tissue ablation and reconstruction of the left atrium. Will the surgeon report code 33254 or 33257 with the CABG code? _____

2. Valvuloplasty of tricuspid valve with ring insertion. _____

Heart (Including Valves) and Great Vessels

This section of the CPT manual provides codes for procedures on the heart, heart valves, and the great vessels of the heart. Always watch for any code description that indicates "without cardiopulmonary bypass" or "with cardiopulmonary bypass." The heart procedures describe repairs for cardiac wounds or cardiac exploration. The great vessel procedures describe suture repair or graft insertions. The great vessels of the heart are the aorta, the pulmonary artery, the pulmonary veins, the superior vena cava, and the inferior vena cava.

Coding for the valve procedures requires knowledge of valve anatomy. The tricuspid valve directs blood flow from the right atrium to the right ventricle and prevents any backflow of the blood into the right atrium (regurgitation). The mitral valve performs the same function on the left side of the heart. The aortic valve is between the left ventricle and the aorta, and the pulmonic valve is between the right ventricle and the pulmonary artery. Regurgitation is one of the conditions that can occur in each of these valves and happens whenever a valve does not close properly. Other conditions are stenosis (narrowing) or congenital anomalies. The types of treatments the surgeons will perform are valve replacement, valvuloplasty, and other repairs.

Transcatheter Aortic Valve Replacement

CPT provides acronyms specifically for transcatheter aortic valve replacements (TAVRs) and transcatheter aortic valve implantations (TAVIs), codes 33361–33369. Both of these procedures require two physicians—a cardiothoracic surgeon and an interventional cardiologist—and each physician will report modifier –62 to indicate that they have provided co-surgery. It is important to note that the services included in these procedures are percutaneous access, placing the access sheath, balloon aortic valvuloplasty, advancing the valve delivery system into position, repositioning the valve as needed, deploying the valve, temporary pacemaker insertion, closure of the arteriotomy site, angiography, radiological supervision and interpretation (RSI), and diagnostic left heart catheterization to provide guidance or aortic or left ventricular outflow tract measurement for the TAVR/TAVI.

The TAVR/TAVI procedures are further defined by criteria associated with diagnostic coronary angiography performed at the time of the TAVR/TAVI. The diagnostic coronary angiography is separately reportable in the following situations:

- No prior catheter-based coronary angiography study is available and a full study is performed, or if a prior study has been done but the patient's condition has changed since the study.
- The prior study has inadequate visualization, or a clinical change occurs during the procedure.
- The diagnostic angiography meets these criteria and is performed during the same session or same day. Report modifier –59 with the angiography code.

■ **CASE SCENARIO**

A 79-year-old male patient presents with aortic stenosis, coronary artery disease, and heart failure. The aortic stenosis is critical and the patient's comorbidities preclude a conventional open-heart aortic valve replacement. A valve team comprised of a cardiothoracic surgeon and interventional cardiologist agree that the open-valve procedure risks outweigh the benefit and a transcatheter aortic valve replacement is performed instead.

Coronary Artery Bypass Grafts

Patients who require a CABG procedure have a blockage in one or more coronary arteries. CABG is an open-heart procedure that requires a sternotomy and cardiopulmonary bypass to accomplish the bypass. When blood flow from the aorta to the heart muscle is blocked, the heart muscle does not receive an adequate blood supply and the patient will likely have a heart attack. The physician uses a vein, an artery, or a combination of both artery and vein to bypass the area of the blockage in the coronary artery and in that way maintain the flow of blood to the heart muscle. There may be only one blockage or several that need the bypass procedure.

There are three ways to report these services:

VEIN ONLY	ARTERY ONLY	COMBINED VEIN/ARTERY
33510–33516	33533–33536	33517 with 33533–33536
		Add-on codes
		Never reported alone
		Always a minimum of two codes

EXAMPLES

- CABG×2, aortocoronary bypass graft using the saphenous vein to bypass the right coronary artery and the left anterior descending artery. Report code 33511, *CABG, vein only; two coronary venous grafts*.
- CABG×2, aortocoronary bypass graft using the internal mammary artery to bypass the right coronary artery and the left anterior descending artery. Report code 33534, *CABG, artery only; two coronary artery grafts*.
- CABG×3, aortocoronary bypass graft using the saphenous vein to bypass the right coronary artery and the left circumflex artery *and* using the left internal mammary artery to bypass the left anterior descending artery. Report code 33533, *CABG×1, artery only; single artery graft*. Also use +33518, *CABG×2, combined vein and artery graft, two venous grafts*.

Procuring the graft material is included in the CABG codes, but there are exceptions:

35500: Upper extremity vein
35600: Upper extremity artery
35572: Femoropopliteal vein segment

If any of these veins or arteries are used in the bypass procedure, their codes can be reported in addition to the bypass code. Code 33530, an add-on code, is reported when the physician has to reoperate on a patient who had a previous CABG or valve procedure. The criteria are that more than 1 month has passed since the previous surgery and it is reported in addition to the CABG or valve procedure. Reporting this code reflects the increased difficulty of an open-heart reoperation: The sternal wires have to be removed, and there are increased risks from scarring and hemorrhage.

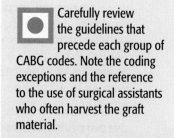 Carefully review the guidelines that precede each group of CABG codes. Note the coding exceptions and the reference to the use of surgical assistants who often harvest the graft material.

CHECKPOINT 20.4

Assign the CPT code(s) for the following situation.

1. A 64-year-old patient has blockages in three coronary arteries. The surgeon will use the saphenous vein as graft material for one of the blocked arteries and the left internal mammary artery (LIMA) will be used to provide graft material for the two remaining blocked arteries. The cardiothoracic surgeon performs CABG×3 using a saphenous vein graft to the right coronary artery (RCA) and left internal mammary artery grafts to the left anterior descending (LAD) and left circumflex arteries. _____

Heart and Lung Transplants

The coding structure for transplant procedures is represented by three types of services throughout the sections of CPT:

1. Harvesting the organ from the donor
2. Backbench work
3. Organ transplantation into the recipient

These services are represented in the cardiovascular system as follows:

1. Donor cardiectomy–pneumonectomy, code 33930
   a. Both the heart and lung are removed from the donor
   b. Includes harvesting the heart and lung and cold preservation
2. Backbench work for a heart and lung transplant, code 33933
   a. Backbench work represents the preparation of the donor organ(s), in this case the heart and lung, including dissection of the organs from surrounding soft tissues, to prepare them for implantation
3. Backbench work for the heart only, code 33944
4. Transplantation of the heart and lung into the recipient with removal of the heart and lung from the recipient, code 33935
5. Donor cardiectomy (only), code 33940
6. Transplant of heart only into the recipient, with or without recipient cardiectomy, code 33945

■ CASE SCENARIOS

• A young man is involved in a motorcycle accident and is brain dead. He is listed as an organ donor. The donor's airways are examined and cultures are taken and during the operation the heart is inspected for any abnormalities. Dissection is performed, and the heart is removed and placed in sterile plastic bags in a container surrounded by ice. The organs are transported to the recipient hospital. Report code 33940, *Donor cardiectomy, including cold preservation.*

- The donated heart is prepared for transplant by dissecting free any residual soft tissue with specific attention to the aorta, superior vena cava, inferior vena cava, and left atrium. Report code 33944, *Backbench standard preparation of cadaver donor heart allograft.*

- The recipient is placed on cardiopulmonary bypass. The recipient heart is opened and the atria, aorta, and pulmonary artery are anastomosed (joined) to the donor heart. The sinoatrial nodes of both hearts are left intact. Report code 33945, *Heart transplant, with or without recipient cardiectomy.*

There is also a coding structure available for implantation of an artificial heart. Code 33927 represents the services required to implant the artificial heart, including a recipient cardiectomy. Code 33928 is reported for removal and replacement of the artificial heart. Additionally, there is a code for removing the artificial heart to perform a heart transplant (+33929). Code +33929 is reported with the heart transplant code 33945, with or without a recipient cardiectomy.

Cardiac Assist

Extracorporeal Membrane Oxygenation or Extracorporeal Life Support Services
Codes 33946–33989 represent services to patients who need cardiac and/or respiratory support to the heart and/or lungs due to illness or injury. Such patients may require extracorporeal membrane oxygenation (ECMO) or extracorporeal life support services (ECLS). ECMO/ECLS will support the function of the heart and/or lungs by pumping some of the patient's blood into an oxygenator where oxygen is added to the blood and carbon dioxide is removed. These two methods require placement of cannulae to accomplish the procedure. These services are distinct from the daily management of the patient while under ECMO/ECLS. CPT provides separate codes for the daily management services.

Intra-Aortic Balloon Assist Device
Intra-aortic balloon (IAB) procedures are represented by codes 33967–33974 and are performed in one of three ways: (1) percutaneously, (2) through the femoral artery as an open procedure, or (3) through the aorta. These procedures are provided most commonly for cardiothoracic postoperative patients who need to be weaned from cardiopulmonary bypass, but such use is by no means exclusive. There is a code for each method of insertion of the IAB followed by a code for the removal of the IAB correlating to the insertion method.

Ventricular Assist Device
Ventricular assist device (VAD) codes (33975–33983) are for VAD procedures performed transthoracically and are based on whether the insertion is extracorporeal or intracorporeal and whether or not the device is placed in a single ventricle or in both. Codes 33990 and 33991 are performed percutaneously and based on the access—arterial only or both arterial and venous. The VAD is a mechanical circulatory device that can partially or completely replace the function of a failing heart. They can be for short-term or long-term use. Originally, they were considered to be a method for keeping patients alive while they waited for a heart transplant. More and more they are considered as a bridge to recovery, meaning the patient is not going to get a heart transplant but is able to recover through the use of the VAD. The guidelines for these procedures require careful review by the coder.

Procedures on Arteries and Veins

Codes under the main heading Arteries and Veins describe treatment for aneurysms, angioplasty, bypass surgery, embolectomies, thrombectomies, varicose veins, and hemangiomas. An embolectomy is a procedure for the removal of a blood clot. A thrombectomy is a procedure for the removal of a thrombus. Varicose veins, dilated/enlarged veins, are most commonly seen in the legs and are often a congenital condition or the result of jobs that require long periods of standing. This condition is also common in pregnant women. Hemangiomas are a proliferation of blood vessels that give the appearance of a neoplasm.

Coding for procedures performed on blood vessels requires a strong knowledge of the vascular anatomy (Fig. 20.4) because the subsection is arranged by artery or vein and the approach. The section provides instructional notes throughout. The notes at the beginning are very important to the coder. They indicate that procedures performed on arteries and veins include establishment of both inflow and outflow, and that arteriograms performed intraoperatively by the surgeon are also included. An arteriogram is the process of viewing dye/contrast as it is injected into an artery to determine if there are any blockages or other abnormalities. Arteriograms are commonly performed by the surgeon after doing a procedure on an artery to be sure that the condition has been corrected and no abnormality remains.

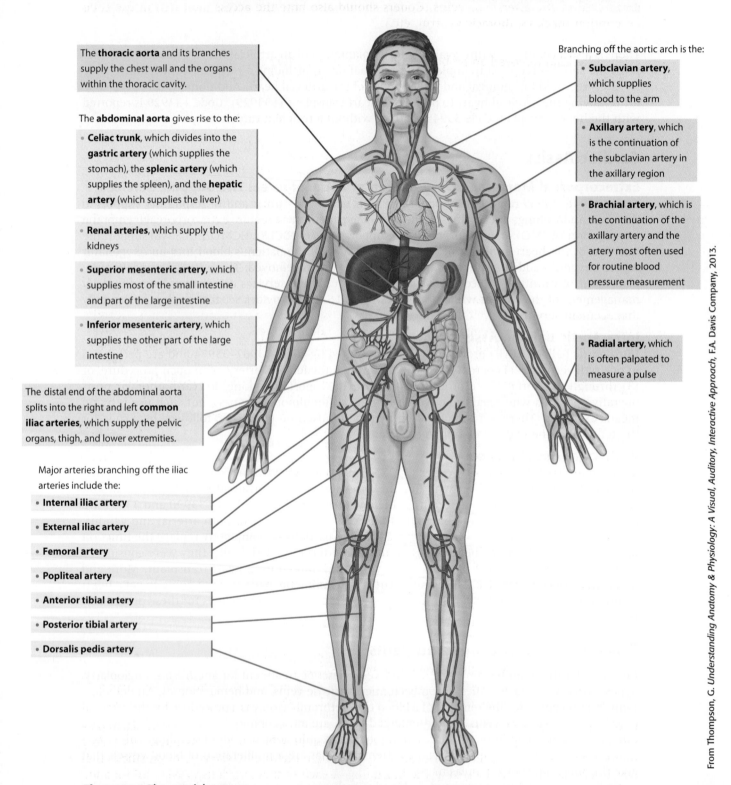

The **thoracic aorta** and its branches supply the chest wall and the organs within the thoracic cavity.

The **abdominal aorta** gives rise to the:

- **Celiac trunk**, which divides into the **gastric artery** (which supplies the stomach), **splenic artery** (which supplies the spleen), and the **hepatic artery** (which supplies the liver)

- **Renal arteries**, which supply the kidneys

- **Superior mesenteric artery**, which supplies most of the small intestine and part of the large intestine

- **Inferior mesenteric artery**, which supplies the other part of the large intestine

The distal end of the abdominal aorta splits into the right and left **common iliac arteries**, which supply the pelvic organs, thigh, and lower extremities.

Major arteries branching off the iliac arteries include the:

- **Internal iliac artery**
- **External iliac artery**
- **Femoral artery**
- **Popliteal artery**
- **Anterior tibial artery**
- **Posterior tibial artery**
- **Dorsalis pedis artery**

Branching off the aortic arch is the:

- **Subclavian artery**, which supplies blood to the arm

- **Axillary artery**, which is the continuation of the subclavian artery in the axillary region

- **Brachial artery**, which is the continuation of the axillary artery and the artery most often used for routine blood pressure measurement

- **Radial artery**, which is often palpated to measure a pulse

From Thompson, G. *Understanding Anatomy & Physiology: A Visual, Auditory, Interactive Approach*, F.A. Davis Company, 2013.

Figure 20.4 The arterial system.

The surgeon removed an embolus from the brachial artery through an incision in the arm. After the successful removal, the surgeon did an arteriogram of the brachial artery to confirm that there was no leak or injury in the surgical area. The surgeon would report code 34101 but would not report a code from the radiology section for the intraoperative arteriogram because it is included in the embolectomy procedure.

Embolectomy and thrombectomy procedures are defined by whether the procedure is performed in the arteries or veins. Coders should also note the access indicated in the code description (neck vs. thoracic vs. arm, etc.).

EXAMPLE

The physician removed an embolus from the aortoiliac artery via a leg incision. The code is 34201, *Embolectomy or thrombectomy, with or without catheter; femoropopliteal or aortoiliac artery, by leg incision.*

Aneurysms

An aneurysm is a localized bulge in a blood vessel caused by disease or weakening of the vessel wall. Aneurysms can occur in any blood vessel, but these typically occur in the vessels of the heart, the base of the skull, or in the abdominal aorta (AAA) or thoracic aorta (TAA). Aneurysms are caused by hypertension, atherosclerosis, infection, injury, and congenital malformation. Blood vessels have three layers. In order to be diagnosed with an aneurysm, all three layers must be bulged. If only one or two of these three layers are bulged or if there is a slow leak of blood through the blood vessel wall, it is classified as a pseudoaneurysm (false aneurysm).

Treatment for aneurysms consists of surgical repair performed by a vascular surgeon. A vascular surgeon specializes in the surgical intervention of arteries and veins of the peripheral vascular system. These procedures include "open" aneurysm repair and endovascular repair, sometimes called *stent graft aneurysm repair*. The open method entails making a large incision through the abdomen or thoracic wall to access the aneurysm site and then incising or excising the artery. This is a lengthy procedure and very risky to the patient, requiring an extensive recuperative period. The endovascular repair requires a small incision, usually in the femoral artery, in order to insert a catheter that has a prosthesis encased within it, which is deployed in the area of the aneurysm through the vascular system. The prosthetic device is advanced into position using fluoroscopic guidance. In open repair, the prosthesis or graft is sutured to the proximal and distal artery, whereas in endovascular repair, the prosthesis is anchored above and below the aneurysm with framework. The best method to repair each aneurysm depends on several factors, including the location and shape of the aneurysm and the condition of the patient. Codes for aneurysms are designated by location (i.e., thoracic or abdominal), type of aneurysm (i.e., false, ruptured, dissected), type of repair (i.e., endovascular), and whether cardiopulmonary bypass is used.

> **INTERNET RESOURCE:** The following website provides additional information related to endovascular aneurysm repairs. Many websites like this are available and can provide more insight into this complex surgical concept. www.nlm.nih.gov/medlineplus/ency/article/007391.htm

The following subsections contain the codes for aneurysm repair:

- Thoracic Aortic Aneurysm: 33860–33877
- Endovascular Repair of Descending Thoracic Aorta: 33880–33891
- Endovascular Repair of Abdominal Aortic Aneurysm: 34701–34706
- Fenestrated Endovascular Repair of the Visceral and Infrarenal Aorta: 34841–34848
- Endovascular Repair of Iliac Aneurysm: 34707–34708
- Direct Repair of Aneurysm or Excision (Partial or Total) and Graft Insertion for Aneurysm, Pseudoaneurysm, Ruptured Aneurysm, and Associated Occlusive Disease: 35001–35152

Coding of these procedures requires paying close attention to the services that are included in providing the endovascular repair and knowing what services can be reported separately. For coding the endovascular repairs, the coder should pay particular attention to the type of prosthesis that was inserted. Guidelines located at the beginning of each of these sections provide information on what services are included in the codes in that subsection as well as what should be reported separately. Examples of the services that are reported separately for the endovascular aortic aneurysm repairs are the add-on codes for artery exposure such as 34713–34716. Note the extensive number of services that are reportable with these add-on codes.

Fenestrated Endovascular Repair of the Visceral and Infrarenal Aorta

A fenestrated endovascular prosthesis has openings in the graft device that allow for incorporation of other arteries that branch off the aorta. If the prosthesis needs placement in the renal or visceral artery area of the aorta, the fenestrated prosthesis has openings for those arteries to be incorporated within the prosthesis to maintain blood flow. The visceral aorta contains the celiac, superior mesenteric, and renal arteries:

- The codes for the visceral aorta specifically are 34841–34844.
- The codes for the visceral aorta and the infrarenal (below the renal arteries) abdominal aorta are 34845–34848.
- Each of the above code groups is based on the number of arteries treated by use of endoprosthesis(es) in addition to the aorta.

EXAMPLE

Code 34841 represents fenestrated endovascular repair of the visceral aorta and one visceral artery endoprosthesis. Code 34842 changes to the visceral aorta and two visceral artery endoprostheses.

The CPT guidelines indicate the included services and the separately reportable services for coding these procedures. Included services are as follows:

- Introduction of guidewires and catheters
- Balloon angioplasty within the target treatment zone
- Fluoroscopic guidance
- Radiological supervision and interpretation
- Diagnostic imaging of the aorta and its branches
- Intraprocedural arterial angiography for confirmation of completion

Separately reportable services are as follows:

- Catheterization of the hypogastric artery(s) and/or arterial families outside the treatment zone of the graft
- Exposure of the access vessels (e.g., 34812)
- Extensive repair of an artery
- Other interventional procedures outside of the target zone

Coders will need to review carefully the guidelines and code descriptions, and the parenthetical notes below the codes.

Direct Repair of Aneurysm or Excision (Partial or Total) and Graft Insertion for Aneurysm, Pseudoaneurysm, Ruptured Aneurysm, and Associated Occlusive Disease

Aneurysms and pseudoaneurysms may also be repaired as a direct (open) procedure. These procedures include preparation of the artery for anastomosis (rejoining) and endarterectomy (removal of the inner lining of the artery). Note that some of these procedures specify the incision site and are differentiated by whether or not the aneurysm has ruptured. Treatment consists of placing a synthetic graft around the vessel to prevent it from bursting, excising the portion of artery that contains the aneurysm, and repairing the hole (endarterectomy), or bypassing the vessel all together. If grafting is performed, the surgeon may cut through the wall of the weakened artery and open it like a butterfly, then insert a graft that is the same size and shape of the artery. The surgeon will attach one end of this graft by sewing it to the healthy artery just above where the aneurysm begins and sewing the other end to the normal artery below the end of the aneurysm.

EXAMPLE

The physician makes an incision in the neck. The blocked section of the vertebral artery is isolated and vessel clamps are affixed above and below the defect. The segment of the artery containing the aneurysm is removed, the artery is anastomosed (rejoined), and the clamps are removed. Report code 35005.

Bypass Grafts

Bypass grafts (35501–35587) are performed in areas other than the coronary arteries, such as the aortic arch arteries (subclavian, carotids, brachiocephalic) and the peripheral arteries (brachial, femoral, popliteal, etc.). They are accomplished in one of three ways based on the material used to perform the bypass procedure:

1. Using a vein as the bypass material
2. Using an in situ vein for the bypass
3. Using material other than vein as bypass material

Because many of the code descriptions look similar under each type of bypass, coders must be aware of the bypass material being used. The in situ method has fewer codes than the other types and is a very different method. For the in situ method, the saphenous vein is clamped off at the upper thigh and at the knee. It is divided and the upper end is sutured to the femoral artery and the lower end is sutured to the popliteal artery. The clamp is removed and blood flows to the foot. In effect, the vein is left in place (in situ) rather than being cut away and moved.

The code descriptions provide a *from-to relationship* with the use of a hyphen (-) in the description.

EXAMPLE

Code 35506, *Bypass graft, with vein; carotid-subclavian or subclavian-carotid*, would be used when a surgeon does a bypass graft from the carotid artery to the subclavian artery *or* from the subclavian artery to the carotid artery.

CHECKPOINT 20.5

Assign the CPT code(s) for the following situations.

1. A patient with severe finger pain and diminished finger blood pressures needs a bypass graft from the brachial artery to the ulnar artery using a vein for the graft. _____

2. Patient is placed on heart/lung bypass and the main pulmonary artery is opened in order to remove the blockage and interior lining of the artery. The artery was then sutured closed and the pulmonary endarterectomy was accomplished. _____

Vascular Injections

Coders need to understand the anatomy of the vascular system and its relationship to the vascular families. The system is complex and does not have equal anatomy bilaterally, which affects the coding of vascular injections. There are five vascular systems in the body: venous, arterial, pulmonary, portal, and lymphatic. VAPPL can be a useful acronym for remembering these five systems. Each vascular system has vascular families associated with it. A vascular family is a group of vessels fed from the main conduit of the vascular system, such as the aorta in the arterial system. The primary branch and all its secondary and tertiary branches comprise a vascular family and they have a common point of origin—the main conduit.

The arterial system's main conduit is the aorta (see Figure 20.4). In the abdominal aorta, for example, the common iliac artery feeds off the aorta on the right and left. Each common iliac artery is a first-order catheterization once the catheter is moved from the main conduit (the aorta) into the primary branch (common iliac) and each is a separate family. Each primary branch (first order) has its own branches that feed off of it. In the common iliac family are the internal iliac, external iliac, and common femoral arteries, and they are considered second-order catheterizations.

Because vascular injections are a complex area of coding, our illustration will focus on the arterial system, specifically in the abdominal aorta, to provide a picture of the process. Vascular injections are performed when a symptomatic patient is evaluated and the physician determines that it is necessary to view the affected vascular system to determine what is causing the problem. When vascular injections are performed, the process may start with a puncture into the femoral artery (although other sites can be accessed instead) through which a catheter is fed into the aorta. Dye is injected and the physician views the movement of the dye to determine if there is any type of anomaly. This is considered a nonselective catheterization, meaning the catheter is placed into the main conduit and *not* moved into one of the families/branches off the main conduit. The catheter may then be placed into one of the families/branches off the aorta, for example, the left common iliac, and dye is then again injected to look for anomalies. Once the catheter leaves the aorta and goes into one of the families, the catheterization is considered selective. Selective catheterizations represent placement of the catheter into a blood vessel other than the main conduit. Selective catheterizations include nonselective catheterizations. The nonselective catheterization codes are not reported with selective catheterization codes.

Some vascular injection procedures require an RSI code, and some codes include the RSI. For example, codes 36221–36228 include the RSI. In each family off the main conduit, the coding rule is that you code to the highest order in each family. The lower-order branches are not reported, but every time an RSI is performed the appropriate RSI code will be reported; therefore, it is important to understand that there is no one-to-one relationship between the catheterization codes and the RSI codes. Most likely coders will report more RSI codes than catheterization codes. For example, consider the following situations:

- If the catheter is placed into the abdominal aorta (main conduit), it is nonselective catheterization.
- If the catheter is placed into the left common iliac family/branch (first order), the catheterization is considered selective.
- If the catheter is placed into any of the following branches, the catheterization is considered a second-order catheterization:

  - Left internal iliac
  - Left external iliac
  - Left common femoral

To understand the different orders in each family, remember the following (you can also refer to Appendix L in the CPT book):

- *First-order catheterization*: Each major branch off the aorta is a primary branch.
- *Second-order catheterization*: Each branch off the primary branch is a secondary branch.
- *Third-order catheterization*: Each branch off the secondary branch is a tertiary branch.

Coders must code to the highest-order vessel catheterized within the same vascular family; therefore, lesser-order vessels within the same vascular family are included in the highest-order vessel codes and not coded separately.

EXAMPLE

The catheter is placed through the left femoral artery to the aorta (main conduit) and dye is injected. The catheter is then placed into the right common iliac (first order) and dye is injected. Report code 36245, *Selective catheter placement, arterial system; each first-order abdominal, pelvic, or lower extremity artery branch within a vascular family*. The catheterization of the aorta is nonselective and included in the selective catheterization of the common iliac.

If the catheter was then placed into the right internal iliac artery and dye was injected, the coder would report code 36246 for the second-order catheterization within the same family. Code 36245 *would not be reported* because it is a first-order code and is included in the higher-order code 36246. There would also be RSI codes associated with these catheterizations. In this scenario, because the RSI services were provided in the aorta, the right common iliac, and the right internal iliac, there would be three RSI codes.

Cervicocerebral Arteries

Another area of study for vascular injections is the cervicocerebral arteries. This arterial area shares many of the other vascular injection coding guidelines but also has its own specific criteria. An American Medical Association (AMA)/CPT work study determined that there was duplication of work among the various carotid angiography services provided during the same session; therefore, the coding structure for these services includes more services than other vascular injection codes. These codes are built on progressive hierarchies where the more-intensive services include the less-intensive services. The codes 36221–36228 still follow the guidelines that nonselective catheterization includes selective catheterization and coding to the highest order but now combines a grouping of services. To understand this area of vascular injection coding, it is important to study the aortic arch vascular families.

> **INTERNET RESOURCES: You will find it useful to research this area of coding. It is very complicated and the more you read about it, the better your understanding will be. One useful website among many is:**
> www.evtoday.com/2013/08/bundled-cervicocerebral -angiography-and-intervention-codes
>
> **Another helpful website is the Society for Cardiovascular Angiography and Interventions. This website can provide illustrations for the cervicocerebral arteries. www.scai.org**

In normal head and neck anatomy, three vascular families originate at the aortic arch:

1. Brachiocephalic (innominate) family
2. Left common carotid family
3. Left subclavian family

These families can be further divided as follows:

1. Brachiocephalic (innominate) family includes all its "branches"—first order
   Right common carotid (RCC)—second order
   Right internal carotid (RIC)—third order
   Right external carotid (REC)—third order
   Right subclavian—second order
   Right brachial—second order
   Right vertebral—third order
2. Left common carotid family includes all its "branches"—first order
   Left internal carotid (LIC)—second order
   Left external carotid (LEC)—second order
3. Left subclavian family includes all its "branches"—first order
   Left vertebral—second order
   Left internal mammary—second order

Codes 36221–36226 include the following:

- Accessing the vessel (same as the noncervicocerebral vascular injections)
- Placing the catheter(s) (same as the noncervicocerebral vascular injections)
- Contrast injection(s) (same as the noncervicocerebral vascular injections)
- Fluoroscopy (now included in codes 36221–36226)
- RSI (now included in codes 36221–36226)
- Closure of the artery incision (arteriotomy; same as the noncervicocerebral vascular injections)

NOTE: If an interventional procedure such as placement of a stent follows a diagnostic vascular injection procedure, report the intervention separately.

Code +36227 is an add-on code for selective catheterization of the external carotid artery:

- Unilateral

Code +36228 is an add-on code for selective catheterization of the initial intracranial branch *and* each additional intracranial branch of the internal carotid or vertebral arteries:

- Unilateral
- Report with 36223, 36224, 36225, or 36226
- Includes any additional second- or third-order selective catheter placement in the same primary branch of the following:

    - Internal carotid
    - Vertebral
    - Basilar artery

Code +36228 includes the following:

- Accessing the vessel
- Placing the catheter(s)
- Contrast injections(s)
- Fluoroscopy
- RSI
- Closure of the artery incision (arteriotomy)

Bilateral Services for Codes 36222–36228. If performed bilaterally, use modifier −50.

EXAMPLE

A physician performs bilateral extracranial carotid angiography with selective catheterization of each common carotid (right and left). Report code 36222–50.

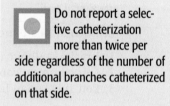
Do not report a selective catheterization more than twice per side regardless of the number of additional branches catheterized on that side.

Separate and Distinct Services for Codes 36222–36228. If different territories are studied in the same session on both sides of the body, use modifier −59 to show that different carotid and/or vertebral arteries are being studied.

EXAMPLE

A physician performs selective right *internal* carotid catheterization with right extracranial and intracranial carotid angiography followed by selective left *common* carotid artery catheterization with left extracranial carotid angiography. Report code 36224 for the right side and 36222–59 for the left side.

Dialysis Circuit

The dialysis circuit allows for easy and repeated access for dialysis. The circuit is created via an arteriovenous fistula or an arteriovenous graft and has two segments, a peripheral dialysis segment and a central dialysis segment. The code range is 36901–36909.

The peripheral segment refers to the upper and lower extremities beginning at the arterial anastomosis and ending at the central dialysis segment. The central dialysis segment represents the draining veins central to the peripheral dialysis segment. For the upper extremity, those draining veins are either the axillary vein or the entire cephalic vein when there is cephalic venous outflow. For the lower extremity the segment extends through the common femoral vein which includes the perianastomotic region. *Perianastomotic* is considered an historic term that refers to the area of the dialysis circuit near the arterial anastomosis and encompassing a short segment of the parent artery, the anastomosis and a short segment of the dialysis circuit immediately adjacent to the anastomosis.

Code 36901 is reported when a diagnostic procedure is performed to determine if therapeutic intervention is required. Give close attention to all the included services in this code. An example of code 36901 is a 70-year-old male with end-stage renal disease having difficulty with access to his arteriovenous shunt for dialysis. The diagnostic procedure is done to determine if he has stenosis at the access site that will require balloon angioplasty or some other intervention.

Codes 36902 and 36903 are reported when the diagnostic procedure as described above shows that either balloon angioplasty or stent(s) are required to clear the access for dialysis in the *peripheral dialysis segment*. Codes 36902 and 36903 include the services provided in code 36901. Coders should review the parenthetical notes provided in CPT below codes 36901–36903.

Code 36904 is reported when a blockage such as a thrombus is removed percutaneously via catheter or a lysis infusion is injected to remove the thrombus. If the thrombectomy procedure determines that balloon angioplasty is required in the peripheral dialysis segment then code 36905 is reported. Code 36905 is an indented code under 36904 and it includes the services in code 36904. If the thrombectomy procedure determines that a stent(s) is required in the peripheral dialysis segment, then code 36906 is reported. Code 36906 is an indented code under 36904 and it includes the services in code 36904.

This coding area has extensive guidelines in the CPT book and all should be carefully reviewed prior to coding the services.

Coding Venous Access Devices and Procedures

Implantable venous access devices provide easy access to the venous system. This avoids having to repeatedly perform venipuncture. The devices come in two types: completely implanted and partially implanted. Central venous access devices (CVADs) or central venous catheters (CVCs) are tubes placed in large veins for patients who require frequent access to their bloodstream for administration of medication (e.g., chemotherapy), administration of fluids, transfusion of blood products, multiple blood draws for diagnostic testing, and administration of total parenteral nutrition (TPN).

Completely implanted central venous devices include Port-a-Cath, Permcath, Medi-Port, Infuse-a-port, and Groshong port. Pinpoint the Code 20.2 illustrates the code assignment based

PINPOINT THE CODE 20.2: Venous Access

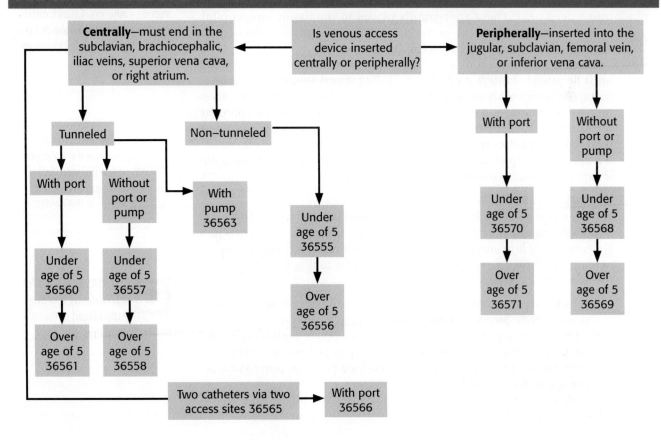

on whether the device is completely or partially implanted. Partially implanted access devices have a visible external catheter that is not near the venous entry site. The catheter is inserted into the subclavian or the internal jugular vein and tunneled and brought out through the subcutaneous tissue and sutured to the skin. Common partially implanted devices are Hickman, Broviac, Leonard, and Ventra.

Central Venous Access Procedures

Catheters have one end that remains outside the body while the other end is in a large vein near the heart. Venous access catheters are typically inserted into a vein of the neck, chest, or upper arm and occasionally the upper leg. The first thing to ask when trying to understand which device is being used is whether it has been placed in a peripheral (superficial) or central (deep) vein. Centrally inserted means that the insertion point is in the jugular, subclavian, or femoral vein or the inferior vena cava. The catheter is inserted and the vein entry site is created. To be classified as a CVC, the tip of the catheter must end in the subclavian veins, brachiocephalic veins, iliac veins, superior vena cava, or right atrium.

The devices are classified by whether they are tunneled or nontunneled. Nontunneled catheters are used for up to 30 days. A CVC is also called a *central line* or *triple lumen*. The most common CVC is the triple lumen. These can be placed by two methods:

- *Percutaneous placement*: The catheter is inserted into a vein through a puncture wound.
- *Cutdown placement*: A surgical incision is made in the skin to expose a vein. Then the catheter is inserted into the vein.

Tunneled CVCs are placed through a puncture in the skin, and then tunneled some distance underneath the skin before being introduced into the vein. Tunneled catheters are typically for long-term use. Examples of commonly used tunneled catheters include Hickman, Broviac, dual-lumen, triple-lumen, and Groshong catheters.

Peripherally inserted means the insertion point is not one of the four areas where a centrally inserted catheter would be placed. Peripherally inserted central venous catheters (PICC lines) are inserted directly into a peripheral vein, but they have a very long catheter that can be fed into a deep vein. These are typically placed in the basilic, antecubital, brachial, or cephalic veins in the arm. PICC lines can be placed by a nurse who is trained in performing this procedure.

To code an insertion of a central venous access device, the catheter must be placed through a newly established access site. Repair involves fixing the device without replacing the catheter, pump, or port. Replacement of a catheter is determined by whether it is a partial or complete replacement. Partial replacement involves the catheter only. Complete replacement requires replacing the entire device using the *same access site*. If a device is completely removed and a new device is inserted into a different access site, two codes would be reported.

> The terms *vascular access device* and *Port-a-Cath* are sometimes used by physicians to describe partially implanted venous access devices, completely implanted devices, or central venous catheters. Coders must read the procedure note or operative report in order to assign the correct CPT code.

> Codes are assigned based on the location where inserted and the technique employed, not by brand name of the device.

Venous Access Ports

Venous access ports are implanted into the subcutaneous tissue. These can be completely implanted or partially implanted under the skin. Ports that are completely implanted have a subcutaneous reservoir. Those that are partially implanted have an external device and tubing tunneled under the skin before it enters a vein.

> Code 36597 is used for repositioning a previously placed catheter under fluoroscopic guidance.

- To properly code CVADs, the coder must read the instructions that precede code 36555 and determine the following: Is this procedure an insertion, repair, partial replacement, complete replacement, or removal? Is the catheter inserted centrally or peripherally? Is the catheter tunneled or nontunneled? Is this a pump or port? What is the age of the patient?

Generally, removal of a CVC is reflected in the evaluation and management (E/M) code that is assigned for the patient visit. This usually entails only suture removal and withdrawal of the catheter and should not be coded separately. Should the catheter be embedded and involve more work in removal, use 37799.

If image guidance is used to place a catheter or port, assign code 76937 or 77001 in addition to the venous access code.

■ **CASE SCENARIO**

A patient is status post–right radical mastectomy and is planning to undergo several courses of chemotherapy. Patient is admitted for insertion of a Groshong catheter for chemotherapy administration. The guidewire was inserted into the right subclavian under fluoroscopic guidance. The Groshong catheter was pulled through the catheter assembly and into the superior vena cava. A subcutaneous pocket was created and the Groshong catheter was pulled subcutaneously downward into the pocket. The end of the catheter was connected to the port. Report codes 36561, 77001.

Ports are surgically implanted so the device is entirely under the skin. Ports do not have any parts projecting from the body. These are for long-term use in chemotherapy or dialysis. Examples are Port-a-Cath, Hemo-Cath, and Permcath. Pumps are placed under the skin to allow continuous intravenous delivery of medication such as pain meds or chemotherapy. Subcutaneous pumps are also used in addition to ports for continuous infusion of insulin and terbutaline for preterm labor.

The most common problem associated with venous access devices are infection and thrombus development. Revision of an access device is coded to 36534. Removal of a catheter is coded to 36589–36590. Declotting of a venous access device is coded to 36593.

CHECKPOINT 20.6

Assign the CPT code(s) for the following situations.

1. Due to the need for repeated IV infusions, a 64-year-old patient requires placement of a central venous access device. Local lidocaine is administered and the subclavian/jugular vein is punctured. The guidewire is passed centrally and the central venous catheter is placed. The catheter is sutured in position, dressed in standard fashion, and attached to IV infusion fluids. _____

2. A central venous catheter is inserted in a 40-year-old patient for chemotherapy treatment. _____

Hemodialysis Access, Intervascular Cannulation for Extracorporeal Circulation, or Shunt Insertion

Codes for shunt and cannulization procedures for hemodialysis patients can be confusing to coders because of the terms used such as *shunt, graft, cannula,* and *fistula.* The documentation must be read to determine which of these was created before assigning a code. An external arteriovenous shunt is an external catheter that connects an artery and a vein. The access point is on the outside of the body. A Scribner shunt is an example. A cannula is an external tube inserted between two veins to remove blood from one vein routing it through a dialysis machine and reinfusing through the other vein. The cannula is inserted for short-term dialysis of several days' duration. Cannula insertion is assigned to 36800. A fistula is an internal surgically constructed connection between an artery and vein allowing blood to flow from the vein through the graft for dialysis and then back to the artery. Fistulas are placed in the wrist or forearm. A direct AV anastomosis (or fistula) is coded 36821. The fistula requires weeks or months to mature before it can be accessed for dialysis.

An arteriovenous graft is done when the patient's veins are too small or too far apart or when there is not enough time to wait for a fistula to heal to perform the direct anastomosis. An AV graft is not direct and requires tube insertion or a donor vein to create a loop connection between an artery and a vein. The graft may be from an autogenous source (36825) or nonautogenous source (36830) such as Gore-Tex or Cimino. AV grafts are most commonly placed in the upper arm or thigh.

A 47-year-old female with chronic renal failure is admitted for arteriovenous fistula placement between the brachial artery and vein using a Gor-Tex graft. Report code 36830.

Complications of AV fistulas and grafts include clotting, obstruction, and narrowing of the access (stenosis). Several methods are used to treat stenoses: angioplasty, stent placement, and thrombectomy. Thrombectomies can be performed with or without revision of the graft. Declotting of a fistula or cannula is coded with 36860 and 36861. Although the code description states "external" cannula, these two codes may be assigned for internal or external cannula. Do not confuse "percutaneous" declotting procedures (36904–36906) with the open thrombectomy procedure described in 36831. Open revision of the AV fistula may or may not include thrombectomy (36832–36833). A portion of the fistula wall is removed and the remaining tissue sutured together. Code 36904 is assigned for a thrombectomy, percutaneous. It includes all the work required to remove the thrombus from the access, declot the graft, and restore flow to the access. Many methods are used to percutaneously remove a thrombus. Some examples are pharmaceutical thrombolysis (pulsed-spray, lyse and wait, short infusions, and longer infusions) and various types of mechanical maceration or clot removal (AngioJet, small Fogarty-type balloons).

> ▣ Thrombectomy of a nonhemodialysis graft has a separate code from dialysis graft thrombectomy. Report this by assigning 35875–35876.

INTERNET RESOURCE: Follow this link to see pictures of an AV fistula and graft: http://kidney.niddk.nih.gov/KUDiseases/pubs/glossary/a-d.aspx

CHECKPOINT 20.7

Assign the CPT code(s) for the following situations.

1. A 56-year-old patient is diagnosed with bladder and prostate carcinoma and must undergo chemotherapy. A Hickman catheter venous access device is inserted for anticipated chemotherapy administration. A guidewire was placed at an entry point in the skin and a tunneling tool was used to reach the venotomy site. The catheter was brought out through the skin near the left collarbone. _____

2. A dialysis patient is experiencing loss of bruits in the right AV fistula. Doppler demonstrates presence of a thrombus. The patient undergoes an open AV fistula revision with thrombectomy.

   _____

Transcatheter Procedures

Transcatheter procedures (37184–37188) are therapeutic services delivered via catheter placement. Report codes for the placement of the catheter and the therapeutic procedure. The RSI services, such as fluoroscopic guidance, are included. For the coder, this means that a minimum of two codes will be reported.

EXAMPLE

A percutaneous catheter was placed into the right common iliac artery for removal of a thrombus, and with a thrombolytic injection, using fluoroscopic guidance. Report 37184 for the thrombectomy and thrombolytic therapy, and 36245 for the selective catheter placement into the right common iliac artery. No code is used for the fluoroscopic guidance because it is included in this procedure.

Other Transcatheter Procedures

Careful review of the code descriptors for other transcatheter procedures (37191–37218) and their parenthetical notes are important because many of these procedures have inclusions such

CPT © 2017 American Medical Association, All Rights Reserved.

as fluoroscopy, selective catheterization, and radiological supervision and interpretations, which contradict the short introductory paragraph at the beginning of this section in CPT. For example, code 37215, *Transcatheter placement of intravascular stent(s), cervical carotid artery, open or percutaneous, including angioplasty when performed and radiological supervision and interpretation; with distal embolic protection,* has an extensive parenthetical note indicating that "37215 and 37216 include all ipsilateral selective carotid catheterization, all diagnostic imaging for ipsilateral, cervical and cerebral carotid arteriography, and all related radiological supervision and interpretation."

Throughout this section of the CPT, there are also references to "other than coronary." This clarification notes that the coronary-related transcatheter services are in the Medicine section of CPT. Examples are codes 37211 and 37213.

Endovascular Revascularization, Lower Extremity

This section provides guidelines for coding *lower extremity* endovascular revascularizations (37220–37235) for occlusive disease. The more-intensive services include the less-intensive services and only one code should be reported for each lower extremity vessel treated. The levels of intensity are as follows:

- Angioplasty is considered the least-intensive service.
- It is included when either an atherectomy or stent placement is performed.
- Atherectomy is the next level of intensity and is included in stent placement.
- The highest level of intensity is the stent placement and it includes atherectomy and angioplasty.

Coders should note that when more than one stent is placed in the same vessel, the code is reported per vessel, not per stent. These services also include accessing and selectively catheterizing the vessel, traversing the lesion, any RSI directly related to the intervention(s) performed, embolic protection, and closure of the arteriotomy site. If an extensive repair or replacement of the arteriotomy site is required, report those services.

These procedures may be performed as open or percutaneous. Three territories were created to represent the coding structure:

1. The iliac vascular territory is divided into three vessels: common iliac, internal iliac, and external iliac arteries.
2. The femoral/popliteal territory is considered a single vessel for reporting purposes.
3. The tibial/peroneal territory is divided into three vessels: anterior tibial, posterior tibial, and peroneal arteries. The common peroneal is considered part of this territory and is not reported separately.

When more than one vessel in a territory is treated, report the add-on code provided. The add-on code is not used for distinct lesions within the same vessel. Report the code per vessel, not per lesion. Note that there is no add-on code for the femoral/popliteal territory because it is considered a single vessel. If a lesion extends across the margins of one vessel within a vascular territory into another but is treated with a single therapy, report a single code for the service.

■ **CASE SCENARIO**

A patient has a stenosis that extends from the common iliac into the external iliac and is treated with placement of one stent; it is to be coded as one vessel in that territory. Report code 37221.

Question: How do you report endovascular revascularization of the iliac artery, unilateral with transluminal angioplasty?

Endovascular Revascularization

The endovascular revascularization codes (37236–37239) represent services for *other than* the lower extremity. These codes would not be used for cervical carotid, intracranial, intracoronary, extracranial vertebral, or intrathoracic carotid endovascular revascularization. They are codes for stent placement in artery(s) (codes 37236, +37237) and in veins (codes 37238, +37239). The primary code represents the initial artery or vein; the add-on codes represent each additional artery or vein. Even if multiple stents are placed, only one code is reported.

If angioplasty is provided during the stent procedure, it is included and would not be reported separately. Do not report the angioplasty if

- Provided in the same vessel as the stent
- Provided for predilation or postdilation of the stent vessel
- In the same vessel but outside the stented segment

NOTE: You may report the angioplasty separately if provided in a separate and distinct vessel.

NOTE: If nonselective or selective catheterization is provided, it is separately reportable—for example, with codes 36005, 36010–36015, 36200, 36215–36218, and 36245–36248.

Another important issue for stent coding is the use of stents for embolization. If the stent is placed for embolization purposes, report the embolization procedure. If the stent is used for management of an aneurysm, pseudoaneurysm, or vascular extravasation, report the stent code and not the embolization code.

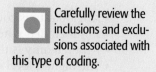
Carefully review the inclusions and exclusions associated with this type of coding.

> **■ CASE SCENARIO**
> A patient presents with abdominal pain and weight loss. Imaging demonstrates stenosis of the mesenteric blood vessels. A stent is placed in the superior mesenteric artery. Report code 37236.

Vascular Embolization and Occlusion

Embolization is the deliberate creation of an embolus or blood clot to obstruct blood flow to an area of treatment. Certain anomalies such as arteriovenous malformations, hemangiomas, and varices can be treated if blood flow to those areas is blocked. CPT codes 37241–37244 are reported in these circumstances. The guidelines for these codes stipulate specific included and separately reportable services. Included services are as follows:

- RSI
- Intraprocedural guidance and road mapping
- Imaging done to document completion of the procedure

Separately reportable services are as follows:

- Embolization/occlusion procedures in the head and neck (report 61624, 61626, 61710, 75894)
- Ablation/sclerotherapy procedures for venous insufficiency/telangiectasia of the extremities/skin (report 36468 for telangiectasia and 36470, 36471 for other than telangiectasia)
- Catheter placement(s)
- Diagnostic angiography

If ultrasound guidance is provided during procedures 36468, 36470, 36471, it may be reported separately. If these same procedures are provided in the office setting, all supplies and equipment are included.

Coders must refer to the diagnostic angiography guidelines in this book and/or the Radiology section of CPT to determine if the diagnostic angiography is allowed in addition to the embolization/occlusion procedures. If it is, use modifier –59 with the diagnostic angiography code.

As with all CPT procedural coding, carefully review guidelines and code descriptions for accurate reporting. Note that code 37241 is specific to venous anomalies other than hemorrhage, code 37242 is specific to arterial anomalies other than hemorrhage, and code 37243 relates to specific anomalies such as tumors, organ ischemia, or infarction. Code 37244 is reported for hemorrhage (arterial or venous) or for lymphatic extravasation.

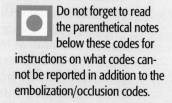
Do not forget to read the parenthetical notes below these codes for instructions on what codes cannot be reported in addition to the embolization/occlusion codes.

> **■ CASE SCENARIO**
> A patient complains of back pain. Based on prior history the patient is sent for a CT scan, which shows an arterial aneurysm. The patient is scheduled for embolization, and code 37242 will be reported on completion of the procedure.

Varicose Veins

Varicose veins are large, painful, and sometimes twisted veins that bulge from the legs because the valves in the veins have stopped working. They plague many people who must stand on their feet for great lengths of time. They may also occur in pregnant women. Spider veins are very small varicose veins that lie close to the surface of the skin. These veins are typically hormonally induced and associated with pregnancy and menstruation. Spider veins grow from reticular veins, also known as "feeder" veins. These are treated more for cosmetic purposes than because of pain.

The long saphenous vein (Fig. 20.5) runs just in front of the inner ankle and then up the medial or inner surface of the leg where it empties into the deeper femoral vein at the

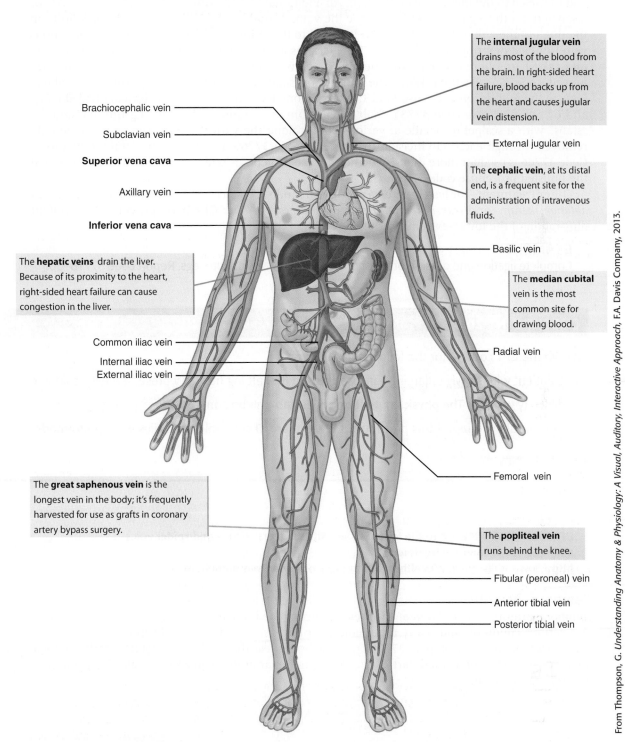

The **internal jugular vein** drains most of the blood from the brain. In right-sided heart failure, blood backs up from the heart and causes jugular vein distension.

Brachiocephalic vein

Subclavian vein

Superior vena cava

Axillary vein

Inferior vena cava

External jugular vein

The **cephalic vein**, at its distal end, is a frequent site for the administration of intravenous fluids.

Basilic vein

The **hepatic veins** drain the liver. Because of its proximity to the heart, right-sided heart failure can cause congestion in the liver.

The **median cubital** vein is the most common site for drawing blood.

Common iliac vein

Internal iliac vein

External iliac vein

Radial vein

The **great saphenous vein** is the longest vein in the body; it's frequently harvested for use as grafts in coronary artery bypass surgery.

Femoral vein

The **popliteal vein** runs behind the knee.

Fibular (peroneal) vein

Anterior tibial vein

Posterior tibial vein

Figure 20.5 The venous system.

From Thompson, G. *Understanding Anatomy & Physiology: A Visual, Auditory, Interactive Approach*, F.A. Davis Company, 2013.

saphenofemoral junction. The short saphenous vein begins at the base of the little toe, runs just behind the outer ankle, and then up the back of the calf where it usually joins the deeper popliteal vein at the saphenopopliteal junction. You may see the word "tributary" used here to indicate secondary veins.

Treatment for severe varicose veins involves ligating and stripping the diseased veins. During ligation, incisions are made over the problem vein, and the vein is tied off in an effort to cut off blood flow, hence making the vein less visible. This technique is becoming less common because the recurrence rate of varicose veins is high and there have been recent advances in vein therapy. Vein stripping utilizes a similar approach by making small incisions in the upper thigh and the area over the varicose vein. An instrument called a *stripper* is inserted through the incision in the thigh and tunneled to the incision over the vein. An additional incision can also be made at the ankle or elsewhere on the leg if necessary to locate the vein. A guidewire is passed through the vein from the thigh to the ankle. The end of the vein is tied to the guidewire, and the entire long saphenous vein is pulled or stripped out (37722). The incisions are closed with suture. The entire procedure may take 1 to 3 hours. When only the upper or lower portion of the long saphenous vein is removed, code 37700 is used. When the entire short saphenous vein (extending from the popliteal fossa to the foot) is removed, use 37718. When secondary varicose veins are ligated, divided (cut), and/or removed, use code 37785. Stab phlebectomy is conducted by creating tiny incisions or "stabs" with a scalpel or needle at various points along the varicose vein. The vein is gradually removed through each stab incision to the next. Code 37765 describes using 10 to 20 incisions. Code 37766 is used for more than 20 incisions. If the surgeon uses less than 10 stab incisions, assign the unlisted procedure code 37799.

Other treatments for less-severe varicosities include *sclerotherapy, electrodessication, endovenous ablation therapy,* and *transilluminated powered phlebectomy.* The CPT book provides an excellent illustration of the lower-extremity arteries.

EXAMPLE
Complete ligation and division of the short saphenous veins of both legs. Report code 37718–50.

CHECKPOINT 20.8

Assign the CPT code(s) for the following situations.

1. A patient with slowly enlarging varicose veins in the left leg has now presented with pain and difficulty walking. The physician performed 15 stab phlebectomies. _____

2. How would you report this procedure if fewer than 10 stab phlebectomies were performed?

   _____

INTERNET RESOURCE: Go to the following website to view varicose and spider veins and read about common treatments:
http://www.nhlbi.nih.gov/health/health-topics/topics/vv/treatment.html

Temporal Arteritis

Temporal arteritis is an inflammatory disease affecting medium and large arteries of the head. This is a serious condition and many times emergent because a patient can abruptly lose his or her vision. Temporal artery biopsy (37609) is a diagnostic test that is done to detect arteritis, which involves removing of a small part of the vessel and examining it microscopically for giant cells infiltrating the tissue.

HEMIC AND LYMPHATIC SYSTEMS ORGANIZATION

Codes in the hemic (blood-producing) and lymphatic systems' subsections encompass procedures on the spleen, bone marrow, lymph nodes, mediastinum, and diaphragm. Common procedures are splenectomy, lymph node biopsy, and bone marrow transplants.

The hemic and lymphatic systems headings include Spleen, General, and Lymph Nodes and Lymphatic Channels.

HEMIC AND LYMPHATIC ANATOMY

The hemic system is the blood that consists of plasma, white blood cells, red blood cells, and platelets. The lymphatic system aids in homeostasis by transporting fluid and nutrients and reabsorbing excess fluid, thus maintaining blood volume levels. It also triggers the immune response by developing lymphocytes, which monitor the blood and interstitial fluid for bacteria, viruses, and cancer cells. Once the immune response is sent into motion, antibodies are produced that bind to these foreign bodies.

The lymphatic system is a complex system made up of a vast highway of vessels, lymph nodes, and organs such as the spleen, thymus, red bone marrow, tonsils, and mucosa-associated lymphatic tissue in the small intestine (Fig. 20.6). All of these vessels and structures work together to transport interstitial fluid, called *lymph*, back to the blood, filter the fluid for foreign or pathological material, and initiate the immune response.

The spleen produces lymphocytes and destroys old red blood cells. The thymus in children and young adults produces T lymphocytes, which are essential to the body's immune function. The tonsils are located in the back of the throat and aid in fighting infection. Lymph nodes are bean-shaped nodes that are located in clusters around the body. Their purpose is to filter the lymph, removing wastes and excess fluid. Lymph nodes cluster in three superficial regions on each side of the body: the inguinal nodes in the groin, the axillary nodes in the armpit, and the cervical nodes in the neck. About 30% of the body's lymph nodes are located in the head and neck. The lymph nodes in the neck are in the following regions:

- Region I—the submental and submandibular group (nodes within the triangular boundary of the anterior belly of the digastric muscle and hyoid bone)
- Region II—the upper jugular group (nodes extending from the skull base to the carotid bifurcation)
- Region III—the middle jugular group (nodes extending from the carotid bifurcation to the omohyoid muscle)
- Region IV—the lower jugular group (nodes below the omohyoid and above the clavicle)
- Region V—the posterior triangle group (all lymph nodes in the posterior triangle of the neck, from the skull base to the clavicles and from the anterior border of the trapezius to the posterior border of the sternocleidomastoid muscles)

Lymph nodes are also located in the chest (supraclavicular region) and abdomen (retroperitoneal region). Superficial nodes are located in the subcutaneous tissue. Deep nodes are located by or below the muscle.

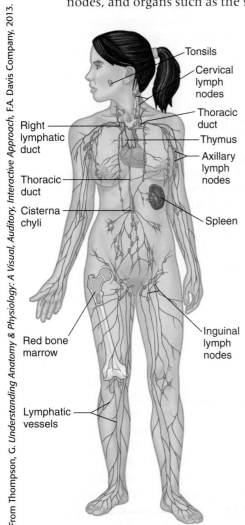

Tonsils

Cervical lymph nodes

Thoracic duct

Thymus

Axillary lymph nodes

Spleen

Right lymphatic duct

Thoracic duct

Cisterna chyli

Inguinal lymph nodes

Red bone marrow

Lymphatic vessels

Figure 20.6 The lymphatic system.

COMMON CONDITIONS OF THE HEMIC AND LYMPHATIC SYSTEMS REQUIRING TREATMENT

Lymphadenopathy

Lymphadenopathy is the enlargement of one or more lymph nodes as a result of normal reactive effects of the cleansing of the lymph and immune response.

Lymphoma

Lymphoma is a cancer that originates in the lymphatic system and is made up of lymphocytes. There are many types of lymphomas, including Hodgkin's disease.

Lymph Node Biopsy

Lymph node biopsy is usually one of the first diagnostic tests performed when determining the cause of the enlarged lymph node and in ruling out lymphoma. Not all swollen or painful lymph nodes are cancerous. Some may be a result of poor lymphatic vessel drainage or infection. Lymph node biopsy is carried out in two ways: needle or open incision. Needle biopsy involves inserting a needle under local anesthetic into a node to obtain the sample. An open biopsy consists of surgically removing all or part of a node under local or IV sedation (38500–38542). A small incision is made and the lymph node or part of the node is removed. Biopsy can be done laparoscopically (38570). Codes are selected based on the lymph node region (cervical, axillary, inguinal, etc.) and whether the lymph nodes are superficial or deep. The coder also needs to determine if the biopsy was via needle aspiration or skin incision. Fine-needle aspiration (as opposed to needle biopsy) is coded 10021.

Lymphadenectomy

Lymphadenectomy refers to removal of more than one lymph node. It is also referred to as *lymph node dissection*. This is a surgical procedure in which lymph glands are removed from the body and evaluated by a pathologist for the presence of cancerous cells. A limited or modified lymphadenectomy (38562–38564) removes only some of the lymph nodes in the area around a tumor; a total or radical lymphadenectomy (38700–38780) removes all of the lymph nodes in the area.

When you see the term *complete* when describing neck dissection, this is synonymous with "radical." When a radical dissection is carried out, all lymph nodes in that area are removed. If a complete cervical lymphadenectomy is performed, all lymph nodes in the five regions listed earlier would be removed. Lymphadenectomy is different from excision of lymph nodes in the range 38500–38555.

Sentinel node injection with biopsy is done to determine the spread of breast cancer or other types of cancers. Usually, four injections with a gamma probe are done. If the sentinel nodes have positive uptake of dye, that means that the cancer has spread.

Lymphedema

Lymphedema is swelling of the extremities from accumulation of interstitial fluid as a result of ineffective lymphatic drainage. The affected area becomes very swollen and painful. Most cases of lymphedema are caused by a blocked lymph vessel but can be a result of lymphadenectomy, trauma, infection, radiation therapy, or malignant disease. Lymphedema is not unusual after breast cancer surgery, particularly among those who undergo radiation therapy following axillary lymphadenectomy. It is diagnosed by using CT, Doppler ultrasonography, and lymphoscintigraphy. Treatments for lymphedema are massage, compression dressings, and drainage (38300). Intermittent pneumatic pump compression therapy may also be instituted on an outpatient basis or in the home. These devices provide sequential active compression from distal to proximal, effectively milking the lymph from the extremity.

Splenomegaly

A splenectomy is the complete or partial removal of the spleen due to extensive disease or trauma. Code selection is based on whether the excision is an open procedure or performed

CPT © 2017 American Medical Association, All Rights Reserved.

laparoscopically and whether the entire spleen is removed or a portion of it. The term *en bloc* in code 38102 means the whole spleen is removed; however, note that this is not a stand-alone code and must be reported with another procedure. In some trauma cases, the spleen can be repaired by suturing the lacerations and removing any damaged segments. Splenoportography requires instilling radiopaque dye into the spleen to radiographically visualize the spleen and portal veins. It is used to diagnose or assess portal hypertension and to stage cirrhosis to determine how far the disease has progressed. Instructions in CPT state that when reporting 38200, also report RSI code 75810.

Bone Marrow Diseases

Bone marrow is the soft spongy tissue found in the hollow interior cavity of bones. All bones have two types of marrow. Red marrow produces red blood cells, platelets, and white blood cells. Yellow marrow is high in fat and contains some white cells. Red marrow is found mainly in the flat bones. Yellow marrow is found in the hollow interior of the middle portion of long bones. In adults, marrow in large bones produces new blood cells. Diseases such as leukemia and tuberculosis, along with the treatments for these diseases such as chemotherapy and radiation, destroy stem cells and marrow, leaving the patient with a weak immune system. Treatments for bone marrow disease primarily consist of bone marrow and stem cell transplantation.

Bone marrow contains two types of stem cells: hematopoietic and mesenchymal stem cells. Hematopoietic or blood-forming stem cells are cells that can mature into blood cells—red blood cells (erythrocytes), white blood cells (leukocytes), or platelets (thrombocytes). These stem cells are found in the bone marrow, bloodstream, or umbilical cord blood. Mesenchymal stem cells are found arrayed around the central sinus in the bone marrow. They have the ability to produce osteoblasts to form bone, chondrocytes to create cartilage, and myocytes to create nervous tissue.

Bone Marrow and Peripheral Stem Cell Transplantation

Bone marrow transplantation (BMT) involves placing the donor under anesthesia and inserting a large-bore needle into the ilium or sternum. It consists of taking hematopoietic stem cells from one person and then infusing them into another person, or into the same person at a later time. Transplantation from one person to another is performed in severe cases of disease of the bone marrow: The patient's marrow is first killed with drugs or radiation, and then the new stem cells are introduced.

■● Transplant preparation codes are reported on a per diem basis, regardless of the quantity of bone marrow or stem cells that are manipulated.

Before radiation therapy or chemotherapy in cases of cancer, sometimes some of the patient's hematopoietic stem cells are harvested and later infused back when the therapy is finished to restore the immune system. *Harvesting* is the term used to describe obtaining the stem cells from the bone marrow or peripheral bloodstream. The stem cells can be harvested directly from the red marrow in the crest of the ilium (38230). The harvested bone marrow is processed to remove blood and bone fragments. The bone marrow is then combined with a preservative and frozen to keep the stem cells alive until they are needed. This technique is known as *cryopreservation*. Stem cells can be cryopreserved for many years.

Bone marrow aspiration (38220) is not the same as a bone marrow biopsy (38221). Aspiration uses a needle to remove some of the liquid bone marrow for analysis, as seen in Figure 20.7. Bone marrow biopsy removes bone and marrow for examination under a microscope. If these procedures are both done at the same biopsy site through the same incision, only report the biopsy. However, if they are done at *different* sites (different bones or different sections of the same bone) report code 38222. You cannot report 38220 with 38221.

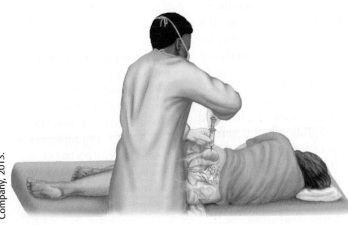

Figure 20.7 Bone marrow aspiration.

Peripheral blood stem cell transplantation (PBSCT) utilizes a process called *apheresis* or *leukapheresis* to obtain peripheral blood stem cells for transplantation. In apheresis, blood is removed through a central venous catheter. The blood goes through a machine similar to that of a dialysis machine that removes the stem cells. The blood is then returned to the donor and the collected cells are stored. The stem cells are frozen or cryopreserved until they are transplanted.

There are three types of transplants:

- Autologous: Patients receive their own stem cells.
- Syngeneic: Patients receive stem cells from their identical twin.
- Allogeneic: Patients receive stem cells from their brother, sister, or parent. A person who is not related to the patient (an unrelated donor) also may be used.

If donor and recipient are compatible, these infused cells will then travel to the bone marrow and stimulate blood cell production.

The code range provides codes for managing the procedures and for each specific type of transplant preparation.

MEDIASTINUM AND DIAPHRAGM ANATOMY

The mediastinum is the median space in the thoracic cavity that contains the heart, thymus, esophagus, trachea, and vasculature that connects to the heart. Codes 39000–39499 are submitted for procedures performed on the mediastinum. The diaphragm is a muscle that extends across the rib cage that divides the thoracic cavity and abdominopelvic cavities. The diaphragm has three large openings to allow for the passage of the aorta, esophagus, and vena cava. It contracts during respiration, causing the chest to expand when breathing in.

COMMON CONDITIONS OF THE MEDIASTINUM AND DIAPHRAGM REQUIRING TREATMENT

Hiatal Hernia

In a hiatal hernia (also called *hiatus hernia*) the stomach bulges up into the chest through an opening (hiatus) that allows the passage of the esophagus. There are two types of hiatal hernia: sliding and paraesophageal. In a sliding hiatal hernia, the stomach and the portion of the esophagus that joins the stomach slide up into the chest through the opening. The paraesophageal hernia is less common. In this condition, the esophagus and stomach are stationary but part of the stomach squeezes through the opening, where it sits next to the esophagus.

Hiatal hernia surgery can be performed laparoscopically. During surgery for a paraesophageal hernia, the stomach is pulled down into the abdomen, the esophageal opening in the diaphragm is made smaller, and the esophagus is attached to the diaphragm. Because sliding hiatal hernias rarely cause problems other than acid reflux, surgery is less likely. If surgery is required, it is carried out similar to the repair of paraesophageal hernias. However, in addition, part of the upper stomach is wrapped around the lower sphincter to augment the pressure at the sphincter and further prevent acid reflux.

> Codes for hiatal hernia repair are not located in the Index under hernia, hiatal. The coder must refer to diaphragmatic hernia and read the code descriptions for esophageal hiatal.

> If a prosthetic patch is required to repair a defect in the diaphragm, don't forget to assign a HCPCS code for the supply. Code 39561 is only applicable in cases where a portion of the diaphragm is removed and would not apply to hernia repairs.

Diaphragmatic Hernia

A diaphragmatic hernia is an opening or defect in the diaphragm, occurring before birth, which allows abdominal organs such as the stomach, small intestine, spleen, part of the liver, and the kidney to move into the chest cavity, crowding out the lungs. This is a medical emergency and must be repaired at birth. On rare occasions as a result of traumatic injury, a diaphragmatic hernia may result, requiring suturing or insertion of a patch to repair the defect. Codes 39540–39541 would apply.

Trauma

Code 39503 is reserved for neonates only. For children and adults, use 39540–39541.

Blunt trauma produces large radial tears of the diaphragm. In contrast, penetrating trauma usually creates only small linear incisions or perforations that result in diaphragmatic hernias. Any tears or injuries to the diaphragm must be repaired because these do not heal spontaneously. Codes 39501–39599 are submitted for procedures on the diaphragm.

CHECKPOINT 20.9

Assign the CPT code(s) for the following situations.

1. A patient presents for a persistently enlarged left posterior (deep) cervical lymph node. The complete node was excised by sharp dissection and sent to pathology. _____

2. A patient sustained an impelling injury to the diaphragm. Surgeon performed an emergent acute diaphragmatic hernia repair. _____

3. A patient sustained a severe injury to the diaphragm necessitating resection with muscle flap. _____

Chapter Summary

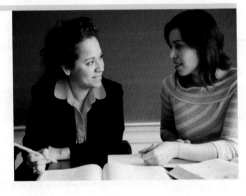

1. The anatomical structures of the cardiovascular system are the heart and its four chambers, arteries, veins, and the pericardium, a membrane that surrounds the heart. The four chambers of the heart are the right and left atria and the right and left ventricles. The arteries and veins are the circulatory system. Arteries carry blood from the heart to the rest of the body, while veins return blood from the body to the heart. The heart is made up of three muscle layers: endocardium, which is the innermost layer of muscle; myocardium, the middle layer; and epicardium, the outermost layer.

2. The most common conditions requiring treatment are bradycardia and tachycardia treated with pacemakers or cardiodefibrillators, coronary artery disease treated with coronary artery bypass grafts, heart valve disorders treated with TAVR/TAVI or more traditional valve repair or replacement methods, aneurysms treated with open or endovascular repairs, and artery or vein occlusions treated with bypass grafts.

3. A pacemaker treats arrhythmias in the heart function, most commonly bradycardia. Cardioverter defibrillators treat ventricular fibrillation, an erratic heartbeat that can cause sudden cardiac death. The cardioverter defibrillator uses electric shock to stop the fibrillation and restore a normal heart rhythm.

4. The more common acronyms in cardiovascular coding as indicated in this chapter are as follows: AAA, abdominal aortic aneurysm; AV, arteriovenous; AVG, arteriovenous graft;

CABG, coronary artery bypass graft; CAD, coronary artery disease; ECMO, extracorporeal membrane oxygenation; IAB, intra-aortic balloon; ICD, implantable cardioverter defibrillator; PCR, pacemaker; TAA, thoracoabdominal aneurysm; TAVI, transcatheter aortic valve implantation; TAVR, transcatheter aortic valve replacement; and VAD, ventricular assist device.

5. The three methods of coronary artery bypass graft are vein only, artery only, and combined artery and vein.

6. Open cardiovascular procedures require making an incision into the operative field to treat a coronary condition. The endovascular procedure allows the problem to be treated by placing a catheter into the arterial system and deploying a prosthetic device, for example, a balloon or an electrode, without making a large incision into the operative field.

7. The three most common types of heart transplant services are obtaining the donor heart, preparing the heart for transplant (backbench work), and placing the heart into the recipient. Placement of an artificial heart is less common.

8. The five vascular systems are venous, arterial, pulmonary, portal, and lymphatic. Each system has a main trunk such as the aorta in the arterial vascular system. Each artery that branches off the main trunk starts a vascular family.

9. Central venous access devices (catheter or device) must terminate in the subclavian, brachiocephalic, or iliac veins; or the superior or inferior vena cava; or the right atrium to qualify as central venous access devices. They can be centrally or peripherally inserted, tunneled or nontunneled.

10. The hemic and lymphatic systems are complex systems made up of vessels, lymph nodes, and organs such as the spleen, thymus, red bone marrow, tonsils, and mucosa-associated lymphatic tissue in the small intestine that work together to transport interstitial fluid, called *lymph*, back to the blood; filter the fluid for foreign or pathological material; and initiate the immune response. The spleen produces lymphocytes and destroys old red blood cells. The thymus in children and young adults produces T lymphocytes, which are essential to the body's immune function. The tonsils aid in fighting infection, and lymph nodes are located in clusters around the body to filter the lymph and remove wastes and excess fluid.

11. The most common conditions requiring treatment in the lymphatic and hemic systems are lymphadenopathy, the enlargement of the lymph nodes; lymphoma, cancer of the lymphatic system; lymphedema, a swelling of the extremities from the accumulation of interstitial fluid; splenomegaly, the enlargement of the spleen; bone marrow diseases such as leukemia and tuberculosis, which weaken the immune system as a result of both the disease and its treatment; hiatal hernia; and diaphragmatic hernia.

Review Questions

Matching

Match the key terms with their definitions.

1. __C__ Reestablishing the blood supply to the heart or within a blood vessel

A. arteriovenous graft
B. arteriovenous fistula
C. anastomosis
D. cannula
E. angioplasty

F. revascularization
G. CABG
H. nonselective catheterization
I. selective catheterization
J. ligation

2. __D__ An external tube used in dialysis and ECMO procedures

3. __A__ An external catheter that connects an artery and a vein

4. __I__ Placement of a catheter into a branch off the main vascular conduit

5. __J__ Vein tied off to cut off blood flow, making the vein less visible

6. __F__ Rejoining a blood vessel

7. __G__ Coronary bypass procedure using a vein and/or artery graft

8. ___E___ The surgical repair or reconstruction of a blood vessel

9. ___H___ Placement of a catheter into the main vascular conduit

10. ___B___ Surgically created connection between an artery and a vein

True or False

Decide whether each statement is true or false.

1. _____ When reporting placement of a transcatheter intravascular stent into a lower extremity artery, report code 37236.

2. _____ A left ventricular electrode must be placed at the time of the insertion of the pacemaker or implantable defibrillator.

3. _____ A needle bone marrow biopsy from the left iliac crest is coded with 38221–LT.

4. _____ If a catheter is placed into the femoral artery, then into the aorta, and then into the left common carotid artery, it is considered a selective catheterization.

5. _____ Coders can report a mitral valve replacement procedure without cardiopulmonary bypass.

6. _____ Always remember to report modifier –51 with the combined CABG codes 33517–33523.

7. _____ The inferior and superior venae cavae carry de-oxygenated blood to the heart.

8. _____ The endovascular revascularization codes 37220–37235 are divided into three territories and each territory is divided into three vessels.

9. _____ The central venous access codes are all age based.

10. _____ Report code 37216 when placing a stent into the cervical carotid artery with distal embolic protection.

Multiple Choice

Select the letter that best completes the statement or answers the question.

1. A patient has a long-standing history of varicose veins and elects to have ligation, division, and stripping of the greater saphenous vein from the saphenofemoral junction of the left leg. Additionally, the physician performed ligation, division, and stripping of the short saphenous vein of the right leg. Which codes are reported?
   A. 37700 LT, 37780–RT–59
   B. 37718–RT, 37722–LT, 37785–LT
   C. 37700–LT, 37718–RT–59
   D. 37722–LT, 37718–RT–59

2. A patient is evaluated for anemia and the blood work and evaluation show that the patient needs a bone marrow biopsy. Multiple passes of the needle are taken from the iliac crest. Report the bone marrow biopsy. Which code or codes are reported?
   A. 38221
   B. 38220, 38221–59
   C. 38220
   D. 38230

3. A 75-year-old patient is seen today for an enlarged deep cervical lymph node. The patient has had the problem for 2 weeks. Open excision of the lymph node is performed and a sample is sent for four-color flow cytometry. Which code is reported?
   A. 38500
   B. 38520
   C. 38510
   D. 38562

4. A patient with a dual-chamber pacemaker that was inserted 9 days ago now needs the atrial electrode repositioned. Which code is reported?
   A. 33216
   B. 33212
   C. 33218
   D. 33215

5. A 73-year-old patient with an existing dual-chamber pacemaker now requires a biventricular pacemaker. The right atrial and ventricular leads are retained and a left ventricular lead is inserted. Which code or codes are reported?
   A. 33216, +33225
   B. 33224
   C. 33224, +33225
   D. 33214, 33224

6. A patient received a heart/lung transplant at a hospital in New York. The donor heart was obtained at a hospital in Missouri. Code for the services of the donor cardiectomy–pneumonectomy.
   A. 33930, 33933, 33935
   B. 33935, 33933
   C. 33940
   D. 33930

7. Which term describes a slow heartbeat?
   A. Tachycardia
   B. Cardiomegaly
   C. Bradycardia
   D. Myocardial infarction

8. Which valve is located between the right atrium and right ventricle?
   A. Tricuspid
   B. Mitral
   C. Aortic
   D. Pulmonary

9. A patient undergoes a coronary artery bypass graft times three using the saphenous vein, an upper extremity vein, and the left internal mammary artery. Which codes are reported?
   A. 33533, +35500
   B. +33518, +35500
   C. 33533, +33518, +35500
   D. 33533, 33511, +35500

10. A patient with aortic stenosis needs a valve replacement procedure using a mechanical valve and cardiopulmonary bypass. Which code is reported?
    A. 33405
    B. 33411
    C. 33406
    D. 33400

CHAPTER 21

CPT: Digestive System

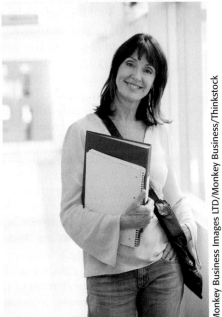

Monkey Business Images LTD/Monkey Business/Thinkstock

CHAPTER OUTLINE

Digestive System Anatomy

Endoscopy Rules

Definitions of Surgical GI Endoscopy Terms

Organization

Common Procedures

Common Endoscopic-Only Procedures

Common Diseases of the Colon

Bariatric Procedures

LEARNING OUTCOMES

After studying this chapter, you should be able to:

1. Identify anatomical structures of the lips, mouth, esophagus, stomach, intestines, and anus.
2. Determine when multiple endoscopy codes can be assigned.
3. Describe different types of hernias and how they are repaired.
4. Differentiate between esophagoscopy and esophagogastroduodenoscopy.
5. Recognize the difference between a screening and a diagnostic colonoscopy.
6. Describe the most common diseases and disorders of the digestive system.
7. Describe the various bariatric procedures available for weight reduction and assign codes for each.

This chapter presents the anatomical structures, common conditions surgically treated, and surgical techniques of the CPT Digestive System section. This chapter covers surgical services of low surgical complexity to high complexity of the mouth, esophagus, stomach, intestines, liver, pancreas, anus, omentum, and peritoneum.

DIGESTIVE SYSTEM ANATOMY

The digestive system is made up of two categories of organs: digestive organs and accessory digestive organs (Fig. 21.1). Digestive organs collectively called the *gastrointestinal (GI) tract* include the oral cavity, pharynx, esophagus, stomach, small intestine (duodenum, jejunum, and ileum), and large intestine (cecum, colon, rectum, and anus). These organs essentially form a continuous tube from the mouth to the anus. The accessory organs are teeth, tongue, salivary glands, liver, gallbladder, and pancreas. The Digestive System section of *CPT Professional Edition* has several anatomical illustrations to assist in visualizing various areas throughout the GI tract. Refer to an anatomy reference or search online for illustrations of the digestive tract.

> The Medicine section of CPT also includes digestive system diagnostic tests (91010–91299). Likewise, there are Category II and III codes as well as HCPCS codes available for procedures performed within the digestive system.

The digestive process begins in the mouth. The aroma of food causes the salivary glands in the mouth to secrete saliva. Saliva contains antibacterial compounds and various enzymes that aid in the breakdown of food particles and soften the food—enabling the tongue to form it into a bolus or ball and push the food to the back of the throat for swallowing. Think about it: Without a tongue, a person cannot swallow. Teeth chop and grind food, breaking the food down into pieces small enough to be digested.

Food is then swallowed and passes into the pharynx, or throat. Food is pushed through the esophagus and into the stomach by peristalsis, sequential muscular contractions. At the bottom of the esophagus, just before the opening to the stomach, is a ring-shaped muscle known as the lower esophageal sphincter (LES). This muscle relaxes (opens) to let food into the stomach and then tightens (closes) to prevent backflow. When the LES malfunctions and allows food in the stomach to reenter the esophagus, it causes gastroesophageal reflux disease (GERD), erosion or irritation of the esophagus characterized by heartburn, bloating, and/or regurgitation.

The stomach is a muscular pouch that acts as a food processor. The strong walls of the stomach churn the food into chyme, a semifluid mixture of partially digested food. Hydrochloric acid and digestive enzymes are released from the gastric walls to help digest foods such as protein, fats, some carbohydrates, and alcohol. Chyme slowly exits the stomach and passes into the small intestine.

The small intestine is approximately 17 feet in length and made up of three sections: the duodenum, jejunum, and ileum. As the chyme enters the duodenum from the stomach, the duodenal lining releases intestinal hormones that stimulate the gallbladder and pancreas to release bile and pancreatic enzymes, which help to further break down food particles. The small intestine is where most of the nutrients are digested and absorbed. The chyme is broken down in the duodenum and jejunum and nutrients are absorbed into the bloodstream through the ileum.

The large intestine, also referred to as the *large bowel*, is approximately 5 feet long and consists of three sections—the cecum, colon, and rectum. It serves two functions: to absorb all remaining water from the food waste and to compress the remaining material into feces or stool for excretion. The cecum is a short pouch containing a valve that opens to receive chyme from the ileum. The colon absorbs water and through bacterial action reduces the bulk of fiber in the feces. The rectum is the holding compartment for stool until it is passed through the anus. The anus comprises two sphincter muscles—the internal sphincter and the external sphincter. The internal sphincter is always tight, except when feces enter the rectum, to maintain continence. The external sphincter can be voluntarily controlled when one gets an urge to defecate. It takes approximately 36 to 48 hours for stool to pass through the large intestine.

Why are the liver and pancreas considered part of the digestive system? When food reaches the small intestine, the pancreas releases a bicarbonate liquid that mixes with the food to neutralize the stomach acid in the food as it enters the intestine. The enzyme produced by the pancreas breaks down the carbohydrate, fat, and protein in food. The liver produces a different digestive

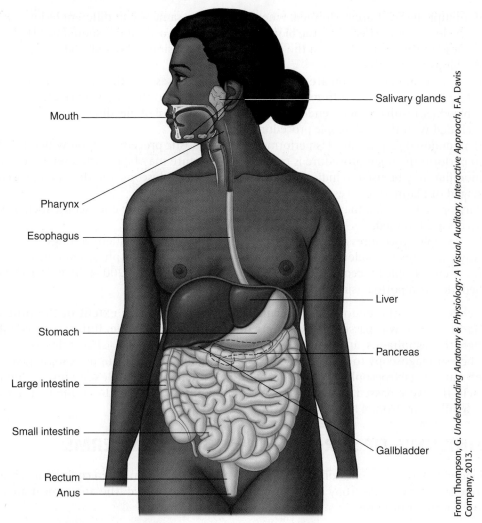

Figure 21.1 The digestive system.

From Thompson, G. *Understanding Anatomy & Physiology: A Visual, Auditory, Interactive Approach*, F.A. Davis Company, 2013.

enzyme—bile. It also cleanses and purifies blood coming from the small intestine that contains the nutrients just absorbed. Bile is stored in the gallbladder, and during meals the gallbladder contracts and forces the bile through the bile ducts and into the intestine to dissolve the fat in the food.

ENDOSCOPY RULES

Query third-party payers to determine their specific guidelines on payment policies for multiple endoscopies.

Because so much of the work done in the digestive system involves endoscopy, it is helpful to recap general rules to master when coding endoscopic procedures. Guidelines indicate it is appropriate to separately report multiple *therapeutic* endoscopic procedures in the same family when performed by the same provider at the same operative session. This is *not* the case if one of the endoscopies is diagnostic. General endoscopy coding points include the following:

- Code selection is based on (1) the location or site of the procedure, (2) the scope entry method (i.e., transnasal, transoral, stoma, transrectal), (3) whether it is diagnostic (used to see an abnormality or to decide the extent of disease) or therapeutic, and (4) the type of instrument used.
- If more than one endoscopic procedure is performed, use the –51 modifier on the second procedure.
- Remember that a diagnostic endoscopy is always included in a surgical endoscopy.

- If multiple biopsies are performed, whether from the same site or different lesions, and none of the lesions is excised, only the biopsy code should be used and it should be listed only once.
- If a lesion is biopsied and then the remainder of the lesion is excised, code only the excision; the biopsy is bundled.
- If a biopsy and an excision are performed at the same session, the biopsy can be coded separately *only if* it was taken from another lesion or site than the one(s) excised.
- If bleeding results from an endoscopic procedure, control of bleeding at the time of service is included with the endoscopic procedure.
- If an endoscopic procedure is performed as a diagnostic procedure upon which the decision to perform the open procedure is made, the procedure may be reported separately. A –58 modifier may be used to indicate that the diagnostic endoscopy and the open procedure are staged or planned services.
- Any procedures that may be normally performed as part of the endoscopy, such as venous access are bundled.
- Endoscopic procedures are done in various inpatient and outpatient settings.
- Any conscious or moderate sedation administered by the same physician performing one of these endoscopic procedures should be reported separately: 43200–45398, G0105, G0121. Sedation is reported using codes G0500 or 99151–99153.

To code any of the endoscopy procedures in this section, the extent of the procedure (or how far the scope was passed) is extremely important. For example, if the scope is only passed through the esophagus, it is an esophagoscopy (43180–43232). CPT endoscopy guidelines describe esophagoscopy to begin at the cricopharyngeus muscle or upper esophageal sphincter and end at the gastroesophageal junction and may include a retroflexed view of the proximal stomach. If it were passed into the stomach, duodenum, or farther down the GI tract, the code range would start from 43235–43259.

DEFINITIONS OF SURGICAL GI ENDOSCOPY TERMS

The following terms are commonly seen in medical documentation when coding for services in the digestive system. GI endoscopy codes specify the instrument used, the anatomical area, and the purpose for the procedure.

Snare Technique
In the snare technique, a wire loop attached to the end of the scope is secured around the growth (such as a polyp), and an electrical current is used to create pressure and sever it.

Hot Biopsy
Hot biopsy is carried out using hot biopsy forceps that simultaneously biopsy tissue and fulgurate or excise the site using electrocoagulation.

Biopsy (Cold)
Biopsy is carried out by introducing forceps through the scope to remove a specimen, whether it is a portion of a tumor or polyp or suspicious lesion of the intestinal wall. This is also referred to as a *cold biopsy*. A cytology brush may be passed through the scope to obtain cells from the surface of the lesion. You may see the term *stacked biopsy* where the physician takes multiple biopsy "bites" of a lesion with a thickened margin base to get a deeper margin to the edge of the wound.

Ablation
Ablation uses hot biopsy forceps, electrocautery, or a laser to disintegrate a lesion rather than remove it. This is done to polyps that are too small to remove (usually smooth sessile polyps of the intestine wall).

For endoscopy with a balloon dilator 30 mm or larger, assign 43214; if the balloon is less than 30 mm, use 43220. Review the operative note for dilations of the esophagus to determine if the scope was left in or removed.

Balloon Dilator
The term *dilation* refers to the process of stretching or widening. This is also referred to as *dilatation*. A balloon dilator is a balloon-tipped catheter that is inserted and then inflated at a narrowed area of the esophagus to dilate the narrowing. In this technique, similar to an angioplasty, force is exerted against the wall of the esophagus for a period of time to open a narrow passage. It can be done with or without an endoscope.

Guidewire

Guidewires are used as part of endoscopic procedures. A small, flexible-tipped guidewire is passed through the endoscope and left in place. The endoscope is withdrawn and dilators are passed over the guidewire to the area of treatment.

Weighted Bougie

A bougie is a metal or rubber device with two compartments. It is weighted (usually with mercury), which pulls it through a narrowed area in the esophagus. Think of it like a sinker used for fishing. This is attached to a balloon or over a guidewire and is used in dilating the esophagus during an upper endoscopy. A guidewire is passed into the stomach past the obstruction. Bougies are introduced over the guidewire in sequentially increasing sizes. The most commonly used bougie-over-guidewire dilators are the Savary or Savary-Gilliard dilators.

Unguided Bougie

Dilation of the esophagus may be accomplished without an endoscope using an unguided sound or unweighted bougie, in a single pass or multiple passes of the bougie. The physician blindly inserts the bougie into the esophagus. With an unguided bougie, no guidewire or dilator is used. Bougies are passed in sequentially increasing sizes to dilate the obstructed area. The Maloney and the Hurst are the most commonly used weighted bougie dilators.

> **INTERNET RESOURCE: Visit the Medovations website to view the various types of dilators.**
> **www.medovations.com/pdf/Esophageal_Dilatation.pdf**

French Size

Catheters and sounds are measured using the French catheter scale. The scale's commonly-used units range from 3Fr to 34Fr to indicate the outside circumference of these and other medical instruments such as endoscopes. Each French unit is equal to 1/3 mm. The diameter in millimeters of the catheter can be determined by dividing the French size by 3. A 24 French sound is equal to 8 mm in diameter. These sizes are often referenced in endoscopic procedures and help determine the size of the narrowing or size of catheter needed to perform procedures.

ORGANIZATION

Specific coding instructions for the digestive system are located in notes below subheadings and codes throughout this section. The organization follows the digestive tract beginning from the top and going down, as shown in Box 21.1, to the liver and biliary tract.

BOX 21.1 Digestive System Headings

Lips	Appendix
Vestibule of Mouth	Colon and Rectum
Tongue and Floor of Mouth	Anus
Dentoalveolar Structures	Liver
Palate and Uvula	Biliary Tract
Salivary Gland and Ducts	Pancreas
Pharynx, Adenoids, and Tonsils	Abdomen, Peritoneum, and Omentum
Esophagus	
Stomach	
Intestines (Except Rectum)	
Meckel's Diverticulum and the Mesentery	

COMMON PROCEDURES

Excision of the Tonsils and Adenoids

Tonsillitis and adenoiditis occur in both children and adults. Recurrent acute or chronic disease usually warrants removal. Age-specific codes are available for excision of tonsils and adenoids together and codes for tonsils and adenoids separately. The structures removed should be documented in the operative report and verified with the pathology report. After codes 42825–42836, the words *primary* or *secondary* appear. A primary procedure is when the designated procedure has not been performed prior to the current episode of care. Secondary means that this procedure has been performed in the past and must be redone because the tissue has regrown.

> ● Many of the digestive NCCI edits have the modifier indicator of "1," so the use of an appropriate modifier (usually –59) can override them.

Excision to Treat Tongue Tie

Tongue tie, or ankyloglossia, is classified by an unusually short, thick lingual frenulum (or frenum), a membrane connecting the underside of the tongue to the floor of the mouth. If you look at yourself in the mirror and curl your tongue back, you will see a strip of connective tissue that connects the tongue to the floor of the mouth. In children with tongue tie, the tip of the tongue or a significant portion of the tongue is "glued" or "tied down," affecting eating, swallowing, and speech. This condition is repaired by frenectomy (41115) or frenuloplasty (41520). With frenectomy, incisions are made in the frenum near where it attaches to the tongue and also where it attaches to the floor of the mouth. The frenum is then excised. In frenuloplasty, an incision in the shape of a "Z" is made through the frenum and the tissue is rearranged. This procedure is different from the simple incision with a blade or laser of surface tissue that characterizes the frenectomy. The frenuloplasty involves muscle repositioning with scar elongation (z-plasty) of a frenuloplasty that reduces the chance of relapse.

> ● Tonsillectomy and adenoidectomy codes are considered bilateral so do not use a –50 modifier.

> ● The words *frenulum* and *frenum* are both used, and these structures are located elsewhere, not just under the tongue. Read the operative report before assigning a code for frenectomy (excision) or frenotomy (incision). Do not rely on the term listed in the CPT Index, *frenulectomy*, which refers to the lips (code 40819). If the procedure is performed on the tongue (lingual), code 41115 is appropriate.

> **INTERNET RESOURCE:** Dr. Bechara Y. Ghorayeb's website has more information about tongue tie and its treatment. www.ghorayeb.com/TongueTie.html

Treatment of Lip Lesions and Injuries

Procedures on lips include biopsy, excision, and repair, and are located in code range 40490–40654. (Reconstructive procedures for cleft lip are discussed separately.) The operative report must be available in order to properly assign codes for excision of lip lesions due to varying techniques and anatomical landmarks. Documentation is important when choosing the correct code for repairs, which are based on the thickness of the laceration and whether the skin or the fleshy part of the lip is involved.

Coders must be careful when coding procedures involving lips. If the incision or repair crosses the vermilion border, a code from the digestive category is assigned. If it does not cross this border, it is considered an Integumentary System procedure. The vermilion border is a raised ridge of collagen along the upper and lower lips. It is composed of firm collagen, which shapes and contours the lip. Procedures done on the "pout" or the pink flesh-colored full lip are considered a digestive procedure. Most lip reconstructions are coded with integumentary surgery codes. Watch for parenthetical references to codes located in the Integumentary System section.

> **INTERNET RESOURCE:** Visit Body Cosmetica's *What Are Perfect Lips?* plastic surgery blog to view illustrations of the vermilion and other landmarks. www.cosmeticsurgeryforums.com/images/bigstockphoto_Lips888_30352.jpg

Repairs of Mouth Disease and Injuries

Tongue and gum lacerations are the most common injuries inside the mouth. Codes for repair of lacerations of the tongue or floor of the mouth are based on size of the laceration and location. The vestibule of the mouth is the oral cavity outside of the teeth. It includes the mucosal and submucosal tissue of the inside of the lips and cheeks. This tissue is often susceptible to oral cancers from smoking and chewing tobacco, and it is often biopsied or lesions are excised from it. The mouth is commonly injured in motor vehicle accidents, brawls, and while playing sports. Repairs to the vestibule (40830–40831) are performed by suturing the mucosa or with a more complex repair that involves tissue rearrangement and/or retention sutures. If a laceration is greater than 2.5 cm, code 40831 is assigned. Repairs to the gums are assigned by the quadrant in which the procedure is performed. The code description contains the phrase *specify*, which is the coder's clue to send the operative report along with the claim. Tongue repair codes are assigned based on size of the laceration (2.5 cm or less or longer than 2.6 cm) and location (anterior two-thirds or posterior one-third), if the repair is complex. A complex repair would involve complex closure techniques such as tissue rearrangement, extensive submucosal suturing, or repair of through-and-through lacerations. If the documentation describes debridement of grossly contaminated lacerations, this would also qualify as a complex repair.

> Codes 40840–40845 describe vestibuloplasty performed for reconstructive purposes or to deepen the vestibule to make room for properly fitted dentures.

> If injuries to the mouth require removal of teeth, there is no specific code for teeth extraction. Assign code 41899, *Unlisted procedures, dentoalveolar structures* or search for a HCPCS D code maintained by the American Dental Association.

> ■ CASE SCENARIO
> A pitcher was hit in the face with a line drive and suffered lacerations of the right inside of the mouth. Several teeth were also fractured. The surgeon examined the oral cavity and vestibule. Two lacerations were identified. A 3.0-cm laceration was located in the right posterior surface and a 4.0-cm laceration was found anteriorly behind the upper lip with obvious mucosal tissue absent. Under conscious sedation, the surgeon repaired the posterior submucosal tissue using submucosal retention sutures. He then performed a tissue rearrangement in the anterior region to close the defect. Report code 40831.

Cleft Lip and Palate

Cleft lip is a birth defect with a separation of the upper lip where the left and right sides of the lip do not meet. Clefts can occur on one or both sides of the upper lip. There is also varying severity of the cleft ranging from a notch in the vermilion to a complete separation running up into the nostril. To repair a cleft lip, the surgeon will perform a cheiloplasty, or lip repair, by making an incision on either side of the cleft from the mouth into the nostril. The vermilion is turned downward to pull the muscle and the skin of the lip together to close the separation and restore normal shape. Muscle function is restored and the "cupid's bow" shape of the mouth is realized. The nostril deformity may also be improved at the time of lip repair but commonly requires additional surgery.

Cleft lip and palate repair are performed by oral maxillofacial surgeons or plastic reconstructive surgeons. Codes for cleft lip (40700–40761, 42200–42225) are determined by whether the cleft surgery is unilateral or bilateral and the number of stages of surgery. *Primary* is considered the first surgery. As in code 40702, *primary, bilateral,* or *one of two stages* infers that there is going to be a second staged surgery to fix the cleft lip, which is not indicated in code 40701. A *secondary* surgery in this case is not necessarily a planned or staged procedure. It is a repeat of the primary surgery when unfavorable results remain from the first surgery, which may be due to infection, scarring, or a nonhealing wound. Cleft reconstruction may also require additional repair to the nose and nasal septum, in which case codes from 30400–30630 may be reported in addition to the cleft repair.

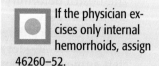

If repair of the nasal deformity is performed at the same time as the cleft lip, assign codes 30460 or 30462 in addition.

Because the lip and the palate develop separately, it is possible for a child to have a cleft lip with or without a cleft palate. A similar birth defect in the roof of the mouth, or palate, is called a *cleft palate*. In some children, a cleft palate may involve only a tiny portion at the back of the roof of the mouth; for others, it can mean a complete separation that extends from front to back. Cleft palate may involve the alveolus, anterior/posterior hard palate, and soft palate. Just as in cleft lip, cleft palate may appear on one or both sides of the upper mouth. Repairing a cleft palate involves more extensive surgery. The size of the cleft, exact location, and whether it is the primary procedure or a revision determine the type of repair performed. To repair a cleft palate, the surgeon will make an incision on both sides of the separation, moving tissue from each side of the cleft to the center or midline of the roof of the mouth. This rebuilds the palate, joining muscle together and providing enough length in the palate to improve eating, swallowing, and speaking. Some of the deformities require complete reconstruction of the alveolar ridge and lengthening of the soft palate. Bone grafting may be necessary to reconstruct the palate or augment the alveolar ridge.

To report a bone graft to an alveolar cleft as a secondary procedure for ridge augmentation, without a palatoplasty, use code 21210. For example, a child had a successful alveolar graft at 7 years old. Patient is now 12 years old and ready for a dental implant. Additional bone is required to properly support the dental implant.

NOTE: Remember to check the NCCI edits when reporting multiple codes for cleft lip or palate repair. Bundling edits exist and may require the use of a modifier to override the edit.

Prosthetic devices may also be used as adjuncts in cleft lip and palate treatment. Prosthetics are custom made to fit the individual from impressions obtained in the office. Assign code 42280 if the impressions are obtained in the office. Code 42281 is reported for insertion of the palatal prosthesis.

Code 21085 is reported for impression and custom preparation of an oral surgical splint. Do not report this code for a cleft palate prosthesis. Code 21076 is reported for preparation of a facial/oral prosthesis and includes taking impression(s), custom preparation, and delivery/insertion for the prosthesis—for example, a presurgical nasoalveolar moulding (NAM).

Hemorrhoids

Hemorrhoids, which affect about half of the population of the United States, are varicose veins in the anorectal region located inside (internally) or outside (externally) the anus. They are caused by increased abdominal pressure, and can become quite large and painful, requiring surgical treatment or removal. Hemorrhoids are treated using five methods: excision, injection, destruction, ligation, and stapling. Hemorrhoidectomy, the removal of hemorrhoids, can be achieved by several techniques: surgically excising the hemorrhoid, attaching rubber bands (ligation), or using a laser (destruction). Rubber band ligation involves tying a rubber band around the base of the hemorrhoid inside the rectum. The band cuts off circulation, and the hemorrhoid withers away within a few days. The terms *simple* and *complex* appear in these code descriptions. Complex hemorrhoids are described as bleeding, prolapsed, thrombosed, or requiring plastic skin closure (i.e., anoplasty). Hemorrhoids can also be treated with sclerotherapy, in which a chemical solution is injected around the blood vessel to shrink the hemorrhoid. Hemorrhoidopexy is used to treat internal prolapsing hemorrhoids and is accomplished by placing two rows of staples while at the same time a circular knife removes redundant mucosa.

If the physician excises only internal hemorrhoids, assign 46260–52.

Anal Fistula

Anal fistulas are caused by infection of an anal gland in the area where the rectum becomes the anus. An abscess forms and creates a tunnel or fistula tract to the outside buttocks or inside to the anus to drain pus. Complex fistulas may have twisting tracts or involve a significant part of the anal sphincter muscle. Treatment depends on the depth of the fistula and whether it involves the anal sphincter muscles. To treat an anal fistula, the surgeon explores the anus to determine the location of the fistula tract. At the time of surgery, a probe is placed in the fistula tract opening on the outside of the buttocks to the inside opening at the origin of the abscess. If the fistula involves only a small amount of sphincter muscle, then the tract is incised (also referred to as *divided*) or fileted open over the probe, exposing the tunnel or tract. The open tract is left open to heal from the inside out over the course of 2 to 4 weeks. If the fistula involves a large amount of anal sphincter muscle, then only part of it will be divided. The remaining portion of the muscle will be surrounded by a seton, which is thread, silk, or gauze that is placed in the fistula tract to allow it to drain to the outside and not trap in pus. If there are multiple fistulas or if they are complex, the surgeon may place a seton to preserve continence once the fistula tract has been dissected. Two types of setons are used: cutting and loose. A cutting seton is tightened over time to eventually erode or cut through the fistula tract, fileting it open gradually to heal from the inside out. Over time these eventually fall out by themselves. A loose seton works exclusively as a mechanism to keep the tract patent, allowing all infection to drain out.

Codes are assigned depending on the following factors: (1) whether an incision and drainage (I&D) of an abscess is performed along with the fistulectomy or fistulotomy (46060), (2) whether a hemorrhoidectomy is also performed (46262), (3) the complexity of the fistula or involvement of the anal sphincter muscle, (4) whether the treatment is staged (46285), (5) whether a fistulotomy/fistulectomy is performed or if fibrin glue (46706) or a fistula plug is placed (46707), or (6) whether the fistula is closed with an advancement flap (46288). Closing a fistula using a flap is accomplished by developing a flap composed of the inner lining of the rectum. This flap is pulled over the internal opening at the source of the anal gland infection and sutured beyond by transposing the skin, covering the internal opening with the flap. Subcutaneous fistulectomy is reported with 46270. Codes 46275–46280 describe treatment involving the specific sphincter muscle.

Varices

Varices are enlarged, dilated, tortuous blood vessels within the wall of the esophagus, stomach, duodenum, and rectum. These are typically caused by portal hypertension from liver disease such as hepatitis or cirrhosis due to alcoholism. These can be life threatening because the vessels can continue to fill with blood and eventually rupture. If bleeding occurs, patients could bleed to death. Surgical treatments include transection, ligation (banding), and sclerotherapy. Transection involves stapling the vessel to cut off blood supply. Ligation utilizes a rubber band that is placed around the base of the vessel. The objective here is to cut off blood supply whereby the vessel will shrivel up. During sclerotherapy, the physician injects the vessel with a chemical sclerosing agent that causes scarring in the vessel. These procedures can be carried out endoscopically. Codes for treatment of esophageal varices are based on whether an esophagoscopy or esophagogastroduodenoscopy (EGD) is performed and the technique used.

Achalasia

Achalasia, also referred to as *cardiospasm*, is an esophageal disorder where the lower esophageal sphincter spasms severely and fails to relax during swallowing. This condition can be treated endoscopically by stretching the sphincter with a balloon via esophagoscopy or EGD. It can also be treated by manipulation (43214). In achalasia treatment, larger balloons are used to apply more pressure to stretch the sphincter than in other balloon procedures.

> **INTERNET RESOURCE:** Visit the El Salvador Atlas of Gastrointestinal Video page to view endoscopic pictures of common gastrointestinal disorders and learn more about corresponding treatments.
> www.gastrointestinalatlas.com/english/hiatus_hernia_.html

Repair of Hernias

Hernias are weaknesses in the muscle wall of the abdomen that allow a sac of abdominal contents to protrude through. Almost all hernias in the muscle of the abdominal wall are the same thing, an area that has thinned out or weakened enough to form an orifice in the abdominal wall tissue. Surgical repair, sometimes with mesh insertion, is the corrective procedure.

There are several types of abdominal hernias. The name of the hernia relates to its location, as follows:

- *Inguinal*—common hernia of the inguinal canal in the groin; includes a "sliding inguinal" in which the hernia contents move down the posterior abdominal wall into the inguinal canal
- *Lumbar*—a very rare hernia occurring in the lumbar region of the torso
- *Incisional*—hernia occurring at the site of a previous incision
- *Femoral*—common hernia occurring in the femoral canal in the groin
- *Epigastric* (umbilical)—hernia located above the naval or inside of the belly button indentation
- *Spigelian*—usually located above the inferior epigastric vessel along the outer border of the rectus muscle
- *Sliding*—has the colon or cecum as part of the hernia sac (and in some cases, the bladder is involved)

Each type of hernia has its own separate code assignment, some differing by the age of the patient. (CPT has approximately 30 hernia repair choices!) Coders need to answer the following questions to choose correctly:

- Where is the hernia located?
- Is the hernia initial or recurrent? Initial hernias refer to the first time a hernia has been detected in any one location. Recurrent hernias are those that were repaired at some point and returned in the same location.
- Is the hernia strangulated/incarcerated or reducible? *Strangulated* hernias have part of the blood supply impaired by the herniation. This can be life threatening. *Incarcerated* (irreducible) hernias are imprisoned in the sac and cannot be manually reduced. It may be necessary to excise a portion of the incarcerated tissue in order to free the contents of the hernia sac. Reducible hernias allow the organs to be returned to normal position by the surgeon manipulating the viscera.
- Is the repair open (laparotomy) or laparoscopic? Hernias can be repaired either via open or laparoscopic surgery.

In the case of strangulated hernias, any repair of the strangulated or obstructed organs should be reported in addition to the hernia repair.

EXAMPLE

In the case of a 59-year-old patient with an incarcerated femoral hernia, the portion of the intestine that is strangulated requires repair. Two codes are reported: 49553 and 44120–51.

Postconception Age

To code for hernia repairs specific to preterm infants and children younger than 6 months at the time of the hernia repair, coders need to understand the concept of postconception age. Postconception age equals the child's gestational age at birth plus his or her age at the time of the repair. This relates to initial inguinal hernia repairs.

EXAMPLES

- A preterm infant is born at 35 weeks and requires hernia repair at 4 weeks of age. The postconception age is 39 weeks and the repair would be coded with 49491.
- A child is born full term and requires hernia repair at 2 months. The repair is coded with 49495.
- A child requires hernia repair at 7 months of age. The repair is coded with 49500.

When coding hernia repairs, follow the steps outlined in Pinpoint the Code 21.1.

> ● Do not code insertion of mesh for any hernia repair other than the incisional or ventral hernia. A separate code for the mesh (49568) is used in addition to the code for incisional and ventral hernia repairs only. Physician coders do not report 49568 with laparoscopic hernia repairs. Facilities are still permitted to report a HCPCS code for the supply of the mesh. Facility coders must check what is bundled into the APC payment for hernia procedure before assigning a code for the supply.

> ● A laparoscope is a thin, tube-like instrument used to look at tissues and organs inside the abdomen. A laparoscope has a light and a lens for viewing and may have a tool for removing tissue.

CPT © 2017 American Medical Association, All Rights Reserved.

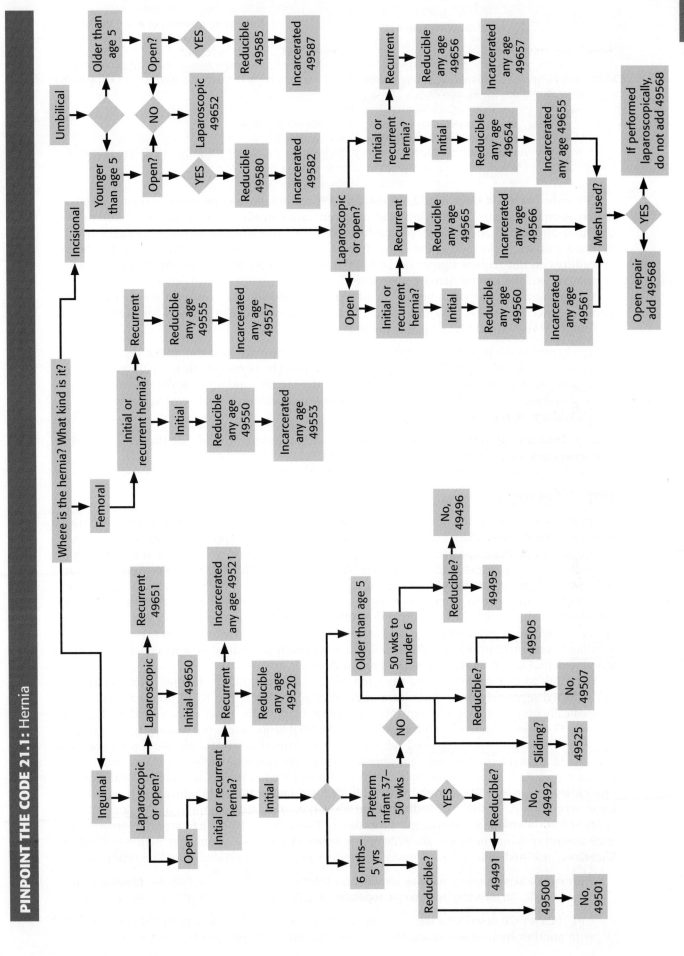

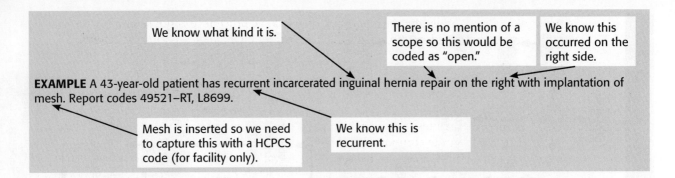

We know what kind it is.

There is no mention of a scope so this would be coded as "open."

We know this occurred on the right side.

EXAMPLE A 43-year-old patient has recurrent incarcerated inguinal hernia repair on the right with implantation of mesh. Report codes 49521–RT, L8699.

Mesh is inserted so we need to capture this with a HCPCS code (for facility only).

We know this is recurrent.

CPT codes 49560, 49565, 49652, 49654, and 49656 for laparoscopic or open repair of reducible incisional or ventral hernia, initial or recurrent, are considered incidental to a more definitive intra-abdominal operative service performed at the same site. Incidental procedures are not planned and are performed at the same time as a more comprehensive procedure. Incidental procedures do not require significant additional surgeon work and/or are integral to the work of carrying out the comprehensive procedure.

It is appropriate to report a hernia repair performed during the course of another open abdominal procedure if it is performed at a different incision site. The Centers for Medicare and Medicaid Services (CMS) NCCI policy manual says:

> If a hernia repair is performed at the site of an incision for an open abdominal procedure, the hernia repair is not separately reportable. The hernia repair is separately reportable if it is performed at a site other than the incision and is medically reasonable and necessary. An incidental hernia repair is not medically reasonable and necessary and should not be reported separately.

If the hernia is separately reportable, modifier –59 is required to indicate that it is extensive and separately identifiable in a different location.

Appendectomy

Appendicitis is inflammation of the appendix that if left untreated can result in the spread of infection throughout the abdomen or even gangrene of the appendix. Appendectomy, removal of the appendix, can be done open or laparoscopically. Incidental appendectomies are not coded separately with other open abdominal procedures. Based on CPT guidelines, appendectomy procedure code 44950, *Appendectomy*, and laparoscopic appendectomy code 44970, *Laparoscopy, surgical, appendectomy*, are included in other more extensive intra-abdominal or laparoscopic operative services performed at the same time. Add-on code +44955, *Appendectomy; when done for indicated purpose at time of other major procedure (not as separate procedure) (List separately in addition to code for primary procedure)*, is reported instead of 44950 for an appendectomy performed for a specific reason, other than incidentally, at the time of another open abdominal surgery.

According to CPT guidelines and the CMS NCCI policy manual, incidental appendectomy is not reported separately from other intra-abdominal procedures. The NCCI policy manual says, "A medically necessary appendectomy may be reported separately. However, an incidental appendectomy of a normal appendix during another abdominal procedure is not separately reportable.''

CPT code 44970, when reported with another laparoscopic intra-abdominal procedure, is considered an incidental laparoscopic appendectomy and not separately reportable. It is incorrect to report 44970 for laparoscopic removal of a diseased appendix at the same time as another intra-abdominal laparoscopic procedure. *CPT Assistant* provides guidance about reporting a laparoscopic appendectomy for indicated purposes (i.e., diseased appendix) at the same time of another intra-abdominal laparoscopic procedure: "There is no CPT code to report a laparoscopic appendectomy when done for an indicated purpose at the time of another major procedure. Therefore, unlisted code 44979, *Unlisted laparoscopy procedure, appendix,* would be reported."

NOTE: Before assigning appendix codes, identify the patient's insurance provider. CMS (i.e., Medicare) has a different policy for reporting laparoscopic appendectomy. Their policy conflicts with CPT where it states:

> CPT code 44970 describes a laparoscopic appendectomy and may be reported separately with another laparoscopic procedure code when a diseased appendix is removed. Since

removal of a normal appendix with another laparoscopic procedure is not separately reportable, this code should not be reported for an incidental laparoscopic appendectomy.

Cholecystectomy

Gallbladder disease is one of the most common gastrointestinal disorders in the United States. Cholecystitis is inflammation of the gallbladder caused by a blockage of the cystic duct. Cholelithiasis describes the presence of stones in the gallbladder, a painful condition that occurs when there is an imbalance or change in the composition of bile.

Cholecystectomy (47562-47579, 47600–47620), removal of gallbladder, the only effective treatment for these conditions, can be done open or laparoscopically. Most gallbladder surgery is performed laparoscopically; an open procedure is required only if surgical complications arise or the gallbladder is too big to remove through the portal. Removal includes destruction by morcellation, coagulation, laser technique, cystic artery and cystic stump inspection, and insertion of drains. The operative note must be read before assigning a code to first determine if the procedure was performed laparoscopically or open, and to determine if cholangiography, or exploration of the common duct, was performed.

■ CASE SCENARIO
A patient has chronic cholecystitis with cholelithiasis. Patient is scheduled for laparoscopic cholecystectomy. A 5-mm trocar was placed in the umbilicus and a 5-mm, 30-degree scope was used to inspect the abdominal cavity. The gallbladder was grasped and lifted. Blunt dissection was carried out around the cystic duct, which was then clipped and divided. The gallbladder was taken off the liver bed. It was pulled out of the 12-mm trocar site. Incisions were closed with 0 Vicryl suture. Report code 47562.

CHECKPOINT 21.1

Assign the CPT code(s) for the following situations.

1. A 4-year-old boy suffers from left inguinal hernia and left scrotal hydrocele. Procedure: Hernia repair. An incision was made in the left groin. The external oblique aponeurosis was opened and the hernia sac identified. The sac was opened and transected and ligated high. The tunica vaginalis was opened and a small amount of hydrocele fluid was removed. A small portion of the hydrocele sac was removed. A trocar was inserted and the abdomen was filled with CO_2. A 120-degree lens was inserted and the right groin appeared normal. The CO_2 was removed. An ilioinguinal nerve block was applied using 10 cc of 0.25% Marcaine with 1:200,000 epinephrine.

   _____

   Check the NCCI edits and indicate if you are permitted to code for the ilioinguinal nerve block. Yes or no? _____

2. The patient presents with a gallstone. Procedure: Laparoscopic cholecystectomy. Trocar was inserted and the patient had dense adhesions around the gallbladder, making it difficult to reach and requiring dissection. Cholangiogram was attempted. I could not get any flow of contrast out of the gallbladder itself. The gallbladder was manipulated and dye still would not spill. The plan changed to dissect the gallbladder out and then do a transcystic cholangiogram. The gallbladder was freed and the cystic duct was opened. Cholangiogram was performed. The gallbladder was taken out through one of the trocar sites. _____

3. The patient is a 65-year-old man who for at least the past 30 years has experienced intermittent hemorrhoidal symptoms, which have become progressively worse. On examination, he was

Continued

found to have moderate-sized edematous left lateral external hemorrhoid with a large prolapse, left lateral internal hemorrhoidal column, containing several small thromboses. A hemorrhoido-pexy by stapling was indicated. Beginning posteriorly, a #2-0 Prolene suture was placed in a purse-string fashion along the submucosal plane approximately 4 to 5 cm above the dentate line. When this was completed, the Fansler retractor was removed and the PPH anal canal dilator and obturator were then placed over the purse-string suture and carefully positioned to protect the anal sphincter complex. The PPHO3 stapler was then fully opened and the purse-string suture was secured around the shaft of the anvil, then retrieved through the barrel of the stapler with a suture threader. The suture was secured upon itself and retracted as the stapler was then fully closed. The stapler was kept closed for 30 seconds, fired, released, removed, opened, and inspected. _____

4. The patient was seen in the ambulatory surgery center (ASC) for removal of tongue mass. A submucosal mass was located on the left anterior third of the tongue. 1% Xylocaine with epinephrine was used to infiltrate the tongue. An incision was made, the submucosal tissue was divided, and the lesion was bluntly dissected. The wound was then closed with 4-0 chromic. _____

5. Diagnosis: A 25-year-old patient with chronic hypertrophic adenotonsillitis. Procedure: Adenotonsillectomy. The nasopharynx was visualized with laryngeal mirror. The adenoids were removed with Barnhill Jones curette. The tonsils were removed by blunt dissection and snare technique. Bleeding was controlled with 2-0 gut loop ties. _____

6. A 2-year-old boy fell and hit his mouth on the coffee table, sustaining a traumatic mucocele. An 8-mm firm mucocele was located on the midportion of the mucosal surface of the lower lip. The lesion was excised sharply with scissors. The base was cauterized with the Bovie. _____

7. The patient is experiencing anal pain in the posterior midline. She was diagnosed with fistula in ano in the posterior midline. The anus was examined and there were Grade I internal hemorrhoids without significant external hemorrhoidal tissue. She had a fistulous opening that was probed. It was superficial above the sphincter muscle. Fistulotomy was performed, opening this area with Bovie cautery. _____

8. Diagnosis: A 36-year-old male with umbilical hernia. Procedure: Umbilical hernia repair. There was a 1-cm umbilical hernia fascial defect. No incarceration was noted. An infraumbilical incision was made, and the umbilical skin was elevated from the hernia sac, which was excised. The fascia was closed with interrupted sutures of 3-0 silk. _____

9. The patient has a recurrent femoral hernia that is strangulated this time. Ten years ago, the patient underwent repair. Physician performs this by making a 4-cm incision in the femoral area and inserting a PerFix mesh patch. _____

COMMON ENDOSCOPIC-ONLY PROCEDURES

Per the CMS NCCI policy manual, procedures for the control of bleeding are included in any invasive procedure in the same anatomical area.

Control of bleeding is an integral component of endoscopic procedures and is not separately reportable. If it is necessary to repeat an endoscopy to control bleeding at a separate patient encounter on the same date of service, the HCPCS/CPT code for endoscopy for control of bleeding is separately reportable with modifier –78 indicating that the procedure required return to the operating room (or endoscopy suite) for a related procedure during the postoperative period.

Endoscopic Retrograde Cholangiopancreatography

When a sphincterotomy of the bile duct or pancreatic duct is performed, it includes a diagnostic ERCP.

Endoscopic retrograde cholangiopancreatography (ERCP) is a diagnostic and therapeutic procedure to evaluate and treat pancreatitis, jaundice, and gallstones. ERCP uses an endoscope to examine and x-ray the pancreatic duct, hepatic duct, common bile duct, duodenal papilla, and gallbladder. The endoscope is passed through the mouth and down into the first part of the small intestine (duodenum). A smaller tube (catheter) is then inserted through the endoscope into the bile and pancreatic ducts. A dye is injected through the catheter into the ducts, and an x-ray is taken.

Code assignment is based on associated procedures performed such as biopsy, sphincterotomy/papillotomy, removal of stones, insertion of stent, removal of foreign body, dilation of ducts, and ablation of tumors. Code the associated sphincterotomy (43262) if performed in addition to the primary procedures 43261, 43263–43265, 43275, 43278, ERCP with removal of foreign body or stones or insertion of stents. ERCP is not considered a component of these procedures and is reported separately.

Esophagoscopy

Esophageal biopsy (43202) can be reported separately from 43216, 43217, and 43229 if the biopsy site is different from the site of tumor removal or ablation. However, 43202 should only be reported once without modifiers regardless of the number of biopsies performed.

Esophagoscopy is an endoscopic examination of the 25-cm esophagus, stopping before the pylorus. It can be performed using a rigid scope under general anesthesia or a flexible scope with topical spray anesthesia and light sedation. It can be either diagnostic or therapeutic using either a rigid or flexible scope and codes are differentiated as such. It is routinely performed to evaluate swallowing difficulties and to diagnose esophageal cancer, Barrett's esophagus, and Schlotzki's ring; to remove foreign bodies; and to treat esophageal strictures. Codes range from 43180–43232. The flexible scope esophagoscopy base code 43200, *Esophagoscopy, flexible, transoral; diagnostic, including collection of specimen(s) by brushing or washing, when performed (separate procedure)*, is not reported with codes 43202–43232, because these codes each include the base code.

Stomach endoscopy is included in a UGI endoscopy.

Esophagogastroduodenoscopy

If an endoscope is passed through only as far as the diaphragm it is an esophagoscopy or esophagogastrostomy (series 43200). If the the scope is passed through the pyloric channel it is an esophagogastroduodenoscopy or EGD or UGI (series 43235). The documentation must indicate that the scope reached into at least the duodenum to code for an EGD.

Esophagogastroduodenoscopy (EGD) is the endoscopic examination of the esophagus, stomach, and duodenum (the upper GI, or UGI). It is also referred to as an upper GI or a gastroscopy. EGDs are performed to evaluate epigastric pain, ulcers, gastroesophageal reflux, dysphagia, hematemesis, and dyspepsia.

The flexible endoscope used is 120 cm long. During this procedure, the scope is inserted into the mouth and moved into the stomach. The various portions of the stomach are inspected, and then the tip is passed through the pylorus, into the duodenal bulb, and sometimes as far as the descending portion of the duodenum. Before the scope is backed out of the stomach, it is *retroflexed* to allow visualization of the gastric fundus.

The EGD code is chosen based on whether the procedure was a simple primary exam, diagnostic, or surgical procedure. Codes for EGD do not all fall within a clean range of codes; they include 43210, 43235–43259, 43266, 43270. The base code for EGD 43235, *Esophagogastroduodenoscopy, flexible, transoral; diagnostic, including collection of specimen(s) by brushing or washing, when performed (separate procedure)*, would not be reported with other codes from 43210, 43239–43259, 43266, 43270, because these codes include the examination. Fluoroscopy may be used to verify positioning of devices introduced into the esophagus and is reported as indicated in CPT. Code 43247, *EGD, flexible, transoral; with removal of foreign body*, includes removal of anything not native to the tissue of the esophagus, stomach, or duodenum such as paper, food, foreign objects from trauma, and percutaneous endoscopic gastrostomy tubes.

EGD With Dilation

Esophageal dilation can be performed either by using a balloon, by using dilators, or by simply passing the scope through the esophagus. Code 43220, *Esophagoscopy flexible, transoral; with transendoscopic balloon dilation (less than 30 mm diameter)*, describes inserting a balloon up to 30 mm in diameter. While viewing through the scope, the balloon is inflated several times. CPT notes that if a balloon larger than 30 mm is used, assign code 43214. Also, if imaging guidance is used, assign code 74360.

A guidewire may also be used for esophageal dilation. Code 43226, *Esophagoscopy flexible, transoral; with insertion of guidewire followed by dilation over guidewire*, works in much the same way as 43220 except dilators such as the Savary-Gilliard are used instead of balloons. After dilation for an obstruction, if a stent is placed, also assign code 43212, *Placement of a plastic tube or stent*. Esophageal dilation without visualization through the scope is coded from the 43450–43460 codes listed under the manipulation header.

Code selection depends on whether a balloon or guidewire was used. The most common code is 43220 for the Maloney dilator attached to a balloon and used endoscopically. If this was done with an EGD, the code would be 43249. If the dilator was *not* attached to the balloon, the codes would be 43200 and 43450. If the Maloney was *not* attached to the balloon used with an EGD, the codes would be 43235 and 43450.

Manipulation. Dilations without endoscopy are typically referred to and coded as manipulations. These codes are found in the Digestive System subsection titled Manipulation. Believe it or not, codes 43450–43460 for manipulation of the esophagus do not indicate that an endoscope is used, so two codes must be reported if an endoscope is used at all during the procedure. Dilation with a bougie is reported with 43450, *Dilation of esophagus, by unguided sound or bougie, single or multiple passes*. If the physician performs endoscopy first, the endoscopy should be reported with 43235, and then the dilation code (43450) with a –51 modifier. For example, the provider performs esophagoscopy followed by dilation of the esophagus. The endoscopy is not included in code 43453, *Dilation of esophagus, over guidewire*; therefore, assign code 43200 in addition.

Percutaneous Endoscopic Gastrostomy

The percutaneous endoscopic gastrostomy (PEG) procedure is performed by placing a tube through the abdominal wall to facilitate feeding and nutrition in patients who have difficulties swallowing from conditions such as oral and esophageal cancer, stroke, spinal cord injuries, and dementia or those on a ventilator. Codes are assigned based on where the tube is placed (stomach, duodenum, cecum), how it is placed (with or without endoscopy), and whether it is an initial insertion or

The CLOtest rapid urease test is often performed in patients with chronic gastritis and peptic ulcer disease. The CLOtest detects urease, which is produced by the bacterium *H. pylori*. *H. pylori* eats through the stomach mucosa and burrows into the lining of the stomach and duodenum causing infection and ulcers. A sample of tissue is obtained from the antrum of the stomach during an EGD. Assign 43239 and 87076 or 87077 *only if* the physician or the endoscopy center has the facilities to perform the actual analysis of the sample. If the specimen is sent to an outside lab, codes 87076 or 87077 cannot be reported by the physician. If the test is positive for *H. pylori*, then the patient is placed on a course of antibiotic therapy.

Esophageal and gastric washings for cytology are part of an upper GI, so do not report codes 91000 or 91055 separately.

In the unlikely event that an esophagoscopy and upper GI endoscopy are performed at the same time, the multiple-endoscopy rule does not apply because the procedures are in different endoscopic families.

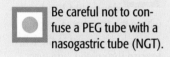

Be very careful when coding esophageal dilations. The extent of the scope will drive the code selection. For example, esophagoscopy with dilation with balloon is coded to 43220; however, the same procedure carried out via EGD is coded 43249.

When endoscopic esophageal dilation is performed, the appropriate endoscopic esophageal dilation code is billed. The CPT codes 43450–43453 are not used in addition even if attempted unsuccessfully prior to endoscopic dilation.

Be careful not to confuse a PEG tube with a nasogastric tube (NGT).

conversion, replacement, or repositioning. Feeding tubes can be placed laparoscopically, endoscopically, or by open incision with direct visualization using fluoroscopic guidance. The documentation should state the method of placing the tube.

Cross-references are located throughout the section directing the coder to endoscopic and nonendoscopic percutaneous tube placement. All codes for placement of the PEG tube include fluoroscopic guidance; therefore, fluoroscopic guidance is not reported separately.

Endoscopic placement of the PEG tube is coded to 43246. The scope is passed through the mouth and esophagus into the stomach. A needle is inserted through the abdomen, visualized within the stomach by the endoscope. A suture passed through the needle is grasped by the endoscope and attached to the end that will be outside the abdomen and pulled out through the abdominal wall.

■ CASE SCENARIO

An 87-year-old nursing home resident has lost weight, has been experiencing an increasing inability to swallow, and is recovering from aspiration pneumonia. Physician felt a PEG tube was necessary to continue to provide adequate nutrition. Physician inserted a nasogastric tube into the stomach under imaging guidance. The stomach was inflated with air. An incision was made to puncture the stomach wall using fluoroscopic guidance. He introduced a needle into the stomach and passed a wire. A gastrostomy tube was inserted and secured to the skin externally. Report code 49440.

There may be times when an existing gastrostomy tube needs to be exchanged because the tube becomes blocked or the stoma site becomes enlarged and enteral fluid leaks out around the tube during feedings. If the tube is removed and replaced with a new one at the same site, report codes 49450–49452. If an existing gastrostomy, duodenostomy, jejunostomy, or gastrojejunostomy tube is removed and a new tube is placed via a separate percutaneous access site, the placement of the new tube is not considered a replacement and would be reported using the appropriate initial placement codes: 43246 for endoscopic placement and 49440–49442 for a nonendoscopic approach.

Anoscopy, Proctoscopy, and Proctosigmoidoscopy

The key to determining which set of codes to apply lies in understanding the differences between anoscopy, proctoscopy, and proctosigmoidoscopy. Coders must identify the specific diagnostic or therapeutic services provided to establish which code within the set to assign. To correctly code sigmoidoscopy versus colonoscopy, coders must find out how much of the bowel was visualized and where/how the scope was inserted.

Anoscopy is the endoscopic examination of the rectal area, including the anus, anal canal, and lower rectum. The scope is passed up to 5 cm into the rectal area. A digital rectal exam is always performed prior to the exam and is not reported separately from the endoscopy. Anoscopy is performed to diagnose hemorrhoids, rectal prolapse, rectal cancer, perianal abscess, and anal fissures. If the procedure is done by manipulation as opposed to endoscopy, using anesthesia (general, spinal, or epidural), code 45990 is reported; CPT specifies the elements this code includes.

Proctoscopy is the endoscopic examination of the anal cavity, rectum, or sigmoid colon using a proctoscope (or rectoscope) to examine 6 to 25 cm of the rectal area and sigmoid colon. According to the CPT index, proctoscopy is reported using the same codes as anoscopy.

Proctosigmoidoscopy is reported using codes 45300–45327. Proctosigmoidoscopy, also called *rigid sigmoidoscopy*, is performed to examine the most distal portions of the GI tract, the rectum and sigmoid colon. Code 45300 is performed as a diagnostic measure when patients exhibit symptoms indicating hemorrhage of rectum and anus, anal or rectal polyp, or anal or rectal pain. Codes 45303–45327 represent therapeutic procedures.

INTERNET RESOURCE: More information on proctoscopy is available at: www.steinergraphics.com/surgical/002_05.6D.html

Flexible Sigmoidoscopy

Sigmoidoscopy uses a flexible endoscope to view the rectum and sigmoid colon up to 60 cm. It is performed with a fiber-optic scope that can be used to view the colon and take biopsies of the mucosa. The length of the scope allows the physician to also examine the descending colon and part of the transverse colon not visible with the rigid scope. Typically, it is performed to find the cause of bright red blood per rectum (BRBPR), abdominal pain, or chronic constipation, and to look for early signs of cancer in the descending colon and rectum. Flexible sigmoidoscopy is not sufficient to detect polyps or cancer in the ascending or transverse colon. A colonoscopy is needed to view beyond 60 cm of intestine.

Colonoscopy

Colonoscopy is the endoscopic examination of the large colon and the distal part of the small bowel. Colonoscopies include examination of the entire colon from rectum to the distal part of the small bowel, the cecum, and may advance into the ileum itself. Colonoscopies are performed with a larger and longer scope that can reach the entire colon. Colonoscopies can become complex—maneuvering the scope through the length of the intestines—and are performed under conscious sedation. The scope can be inserted through the rectum, a colostomy, or a colotomy. A colonoscopy is coded if the scope is passed beyond the splenic flexure or more than 60 cm of colon (Pinpoint the Code 21.2). There is great debate about this issue. General coding rules have always indicated that you code to the extent that the procedure is performed. Technically, if the scope is not passed through the splenic flexure, it is not a colonoscopy—it is a sigmoidoscopy. CPT provides specific instructions for this and we must follow these guidelines. The *CPT Professional Edition* contains a colonoscopy decision tree to help guide coders with decision points for both diagnostic and therapeutic procedures.

The splenic flexure is the area of the downward bend where the transverse colon passes horizontally to the left, toward the spleen, and turns down.

According to CPT, if a patient is scheduled for and fully prepped for a diagnostic colonoscopy and due to unforeseen circumstances the scope is not passed beyond the splenic flexure, report code 45330. If the scope passes the splenic flexure but does not reach the cecum, report 45378 with a –53 modifier. However, for Medicare patients, Medicare carriers require reporting 45378 with the –53 modifier instead. For a therapeutic colonoscopy that does not reach the splenic flexure, report a code from 45331–45347. If the scope reaches beyond the splenic flexure but not to the cecum, report 45379–45398 with a –52 modifier. For Medicare patients, Medicare requires the –53 here, too. Check your local Medicare payer for specific payment policies.

Screening Versus Diagnostic Colonoscopy

Medicare (and possibly some private payers) defines and regulates screening procedures—those performed in the absence of a reason to do them, such as signs and symptoms of a disease. The *ICD-10-CM Official Guidelines for Coding and Reporting* defines screenings as "the testing for disease or disease precursors in seemingly well individuals so that early detection and treatment can be provided for those who test positive for the disease." A screening colonoscopy is done when the patient exhibits no intestinal problems or complaints (such as bleeding or constipation). A screening colonoscopy code is also assigned when a patient has a strong personal or family history of colon cancer but has no signs or symptoms at that time. The screen is performed to detect asymptomatic polyps/cancers. The first-listed diagnosis code will always be ICD-10 code Z12.11, *Encounter for screening for malignant neoplasm of colon,* for a Medicare colon screening followed by any diagnoses for conditions or abnormalities discovered or treated during the colonoscopy.

The rules governing Medicare prohibit coverage of a screening procedure unless it is approved as an exception by Congress. But because they are so effective in keeping people healthy, Medicare has gradually received authorization to cover some screening services, such as colonoscopies. The coding and billing must carefully follow Medicare guidelines for reimbursement.

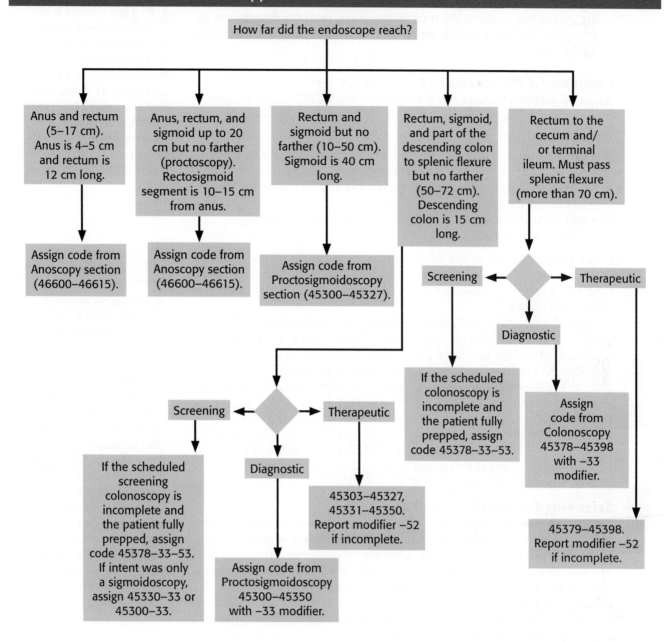

How far did the endoscope reach?

Anus and rectum (5–17 cm). Anus is 4–5 cm and rectum is 12 cm long.
→ Assign code from Anoscopy section (46600–46615).

Anus, rectum, and sigmoid up to 20 cm but no farther (proctoscopy). Rectosigmoid segment is 10–15 cm from anus.
→ Assign code from Anoscopy section (46600–46615).

Rectum and sigmoid but no farther (10–50 cm). Sigmoid is 40 cm long.
→ Assign code from Proctosigmoidoscopy section (45300–45327).

Rectum, sigmoid, and part of the descending colon to splenic flexure but no farther (50–72 cm). Descending colon is 15 cm long.

Rectum to the cecum and/or terminal ileum. Must pass splenic flexure (more than 70 cm).

Screening ↔ Therapeutic

Diagnostic

If the scheduled colonoscopy is incomplete and the patient fully prepped, assign code 45378–33–53.

Assign code from Colonoscopy 45378–45398 with –33 modifier.

45379–45398. Report modifier –52 if incomplete.

Screening ↔ Therapeutic

Diagnostic

If the scheduled screening colonoscopy is incomplete and the patient fully prepped, assign code 45378–33–53. If intent was only a sigmoidoscopy, assign 45330–33 or 45300–33.

45303–45327, 45331–45350. Report modifier –52 if incomplete.

Assign code from Proctosigmoidoscopy 45300–45350 with –33 modifier.

For private payers, a screening or diagnostic colonoscopy is reported with the same CPT code. The diagnoses submitted will be one for screening colonoscopy and a second for any abnormality found on examination. For Medicare, assign the same diagnosis code for screening. As long as no abnormality is treated, use the HCPCS G code for the screening colonoscopy instead of the CPT code.

If the patient presents with any gastrointestinal complaints such as diarrhea or constipation and the physician orders a colonoscopy, it is not a screening service, it is a *diagnostic* colonoscopy. The aim of the procedure is to uncover the cause of the symptoms—that is, to detect any malignancies and treat them. The coder would code the procedure and assign the diagnosis codes for the presenting symptoms if there were no significant findings on endoscopy. Making this determination is paramount in assigning the correct diagnosis codes to Medicare patients specifically.

EXAMPLE

For a 55-year-old patient not on Medicare, a diagnostic colonoscopy code (45378) is assigned along with the diagnosis code Z12.11 for the screening. If the patient is having diarrhea and a colonoscopy is performed, 45378 is assigned with the diagnosis code R19.7, along with any other incidental findings. In contrast, a Medicare patient code

G0105 or G0121 is submitted depending on whether the patient is high risk along with diagnosis code Z12.11. If the patient is complaining of diarrhea, code 45378 is submitted along with the diagnosis code R19.7. No screening code is reported because the patient is exhibiting symptoms.

Medicare HCPCS Screening Colonoscopy Codes

As stated earlier, Medicare often assigns its own HCPCS codes for procedures. The specific colorectal screening codes required by Medicare for reporting patients who are at high risk are as follows:

- G0104, *Colorectal screening; flexible sigmoidoscopy*
- G0105, *Colorectal cancer screening; colonoscopy on individual at high risk*
- G0106, *Colorectal cancer screening; alternative to G0104, screening sigmoidoscopy, barium enema*
- G0120, *Colorectal cancer screening; alternative to G0105, screening colonoscopy, barium enema*

A high-risk patient is one who has had colon cancer before, has had colon polyps, has a history of inflammatory bowel disease (ulcerative colitis or Crohn's disease), or has a family history of colon cancer or adenomatous polyps.

Code G0121, *Colorectal cancer screening; colonoscopy on individual not meeting criteria for high risk*, is used when performing a screening on a patient who does not have any high-risk factors. An example is a 69-year-old person who is concerned about cancer and just wants to have the procedure done for early detection. This is a special coverage service by Medicare, and the beneficiary may be liable for payment. For example, Medicare will allow G0121 to be reported once every 10 years. An Advance Beneficiary Notice (ABN) should be obtained prior to services being rendered. Code G0122, *Colorectal cancer screening; barium enema*, is not covered and is submitted when performed on a patient who is not high risk.

Screening Converted to Surgical

Coders are often confused about what to do when a screening colonoscopy is performed and there are incidental findings such as hemorrhoids. Is the procedure still considered a screening colonoscopy? The answer is yes, it is. The intent of the procedure and whether the patient is high risk drive the code. The code for the screening (CPT 45378) along with the diagnosis code Z12.11 and the code for the hemorrhoids (internal versus external) are assigned. The only time Z12.11 is not used as the principal diagnosis code is when a malignancy is found.

If a screening colonoscopy is scheduled and initiated, and there is need to perform a biopsy or polypectomy, the procedure is no longer considered a screening colonoscopy. Because of the additional procedures, it is converted to a surgical colonoscopy that includes the screening. In this case, no G code is submitted. The coder assigns a code from the range 45379–45392. To help differentiate between diagnostic and screening colonoscopies for Medicare patients, use the decision tree provided in Pinpoint the Code 21.3. When the screening endoscopy is converted to a surgical endoscopy, append modifier –33 to the surgical endoscopy code (for commercial plans). Medicare requires modifier –PT in lieu of modifier –33.

Colonoscopy With Biopsy

Code 45380, *Colonoscopy, flexible, proximal to splenic flexure; with biopsy, single or multiple,* should be reported for the removal of a portion of the polyp by cold biopsy forceps. Code 45380 is also used when the entire polyp is removed by cold biopsy forceps. As in all endoscopic procedures, if a biopsy is performed at a different site from a polyp removal or destruction of a lesion, it can be reported separately using a –59 modifier.

Section G of HCPCS has Medicare professional services codes that may or may not be used by commercial insurance plans. In many cases, G codes are used in lieu of CPT codes for Medicare patients. For example, G0105, *Colorectal cancer screening; colonoscopy on individual at high risk*, is required instead of CPT code 45378.

- Medicare covers screening colonoscopies in an individual of average risk every 120 months (10 years); for persons at high risk for colon cancer, every 2 years; and flexible sigmoidoscopies are covered every 4 years for beneficiaries who have reached age 50.
- Start counting with the month after the patient received the last test/service. For example, if a high-risk patient is seen in March for a screening colonoscopy, start counting 24 months beginning with April. The patient would be eligible for another screening colonoscopy in April 2 years following.

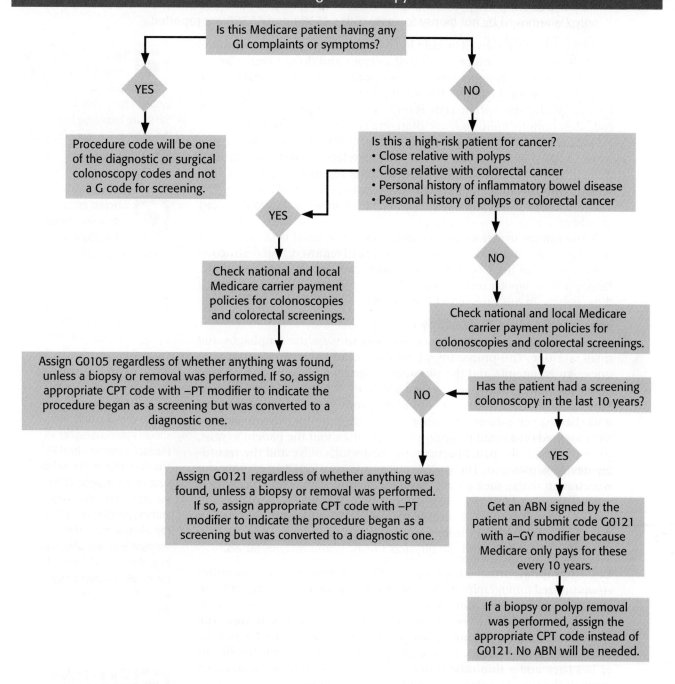

Is this Medicare patient having any GI complaints or symptoms?

YES

Procedure code will be one of the diagnostic or surgical colonoscopy codes and not a G code for screening.

NO

Is this a high-risk patient for cancer?
• Close relative with polyps
• Close relative with colorectal cancer
• Personal history of inflammatory bowel disease
• Personal history of polyps or colorectal cancer

YES

Check national and local Medicare carrier payment policies for colonoscopies and colorectal screenings.

Assign G0105 regardless of whether anything was found, unless a biopsy or removal was performed. If so, assign appropriate CPT code with –PT modifier to indicate the procedure began as a screening but was converted to a diagnostic one.

NO

Check national and local Medicare carrier payment policies for colonoscopies and colorectal screenings.

NO

Has the patient had a screening colonoscopy in the last 10 years?

Assign G0121 regardless of whether anything was found, unless a biopsy or removal was performed. If so, assign appropriate CPT code with –PT modifier to indicate the procedure began as a screening but was converted to a diagnostic one.

YES

Get an ABN signed by the patient and submit code G0121 with a –GY modifier because Medicare only pays for these every 10 years.

If a biopsy or polyp removal was performed, assign the appropriate CPT code instead of G0121. No ABN will be needed.

EXAMPLE
Colonoscopy is performed and random biopsies are performed at 50 and 35 cm. A 5-mm polyp is fulgurated at the distal sigmoid. Codes 45378 and 45380–59 would be reported.

Colonoscopy With Polyp Removal
Colon polyps are described as either pedunculated or sessile. Pedunculated polyps grow from a stalk on the wall of the bowel. Sessile polyps are wart-like growths that are attached directly to the wall of the colon. Sessile polyps by nature are more difficult to remove because of this attachment. Codes are assigned based on the technique used and whether the polyp was partially or completely removed, destroyed, or biopsied. When multiple techniques are used to remove a *single* polyp, only the most comprehensive or complex code that accurately describes the procedure is reported. When different polyps are removed by different techniques/methods, both techniques are reported.

If a polyp is completely removed from the ascending colon by snare technique and a second polyp is removed by hot biopsy forceps, codes 45384 and 45385 are reported.

Polyps may be removed by cold biopsy forceps or by snare technique. Cold biopsy forceps utilize no electric current and do not cauterize. In contrast, snare technique uses an electrocautery snare (a heated wire loop) to shave off the polyp. If several polyps are removed by the same technique, the appropriate code is only reported once, because the CPT code descriptions indicate more than one tumor, polyp, or lesion.

At times, the physician may want to "mark" the inside of the intestine where a polyp once was removed for future reference and tracking. This is described by the physician in the endoscopy report as "inking" or "tattooing" with India ink. If this is done, also assign code 45381, *Colonoscopy, flexible, proximal to the splenic flexure; with directed submucosal injection(s), any substance*.

Some tumors or lesions are not amenable to removal because of their size, type, or location and are destroyed instead of removed. This destruction is done by using hot biopsy forceps, bipolar cautery, or snare technique. Heater probes, bipolar probes, or argon lasers may also be used in treating these polyps. In this case, report code 45388.

> If one polyp, tumor, or lesion is removed with both snare and hot biopsy, report only the code for the snare technique because the snare is the more complex procedure.

> Wireless endoscopy is only reimbursable in the physician office (place of service 11).

Wireless Capsule Endoscopy

Wireless capsule endoscopy is another way to view the esophagus and small intestine. This procedure is typically performed when a patient has unexplained anemia and the physician suspects GI bleeding. A capsule no bigger than a multivitamin called a PillCam is swallowed and with its cameras takes 14 pictures per second as it moves through the digestive tract. During the 8-hour exam, the images are continuously transmitted and captured on a small recording device worn about the patient's waist. After the exam, the patient returns to the doctor's office and the recording device is removed. The stored images are transferred to a computer workstation where they are reviewed by the physician. This procedure is not a replacement for colonoscopy, because the PillCam's battery does not last long enough to take pictures of the colon. This procedure is coded by using codes 91110–91111 from the Medicine section. These codes include the cost of the capsule and the physician reading and interpretation.

> If the physician uses an endoscope to place the PillCam for the capsule study, you should append modifier –52 (Reduced services) to 91110. The descriptor of 91110 clearly states the evaluation is from the esophagus to the ileum. The endoscopic placement of the capsule makes it technically impossible for the physician to perform the assessment of the esophagus depending on where the physician releases the capsule.

Colonography. Virtual colonoscopy (VC), or colonography, uses either computerized tomography (CT) or magnetic resonance imaging (MRI) to produce two- and three-dimensional images of the colon from the lowest part, the rectum, all the way to the lower end of the small intestine. The procedure is used to diagnose colon and bowel disease, including polyps, diverticulosis, and cancer. During the procedure, the patient lies on his or her back and a thin tube is inserted into the rectum. Air is pumped through the tube to inflate the colon for better viewing.

Gastroenterologists may order a CT colonography (74261–74262) as a diagnostic procedure when traditional colonoscopy fails. Patients with documented signs or symptoms of GI disease that undergo an incomplete diagnostic colonoscopy due to obstruction from neoplasm, stricture, tortuosity, spasm, redundant colon, diverticulitis, extrinsic compression, or scarring from prior surgery require further workup to determine the extent of disease and treatment options.

Colonography is not reimbursable when used as an alternative to standard colonoscopy, for screening, or in the absence of signs or symptoms of disease.

> Virtual CT colonoscopy may be reimbursed when performed following a fiber-optic colonoscopy that was incomplete due to obstruction. Results of a previous incomplete fiber-optic colonoscopy must be documented and available for review if requested by the carrier.

Assign the CPT and HCPCS code(s) if necessary for the following situations.

1. A 65-year-old is admitted for a screening colonoscopy. The patient had no symptoms but does have a family history of colon cancer. The physician finds diverticulosis on exam. Assign the procedure code. _____

2. A patient had been experiencing chronic constipation, nausea and vomiting, and left lower quadrant abdominal pain. Upon testing, there was blood in the stool and upper GI x-ray showed sigmoid volvulus. A flexible sigmoidoscopy with decompression of the volvulus was carried out.

   _____

3. A 3-year-old boy is seen in the emergency department (ED) for suspected foreign body in the throat. His parents state that he was playing with his army action figure and put the figure in his mouth, swallowing the helmet. A flexible esophagoscopy with foreign body removal is performed.

   _____

4. A 4-year-old child is operated on for her second-stage operation for a bilateral cleft lip. Her first primary repair was performed at 1 year of age. _____

5. A patient is seen in follow-up for Barrett's esophagus. A scope was passed into the esophagus under direct visualization to the gastroesophageal (GE) junction at 37 cm in the distal esophagus. Barrett's was seen. Multiple biopsies were obtained. The scope was passed into the stomach, which appeared normal. The scope was then advanced into the duodenum, which was also normal.

   _____

6. A patient is seen for screening colonoscopy. The patient is complaining of hematochezia. Scope is inserted and two sessile polyps are located in the ascending colon, each measuring 2 mm in size. Biopsies were taken with cold biopsy forceps, essentially removing the polyps. One additional polyp was found in the transverse colon. This polyp measured 5 mm and was removed by hot snare. _____

7. A patient with rectal cancer was seen in follow-up for flexible sigmoidoscopy with submucosal tattooing (10 mL of India ink) of mid to upper rectal cancer. It was recommended to him that he undergo flexible sigmoidoscopy with tattooing of the cancer to facilitate proper identification and subsequent laparoscopic resection. The scope was passed proximal to the lesion into the distal sigmoid colon at approximately 25 cm and slowly withdrawn, where at 12 cm a sessile villous-appearing lesion was located. Multiple photographs were taken. Ten milliliters of India ink were injected in three separate quadrants just distal to the lesion. The scope was withdrawn.

   _____

8. The patient underwent colonoscopy for chronic constipation. The patient was fully prepped for the study. A scope was inserted and advanced to the sigmoid colon. The prep was totally inadequate. The scope was unable to pass beyond the sigmoid due to obstruction with firm stool. _____

COMMON DISEASES OF THE COLON

Colon and rectal diseases encompass a broad range of conditions and ailments. Some conditions may be mildly chronic, but when flare-ups occur, they can be debilitating and painful, while others are acute and potentially life threatening. Diseases or disorders of the colon primarily fall into three categories: (1) structural, (2) autoimmune, and (3) functional. Structural conditions may be congenital or develop over time and involve an abnormality that may need to be removed (e.g., polyp, mass), altered, or repaired (e.g., perforation). Structural conditions also include blockages and twisting of the intestine. Colitis is classified as an autoimmune inflammatory bowel disease of the colon where the patient's body attacks its own intestinal tissue. The two main types are ulcerative colitis and Crohn's disease. Bowels that are formed appropriately but don't function properly are attributed to functional disorders. These disorders consist of chronic constipation, diarrhea, irritable bowel syndrome (IBS; also referred to as *spastic colon*), and so forth.

The following is a short list of common diseases and disorders of the colon that may require surgical intervention:

- *Cancer*: According to the American Society of Colorectal Surgeons, colorectal cancer strikes about 140,000 people and causes 60,000 deaths annually. Colon cancer has a high cure rate if it is detected in its early stages.
- *Colitis*:
  - *Ulcerative colitis*: This is an inflammatory disease that affects people under the age of 30 that consists of bleeding with bowel movements, abdominal pain or bloating, constipation, diarrhea, or a combination of all of these symptoms.
  - *Crohn's disease*: Like ulcerative colitis, Crohn's affects people under the age of 30 and carries many of the same symptoms. Patients experience abdominal pain, bloody diarrhea, and mucus in the stools. It is treated with anti-inflammatories and immunosuppressants with the vast majority of patients requiring surgery to remove the diseased portion of the colon.
- *Diverticulosis*: Afflicting about 50% of Americans, diverticulosis is the formation of pockets or sacs (called *diverticula*) in the lining of the bowel that occur when the lining is pressed through weak spots in the muscle of the bowel wall. They usually occur in the sigmoid colon, where the large bowel exerts the highest pressure. When the pockets become inflamed or infected, the patient is said to have diverticulitis. This condition doesn't always require surgery and can be managed with dietary changes and medications.
- *Intussusception*: This occurs when the bowel folds into itself, causing obstruction.
- *Volvulus*: This is a twisting or displacement of the intestines resulting in obstruction.

Treatment of these conditions often results in bowel diversion surgery such as ileostomy and colostomy. Ileostomy diverts the ileum to a stoma. Colostomy is similar to an ileostomy, except the colon is diverted to a stoma.

Colectomy

Colectomy is a surgical procedure to remove all or part of the colon. Depending on the extent of disease or injury to the colon, either partial or complete colectomy is performed. When the bowel is resected, bowel diversion is then necessary to restore the defecation process. Colectomy is performed via open (44139–44160) or laparoscopic (44204–44213) approaches. Colectomy is performed by a colorectal surgeon for any of the following reasons:

- Bleeding from the colon—especially if it cannot be controlled—that may be caused by disease or trauma
- Bowel obstruction
- Colon cancer
- Ulcerative colitis
- Trauma from accidents such as motor vehicle collisions, crushing injuries, gunshots, stabbing, and so forth

Total colectomy involves removing the entire colon. Partial colectomy entails removing a portion of the colon and may also be referred to as *subtotal colectomy*. Hemicolectomy involves removing the right or left portion of the colon. In a proctocolectomy, both the colon and rectum are removed. Once a section of colon is removed, it has to be reattached (anastomosed) to the remaining colon.

Ileostomy and Colostomy

Some of the colectomy procedures involve creating an ileostomy, while others do not require it because the colon is immediately anastomosed. An ileostomy is an opening from the small intestine to the outside of the body and bypasses the colon, rectum, and anus. To create the ileostomy, the surgeon makes a small incision in the abdomen, and the end of the small intestine that is farthest from the stomach (ileum) is brought up through the incision and cuffed back over itself (like folding a sock down over the ankle) and secured to the outside of the abdomen, creating a stoma. The ostomy pouch can then be connected to the stoma to collect stool. Ileostomies may be used in the short term after a colectomy where the large intestine was removed but the rectum remains intact. This is done to allow the remaining intestine time to rest and heal. A second surgery is later conducted to reattach the small intestine and close the ileostomy. Ileostomies are permanent if all of the large intestine and rectum are removed. Colostomy is similar to an ileostomy, with the colon used instead of the ileum to create the stoma, which bypasses the rectum and anus. Some patients prefer not to wear an ostomy bag that is connected to the stoma and can opt for a continent ileostomy/colostomy (44151, 44156). A stoma is still created, but after the large intestine is removed a pouch that resembles a colon is created using the end of the ileum. The patient inserts a tube each day to drain this pouch in lieu of wearing a bag that must be changed several times a day. When the entire colon is removed but the anus remains intact, an ileoanal reservoir is an alternative to an ileostomy (44158). The surgeon creates a pouch or reservoir from the last several inches of the ileum and attaches it to the anus. Stool collects in the pouch and then exits though the anus as in a normal bowel movement. The ileoanal reservoir is also called a *pelvic pouch* or *J-pouch*.

Colorectal cancer is surgically treated by removing the diseased tissue by any number of surgical techniques. Laparoscopic abdominoperineal resection is performed for cancers in the rectum or anus and involves removing the anus, rectum, and sigmoid colon. Once they are removed, a stoma is created (usually through a portal incision made for the scope on the left side) for the colostomy access.

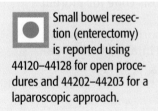
Small bowel resection (enterectomy) is reported using 44120–44128 for open procedures and 44202–44203 for a laparoscopic approach.

Code descriptors in this section must be read carefully. Codes are selected based on (1) which intestine was removed—small or large, (2) whether partial or complete removal of the intestine was performed, (3) whether the procedure was open or laparoscopic, (4) whether an ileostomy or colostomy was performed and whether it is continent, (5) whether an ileoanal reservoir was created, and (6) whether intestines were anastomosed.

BARIATRIC PROCEDURES

Obesity is one of the greatest public health dilemmas in the United States, because it is driving up the cost of health care, shortening life expectancy, and decreasing the overall quality of health for people with a body mass index (BMI) greater than 30. Individuals who are obese succumb to more than 40 obesity-related diseases and conditions including type 2 diabetes, heart disease, and cancer and require ongoing medical intervention, which could be avoided if the patient sustained a healthy weight. According to the CDC, nearly 79 million Americans are obese, and it has been estimated that 220,000 people undergo weight loss surgery each year in the United States.

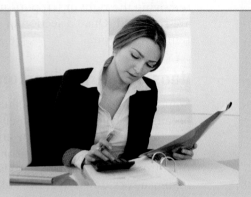

Medicare publishes all of their medical coverage policies at the national level in the *Internet-Only Manual (IOM) Medicare National Coverage Determinations Manual*, Publication 100-03, and the *Medicare Claims Processing Manual (MCPM)*, Publication 100-04. Policies specific to bariatric surgery are located in 100-03, Sections 100.1 and 100-4, Chapter 32, Section 150. Local Coverage Determinations (LCDs), however, supersede any national policy and should be reviewed.

Procedures for weight loss range from less-invasive restricting procedures to extensive gastric bypasses involving reconstruction of the small intestine. Bariatric surgery may involve the stomach, duodenum, jejunum, and/or ileum.

"Stomach stapling" is a slang term used broadly to refer to weight loss surgery; however, it is just one of the methods of weight reduction surgery available. The most common methods of surgery are described as follows.

According to the American Society for Metabolic and Bariatric Surgery, bariatric surgery has been proven to improve the overall health of patients with obesity, achieving remission of type 2 diabetes, kidney diseases, and high blood pressure. Because of this success, insurance carriers provide coverage for these procedures. Each carrier has policies pertaining to bariatric surgery with specific coverage criteria such as age, BMI, supervised physician nutrition counseling, presence of system diseases, and psychological counseling that must be met before surgery is authorized.

INTERNET RESOURCE: This link provides a snapshot in time of bariatric policies for carriers across the United States:
http://obesitycoverage.com/insurance-and-costs/am-i-covered/check-my-insurance

Medicare covers obesity screening and counseling with no copay required if the patient has a BMI greater than 30. When submitting claims for bariatric surgery, a diagnosis code for morbid obesity and a status code for the patient's BMI must be on the claim.

Bariatric procedures are divided into two types: restrictive and malabsorptive. Restrictive procedures create a smaller gastric pouch that restricts the amount of food intake, making patients feel fuller sooner. Malabsorptive procedures require surgically altering and bypassing the intestines so fewer calories are absorbed into the body.

INTERNET RESOURCE: Visit WebMD to see animations of the various bariatric surgery techniques, including a biliopancreatic diversion.
www.webmd.com/diet/obesity/ss/slideshow-weight-loss-surgery

Codes for bariatric procedures are located in the Bariatric Surgery subsection within the Digestive System section. Unfortunately, this section is not complete and there are two codes *not* located within this section: 43644 and 43645.

Revision of bariatric surgery may be required in severe cases where the patient experiences one of the following problems: staple-line malfunction, obstruction, stricture, nonabsorption resulting in hypoglycemia or malnutrition, band dislodgement/failure, weight loss of 20% or more below ideal body weight. Should revisional surgery be performed, report a code from 43848–43865.

Gastric Restrictive Procedures

Gastric restrictive procedures are considered the safest, least invasive weight loss surgery. This type of surgery is not permanent—the band can be removed if necessary, allowing the stomach to return to its normal size. Restrictive procedures may be utilized as a phase I approach to weight loss surgery. If a patient is not successful in losing the desired amount of weight with the banding, he or she may have the band removed and undergo a permanent gastric bypass.

Laparoscopic Gastric Silicone Band

The most common restrictive procedure is the laparoscopic gastric silicone band (LASGB) procedure (43770–43774, 43843), more commonly known as the "lap band." A silicone band is placed around the upper stomach to form a smaller pouch with a funneled narrow outlet called a *stoma*. A small port, or reservoir, is then placed under the skin connected to the silicone band with tubing. The advantage to banding is that the stomach is not cut and there are no structural changes to the stomach.

The band is adjusted periodically in the months following surgery by either adding or removing saline from the port. The first adjustment is usually done 4 to 6 weeks after surgery and is included in the global period of the surgery. Saline is injected to fill the port if the patient is not experiencing the level of fullness or the expected amount of weight loss. Saline is removed if the patient is reaching the achieved weight loss goal or is having problems with heartburn or regurgitation.

The lap band is adjusted in the physician office and does not require anesthesia. The physician palpates the abdomen to locate the port then inserts a saline-filled syringe. Depending on the patient's insurance, lap band adjustments are reported with CPT code 43771 or HCPCS code S2083 or unlisted code 43999. Medicare does not recognize or reimburse services reported with HCPCS S codes.

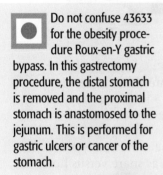

Do not report an E/M code along with the adjustment service (S2083 or 43999) unless a separately identifiable E/M service was performed that warrants appending modifier –25 to the E/M code. If the reason for the visit is for the adjustment, report only the adjustment code.

Vertical Banded Gastroplasty

The vertical banded gastroplasty (VBG) (43842) also involves placing a plastic band around the stomach. However, in addition to the band placement, the surgeon staples the stomach above the band into a small pouch. The stomach is split into segments along its vertical axis. To create a durable, reinforced, and rate-limiting stoma at the distal end of the pouch, a plug of stomach is removed, and a propylene collar is placed through this hole and then stapled to itself.

Longitudinal Sleeve Gastrectomy

The longitudinal sleeve gastrectomy (43775, 43843) is a restrictive procedure that requires removing about 50% of the stomach. A vertical incision is made into the stomach, and the remaining portion of the stomach is stapled closed and resembles the size and shape of a banana. This procedure can be done laparoscopically or via open incision. Unlike the other restrictive procedures, this procedure cannot be reversed because part of the stomach is removed. For some patients, this procedure is phase I of a more extensive Roux-en-Y gastric bypass or duodenal switch.

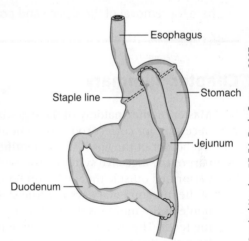

Gastric Bypass

The Roux-en-Y gastric bypass (43644, 43846–43847) is the most common type of bypass performed and is considered to be both a restrictive and malabsorptive procedure. It consists of two steps: (1) creating a small stomach pouch and (2) bypassing part of the small intestine. The small pouch that remains restricts the amount of food a patient can eat, and the patient quickly feels full on a cup of food or less. None of the stomach is removed during this procedure. Most times, the gastric bypasses are performed laparoscopically (Fig. 21.2).

Do not confuse 43633 for the obesity procedure Roux-en-Y gastric bypass. In this gastrectomy procedure, the distal stomach is removed and the proximal stomach is anastomosed to the jejunum. This is performed for gastric ulcers or cancer of the stomach.

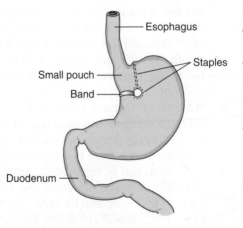

Figure 21.2 Bariatric surgery.

From Williams, L. and Hopper, P. *Understanding Medical Surgical Nursing, 3E,* F.A. Davis Company. 2007.

During the first step of the procedure, the stomach is divided into two sections by either sewing or stapling through the stomach at the lesser curvature, forming a small pouch at the proximal end of the stomach. Step 2 of the surgery entails creating the bypass. A short limb of the proximal small bowel is divided into a Y-shaped section and attached to the pouch so food bypasses the rest of the stomach, duodenum, and the first portion of the jejunum. Postsurgery, food passes directly from the stomach into the jejunum, bypassing the duodenum, which decreases fat absorption and the amount of calories and nutrients absorbed into the body.

INTERNET RESOURCE: Watch this animated video of the Roux-en-Y bypass:
www.youtube.com/watch?v=WN6pECaL3Fw

CHECKPOINT 21.3

Assign the CPT codes—and HCPCS code(s), if necessary—for the following situations.

1. A 37-year-old patient suffers from morbid obesity and despite 10 years of various diets, his condition remains the same. He also suffers from hypertension, hypercholesterolemia, and diabetes. The surgeon has decided to perform a vertical banded gastroplasty. _____

2. A 40-year-old female patient presents with a body mass index of 48. She is hypertensive and diabetic. She has a history of dieting that has been unsuccessful. She is here today for laparoscopic adjustable gastric band and subcutaneous port placement. _____

3. The patient from Question 2 returns 1 year after placement of the adjustable gastric band. She has not had a good result from the procedure and has not felt well since its placement. She is here for removal of the device and port components. _____

Chapter Summary

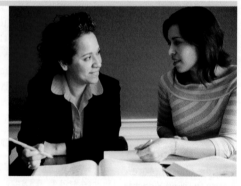

1. Mastering the anatomy of the digestive system is necessary for correct code assignment. The vermilion border of the lips is what identifies the lips as part of the digestive system; otherwise, procedures performed outside the vermilion border are part of the integumentary system (the skin). The vestibule of the mouth is the oral cavity other than the teeth. The esophagus is 25 cm long, running from the throat to the pylorus opening into the stomach. The stomach sits between the esophagus and the small intestines, providing the digestive process (peristalsis) that allows food to be eliminated through the intestines. The intestines are divided into the small intestines, 17 feet in length—duodenum, jejunum, ileum—and the large intestines or colon, 5 feet long—cecum, ascending, transverse, descending, sigmoid, rectum. The anus is at the terminus of the intestines.

2. Multiple therapeutic endoscopies can be reported separately if within the same family when different methods are used within the same endoscopic procedure, such as snare versus hot biopsy forceps. This is not the case if one of the endoscopies is a diagnostic one. Also, if the same method is used to remove multiple growths, only one endoscopy code is reported.

3. All hernias can be repaired via an open approach. Likewise, with the exception of femoral and sliding hernias, they can also be repaired laparoscopically. Depending on the size of the defect, mesh may also be used. The types of hernias are the hiatal, diaphragmatic, inguinal, incisional, femoral epigastric, and spigelian.

4. Coders need to differentiate between esophagoscopy and esophagogastroduodenoscopy to correctly assign codes. Esophagoscopy procedures include viewing and treating the esophagus and stomach up to the pyloric sphincter. Esophagogastroduodenoscopy procedures include everything that is done via esophagoscopy, but the key difference is that the scope advances beyond the pyloric sphincter and into the duodenum.

5. Recognizing the difference between a screening colonoscopy and a diagnostic colonoscopy impacts code assignment, particularly for Medicare members. A screening colonoscopy is scheduled and performed as a preventive service for asymptomatic patients over the age of 50 who may or may not have a family history of colon cancer or polyps. A diagnostic colonoscopy is performed exactly the same way as a screening colonoscopy, except the purpose is to diagnose what is causing the patient's pain, bleeding, or other GI symptom.

6. The bariatric procedures are the gastric band, vertical band, sleeve gastrectomy, and gastric bypass.

Review Questions

Matching

Match the key terms with their definitions.

A. cholecystectomy
B. esophagoscopy
C. diagnostic
D. incidental appendectomy
E. colonoscopy

F. bariatric surgery
G. polyp
H. snare
I. volvulus
J. cleft lip

1. _____ A wire loop with an electric current

2. _____ A type of birth defect involving a separation of the lip

3. _____ A twisting of the intestines

4. _____ Surgical removal of the gallbladder

5. _____ The type of endoscopy that is included in a surgical endoscopy

6. _____ Placing a scope into the esophagus

7. _____ May or may not be separately reportable from other intra-abdominal procedures

8. _____ A tumor on a pedicle

9. _____ A gastric restrictive procedure

10. _____ Scope placement from the anus to the cecum

True or False

Decide whether each statement is true or false.

1. __T__ EGD is the abbreviation for esophagogastrodilation.

2. __F__ With respect to polyps, biopsy and polypectomy are synonymous.

3. __T__ If an esophageal dilation using a Savary dilator was performed, the dilation was carried out using a guidewire.

4. __T__ If a screening colonoscopy is scheduled but during the procedure a polyp is found and removed, a code for the screening should still be submitted because this was why the case was originally scheduled.

5. __F__ To report a colonoscopy, the physician passes the scope beyond 50 cm of the large intestine.

6. __F__ An EGD with Maloney dilation is reported with 43235 and 43450.

7. __F__ An incidental appendectomy is coded separately when performed with other abdominal procedures on the digestive system.

8. __F__ Placement of an anal seton cannot be reported separately from other rectal procedures.

9. __F__ The use of hot biopsy forceps does not constitute an ablation technique.

10. __T__ Medicare accepts either the diagnostic colonoscopy CPT code or the HCPCS code for screening colonoscopies.

11. __F__ Suture of the diaphragm due to traumatic multiple stab wounds is assigned to 39501.

12. __T__ Inflammation of the bile ducts is referred to as cholangitis.

Multiple Choice

Select the letter that best completes the statement or answers the question.

1. A patient is seen for a screening colonoscopy. The patient is 75 years old and has a family history of colon cancer. During the colonoscopy, a polyp is discovered in the proximal sigmoid. The polyp is snared with cold biopsy forceps. Which code(s) should be reported?
   A. 45385, G0105
   B. 45385
   C. 45338
   D. G0105

2. Colonoscopy is performed in a 46-year-old patient. A biopsy was taken of the terminal ileum. A scope was withdrawn into the cecum and multiple biopsies were taken of several suspicious-looking areas. At the area of the hepatic flexure, a polyp was removed with the snare technique. Which code(s) should be reported?
   A. 45385, 45380, 45385–59
   B. 45385, 45380-59
   C. 45385 ×2, 45380–59
   D. 45385, 45380 ×2

3. A 53-year-old patient exhibits hernias of the left inguinal canal and of the umbilicus. The inguinal canal was repaired 5 years ago. At this episode, the physician uses mesh to repair the inguinal hernia. Both hernias are repaired laparoscopically under general anesthesia. Which codes should be reported?
   A. 49520, 49585
   B. 49650, 49659, 49568
   C. 49585, 49651–51
   D. 49651, 49652

4. A 47-year-old patient complaining of persistent right upper quadrant nagging pain undergoes an ERCP with removal of stent and sphincterotomy. Which code(s) should be reported?
   A. 43260, 43262–51
   B. 43274
   C. 43275, 43262–51
   D. 43275, 43260–59

5. A 56-year-old patient complaining of difficulty swallowing and persistent indigestion undergoes an endoscopy with biopsies and dilation of an esophageal stricture. The physician inserted the scope into the esophagus and at 20 cm noted esophagitis. The scope was advanced into the stomach and to the second portion of the duodenum. Biopsies were taken of the stomach and esophagus. A 20-mm balloon was used to dilate the esophagus. Which codes should be reported?
   A. 43249, 43239–59
   B. 43213, 43239–51
   C. 43202, 43220–51
   D. 43249, 43239–51

6. A 47-year-old patient with a 10-year history of chronic alcoholism reported to the physician-owned endoscopy suite with abnormal liver function tests and vomiting blood. The physician performed an endoscopy with injection of esophageal varices. Once the endoscopy procedure was completed, under fluoroscopic guidance, a hollow-bore needle was inserted between the ribs on the patient's right side and the liver was biopsied. Which codes should be reported?
   A. 43204, 47000, 77002
   B. 43243, 47001–51
   C. 43201, 47000
   D. 43204, 47000–51, 77003

7. A patient had a right recurrent ventral hernia repaired with Marlex mesh. Which codes should be reported?
   A. 49550, C1781
   B. 49565, 49568
   C. 49560, 49568
   D. 49565, C1781

8. A patient is seen in follow-up for polypectomy. A polyp was removed 1.5 years ago. She is scheduled for a colonoscopy. A scope was inserted and at about 38 cm a polyp was found. It was removed with a snare. Which code should be reported?
   A. 45378
   B. 45385
   C. 45338
   D. 45315

9. An elderly patient has a history of pancreatic cancer and now needs an ERCP procedure to place a biliary stent due to recurrent jaundice 4 months after a previous ERCP procedure. Which code(s) should be reported?
   A. 43266
   B. 43274
   C. 43275
   D. 43260, 43274–51

10. A 41-year-old female patient has been experiencing right flank pain radiating to the shoulder and irregular bowel movements. Ultrasound showed a 4+ gallbladder with two large stones. Patient undergoes a laparoscopic cholecystectomy with common bile duct exploration. Which code should be reported?
    A. 47562
    B. 47563
    C. 47564
    D. 47579

11. A patient presents with a long-standing history of abdominal pain and now presents with acute rebound tenderness of the right lower quadrant. Exploratory laparotomy with appendectomy is performed. Which code(s) should be reported?
    A. 49000, 44955
    B. 49010, 44950
    C. 44970
    D. 44950

12. A 4-year-old boy presents with a bulge in the left inguinal area and an associated hydrocele on examination. The surgeon performs an open inguinal hernia repair with hydrocelectomy. Which code(s) should be reported?
    A. 49505, 55500
    B. 49520, 55000
    C. 49495
    D. 49500

13. A 4-year-old swallowed a small toy that got stuck in her throat. A flexible esophagoscopy was performed to remove the toy. Which code should be reported?
    A. 43200
    B. 43235
    C. 43247
    D. 43215

14. Assign the appropriate code(s) for EGD with biopsies of the stomach and duodenum and injection of implant material into the muscle of the lower esophageal sphincter.
    A. 43235, 43239
    B. 43239, 43236
    C. 43239, 11900
    D. 43239

15. A 40-year-old male has had severe GERD for almost a year. After a previous endoscopy of the esophagus and a barium swallow, the physician determines that he will perform a laparoscopic Nissen procedure. Code for the Nissen procedure. Which code(s) should be reported?
    A. 43280
    B. 43328
    C. 43327
    D. 43279, 43280–51

16. A 48-year-old man went to the ED complaining of vomiting coffee-ground material several times within the past hour. He had abdominal pain and had been unable to eat for the past 24 hours. He was dizzy and light-headed. His stools today have been black and tarry. While in the ED he vomited bright red blood and some coffee-ground material. After evaluating the patient, a consult was requested. The GI physician took the patient to the endoscopy suite and performed an upper GI endoscopy for diagnostic purposes. Which code(s) should be reported?
    A. 99255–57, 43235
    B. 43235
    C. 43200, 43235
    D. 43243

17. An endoscope was inserted into the esophagus, and the stomach was entered. The pyloric channel was traversed, showing a pyloric stenosis. The endoscopy was then introduced into the second portion of the duodenum, which showed normal mucosa. A 15-mm balloon was placed across the stenosis and dilated and then withdrawn. Which code should be reported?
    A. 43205
    B. 42400
    C. 43204
    D. 43245

18. A diagnostic colonoscopy and a diagnostic EGD are performed on the same patient by the same physician on the same day but not during the same session. Which code(s) should be reported?
    A. 45378, 43235–59
    B. 45378, 43235–51
    C. 45330, 43200–51
    D. 45330, 43200–59

19. A child's gestational age at birth was 34 weeks. Fourteen weeks later, she had an initial inguinal hernia repair done. Which code should be reported?
    A. 49491
    B. 49491–63
    C. 49495
    D. 49495–63

20. A patient with Crohn's disease has been on drug therapy to treat the condition. She is now seen for extreme pain. An x-ray is taken, showing small-bowel obstruction. The patient is taken immediately to surgery and a partial colectomy is performed with an end-to-end anastomosis. Which code(s) should be reported?
    A. 44020, 44120–51
    B. 44020
    C. 44120
    D. 44120, 45136

CHAPTER 22

CPT: Urinary System

CHAPTER OUTLINE

Urinary System Anatomy

Organization

Endoscopy

Urodynamics

Diseases and Disorders of the Urinary System and Surgical Therapies

LEARNING OUTCOMES

After studying this chapter, you should be able to:

1. Describe the coding process used to assign the correct codes for urethral dilation.
2. Differentiate among laparoscopic, cystourethroscopic, and open surgical procedures.
3. Discuss the purpose of urodynamic testing.
4. Compare the three common methods of treating kidney stones via lithotripsy.

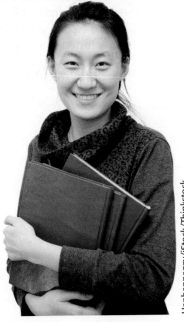

Hanhanpeggy/iStock/Thinkstock

This chapter focuses on terminology and coding of urinary system procedures. *Genitourinary* is a collective term used to describe the male and the female reproductive organs as well as the organs that create and excrete urine. These organs and anatomical structures are grouped together in CPT because of their proximity in the body and the fact that they share common viaducts. This chapter focuses on diseases and disorders of the urinary system and associated surgical treatments.

Urologists specialize in the diagnosis and medical/surgical treatment of diseases and injuries of the urinary tract for both male and female patients. Urology is closely related to, and in some cases overlaps with, the medical fields of oncology, nephrology, gynecology, andrology, pediatric surgery, and endocrinology. The organs covered by urology include the kidneys, ureters, urinary bladder, and urethra. Both urologists and general surgeons operate on the adrenal glands, remove kidneys, transplant kidneys, and perform hernia operations.

A wide range of clinical conditions is managed by this specialty, so knowledge of internal medicine, pediatrics, gynecology, and oncology is necessary. Some urologists specialize in the treatment of the male reproductive system. Urologists and gynecologists routinely assist one another in complex gynecology (GYN) procedures that involve a prolapsed bladder or urethra. Chapters 23 and 24 of this text discuss the male and female genital systems. Some of the surgical specialty overlap is discussed in those chapters.

Urologists are often confused with nephrologists, internal medicine physicians who obtained additional training in treating kidney disease. Nephrologists specifically treat patients with damaged or weak kidneys due to chronic conditions such as diabetes and hypertension and are the only physicians trained to provide dialysis for patients in kidney failure. Dialysis is discussed in Chapter 29 of this text. Nephrologists also are part of the kidney transplant team managing the patient through the transplant process, placing the patient on the donor list, and monitoring the patient post-transplant. Nephrology is considered an internal medicine subspecialty and not a surgical subspecialty; nephrologists do not operate.

INTERNET RESOURCE: The American Urology Association
www.auanet.org/resources/aua-coding-resources.cfm

URINARY SYSTEM ANATOMY

The body's urinary system maintains a steady balance in the fluid and chemical composition of the blood (homeostasis) and disposes of waste products from the blood. The urinary system coordinates with the lungs, skin, and intestines—all of which also eliminate wastes—to maintain the delicate balance of chemicals and water in the body.

The anatomical components of the urinary system are the kidneys, ureters, urinary bladder, sphincter muscles within the bladder, and urethra (Fig. 22.1). The kidneys filter the blood and produce urine. The kidney is a layered organ. The outermost layer is called the cortex. Inside the cortex is the medulla, which contains drainage channels called the renal calyx. The urine collects in the renal pelvis from the

> Remember that the abdomen can be surgically accessed by several approaches: via laparotomy with a large open incision; percutaneously with a small incision; endoscopically via the urethra, vagina, or esophagus; or laparoscopically. Assign codes based on the approach.

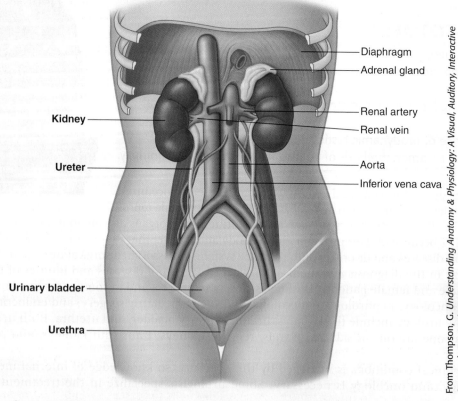

Diaphragm
Adrenal gland
Renal artery
Renal vein
Aorta
Inferior vena cava
Kidney
Ureter
Urinary bladder
Urethra

From Thompson, G. *Understanding Anatomy & Physiology: A Visual, Auditory, Interactive Approach*, F.A. Davis Company, 2013.

Figure 22.1 The urinary system.

calyx, which is similar to a "lobby." From the renal pelvis (lobby), the urine is channeled into the ureter, which acts like a 16- to 18-cm-long "moving sidewalk" to carry the urine to the bladder.

The bladder is a muscular sac that can hold approximately 2 cups of urine before urinating (*voiding*) becomes necessary (Fig. 22.2). The bladder muscle contracts and the sphincter muscles open, allowing for urine to flow out of the urethra. The area where the bladder narrows to connect to the urethra is called the bladder neck. The top of the bladder is referred to as the bladder dome. The trigone of the bladder is a triangular area of the posterorinferior bladder wall where the ureteral openings are located. This area has no elasticity and therefore does not stretch. The trigone acts like a funnel channeling urine into the urethra. The urethral meatus is the external opening of the urethra at the end of the penis. The ureters, bladder, and urethra are referred to collectively as the *urinary tract*.

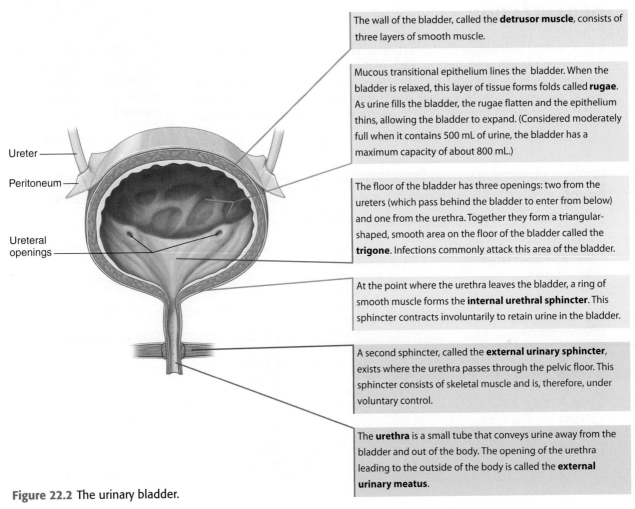

The wall of the bladder, called the **detrusor muscle**, consists of three layers of smooth muscle.

Mucous transitional epithelium lines the bladder. When the bladder is relaxed, this layer of tissue forms folds called **rugae**. As urine fills the bladder, the rugae flatten and the epithelium thins, allowing the bladder to expand. (Considered moderately full when it contains 500 mL of urine, the bladder has a maximum capacity of about 800 mL.)

The floor of the bladder has three openings: two from the ureters (which pass behind the bladder to enter from below) and one from the urethra. Together they form a triangular-shaped, smooth area on the floor of the bladder called the **trigone**. Infections commonly attack this area of the bladder.

At the point where the urethra leaves the bladder, a ring of smooth muscle forms the **internal urethral sphincter**. This sphincter contracts involuntarily to retain urine in the bladder.

A second sphincter, called the **external urinary sphincter**, exists where the urethra passes through the pelvic floor. This sphincter consists of skeletal muscle and is, therefore, under voluntary control.

The **urethra** is a small tube that conveys urine away from the bladder and out of the body. The opening of the urethra leading to the outside of the body is called the **external urinary meatus**.

Ureter

Peritoneum

Ureteral openings

Figure 22.2 The urinary bladder.

From Thompson, G. *Understanding Anatomy & Physiology: A Visual, Auditory, Interactive Approach*, F.A. Davis Company, 2013.

Urinary system problems can be caused by normal aging, illness, or injury. The aging process induces changes in the kidneys' structure, causing them to lose some ability to remove wastes from the blood. Muscles in the ureters, bladder, and urethra tend to lose some of their strength and become less taut. Urinary tract infections (UTIs) become more frequent because the bladder muscles do not tighten enough to empty the bladder completely, and the residual waste harbors bacteria. A decrease in strength of the sphincter muscles and the pelvic floor can cause *incontinence*, or leakage of urine. Illness, such as diabetes or congenital deformities, can also prevent the kidneys from filtering the blood completely or block the passage of urine.

Knowledge of the urinary anatomy is important. The layers of the kidney, the differentiation of ureter versus urethra, and their functions are examples. Coders will use anatomy and their surgery coding skills to understand the various methods for diagnosis and treatment such as endoscopy, laparoscopy, cystourethroscopy, and the open surgical techniques. Guidelines in this section indicate that there are minor included services for the more major urinary surgeries, and knowledge of the professional and technical components is necessary to accurately code these services. Stents are also important, and coders must read documentation carefully to determine if the stent is temporary or indwelling. Urodynamics is also an area of coding specific to the urinary system and should be studied carefully.

The urinary system is evaluated and monitored by conducting urinalysis (UA) tests, taking diagnostic x-rays such as intravenous pyelograms (IVPs), and urodynamic testing. Such testing is performed to identify blockages in the ureters, back flow of urine into the ureters and kidneys, kidney functioning, and bladder abnormalities. Patients with kidney disease typically experience hypertension because the kidneys control the volume of blood and interstitial fluid. If a urologist determines that a patient has kidney failure, the patient is referred to a nephrologist for further management of this disease.

ORGANIZATION

The urinary subsection of CPT lists codes under four anatomical sites: kidney, ureter, bladder, and urethra. Each of these sites has headings covering the common general procedures plus site-specific treatments as appropriate, as shown in Box 22.1. Code descriptors often refer to specific sizes, such as of stones or tumors, so code selection is based on these findings.

> ◉ Note that male prostate procedures are located in the bladder codes section under Vesical Neck and Prostate, in the urethra codes section under Other Procedures, and in the Male Genital subsection. Prostate procedures are discussed in Chapter 23 of this text.

BOX 22.1 Urinary Subsection Headings

KIDNEY
Incision
Excision
Renal Transplantation
Introduction
Repair
Laparoscopy
Endoscopy
Other Procedures

URETER
Incision/Biopsy
Excision
Introduction
Repair
Laparoscopy
Endoscopy

BLADDER
Incision
Removal
Excision
Introduction
Urodynamics
Repair
Laparoscopy
Endoscopy—Cystoscopy, Urethroscopy, Cystourethroscopy
Transurethral Surgery
Vesical Neck and Prostate

URETHRA
Incision
Excision
Repair
Manipulation
Other Procedures

The terms *simple* and *complicated* have specific meanings in the urinary subsection. A code for a complicated procedure would be considered if the patient had prior surgery of a site that resulted in scar tissue that must be handled during the present procedure. A large-size lesion or stone, the presence of a foreign body (FB), or the requirement for placement of a urinary stent (a device used to hold open a structure) may also justify choosing a complicated code over a simple code.

Acronyms

The predominant types of documentation for urology procedures and services include notes covering office visits, operative reports, and related pathology/radiology reports. Box 22.2 lists the key acronyms and their meanings.

BOX 22.2 Common Acronyms for Urology

BNO	Bladder neck obstruction
BOO	Bladder outlet obstruction
Cath	Catheter
CKD	Chronic kidney disease
CRF	Chronic renal failure
CUG	Cystourethrogram
ESRD	End-stage renal disease
ESWL	Extracorporeal shock wave lithotripsy
GU	Genitourinary
IC	Interstitial cystitis
IVP	Intravenous pyelogram
OAB	Overactive bladder
UA	Urinalysis
UPJ	Ureteropelvic junction
US	Ultrasound
UTI	Urinary tract infection
UUO	Unilateral urethral obstruction

ENDOSCOPY

Endoscopic procedures are located not only under the subheadings Endoscopy and Laparoscopy but also under the subheadings Transurethral Surgery and Endoscopy—Cystoscopy, Urethroscopy, Cystourethroscopy. Endoscopic procedures of the urinary tract may be diagnostic or therapeutic in nature. Procedures range from visually examining the structures, to removing lesions and inserting radioactive material into the bladder, to everything in between.

Cystourethroscopy

Codes for cystoscopy and urethroscopy are combined under the term *cystourethroscopy*, the radiographic imaging procedure of the bladder and urethra. Most of the procedures on the urinary system can be done via the cystourethroscope, so the coder must choose carefully among the many codes available. The location of the semicolon must be noticed in the code descriptions for endoscopic procedures to accurately assign codes. As in all endoscopy codes, the common portion of the code reflects the *approach* and the unique portion describes the *intent* of the procedure. The destination of the scope or the site of the cystourethroscopy (e.g., the bladder, urethra, or ureter) must be known in order to assign these codes. Note that the cystoscopy code 52000 is designated as a separate procedure and is therefore always bundled into a surgical cystoscopy procedure and not reported separately.

> The terms *cystoscopy*, *urethroscopy*, and *cystourethroscopy* are used interchangeably.

Scopes can be inserted into any natural orifice of the body or those created by the surgeon. Read the documentation carefully to determine how the scope was inserted. Was it inserted transurethrally (through the urethra), via an existing stoma (a surgically created opening in the body that connects a body part or cavity to the outside environment), or via a new incision? Examine these two code descriptors:

> Cystoscopic procedures include several minor procedures, such as dilation. These secondary procedures may be reported with a –22 modifier only if significant additional time and effort are documented.

50980, *Ureteral endoscopy through ureterotomy, with or without irrigation, instillation, or ureteropyelography, exclusive of radiologic service; with removal of foreign body or calculus*

52320, *Cystourethroscopy; with removal of ureteral calculus*

These codes appear to be similar, but the approach to the calculus removal is dramatically different. With 50980, an incision is made in the flank (the ureterotomy) and the scope is inserted into the ureter; in 52320, the scope is inserted through the urethra and fed up to the ureter.

As noted in CPT, cystoscopic procedures include the required associated minor procedures. For example, the main procedure transurethral resection of the prostate (TURP), which is endoscopic removal of the prostate gland, requires a meatotomy, urethral calibration and/or dilation, urethroscopy, and a cystoscopy in preparation for the procedure. Those associated procedures are not reported unless they are documented as being unusually demanding of the surgeon. Carefully review the guidelines that precede code 52000. These guidelines specify three important instructions regarding included services for TURP, extraction of ureteral calculus, and cystourethroscopy for the female urethral syndrome. A fourth instruction directs the coder to report the major service with modifier –22 if any of the included services require additional time and effort. The example given is for a cystourethroscopy for the female urethral syndrome with urethrotomy (the included service) for a preexisting stricture or bladder neck contracture. Code 52285 would be reported with modifier –22.

Endoscopic coding rules are consistent regardless of body system:

- Biopsies, fulguration, and lesion removal cannot be reported simultaneously unless the biopsy site is different from the site of lesion removal and fulguration. Modifier –59 is needed to differentiate separate locations.
- If an excisional biopsy is performed along with a therapeutic excision of the same site, only the excision is reported; the biopsy is included in the excision. Watch for code descriptor language. Cystourethroscopy with biopsy(s) (CPT code 52204) includes all biopsies during the procedure and should only be reported once, no matter how many biopsies were obtained.
- When multiple endoscopic procedures are performed at the same patient encounter, assign the most comprehensive code that fully describes the service(s) performed. If several endoscopic procedures are performed at the same session and these individual services are not part of a more comprehensive procedure (reported in one code), multiple CPT codes may be reported with modifier –51.

Catheter Insertions

Urinary catheters can be either nonindwelling or indwelling. Nonindwelling catheters are inserted into the urethra to drain the bladder of residual urine and are not intended to be left in long term. Use of this type of catheter is commonly referred to as an *in-and-out catheterization*. Another type of nonindwelling catheter, called a *condom catheter*, can be attached to the external penis (not actually inserted into the urethra) with a "suction cup" effect. Indwelling catheters such as a Foley catheter are left in the bladder for extended periods of time, such as after major surgery or in the case of stroke or spinal cord injuries.

> **■ CASE SCENARIO**
> A patient has severe benign prostatic hypertrophy (BPH) and requires a temporary dwelling catheter. Patient will have the catheter in place for 2 weeks and will return to the office to have it removed. Code: 51702.

It is quite common for a physician to perform an x-ray procedure called *retrograde pyelogram*—used to detect abnormalities of the urinary tract—during a cystoscopy procedure. The patient is placed under general anesthesia and a catheter is inserted into the urethra, bladder, and ureters. Dye is injected and x-rays are taken to examine the ureters and kidneys to identify possible blockages, filling defects, and tumors. When a retrograde pyelogram (ureteropyelography) is performed by ureteral catheterization through a cystoscope, code 52005 is appropriate. Because such ureteropyelography is used routinely in endoscopic procedures of the ureter, it is usually bundled into the surgical procedure and is not reported separately.

Some code descriptors in this section state *exclusive of radiologic service*, meaning that an additional code from the Radiology section is required to report radiological supervision and interpretation. However, cystourethroscopy and transurethral procedures include fluoroscopy and fluoroscopic guidance when performed (e.g., 76000, 76001, and 77002) and should not be reported separately.

Cystourethroscopy procedures performed on the *ureters* are inherently unilateral. If the same procedure is performed on both ureters, report a –50 modifier. Likewise, if two different procedures were performed on each of the ureters, use the –RT and –LT modifiers to designate which procedure was performed on which ureter. Do not report this modifier with codes 52005, 52007, or the range 52320–52356. These procedures include services provided on one or both ureters.

When catheters are inserted before surgery, or if urethral catheterization or urethral dilation is required to accomplish a more extensive procedure, do not report it separately because it is included in the global service.

Be careful! The word *pyeloscopy* does not indicate that a retrograde pyelogram was performed. Pyeloscopy is merely looking into the renal pelvis with a pyeloscope and does not use x-rays.

URODYNAMICS

Urodynamics encompasses several tests to assess bladder functioning, including the filling, storage, and emptying of urine as well as urethral sphincter function. Tests include cystometrogram, uroflowmetry, urethral pressure profile (UPP), neuromuscular studies, and voiding pressure (VP) studies. By performing these diagnostic studies, the physician can determine the strength of the bladder wall, bladder volume, urine flow, and the volume of residual urine (urine that has not been voided). These tests are interactive between the patient and provider.

CPT guidelines state that all of the procedures performed in this code range (51725–51798) are either performed by or under the direct supervision of a physician. If the physician only interprets the results of a technician's work, modifier –26 must be appended to the code. The facility or entity providing the equipment and supplies will report the same codes with a –TC modifier. All supplies, medications, instruments, fluids, and gases provided by the physician are part of the surgical package and are not coded separately.

There are urodynamic procedures that include both the technical and professional components. Offices reporting these codes are expected to provide all equipment and instruments, supplies, and technician services. If an office or physician does not own the urodynamic equipment, append a –26 modifier to the procedure codes.

Cystometrogram

A cystometrogram (CMG) (51725, 51726) measures how much urine the bladder can hold, how much pressure builds up inside the bladder as it stores urine, and how full it is when the patient feels the urge to urinate. This test displays a graphic recording of bladder pressure at various volumes. A catheter is inserted to empty the bladder completely. A smaller catheter with a pressure-measuring tube called a *cystometer* is used to fill the bladder slowly with warm water. An anal probe may be placed into the rectum to record intra-abdominal pressure as well. Patients are asked how full the bladder feels and when they feel the urge to urinate. The volume of water and the bladder pressure are recorded.

This test is useful in differentiating bladder outlet obstruction from other voiding problems. A complex CMG includes placement of a transurethral catheter and an anal probe for measuring intra-abdominal pressure, use of voiding cystometry and infusing agents, and repositioning of the patient. Patients may be asked to turn on their side, cough, and exhale or hold their breath to identify leakage pressure or involuntary bladder contractions.

> ■ **CASE SCENARIO**
> A 72-year-old woman complains of urinary urgency and frequency throughout the day and night. A complex cystometrogram was performed along with a post-voiding residual urine US revealing a residual urine volume of 100 ml. Codes: 51726, 51798–51.

Uroflowmetry

A uroflowmetry study (51736–51741) is typically performed immediately after the CMG to measure urine speed and volume. A patient is requested to void into a collection device that measures the amount of urine that flows from the bladder per second. It is sensitive enough to determine the "peak flow" of urine and how long it took to reach the peak. The amount of urine voided is divided by the time it takes to urinate from start to finish to establish an average flow rate. During typical urination, the initial urine flow starts slowly but immediately speeds up until the bladder is nearly empty. The urine flow then slows again until the bladder is empty. In people with a urinary tract obstruction, BPH, or frequent UTIs, this pattern of flow is altered and increases and decreases more gradually. The uroflowmeter graphs this information, taking into account the person's gender and age.

Urethral Pressure Profile

To conduct a UPP (51727, 51729), fluid is infused into the bladder and the catheter is pulled back into the urethra. Bladder contractions and abdominal volume are recorded. Each rise in urethral pressure is noted. This is an interactive test between the patient and provider. The patient may be asked to cough, laugh, and so forth to test the competence of the urethral sphincter. It is much like testing the "dam" to see how much water and pressure it can sustain before it leaks. A graph is recorded indicating the intraluminal pressure along the length of the urethra.

Neuromuscular Studies

Neuromuscular studies (51784, 51785, and 51792) are performed on patients with voiding dysfunction. Voiding dysfunction can be a congenital or an acquired condition in diseases such as cerebral palsy and multiple sclerosis. The studies measure electrical activity in the anal and/or urethral sphincter muscles. An electromyography needle is placed into the anal and/or urethral sphincter or by placing electrodes perianally. Electrical activity is measured while the bladder is filled and during urination. The urologist interprets the graphic recordings and determines if the muscle activity is appropriately increasing and decreasing at proper intervals.

Voiding Pressure Studies

VP studies (51728–51729, 51797, 51798) can detect outlet pressure obstructions if the patient is unable to void. A transducer is placed into the bladder and measures urine flow rate and pressure during bladder emptying. Abdominal pressure is also measured, which indicates the level of strain required by the patient to void. The postvoiding measurement determines how much urine is left (residual) in the bladder after voiding. This is measured using an ultrasound scanner. If more than a few ounces of urine are remaining, it indicates that the detrusor muscle is not contracting strongly enough to force all of the urine out.

CHECKPOINT 22.1

Answer the following questions.

1. What are the six major anatomical sites associated with the urinary system? _____

2. What are the minor related procedures included in cystourethroscopy for the female urethral syndrome? _____

3. What is the code for a complex cystometrogram with urethral pressure profile studies?

_____

DISEASES AND DISORDERS OF THE URINARY SYSTEM AND SURGICAL THERAPIES

Hematuria

Blood in the urine (hematuria) can be the first sign of any of several different problems in the urinary tract. The urinary tract is susceptible to inflammation as a result of chronic infection. Some common inflammatory problems include cystitis, urethritis, and chronic interstitial cystitis. Urologists will often perform a diagnostic cystoscopy (52000) to determine where bleeding originates and the extent of inflammation. Diagnostic cystoscopies can be performed in the office setting. The patient lies flat on an exam table with legs placed in leg rests or stirrups, and the genital area is cleaned. A topical anesthetic jelly is used to numb the urethra and act as a lubricant. The flexible cystoscope is passed into the urethra and bladder for visual inspection. During the procedure the bladder is filled with sterile fluid to expand it, making it possible for the bladder walls to be inspected. The procedure takes less than 5 minutes to perform. With the flexible cystoscope, no biopsies are obtained and no therapeutic treatment is carried out.

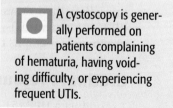

A cystoscopy is generally performed on patients complaining of hematuria, having voiding difficulty, or experiencing frequent UTIs.

Urethral Strictures

Strictures within the urethra narrow the passage of urine. The urethra is especially susceptible to stricturing as a result of infection, trauma, or after gynecological surgery, although strictures may also occur anywhere along the ureter or within the kidney. Codes for treatment of strictures are assigned based on the location of the stricture and how the stricture is dilated. Endoscopic stricture therapy codes range from 52270–52346.

Urethral Dilation

Urethral dilation, generally performed in the office setting, involves stretching of the stricture using progressively larger instruments, such as a balloon dilation instrument. Balloon therapy (52281), in which a scope is inserted and a balloon is inflated at the stricture site, may be used. Laser and electrocautery are also treatment options. At times, the patient may go home with a temporary urinary catheter in place to maintain the opening of the stricture. Internal urethrotomy (52270 female, 52275 male) is generally performed if initial balloon dilation treatment fails. An endoscope is inserted and an incision is made in the site of the stricture. It is very common to place a stent at the stricture site to maintain the opening and prevent it from narrowing again. The urethra can also be injected with a steroid at the stricture site (52283), or a urethral stent can be inserted at the stricture site once it is dilated (52282).

As shown in Pinpoint the Code 22.1, when coding urethral dilation, the coder must answer these questions:

- Was the procedure performed on a male or female?
- Was general or spinal anesthesia administered?
- Was it done endoscopically or nonendoscopically?
- Was it an initial or subsequent procedure?
- Was a permanent stent placed?

> Urethral dilation is not coded separately if it is necessary to accomplish a more extensive procedure because the urethra is too small to insert instrumentation.

> It is easy to confuse stent insertion of the ureter with the urethra. Pinpoint the Code 22.1 describes the thought process for urethral dilation. If this procedure is not done endoscopically, there currently is no code for urethral stent insertion so the unlisted procedure code 53899 is also assigned.

> ### ■ CASE SCENARIO
> A male patient is seen in the office for complaints of painful urination and decreased urine flow. It is determined after examination and testing that the patient has an anterior urethral stricture. The patient elected to have a cystourethroscopy with urethral dilation under general anesthesia, along with internal urethrotomy at the surgery center. Codes: 52281, 52276–51.

Ureter Stricture

A stricture in the ureter causes a functional blockage of urine from the kidney to the bladder, which may cause urine to back flow into the kidney. The most common cause of ureteral stricture is ureteropelvic junction (UPJ) obstruction, which is a congenital or acquired narrowing at the level of the UPJ. Stents are also placed to keep the ureter open for passage of urine. Stents can be inserted percutaneously through the renal pelvis, laparoscopically, by open surgical ureterotomy, or endoscopically using the cystourethroscopic technique. The coding guidelines in this CPT section explain the difference between a temporary and an indwelling stent and when it is appropriate to code separately. If a stent is placed temporarily during a procedure, this placement is *not* coded, because it is removed after the procedure. Insertion of an indwelling/self-retaining ureteral stent (double J stent) is coded separately in addition to the primary procedure performed. Use modifier –51 on the stent code. If stents are placed in both ureters, a –50 modifier is appended.

Ureteral strictures are treated in the same manner by incision (52290), balloon, laser, and electrocautery (52341–52346), and stent insertion (52332, 50693–50695).

> Codes 52320–52356 do not include the insertion of an indwelling stent. Assign 52332 along with the applicable modifier (–RT, –LT, or –50) in addition to the procedure code.

EXAMPLE
Cystourethroscopy was performed. Significant cystitis was appreciated. Ureteral stents were placed at the junction of the ureter and kidneys, bilaterally. Code: 52332–50.

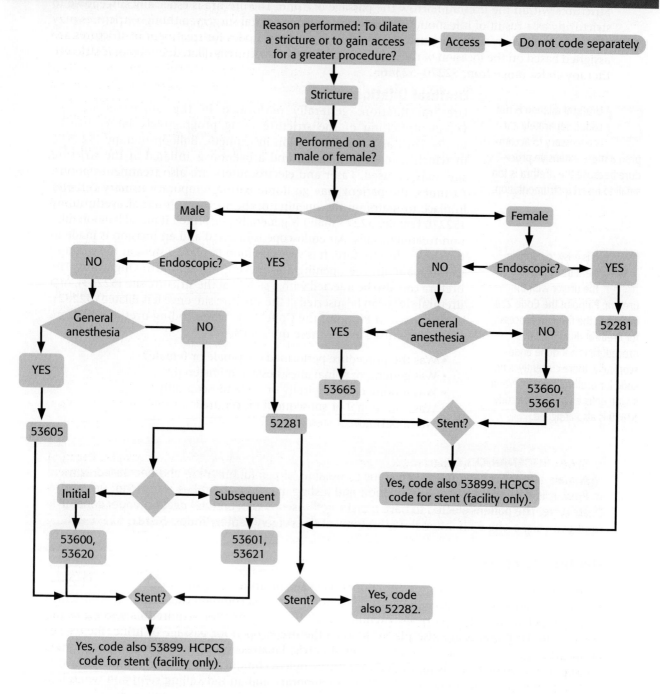

To code an endoscopic ureteral stent removal, report either code 52310 or 52315 and append modifier –58 for a planned or staged procedure. However, if a stent is removed and a new ureteral stent is inserted during the same operation, only the stent insertion should be reported. In this case, the stent removal is a "separate procedure" and is not reported at the time of a more definitive surgical procedure. Code 50382 or 50384 is assigned if the stent is removed percutaneously. Codes 50385 and 50386 are reported for transurethral removal of the ureteral stent without the use of cystoscopy. One of these codes would be assigned if the stent is removed without cystoscopy, most likely in the physician office setting. The physician uses a clamp or other instrument and passes it through the urethra to grasp the stent and facilitate its removal or exchange. Most often, the physician would perform this under radiological guidance, which is included in the new CPT codes.

- Read the operative report to determine the approach (how the stent was inserted) before assigning a code.
- Pay close attention to the anatomical site where the procedure is being performed. It is easy to confuse *urethra* and *ureter*.

Incontinence

When injections are performed, also assign a HCPCS code for the medication provided.

Urinary incontinence is the partial or complete loss of bladder control. Treatment for incontinence depends on the type of incontinence, the severity, and the underlying cause. Some conservative treatments involve medications, Kegel exercises, physical therapy, and bladder training. The urologist may inject bulking material (51715)—such as carbon-coated zirconium beads (Durasphere), calcium hydroxylapatite (Coaptite), or collagen—into the tissue surrounding the urethra to provide support and reduce urine leakage. IV sedation or local anesthesia is administered, and a 21 French rigid cystoscope is inserted into the urethra and advanced to the level of the bladder neck. Injections are performed at various locations (6 and 3 o'clock positions, for example) until bulking is noted. This is commonly performed in the office setting. Repeat injections are required.

Bladder and Urethral Suspension

If the bladder has moved out of the correct anatomical location, surgical intervention is required. Three types of suspension procedures are available: sling, retropubic suspension, and midurethral suspension.

Sling. A sling procedure uses strips of the body's connective tissue (fascia), synthetic material, or mesh to create a pelvic sling or hammock around the bladder neck and urethra. The sling helps keep the urethra closed, especially during sudden strenuous activities such as laughing, coughing, or sneezing. There are many types of slings, including tension free, adjustable, and conventional.

The surgeon attaches both ends of the sling to the pubic bone or ties them in front of the abdomen just above the pubic bone. This can be done vaginally (57288 in the female genital system) or laparoscopically (51992). CPT has separate procedure codes for male sling procedures (53440, 53442).

> ■ **CASE SCENARIO**
> A patient is 10 years post-hysterectomy and now suffers from stress urinary incontinence. Physician performs a laparoscopic sling operation. Code: 51992.

Retropubic Suspension. Retropubic suspension uses sutures to support the bladder neck. The most common retropubic suspension procedure is the Burch procedure (51840, 51990). This treatment is used when the bladder or urethra has dropped out of position. The Burch procedure can be performed through an incision in the abdomen or with laparoscopy. In this operation, an incision is made in the abdomen a few inches below the navel, and sutures are placed through the tissue surrounding the urethra. The bladder neck is raised back to the correct position using a few stitches placed in the anterior wall of the vagina and the pelvic tissues. The goal of this surgery is to elevate and stabilize the urethra by using the anterior vaginal wall; that tissue is then suspended to the Cooper's ligament. These stitches keep the bladder neck in place and help support the urethra. This common procedure is often done at the time of another open abdominal procedure such as a hysterectomy.

The abdominovaginal suspension (51845) uses the same suspension procedure as the Burch but is done via a vaginal approach by allowing sutures to be passed up to the base of the bladder. A small incision is made in the suprapubic area. On both sides of the bladder neck, a needle is passed down through the vaginal incision and pulled back through the suprapubic incision. This is repeated on both sides, and upward traction is used to tighten the bladder neck. An endoscope may be used to confirm proper placement of the sutures.

Several surgical techniques are available for treating stress urinary incontinence (tension-free vaginal tape, suprapubic urethral support sling, transobturator tape, pubovaginal sling placed at the bladder neck). Only one code exists when performed vaginally: 57288.

Midurethral Suspension. The newer midurethral sling procedures use synthetic mesh materials that the surgeon places midway along the urethra. There are two types of midurethral slings: retropubic (i.e., transvaginal tape [TVT]) and transobturator (TOT). The surgeon makes small incisions behind the pubic bone or just by the sides of the vaginal opening, as well as a small incision in the vagina. Specially designed needles are used to position a synthetic tape under the urethra. The surgeon pulls the ends of the tape through the incisions and adjusts them to provide the right amount of support to the urethra. The tape is then attached to the rectus fascia or to the pubic bone by using bone screws. Stabilization and support of the urethra are the goals of this procedure.

Artificial Urinary Sphincter

An artificial sphincter is used to treat incontinence in men. This device is often used for men who have weakened urinary sphincters from treatment of prostate cancer. The fluid-filled ring, shaped like a doughnut, is implanted around the bladder neck. The ring keeps the urinary sphincter closed. To urinate, he presses a valve implanted under the skin that causes the ring to deflate and allows urine to flow from the bladder. Assign code 53445 for insertion of the inflatable ring and the component parts. Codes 53446–53448 are assigned for removal and removal/replacement, depending on the circumstance and if infection is present requiring debridement.

CHECKPOINT 22.2

Answer the following questions.

1. Which part of the urinary system is particularly susceptible to structuring as a result of infection, trauma, or previous surgery? _____

2. Code for the complicated removal of a ureteral stent via cystourethroscopy. _____

3. Which code represents the most common retropubic suspension procedure for supporting the bladder neck (also known as the *Burch procedure*)? _____

Bladder Neoplasms

Tumors can occur anywhere along the urinary tract but are most common in the bladder. Such tumors may be biopsied, fulgurated (destroyed by means of high-frequency electric current), or excised (terms include *resection, removal,* or *ablation*). The operative and pathology reports must be available to accurately code for these procedures. A biopsy can be coded separately only if the biopsy was taken from another site other than the one that is excised or fulgurated. If multiple lesions are excised, the size of the largest lesion is the basis for code selection.

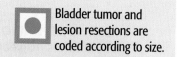 Bladder tumor and lesion resections are coded according to size.

Bladder tumors are staged and classified by how deeply a tumor has penetrated the bladder wall. Tumors that are not located in the bladder wall are removed cystoscopically in a procedure called *transurethral resection of the bladder* tumor (TURBT). The lesion or tumor not involved in the deeper muscle wall is removed. Laser therapy is an alternative method to TURBT where, after a sample of tumor tissue is obtained, a laser is used to destroy the cancerous tissue. Code 52214 is assigned for fulguration of the bladder trigone, bladder neck, prostatic fossa, urethra, or periurethral glands, which may be used to report conditions other than neoplasm. Code 52224 is assigned for fulguration of minor lesions (less than 0.5 cm) of the bladder. CPT code assignment is the same despite the different methods of treatment for lesions or tumors 0.5 cm or larger. Codes 52234–52240 are assigned for fulguration or resection of bladder tumors based on tumor size: small, medium, or large.

EXAMPLE

Cystoscopy with fulguration of 1.0-cm lesion of the bladder. Code: 52234.

Following removal of a bladder tumor, intravesical chemotherapy or intravesical immunotherapy may be used to try to prevent tumor recurrences. Intravesical means "within the bladder." The bladder is flushed or lavaged, and the medication is instilled through the catheter into the bladder within a few minutes. Instillation refers to delivering the liquid one drop at a time into a body part.

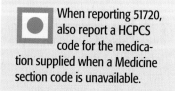 When reporting 51720, also report a HCPCS code for the medication supplied when a Medicine section code is unavailable.

The therapeutic agents are retained for 1 to 2 hours, and then urinated out (51720). The chief intravesical agents currently available are thiotepa, doxorubicin, mitomycin C, and bacillus Calmette-Guerin (BCG). The first three are chemotherapy drugs. The fourth, BCG, is a live but weakened vaccine strain of bovine tuberculosis. It is one of the most effective agents for treating bladder cancer and especially for treating carcinoma in situ (CIS) of the bladder.

EXAMPLE

51720 Bladder instillation of anticarcinogenic agent BCG. Code: 90586, *Bacillus Calmette-Guerin vaccine (BCG) for bladder cancer, live, for intravesicular use.*

Cystectomy

Cystectomy involves removing all or part of the urinary bladder (51550–51596) and is performed for patients who have bladder cancer (transitional cell carcinoma), cancer of the surrounding pelvic structures, or incontinence. Code descriptors vary depending on whether a partial or complete cystectomy is performed and by the extent of reconstructive work performed at the time of the bladder removal. During cystectomy, it is necessary to divert urine from the ureters, which can be accomplished by ureterostomy, an opening or stoma in the skin where a bag is attached to the outside of the patient's abdomen to collect urine. Other methods of diversion are uretero-sigmoidostomy (51580); the creation of a connection between the ureters and the sigmoid colon; ureteroileal conduit (51590); the connection of the ureters to the ileum, which is the last section of the small intestines; or the creation of a neobladder (51596), which is the construction of a replacement bladder usually using the stomach or intestines.

If bilateral pelvic lymph node dissection is also performed with cystectomy, it is included by reporting the indented codes 51585 and 51595. Both codes include the cystectomy and bilateral pelvic lymphadenectomy.

Interstitial Cystitis

Interstitial cystitis (IC) is classified as recurring or constant inflammation of the bladder, which causes pain and discomfort of the bladder and surrounding pelvic area. The cause of IC is unknown. Chronic inflammation with IC causes the bladder lining to scar, leading to stiffening of the bladder wall, which affects the way the bladder expands. People with IC may urinate 60 times a day compared to healthy people at 7 to 10 times a day. There is no cure for this condition; however, bladder dilation seems to help patients manage by stretching the bladder back to normal size to decrease the urinary frequency (52260–52265). This procedure is usually done hydrostatically with water instilled into the bladder to stretch it and break up inflammation caused by chronic IC. If the patient does not have IC, these codes should not be used. If the bladder is dilated for any other purpose, the unlisted code 53899 should be assigned instead. This code is assigned for current or past history of IC.

Another common treatment for IC involves instilling medication (such as dimethyl sulfoxide [DMSO]) into the bladder through a catheter (51700). This is usually done once a week for 6 weeks. Some patients continue this treatment for maintenance therapy, with longer intervals in between treatments. This medication works to block inflammation, decrease pain, and remove toxins that can damage tissue.

Kidney Tumors

A kidney tumor is an abnormal mass that develops in a kidney and can form when old cells do not die off and new cells grow when they are not needed, creating a tumor. A benign kidney tumor is not cancerous and does not spread to other areas of the body, but it can impair kidney function. Malignant kidney tumors are more serious and potentially life threatening. Renal cell carcinoma, transitional cell carcinoma, and Wilms' tumor are the more common malignant tumors in the kidney. The risk of renal cell carcinomas increases with age and is most common in patients 60 and older. Kidneys are also susceptible to cysts and masses. Tumors, cysts, and masses can be excised or ablated via laparoscopic, percutaneous, or open surgical technique. Use code 50250 for open ablation of renal mass lesion(s). To report laparoscopic ablation of renal cysts, use 50541 or 50542 for laparoscopic ablation of renal mass lesion(s). Codes 50592 and 50593 are reported for percutaneous ablation of renal tumors based on the method of ablation: radio-frequency versus cryosurgery.

Kidney Stones

Urolithiasis is the process of stones (called *calculi*) forming in the urinary tract. These calculi can be wedged anywhere in the kidney, bladder, or ureter. The incidence of kidney stones is significant: They occur in about 12% of males by age 70 and 5% of females in the United States. Once a stone is confirmed, either via x-ray, IVP, or CT scan, lithotripsy, litholapaxy, or extraction of the calculus may be performed if the stone will not pass through the urethra on its own. Stone size, the number of stones, and their location are very important factors in deciding the appropriate treatment. The composition of a stone, if known, can also affect the choice of treatments.

Treatment of Calculi in the Bladder

Litholapaxy is a method of treating stones in the bladder that involves the crushing of a calculus (52317–52318). This may be done by using ultrasound to fragment the stones, which are then flushed and suctioned out. Sometimes stones are too big to be flushed and must be manually crushed by using a lithotriptor or lithotrite. These instruments act like nutcrackers that grasp the stone and apply even force on both sides of the stone until it breaks.

Treatment of Calculi in the Kidneys, Ureter, and Urethra

A number of approaches are used to treat stones located in the kidneys, ureter, or urethra: (1) open method, (2) extracorporeal shock wave *lithotripsy*, (3) percutaneous *lithotripsy*, (4) laparoscopic removal, (5) endoscopic removal, (6) transurethral endoscopic stone removal, and (7) transurethral endoscopic *lithotripsy*. (Note the three approaches using lithotripsy.) Coders must read the operative report closely to determine where the stone is located, how it is accessed, and whether it is removed or crushed.

Open Approach. Some stones are too large to be crushed by lithotripsy and require surgical removal. Lithotomy refers to incising a structure to remove a stone. Each subsection has codes designated for an open lithotomy approach. For the kidney, codes 50060–50075 are assigned. For the ureter, assign codes 50610–50630 based on which segment of the ureter the stone is lodged. For the bladder, assign codes 51050–51065.

> ● Do not confuse lithotripsy with litholapaxy. Litholapaxy is the crushing of stones located in the bladder. Lithotripsy involves crushing stones located in the ureter, renal pelvis, or urethra.

Extracorporeal Shock Wave Lithotripsy. Extracorporeal shock wave lithotripsy (ESWL) is coded to 50590. This procedure is considered non-operative in that it is not carried out in an operating room. The patient is heavily sedated and placed in a lithotripsy tub where shock waves are directed via radiological guidance (either ultrasound or fluoroscopy) through deionized water surrounding the patient to a specified area. Lithotripsy can also be conducted by having the patient lie down on a water-filled cushion that is placed against the skin. The repeated force caused by the shock waves fragments the stone into small pieces, and the patient will void the stone fragments in the urine.

> ● Urologists will treat bilateral kidney stones with ESWL at different times. If the second side is done within the global period of the first, add the –58 modifier to indicate that the ESWL is staged with one kidney treated initially and another later.

The urologist performs ESWL to break up one or more stones in the kidney; it does not permit the urologist to target just one stone. The ESWL procedure is the same regardless of the number of stones in the kidney, so there is no justification for extra billing or applying the –22 modifier for multiple stones. Whether the stones are in the renal pelvis, calyx, UPJ, ureter, or all four locations, use 50590 only once per kidney. The code is valued at a high rate because it is intended to cover instances when multiple stones are treated.

Sometimes stones are treated more than once. For example, the left kidney is treated in June and again in July, and the right is treated in September. Code 50590–LT for June, 50590–LT–58 for July, and 50590–RT–58 for September.

Percutaneous Lithotripsy. Percutaneous lithotripsy (50080–50081) uses ultrasonic, electrohydraulic, or mechanical lithotripsy to treat large stones located within the kidney such as a staghorn that involves the renal pelvis and extends into at least two calyces. This method is chosen when stones cannot be fragmented by ESWL or when ESWL treatment

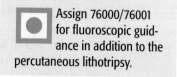

> ● Assign 76000/76001 for fluoroscopic guidance in addition to the percutaneous lithotripsy.

fails, when stones are impacted in the ureter, or in the case of cystine stones. Rather than making a large incision with open surgery, a 1-cm incision is made over the flank. The urologist places a guidewire through this incision. The wire is inserted into the kidney under fluoroscopic guidance and directed down the ureter. A passage is then created around the wire using dilators to provide access into the kidney. A nephroscope is passed into the kidney to visualize the stone. The stone is fragmented by using a laser or an ultrasonic probe. The surgeon can then grasp or suction out the fragments of stone.

Laparoscopic Removal. For laparoscopic removal of a ureteral calculus, assign 50945.

Endoscopic Removal. Endoscopic removal involves inserting a scope into the affected area that is already accessed by an open abdominal or pelvic incision. This can prove confusing to coders because many of the procedure descriptions end in the suffix "oscopy," meaning an endoscope was used. A scope is also used to access stones by entering the urethra (transurethral) with no open incision to the abdomen. Codes for endoscopic removal of stones are located under the subheading Endoscopy within each subsection of the Urology chapter. For endoscopic ureteral stone removal, assign code 50961 or 50980.

Transurethral Endoscopic Stone Removal. Transurethral endoscopic stone removal procedures include inserting the scope into the urethra to the destination of the stone to grasp it and remove it. Once a stone is seen through the ureteroscope, a small device called a *basket extractor* can be used to grasp smaller stones and remove them. Codes are assigned based on where the stone is located. Assign 52310–52315 for removal of stones from the urethra or bladder. CPT code 52320 is assigned for removal of ureteral calculus without ureteroscopy and 52352 if ureteroscopy is also performed.

Transurethral Endoscopic Lithotripsy. Transurethral endoscopic lithotripsy procedures include inserting the scope into the urethra to the destination of the stone to break it up (crush it) and remove the fragments. Transurethral lithotripsy is used to treat stones in the ureter or kidney that are greater than 2.5 cm and are too large to successfully treat with other methods of lithotripsy because the stone fragments would still be too large to pass through the ureters and urethra. For stones that are too large to remove, a laser, spark-generating probe, or air-driven (pneumatic) probe is passed through the scope to fragment the stone, allowing for basket extraction. Codes are assigned based on where the calculus is located and subsequently fragmented and if ureteroscopy was also performed. Code 52325 is assigned for *ureteral* calculus fragmentation (without ureteroscopy). Code 52353 is assigned when ureteroscopy and/or pyeloscopy is used during fragmentation in the *ureter* or *urethra*. For *bladder* stone fragmentation, assign 52317–52318 based on the size of the calculus (Pinpoint the Code 22.2).

PINPOINT THE CODE 22.2: Lithotripsy

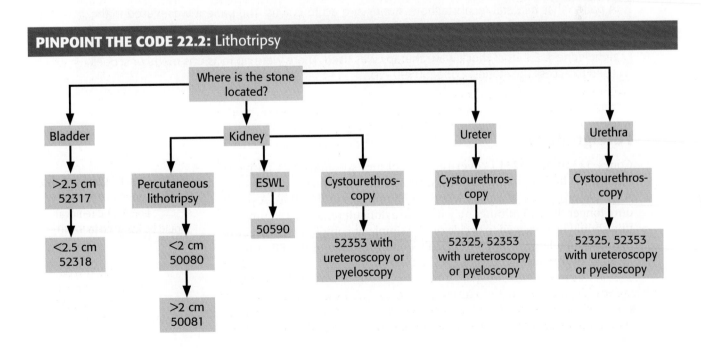

EXAMPLE

Preoperative diagnosis: multiple large left ureteral stone fragments post-ESWL with indwelling left ureteral stent.

Procedure performed: cystoscopy with left ureteroscopic laser lithotripsy.

A 19 French cystourethroscope was passed under direct vision into the bladder, and forceps were used to grasp the distal end of the indwelling left ureteral stent and remove it. The ureteroscope was then passed under direct vision into the bladder and into the left ureter. Within the ureter, the distal-most stone fragment was encountered, which was noted to have a very irregular surface. The stone was pushed somewhat distally with the ureteroscope to reach a more suitable stone position for lithotripsy. While doing so, the second stone fragmented directly proximal to the first.

A small holmium laser fiber was passed through the ureteroscope, and laser disintegration of both large stone fragments was accomplished. The stone fragments broke into smaller pieces but never disintegrated as expected.

When all fragment sizes had been reduced to 2 mm or less, lithotripsy was terminated. The laser fiber was withdrawn, and a 4-wire stone basket was passed through the ureteroscope and up above the stone fragments, grasping them and dropping them into the bladder. Code: 52353.

INTERNET RESOURCE: View a brief video clip from Duke University demonstrating kidney stone dusting at: www.youtube.com/watch?v=ooj9d_f81MY

Lithotripsy Coding Steps. Three elements must be determined before assigning a code:

1. **Where** is the stone?
2. **Which** approach is used?
3. **How** is the procedure performed?

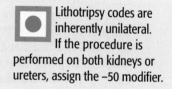
Lithotripsy codes are inherently unilateral. If the procedure is performed on both kidneys or ureters, assign the −50 modifier.

■ CASE SCENARIO

A patient has bilateral renal staghorn stones and acute cystitis. The patient was placed in the lithotripsy unit and the gantry lowered into the bath. Under fluoroscopy, both stones were located and treated during the same session. 2400 22-kV shocks were given to the left and right kidneys. External shock wave therapy was used. There were no incisions made or scopes used to access the stones. Code: 50590–50.

Foreign Body

Codes 52310 and 52315 cover removal of any substance not native or natural to the urethra or bladder, such as a stone, catheter tip, or stent. A simple procedure is usually less than 15 minutes in duration. A procedure longer than 15 minutes may indicate a difficult removal. Documentation should be reviewed to decide on the simple or complicated procedure, mentioning a large, numerous calculus, the condition of the FB, and the location of the stent.

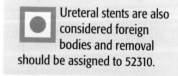
Ureteral stents are also considered foreign bodies and removal should be assigned to 52310.

Assign codes to the following procedures. Include any necessary modifiers. In some cases, more than one code is required.

1. EMG studies of urethral sphincter _____

2. Cystourethroscopy with double J stent _____

3. Simple bladder irrigation _____

4. Renal endoscopy through nephrotomy, right _____

5. The patient was placed on his right side on a water cushion and shock waves were used to crush a right renal calculus. _____

6. The surgeon performed a cystoscopy with biopsy of the trigone and dilation of the ureteral stricture. _____

7. A urologist needs to examine both ureters and the bladder. She inserts a scope into the ureter(s), making an incision in the opening of the ureters to the bladder (meatotomy), and completes the examination. _____

8. Repair hypospadias second stage, greater than 3-cm diversion _____

If the patient had prior surgery of the bladder or urethra, FB removal may be complicated because of scarring adhesions, or anatomical changes. Check the documentation for wording to indicate this situation.

INTERNET RESOURCE: BroadcastMed allows viewing of urological procedures. Click on the procedure to see the video. You are required to register at no charge before the video is played. www.broadcastmed.com

INTERNET RESOURCE: Medline Plus offers interactive tutorials and videos demonstrating urological procedures, as well as valuable reference material and links to organizations. www.nlm.nih.gov/medlineplus/kidneysandurinarysystem.html

Renal Transplants

Technological and surgical advancements allow physicians to salvage organs that would have been discarded previously. In coding for these surgeries, it is important to understand the three basic services involved in transplantation:

1. Harvesting the organ from either a cadaver or living donor, which includes cold preservation of the organ
2. Backbench work, which includes standard preparation of the organ prior to transplantation to make it transplantable
3. Transplantation, which may include removal of the existing organ from the recipient

These are the general components of a transplant that apply to renal transplants as well. The code range is 50300–50382. There is also a laparoscopic code for a donor nephrectomy from a living donor (50547). Review the following example for the coding structure for renal transplants.

- A man was in a motor vehicle collision resulting in brain death. Documentation exists that this patient is an organ donor, but only one kidney is viable. Blood work is done, along with an extensive review of the family and social history. The procurement team arrives at the hospital to remove the kidney, which is placed in a sterile plastic bag housed in a container with ice to keep the kidney cold. The code for this service is 50300.

- The kidney is transported to the recipient's hospital, where backbench preparation is performed. Backbench work may include dissection of fat from around the kidney, excision of any adrenal glands, and preparation of the ureter, renal vein, and renal artery. This service is reported with code 50323.

- Finally, the recipient patient is taken to the operating room and, if necessary, the recipient's kidney may be removed. If both the transplant and the recipient's kidney removal are done during the same session, the code reported is 50365.

NOTE: Another area of importance is when the donated kidney requires extension grafts to be fully viable. This is considered backbench work and is reported with code range 50327–50329 based on whether the extension grafts are venous, arterial, or ureteral.

Keep in mind that the transplant codes break down based on whether the three basic services are related to kidneys from a cadaver or a living donor, and whether the recipient patient's nephrectomy is performed at the time of the transplant or was performed previously.

Chapter Summary

1. To determine code selection for the urethral dilation procedure, the coder assesses whether the procedure was performed on a male or female, whether general or spinal anesthesia was administered, whether the procedure was done endoscopically or nonendoscopically, whether it was an initial or a subsequent procedure, and whether a permanent stent was placed.

2. Laparoscopic and cystourethroscopic procedures use an endoscope and shorten recovery time. Open surgical procedures are declining with technological advancements. With a laparoscope, used to inspect the pelvic organs, two to three small abdominal incisions are made in the abdomen allowing for passage of the scope and instruments. A cystourethroscope is inserted through the urethra for visualization of the lower urinary tract and bladder.

3. Urodynamics testing is performed to determine the strength of the bladder wall, bladder volume, urine flow, and the volume of residual urine used in diagnosing and treating urinary disorders.

4. There are three approaches for the treatment of kidney stones with lithotripsy. First, ESWL uses shock waves delivered via a lithotripsy tub to break up the calculus. The repeated force caused by the shock waves fragments the stone into small pieces. The patient will void the stone fragments in the urine. Second, percutaneous lithotripsy uses ultrasonic, electrohydraulic, or mechanical lithotripsy delivered via a small incision in the flank. A guidewire is inserted into the kidney. A nephroscope is passed into the kidney to visualize the stone, which is fragmented by using a laser or an ultrasonic probe. The surgeon can then grasp or suction out the fragments. Third, transurethral ureteroscopic lithotripsy uses the cystoscope, which is inserted through the urethra and into the bladder and ureters.

Matching

Match the key terms with their definitions.

A. litholapaxy
B. cystourethroscopy
C. cortex
D. extracorporeal shock wave lithotripsy
E. urodynamics

F. incontinence
G. bladder neck
H. calculus
I. stricture
J. stent

1. _____ The crushing of a calculus located in the bladder

2. _____ Where the bladder narrows to connect to the urethra

3. _____ Stones that form in the urinary tract

4. _____ Endoscopic procedure where the scope is inserted into the urethra and the bladder, ureters, and kidney

5. _____ Used to keep the ureter open for the passage of urine

6. _____ The assessment of bladder function

7. _____ A method of treatment for kidney stones (nonoperative)

8. _____ Outermost layer of the kidney

9. _____ Functional blockage urine

10. _____ Loss of bladder control

True or False

Decide whether each statement is true or false.

1. _____ Lithotripsy is assigned to 50590 regardless of where the stones are located or the approach.

2. _____ The fact that a patient has had prior surgery on the bladder with scarring present would justify choosing a complicated removal of ureteral stent code (52315).

3. _____ Cyst and vesic are both prefixes for the bladder.

4. _____ Urethral calibration can be reported separately from transurethral resection of the prostate.

5. _____ The placement of an indwelling ureteral stent is included in cystourethroscopy.

6. _____ Nephrolithotomy represents the services of removing a stone from the kidney.

7. _____ Hematuria is a urinary tract infection.

8. _____ The backbench work during a kidney transplant includes cold preservation.

9. _____ TURP is the acronym for transurinary resection of prostate.

10. _____ The code range for a laparoscopic nephrectomy is 50220–50240.

Multiple Choice

Select the letter that best completes the statement or answers the question.

1. Contrast is instilled and a voiding urethrocystography is conducted in the outpatient department. Which code should be reported?
   A. 51610
   B. 51600
   C. 51728
   D. 74430

2. A 29-year-old female with interstitial cystitis, frequency, and urethral itch diagnosed with urethral syndrome undergoes cystoscopy with urethral dilation, urethral meatotomy, and hydrodistention of the bladder under general anesthesia. Which code(s) should be reported?
   A. 52260
   B. 52260, 52285
   C. 52270, 52260, 52281
   D. 52281, 52260

3. The urologist performed a cystourethroscopy to remove two bladder tumors by fulguration. The tumors measured 1.7 cm each. Which code should be reported?
   A. 52234
   B. 52234–50
   C. 52234 x 2
   D. 52234–22

4. The surgeon performed a nephrolithotomy and removed a large staghorn calculus. Which code should be reported?
   A. 50060
   B. 50070
   C. 50065
   D. 50075

5. The urologist performed a cystectomy with urinary diversion by connecting the ureters to a ureteroileal conduit on a patient with a malignant neoplasm of the bladder. Which code should be reported?
   A. 51595
   B. 51580
   C. 51590
   D. 51565

6. A physician dilates a male patient's urethra under local anesthesia using a urethral dilator. This is the initial session for this patient. Which code should be reported?
   A. 53600
   B. 53660
   C. 53605
   D. 53620

7. A male patient with urinary retention, urinary stenosis, and vesical neck stenosis. The urologist performs a meatotomy, urethral dilation, and TURP. Which code(s) should be reported?
   A. 52500, 53605–51
   B. 52601, 52501–51
   C. 52500, 52601
   D. 52601

8. A patient presents with vesicouterine fistula and the urologist performs a closure of the fistula. Which code should be reported?
   A. 51920
   B. 51900
   C. 51925
   D. 51900–50

9. The urologist performs a cystourethroscopy with removal of ureteral calculus and insertion of indwelling right ureteral stent. Which code(s) should be reported?
   A. 52332
   B. 52320
   C. 52320, 52332–59
   D. 52320, 52332–51

10. A patient has been on dialysis for 3 years and his sister has agreed to donate a kidney. The transplant team is sent to the donor's hospital to retrieve the kidney. They transport it to the recipient's hospital where backbench work is provided and the kidney is transplanted into the recipient. The recipient's own kidney was removed several years ago. Provide the codes that represent this set of services.
    A. 50320, 50325, 50360
    B. 50320, 50323, 50365
    C. 50300, 50325, 50365
    D. 50300, 50323, 50360

CHAPTER 23

CPT: Male Genital System

CHAPTER OUTLINE

Male Anatomy

Organization

Male Preventive Services

Common Problems of the Male Genital System and Surgical Therapies

LEARNING OUTCOMES

After studying this chapter, you should be able to:

1. Identify anatomical structures of the male genital system.
2. Compare newborn versus adult circumcision.
3. Understand the techniques associated with hypospadias repair codes.
4. Describe the various techniques for prostatectomy.

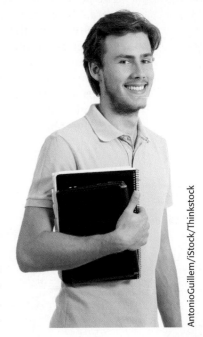

AntonioGuillem/iStock/Thinkstock

This chapter focuses on the procedural coding and terminology of surgical cases of the male genital system. The *genitourinary system* is a collective term used to describe all of the reproductive organs and the organs responsible for creating and excreting urine. These organs and anatomical structures are grouped together in CPT because of their proximity to each other and the sharing of common viaducts, like the male urethra. Urologists are physicians who specialize in diagnosing and treating diseases and injuries of the genitourinary system and the male reproductive system. A wide range of clinical conditions is managed by this specialty, so knowledge of internal medicine, general surgery, and pediatrics is necessary. Urologists specialize in endoscopic surgery to diagnose problems and provide surgical treatment. Urology is classified as a surgical subspecialty and covers surgery on the urinary system and on the male genitalia and prostate.

INTERNET RESOURCE: The American Urological Association website is helpful for learning about male genital and prostate procedures. **www.auanet.org/resources/coding-tips.cfm**

MALE ANATOMY

The male reproductive system consists of the penis, testicles (epididymis, scrotum, vas deferens, spermatic cord, seminal vesicles), and prostate (Figs. 23.1 and 23.2). The scrotum is a sac that houses the testicles (or testes). The testes have two primary functions—to produce sperm and androgens (testosterone). They are covered in two protective membranes: the tunica vaginalis and the tunica albuginea. The tunica vaginalis is an extension of the peritoneum and the outermost membrane. The tunica albuginea is the inner serous membrane layer that extends between the lobules acting like an insulator where lymphatic vessels, blood vessels, and nerves are connected to the testes. Each testicle contains between 200 and 300 lobules. Each lobule contains seminiferous tubules (where spermatogenesis takes place) and interstitial cells of Leydig (which secrete testosterone). The hypothalamus and pituitary gland control how much testosterone the testes produce and secrete. Testosterone is required for physical development of boys. In adulthood, testosterone maintains libido, muscle strength, and bone density.

The spermatic cord is a multilayered structure that acts like a tunnel where blood vessels and nerves travel from the abdomen to the scrotum. The epididymis is located outside the testes and stores the sperm until they are mature enough to be mobile. Sperm need nutrition to survive the trip through the female reproductive tract. They are provided nutrients from the seminal fluid, which is produced by seminal vesicles, the prostate, and bulbourethral glands. The sperm leave the epididymis and enter the vas deferens (also called the *ductus deferens*). The vas deferens travels through the spermatic cord, moving the sperm along and into the ejaculatory duct. The ejaculatory duct steers the sperm along with seminal fluid into the urethra. The tip of the penis is called the *glans*. At birth, the glans is covered by foreskin called the *prepuce*.

The penis is made of several components: glans, corpus cavernosum, corpus spongiosum, and urethra. The glans is the head or tip of the penis that is covered with pink, moist mucosa. In uncircumcised men, the foreskin (prepuce) covers the glans. In circumcised men, the foreskin has been surgically removed and the mucosa on the glans is exposed to air and becomes dry skin.

The penile shaft is composed of three erectile columns—two corpora cavernosa and the corpus spongiosum, which fill with blood during erection. The urethra runs through the corpus spongiosum, conducting urine out of the body. These columns are surrounded by a very strong deep penile fascia (Buck's fascia) and dartos fascia. Additional columns encircle fascial layers, nerves, lymphatic vessels, and blood vessels.

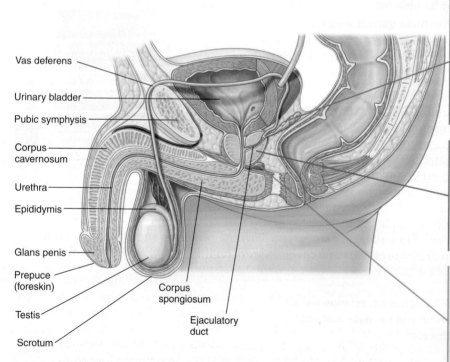

Located at the base of the bladder, a pair of **seminal vesicles** (one for each vas deferens) secretes a thick, yellowish fluid into the ejaculatory duct. The fluid—which comprises about 60% of semen—contains fructose (an energy source for sperm motility) as well as other substances that nourish and ensure sperm motility.

The **prostate gland** sits just below the bladder, where it encircles both the urethra and ejaculatory duct. It secretes a thin, milky fluid into the urethra; besides adding volume to the semen (it comprises about 30% of the fluid portion of semen), the fluid also enhances sperm motility.

Two pea-shaped **bulbourethral glands** (also called **Cowper's glands**) secrete a clear fluid into the penile portion of the urethra during sexual arousal. Besides serving as a lubricant for sexual intercourse, the fluid also neutralizes the acidity of residual urine in the urethra, which would harm the sperm.

Labels (left, top to bottom): Vas deferens · Urinary bladder · Pubic symphysis · Corpus cavernosum · Urethra · Epididymis · Glans penis · Prepuce (foreskin) · Testis · Scrotum

Labels (center): Corpus spongiosum · Ejaculatory duct

Figure 23.1 The male genital system.

From Thompson, G. *Understanding Anatomy & Physiology: A Visual, Auditory, Interactive Approach*, F.A. Davis Company, 2013.

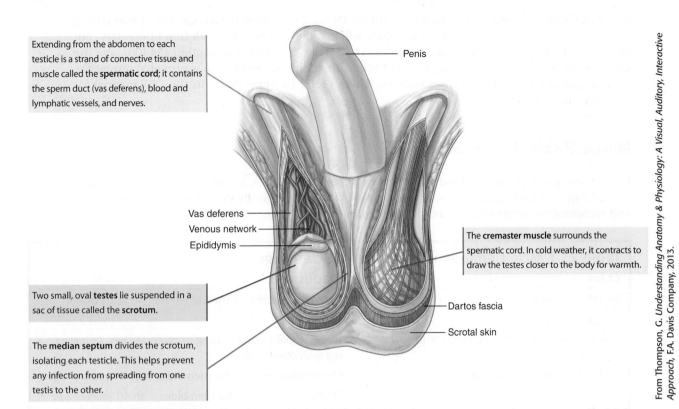

Extending from the abdomen to each testicle is a strand of connective tissue and muscle called the **spermatic cord**; it contains the sperm duct (vas deferens), blood and lymphatic vessels, and nerves.

Penis

Vas deferens
Venous network
Epididymis

The **cremaster muscle** surrounds the spermatic cord. In cold weather, it contracts to draw the testes closer to the body for warmth.

Two small, oval **testes** lie suspended in a sac of tissue called the **scrotum**.

Dartos fascia

Scrotal skin

The **median septum** divides the scrotum, isolating each testicle. This helps prevent any infection from spreading from one testis to the other.

From Thompson, G. *Understanding Anatomy & Physiology: A Visual, Auditory, Interactive Approach*, F.A. Davis Company, 2013.

Figure 23.2 The scrotum and testis.

The prostate is a butterfly-shaped structure that is partly glandular and partly muscular that helps make semen. The urethra runs through the center of the prostate where it is situated in the pelvic cavity, below the lower part of the symphysis pubis bone and in front of the rectum and can be felt through the rectal wall. (For this reason, a digital rectal exam is performed to diagnose prostate enlargement.) It is normally about the size of a walnut with multiple surfaces.

BOX 23.1 Male Genital System Sections	
Penis	Vas Deferens
Testis	Spermatic Cord
Epididymis	Seminal Vesicles
Tunica Vaginalis	Prostate
Scrotum	

BOX 23.2 Male Genital System Subsections	
Incision	Repair
Destruction	Manipulation
Excision	Laparoscopy
Introduction	Suture

ORGANIZATION

The Male Genital System section is arranged by anatomical site and category of procedure. It follows the same schematic as all of the other surgery sections. There are nine main headings (Box 23.1). These sections are further broken down into subheadings or categories (Box 23.2).

Some of the procedures in this section of CPT are differentiated by age. Many of the procedures on the male anatomy are found in the Urinary System section of the manual. Coding procedures on the male genitourinary system may require combination coding, with codes being assigned from both the Urology and Male Genital System sections.

Coding guidelines and instructional notes are located throughout the chapter and should be reviewed before assigning codes from this section. Careful attention also should be given to modifiers –50, –52, –58, and –63. In using modifier –50, the coder explains that a unilateral procedure such as orchiopexy (54640) is being provided bilaterally. For modifier –52, the reduced service modifier, a circumcision that includes a dorsal penile or ring block (54150) is provided without the dorsal or penile block. Modifier –63 also applies to this code. Modifier –63 should not be reported for procedures that are already indicated for neonates and infants with a present body weight of 4 kg. The use of modifier −58 represents staged procedures. Often, coders who see a code description stating that the procedure is a second-stage procedure will assume that modifier −58 is not necessary, but that is not the case. The code description of "second stage" is a clinical indication (54308), and the use of modifier −58 is a coding requirement when an additional procedure is provided during the surgical global period of a previous surgery. Always refer to Appendix A in the CPT manual for complete descriptions of modifiers.

MALE PREVENTIVE SERVICES

Until recent years, the focus of preventive care has been on females, who were encouraged to have annual Pap tests and breast exams. The American Academy of Family Practitioners, however, now also recommends screenings for male genitourinary health (Table 23.1).

Table 23.1 Male Genitourinary Preventive Screenings

EXAM	FREQUENCY
Rectal/prostate exam	Low risk: annually for men older than 40 years of age
Testicular exam	Every 3 years
Sexually transmitted disease (STD) screening	When sexually active, having unprotected sex, or having sex with other males
Prostate-specific antigen (PSA)	FH negative: annually for men older than 50 years of age
	FH positive: annually for men older than 40 years of age

Prostate cancer ranks in the top 10 causes of death in men over the age of 45. Prostate cancer screening is looking for early-stage disease when treatment may be more effective. The main screening tools for prostate cancer are the digital rectal examination (DRE) and the prostate-specific antigen (PSA) test. The DRE is a quick exam for checking the health of the prostate. For this test, the doctor inserts a gloved finger into the rectum. This allows the doctor to feel the back portion of the prostate for abnormal size and any irregular areas. The PSA test measures the prostate-specific antigen level in the blood; the higher the value, the greater the risk of prostate cancer.

Medicare has expanded its coverage of preventive services. Prostate cancer screening tests, in the form of DRE (G0102) and the PSA test (G0103), are covered once a year for male beneficiaries 50 years of age or older (coverage begins the day after the 50th birthday).

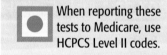 When reporting these tests to Medicare, use HCPCS Level II codes.

COMMON PROBLEMS OF THE MALE GENITAL SYSTEM AND SURGICAL THERAPIES

Penis

Phimosis and Balanitis

Phimosis is the inability of the foreskin to be retracted behind the head of the penis. This is a congenital condition for all newborn males. Balanitis is the inflammation of the glans penis caused by phimosis or redundant foreskin. Circumcision is the treatment of choice for these conditions. The surgeon removes the foreskin by excising the foreskin and, if present, removing redundant foreskin. According to the Centers for Disease Control and Prevention, circumcision lowers the risks of penile cancer, HIV, and urinary tract infection. Phimosis and balanitis codes are in the 54160–54164 range. Infant/child circumcisions are assigned codes 54000, 54150, and 54160.

Adult circumcision is performed using one of three techniques.

Guided Forceps. The guided forceps technique (54150) is the simplest technique. In this procedure, the foreskin is pulled forward over the glans with a pair of forceps, and the foreskin is then snipped and excised.

Dorsal Slit. The dorsal slit technique (54001) is the method of choice when treating phimosis or paraphimosis. In this procedure, the foreskin is pulled taut, and artery forceps are placed at the 1 and 3 o'clock and 11 and 9 o'clock positions to separate the glans from the prepuce. Keeping the skin taut, an incision (slit) is made through the dorsal side of the prepuce (foreskin) to loosen the constriction and carried down a few centimeters and then around in a circle about the glans. The skin is trimmed and sutured circumferentially around the base of the frenulum.

> ● Adult circumcisions are predominantly performed under anesthesia. In addition, anesthetic topical cream and a local anesthetic is injected into the base of the penis.

Sleeve Resection. A sleeve resection (54160) is more complicated than the other two procedures, but often preferred when there is a risk for excessive bleeding. In this procedure, two parallel cuts are made along the shaft of the penis, one at the base of the glans and the second further down the shaft, resulting in a thin band or sleeve of detached foreskin. When this is removed, the top and bottom portions of the frenulum are reattached with dissolving sutures.

When assigning a code, the coder must read the operative note to determine the method used to carry out the circumcision. The age of the patient also plays a role in correct code choice. A dorsal slit (54000–54001) can be assigned for phimosis and falls outside the range of codes for circumcision.

■ **CASE SCENARIO**

A 2-day-old baby undergoes an excisional circumcision in the hospital nursery. A penile anesthetic block is administered. Report codes 54160, 64450. Had the physician used a clamp or other device instead of surgical excision, code 54150 would apply and there would be no need to assign 64450 because the code description includes penile block.

> ● If the physician performs a dorsal penile nerve block on a newborn while performing the circumcision, report code 64450 in addition to the circumcision. A newborn is a baby up to 28 days old.

EXAMPLE
A 24-year-old male was not circumcised as an infant. Excisional circumcision is performed. Report code 54161.

INTERNET RESOURCE: Visit the Net Doctor website to learn more about balanitis.
www.netdoctor.co.uk/menshealth/facts/balanitis.htm

Penile Adhesions

There are instances when a circumcision "fails." A failed circumcision is a somewhat broad term used to describe when the post-circumcised penis may have a distorted appearance, when penile adhesions are present, or when the physician documents redundant prepuce, phimosis, or balanoposthitis. Sometimes the circumcision procedure fails because not enough foreskin is excised, allowing skin bridges (or adhesions) to attach the side of the glans penis to the penile shaft skin. Lysis of post-circumcision adhesions is reported with 54162 (*Lysis or excision of penile post-circumcision adhesions*). This procedure is done under general anesthesia and releases preputial post-circumcision adhesions and cleanses the glans. The physician may place two vertical incisions directly over the fibrous ring, and the fibrous bands are divided to expose the Buck's fascia.

Repair of an incomplete circumcision is assigned code 54163. This code is reported when a patient with a failed circumcision requires a plastic surgical correction because of scarring or completion of the circumcision excision to remove any remaining prepuce. This procedure is painful and requires quite a bit of cutting, warranting general anesthesia. The surgeon typically uses loop magnification to be able to visualize adhesions. The adhesions are freed up between the foreskin and the glans. The skin bridges (areas from previous circumcision that healed incorrectly, leaving the glans attached to the penile shaft) are incised. Any excess foreskin remaining is excised with scissors. Multiple absorbable sutures are placed to close the penile shaft skin incision.

Repair of Hypospadias

Hypospadias is a congenital condition in which the urethral opening is not located at the tip of the penis, but rather on the underside of the penis. It occurs in about 1 in 250 male births. The urethral opening can be located anywhere along the urethra. Most commonly, the opening is located along the underside of the penis, near the tip. Epispadias is another congenital abnormality in which the urethral opening is on the upper surface of the penis. If this condition is not treated, it may lead to a deformity of the penis called *chordee,* which is an unnatural curving of the penis. If the opening is close to the perineum, it could also lead to fertility problems.

Surgical repair is usually done when the child is between 6 and 18 months. Various techniques are used to treat this condition. The coder must pay particular attention to the description of the operation to determine if a staged procedure or a one-stage procedure was carried out. Mild defects are corrected in one stage, whereas more severe defects necessitate more procedures. For the more distal defects where the openings are closer to the normal position at the end of the penis, a new tube can be created from the surrounding skin. This technique is known as a *Thiersch-Duplay repair.* Snodgrass and MAGPI are also names of common procedures. Descriptions are similar yet very different in method and location of the hypospadias. Coders should report 54322 for the meatal advancement and glanuloplasty (MAGPI) procedure for distal hypospadias.

In less serious cases, in which the hypospadias meatus is in the zone of the glans, a MAGPI procedure may be selected to reposition the meatus near the glans without creating a new urethral canal from skin. This is a one-step procedure, whereas other methods may require two or more staged operations. A vertical incision between the tip of the glans and the meatus is created. This incision is then closed transversely, advancing the meatus. A circumferential incision is made in the skin below the corona and the meatus. The glanuloplasty is then performed in two layers, making sure there is glans-to-glans approximation. Finally, the penis is circumcised and the skin closed.

The Snodgrass technique is used for proximal and distal hypospadias. A new urethral canal is created by a technique called a *tubularized incised plate (TIP) urethroplasty* (or *Snodgrass repair*), forming a vertical slit-like meatus. Of the various procedures, TIP urethroplasty most reliably creates a normal-appearing penis. This technique creates a vertical slit like a normal-appearing meatus, unlike a horizontally oriented and rounded meatus ("fish mouth") produced by the meatal-based (Mathieu and MAGPI) and onlay island flap repair techniques. In addition, the TIP urethroplasty procedure allows construction of a neourethra from the existing urethral plate without additional skin flaps. A circumferential incision is made in the skin below the corona and the meatus to deglove the penis. Incisions are made along the lateral margins of the urethral plate. The urethral plate is tubularized by a two-layer suture, running subepithelial absorbable suture, beginning at midglans level. The new meatus is large and oval.

A pedicle flap obtained from dorsal prepuce and shaft skin is button-holed and transposed ventrally to cover the whole new urethra. Glanuloplasty begins with approximation of the lateral incisions made along the glans, creating wings at the corona. The new meatus is sewn to the glans at the 5 and 7 o'clock positions. Closing of skin is completed by use of subepithelial stitches.

EXAMPLE

Code 54308, *Urethroplasty for second-stage hypospadias repair (including urinary diversion); less than 3 cm.*

INTERNET RESOURCE: Visit the MedlinePlus website for more information about hypospadias and to view before and after correction illustrations. www.nlm.nih.gov/medlineplus/ency/article/003000.htm#Description

Chordee

Chordee (54300–54304, 54328–54336) is a birth defect consisting of the unnatural curving of the penile shaft downward. It is routinely present in babies with hypospadias where the urethral opening may be located on the underside or topside of the penis. Hypospadias is discussed further in the Urinary System chapter. Chordee without accompanying hypospadias occurs in about 1 in 200 males. In adulthood, chordee may cause pain with erection, because the penile shaft is filling with blood but cannot straighten. Discomfort during sexual intercourse may also result.

Surgery is the only treatment to correct chordee and is preferably performed on toddlers but may go undiagnosed until puberty or adulthood. Depending on the severity of the chordee, it may be surgically corrected in one operation. All chordee surgical techniques consist of phalloplasty, release of chordee, correction of penile torque, correction of penile angulation (if present), and circumcision.

Techniques vary, but all chordee procedures require creation of an artificial erection and a circumcising incision, reflecting the skin down to expose the shaft of the penis. This portion

> Chordee differs from penile angulation in that chordee is the downward curvature of the penis when erect, whereas penile angulation is more severe where the curve may occur laterally, ventrally, or dorsally. The CPT code for penile angulation correction is 54360.

of the procedure is referred to as penile "degloving." From here, techniques vary and are influenced by whether or not hypospadias is present. The elastic corpus spongiosum containing the urethra is mobilized by resecting tissue in the dartos and Buck's fascia layers. Some techniques involve mobilizing the dorsal bundle of vessels and nerves and removing ellipses of tunica albuginea to even out the lengths of the ventral and dorsal aspects of the corpora cavernosa.

INTERNET RESOURCE: Watch a single-stage chordee repair in a male with torsion.
www.youtube.com/watch?v=kPvNTv56j8Y

Viral Infections

A number of lesions can develop on the penis (and/or anogenital area). The most common ones are condyloma acuminata, herpetic vesicles, and molluscum contagiosum. Condylomas are caused by the HPV virus. Molluscum contagiosum appears as multiple, small, dome-shaped papules, often with a central depression or plug. Freezing or cautery is typically performed. Electrodesiccation can also be performed by using a small needle that is connected to an electrical source to destroy the growth. Some warts are more amenable to destruction by laser.

Codes are described as simple or extensive. There are no quantity qualifiers in these code descriptions, making the choice between simple and complex somewhat subjective. The code descriptor says "lesion(s)." The extensive code can be assigned if one or more of the following applies:

- If there were more than just a few lesions
- If more time was taken than usual
- If the lesions were large
- If different methods of destruction were used
- If the warts were on different parts of the penis and not localized in one area

As a rule, when assigning destruction of lesions on male or female genitals, assign a code from the M/F Genital section and not the Integumentary section.

> **■ CASE SCENARIO**
> A patient has six genital warts. Three were removed by cryosurgery, and the other three were electrodesiccated. Code 54065 is assigned because of the number of warts and the two different methods used.

Peyronie's Disease

Peyronie's disease is a painful condition of the penis in which the corpora cavernosa (see Fig. 23.1) becomes hardened with scar tissue that causes painful erections and significant curvature of the penis. A man's penis may actually become shortened and the pain significant. Causes are not entirely understood, but researchers believe it may be caused by ruptures in small blood vessels inside the penile shaft from injury. The corpus cavernosum and the tunica albuginea are spongy and flexible and expand during erection. If a segment of this chamber becomes injured or damaged, cells and tissue become trapped at the site and scar tissue forms. Surgery is indicated in severe cases where the male is unable to obtain and sustain erection or when intercourse is too painful. Treatment consists of either injecting the area with an antisclerosing medication to break up the scar tissue or plaque (54200) or surgically incising the affected area and excising the scar tissue or plaque (54205, 54110–54112). Extensive excisions requiring skin graft closure are reported with 54111–54112. According to *CPT Assistant*, if a graft is obtained from a separate site through a separate incision, a second code for procurement (obtaining or harvesting) of the graft is reported in addition to 54111, but not specified as such with 54112. Grafts may be procured from multiple sources (e.g., fascia, tunic of testis, and cadaver sources). In this case, an additional code from the Musculoskeletal System section and not the Integumentary System section of CPT is assigned. For example, code 20920 may be reported for procuring a fascia graft, or code 20926 for the tunic of testis. Unfortunately, the CPT manual does not direct the coder to assign a second code, and this will oftentimes be omitted.

Testes

The following are common diseases and conditions involving the testicles (testes).

Undescended Testicle

The testicles develop inside the abdomen and usually move down into the scrotum before birth. Sometimes, this does not occur. Undescended testicle is a congenital condition in which the testicle does not descend into the scrotum but instead remains in the pelvis. Most undescended testes are associated with a hernia that must be repaired. According to medical research, 3% to 4% of full-term male births exhibit this condition. However, in most cases, the testicles descend by the child's first birthday. An undescended testicle that remains outside the scrotum throughout childhood can result in abnormal testicular development with an increased risk of the undescended testicle developing cancer regardless of whether or not they are brought down into the scrotum. A surgical procedure called an *orchiopexy* (codes 54640–54650, 54692) is performed to pull the testicle down into the scrotum and permanently secure it.

If the testicle is located high in the inguinal canal or abdomen, the surgeon may perform an exploratory procedure of the inguinal canal (54550) or of the abdomen (54560). These are exploratory procedures only and involve no excision. If the testis is located and deemed viable, the surgeon may attempt to pull the testis down into the intended anatomical destination—the scrotum. If this orchiopexy is performed, the exploration codes are an inherent component of the therapeutic surgery and not separately reported. If the testis is known to be located high up in the canal or abdomen, the laparoscopic orchiopexy approach is indicated.

Read the operative report closely and pay close attention to the surgical approach. Various techniques and approaches are used with this procedure. Orchiopexy code descriptors vary by approach (inguinal, abdominal, laparoscopic) and by whether a hernia repair is also performed.

Torsion

Within the scrotum, the testicles are secured at one end by the spermatic cord. Sometimes, this cord gets twisted, cutting off the testicle's blood supply. Torsion, twisting of the spermatic cord within the testicle, is considered a urological emergency. A patient experiencing torsion must seek medical attention within the first 6 to 8 hours of pain to preserve the testicle. If a patient delays treatment too long, the testis may become permanently damaged and require removal. This disorder, which occurs most often in young males between the ages of 12 and 18, can result from an injury to the testicles or from strenuous activity. It also can occur for no apparent reason. One out of every 4,000 males under the age of 25 will experience this painful condition.

Surgical treatment is required to correct the torsion where the testicle must be tacked in place within the scrotum (54600–54620). The surgeon makes an incision in the affected testis to view the twisted spermatic cord. The spermatic cord is untwisted, and if the testis is viable, the surgeon then "tacks" or "anchors" the testis to the scrotum with sutures. The surgeon may prophylactically anchor the testis in the contralateral testis to prevent torsion on that side. When reporting 54600, *Reduction of torsion of testis, surgical, with or without fixation of contralateral testis,* report the appropriate anatomical modifier, –LT or –RT, for the side treated. Do not report 54620 (*Fixation of contralateral testis*) with 54600, because it is an inherent part of that procedure.

> ● If the surgeon performs fixation of a contralateral testis during reduction of torsion, *do not* append modifier –50 unless both testes were twisted.

> **INTERNET RESOURCE: Visit BroadcastMed and view the urological procedures.**
> **http://uro.broadcastmed.com**

Testicular Trauma

The testes, located within the scrotum, hang outside of the body and do not have the protection of muscles and bones. The testes may be injured during contact sports or in an assault where they may be hit, kicked, or crushed. Trauma causes severe pain, bruising, and/or swelling. Most often because of the spongy serous medium of the tunica albuginea and the many lobules, the testes can absorb the shock without serious damage. Testicular rupture occurs rarely when the testis receives a direct blow such as a kick or is squeezed against the hard surface of the pelvis from a crush injury. This injury can cause blood to leak into the scrotum. In severe cases, surgery to repair the rupture may be necessary. Surgery may involve simply draining a hematoma (54700) or suture repair of the tunica vaginalis or scrotum (54670).

Testicular Cancer Requiring Orchiectomy

Testicular cancer accounts for 1% of all cancers in men in the United States between the ages of 15 and 39. The exact causes of testicular cancer are not known, but there are certain risk factors for the disease, such as age, race, family history, and undescended testis.

Testicular cancer is highly treatable and usually curable. Surgery is the most common treatment for testicular cancer. Surgical treatment involves removing the cancerous testicle. Lymph nodes may also be removed from the immediate area. Orchiectomy is the surgical removal of a cancerous or damaged testicle. Radiation therapy and/or chemotherapy typically follow. At times, prophylactic removal of a testicle is required because of cancer of other parts of the male reproductive system (prostate). For noncancerous testicular conditions, sometimes only a partial orchiectomy (54522) is required.

The testis may be accessed by making an incision in the scrotum or inguinal region. For the scrotal approach, an incision is made in the side of the scrotum and the spermatic cord is identified and isolated. The cord is then clamped, cut, and sutured. The testis is then removed. The patient may elect to have a testis prosthesis inserted at the time of the orchiectomy, at a later interval, or never. Report 54520 if the testis is removed via scrotal or inguinal approach, with or without prosthesis insertion. Radical orchiectomy codes (54530–54535) are reported if the testis is removed en bloc, meaning the entire contents of half of the scrotum.

**INTERNET RESOURCE: Visit
www.urologymatch.com Search for "Radical orchiectomy"
to read the step-by-step procedure and view images of a radical orchiectomy.**

Hydrocele

Hydrocele is fluid collection in the scrotum around the testicle. There are three types of hydroceles: communicating, noncommunicating, and cord hydroceles. Hydroceles typically are present at birth or in the early years of life. Late-onset hydroceles in adulthood may result acutely from local injury, infections, and radiotherapy. Hydrocele can adversely affect fertility. Hydrocele must be treated either by aspiration of the fluid or by surgical correction. The surgeon makes an incision in the scrotum or inguinal area. The hydrocele sac is dissected free from any attachments and then the sac is opened and partially excised, leaving only remnant tissue.

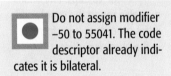 **Do not assign modifier –50 to 55041. The code descriptor already indicates it is bilateral.**

The coder must determine if the procedure was unilateral or bilateral. If the hydrocele is excised at the same time that an initial hernia repair is done, the coder will assign a code from the Digestive System section and should take into consideration the patient's age, because age influences code assignment. Codes are broken into three age categories—under 6 months, age 6 months to under 5 years, and age 5 years and older. If the patient is under the age of 5 years, hydrocelectomy is not separately reportable, because it is considered included in the hernia repair. See codes 49491–49501.

Spermatocele

Spermatoceles are most often found in men between the ages of 40 and 60 years. A spermatocele is a cystic accumulation of fluid that usually contains dead sperm arising from the epididymis. It is a common benign finding on routine physical examination and is usually smaller than 2 to 3 cm. Less commonly, these enlarge to several centimeters and cause significant discomfort or scrotal distortion requiring surgical intervention. The physician may use a light to shine through the testicle to determine if the cyst is fluid filled. Ultrasound may also be performed to confirm the diagnosis. The cyst can be drained and injected with sclerotherapy agents to help prevent recurring cysts. If surgery is prompted, the cyst is excised by making an incision into the scrotum and separating the cyst from the testicle and epididymis.

Varicocele

A varicocele is a mass of varicose veins that develop in the spermatic cord, usually during puberty. In 85% of cases, this develops in the left testicle. The circulation of blood to the testis is impaired;

therefore, the blood does not cool as it does normally. The temperature in the testis then rises, which impedes sperm production. If a varicocele suddenly develops in an older man, there may be a tumor blocking the spermatic vein. Varicoceles can be treated via the scrotum or an abdominal approach. Code 55540 is assigned if a hernia repair is also performed. The surgical approach and procedure are much like that for a hydrocele but with the varicose vein ligated and dissected. Code 55550 is assigned if the procedure is carried out laparoscopically.

Epididymitis

Epididymitis is inflammation of the epididymis and is often caused by the sexually transmitted disease chlamydia. Symptoms of epididymitis include scrotal pain and swelling. In severe cases, the infection can spread to the adjacent testicle, causing fever and abscess. Treatment for epididymitis includes antibiotics and anti-inflammatory medicines. Biopsy of the epididymis (54800, 10021–10022) may be necessary to determine the specific infectious process. For severe infection and scarring, local excision of the epididymis may be required (54830) or complete removal of the structure (54860–54861).

Sterilization

Sterilization is a medical term used to describe permanent birth control status, better known as *vasectomy* in males. Once an individual has elected to become surgically "sterilized," he or she is no longer capable of procreation. According to the National Institutes of Health, the number of men who undergo a vasectomy each year in the United States is approximately 500,000. A urologist performs a vasectomy on an outpatient basis, frequently in the office setting. A traditional vasectomy requires that the vas deferens be cut to permanently sterilize the male by interrupting the passage of sperm. The scrotum is numbed with one or more injections of local anesthetic (Lidocaine), and a small incision is made. The vas deferens is then pulled out slightly through the incision and is cut in two places. A segment is removed and the remaining ends are tied off. Another technique is called a "no-scalpel vasectomy" that uses a clip to hold the vas deferens while the physician uses a special forceps to puncture the scrotum and stretch the skin. The rest of the remaining procedure is virtually the same, with the exception that no sutures are required to close the skin.

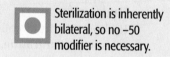 Sterilization is inherently bilateral, so no –50 modifier is necessary.

Vasclip®

The Vasclip works very much like the Hulka clips used in female "tube tying." It is an alternative to traditional vasectomy and does not involve cutting the vas deferens. A small plastic device is clamped around the vas deferens to prevent sperm from entering the semen.

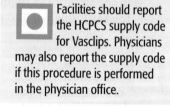 Facilities should report the HCPCS supply code for Vasclips. Physicians may also report the supply code if this procedure is performed in the physician office.

> INTERNET RESOURCE: Visit the Vasclip website to see what the device looks like and read more about this procedure. http://vasweb.com/vasclip.html

Vasectomy Reversal

Approximately 10% of all men who undergo a vasectomy change their mind and want to be able to procreate again. The vasectomy reversal is considered a self-pay situation because insurance carriers will not cover this elective service. According to statistics, if the vasectomy reversal is performed less than 3 years after the vasectomy, about 97% of men will have success. For every 5 years (give or take) post-vasectomy, the success rate declines, reaching 70% after 15 years. A vasovasostomy or vasovasorrhaphy is performed under general anesthesia to reconnect the vas deferens (55400). These are very complex microsurgical procedures requiring an assistant surgeon and can take up to 3 hours to perform. This code is inherently bilateral, so no –50 modifier is necessary. A second code for the microscope is assigned (69990).

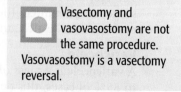 Vasectomy and vasovasostomy are not the same procedure. Vasovasostomy is a vasectomy reversal.

> INTERNET RESOURCE: Visit www.circlist.com/glossarymale/m-glossary.html for a comprehensive list of male anatomy terms and conditions with layman's explanations and illustrations.

Assign codes to the following procedures. Include any necessary modifiers. In some cases, more than one code is required.

1. Spermatocele excision _____

2. Simple electrodesiccation of four lesions on penis _____

3. Bilateral vasectomy _____

4. Incision and drainage (I&D), abscess of epididymis _____

5. Removal of foreign body, scrotum _____

6. Patient presents with symptoms of deformity of his penis and painful erection. The physician diagnosed Peyronie's disease and performed an injection and then excision of penile plaque.

   _____

7. A couple is trying to conceive, and they decide to have a testicular biopsy to extract sperm from the tubules of the epididymis to be artificially inseminated into the wife. The epididymis is isolated through a 0.5-inch incision made in the scrotal skin. An operating microscope is used to open a dilated tubule, and the fluid is collected. All of the sperm-containing fluid is collected and sent to the lab for processing. _____

8. A 2-year-old boy has had a hydrocele that seems to come and go. The patient's mother requests a hydrocelectomy. A small incision is made in the skin fold of the groin. The hydrocele "sac" is identified. The surgeon empties the fluid from the sac. The sac is removed.

   _____

9. A 39-year-old patient noticed a lump in his right testicle. The surgeon recommended removal, because 95% of testicular masses are malignant. A 4-inch incision was made along the "bikini line" through the lower abdomen on the right side. The surgeon pushed the testicle up through the pelvic region and removed it. _____

Prostate

Many surgical procedures of the prostate are performed endoscopically by placing the endoscope into the urethra to access the prostate. Prostate resection is also performed laparoscopically with robotic assistance (55866) and in some cases via the standard open laparotomy approach (55840). Prostate procedures are also performed transperineally (55873, 55874, 55875) or transabdominally (55876). Be sure to check NCCI and read the parenthetical notes for instructions on separately coding ultrasound, cystoscopy, or radioelement placement.

As mentioned previously, urologists are surgeons with specialized training in performing transurethral procedures and in treating prostate disease via procedures such as prostatectomy. For this reason, prostate procedures are located in both the Urinary System and Male Genital System sections of CPT. Prostate procedures are discussed in detail in this chapter for the purposes of keeping content centralized in one chapter.

Prostate Hypertrophy

Prostate enlargement is referred to as *benign prostatic hypertrophy (BPH)*, or *hyperplasia*. Enlargement of the prostate occurs in 30% of men between the ages of 50 and 60 years. The male urethra runs through the prostate gland and penis; therefore, it is much longer than the female urethra. When the prostate gland swells, it constricts the urethra, and the flow of urine is restricted. BPH is diagnosed using three methods: (1) PSA test, (2) DRE, and (3) ultrasound. PSA is a protein produced by the prostate gland. The PSA test measures the blood level of the antigen. The higher the value, the more likely a man has prostate cancer. Biopsies (55700–55706) are done to confirm the diagnosis. Code 55700 is for needle or punch biopsy, and 55705 is reported for incisional biopsy. It is not uncommon for a biopsy to be performed via a cystoscopic approach. If image guidance is used, also assign one of the following radiology codes with the appropriate modifier: 76942, 77002, 77012, 77021.

Dysplasia

Dysplasia of the prostate, or prostatic intraepithelial neoplasia (PIN), is a premalignant condition diagnosed by biopsy. PIN is categorized pathologically similarly to the cervical Pap smear. PIN III is synonymous for carcinoma in situ of the prostate. Prostatectomy can be performed via several methods and varies in the amount of tissue excised. Most commonly, if the prostate requires removal, it is done endoscopically. There are several codes for an "open" prostatectomy specified by approach 55801–55845. Code descriptors do not describe the approach employed, but it is understood that these are performed via an open approach. Codes are differentiated by whether total or subtotal removal was carried out. The perineal method requires an incision in the perineum. The suprapubic method requires an incision in the lower abdomen just above the pubic area. The retropubic approach also utilizes an incision above the pubic area and removes the entire prostate, seminal vesicles, and sections of the vas deferens. Prostatectomy can also be done laparoscopically (55866). Read the documentation carefully to determine the approach applied. Code 55866 includes robotic assistance when performed so there is no need to additionally assign HCPCS code S2900 (*Surgical techniques requiring use of robotic surgical system*).

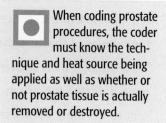 When coding prostate procedures, the coder must know the technique and heat source being applied as well as whether or not prostate tissue is actually removed or destroyed.

Transurethral Resection of the Prostate

Code 52601, *Transurethral electrosurgical resection of prostate, including control of postoperative bleeding, complete,* describes prostate resection via the transurethral approach whereby an electrosurgical device, such as a wire loop or VaporTrode, is inserted into the urethra from the penis. The illustration under this code in the *CPT Professional Edition* demonstrates this procedure. This code does not include the use of a laser. If a laser is used to resect the prostate, another code should be used. If the procedure involves the use of transurethral waterjet ablation, report code 0421T. CPT instructs the coder to report 52601 for first and second-stage partial prostate resections with a –58 modifier on the second procedure. Staged transurethral resection of the prostate (TURP) is a planned approach where work is done in two separate sessions, one side of the prostate at a time. Because it is planned, the –58 modifier is applicable if the second procedure is performed during the global period of the first procedure.

Visual Laser Ablation of the Prostate

A similar procedure, visual laser ablation of the prostate (VLAP), can also be performed. In a VLAP procedure, the endoscope is passed through the urethra and a laser is used to vaporize or destroy the prostate. Code 52647, *Laser coagulation of prostate, including control of postoperative bleeding, complete,* covers the procedure that utilizes laser energy to heat and coagulate the prostate tissue. For weeks following the procedure, prostate tissue will slough off. A probe is placed outside the prostate for destruction.

■ **CASE SCENARIO**
A 63-year-old male has BPH and had been treated with medications with little improvement of his urine flow. He now has severely decreased flow secondary to BPH. A cystoscope is inserted and a laser fiber is placed into the prostatic fossa where laser energy is administered for 90 seconds to all four quadrants and the median lobe of the prostate.

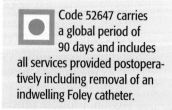 Code 52647 carries a global period of 90 days and includes all services provided postoperatively including removal of an indwelling Foley catheter.

Laser Vaporization

Laser vaporization is similar to laser ablation (described earlier); however, the laser in this procedure is used to vaporize the tissue by placing the laser contact tip or high-power density probe into the prostate. The most significant difference is the amount of electrical current used and the type of contact made with the instrument.

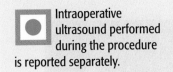
Intraoperative ultrasound performed during the procedure is reported separately.

EXAMPLE

A cystoscope is inserted and a laser is passed through the scope into the prostate. Laser energy is administered for vaporization.

Transurethral Microwave Therapy

The technique for transurethral microwave therapy (TUMT) (53850), is much the same as the other prostate procedures but instead of using a laser to ablate or vaporize the prostate tissue, microwave thermotherapy is administered by using a Prostatron or Targis device. Some of the newer techniques revolve around a catheter that cools the lining of the prostate while the prostate tissue deep inside is heated; thus, this procedure is comparable to inducing hyperthermia.

Radio-Frequency Thermotherapy

Instead of using laser or microwave energy, this procedure uses radio-frequency to heat and destroy tissue. The catheter is inserted into the urethra and needles are placed in the prostate. This procedure is often referred to as "TUNA" for transurethral needle ablation. Code 53852, *Transurethral destruction of prostate tissue; by radiofrequency thermotherapy,* is assigned.

Water-Induced Thermotherapy

Water-induced thermotherapy (WIT) consists of an extracorporeal heat source and a closed-loop catheter system. It is used to treat urinary outflow obstruction secondary to BPH. Water is continuously circulated through the catheter to a treatment balloon, which conducts thermal energy to targeted prostatic tissue. WIT treatment is performed using only topical urethral anesthetic and takes about 45 minutes to complete. This type of therapy has no side effects, is inexpensive, and is commonly performed in physician offices. Code 55899, *Unlisted procedure, male genital system,* is assigned, because no code is available that describes this technique.

CHECKPOINT 23.2

Assign codes to the following procedures. Include any necessary modifiers.

1. Completion (second stage) of transurethral electrosurgical prostate resection during global period of first stage of resection _____

2. Patient had suffered from frequent urination, pressure, and pain in the bladder. Upon examination, the physician found a prostate mass. Due to the size and specific location of the mass, an incisional biopsy of the prostate was performed to determine if the mass was benign or malignant.

   _____

3. A 70-year-old patient was seen for chronic urinary urgency. The urologist's examination revealed an enlarged prostate that was most likely the cause of the problem. Testing determined that the patient did not have prostate cancer, and drug therapy was prescribed initially. The patient's problem was not alleviated and surgery was recommended. The urologist performed an electrosurgical resection of the prostate using a transurethral approach and internal urethrotomy.

   _____

4. Discontinued contact laser vaporization of the prostate _____

5. Incisional biopsy of testis followed by radical orchiectomy for tumor, inguinal approach

   _____

6. Radical perineal prostatectomy _____

Chapter Summary

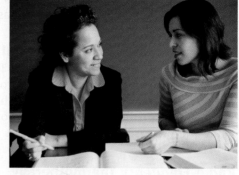

1. Being able to identify anatomical structures of the male genital system and their function while reading operative reports is mandatory to capture independent procedures and accurately assign CPT codes. The interaction of the male genital system structures, such as the correlation between chordee and hypospadias and the vasectomy, prostate, circumcision, and orchiectomy procedures, requires precision in terminology.

2. Adult circumcision uses one of three techniques: guided forceps, dorsal slit, or sleeve resection. Infant/child circumcision uses the dorsal or lateral slit, a clamp or other device, or surgical excision.

3. Hypospadias surgical correction techniques vary depending on how far distal the defect is. The procedure can be staged or carried out in one stage. Mild defects are corrected in one stage, whereas more severe defects necessitate more procedures. For the more distal defects where the openings are closer to the normal position at the end of the penis, a new tube can be created from the surrounding skin. This technique is known as a *Thiersch-Duplay repair*. Snodgrass technique is used for proximal and distal hypospadias. A new urethral canal is created using TIP urethroplasty, which forms a vertical, slit-like meatus.

4. Prostatectomy can be performed by transurethral resection whether done in one or more stages, VLAP, laser vaporization, TUMT, radio-frequency thermotherapy, or surgical removal.

Review Questions

Matching

Match the key terms with their definitions.

A. orchiectomy
B. PSA
C. hydrocele
D. spermatocele
E. BPH

F. PIN
G. undescended testicle
H. TUNA
I. torsion
J. TUMT

1. _____ Twisting of the spermatic cord

2. _____ Uses microwave thermotherapy to destroy prostate tissue

3. _____ Benign prostatic hyperplasia

4. _____ Uses radio-frequency to destroy prostate tissue

5. _____ Prostate-specific antigen

6. _____ Dysplasia of prostate

7. _____ Congenital condition where the testis is not in the correct anatomical location

8. _____ Surgical removal of part of or the entire testis

9. _____ Fluid collection in the scrotum around the testicle

10. _____ Cystic accumulation of fluid that usually contains dead sperm arising from the epididymis

True or False

Decide whether each statement is true or false.

1. __T__ Simple left orchiectomy with insertion of prosthesis using scrotal approach is coded as 54520–LT.

2. __T__ The prostate gland completely encircles the male urethra.

3. __F__ Circumcision involves removal of the glans penis.

4. _____ A retropubic radical prostatectomy is coded as 55831.

5. __T__ Transurethral microwave treatment performed in the office is assigned code 53850.

6. __T__ Dorsal slit is the simplest circumcision technique.

7. __F__ Torsion is the twisting of the spermatic cord.

8. __F__ Chordee is the unnatural curvature of the penis upward.

9. __F__ Orchiopexy is the repair of testicular rupture.

10. __F__ Peyronie's disease is a hereditary disease of the penis.

Multiple Choice

Select the letter that best completes the statement or answers the question.

1. A 15-year-old male with inadequate circumcision undergoes surgical circumcision. Which code should be reported?
   A. 54150
   B. 54160
   C. 54162
   D. 54163

2. The patient has a bilateral vasovasostomy reversal with operating microscope. Which code(s) should be reported?
   A. 55400–50, 69990–51
   B. 55400–50, 69990
   C. 55400, 69990
   D. 55400

3. A sexually active male patient presents with numerous condyloma on the base and shaft of the penis varying in size and shape. Laser destruction of the numerous lesions was performed under general anesthesia. Which code(s) should be reported?
   A. 54057
   B. 54065
   C. 17000, 17003
   D. 54110

4. The patient is seen for transrectal ultrasonic guided prostate biopsy. Two biopsies were taken from each side. Which code should be reported?
   A. 55700×4
   B. 55705
   C. 52450
   D. 55700

5. The _____ is a tunnel-like structure where the nerves and vessels travel from the abdomen to the scrotum.
   A. Spermatic cord
   B. Epididymis
   C. Tunica vaginalis
   D. Seminal vesicle

6. A physician injected the penis on the dorsal side to break up scarring that was causing painful erection. Which code should be reported?
   A. 54235
   B. 54231
   C. 54230
   D. 54200

7. A urologist performs three needle biopsies of the prostate gland using ultrasonic guidance in the hospital. Which code(s) should be reported?
   A. 55700×3
   B. 55700×3, 76942
   C. 55700, 76942-26
   D. 55700, 76942-51

8. A urologist performs a meatotomy, urethral dilation, and TURP on a male patient with urinary retention, urethral stenosis, and vesical neck stenosis. Which code(s) should be reported?
   A. 52500, 53605-51
   B. 52601, 52500-51
   C. 52500, 52601
   D. 52601

9. A physician dilates the urethra, which passes through the prostate, using a urethral dilator under general anesthesia. Which code should be reported?
   A. 53600
   B. 53660
   C. 53605
   D. 52344

10. The patient was born with distal hypospadias and has had two prior surgeries to correct the abnormality. The patient now presents with urethral fistula and urethral diverticulum, both of which are complications of his previous hypospadias condition. During the repair procedure, the urethra was explored and found to be dilated and required tapering. A long urethral plate was ready for tubularization. The proximal urethral plate was at the urethra and was tapered proximal to the fistula. Unroofing the distal urethra and incision on either side of the urethra distally formed the distal urethral plate. Excess shaft skin was trimmed off in order to have sufficient skin to wrap around the penis. Which code(s) should be reported?
    A. 54344
    B. 54304-80
    C. 54344-62
    D. 54304-50

CHAPTER 24

CPT: Female Genital System and Maternity Care and Delivery

CHAPTER OUTLINE

Female Anatomy

Organization

Preventive Exam

Common Problems of the Female Genital System and Associated Therapies

Maternity Care and Delivery

Common Obstetrical Conditions and Procedures

Infertility

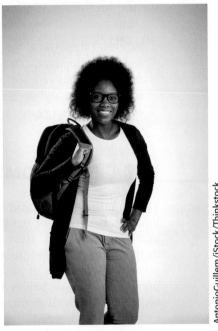

LEARNING OUTCOMES

After studying this chapter, you should be able to:

1. Differentiate among laparoscopic, hysteroscopic, colposcopic, and open surgical procedures.
2. Identify the two major subsections of the female genital system section of CPT.
3. List the procedures that are provided as part of an annual examination.
4. Describe the most common diseases and disorders of the female genital system.
5. Select the appropriate hysterectomy procedure code based on seven criteria.
6. Describe the various surgical methods for repairing vaginal prolapse.
7. Describe the various surgical techniques for vaginal hernias.
8. List services included in the maternity and delivery global package.
9. Differentiate between elective and therapeutic abortions and the various techniques.
10. Describe assisted reproductive technology treatments for infertility.

This chapter focuses on the procedural coding and terminology for surgical cases of the female genital and reproductive systems. Gynecology is classified as a surgical subspecialty that concentrates on the study of diseases of the female reproductive organs, including the breasts. Gynecology encompasses surgical and nonsurgical expertise. Endoscopic procedures are commonly performed to diagnose conditions in the pelvis and provide treatment. Urologists and gynecologists routinely assist each other in complex gynecology (GYN) procedures.

AntonioGuillem/iStock/Thinkstock

The *genitourinary system* is a collective term used to describe all of the reproductive organs and the organs responsible for creating and excreting urine. These organs and anatomical structures are grouped together because of their proximity to each other. Gynecologists specialize in the medical and surgical treatment and diagnosis of female reproductive disorders to include preventive services, family planning, detection of sexually transmitted infections (STIs), and treatment of premenstrual and postmenopausal conditions. Obstetricians are gynecologists who monitor and treat pregnant women from the onset of conception through delivery. An obstetrician/gynecologist (OB/GYN) provides medical and surgical care directed to the female reproductive system as well as prenatal care, delivery, and postpartum services. OB/GYNs can serve as primary care physicians and they often serve as consultants to other physicians. OB/GYNs may choose to specialize in the following areas:

- Adolescent gynecology
- Behavioral conditions associated with premenstrual syndrome (PMS) and hormone irregularity
- Gynecological oncology (cancer treatment of reproductive organs only)
- Endocrinology
- Infertility
- Operative gynecology
- Pregnancy and delivery
- Preventive health
- Urinary tract disorders

Coders should be aware that many procedures can be performed in more than one way. The abdomen can be surgically examined and treated by several approaches: via laparotomy with an open incision, percutaneously with a smaller incision than for a laparotomy, endoscopically via the urethra or vagina, or laparoscopically. Correct code assignment requires determining the approach that was documented.

INTERNET RESOURCE: The American Congress of Obstetricians and Gynecologists (ACOG) is a specialty organization that serves as an authoritative body for OB/GYN practitioners. They publish several clinical and practice management resources along with information geared toward patient education. www.acog.org

FEMALE ANATOMY

The female anatomy and reproduction system consists of the following: uterus, ovaries, fallopian tubes (ostia or oviducts), vagina, vulva, clitoris, vestibule (urethral meatus, Bartholin's and Skene's glands), and the vaginal orifice (Fig. 24.1). All of the internal structures are located in the pelvis. Ovaries are almond shaped and about 1 inch wide and 1 inch tall. The ovaries' physiological role is to produce eggs and hormones that influence menstruation and maintain pregnancy. Female babies are born with two ovaries; each ovary contains about 250,000 eggs at birth. Every month during ovulation, an ovary produces and releases an egg, which is collected by the fimbria located at the open end of the fallopian tube. The ovaries alternate each month, taking turns releasing an egg. The egg then travels through the fallopian tube to the uterus. Fertilization of an egg by a sperm occurs within the fallopian tube.

The uterus is about the size of a fist and is shaped like an upside-down pear. It is suspended in the pelvis by supporting structures—broad ligament, transverse cervical ligament, and suspensory ligaments (uterosacral ligament, round ligament, and cardinal ligament). These structures stabilize the uterus and pelvic wall. The uterus consists of two main areas: the body of the uterus (corpus) and the cervix. The top round portion of the uterus is referred to as the *fundus*. The cervix is the lower portion of the uterus and extends into the upper end of the vagina. Each month, prior to the menstrual cycle, the lining of the uterus (endometrium) prepares to accept a fertilized egg. The hormone estrogen is responsible for building up the endometrium, and progesterone increases after ovulation to assist in keeping the endometrium lining thick. If no egg is fertilized, progesterone and estrogen levels drop, causing the uterine lining to break down and shed. This is when menstrual bleeding (the "period") occurs.

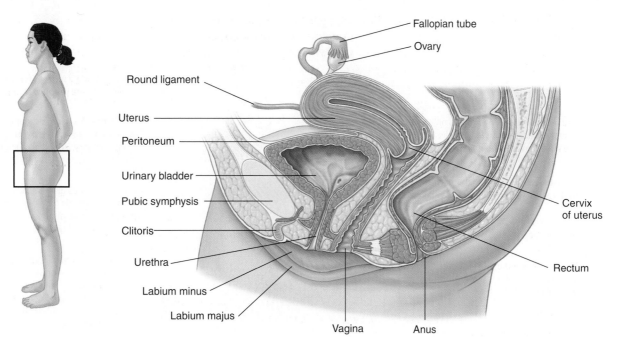

Figure 24.1 The female reproductive system.

> ● It is very important for the coder to be able to recognize the differences between vulva, labia, and vagina for correct code assignment.

The cervical canal, or birth canal, is the passage through the center of the cervix that connects the vagina to the uterus. The transformation zone, also referred to as the *squamocolumnar junction*, is an area of the cervix where columnar epithelium in the cervical canal changes into squamous epithelium. This zone is an area of constant cellular change and the most common place on the cervix for abnormal cells to develop. These abnormal cells can be detected with a Papanicolaou (Pap) test (or smear).

The location of the transformation zone varies based on the woman's age. This zone is located on the outer surface of the cervix in young women and makes them more prone to infection than adult women in whom it is located higher in the cervical canal. The opening of the cervical canal is called the *cervical os*. The vagina is a 5-inch tube that serves as the passageway for birthing babies. This canal is in a collapsed position except for during childbirth or intercourse. The vagina leads from the cervix to the outside body. The entrance to the vagina from the outside is referred to as the *introitus*.

The external sex organs, also referred to as the *vulva* (Fig. 24.2), consist of the labia minora, labia majora, clitoris, and vestibule. The vulva is the area that surrounds the opening of the vagina. The labia are thick skinfolds on both sides of the vaginal orifice. The labia minora are thinner skinfolds immediately internal to the labia majora. The vestibule is the space located between the labia majora and the labia minora. Within this vestibule is the urethral opening and vaginal orifice. Bartholin's glands are located on each side of the vaginal orifice. These glands are also called the *greater vestibular glands*. The perineum is the area between the anus and the vulva.

INTERNET RESOURCE: View more detailed illustrations and review female genital physiology at www.fastbleep.com/wiki/article/495

ORGANIZATION

The female genital/reproductive system is much more complex than the male counterpart. Codes in the female genital system of CPT describe minor surgical services performed in the physician office as well as major hospital inpatient and outpatient procedures. It is not unusual for a GYN physician to diagnose and treat urinary problems because of the proximity of the body systems and the anatomical and physiological impacts as such.

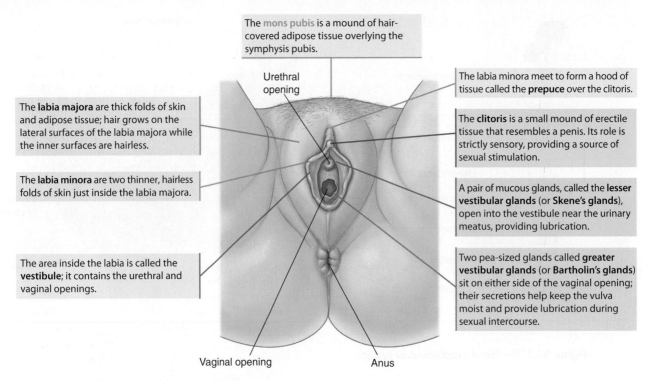

The **mons pubis** is a mound of hair-covered adipose tissue overlying the symphysis pubis.

Urethral opening

The **labia majora** are thick folds of skin and adipose tissue; hair grows on the lateral surfaces of the labia majora while the inner surfaces are hairless.

The **labia minora** are two thinner, hairless folds of skin just inside the labia majora.

The area inside the labia is called the **vestibule**; it contains the urethral and vaginal openings.

The labia minora meet to form a hood of tissue called the **prepuce** over the clitoris.

The **clitoris** is a small mound of erectile tissue that resembles a penis. Its role is strictly sensory, providing a source of sexual stimulation.

A pair of mucous glands, called the **lesser vestibular glands** (or **Skene's glands**), open into the vestibule near the urinary meatus, providing lubrication.

Two pea-sized glands called **greater vestibular glands** (or **Bartholin's glands**) sit on either side of the vaginal opening; their secretions help keep the vulva moist and provide lubrication during sexual intercourse.

Vaginal opening

Anus

Figure 24.2 The female external genitalia.

Many of the procedures performed on the female abdomen can be done via laparoscope, a hysteroscope, or a colposcope, instead of the traditional open method. Hysteroscopy involves the use of a long, lighted tube (endoscope) with an eyepiece on one end and a magnifying lens on the other inserted through the vagina and into the uterus to examine and magnify the cervix and interior of the uterus. It is used as an approach for diagnostic and therapeutic examinations. Colposcopy involves using a low-power microscope to magnify the surface of the vagina, vulva, and cervix.

Females may undergo a laparoscopic and a hysteroscopic procedure during the same operative session. Both would be coded because they are distinctly different procedures using different "scopes" and have different "base" endoscopy codes. Pay close attention to the approach in the operative note.

This CPT section is arranged by anatomical site and then by type of root procedure. The seven main headings are arranged from the outside of the body to the genital structure deepest inside the body (Box 24.1).

The subheadings follow the same outline as the other surgery chapters with the following subheads: Incision, Destruction, Excision, Introduction, Repair, Manipulation, Endoscopy, and Laparoscopy/Hysteroscopy.

> **BOX 24.1 Female Genital System Subsections**
>
> | | |
> |---|---|
> | Vulva, Perineum, and Introitus | Oviduct/Ovary |
> | Vagina | Ovary |
> | Cervix Uteri | In Vitro Fertilization |
> | Corpus Uteri | |

The Maternity Care and Delivery section immediately follows the Female Genital System section. Services are broken into several subheadings (Box 24.2) that differentiate between antepartum, delivery, and abortion. Codes in this section also include procedures carried out on the fetus prior to delivery.

> **BOX 24.2 Maternity Care and Delivery Subsections**
>
> | | |
> |---|---|
> | Antepartum and Fetal Invasive Services | Excision |
> | Introduction | Repair |
> | Vaginal Delivery, Antepartum, and Postpartum Care | Cesarean Delivery |
> | | Delivery After Previous Cesarean Delivery |
> | Abortion | Other Procedures |

PREVENTIVE EXAM

Each year a female should undergo an annual "well-woman" examination. This preventive medicine visit includes vital signs and weight, breast examination, urine dipstick, pelvic exam, and Pap smear. For non-Medicare patients, a code from the Evaluation and Management (E/M) Preventive Medicine section is submitted. Codes from the Female Genital System section would not apply to this annual service because the exam is focused on screening for potential problems of the female anatomy and prevention and does not involve invasive studies or require surgery. If, however, the physician provides care for an illness or diagnoses a new problem significant enough to require additional work (i.e., history, exam, medical decision making), a second code from the office E/M section is also assigned with a –25 modifier. Medicare requires the use of HCPCS code G0101 (Cervical or vaginal cancer screening; pelvic and clinical breast examination) for annual pelvic examination instead of the E/M code.

> ● It is important to check the insurance benefits for patients being seen for this annual exam. Carriers frequently change coverage policies for preventive services and what is covered one year might not be covered the next.

A pelvic examination is an essential component of diagnosing gynecological conditions. It is often performed in conjunction with or prior to most GYN procedures and is not reported separately. When a pelvic examination is performed in conjunction with a GYN procedure, either as a necessary part of the procedure or as a confirmatory examination, the pelvic examination is not separately reportable. If a diagnostic pelvic examination is performed on a symptomatic patient and the determination for surgery is made, this exam is included in the E/M service at the time the decision to perform the procedure is made.

EXAMPLE

External vaginal and pelvic examination prior to hysteroscopy with dilation and curettage (D&C): The pelvic and vaginal exam is considered a component of the hysteroscopic exam, so only the hysteroscopic procedure code is reported.

Pap Smear

> ● Medicare claims for Pap smears must indicate the beneficiary's low- or high-risk status by linking the Q0091 with an ICD-10 status diagnosis code on the claim form.

Screening Pap smears are performed as part of the annual well-woman check. Medicare will only pay for one screening Pap smear every 2 years as long as the patient is of childbearing age, no test has been done in the preceding 3 years, or the patient is at high risk for developing vaginal or cervical cancer. For Medicare patients, report HCPCS code Q0091 for a routine screening Pap smear. Medicare will allow one diagnostic Pap smear every year for high-risk beneficiaries. A high-risk individual would be one with any of the following:

- Early onset of sexual activity (under 16 years of age)
- Multiple sexual partners (five or more in a lifetime)
- History of STI (including HIV infection)
- Fewer than three negative or any Pap smears within the previous 7 years
- Exposed daughters of women who took diethylstilbestrol (DES) during pregnancy

Per the Medicare manual, a diagnostic pap smear and related medically necessary services are covered under Medicare Part B when ordered by a physician under one of the following conditions:

- Previous cancer of the cervix, uterus, or vagina that has been or is presently being treated;
- Previous abnormal or suspicious Pap smear;
- Any abnormal findings of the vagina, cervix, uterus, ovaries, or adnexa;
- Any significant complaint by the patient referable to the female reproductive system; or
- Any signs or symptoms that in the physician's judgment reasonably might be related to a gynecologic disorder.

The American Cancer Society, the American Society for Colposcopy and Cervical Pathology, the American Society for Clinical Pathology, the American Congress of Obstetricians and Gynecologists, and the Society of Gynecologic Oncology (SGO) develop guidelines for routine screening of low-risk patients. These guidelines recommend that women have their first Pap test at age 21 and every 3 years after. Guidelines are specific to patient age, patient medical history, and previous Pap smear findings. Once a woman reaches 30 years of age, these societies also recommend HPV cotesting with cytology. Recommendations from these organizations are located at http://www.cdc.gov/cancer/cervical/pdf/guidelines.pdf.

Diagnostic Pap smears are reported (by the pathologist) using codes 88141–88177.

INTERNET RESOURCES:
Visit the Medicare website and search for "Preventive Services Chart" for coding and billing requirements for female screening pelvic examinations.
www.cms.gov/Medicare/Prevention

> ● Blue Cross and Blue Shield (BC/BS) and some state Medicaid carriers are requiring HCPCS codes S0610–S0612 for reporting annual GYN exams. Check the carriers in your state before submitting preventive screening codes.

COMMON PROBLEMS OF THE FEMALE GENITAL SYSTEM AND ASSOCIATED THERAPIES

Endometriosis

Endometriosis is a condition that occurs when endometrial tissue that lines the uterus is present elsewhere in the abdomen. This tissue that is displaced throughout the pelvis functions the same way it does within the uterus—it thickens, breaks down, and bleeds with each menstrual cycle—but it has no way to exit the body. The ovaries, fallopian tubes, uterosacral ligaments, sigmoid colon, pelvic peritoneum, cul-de-sac peritoneum, and the serosal surface of the uterus are common sites for these ectopic endometrial "implants." Over time, this trapped tissue binds to surrounding tissue and scar tissue or adhesions develop. Surgical treatment for woman of childbearing age involves lysing the adhesions and cauterizing (fulgurating) the endometrial implants with Bovie cautery during a laparoscopic procedure (58662). For women with extensive endometriosis, pelvic pain is severe, fertility is commonly disrupted, and hysterectomy is ultimately performed.

Ovarian Cysts

Cysts can occur on one or both ovaries. Cysts can be drained (aspirated) or excised via vaginal, abdominal, or laparoscopic approach. Cysts can resolve spontaneously; however, some require removal due to their size. Large cysts can cause the ovary to be heavier on one side and "flop" over, causing the fallopian tube to twist, resulting in severe pain. This condition is called *ovarian torsion*. Ovarian cysts are most commonly removed via the laparoscopic technique. Code 58662 is assigned for laparoscopic removal and only reported once, even if cysts are removed from both ovaries. This code lumps the ovaries in with various anatomical parts; therefore, the −50 modifier could not be appropriately applied. Code 58925 is assigned for the open technique. If cysts are removed from both ovaries, whether laparoscopically or by open surgical technique, the −50 modifier is not appended as you would expect. This also applies if the cyst(s) is drained. Code descriptors contain the language *unilateral or bilateral* or *single or multiple;* therefore, modifier −50 would not be appropriate. Cysts are often drained at the same time as other pelvic procedures. For laparoscopic drainage of ovarian cyst(s), report code 49322. Assign codes 58800–58805 for vaginal and open abdominal techniques. Take notice that these codes are designated "separate procedures" and separate procedure guidelines will apply. There are several different types of ovarian cysts, as described in the paragraphs that follow.

Corpus Luteum Cyst

This type of cyst occurs each month after an egg has been released from a follicle. The follicle becomes what is known as a *corpus luteum*. If pregnancy doesn't occur, the corpus luteum breaks down and disappears automatically. Sometimes it will fill with fluid or blood and stay on the ovary.

Dermoid Cyst

Also referred to as a *teratoma*, this type of cyst is similar to the type of cysts that appear on top of the skin and range anywhere between a few millimeters to 6 inches in diameter. They contain sebaceous material such as fat, hair, and sometimes bone.

Follicular Cyst

A follicular cyst can form when ovulation does not occur or when a mature follicle involutes instead of regressing during the second phase of the menstrual cycle. It usually forms at the time of ovulation and can grow to over 2 inches in diameter.

Chocolate Cyst

This cyst is filled with old brown blood or hemosiderin. It is insoluble tissue high in iron.

> Read the documentation carefully, because cysts can be drained, destroyed, or removed laparoscopically, vaginally, or by an open abdominal approach.

Endometrioid Cyst

This cyst occurs in women with endometriosis as the ovaries are invaded. This type of cyst affects fertility and causes severe abdominal pain in women in their reproductive years.

Hemorrhagic Cyst

Hemorrhagic cyst is the name for bleeding that occurs within a cyst.

Hydrosalpinx

Hydrosalpinx occurs when a fallopian tube becomes blocked and fills with fluid. This is caused by residual effects of a prior STI such as gonorrhea and chlamydia, excessive tissue buildup due to endometriosis, or pelvic adhesions. The tube then develops chronic salpingitis (inflammation or infection of the fallopian tube) and occludes the fimbriated end of the tube, causing infertility. The tubal infection may also involve the ovary and develop into an abscess called a *tubo-ovarian abscess*. Surgical treatment of hydrosalpinx is primarily done laparoscopically by making an incision into the tube (salpingostomy, 58673), thus reopening the sealed end. Laparoscopic salpingectomy (58661)—the complete removal of the tube—is another treatment option and provides permanent correction. Women with hydrosalpinx are at higher risk of ectopic pregnancy.

Pelvic Adhesions

Pelvic adhesions are fibrous bands of scar tissue that cause internal organs located within the pelvis to adhere or stick to each other or to the abdominal wall. Adhesions may result from pelvic infection, previous abdominal surgery, or severe cases of endometriosis. Adhesions are a common cause of pelvic or abdominal pain and infertility. Adhesions can be dense and require extensive dissection to free the internal contents, or at times to gain access to a particular anatomical area. Adhesions may be lysed, or "taken down," by using blunt dissection or electrocautery. Sometimes the adhesions are so dense that the surgeon cannot safely or adequately remove them and may have to remove all or part of the fallopian tube or ovary.

Lysis of adhesions is typically bundled into other more extensive surgical abdominal procedures—laparotomy or laparoscopy—because it is considered incidental to carrying out the more extensive procedure (a means to an end, so to speak). It can be coded and billed separately only if the adhesions were in another area of the pelvis from where the other surgery was performed. A –59 modifier is required to indicate this was a separate and distinct service. If the adhesions are located in the same area, if the surgeon states that the adhesions were extensive, if tedious dissection was required—adding significant surgeon work—or if the dissection took an extended amount of time, a –22 modifier may be appended to the procedure code to indicate that extra work was incurred over and above what is routinely performed.

Abnormal Bleeding

Dysfunctional uterine bleeding (DUB) is considered bleeding that does not occur in the 28- to 30-day cycle for premenopausal women or irregular bleeding that is too heavy, too scanty, or delayed that has not been amenable to other treatment. Many women experience menorrhagia, which is excessive bleeding during monthly menstrual cycles. Metrorrhagia is uterine bleeding at irregular intervals between the expected monthly menstrual cycles. Excessive uterine bleeding, during monthly menstrual cycles and at other irregular intervals, is called *menometrorrhagia*. If medication does not regulate bleeding, a hysteroscopy is commonly performed to examine the uterine cavity for abnormalities followed by a D&C to remove the lining of the uterus.

Hysteroscopy is used to visualize the uterine cavity. Diagnostic hysteroscopy and simple operative hysteroscopy can be carried out in an office setting. More complex surgical hysteroscopy procedures are done in an operating room setting under general anesthesia. A routine hysteroscopic procedure includes manual pelvic exam, dilation of the cervix, insertion of the scope into the uterus, diagnostic evaluation, uterine biopsies, uterine polypectomy, and D&C. In the case of abnormal bleeding, a D&C is performed to scrape or remove the lining of the uterine wall.

For some women, D&C does not resolve the abnormal bleeding. The surgeon may elect to perform an endometrial ablation to destroy the lining of the uterus to stop the bleeding. Endometrial ablation ablates or destroys cells of the endometrium using equipment such as a YAG or CO_2 laser, hot cautery, or a heated balloon (THERMACHOICE) or roller ball. The Hydro ThermAblator (HTA) system is another type of tool used to perform this service. Code assignment is based on the type of ablation and whether hysteroscopic guidance is used. If the NovaSure Impedance Controlled Endometrial Ablation system is used to perform the ablation, report 58999. If the Her Option Uterine Cryoablation Therapy System (extreme cold) is applied, report 58356. A hysterectomy may be indicated if these procedures, along with other conservative measures, fail to correct the problem.

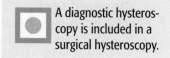
A diagnostic hysteroscopy is included in a surgical hysteroscopy.

Codes for D&C procedures are divided into two categories—obstetrical or nonobstetrical. The reason for the encounter must be known to assign a code from the appropriate category. D&C performed for postobstetrical patients who experience excessive bleeding is reported with 59160.

D&C can be performed with or without a hysteroscope. Read the operative note carefully to identify use of the hysteroscope before assigning a code. Code 58120 is assigned for nonobstetrical D&C without a scope.

Cervical Dysplasia

Cervical cancer is a sexually transmitted infection and the second leading cause of cancer death in women worldwide. More than half of all cervical cancers are caused by human papillomavirus (HPV). Cervical dysplasia is abnormal tissue development or cell growth in the cervix. Cervical dysplasia is considered to be precancerous, but not cancer. At times, the dysplasia converts to carcinoma in situ of the cervix and should be further evaluated and treated to prevent cancer from progressing. Dysplasia is identified initially by performing a Pap smear. If an abnormal Pap smear is returned, the next step is to biopsy the cervix and to determine the depth and level of dysplasia. The physician usually performs a colposcopy with biopsy in the office and sends the specimen to be examined. If for some reason the colposcopic exam and biopsy do not show why the Pap smear was abnormal, a more extensive biopsy may be suggested.

> **INTERNET RESOURCE: Visit MedlinePlus and view an illustration of the cervical punch biopsy technique.**
> **www.nlm.nih.gov/medlineplus/ency/imagepages/17032.htm**

Dysplasia is classified into three categories based on the Bethesda reporting system for Pap smears. Cervical intraepithelial neoplasia (CIN) I is mild dysplasia or abnormal growth of epithelial cells where only a few cells are abnormal. CIN II is moderate dysplasia where the abnormal cells involve about one-half of the thickness of the surface lining of the cervix. CIN III is severe and is also considered to be carcinoma in situ of the cervix. The entire thickness of cells is involved, but the abnormal cells have not yet spread below the surface of the epithelium. The progressive diagnosis would then be squamous cell carcinoma.

Treatment solely depends on the severity of the dysplasia. Laser ablation and cryotherapy are effective treatments for dysplasia; they are not suitable for invasive cancer. The term *paracervical*, meaning "around the cervix," is commonly used when describing the surface of the cervix and when referring to the administration of an anesthetic injected locally around the cervix. A paracervical block is administered locally into the cervix to numb it prior to surgical procedures such as biopsies, laser ablation, or conization. CIN I will normally resolve itself and does not require surgical intervention. CIN II is amenable to laser ablation, in which a CO_2 laser uses a tiny beam of light (LAC) to vaporize the abnormal tissue of the cervix (code 57513), or cold knife conization (CKC)—code 57520. Conization can be performed for diagnostic or therapeutic purposes. With the cone biopsy, a cone-shaped specimen of tissue is excised from the deeper layers of the cervix. If conization was done via a loop electrosurgical excision procedure (LEEP) of the cervix or large-loop excision of the transformation zone (LLETZ), use code 57522. Both names refer to the removal of the outer layer of cervical cells, which are at highest risk of becoming cancerous, by using a loop-shaped electrosurgical wire to glide over the surface of the cervix.

> **INTERNET RESOURCE:** Visit MedlinePlus and view an illustration of the cervical cold knife cone biopsy technique.
> www.nlm.nih.gov/medlineplus/ency/imagepages/17040.htm

CHECKPOINT 24.1

Assign code(s) to the following procedure. Include any necessary modifiers.

1. A 29-year-old female is being treated for CIN II. A speculum is inserted into the cervix. The surgeon bathes the cervix with Monsel's solution. A laser is used to cut around the opening in the cervix and remove a cone-shaped piece of tissue. _____

Sterilization

Sterilization is a term used to describe permanent and irreversible birth control. Tubal ligation, also known as "tube tying," is the most common female method of sterilization and is performed via various techniques. Read the operative note closely to determine which one was applied. Sterilization can be accomplished laparoscopically, hysteroscopically, or via the open method. The laparoscopic method is by far the most common. The fallopian tubes may be clamped with Hulka clamps that close off the tube, blocking the egg from migrating and becoming fertilized (58615, 58671). Another sterilization technique involves cutting the tubes, removing a segment, and fulgurating (cauterizing) the ends of the tube (58600, 58670). The tubes are no longer connected, disrupting the egg's pathway. Sterilization is also accomplished by using a hysteroscope. The surgeon enters the uterus and locates the fallopian tube openings. A catheter is inserted into each fallopian tube and metallic implants are placed to obstruct the tube, achieving a mechanical occlusion (58565). Scar tissue develops around the implant, completely blocking the tube. The most common kind of implant used is the Essure Microcoil implant or Adiana.

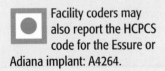 Facility coders may also report the HCPCS code for the Essure or Adiana implant: A4264.

Birth Control Maintenance

Surgical birth control consists of sterilization, insertion of an intrauterine device (IUD) (58300), or insertion of a drug-delivery implant (11981). With the exception of the tubal occlusion, these procedures are performed in the provider's office. Insertion of a contraceptive implant drug-delivery device (e.g., Implanon Rod or Nexplanon) is assigned code 11981. A small incision is made on the inside of the upper arm and the thin rod-like implant is placed subdermally and can be palpated under the skin. The implant can remain up to 3 years and will need to be removed at the end of its useful life. This code does not include the cost of the implant, which should be reported with HCPCS code J7307 or CPT code 99070, depending on carrier requirements. Removal of Norplant implanted contraceptive capsules is reported with code 11976. This code only applies to the removal of the Norplant system. Removal of other drug-delivery implants is reported with code 11982.

Other non-surgical methods of birth control are available as well, such as placement of a cervical cap (diaphragm) (57170). Assign HCPCS code A4261 for the supply of the cervical cap or A4266 for a diaphragm in addition to the code for fitting it.

Bartholin's Gland Abscess

The Bartholin's glands are located in the lips of the labia minora. The glands (normally the size of a pea) provide moisture for the vulva area. A Bartholin's gland cyst or abscess may form in the gland itself or in the duct draining the gland. Options for treatment of a Bartholin's cyst include incision and drainage (I&D), marsupialization, and excision (56420, 56440, 56740). Marsupialization involves I&D of the cyst, turning it inside out, and suturing the cyst wall to the edges of the incision that was made.

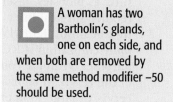 A woman has two Bartholin's glands, one on each side, and when both are removed by the same method modifier –50 should be used.

Lesions of the Vulva

Lesions located on the external genitalia require examination and often biopsy to properly diagnose. Lesions range from genital warts (condyloma), cysts, and sexually transmitted viral infections to cancer. Vulvar intraepithelial neoplasia (VIN) are flesh-colored, hypopigmented, or hyperpigmented lesions that appear anywhere on the vulva. The two types of VIN are usual-type VIN and differentiated VIN. (Previous classification by pathologists was similar to that used in the Bethesda system for the three-grade CIN classification.) Undifferentiated or usual-type VIN is linked with high-risk types of HPV infection. VIN is also commonly referred to as *vulval carcinoma in situ, vulval atypia,* or *bowenoid papulosis.* Women whose Pap smears show HPV infection are prone to develop VIN, as are women who smoke and are sexually active from a young age. Differentiated VIN is not associated with HPV. It is more common in postmenopausal women or women with lichen sclerosus. A diagnosis of VIN is made by visualizing the lesion and performing a biopsy. Surgical excision or destruction is currently the standard treatment for VIN.

When lesions of the vulva are localized and do not require removal of the vulva, assign codes for the excision from the Integumentary System section: 11420–11426, 11620–11626.

Destruction of a lesion is appropriate at times, such as with condyloma. Assign codes 56501–56515 based on whether simple or extensive destruction was applied. Code 56515 is assigned if there are multiple lesions or if any complications were encountered.

CHECKPOINT 24.2

Assign code(s) to the following procedure. Include any necessary modifiers.

1. A 45-year-old patient presents with three vulvar lesions that were previously biopsied and pathology testing has determined they were condyloma. The lesions were removed by laser ablation with no complicating factors. _____

Vulvectomy is the surgical removal of all or part of the vulva. The extent of the excision guides code assignment. A vulvectomy is the recommended treatment for cancer of the vulva and for large skin growths such as condyloma. Refer to the definitions at the beginning of the Vulva, Perineum, and Introitus subsection of CPT for simple, radical, partial, and complete vulvectomy to assist in selecting a vulvectomy code to assign based on depth of excision and amount of vulva excised (56620–56640).

CHECKPOINT 24.3

Assign code(s) to the following procedure. Include any necessary modifiers.

1. The physician performed a radical, partial vulvectomy. Provide the code and a definition of *radical* and *partial* in terms of vulvectomy procedures. _____

CPT © 2017 American Medical Association, All Rights Reserved.

Uterine Fibroids

Uterine fibroids (58140–58146, 58561) are also referred to as *myomas* or *leiomyomata*. Fibroids are fibrous tumors that can form in various layers of the uterine tissue. There are three different types of fibroids: intramural, submucous, and subserous. More than 30% of women are affected by fibroids and experience abnormal bleeding or infertility. These tumors or fibroids can be removed either hysteroscopically, laparoscopically, or via open abdominal technique depending on what type of fibroid, the size, number, and location. Submucous fibroids are the only kind that can be removed hysteroscopically. The other types are surgically removed via laparotomy or laparoscopically.

Myoma

A myoma is a benign fibroid tumor of the uterus. Subserous myomas grow on the outside wall of the uterus and can be connected to the uterus by a stalk (pedunculated myoma). Submucous myomas are located partially in the uterine cavity and partially in the wall of the uterus. Intramural myomas grow in the wall of the uterus itself. Intracavity myomas are located inside the uterine cavity. These fibroids can cause abdominal pain, heavy menstrual bleeding, and pain with intercourse. Myomectomy is performed to remove symptomatic tumors while leaving the uterus intact. This procedure can be performed via an open, laparoscopic, or hysteroscopic approach. Code selection depends on the surgical approach, the number of tumors removed, and the total weight of the tumors. Open abdominal myomectomy is reported with codes 58140, 58146. Laparoscopic myomectomy is reported with codes 58545–58546. Myomectomy via hysteroscope is reported with code 58561.

If the fibroid tumors are too large, or in the case of intramural myomas, which are not always safe to excise, hysterectomy may be required.

CHECKPOINT 24.4

Assign code(s) to the following procedure. Include any necessary modifiers.

1. The patient presented with three intramural myomas weighing 210 grams. The surgeon performed a myomectomy via abdominal approach. _____

Hysterectomy

A hysterectomy is the surgical removal of the uterus, which may or may not also include the fallopian tubes and ovaries. Hysterectomy is often indicated for excessive or dysfunctional uterine bleeding, endometriosis, uterine fibroids, uterine prolapse, or for certain types of pelvic cancer. Hysterectomy codes are dispersed throughout the female genital section so caution is needed. The procedure can be performed via open abdominal approach, vaginally, or laparoscopically (called a *laparoscopically assisted vaginal hysterectomy or LAVH*).

Look up the term *Hysterectomy* in the Index. Take note of the number of entries provided. An understanding of the approach and several other criteria are necessary to select the most appropriate code. Accurate code assignment depends on several factors. Look for the answers to the following questions within the medical documentation and follow the steps in Pinpoint the Code 24.1:

1. Is it performed at the same time as a cesarean section (C section) or vaginal delivery? If so, assign code +59525 in addition to the code for the delivery.
2. What surgical approach was used?
   a. Abdominal (58150–58240) approach: The surgeon makes a 5- to 7-inch incision, either vertical or horizontal; opens the abdomen; and removes the uterus. This is commonly performed through a previous C-section scar.
   b. Vaginal (58260–58294) approach: An incision is made in the vagina, and the uterus is removed through this incision. The incision is closed, leaving no visible scar.
   c. Laparoscopic (58541–58544, 58548) approach: The surgeon uses the laparoscope to examine the pelvis and detach the uterus from the supporting structures and pelvic floor (above or below the cervix depending on technique). The uterus is morcellized and removed through the small portal incisions.

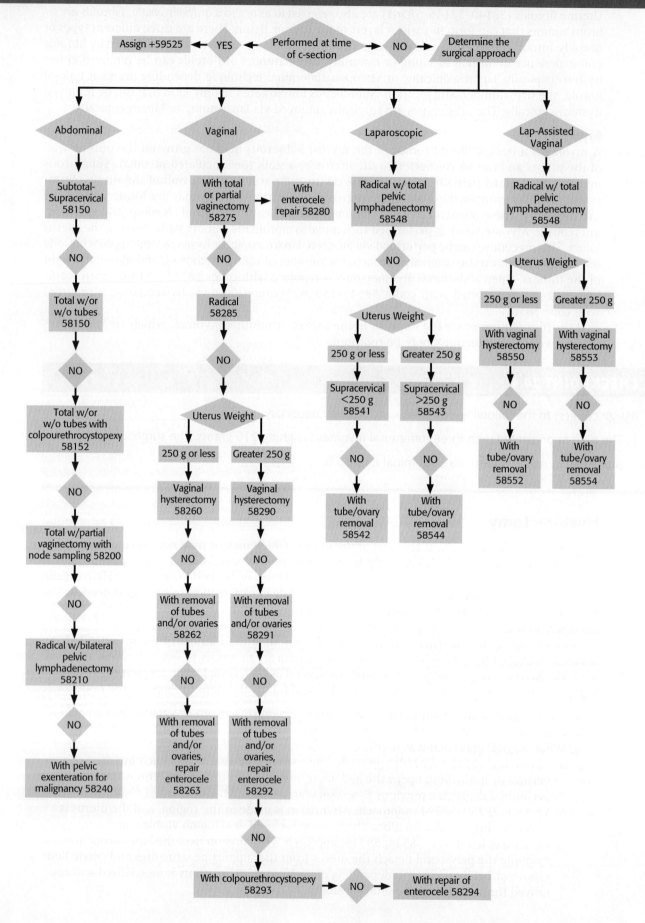

CPT © 2017 American Medical Association, All Rights Reserved.

d. Laparoscopically assisted vaginal approach (58550–58554): The surgeon uses the laparoscope to examine the pelvis and detach the uterus from the supporting structures and pelvic floor (above or below the cervix depending on technique). A separate incision is made in the vagina, and the uterus is then removed through this incision.

3. What was the weight of the uterus? Codes differ based on weight (less than or greater than 250 g).

4. Was it a total or subtotal hysterectomy? Total hysterectomy means removal of uterus and cervix. Subtotal hysterectomy is also referred to as a *supracervical hysterectomy*, which leaves the cervix intact and only removes the corpus uterus.

5. Were the tubes and ovaries also removed? Codes differ for some approaches based on whether or not the tubes and ovaries are also removed.

6. Was a radical hysterectomy performed? The surgeon removes the whole uterus, tissue on the sides of the uterus, the cervix, and the top part of the vagina. This procedure is performed when a patient has some type of pelvic cancer. Additional dissection is often performed. Code assignment depends on what else is removed: lymph nodes, tubes, ovaries, bladder, rectum, colon, and vagina (58200–58240, 58548).

7. Were additional repair or reconstruction procedures performed on the bladder, urethra, or vaginal floor? Some hysterectomy combination code options report additional procedures for urethropexy and enterocele.

CHECKPOINT 24.5

Assign code(s) to the following procedure. Include any necessary modifiers.

1. Code for a total abdominal hysterectomy without removal of tubes and ovaries. _____

Paravaginal Defects

Vaginal Prolapse

Muscles and ligaments located in the pelvis support pelvic viscera and the vagina. A vaginal prolapse occurs when the weight-bearing or stabilizing structures that keep the vagina in place weaken or deteriorate. Female genital or vagina prolapse is a common condition in post menopausal women, women who are obese, and those who have borne multiple children. It is characterized by a portion of the vaginal canal protruding (prolapsing) from the opening of the vagina resulting from defects in the vaginal wall or floor that allow the uterus and vaginal walls to prolapse into the vagina. When supporting structures are weakened or damaged (e.g., from menopause, childbirth, disease, and pelvic surgery), the vagina and surrounding structures lose the support that holds them in place. When this happens, it is referred to as *pelvic floor relaxation*. Menopause is a major contributor to prolapse. After menopause, the estrogen level decreases. Estrogen helps to keep the muscles and tissues of the pelvic support structure strong; when estrogen decreases, support structures weaken. This may cause the supports for the rectum, bladder, uterus, small bladder, urethra, or a combination of these to become less stable. Uterine prolapse occurs when the pelvic floor muscles become weak and the uterine support structures become stretched, allowing the uterus to protrude into the vagina. Hysterectomy is the preferred method of correction for this type of prolapse. The uterus and its surrounding ligature serve as a support mechanism for the vagina. After hysterectomy, the woman's vaginal roof is vulnerable to prolapsing. If it does, this is referred to as *vaginal vault prolapse*.

Depending on the type and severity of prolapse, women have treatment options. A nonsurgical treatment option for vaginal prolapse is placement of a pessary. A pessary is a ring-like device inserted into the vagina to provide structural support to the vaginal walls. The pessary can be removed by the patient, cleaned, and reinserted. Proper fitting of the pessary is important and often requires the patient to try several sizes and/or styles, some of which are developed for specific types of prolapse.

INTERNET RESOURCE: The American Academy of Family Physicians (AAFP) published an informative article about vaginal prolapse and the use of a pessary.
www.aafp.org/afp/2000/0501/p2719.html

Women who have extensive prolapse and failed conservative treatments may require surgical reconstruction to correct the prolapsed vagina. Reconstructive surgery corrects the prolapsed vagina and aims to restore normal anatomy. Colpopexy is defined as the suture repair of a relaxed vagina to the abdominal wall to secure the vagina in the correct anatomical position. The abdominal sacral colpopexy (57425, 57280) is one of the most successful operations for vaginal vault prolapse. It involves making an incision in the abdomen and suturing a synthetic mesh or harvested strip of abdominal fascia to the apex of the vagina connecting it to the sacrum and forming a bridge. By doing this, the vagina is stabilized and will not collapse. This procedure is also carried out transvaginally by entering the vagina and suturing the apex to the sacrospinous or by locating the iliococcygeus muscle, which is located lateral to the rectum and anterior to the ischium, and suturing the apex to the iliococcygeus muscle fascia (57282). Report code 57283 if uterine suspension is performed using the uterosacral ligament or levator musculature.

Women of advanced age who are not candidates for extensive reconstructive surgery may opt for an obliterative surgery to correct vaginal prolapse called *colpocleisis* or *colpectomy* (57120), which involves removing and/or closing off all or a portion of the vagina, resulting in reducing the prolapsed viscera back into the pelvis. This procedure is performed via a vaginal approach and results in complete closure of the vaginal orifice. Women who undergo this procedure can no longer have vaginal intercourse.

Vaginal Hernias

There are four types of paravaginal hernias that require surgical intervention:

- Cystocele (bladder into vagina)
- Rectocele (rectum into vagina)
- Enterocele (small intestine into vagina)
- Urethrocele (urethra into vagina)

When the walls of the vagina become weak, the bladder may also "drop" into the vagina. This condition is called a *cystocele*. With a rectocele, the fascia barrier between the vagina and the rectum weakens, allowing the front wall of the rectum to bulge into the vagina. An enterocele occurs when the muscles and fascia that hold the small bowel in place stretch or weaken along with the vaginal roof, giving way and allowing the small bowel to drop from its original position and protrude through the vaginal wall. Urethrocele is the prolapse of the urethra into the vagina and commonly occurs along with a cystocele.

Repair may be performed using a vaginal or abdominal approach. Anterior vaginal repairs (colporrhaphy) (57240) are performed to treat cystoceles and accomplished by making an incision in the anterior vaginal wall where pubocervical fascia is folded over the defect in the vaginal wall and stitched in place. Posterior vaginal repairs (57250) target rectoceles and are performed in the same manner by making an incision in the posterior vaginal wall. Combined anteroposterior colporrhaphy (57260) entails repair to both the anterior and posterior vaginal walls. Mesh may be inserted to offer additional support at the site of the repair. Report +57267 in addition to the codes for vaginal repairs (57240–57265, 57285). Cystourethroscopy (cystoscopy) is commonly performed during gynecological reconstructive procedures to check the patency of the urethra and to check for urinary tract injury during surgery. The cystoscopy that occurs during these procedures is not separately reportable.

Paravaginal defect repair codes 57284–57285 and 57423 are assigned to repair lateral defects of the vagina where the pubovesical fascia laterally detaches from the arcus tendineus pelvic fascia (ATFP). Repair includes cystocele repair or anterior colporrhaphy. The goal of the repair is to reattach the lateral vagina to the ATFP and involves entering the space of Retzius and using sutures to attach it. The space of Retzius is located between the symphysis, the bladder, and the anterior abdominal wall that is made up of loose connective tissue and fat. CPT parenthetical notes provide a list of procedures that cannot be reported in addition to these paravaginal defect procedures.

INTERNET RESOURCES: Visit the OR-Live Surgical Archives website and view videos of OB/GYN procedures.

There is opportunity for code confusion here. Careful review of the terminology and the different approaches is needed before selecting codes because the words are similar.

CPT Assistant states that code 57284 is considered inherently bilateral. The guidelines also indicate that if an enterocele repair (vaginal approach) is performed in addition to the paravaginal defect (abdominal approach), it should also be reported despite the fact that 57268 (enterocele repair, vaginal approach) is a "separate procedure" because of the two different approaches. Report modifier −59 with the enterocele repair.

Click on the procedure to see the video. You are required to register at no charge before the video is played.
obgyn.broadcastmed.com/procedures

Pelvic exenteration code 51597 is not a gender-specific code. This is in contrast to the pelvic exenteration code 58240, which is specifically for gynecological malignancy.

Visit the Pelvic Floor Institute's website and participate in the interactive activities. The site requires you to register and create a password but it is free. The site simulates a clinic and takes the viewer on a tour through the exam room, doctors' lounge, auditorium, operation room, and health provider resources. Users can watch videos, view interactive three-dimensional models, obtain reimbursement information, and learn more about the various techniques and mesh systems used to repair pelvic floor defects.
www.bostonscientific.com/templatedata/imports/HTML/PFI/PFI_bridge.html?cid=ps51961

MATERNITY CARE AND DELIVERY

OB/GYN physicians specialize in the care of pregnant females including treating infection, management of chronic conditions such as hypertension, and fetal monitoring for the duration of the 9-month pregnancy and the 6-week puerperium. The estimated date of delivery (EDD), also known as the *estimated date of confinement (EDC)*, is calculated from the last menstrual period (LMP) out 280 days. This time period of 9 months (40 weeks) is referred to as *gestation*. Physicians refer to the growth of the embryo and fetus in terms of gestational age.

The antepartum period is the time period between the EDD and delivery. The time period from the EDD to delivery is also referred to as the *prenatal period*. Pregnancy is separated into three trimesters. Physicians refer to a patient's OB history by gravidity and parity and abortions. Gravidity (gravida) is the number of pregnancies the patient has had. Parity indicates the number of pregnancies where a fetus reached a viable age (approximately 22 weeks) and the patient delivered a newborn. Abortus indicates the number of pregnancies that were terminated before 22 weeks, whether by induced abortion or miscarriage. Documentation in the obstetrical record would look like this, for example: P2G3A1. In this example, the patient delivered 2 live newborns, had 3 pregnancies, and had 1 miscarriage or abortion. The puerperium (postpartum) period begins immediately after delivery through the recovery period of approximately 6 weeks after vaginal or C-section delivery.

Organization of Section

The beginning of this CPT section contains detailed notes and instructions describing the various services that are "packaged" according to period of pregnancy when services are rendered—antepartum, delivery, or postpartum. The services in this section are categorized by the timing of the service provided as well as by who provided the care. All the procedure codes located pertain to pregnancy services whether antepartum, delivery, postpartum, or abortion.

Routine Obstetrical Care

Uncomplicated maternity care is billed as a "package" that includes antepartum care, delivery (either vaginal or via C-section), and postpartum care (Box 24.3). Definitions are located at the beginning of the Maternity Care and Delivery section. To properly interpret maternity care services, the following definitions must be mastered.

- *Antepartum care/period* includes initial and subsequent history and physical (H&P), measurement of weight, monitoring of blood pressure (BP) and fetal heart tones, routine chemical urinalysis, monthly visits up to 28 weeks, biweekly visits up to 36 weeks, and weekly visits until delivery. All E/M services pertaining to these services are included. Any visits during this period other than those listed would be reported separately. About 41% of the physician work is performed in the antepartum period.
- *Delivery services* include admission to the hospital, admission H&P examination, fetal monitoring, management of uncomplicated labor, and vaginal delivery or C-section.

Delivery of placenta, venipuncture, IV placement, postoperative pain management (after C-section), induction of labor with Pitocin, artificial rupture of membranes (AROM), episiotomy, forceps delivery, vacuum extraction, and episiorrhaphy are all considered part of the delivery package and are not coded separately. Episiotomy involves incising the perineum to aid in delivery. It prevents tearing or deeper lacerations to the perineal tissue or anal sphincter. Episiorrhaphy is the surgical suturing of the perineum and the vagina following episiotomy.

The admission H&P and labor management make up approximately 36% of the work of the global maternity care package. Vaginal delivery equates to approximately 15% of the package.

- *Postpartum care/period* includes hospital stay and office visits during the 6 weeks following delivery. Postpartum care consists of approximately 8% of the work of the global package.

BOX 24.3 Maternity Package

Initial and subsequent history	Fetal monitoring during delivery
All physical exams	Biweekly visits up to 36 weeks
Monitoring of vital signs (BP, weight, fetal heart, uterine measurements)	Weekly visits from 36 weeks until delivery
	Delivery services for uncomplicated labor
Routine urinalysis	Postpartum care
Monthly visits up to 28 weeks	

When complications arise and extra visits or hospitalizations are necessary, these are billed separately and in addition to the obstetrical package. Services that are performed during pregnancy but not included in routine obstetrical services are as follows:

- Fetal stress tests
- Amniocentesis
- Genetic testing
- Ultrasound
- Laboratory studies
- High-risk illness services
- Chorionic villus sampling
- Administration of Rh immunoglobulin
- Fetal scalp blood sampling
- External cephalic version

A complete, thorough level 2 ultrasound performed in the second or third trimester is time consuming and requires a high level of skill and expertise to interpret; therefore, it is separately reimbursable.

The greater part of OB services is provided without obstacles and can be reported using 59400, *Routine obstetric care including antepartum care, delivery, and postpartum care*. Before assigning any vaginal delivery codes, the coder needs to determine if the patient had a previous C-section or not. If so, there are very specific codes in the 59610–59622 range that must be used to indicate this. They are used to indicate a vaginal birth after a previous C-section (VBAC) (59610) or an attempted vaginal delivery after C-section completed by C-section (59618), for example. A *repeat C-section* is the term used to describe C-sections performed on women who had previous C-section deliveries and either elect to forgo a vaginal birth attempt or have a clinical reason for needing a C-section for a present or future delivery. Unlike vaginal delivery after C-section, there isn't a separate designation of codes for repeat C-sections.

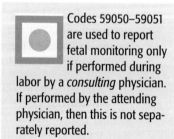 Codes 59050–59051 are used to report fetal monitoring only if performed during labor by a *consulting* physician. If performed by the attending physician, then this is not separately reported.

> Do not confuse yourself with the ICD-10 rules for complicated OB care. Use of forceps and vacuum extractors is considered a complicated delivery in CPT.

NOTE: In rural, underserved areas family practitioners may provide obstetrical care and deliver babies in uncomplicated cases; however, they do not perform C-sections.

Episiotomy or vaginal repair performed by a *consulting* physician is reported with 59300. If performed by the attending physician, it is included in the OB package for the vaginal delivery. Small vaginal tears are not considered a complication. If an extensive laceration occurs, the –22 modifier can be appended to the code for the vaginal delivery to indicate the additional effort incurred by the physician to repair the perineum.

Medical complications of pregnancy may require the necessity of additional E/M codes or services from the Medicine section. Pregnant females who develop preeclampsia or anemia, or patients with poor control of their diabetes are considered high risk. These conditions would qualify as a complication of pregnancy and may require hospitalization. If these complications require any additional services beyond those listed in the maternity care and delivery guidelines, these services are reported separately. At times, medical conditions requiring surgical intervention such as hernias, ovarian cysts, cholecystitis, appendicitis, fractures, kidney stones, and so forth occur during pregnancy. Treatments for these conditions are coded separately from their respective surgery sections of CPT.

In some instances, a physician may only provide care in one or two of the three phases of obstetrical care (antepartum, delivery, postpartum). Circumstances do arise that could potentially warrant three different care providers during the pregnancy, delivery, and after care. In such a case, assign the code as appropriate for the extent of the care provided for each provider. Per CPT, if a physician saw a patient for fewer than four antepartum visits, E/M codes should be submitted in lieu of codes from the Maternity Care and Delivery section. Codes can be located and assigned specific to the stage of pregnancy and the number of visits in which a provider participated. Codes 59425–59426 are specific to antepartum care. Code 59430 is assigned when only postpartum care is provided. If a provider only participated in the delivery of the baby, 59409 is assigned for the vaginal delivery and 59514 is reported for a cesarean delivery.

> ■ **CASE SCENARIO**
> Mrs. Quinn saw Dr. Lee for 7 months of her pregnancy, but then her husband got transferred out of state. She resumed her care with Dr. Shaw for the remaining 2 months and subsequent delivery and postpartum visit. Dr. Lee would bill 59426 (antepartum care; seven or more visits) and Dr. Shaw would bill 59425 (antepartum care; four to six visits) and 59410 (vaginal delivery including postpartum care).

COMMON OBSTETRICAL CONDITIONS AND PROCEDURES

Amniotic Fluid

Amniotic fluid within the amniotic sac protects the baby and aids in the development of muscles, limbs, lungs, and the digestive system. In the second trimester, the baby begins to breathe and swallow the amniotic fluid. Amniotic fluid levels continually rise until about 32 to 33 weeks' gestation, and then they taper off. Tests are performed on this fluid to diagnose congenital defects, fetal distress, and fetal lung development. Amniocentesis (often abbreviated as "amnio") is the most common prenatal test used to diagnose chromosomal and genetic birth defects and is performed in the second trimester. Diagnostic amniocentesis (59000) is suggested to women of increased maternal age (over the age of 35), who have had previous babies with birth defects, have a family history of birth defects, or have an abnormal alpha fetal protein (AFP) blood test suggestive of Down syndrome. Amniocentesis is performed by inserting a thin needle into the uterus to withdraw a small sample of the amniotic fluid that surrounds the fetus. The physician uses ultrasound to guide the needle and aspirate fluid surrounding the fetus so as not to injure the fetus. The fluid is sent off to a lab to be analyzed. It can be performed in late pregnancy to assess anemia in babies with Rh disease and to find out if the fetal lungs are mature enough for

> The radiological supervision and interpretation code 76946 is reported separately for diagnostic amniocentesis. Do not report this separately for therapeutic amniocentesis.

the baby to be delivered. Do not confuse therapeutic amniotic fluid reduction (59001) with diagnostic amniocentesis (59000). Therapeutic amnio is performed to treat polyhydramnios, a condition where there is too much amniotic fluid. The higher the fluid level, the increased chance the baby has a congenital defect that hinders swallowing, which can prohibit ingestion of the amniotic fluid, resulting in buildup of fluid.

Incompetent Cervix

An incompetent cervix describes a cervix that prematurely stretches or dilates and is often the cause of premature delivery. Women with incompetent cervix with a history of miscarriages or premature delivery require surgical intervention. Cervical cerclage is a preventive procedure performed to prevent premature dilation by sewing the cervix closed using a McDonald's suture through the cervical epithelium or a Shirodkar suture, which is buried beneath the cervical epithelium. When the procedure is performed vaginally, assign 59320. Abdominal cerclage involves placing a band around the cervical os or opening (59325).

Cesarean Section Delivery

C-section is performed by making an incision through the abdomen into the uterus (59510–59525). C-sections are very common and are often required in cases where the baby's head is too big to pass through the pelvis. This may be a result of a large baby or a congenital abnormality of the mother's pelvis. There may be times when the baby is not in the correct position in the birth canal. A baby presenting in the breech position (feet, legs, or buttocks first) is hazardous to the mother and baby and will complicate delivery. The physician will attempt to perform an external cephalic version (59412), which entails manipulating the fetus into the head-down position by pushing on the abdomen. If this effort fails, a C-section is indicated. A C-section is also indicated if labor is slow to progress or if there are any indications of fetal distress or umbilical cord tangling. Planned C-sections are scheduled in advance and carried out in the following circumstances:

- Multiple gestations
- Placental problems
- Prior C-section in previous pregnancy
- Large babies
- Birth defect
- Maternal HIV or genital herpes

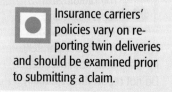
If a tubal ligation is performed at the same session as a C-section, +58611 is also assigned.

CHECKPOINT 24.6

Assign code(s) to the following procedure. Include any necessary modifiers.

1. Cesarean delivery, including postpartum care, and total hysterectomy following attempted vaginal delivery; patient had previous cesarean delivery. _____

Delivery of Twins

The use of fertility drugs and reproductive medicine procedures commonly results in more than one fertilized egg. Multiple fetuses, however, may not automatically classify as a complicated delivery.

The preferred way to report vaginal delivery of twins by the same physician or physician group is 59400 and 59409–51 for vaginal delivery or 59510 and 59514–51 for cesarean delivery. If one twin is delivered vaginally and the other by C-section and the obstetrical care is provided by the same physician or group, report 59510 or 59618 as appropriate for the C-section and 59409–51 or 59612–51 for the vaginal delivery.

Insurance carriers' policies vary on reporting twin deliveries and should be examined prior to submitting a claim.

Ectopic Pregnancy

Tubal pregnancy and *ectopic pregnancy* are terms used to describe a fertilized egg that has become implanted outside the uterus in one of the fallopian tubes. The fertilized egg may also become lodged in the ovary. This condition must be treated because the risk of rupture and bleeding are too great. If the ovum is ruptured, a more extensive procedure and repair are indicated. Surgical treatment can be performed via an abdominal, laparoscopic, or vaginal approach. Codes in this section are specific to the location of the pregnancy, the approach, and the extent of the repair (59120–59151). Codes 59150–59151 are reported for laparoscopic treatment. The fertilized embryo is removed by inserting the laparoscope and making an incision into the fallopian tube or by removing a segment of the tube and anastomosing the remnants together. Read the operative report carefully to identify these factors.

Watch for *salpingectomy* versus *salpingotomy*. These terms do not mean the same thing! If the complete removal of a tube is required, then 59120 is applied. If not, 59121 should be used.

INTERNET RESOURCE: Visit the Advanced Fertility Center of Chicago's website for illustrations of an ectopic pregnancy. www.advancedfertility.com/ectopfot.htm

Abortion

Abortion (59812–59857) is the premature expulsion of a fetus, embryo, or products of conception (POC) from the uterus. There are two categories of abortion: spontaneous and elective (induced). Codes for abortion are specific to the type of abortion and the stage of pregnancy when it occurred. Spontaneous abortion (SAB), according to *CPT Assistant*, is the natural loss of the products of conception before the 20th week of pregnancy. Several types of abortion fit into this category: (1) missed abortion, (2) incomplete abortion, (3) septic abortion, and (4) complete abortion.

A missed abortion (MAB) (59820) is the retention of the products of conception after fetal death prior to 22 weeks of gestation. A blighted ovum, a fertilized egg that fails to develop, would be considered a missed abortion because the mother did not begin to expel any products of conception. It is not uncommon to have a woman present unknowingly to the office with a blighted ovum. Depending on when prenatal care began, the patient may be far into her first or second trimester before this is diagnosed. On ultrasound, a degenerated or absent embryo with an ova will be seen. An incomplete abortion (59812) is a spontaneous miscarriage where the woman begins to miscarry but does not expel all of the products of conception. Membranes are ruptured but tissue remains in the uterus or vagina. Septic abortion (59830) can occur when uterine contents become infected as a result of a bacterial or sexually transmitted infection that enters the uterus, causing premature rupture of membranes (PROM), severe abdominal pain, and fetal demise. This infection often leads to infection of other pelvic organs and may cause sepsis. Septic abortion may also occur after an elective abortion when some of the uterine contents are left behind. When a spontaneous abortion is a complete abortion, all the uterine contents are expelled or emptied, and no surgical intervention is necessary. Codes 59840–59841 should not be used for the surgical completion of a spontaneous abortion; use 59812 for this service. Code 59812 is used to report D&C (either sharp or suction curette) for the surgical completion of a spontaneous incomplete abortion with exception of a septic abortion or missed abortion. Surgical management of a missed abortion is reported with codes 59820–59821 based on the trimester in which it occurs. Septic abortion is reported with code 59830.

Induced abortion is the elective termination of pregnancy prior to 22 weeks' gestation via D&C, dilation and evacuation (D&E), intra-amniotic injections, or vaginal suppositories. Induced abortions can be either elective for birth control purposes or therapeutic (TAB), because of a medical condition threatening the life of the mother. Abortions can be performed in an outpatient clinic under general anesthesia or in a physician office under conscious sedation if equipment is available.

First-trimester abortions (0 to 14 weeks) are typically performed by using a vacuum aspirator (suction D&C). Code 59840 is reported for abortions where a D&C is performed by dilating the cervix and using a sharp curette to remove all uterine contents. If D&E is performed using a suction catheter, report 59841. Second-trimester abortions (14 to 26 weeks) are typically performed using the same methods as first-trimester abortions up to 20 weeks. Beyond 20 to 22 weeks, other methods are applied. Intra-amniotic hyperosmotic solutions may be injected to stimulate uterine contractions (59850) and cervical dilation simulating birth where the patient delivers the fetus. Solutions of hypertonic urea and prostaglandin are injected into the amniotic sac after partially removing some of the amniotic fluid. The urea kills the fetus and prostaglandin induces labor to expel the contents. Contractions begin within 8 to 12 hours and may last 2 days before the fetus, placenta, and membranes are expelled. If the injection is performed, and the patient does not completely deliver the fetus, thus requiring D&E, report code 59851.

Induced abortion by using vaginal suppositories to soften and dilate the cervix is reported with 59855–59856. With this type of medical abortion, the patient is admitted to the hospital and given an injection of methotrexate or oxytocin and a vaginal prostaglandin suppository (e.g., misoprostol) is inserted. Within 12 to 24 hours, the fetus and placenta are delivered. Be sure to note the inclusion of hospital admission and visits in codes 59850–59857.

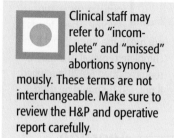

Pay close attention to the stage of the pregnancy (first, second, or third trimester), the category, and the type of abortion before choosing an abortion code.

Clinical staff may refer to "incomplete" and "missed" abortions synonymously. These terms are not interchangeable. Make sure to review the H&P and operative report carefully.

■ **CASE SCENARIO**

A pregnant patient is seen in the OB office for spotting. The patient is currently 9 weeks pregnant. Ultrasound showed a 4-week sac. Diagnosis of missed AB was made and D&C was carried out the following day. Report code 59820.

CHECKPOINT 24.7

Assign code(s) to the following procedure. Include any necessary modifiers.

1. Spontaneous incomplete miscarriage surgically completed in first trimester _____

Multifetal Pregnancy Reduction

When the mother is carrying multiple fetuses, it may be necessary to reduce the number of fetuses in the uterus to protect the health of the mother and the remaining fetuses. Risks of multiple gestations are significant and include an increased chance of miscarriage, birth defects, severely premature birth, and the mental and/or physical problems that can result from a premature delivery. It is extremely difficult for a mother to carry multiple babies to term. The average length of twin pregnancy is 35 weeks, 33 weeks for triplets, and 29 weeks for quadruplets. Multifetal pregnancy reduction (MPR) is typically not performed unless more than three fetuses are present. MPR is usually performed between 9 and 12 weeks' gestation. It is done on an outpatient basis whereby a needle is inserted into the uterus via the abdomen or vagina and potassium chloride is injected into select fetuses. The code for this procedure is 59866.

> **INTERNET RESOURCE:** Visit the ACOG website and read its opinion about multifetal reductions.
> www.acog.org/Resources%20And%20Publications/Committee%20Opinions/Committee%20on%20Ethics/Multifetal%20Pregnancy%20Reduction.aspx

INFERTILITY

Infertility is the inability of a couple to conceive after 12 months of unprotected intercourse in women under 35 years of age, or after 6 months in women over 35. Several conditions are considered known obstacles to fertility such as endometriosis, polycystic ovarian syndrome, irregular menstrual cycles, early menopause, uterine fibroids, blocked fallopian tubes, male factor infertility, and irregular cycles, to name a few. One out of seven couples seeks a reproductive endocrinologist who specializes in assisted reproductive technology (ART), a medical specialty that encompasses medical and surgical treatments for infertility.

Family planning is an integral part of infertility management. Most insurance carriers will cover the diagnostic workup for infertility to determine the cause but limit coverage for fertility treatment. Some carriers allow no payment for fertility services, leaving many couples responsible for the counseling, workup, and treatment.

INTERNET RESOURCE: Visit the American Society of Reproductive Medicine's website to learn about which states have infertility laws.
www.reproductivefacts.org/detail.aspx?id=2850

Blocked Fallopian Tubes

A diagnostic test called *chromotubation* (58350) is performed to determine patency of the fallopian tubes. Dye is injected through the cervix into the uterus and fallopian tubes to view the anatomy and determine if there is a blockage. The surgeon then performs diagnostic laparoscopy (49320) to look for spillage of dye from the fimbriated end of the tube, indicating the tube is not blocked. Because code 58350 is neither a hysteroscopic nor laparoscopic code, it is not bundled into the diagnostic laparoscopy procedure, and both codes are reported to describe the complete service. Most insurance carriers view this as a noncovered elective fertility service and will not pay for this service unless the diagnosis is for other than fertility.

INTERNET RESOURCE: Visit the Advanced Fertility Medical Group of Chicago's website to read more about this service and see illustrations.
www.advancedfertility.com/hsg.htm

In Vitro Fertilization

In vitro fertilization (IVF) is usually performed in a fertility clinic. In IVF, fertilization is achieved outside of the uterus and not in the natural way. IVF is a multistep process. The female's eggs are visualized by ultrasound and retrieved from the ovary by placing a needle through the vaginal wall. The eggs are then kept in the laboratory under physiological conditions. An infertility doctor will place the sperm with the eggs when they are ready for fertilization. They are maintained in laboratory Petri dishes, in a special mixture that acts as a substitute for the environment that would be found in the fallopian tubes. Code 58970 is assigned for the egg (oocyte) retrieval from the ovary. Assign a separate code if ultrasound is provided. The egg is then fertilized outside of the body to be implanted later. Once the egg is fertilized and grows into an embryo, it is inserted into the uterus (58974) by using a special catheter that is passed through the vagina and into the uterus at the time when the pre-embryos would naturally have reached the uterus (3 to 5 days after retrieval). If the embryo is placed into the fallopian tube instead, assign code 58976.

Intrauterine Insemination

An intrauterine insemination (IUI) procedure (58322) takes sperm and inserts it into the cervix or higher in the uterine cavity using a catheter. This procedure is a less complex procedure than IVF in that it is performed during one session. The male provides a semen sample after 2 days of no ejaculation. The sperm are "washed" and separated, leaving a purified fraction of highly motile sperm that is then inserted into the cervix. By doing this, the sperm bypass the acidic environment of the vagina, giving them a greater chance of survival as they swim toward the fallopian tubes.

INTERNET RESOURCE: Visit the American Society of Reproductive Medicine's website to learn more about infertility, risk factors, and treatments.
www.reproductivefacts.org/FactSheets-Booklets

CHECKPOINT 24.8

Assign codes to the following procedures. Include any necessary modifiers. In some cases, more than one code is required.

1. Laser destruction of vaginal lesions (extensive) _____

2. Laparoscopically assisted vaginal hysterectomy (uterus less than 250 grams) _____

3. Routine obstetrical care plus vaginal delivery after previous cesarean delivery _____

4. An elderly woman without any prior history of cancer is diagnosed with an extensive malignant vaginal cancer, requiring vaginectomy and complete removal of the vaginal wall. _____

5. An obstetrician has been seeing this patient starting with her first visit to determine that she was pregnant. She recently performed the vaginal delivery, and the patient is now being seen in the office for her last postpartum visit. How will the obstetrician code for her services? _____

6. A patient has a hysterotomy to remove a hydatidiform mole as well as tubal ligation during the same surgical session. _____

7. A patient is pregnant with her fourth child and is having contractions that are rapidly coming closer together. She and her husband leave for the hospital, but the baby is born in the car before reaching the hospital. Once the baby is secured by emergency medical technicians, the patient is admitted and her physician delivers the placenta. _____

Chapter Summary

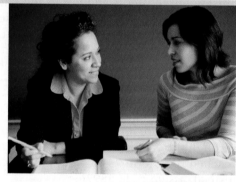

1. Laparoscopic, hysteroscopic, and colposcopic procedures use an endoscope and shorten recovery time compared with open surgical procedures. With a laparoscope, two or three small abdominal incisions are made in the abdomen, allowing for passage of the scope and instruments. Hysteroscopic procedures are performed by using a hysteroscope and inserting it into the vagina through the uterus. A colposcope is used to magnify the surface of the external genitalia and cervix.

2. The female genital section of CPT has two parts, female genital system surgery and maternity care/delivery.

3. A female annual gynecology examination includes vital signs and weight, breast examination, urine dipstick, pelvic exam, and Pap smear.

4. Common diseases and disorders in the female genital system include ovarian cysts, hydrosalpinx, pelvic adhesions, endometriosis, dysfunctional bleeding, cervical dysplasia, abscesses and lesions, and uterine fibroids.

5. Hysterectomy procedure code assignment depends on (1) whether it was done at the same time as a cesarean section, (2) the approach, (3) how much the uterus weighed, (4) whether it was total or subtotal, (5) whether or not the tubes and ovaries were removed, (6) whether it was a radical procedure, and (7) whether additional repair or reconstruction work was done.

6. Colpopexy is performed via vaginal, abdominal, or intraperitoneal approaches to repair vaginal prolapse.

7. Anterior, posterior, or combined colporrhaphy approaches are used to repair vaginal hernias.

8. The maternity and delivery global package includes antepartum, delivery, and postpartum services provided in uncomplicated maternity care. Additional CPT codes should be assigned to capture treatment in complicated maternity cases. Medical conditions can develop warranting additional E/M codes and at times surgical services codes. Codes are assigned outside of the Maternity Care and Delivery section as appropriate. If surgery is performed, codes from the respective surgery chapters are assigned.

9. Elective abortions are performed to terminate a pregnancy as a means of birth control or are therapeutic in nature because of a severe birth defect or maternal condition threatening the life of the mother. Spontaneous abortions are natural miscarriages and do not result in a viable fetus. Missed abortions are classified as fetal demise or death prior to 20 weeks of gestation whereby the body still thinks it is pregnant. The embryo has no heartbeat and the embryo sac shrinks instead of growing. D&C or D&E are performed to remove fetal tissue.

10. Assisted reproductive technology is considered for infertile couples after 12 months of unsuccessful pregnancy. Many steps are involved in the initial workup of an infertile couple. Treatments range from surgically unblocking fallopian tubes to using medication to stimulate or suppress ovulation and insemination. Insemination can be conducted outside the uterus in the laboratory and implanted days later, or sperm can be injected directly into the uterus via a catheter.

Review Questions

Matching

Match the key terms with their definitions.

A. antepartum
B. blighted ovum
C. colpocleisis
D. colpopexy
E. hydrosalpinx

F. hysteroscopy
G. pessary
H. LMP
I. menometrorrhagia
J. endometriosis

1. _____ Last menstrual period

2. _____ Time period between onset of pregnancy and delivery

3. _____ A synthetic or rubber device intended to take up space within the vagina

4. _____ Suture repair of prolapsed vagina

5. _____ Fallopian tube fills with fluid as a result of adhesions

6. _____ The use of a scope that is inserted through the cervix into the uterus, to visualize the uterine cavity

7. _____ Tissue lining of uterus found elsewhere

8. _____ Procedure performed to correct vaginal prolapse

9. _____ A fertilized egg that fails to develop

10. _____ Excessive uterine bleeding during monthly menstrual cycles and at other irregular intervals

True or False

Decide whether each statement is true or false.

1. _____ The inner lining of the uterus is called the *ectometrium*.

2. _____ A pelvic examination performed in conjunction with a gynecological surgery is coded in addition to the surgery.

3. _____ If a physician only sees a pregnant patient for one to three antepartum visits, E/M codes should be assigned instead of a maternity care code.

4. _____ Antepartum care begins with conception and ends at delivery.

5. _____ The maternity package may be broken up when necessary to capture services of multiple providers.

6. _____ Abortions can be initiated by inserting vaginal suppositories.

7. _____ CPT code 59510 is assigned twice in the case of twin delivery.

8. _____ Cryosurgery on nine vaginal warts is assigned 57061.

9. _____ When reporting maternity care services, codes are assigned for antepartum, delivery, and post-partum services in order to capture all components of the maternity package.

10. _____ Complete level ultrasound is considered part of the global maternity package and is not reimbursed separately.

11. _____ The –50 modifier is appended to code 58672.

12. _____ A couple suffers from infertility and physician utilizes electroejaculation to secure a sperm sample from the male to inseminate his partner. Sperm was injected into the cervix after washing. Codes submitted would be 58321, 58323.

Multiple Choice

Select the letter that best completes the statement or answers the question.

1. A LEEP procedure is
   A. A vaginal conization technique
   B. A method of performing cervical conization
   C. A method of removing endometrial polyps
   D. A type of cauterization

2. If a single area is biopsied and excised
   A. Only code the biopsy
   B. Code the biopsy and the excision
   C. Only code the excision
   D. Assign the excision code with a–22 modifier

3. A missed AB refers to
   A. A miscarriage
   B. An incomplete abortion
   C. A missed appointment
   D. Failure to expel a dead fetus

4. The physician performs an exploratory laparoscopy with bilateral salpingo-oophorectomy. What is the correct code assignment?
   A. 58661
   B. 49000, 58661
   C. 49000, 58720
   D. 58720

5. What is the correct CPT code assignment for hysteroscopy with lysis of intrauterine adhesions?
   A. 58555, 58559
   B. 58559, 58740
   C. 58559
   D. 58555, 58559, 58740

6. What is the correct code assignment for version or breech presentation, successfully converted to cephalic presentation with normal spontaneous delivery?
   A. 59400
   B. 59612, 59412
   C. 59409
   D. 59409, 59412

7. A pregnant woman is rushed to the hospital by a friend. While en route, she delivers in the vehicle. The husband cuts the cord before arrival at the hospital, leaving the emergency department (ED) physician to deliver the placenta in the ED. What is the correct code assignment?
   A. 59409
   B. 59430
   C. 59414
   D. 59899

8. The OB who provided Lilly's obstetrical care performed a C-section and ligation of the fallopian tubes at the time of delivery. She also saw Lilly for her 6-week postpartum visit. What is the correct code assignment?
   A. 59515, 58671
   B. 58670, 59510
   C. 59510, 58611
   D. 59510, 59525

9. A perimenopausal patient undergoes a colposcopy with an endometrial biopsy in the office. What is the correct code assignment?
   A. 58100
   B. 57456
   C. 57421
   D. 57420, 58110

10. Routine obstetrical care is provided by Dr. Hugh with subsequent C-section delivery. The patient elected to change physicians and goes to Dr. May in another practice for her post-op follow-up. What code(s) will Dr. Hugh report to the insurance carrier?
    A. 59400
    B. 59426, 59514
    C. 59510
    D. 59514

CHAPTER 25

CPT: Endocrine and Nervous Systems

CHAPTER OUTLINE

Endocrine System: Anatomy and Coding Issues

Nervous System Anatomy

Nervous System Organization

Procedures of the Skull and Brain

Skull Base Surgery

Common Nerve Conditions Requiring Treatment

Spinal Injections and Pain Management

Spinal Decompression Procedures

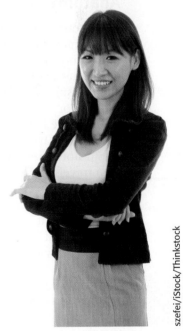

szefei/iStock/Thinkstock

LEARNING OUTCOMES

After studying this chapter, you should be able to:

1. Identify anatomical structures of the endocrine system.
2. Describe nervous system anatomy.
3. Compare and contrast common treatments of nerve pain: neurolysis, neuroplasty, neurorrhaphy, and nerve blocks.
4. Explain when it is appropriate to report nerve blocks separately from the anesthesia provided for the surgery.
5. Describe the various methods of nerve repair: nerve graft, nerve wrapping, and suture repair.
6. Explain the purpose of neurostimulators and list their components.
7. Explain when procedure codes from both the Musculoskeletal System and Nervous System sections are required when reporting services performed on the spine.
8. Describe the purpose of the common spinal procedures: discectomy, decompression, corpectomy, and laminectomy.

This chapter presents the anatomical structures, common surgically treated conditions, and surgical techniques of the CPT Endocrine System and Nervous System sections. These body organs/systems are grouped in the 60000 code range and are related because each is responsible for processing sensory information. Together they allow us to sense and react to our environment through vision, hearing, somatic sensation (touch), taste, and olfaction (smell)—all of which are controlled by the nervous system.

ENDOCRINE SYSTEM: ANATOMY AND CODING ISSUES

The Endocrine System section represents codes for procedures that involve the glands that release their hormones directly into the bloodstream. The ductless glands regulate body functions by secreting their hormones in response to the body's needs and regulating growth, development, mood, and metabolism. The endocrine system glands are the pituitary, thyroid, parathyroid, adrenal, thymus, the islet cells of the pancreas, the ovaries and testes, and the pineal gland (Fig. 25.1).

> NOTE: The codes for ovaries, testes, and pancreas are in different sections of the CPT manual. The ovaries are covered in the female genital system, the testes in the male genital system, and the pancreas in the digestive system section.

Anatomy

The pituitary gland is located at the base of the brain and hangs from a slender stalk that connects with the hypothalamus, which lies above it. It regulates growth, metabolism, milk production, and uterine contractions in pregnant women. Cushing's disease is caused by overproduction of the pituitary hormone adrenocorticotropic hormone (ACTH). This hormone then travels to the adrenal glands, causing them to produce excessive amounts of the steroid hormone cortisol, which leads to many different health problems including the decreased ability to fight infection and difficulties with the body's metabolism. Gigantism is another pituitary gland disorder. If the pituitary produces too much growth hormone, a child's bones and body parts may grow abnormally fast. Conversely, too little growth hormone will cause a child to stop growing in height.

The thyroid is in the lower neck sitting to the right and left of the trachea with an isthmus that lies over the trachea connecting both sides; each side is a thyroid lobe. The thyroid produces two hormones that control metabolism and growth by controlling how the body uses energy and makes proteins: triiodothyronine (T_3) and thyroxine (T_4). If the thyroid produces too much of these thyroid hormones (hyperthyroidism), the result is weight loss, a fast heart rate, sweating, and nervousness. One of the most common causes of an overactive thyroid is Graves' disease. When the thyroid does not produce enough hormones (hypothyroidism), the result is fatigue, dry skin, constipation, depression, and, for some, weight gain.

The parathyroid glands (four) are located on the back surface of the thyroid lobes. These glands control calcium levels, which play a role in bone development, and they control

Figure 25.1 The endocrine system.

From Thompson, G. *Understanding Anatomy & Physiology: A Visual, Auditory, Interactive Approach*, F.A. Davis Company, 2013.

phosphate levels in the blood. The parathyroid hormone is referred to as *parathormone* or *parathyrin (PTH)*.

The adrenal glands sit on top of each kidney. They control carbohydrate metabolism and blood glucose levels and release stress hormones, including cortisol and norepinephrine. The adrenal glands can also restrict the inflammatory process. Too little cortisol causes symptoms such as fatigue, stomach upset, dehydration, and skin changes.

The pancreas is near the lower part of the stomach and its islet cells secrete the insulin and glucagon hormones. These are the hormones that regulate blood glucose levels. The pancreas also has a digestive function of secreting enzymes to the small intestine. One of the most common endocrine disorders is diabetes, which is caused by a breakdown in the production of insulin from the pancreas.

The *carotid body* is not an endocrine gland but CPT locates it in the endocrine section (60600–60605). It is in the neck at the bifurcation or split of the common carotid artery into the internal and external carotid arteries. It helps regulate breathing and blood pressure by detecting changes in the composition of arterial blood flowing through it, mainly the partial pressure of oxygen, but also of carbon dioxide. Furthermore, it is sensitive to changes in pH and temperature.

The ovaries secrete estrogen, progesterone, and testosterone, all of which are released directly into the bloodstream and are responsible for the appearance and maintenance of the reproductive organs in women. Progesterone prepares the uterus for pregnancy and the mammary glands for lactation.

The testes have two functions, to secrete sperm and testosterone. Testosterone is important to the first stages of developing the male reproductive organs in a fetus. It also causes the growth of facial hair, deepening of the voice, and the growth spurt that takes place during puberty. Testosterone is important in maintaining these male characteristics throughout a man's life. From puberty onward, testosterone provides the main stimulus for sperm production.

The thymus is behind the sternum and in front of the heart. It secretes several thymosin and thymopoietin hormones that control the immune function and produce T lymphocytes, or T cells, which are white blood cells. Their function is to help the body fight disease and harmful substances.

The pineal gland is located in the brain above the cerebellum. It produces melatonin, which regulates sleep patterns and stimulates the body's smooth muscle contraction and also inhibits gastric secretions.

Coding Issues

For thyroid gland coding, pay attention to the terminology in the code descriptions. In code 60210, the description indicates a partial lobectomy, unilateral, with or without isthmusectomy. This refers to one side of the thyroid, either the right or left, and only part of the lobe is removed. Code 60212 then indicates partial lobectomy, unilateral with contralateral subtotal lobectomy, including isthmusectomy. If code 60212 is reported, it represents a partial removal of one lobe of the thyroid, with a subtotal removal of the lobe on the opposite side. *Contralateral* refers to the opposite side, and it includes removing the isthmus. If both lobes of the thyroid are removed, CPT designates that as a total or complete thyroidectomy (60240). The remaining codes specify total or subtotal for malignancy, removal of all remaining thyroid tissue after previous removal of part of the thyroid, and then thyroidectomy based on specific approaches.

The parathyroid, thymus, adrenal glands, pancreas, and carotid body codes are grouped together based on removal or exploration, and approach. The last code in this section represents a laparoscopic adrenalectomy.

NERVOUS SYSTEM ANATOMY

The nervous system consists of the central nervous system (CNS), peripheral nervous system, and the autonomic nervous system. The nervous system basically is the body's "electrical system" and consists of wiring, fuses, transmitters, junctions, and a fuse box. The CNS is comprised of the brain, spinal cord, and retina. The brain is considered the fuse box or the switchboard of the body. The brain and spinal cord are cushioned by layers of membranes called *meninges* and cerebrospinal fluid (CSF). CSF helps protect nerve tissue and maintain its health by removing waste products. The meninges comprise three layers: The inner layer is the pia mater, the middle layer is the arachnoid, and the outer layer (the strongest of the three) is the dura mater. These layers will be important to the coder when terms such as *intradural*, *extradural*, and *subarachnoid* are used in surgery on the brain.

The brain is made up of the cerebrum (forebrain), midbrain, and cerebellum (hindbrain). The cerebrum is the largest and most complex of the section and contains the information that is unique to us: our intelligence, memory, personality, emotion, speech, senses, and ability to move. Specific areas (lobes) of the cerebrum process the various types of information received: frontal, parietal, temporal, and occipital.

The outer layer of the cerebrum is called the *cortex* (also known as "gray matter"). Information collected by the five senses comes into the brain from the spinal cord to the cortex. This information is then directed to other parts of the nervous system for further processing.

INTERNET RESOURCE: Visit www.pbs.org/wnet/brain/3d/index.html to view a three-dimensional tour of the brain.

Within the cerebrum are the thalamus, hypothalamus, and pituitary gland. The thalamus carries messages from the sensory organs such as the nose to the cortex. The hypothalamus controls the pulse, thirst, appetite, sleep patterns, and other autonomic functions. Signals are sent to the pituitary gland, which releases hormones that control growth, metabolism, digestion, and so forth.

The cerebellum, pons, and medulla (hindbrain) sit underneath the back of the cerebrum and are responsible for balance and movement. The pons and the medulla are referred to as the *brainstem*. The brainstem is the link to the spinal cord and mother board of the body receiving, sending, and coordinating all of the brain's messages. Another important area is the tentorium, an extension of the dura mater that separates the cerebellum from the occipital lobes of the brain. Documentation for many of the procedures throughout the nervous system section will refer to *supratentorial* or *infratentorial*, meaning the procedure is being done above the tentorium or below the tentorium, respectively.

The spinal cord contains bundles of both sensory and motor nerves. The sensory nerves send and receive signals about pain, temperature, and position of the body to the brain. Motor nerves transmit messages from the brain to the body to control movement.

The peripheral nervous system is comprised of cranial nerves, spinal nerves, and peripheral nerves. As would be expected, cranial nerves are located in the head and neck region. The 12 cranial nerves are commonly referred to by Roman numerals. For example, the seventh cranial nerve—CN VII—is the facial nerve that sends signals to the muscles that control facial expression. The autonomic nervous system is part of the peripheral nervous system and is responsible for controlling body functions we don't need to think about, such as breathing, heartbeat, digestion, sweating, and shivering. The autonomic nervous system has two parts: the sympathetic and the parasympathetic nervous systems.

Refer to an anatomy reference or an online site to view detailed images of the nervous system and nerve groups.

The sympathetic nervous system prepares the body for sudden stress, such as seeing a robbery taking place. When something frightening happens, the sympathetic nervous system makes the heart beat faster so that it can send blood more quickly to the different body parts that might need it. It also causes the adrenal glands at the top of the kidneys to release adrenaline, a hormone that helps give extra power to the muscles for a quick getaway. This process is known as the body's "fight-or-flight" response.

The parasympathetic nervous system does the exact opposite: It prepares the body for rest. It also helps the food move through the digestive tract so our bodies can efficiently take in nutrients from the food we eat.

INTERNET RESOURCE: Visit the University of Washington's Neuroscience for Kids website to learn more about the autonomic nervous system. https://faculty.washington.edu/chudler/auto.html

Spinal nerves are located bilaterally along the length of the spinal cord. Each of the spinal nerves is attached to the spinal cord by spinal nerve roots. Each spinal nerve root has two segments—the dorsal root and the ventral root. The dorsal root is attached to the back of the spinal cord and carries the sensory nerves. The ventral root is attached near the front of the spinal cord and carries the motor nerves. In some areas of the body, several spinal nerve roots join to form a network called a *plexus*—for example, the brachial plexus that innervates the arms and the celiac plexus that innervates the abdominal cavity.

Peripheral nerves, shown in Figure 25.2, supply tissues with sensory and motor fibers. These are the nerves outside the CNS. These include 12 pairs of cranial nerves, 32 pairs of spinal nerves, and sensory, sympathetic, and parasympathetic nerves. Common peripheral nerves that undergo treatment are listed in Table 25.1.

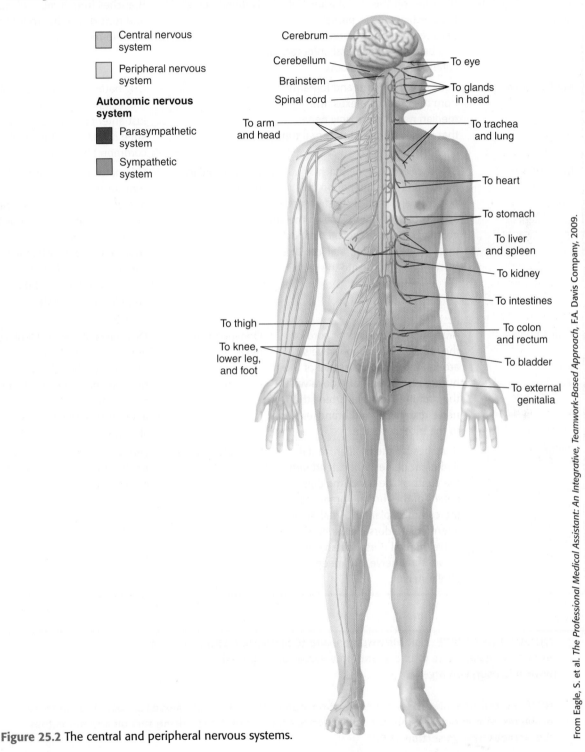

Figure 25.2 The central and peripheral nervous systems.

From Eagle, S. et al. *The Professional Medical Assistant: An Integrative, Teamwork-Based Approach*, F.A. Davis Company, 2009.

Table 25.1 Peripheral Nerves

NERVE NAME	LOCATION	NERVE NAME	LOCATION
Axillary nerve	Branches off the posterior aspect of the brachial plexus axilla (armpit) and carries nerve fibers from C5 and C6	Ilioinguinal nerve	Originates from first lumbar root and passes around posterior abdominal wall, travels under external oblique, enters inguinal canal, and descends to supply sensation to skin of scrotum and root of penis
Musculocutaneous nerve	Branches off the lateral aspect of the brachial plexus, passes between biceps and brachialis, and becomes the lateral antebrachial cutaneous nerve at elbow	Femoral nerve	Branches from lumbar plexus and runs down the front of the thigh to medial side of foot
Median nerve	Runs down the arm and forearm from the brachial plexus; the median nerve is the only nerve that passes through the carpal tunnel	Sciatic nerve	Originates from the sacral plexus and extends into posterior thigh; just anterior to the back of the knee it splits into the tibial and common fibular nerves
Ulnar nerve	Branches off from the brachial plexus, and runs inferior on the posterior and medial (posteromedial) aspects of the humerus down the arm, going behind the medial epicondyle, through the cubital tunnel into the forearm and finally into the palm	Suprascapular nerve	Originates from C5 and C6 nerve roots of the brachial plexus, passes through the suprascapular notch into the supraspinous fossa where it supplies the supraspinatus muscle, then continues around the lateral border of the spine of the scapular to supply the infraspinatus as well
Radial nerve	Arises from the posterior cord of the brachial plexus and travels around the posterior aspect of the humerus in the spiral groove with the profunda brachial artery; the nerve distributes and branches here to the triceps muscle	Iliohypogastric nerve	Originates at the L1–L2 plexus and penetrates the transversalis muscle and then the internal oblique and external oblique muscle groups; it supplies anterior cutaneous branch to skin of suprapubic region
Digital nerve	Branches off the median, radial, and ulnar nerves that extend into the digits of the hand; the digital nerves of the foot are branches of the common plantar digital nerve, intermediate dorsal cutaneous nerve, medial dorsal cutaneous nerve, sural nerve, and deep fibular nerve	Intercostal nerve	Divisions of the thoracic spinal nerves from T1 to T11 located between the ribs

INTERNET RESOURCE: Visit Microsurgeon.org to learn more about the anatomy of nerves, those prone to injury, and how nerves are repaired. www.microsurgeon.org

NOTE: Procedure codes for nerve conduction studies used to assess nerve function and diagnose problems with nerve transmission and speed are located in the Medicine section and not within the Nervous System section of CPT.

The spinal cord is located in the vertebral foramen (spinal canal) and protected by the vertebrae. It is 40 to 50 cm long and 1 to 1.5 cm in diameter. It does not run the entire length of the spine, ending at about the first or second lumbar vertebrae. The spinal cord consists of white matter in the periphery, gray matter inside, and at the center of the canal is a tube filled with CSF (Fig. 25.3). Nerve roots emerge on each of its sides. These nerve roots join distally to form 31 pairs of spinal nerves.

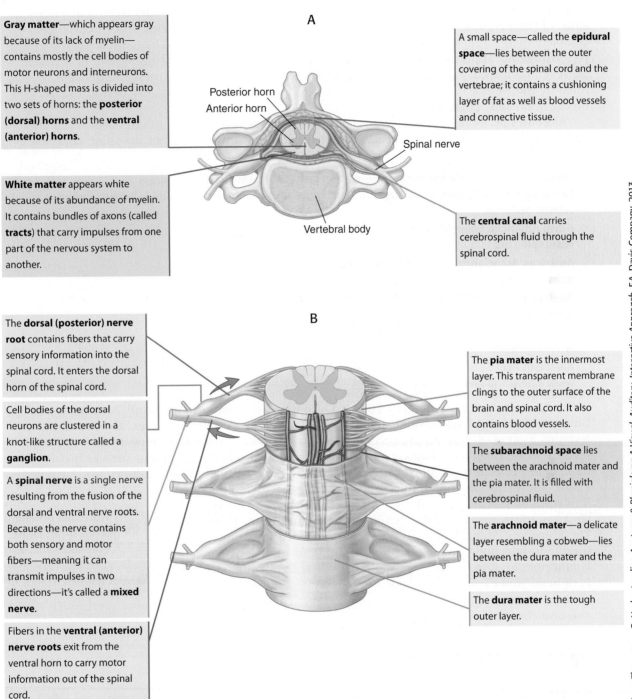

Gray matter—which appears gray because of its lack of myelin—contains mostly the cell bodies of motor neurons and interneurons. This H-shaped mass is divided into two sets of horns: the **posterior (dorsal) horns** and the **ventral (anterior) horns**.

White matter appears white because of its abundance of myelin. It contains bundles of axons (called **tracts**) that carry impulses from one part of the nervous system to another.

A small space—called the **epidural space**—lies between the outer covering of the spinal cord and the vertebrae; it contains a cushioning layer of fat as well as blood vessels and connective tissue.

The **central canal** carries cerebrospinal fluid through the spinal cord.

Posterior horn
Anterior horn
Spinal nerve
Vertebral body

A

The **dorsal (posterior) nerve root** contains fibers that carry sensory information into the spinal cord. It enters the dorsal horn of the spinal cord.

Cell bodies of the dorsal neurons are clustered in a knot-like structure called a **ganglion**.

A **spinal nerve** is a single nerve resulting from the fusion of the dorsal and ventral nerve roots. Because the nerve contains both sensory and motor fibers—meaning it can transmit impulses in two directions—it's called a **mixed nerve**.

Fibers in the **ventral (anterior) nerve roots** exit from the ventral horn to carry motor information out of the spinal cord.

The **pia mater** is the innermost layer. This transparent membrane clings to the outer surface of the brain and spinal cord. It also contains blood vessels.

The **subarachnoid space** lies between the arachnoid mater and the pia mater. It is filled with cerebrospinal fluid.

The **arachnoid mater**—a delicate layer resembling a cobweb—lies between the dura mater and the pia mater.

The **dura mater** is the tough outer layer.

B

Figure 25.3 The spinal cord.

From Thompson, G. *Understanding Anatomy & Physiology: A Visual, Auditory, Interactive Approach*, F.A. Davis Company, 2013.

NERVOUS SYSTEM ORGANIZATION

The Nervous System section covers many procedures on the skull, meninges, brain, spine, spinal cord, and nerves. Some of the procedures in this section are accomplished endoscopically; however, most of them are carried out by open technique. The Nervous System section is not exclusively reserved to reporting for neurologists or neurosurgeons. Orthopedic surgeons and anesthesiologists also commonly report codes from this section.

A neurologist is a medical doctor specifically trained in the diagnosis and treatment of diseases of the nervous system including the brain, spinal cord, and muscles. Once neurologists complete their training, they are certified by the American Board of Psychiatry and Neurology. Neurosurgeons are also trained in the diagnosis and treatment of nervous system disorders; however, their focus is on the surgical treatment of these diseases or injuries, and they are certified by the American Association of Neurological Surgeons. They primarily perform surgery on the brain and spinal column.

Procedures performed on the bony spinal column are performed by both orthopedic surgeons and neurosurgeons. Some orthopedic surgeons specialize in procedures of the spine and pain management.

> **INTERNET RESOURCES:** For coding information, ask physicians to provide access to the appropriate professional organization. Some sites require membership to access coding-related material.
> **North American Spine Society**
> www.spine.org
> **American Association of Neurological Surgeons**
> www.aans.org
> **American Academy of Orthopaedic Surgeons (AAOS)**
> www.aaos.org
> **American Academy of Pain Management**
> www.aapainmanage.org
> **American Pain Society**
> www.americanpainsociety.org

The Nervous System section is subdivided into three main subsections: Skull, Meninges, and Brain; the Spine and Spinal Cord; and Extracranial Nerves, Peripheral Nerves, and Autonomic Nervous System. Subheadings in this section do not follow a standard repeatable format as seen in previous surgery chapters. Some of the familiar headings are present such as Incision, Repair, and Introduction; however, each subsection has its own unique subsections. For example, the Skull, Meninges, and Brain section is further subdivided into sections specific to craniectomy, skull base surgery, neurostimulator insertions (intracranial), aneurysm repair, and shunt insertions. The Spine and Spinal Cord subsection is subdivided into subsections specific to injections, stereotaxis, neurostimulator insertions (spinal), laminectomies, nerve injections, and repairs. The Extracranial Nerves, Peripheral Nerves, and Autonomic Nervous System subsection is categorized by nerve type—Somatic Nerves, Paravertebral Spinal Nerves and Branches, and Autonomic Nerves.

> Procedures performed on the spine may require codes from both the Musculoskeletal System and Nervous System sections of CPT.

PROCEDURES OF THE SKULL AND BRAIN

Several methods are used to access the skull or brain in order to provide treatment: a twist drill, burr holes, trephine, craniotomy, and craniectomy. The twist drill is used to perforate the skull to gain access to the epidural and subdural spaces and the brain. The twist drill can be preset to penetrate no further than the expected thickness of the skull. A burr hole is surgically placed in the skull to allow for a procedure to be done such as allowing a catheter to be placed for drainage. A trephine is a surgical instrument with a circular blade used to create an opening in the skull. Craniotomy and craniectomy are surgical incisions into the skull and are more extensive than the twist drill, burr hole, or trephine. The craniotomy usually results in a bone flap through which the surgeon can operate, whereas a craniectomy involves the removal of a portion of the skull. As you review codes 61105–61576, you will see all these methods in the code descriptions; however, it is important to watch for three pieces of information about each code to accurately report services:

1. Method
2. Purpose
3. Location

For example, for code 61304, *Craniectomy or craniotomy, exploratory; supratentorial*, the method is craniectomy or craniotomy, the purpose is exploratory, and the location is supratentorial. Another example is code 61343, *Craniectomy, suboccipital with cervical laminectomy for decompression of medulla and spinal cord, with or without dural graft*. The method is craniectomy with cervical laminectomy with or without dural graft, the purpose is decompression of medulla and spinal cord, and the location is suboccipital. The nervous system codes related to the skull and brain can become complex, and using this method will assist coders in determining which code most accurately reflects the physician's services.

SKULL BASE SURGERY

The skull base, despite what one may envision as the brain stem, is actually the point of contact between the brain and the floor of the cranium or skull. Contained within the skull base are the following:

- Eye orbits
- Ear canals
- Two carotid arteries
- Two vertebral arteries
- Twelve cranial nerves
- Blood drainage system of the brain

Skull base surgery covers a wide variety of operations, including those on the brain stem where the brain and neck meet. Several surgical techniques can be used to perform skull base surgery, including open surgery and minimally invasive procedures. In open surgery, various surgical approaches are available (craniofascial, orbitocranial, bicoronal, infratemporal, transcochlear, transcondylar, transpetrosal, etc.) where incisions are made in the head (cranium) and/or face, and a small amount of bone is removed to allow access to the area. Minimally invasive techniques, such as endoscopic surgery, enable access through the nose and sinuses using smaller incisions, reducing pain, infection, and postoperative complications.

The skull base has three distinct areas:

- Anterior—the area in front of the ears and behind the eyes and sinuses
- Middle—the area above the ears
- Posterior—the area located behind the ears and above the spine

Skull base surgery is performed to treat brain tumors, pituitary tumors, and vascular lesions such as aneurysms, arteriovenous malformations (AVMs), and fistulas. The codes in this section are divided into stages of the procedure: (1) approach, (2) definitive procedure, and (3) repair/reconstruction. The codes for the approach procedure are differentiated by the anatomical area being accessed (i.e., cranial fossa, middle cranial fossa, posterior cranial fossa, brain stem, or upper spinal cord). Definitive procedure codes describe the surgical intervention: biopsy, repair, resection, or excision. The repair codes are reported separately only if there is extensive repair performed to describe dural grafting, skin grafts, myocutaneous pedicle flaps, and cranioplasty. Not all skull base procedures will require repair or reconstruction. To report primary closures, consider reporting 15733 or 15756–15758.

This type of surgery may involve the work of multiple surgeons from different specialties such as neurosurgery, otolaryngology (ENT), and plastic surgery. Each surgeon reports the stage of the procedure personally performed. Dividing the procedures into stages makes reporting for multiple surgeons clearer. If a surgeon only performs the approach, then only one code from the Approach Procedures subsections (61580–61598) is reported. If a surgeon performs more than one stage (approach and definitive), the code is reported using the –51 modifier on the second.

> ■ **CASE SCENARIO**
> A patient is diagnosed with a meningioma at the base of the middle cranial fossa, in the midline skull base, extradural. The necessary approach for removal of this neoplasm was infratemporal and preauricular including parotidectomy. It was determined that an otolaryngologist should provide the approach and a neurosurgeon should provide the definitive procedure. Report code 61590 for the otolaryngologist and 61607 for the neurosurgeon.

In this example, a coder might question if a modifier is needed. In skull base surgery when more than one surgeon provides a stage of the procedure, no modifier is used. Do not report co-surgery (–62); do not report multiple procedure (–51) or team surgery (–66). The multiple surgery modifier is used only when one surgeon does both the approach and the definitive procedures.

Endovascular Therapy

Codes 61623–61651 represent endovascular procedures, meaning "within" (endo) the blood vessels. Coders will see extensive coding instructions associated with code 61623 versus code 61624 that attempt to provide the applicable inclusions and exclusions, but they can be confusing. Table 25.2 assists in clarifying any confusion. In code 61623, the surgeon is providing temporary balloon occlusion (blockage) of an artery in the head or neck. This is commonly done to prevent bleeding in an extracranial or intracranial artery. Bleeding into the brain is a dangerous condition. In code 61624, the occlusion is permanent.

Surgery for Aneurysm, Arteriovenous Malformation, or Vascular Disease

An aneurysm is a weakening of the arterial wall that allows blood to pool in the artery, causing pressure and leading to rupture. An AVM occurs when arteries and veins become entangled, causing disruption in the flow of blood. Again, watching for methodology, purpose, and location will assist in the coding process. For example, in code 61680 the method is generic "surgery," the purpose is to treat an arteriovenous malformation, and the location is intracranial and then more specifically supratentorial or above the tentorium.

Carefully review the notes associated with codes 61697 and 61698. CPT is clarifying what circumstances define a complex intracranial aneurysm as opposed to a simple intracranial aneurysm. If the documentation does not meet the definition of complex, coders must choose the simple intracranial codes 61680–61692.

Stereotactic Radiosurgery

Codes 61796–61800 represent services to inactivate or eradicate defined targets in the head without making an incision by using high-resolution stereotactic imaging. The neurosurgeon reports the radiosurgery codes and headframe application:

- These services include planning, dosimetry, targeting, positioning, and blocking performed by the neurosurgeon.
- These codes also include computer-assisted planning and application of the stereotactic frame. Do not report code 20660 with these codes.
- Do not report codes 77427–77435 for the neurosurgeon; instead report 61800 with 61796 and 61798.
- Codes 77427–77435 represent radiation oncology treatment management sessions. Those services are included in the 61796–61799 series for the neurosurgeon.

Table 25.2 Endovascular Therapy

61623	61624–61626	61630	61635	61640–61642
Endovascular temporary balloon arterial occlusion	Transcatheter permanent occlusion or embolization	Intracranial balloon angioplasty, percutaneous	Transcatheter placement of intravascular stent(s)	Balloon dilation of intracranial vasospasm, percutaneous
Includes selective catheterization of occluded vessel	Use 75894 for RSI*	Includes selective catheterization of target area	Includes balloon angioplasty	Includes all selective vascular catheterization of target vessel
Includes positioning and inflating the balloon		Includes diagnostic imaging for arteriography of target area	Includes diagnostic imaging for arteriography of target area	Includes contrast injection(s), vessel measurement, roadmapping, postdilation angiography, and fluoroscopic guidance
Includes neurological monitoring				
Includes RSI* for the angiography needed for the balloon occlusion		Includes RSI* for targeted area	Includes RSI* for targeted area	
Includes RSI* for the angiography needed to prevent vascular injury after the occlusion		If diagnostic imaging indicates the need for angioplasty or stent, codes 61630 and 61635 will include the diagnostic imaging and selective catheterization	If diagnostic imaging indicates the need for angioplasty or stent, codes 61630 and 61635 will include the diagnostic imaging and selective catheterization	
		If diagnostic imaging does not indicate the need for angioplasty or stent, report the diagnostic imaging codes. Do not report 61630 or 61635.		

*RSI = radiological supervision and interpretation.

Radiosurgery is most commonly done in a single planning and treatment session, but it can also be done in more than one session:

- Do not report the code more than once per lesion per course of treatment even when the treatment requires more than one session.
- In effect, these codes are assigned per lesion regardless of the number of sessions.

Codes 61796, 61797 equal simple lesions and are as follows:

- Less than 3.5 cm in maximum dimension and/or do not meet the definition of a complex lesion

Codes 61798, 61799 equal complex lesions and are as follows:

- 3.5 cm or greater, or
- Schwannomas, AVMs, glomus tumors, pineal region tumors, cavernous sinus/parasellar/petroclival tumors or
- Any lesion adjacent (within 5 mm) to the optic nerve/optic chasm/optic tract or within the brain stem

Code 61798 is also used for procedures to create therapeutic lesions. When reporting the procedures to create therapeutic lesions, report 61798 only once regardless of the number of lesions created. The radiation oncologist reports the following:

- Clinical treatment planning
- Physics
- Dosimetry
- Treatment delivery
- Treatment management
- Codes 77261–77790

CHECKPOINT 25.1

Assign codes to the following procedures. Include any necessary modifiers. In some cases, more than one code is required.

1. A 63-year-old female patient fell 2 weeks ago and struck her head on a coffee table. She did not lose consciousness but has had headaches and some dizziness. A CT scan showed a subdural hematoma. A burr hole was placed and the hematoma was evacuated. _____

2. A patient has a primary neoplasm in the ethmoid sinus and, due to the many risks associated with this surgery, the craniofacial extradural approach without maxillectomy including lateral rhinotomy will be performed by an otolaryngologist. The definitive procedure, an intradural excision including dural repair of the neoplasm at the base of the anterior cranial fossa, will be performed by a neurosurgeon. _____

3. A coder is attempting to provide the correct code for an endovascular temporary balloon occlusion of an intracranial artery. The surgeon has indicated that the procedure code for the surgery is 61623 and has asked the coder to add a code for the selective catheterization and the RSI for the angiography. The coder is hesitant to do this based on the CPT code description. Is the coder correct? _____

4. Because of an aneurysm in the carotid artery, the surgeon performed intracranial and cervical occlusion of the carotid. _____

5. A 3.5-cm cranial lesion was treated with stereotactic radiosurgery (gamma ray). Report the code(s) for the neurosurgeon. _____

COMMON NERVE CONDITIONS REQUIRING TREATMENT

The nervous system, like any other, is vulnerable to disease and injury, such as trauma, degeneration, infection, autoimmune disorders, and congenital malformations. Acquired structural conditions affecting the nerves, spine, and brain require surgical intervention. Examples are brain or spinal cord injury, Bell's palsy, cervical spondylosis, carpal tunnel syndrome, brain or spinal cord tumors, peripheral neuropathy, and Guillain-Barré syndrome.

Nerve Pain

Neuralgia, or nerve pain, indicates that there is pain in the area fed by one or more nerves. Nerve pain is typically caused by neuritis (inflammation of a peripheral nerve), radiculitis (inflammation of the spinal nerve root), nerve palsy, trauma, or compression. Common treatment of nerve pain consists of neurolysis, nerve block, neuroplasty, neurorrhaphy, and decompression.

Neurolysis

Neurolysis (64702–64726) involves injecting a nerve with a neurolytic agent (e.g., alcohol, phenol, iced saline, ethanol) to destroy the nerve. It is performed in patients with chronic pain, patients with cerebral palsy, and those who have spasms. If fluoroscopic guidance is performed, use code 77003. When internal neurolysis requiring the use of an operating microscope is performed, use add-on code 64727 (do not report the operating microscope code 69990 in addition to +64727).

Nerve Blocks

Nerve blocks relieve pain by interrupting pain sensory pathways and preventing them from reaching the brain. Nerve blocks are performed on peripheral nerves for pain management purposes. The nerves are injected with a mixture of steroids and anesthetics. For example, the greater occipital nerve is injected for chronic or ongoing headaches. Injections are also performed in the sympathetic nerves (stellate ganglions) for analgesia. The goal of these injections is to reduce inflammation and produce anesthesia.

Nine types of nerve blocks are commonly used for pain management:

- *Trigger point injection*—injection of local anesthetic/steroid mixture in the muscle where pain is present (Trigger point injections are not truly nerve blocks; rather, they are muscle blocks.)
- *Epidural steroid injection*—injection of a small amount of anesthetic/steroid mixture near nerves in the cervical or lumbar spine
- *Facet joint injection*—injection of a small amount of anesthetic/steroid mixture near facet joints
- *Stellate ganglion block*—injection of anesthetic/steroid mixture around a group of nerves in the neck area
- *Lumbar sympathetic block*—an injection of anesthetic/steroid mixture around a group of nerves in the lumbar area
- *Intercostal nerve block*—an injection of anesthetic/steroid mixture in the area between the ribs
- *Occipital nerve block*—an injection of anesthetic/steroid mixture at the base of the skull
- *Ilioinguinal nerve block*—an injection of anesthetic/steroid mixture medial to the hip bone to treat groin and abdominal pain
- *Celiac plexus*—injection of anesthetic/steroid mixture into the celiac plexus, which is situated retroperitoneally in the upper abdomen at the level of the T12 and L1 vertebrae

These nerve blocks are not to be confused with blocks used as anesthesia for surgical procedures.

Accurate needle placement is achieved by using fluoroscopic guidance. In difficult cases where the anatomy might be distorted, CT guidance is used.

Refer to Table 25.3 to assist in assigning the appropriate injection code by determining the substance injected.

Table 25.3 Substances Injected for Pain Management

ANESTHETICS	NEUROLYTIC AGENTS	STEROIDS
Lidocaine (Xylocaine)	Alcohol	Aristocort
Bupivacaine (Marcaine, Sensorcaine)	Phenol	Kenalog
Naropin	Iced saline	Aristospan
Duramorph	Ethanol	Depo-Medrol
	Butyl aminobenzoate (Butamben)	Solu-Medrol
		Methylprednisolone

Nerve Blocks for Postoperative Pain. Nerve blocks are not only used for chronic pain therapy but also for postoperative pain management. Coders need to be diligent in reading the operative report and differentiating the nerve blocks used as anesthesia to conduct the procedure versus that used as a postoperative pain control method. Coders should report a code from 64400–64450 when the physician uses a nerve block for postoperative pain management. Nerve blocks are short-term analgesia, which means they are best performed after the procedure is completed and not as a choice for completing the procedure itself. To report a nerve block for the purposes of postoperative pain control, the physician must document that the use of the injection or nerve block was specifically for postoperative pain relief, not the mode of anesthesia for the surgery. A –59 modifier should be appended to the postoperative injection code. Pain management procedures described before, during, or at the end of the operative note performed in conjunction with the operative anesthesia may be additionally reported from the 64400–64530 series in these situations:

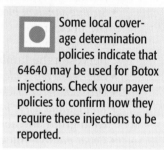
Do not confuse nerve blocks with neurolysis. Look to see what substance is injected and for what purpose before assigning codes.

- The pain management procedure is not the operative anesthesia being utilized for the operative procedure.
- It is administered pre-, inter-, or post-op for the *purpose of pain management*. This must be clearly documented.

Spastic Conditions

Spasticity is found in conditions where the brain and/or spinal cord is damaged by acute injury or disease process or fails to develop normally, as can occur with cerebral palsy, multiple sclerosis, spinal cord injury, and brain injury, including stroke. In spasticity, patients are unable to control the affected muscles, and muscles become stiff and contracted. Chemodenervation is performed to provide relief and relax the muscle. The muscle's nerve supply is disabled by injecting a chemical substance. This is also commonly carried out for treatment of blepharospasm, hemifacial spasm, focal dystonias, migraines, and spastic conditions. Coders should select the chemodenervation code that most accurately describes the anatomical area injected—facial muscles, neck muscles, or extremities/trunk. Botulinum toxin (Botox) is a common choice of substance to inject. The relaxation of the muscles and reduced appearance of wrinkles is affected by blocking impulses from nerves to the small facial muscles that control expression. It does not matter how many injections are performed or how many muscles are injected; the code is only assigned once per session. Currently, codes 64612–64616 and 64642–64647 are used to report botulinum toxin injections. If the physician is also supplying the medication, you should also assign the HCPCS code for the drug.

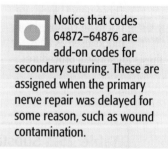
Some local coverage determination policies indicate that 64640 may be used for Botox injections. Check your payer policies to confirm how they require these injections to be reported.

Nerve Injury

Nerves are fragile and can be damaged by pressure, stretching, or cutting. Pressure or stretching injuries can cause the fibers carrying the information to break and stop the nerve from working, without disrupting the insulating cover. When a nerve is cut, both the nerve and the insulation are broken. Injury to a nerve can stop the transmission of signals to and from the brain, preventing muscles from working and causing loss of feeling in the area supplied by that nerve.

Notice that codes 64872–64876 are add-on codes for secondary suturing. These are assigned when the primary nerve repair was delayed for some reason, such as wound contamination.

Nerve Repair (Neurorrhaphy)

Nerve repair can be accomplished by suturing, wrapping, or grafting of the nerve. Neurorrhaphy, or suturing, of the nerve is done by splicing the nerve endings together. This is achievable if there isn't a large gap between the two endings. When assigning codes for neurorrhaphy, the coder must determine the nerve repaired, the site, the number of nerves repaired, and whether the repair is a primary or secondary repair.

Nerve Graft. Nerves are made up of many fibers called axons. Some of the fibers are sensory to allow feeling, while others are motor stimulating for movement of muscles. The body's natural healing process starts when a nerve is injured. The fibers will grow out of the nerve ending and attempt to grow across to the severed nerve ending. Nerves can regenerate about 1 mm a day. However, sometimes the gap between the two nerve endings is too great and the nerve cannot grow across. When the gap is too large, a nerve graft may be required. There are three types of nerve grafts: autograft (64885–64907, 64911), artificial conduit (64910), and allograft (64912, 64913). Autografts are performed by harvesting portions of a sensory nerve from another part of the patient's body to be used as graft (vein, muscle). Muscle grafts consist of taking a sliver of muscle from a donor site that is snap-frozen. The freezing kills the muscle but the structure remains intact to allow the nerves to grow across, similar to a trellis. Artificial conduit grafts look like plastic tubing whereby the nerve ends are placed into the tube, allowing the fibers to grow through it, similar to a viaduct. An allograft is nerve tissue obtained from another human (cadaver). Allografts are often chosen when the area to repair is large or multiple repairs are needed. The advantages of using allografts is that no defect remains from the patient's donor site and, because allografts are human nerves, the body is less likely to reject the graft as it might with the artificial conduit. Once the graft is in place, the regenerating nerve fibers grow from the nerve stump, through the graft, through the distal nerve segment into the target muscles. Without grafting, patients may never recover function in muscles following a nerve injury. To select a code for nerve graft, you must determine the following:

- The type of graft used
- Whether the length of the nerve graft is less than or equal to 4 cm or greater than 4 cm
    - Whether the graft has single or multiple strands
    - The site

○ Do not assign a separate code for obtaining the graft because it is included in the nerve graft code description.

EXAMPLE

64890 *Nerve graft (includes obtaining graft), single strand, hand or foot; up to 4 cm length*

If more than one nerve is repaired by grafting, even if the nerves are bilateral, assign 64901–64902 instead of modifier –50 to describe nerve grafts placed bilaterally. The physician fee schedule does not recognize laterality for this code assignment, so submitting codes 64885–64898 with a –50 modifier would be inappropriate. You can, however, append modifiers –LT and –RT to differentiate the procedures and avoid accusations of double billing.

○ Mention of the operating microscope is a good indicator of a multiple-strand graft, but this alone is not enough to assign a code for multistrand repair. If documentation is unclear as to whether the repair was single strand or multistrand, query the surgeon before assigning a code.

Microsurgery. A microscope may be indicated when microdissection or microrepair of a nerve is required. Assign 69990 for use of the microscope in addition to the code for the procedure unless the code description already includes the use of the operating microscope. CPT and Medicare specifically allow +69990, *Microsurgical techniques, requiring use of operating microscope (list separately in addition to code for primary procedure)*, if performed with 64885–64898. Do not assign 69990 with 61548, 63075–63078, 64727, 64912, or 64913. Code 69990 should be listed separately in addition to 64831–64876.

Intraoperative Neurophysiological Monitoring

CPT guidelines explain that the neurophysiological monitoring performed with +95940, +95941 is distinct from performing baseline neurophysiological studies in the operating room during procedures. Intraoperative neurophysiological monitoring (IOM) is considered reimbursable as a separate service *only* when a licensed health-care practitioner, *other* than the operating surgeon or anesthesiologist, interprets the monitoring. The monitoring is performed by a health-care practitioner or technician who is in attendance in the operating room throughout the procedure. CPT guidelines emphasize this: "When the service is performed by the surgeon or anesthesiologist, the professional services are included in the surgeon's or anesthesiologist's primary service code(s) or the anesthesiologist's primary service code(s) for the procedure and are not reported separately."

○ Prior to performing monitoring, research payer policies and coding guidelines for IOM. Codes +95940 and +95941 are add-on codes and the primary codes listed in the parenthetical notes are for the baseline neurophysiological test (e.g., electromyography) and not surgical codes. Carriers consider monitoring with an automated device integral to the surgery performed and will not reimburse for these services separately.

Neuroplasty. Neuroplasty, or repair of the nerve, is accomplished by transposing, wrapping, or decompressing the nerve. Nerve decompression and transposition involve the freeing of an intact nerve from scar tissue or entrapment.

Wrapping is performed for revision surgeries or secondary repairs whereby a vein is harvested (primarily the saphenous vein) and is wrapped around the nerve to protect it and act as a buffer to decrease nerve sensitivity. This procedure is typically performed on the median and ulnar nerves. Wrapping can also be accomplished by using a synthetic material that acts as a conduit to avoid having to harvest a vein from the patient's leg. Pay close attention to what the nerve is wrapped in for proper code assignment.

Nerve Repair Coding Steps. To assist in assigning codes for nerve repair, refer to Pinpoint the Code 25.1.

> Nerve decompression can also be called *neurolysis* so be careful. You must read the operative note to determine if the nerve was moved or if it was injected.

PINPOINT THE CODE 25.1: Nerve Repair

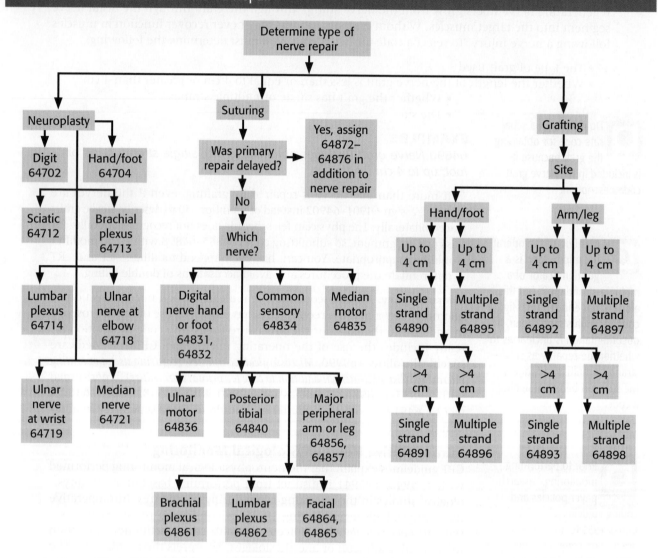

Continuous Infusion Nerve Block

Nerve blocks can be performed by a single injection, as previously described for short-term pain control, or by inserting a catheter with continuous infusion of analgesic for extended pain control. Physicians may utilize continuous infusion after surgery for pain management to help tolerate physical therapy or to allow the patient to ambulate sooner. The following codes are assigned for continuous infusion:

64416: *Injection, anesthetic agent; brachial plexus, continuous infusion by catheter (including catheter placement)*

64446: *. . . sciatic nerve, continuous infusion by catheter (including catheter placement)*

64447: *. . . femoral nerve, single*

64448: . . . femoral nerve, continuous infusion by catheter (including catheter placement)

64449: . . . lumbar plexus, posterior approach, continuous infusion by catheter (including catheter placement)

CHECKPOINT 25.2

Assign codes to the following procedures. Include any necessary modifiers. In some cases, more than one code is required.

1. A patient experiences chronic unilateral muscle spasms of the face. The patient is injected with Botox type A, 1 unit. _____

2. A patient suffers from intractable hiccups caused by his advanced lung cancer. The physician performs a phrenic nerve block. Five milliliters of 0.5% bupivacaine were injected.

   _____

3. A patient lacerates her finger on a windowsill. She follows up with her doctor and is found to have numbness in the right index finger. She is referred to a surgeon, and neuroplasty of the finger is performed. _____

4. A patient has carpal tunnel syndrome and undergoes left carpal tunnel release and left ulnar nerve decompression. _____

5. The anesthesiologist performs a bilateral femoral nerve block. Check the physician fee schedule to determine if this code is reportable as a bilateral code (see www.cms.hhs.gov/pfslookup). Choose Medicare *Physician Fee Schedule Look-up Tool, Start Search,* and then select *Payment Policy Indicators.* Enter the code for femoral nerve block. Can this code be reported with a −50 modifier?

   _____

For each of these codes, CPT clarifies that the daily hospital management code 01996 should not be reported with these services.

> ■ **CASE SCENARIO**
> A patient undergoes complete rotator cuff tear reconstruction. The physician administers an interscalene block for post-op pain control. The catheter is placed and left in for 10 days. Report code 64416.

Pain Pumps

Pain pumps are implanted either in the spine or subcutaneously for patients with chronic intractable pain, patients with pain from malignancy who have a life expectancy of greater than 3 months, or patients who have been unresponsive to less invasive therapy. The patient's medical record should state that a preliminary trial of intraspinal opioid drug administration was completed with a temporary intrathecal/epidural catheter to substantiate adequately acceptable pain relief and degree of side effects.

Pain pumps are inserted for long-term pain relief. Medication is released at a prescribed dose and rate over a period of time. External pain pump insertion following a surgical procedure for post-op, short-term pain relief is not billed separately unless it is a cardiovascular procedure. If a patient has knee surgery or shoulder surgery during which the surgeon places a pump for short-term use, the insertion of the pump cannot be billed separately, but the pump itself can be billed with a HCPCS code (E0781, E0782, E0783) to capture the cost of the supply.

The insertion of a catheter and implantation of a pump are covered by Medicare. Refer to Table 25.4.

Table 25.4 Spinal Catheters, Pumps, and Stimulators

PROCEDURE INTENT	CATHETER	PUMP	STIMULATOR
Trial	62324–cervical/thoracic 62326–lumbar/sacral	N/A	63650–without laminectomy 63655–with laminectomy
Implantation	62350–without laminectomy reservoir 62351–with laminectomy	62360–subcutaneous 62361–nonprogrammable pump 62362–programmable pump	63685–pulse generator or receiver
Revision	N/A	N/A	63663–electrode percutaneous array 63664–electrode plate/paddle 63688–revision or removal of pulse generator or receiver
Removal	62355	62365	63661–electrode percutaneous array 63662–electrode plate/paddle 63688–revision or removal of pulse generator or receiver
Analysis	N/A	62367	95970–95975
Reprogramming	N/A	62368	N/A
Refilling	N/A	62369–reprogram and refill (nonphysician or qualified provider) 62370–reprogram and refill (physician or qualified provider)	N/A

If the physician supplied the pain pump, the pump and the catheter can be reimbursed by submitting a separate claim to the durable medical equipment regional carrier (DMERC) by supplying the appropriate HCPCS supply code (i.e., E0782–E0786) for the pump and J codes for the medication used to refill the pump. Codes for the drugs used depend not only on the drug but also on the amount needed for refilling.

Spinal Neurostimulators

Neurostimulators are devices that deliver electrical impulses to a specific area of the nervous system. These impulses keep the nerve "busy" so that it is unable to send messages to the brain. Stimulators can be inserted directly into the brain, spinal cord, or nerve. Neurostimulation refers to spinal cord and peripheral nerve stimulation. Both forms of neurostimulation use an implantable neurostimulator that is surgically placed under the skin to send mild electrical impulses to the spinal cord or to a specific nerve. The electrical impulses are delivered through a lead and interfere with pain signals traveling to the brain, providing pain relief for the patient. Neurostimulators are not only used to treat patients with chronic pain but also to treat tremors, Parkinson's, paralysis, epilepsy, obesity, and depression.

Neurostimulation uses either a fully implantable neurostimulation system or an external radio-frequency system. Peripheral nerve stimulation uses an external radio-frequency system. Codes 63650–63688 describe the placement, revision, and removal of percutaneous or subcutaneous spinal neurostimulators. Codes 64553–64595 describe peripheral nerve neurostimulators.

A neurostimulator system includes an implanted neurostimulator, external controller, extension, and collection of contacts. These can be placed percutaneously or via open surgical incision. The associated CPT codes cover the placement and revision of the stimulator but require a HCPCS code to designate the supply of the implant itself. These codes do not, however, include evaluation, testing, programming, or reprogramming. To report neurostimulator insertion or revision, codes from the nervous system section and the medicine section are assigned. Codes for neurostimulator testing, programming, and so forth fall in the Medicine section.

A pulse generator is placed after the electrodes are placed and is coded separately. The use of the stimulator may begin 4 to 6 days after the implantation of the generator and electrodes. Code 63685 describes the placement of a neurostimulator pulse generator, which is attached to the electrodes. For percutaneously placed neurostimulators (63650), the contacts are on a catheter-type lead. An array is a collection of contacts on one catheter.

Neurostimulator insertion and removal codes apply to both simple and complex device components. Codes for neurostimulator analysis and programming located in the Medicine section are described as simple or complex. CPT says that a simple neurostimulator is one capable of affecting three or fewer of the following:

- Pulse amplitude
- Pulse duration
- Pulse frequency
- Eight or more electrode contacts
- Cycling
- Stimulation train duration
- Train spacing
- Number of programs
- Number of channels
- Phase angle
- Alternating electrode polarities
- Configuration of wave form
- More than one clinical feature (e.g., rigidity, dyskinesia, tremor)

A complex neurostimulator is one capable of affecting more than three of the above.

Pinpoint the Code 25.2 shows a decision tree for making neurostimulator insertion code assignments.

PINPOINT THE CODE 25.2: Spinal Neurostimulator Insertion

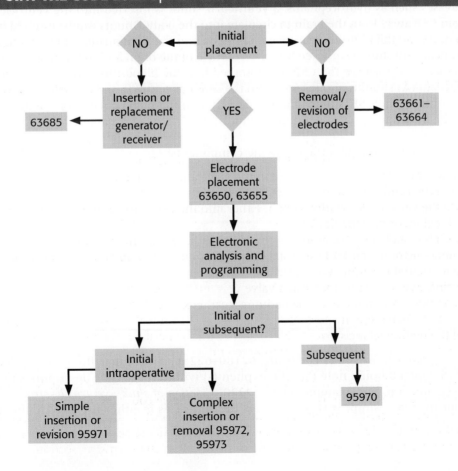

Transcutaneous Electrical Nerve Stimulation

Transcutaneous electrical nerve stimulation (TENS) (64550) is a noninvasive treatment used routinely for sprains and strains of the back and neck. Electrodes attached to a battery pack are placed on the skin to stimulate the muscles and nerves. In addition to the therapy, the coder must also capture the HCPCS code for the actual unit: E0720, E0730, A4595. The surface (transcutaneous) neurostimulator can be used on any body site, unlike the percutaneous implantation of neurostimulator electrodes (PENS). During a PENS procedure, the physician introduces needles through the skin to place electrode arrays over the sensory nerves to decrease pain. (64553, 64555, 64561, 64999).

Blood Patch

A blood patch is performed to treat the effects of spinal fluid leakage following a lumbar puncture or epidural injection. CSF leaks out of the hole where the dura was punctured, and when the patient stands up gravity pulls more CSF from around the brain, resulting in an intractable headache. Blood is drawn from the patient's arm and injected into the epidural space to clot or patch the hole in the dura. Patients often develop a postdural puncture headache after having a myelogram or an epidural placed for labor and delivery. Assign code 62273.

> ■ Do not confuse therapeutic and diagnostic lumbar punctures. Thoroughly review the documentation to determine the reason for the procedure before assigning a code.

Lumbar Puncture

Lumbar puncture, also known as a spinal tap, is a diagnostic and at times therapeutic procedure that is performed in order to collect a sample of CSF for biochemical, microbiological, and cytological analysis, or occasionally as a treatment ("therapeutic lumbar puncture") to relieve increased intracranial pressure. A needle is inserted into the subarachnoid space in the lumbar region. The color of the fluid can indicate hemorrhage, infection, and so forth. Sometimes, a therapeutic spinal puncture to drain excess fluid off the spine is required for a condition known as pseudotumor cerebri; in this case, assign 62272.

Shunts

A shunt is a hole or passageway that directs movement of fluid from one part of the body to another. In cases such as hydrocephalus, a ventricular shunt is inserted into the ventricle of the brain to drain CSF away from the brain to circulate into the body. Shunts can be inserted into the cranium to drain the fluid into the peritoneal cavity or into the right atrium of the heart. A ventriculoperitoneal (VP) shunt is inserted into the ventricle of the brain and the catheter is tunneled to the peritoneal cavity where the CSF is reabsorbed into the blood through the peritoneum. A ventriculo-atrial (VA) shunt is also inserted into the cerebral ventricle and tunneled into the right atrium of the heart. The CSF is then shunted directly into the blood circulation. Neurosurgeons will choose the most appropriate operating method and valve for each patient depending on their experience.

The shunt procedure includes the following components:

- Making several small incisions to position the valve and catheters under the skin
- Tunneling the catheters into the subcutaneous tissue
- Inserting the valve underneath the skin, either into the cranium behind the ear, into the pectoral region, or into the flank
- Creating a burr hole in the cranium to insert the catheter into the ventricles
- Positioning one of the ends of the distal catheter into the abdominal cavity or in a neck vein, leading to the right atrium of the heart
- Connecting a ventricular catheter to a valve
- Checking the flow at the end of the peritoneal catheter
- Closing the cranial incision
- Closing the peritoneal incision

The cerebrospinal fluid shunt codes are 62180–62258. The spinal fluid shunt codes are 63740–63746. Coders should note that the hyphen (-) within these code descriptions indicates a from/to relationship. For example, code 62220, *Creation of shunt; ventriculo-atrial, -jugular, -auricular*, means that a shunt was created *from* the ventricles *to* either the atrium, the jugular vein, or the ear.

Assign codes to the following procedures. Include any necessary modifiers.

1. A patient has long-standing chronic back pain. Conservative measures only provide limited relief. The neurosurgeon feels that neurostimulator insertion for long-term therapy is a viable option. The patient is placed in the prone position and a laminotomy midline incision is made overlying the affected vertebrae. The surgeon places the inductive electrode pads in the epidural space proximal to the damaged spinal segment. The pulse generator is sutured over the muscles and the skin is closed. _____

2. A patient is being followed for suspected multiple sclerosis. A diagnostic lumbar puncture is performed. _____

3. A patient with cerebral palsy has received many treatments for spasticity with no significant relief. He agrees to proceed with implantation of a nonprogrammable baclofen spinal cord pump. The patient's back was prepped and the incision was made in the skin at the L3–L4 level. A catheter was inserted into the subarachnoid space. The catheter tubing was then anchored to the fascia with 2-0 silk. A second incision was made in the right lower quadrant of the abdomen 1 inch below the skin. The pump was placed into this pocket. The tubing was connected to the pump and anchored with sutures. _____

4. A 6-month-old infant is brought to the emergency department. It is determined that she is suffering from hydrocephalus secondary to subarachnoid hemorrhage associated with shaken baby syndrome. A VP shunt was placed to drain the fluid from her brain. _____

SPINAL INJECTIONS AND PAIN MANAGEMENT

Spinal injections may be performed by orthopedic surgeons, neurosurgeons, or anesthesiologists specializing in pain management. These types of injections may be performed in the office or in an outpatient surgery center.

Spinal injections are commonly performed for diagnostic and therapeutic purposes for patients with chronic back pain. Diagnostic injections are performed to differentiate between peripheral nerve and central nerve pain and assist the physician in identifying the source of the patient's pain. Therapeutic injections are performed to ease the pain and symptoms for patients with chronic back or neck pain, spinal stenosis, sciatica, degenerative disc disease, disc herniation, radiculopathy, sciatica, and post-laminectomy syndrome (failed back syndrome). Injections are typically performed after all conservative measures have been taken but the pain persists. Types of injections include trigger points, hypertonic saline injection for epidural lysis of adhesions, epidural steroid injections, spinal nerve blocks, and facet joint injections. Codes are selected based on the purpose of the injection, location, and approach. Detailed documentation and familiarity with the intricate anatomy of the spine are required to precisely code these services.

Epidural injections involve placing the needle into the epidural space (outside the dura mater). In subarachnoid injections, the needle is placed into the subarachnoid space. Physicians may use the terms *intrathecal* or *subdural* to describe subarachnoid injections.

Fluoroscopic Guidance

Fluoroscopy guidance is only assigned when the fluoroscope (C-arm) is used for guiding the needle or locating the site, and a parenthetical instruction, code descriptor, or National Correct Coding Initiative (NCCI) edit indicates it is separately reportable. A modifier –TC is applied for facility coders when performed in a facility to capture the technical component of the equipment use. Code 77003–26 is reported by the physician if the procedure is performed in a facility. Code 77003 does not indicate a formal contrast study (arthrography, myelography, and epidurography). No formal arthrogram is performed, so no radiology report is generated. Injection of the contrast material is not separately reportable. Some of the spinal injection codes include the use of fluoroscopic assistance, so read the code descriptions carefully.

> Code 72295 is used when an epidurogram is recorded, performed, and a formal radiological report issued.

Percutaneous Epidurolysis (RACZ Procedure)

Percutaneous epidurolysis targets scar tissue caused by failed back surgery, herniated discs, compression fractures, and infection. The purpose of this procedure is to dissolve scar tissue from around entrapped nerves in the epidural space so that medications such as steroids can reach the affected areas. A catheter is inserted into the epidural space to the area of scarring using fluoroscopic guidance. The catheter is then sutured to the skin and used to perform subsequent injections. This procedure involves a series of three injections performed over a 3-day or longer period. Injection consists of a mixture of local anesthetic and a steroid as well as contrast material to visualize the scar tissue and hyaluronidase, a concentrated salt solution, to soften the scar tissue. Code 62264 is reported if the procedure is performed exclusively over 1 day. Code 62263 is only reported once even though the procedure occurs over several days. Do not report codes 77003 or 72275 in addition to this code. It is an inherent part of the procedure and is not reported separately.

> Endoscopic lysis of epidural adhesions is reported with code 64999. An endoscope may be inserted into the epidural space. When the scope is manipulated through the epidural space but no instruments are passed through the scope, this is not considered an endoscopic lysis of adhesions. The scope in this scenario acted like a blunt instrument to break the adhesions apart. If instruments are passed through the endoscope to mechanically lyse adhesions or for dissection after visualization, this constitutes an endoscopic lysis and is reported with 64999.

Provocative Discography

Discography (62290–62291) is a minimally invasive procedure used to evaluate and localize the etiology of back pain. This procedure involves inserting a needle into the nucleus of an intervertebral disc. Dye is injected and may reveal tears in the annulus fibrosus, the tough outer shell of a disc. If the disc is diseased, the patient should experience a reproduction of his or her chronic pain when the injection is performed. This is strictly a diagnostic test to determine the source of pain.

Chemonucleolysis

In chemonucleolysis, code 62292, an enzyme or other agent is injected to dissolve the soft central portion of the intervertebral disc, resulting in relief of pressure on the spinal cord and nerves. Report this code only once regardless of how many levels were injected. X-ray (fluoroscopy) is used to confirm needle placement and is included in this code.

Spinal Blocks (Pain Blocks)

Spinal blocks or injections are performed to block pain receptors in the nerves surrounding the spinal canal. These are unilateral codes and if performed on both sides of the spine, a –50 modifier is reported. If one needle is used and manipulated for multiple injections, report the code once. If the needle is removed and repositioned, the code can be listed twice. These codes are specific to the purpose of the injection, the approach (epidural, subarachnoid), the site (cervical, lumbar), and the substance injected.

Lumbar or Cervical Epidural Injections—Single Injection

Codes 62320 and 62322 describe a single injection of steroids and anesthetic into the epidural or subarachnoid space. Codes 62321 and 62323 include imaging guidance, so no additional radiology code is required.

EXAMPLE

The patient was prepped and draped lying in the supine position. Fluoroscopy was used to identify the L3–L4 interspace. The subcutaneous tissue at this site was infused with 2 cc of lidocaine followed by placement of a Touhy catheter. The catheter was advanced in the L3–L4 epidural space and identified with fluoro by instilling 1 cc of contrast. Aspiration of CSF and blood was negative. 2 cc of triamcinolone, 4 cc of sterile saline, and 1 cc of lidocaine were injected into the epidural space. The catheter was removed and a sterile dressing was applied. Report codes 62323.

Lumbar or Cervical Epidural Injections—Continuous

Codes 62324 and 62326 describe a continuous infusion or intermittent bolus injection via a catheter. The drug is infused in small quantities over a period of time (similar to an IV). A catheter may be placed as a trial catheter prior to permanent insertion of a pain pump to assess the patient's tolerance of the drug, adequate pain relief, and any side effects. Catheter placement and the injection are reported using one code. Additional codes are assigned for services associated with refilling and maintenance of an implantable reservoir or infusion pump. Codes for these services are located in the Medicine section of CPT.

Transforaminal Epidural Injections

Codes 64479 and 64484 report epidural injections.

Facet Joint Injections

In a facet joint injection, codes 64490 through 64495, the destination of the injection is the facet joint. The procedure is reported per *level*, not by the number of injections. A level in this service refers to the area between adjacent nerves (the joint) that is the target of the injection, which involves two nerves. Coders must determine the targeted nerve and whether a single nerve or multilevel injection was done. A provider may choose to administer a right-side intra-articular injection using a single injection (needle puncture) or to administer two separate injections to the nerves supplying the facet joint. In either case, only one code is reported per level.

For example, a provider administers nerve blocks at T1, T2, and T3. He is addressing three nerves but only two levels (the joint between T1/T2 and T2/T3). Report code 64490 for the first level and +64491 for the second level. Pay attention to the code descriptions to determine if they are unilateral or bilateral. If the provider administers injections bilaterally *at the same level*, append modifier –50. CPT includes parenthetical instructions for reporting bilateral injections. The facet injection codes already include fluoroscopy and any injection of contrast as inclusive components; therefore, reporting 77003 with this service is not allowed.

Transversus Abdominis Plane Block

The transverse abdominis plane (TAP) block (codes 64486–64489) is a peripheral nerve block that anesthetizes the nerves supplying the anterior abdominal wall (level of T6 to L1). This block controls postoperative pain following abdominal, gynecological, and urological procedures. This may also used instead of epidural anesthesia in patients who because of medical contraindications are not candidates for an epidural.

Rhizotomy

Rhizotomy is a radio-frequency (RF) ablation technique used to destroy tissue or denervate the median branch of the facet nerve. Like other spinal injection procedures, it is done to alleviate lower back pain caused by degenerative changes in the facet joints. Codes for this procedure are determined by the nerve or branch involved, not the technique used.

Some payers may require reporting HCPCS code S2348 (*Decompression procedure, percutaneous, of nucleus pulposus of intervertebral disc, using radiofrequency energy, single or multiple levels, lumbar*) instead of the CPT code.

EXAMPLE

The median branches of the facet joint nerves L3–L4 and L4–L5 are identified using fluoroscopic guidance. Lidocaine is infiltrated over each level. A radio-frequency cannula is introduced at L3–L4 on the right side and delivers a pulsed RF lesion for 120 seconds. The cannula is then positioned on the left side to deliver RF for 120 seconds. The procedure is repeated bilaterally for the L4–L5 nerves. Report codes 64635–50, 64636–50.

Intradiscal Electrothermal Therapy

The intradiscal electrothermal therapy (IDET) procedure describes a percutaneous intradiscal electrothermal annuloplasty in which a catheter is placed in a diseased disc using fluoroscopic guidance. The catheter is then heated. Targeted thermal energy directed to the posterior disc annulus causes contraction of collagen fibers and destruction of receptors to treat chronic low back pain related to degenerative disc disease. The theory is that the disc shrinkage may result in less nerve compression and pain. Codes 22526–22527 are reported for this procedure.

> **INTERNET RESOURCE: Visit**
> **www.bayareapainmedical.com/Animations.html**
> **for animations of spine injections and disorders of the spine.**

Assigning Spinal Injection Procedure Codes

The following information should be available in the operative note or procedure note. To correctly code spine injections or pain blocks, the coder must answer the following questions before selecting codes:

1. Why was the injection being done: for therapeutic or diagnostic purposes (destruction of nerve, short-term pain relief, long-term anti-inflammatory effect of steroid, etc.)?
2. What was the approach? The vertebral injection site (epidural, transforaminal, facet) must be known and drives code assignment.
3. What was injected (steroid, anesthetic, contrast, neurolytic agent)? Knowing what was injected defines the purpose of the injection. A list of common steroids and anesthetics was provided earlier in Table 25.3.
4. Where was the needle inserted (cervical, thoracic, lumbar, or sacral region)?
5. Was this a single injection, a continuous infusion, or a regional injection?
6. How many levels were treated? Assign a code for each level injected.
7. Was the injection unilateral or bilateral? If performed on both sides of the spine, append the −50 modifier.
8. Was fluoroscopy used? If so, also report 77003 if allowed.

The documentation needs to support the reported codes.

SPINAL DECOMPRESSION PROCEDURES

Learning the terminology used in the Nervous System section can become overwhelming. Coding complex surgeries involving the vertebrae, nerves, and discs of the spine requires strong knowledge and understanding of spinal anatomy, and detailed procedural documentation is required to properly assign procedure codes for spinal decompression surgeries. Refer to Box 25.1 for descriptions of the decompression procedures covered in this section.

BOX 25.1 Decompression Techniques

Laminectomy	Removal of the entire bony lamina, a portion of the facet joints, and the ligaments overlying the spinal cord and nerves.
Laminotomy	Removal of a small portion of the lamina and ligaments, usually on one side. This method keeps the natural support of the lamina intact.
Foraminotomy	Removal of bone around the neural foramen. This method is used when disc degeneration causes the height of the foramen to collapse, pinching nerves.
Laminoplasty	Enlargement of the spinal canal opening by cutting the lamina on one or both sides, creating hinges in the bone so they swing open like a door, taking pressure off the spinal cord. The spinous process projections are removed, making room for the hinged lamina to remain open. It is used only in the cervical area.
Corpectomy	Removal of the vertebral body or a substantial portion thereof (usually one-third to one-half of the body), reconstructing it with bone graft. This procedure is used to treat cervical spinal stenosis or spurs compressing the spine.
Discectomy	Removal of herniated disc material pressing on a nerve root or the spinal cord.

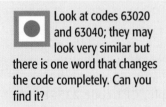

Careful note should be made of the instruction below the vertebral corpectomy code 63091. CPT indicates that the vertebral corpectomy codes 63081–63091 include discectomy above and/or below the vertebral segment. For this reason, a discectomy code would not be reported in addition to the vertebral corpectomy codes.

Codes for decompression surgery are grouped by approach and technique, as follows:

63001–63050: Posterior extradural laminotomy or laminectomy for exploration/decompression of neural elements or excision of herniated intervertebral discs

63055–63066: Transpedicular or costovertebral extradural exploration/decompression

63075–63091: Anterior or anterolateral approach for extradural exploration/decompression

63101–63103: Lateral extracavitary approach for extradural exploration/decompression

Careful consideration of the code descriptor and technique must take place before selecting a code because many procedures appear similar. Combination codes are common in this section, making reporting easier.

EXAMPLE

63020 *Laminotomy (hemilaminectomy), with decompression of nerve root(s), including partial facetectomy, foraminotomy and/or excision of herniated intervertebral disc; 1 interspace, cervical.*

Procedures on the spine may be performed on either side or bilaterally. Pay close attention to the code descriptor for the terms *unilateral* or *bilateral* before appending modifiers –RT, –LT, or –50. Also review the parenthetical notes below the codes. For example, the note under 63020 states, "For bilateral procedure, report 63020 with modifier –50." As you review this group of codes, do you see that note repeated?

Look at codes 63020 and 63040; they may look very similar but there is one word that changes the code completely. Can you find it?

EXAMPLE

63047 *Laminectomy, facetectomy and foraminotomy (unilateral or bilateral with decompression of spinal cord, cauda equina and/or nerve root(s) (e.g., spinal or lateral recess stenosis)), single vertebral segment; lumbar.* The code may only be reported once per segment regardless of whether it is performed bilaterally, because the code descriptor says "unilateral or bilateral."

Spinal Decompression Procedure Components

Spinal decompression can be performed anywhere along the spine. The procedure is performed in five steps through a posterior surgical incision, as follows:

- *Step 1: Make a posterior incision over the appropriate vertebra(e).* The length of the incision depends on how many vertebrae require decompression. The muscles are divided down the middle and retracted aside, exposing the lamina of each vertebra. The lamina is the bone that forms the backside of the spinal canal and makes a roof over the spinal cord. Removing the lamina and other soft tissues gives more room for the nerves and allows for removal of bone spurs. Depending on the extent of stenosis, one vertebra (single level) or more (multilevel) may be involved.
- *Step 2: Laminectomy or laminotomy.* Once the affected bone is exposed, x-ray confirmation is obtained of the correct vertebra. If a laminectomy is performed, the surgeon removes the bony spinous process. Using a drill or bone-biting tools, the bony lamina is then removed. The ligamentum flavum that connects the laminae of the vertebra directly below with the vertebra directly above is removed. Some circumstances may not require complete removal of the bony lamina, in which case a laminotomy is carried out by creating a small opening in the lamina above and below the affected spinal nerve to relieve compression. Laminas are located on each side of the spine and may be performed unilaterally or bilaterally. An endoscope may be used for this procedure, allowing for a smaller, less invasive approach.
- *Step 3: Decompress the spinal cord.* Once the lamina and ligamentum flavum have been removed, the dura mater of the spinal cord is visible. The surgeon can gently retract this protective layer of the spinal cord and nerve root to remove bone spurs.

- *Step 4: Decompress the spinal nerve.* Foraminotomy, trimming the facet joints located directly over the nerve, enlarges the neural foramen (site where spinal nerves exit the spinal column), freeing up the nerve roots, which results in decompression of the nerve. If a herniated disc is causing compression, the surgeon will perform a discectomy.
- *Step 5: Arthrodesis.* In some cases, spinal fusion may be done at the same time to help stabilize sections of the spine treated with laminectomy, particularly if multiple vertebrae are treated. Fusion uses a combination of bone graft, screws, cages, and rods to connect two separate vertebrae into one new piece of bone. By fusing the joint, the bones become one, which prevents recurrence of spinal stenosis and eliminates pain from an unstable spine. The most common type of fusion is called *posterolateral fusion,* in which a layer of bone from the transverse process is removed and replaced with a bone graft.

Discectomy, arthrodesis, and decompression procedures are often miscoded because of the number of similar code choices in this section. Codes from both the Musculoskeletal System and Nervous System sections may be required to capture all of the procedures performed on the spine. Case in point, a surgeon performs a discectomy with decompression of the spinal cord along with arthrodesis and insertion of spinal instrumentation.

The global service package for decompression surgeries does not include the following:

- Harvesting and/or preparation of grafts for arthrodesis
- Harvesting and placement of soft tissue graft, muscle, or fat obtained through a separate incision
- Application of spinal instrumentation
- Preparation and insertion of bone grafts or other devices into areas of bone resection or instability

INTERNET RESOURCE: Visit the University Spine Associates website to view animations of procedures discussed in this section. www.universityspine.com

> Fluoroscopy is used to verify the location of a vertebral segment or to confirm placement of hardware. Intraoperative fluoroscopy (77003, 76000) during open spine procedures (i.e., laminectomy, discectomy, or arthrodesis) is considered an integral part of the procedure and is not separately reportable.

Coders make code selections for spinal procedures based on diagnosis and approach. This concept is reinforced when assigning codes for decompression. For example, CPT code 22551 combines arthrodesis and discectomy. In this case, no additional code from the 63000 series of CPT is reported. Parenthetical instructions for code 22554 state not to report 22554 with 63075 and to report 22551 if cervical discectomy and interbody fusion are performed at the same level during the same session. When reporting code 22630, however, a code for discectomy will be reported unless the discectomy was minimal and done only to prepare the interspace for the arthrodesis procedure. Codes from the 63000 series of CPT are reported when, in addition to removing the disc, preparing the vertebral endplate, and performing interbody fusion, the surgeon removes posterior osteophytes and decompresses the spinal cord or nerve root, which involves work above and beyond that. The coder selects the code for the reason or intent of the procedure—differentiating between procedures located in the Musculoskeletal System and Nervous System sections of CPT. Distinction between similar codes located in both of these sections is ultimately based on whether or not decompression was the goal and if additional work such as a facetectomy(ies) and/or foraminotomy(ies) was required to adequately decompress the affected nerve root. Documentation of decompression is crucial here.

Category III CPT codes 0274T and 0275T are available for reporting endoscopic, CT, or fluoroscopic-guided laminotomy/laminectomy (interlaminar approach) for decompression of neural elements, with or without ligamentous resection, discectomy, facetectomy, or foraminotomy. Category III codes are updated regularly with advances in surgical technology.

Steps to Spinal Decompression Coding

Look for the answers to the following series of questions in the operative report to assist in selecting the appropriate codes and identifying and capturing all reportable components of this complex procedure:

1. What was the reason for the procedure? Was the goal decompression?
2. What was the diagnosis? Code descriptors help guide the coder by using example diagnoses in the descriptors (e.g., spinal stenosis, herniated disc, spondylolisthesis).
3. What approach and technique were used?

CPT © 2017 American Medical Association, All Rights Reserved.

4. What procedure(s) was performed: laminectomy, laminotomy, discectomy, facetectomy, foraminotomy with decompression?
5. For laminotomy, was the procedure performed unilaterally or bilaterally?
6. If fusion was performed, how many interspaces were fused?
7. Were any interspinous fusion devices (IFDs) or biomechanical devices (e.g., cages, threaded dowel) inserted? The code is reported once per interspace regardless of how many cages are used per level.
8. Were bone grafts used? If so, what kind: autograft local (same incision), autograft morselized, autograft structural, bicortical, or tricortical, allograft structural, or autograft morselized?
9. Was any instrumentation used? If so, was it segmental or nonsegmental?
10. Was any microdissection performed using an intraoperative microscope? If the documentation is appropriate and CPT allows, report +69990.

In addition, check the NCCI edits to be sure codes are not bundled or part of the global surgical package.

INTERNET RESOURCE: Visit www.spine-health.com/video to learn more about the spine.

Let's Code It

The following operative report is dissected using colored highlighting to help you identify the reportable components.

Diagnosis: Cervical disc herniation C6–C7.
Operation: Anterior cervical discectomy, microdissection, microdiscectomy, removal of spur C6–C7, fusion with bone plug, DBX bone putty, and 18-mm Globus plate with 4 pedicle screws.
Procedure: Incision was made in the skin crease opposite C6–C7. Platysma was opened and divided. An interval was developed between the sternocleidomastoid and strap muscles down to the pre-vertebral fascia. The fascia was opened, and the C6–C7 interspace was identified. X-ray was taken confirming correct position. The operating microscope was brought in and the remainder of the operation until the time of closure was done under use of the microscope. The patient had a large spur and this was removed. The disc space was entered and degenerated disc material was removed. Synthes distraction pins were placed in the body of the C6–C7 interspace to distract the space. Additional disc material was removed. The posterior osteophyte was thinned down with an Anspach drill and removed. The spur that was compressing the spinal cord was trimmed. At the end of the procedure, the C6–C7 nerve roots were palpated and were well decompressed. A bone plug was taken and its central canal was filled with DBX bone putty. It was impacted into position. DBX was applied in the lateral gutters on both sides as well. The anterior osteophyte from C6–C7 was removed. A plate was secured into position with four 4-by-4 mm screws.

Preliminary Codes: 63075, 22554–51, 22845, 20931.
Final Codes: CPT provides parenthetical instructions that clearly state that 22554 should not be reported with 63075, directing the coder to report 22551 instead. Report codes 22551, 22845, 20931.

CHECKPOINT 25.4

Assign codes to the following procedures. Include any necessary modifiers.

1. The neurosurgeon performed a laminotomy with partial facetectomy and excision of a herniated disc for C3–C4 and C5–C6. _____

2. A vertebral corpectomy procedure with decompression of the cauda equina was performed on three segments, using a thoracolumbar approach. _____

3. Code for a laminectomy with facetectomy and foraminotomy, bilateral, with decompression of the spinal cord, two thoracic segments. _____

4. Code for a laminotomy, decompression of nerve root, foraminotomy, and excision of the intervertebral disc for L1–L2. _____

Chapter Summary

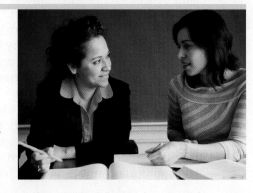

1. The endocrine system glands are the pituitary, thyroid, parathyroid, adrenal, thymus, the islet cells of the pancreas, the ovaries and testes, and the pineal gland.

2. The nervous system comprises the central nervous system and the peripheral nervous system. The central nervous system is the brain and spinal cord, both of which are covered by the meninges. The basic anatomy of the brain is the cerebrum, the midbrain, and the cerebellum, and the brain is also divided into lobes. The peripheral nervous system is comprised of the cranial, spinal, and peripheral nerves. The autonomic nervous system is part of the peripheral nervous system and controls body functions that we do not have to think about.

3. Nerve blocks are performed on peripheral nerves for pain management purposes. The nerves are injected with a mixture of steroids and anesthetics. Neurorrhaphy, or suturing, of the nerve is done by splicing the nerve endings together. This is achievable if there isn't a large gap between the two endings. Neuroplasty is accomplished by transposing, wrapping, or decompressing the nerve. Nerve decompression and transposition is the freeing of an intact nerve from scar tissue or entrapment.

4. It is appropriate to report nerve blocks separately from the anesthesia provided for the surgery when the pain management procedure is not the operative anesthesia being utilized for the operative procedure and documentation states that it is administered pre-, inter-, or post-op for the purpose of pain management.

5. Nerve repair is accomplished by three various methods: nerve graft, nerve wrapping, and suture repair. Wrapping involves harvesting a vein (primarily the saphenous vein) and wrapping it around the nerve to protect it and to act as a buffer to decrease nerve sensitivity. When nerves are severed and the gap between the two nerve endings is too great, the nerve cannot grow across. A nerve is harvested and sewn to the two nerve endings, bridging the gap between them. Neurorrhaphy, or suturing, of the nerve is done by splicing the nerve endings together.

6. Neurostimulators are surgically placed under the skin to send mild electrical impulses to the spinal cord or to a specific nerve. The electrical impulses are delivered through a lead and interfere with pain signals traveling to the brain, providing pain relief for the patient. Neurostimulation uses either a fully implantable neurostimulation system or an external radio-frequency system. Peripheral nerve stimulation uses an external radio-frequency system. Neurostimulators are not only used to treat chronic pain but also to treat tremors, Parkinson's, paralysis, epilepsy, obesity, and depression.

7. The musculoskeletal system codes are used for spinal arthrodesis (spinal fusion), and in many circumstances other codes from the nervous system section are also required. An example would be when the surgeon performs spinal arthrodesis and vertebral corpectomy.

8. Discectomy is performed to alleviate compression of the spinal cord caused by displacement or deterioration of the intervertebral disc. Decompression is the same type of service; removal of the disc decompresses the spinal cord. Vertebral corpectomy is performed when the body of the vertebra has been damaged or impacted by a lesion or tumor and it requires removal. Laminectomy is done when testing reveals spinal stenosis caused by encroachment of the lamina requiring removal of a portion or all of the lamina to enlarge the area where the spinal cord passes through.

Matching

Match the key terms with their definitions.

A. meninges
B. neurorrhaphy
C. plexus
D. cerebrum
E. corpectomy

F. islet cells of pancreas
G. nerve block
H. skull base surgery
I. rhizotomy
J. discectomy

1. _____ Partial or complete removal of solid round portion of the vertebra

2. _____ Suture of the nerve

3. _____ Procedure performed to decompress the spinal cord

4. _____ A network of nerves

5. _____ The largest portion of the brain

6. _____ Lining of the brain and spinal cord

7. _____ Procedure performed on an area between the brain and the floor of the skull

8. _____ Procedure performed for pain control

9. _____ Radio-frequency ablation technique

10. _____ A gland within the endocrine system

True or False

Decide whether each statement is true or false.

1. _____ The neurostimulator insertion/removal codes 63661–63664 do not include evaluative testing, programming, or reprogramming.

2. _____ Destruction of the trigeminal nerve with iced saline is coded as 64600.

3. _____ Secretion of hormones is a function of the endocrine system.

4. _____ Nerve blocks can be performed by a single injection and continuous infusion of analgesic and are both administered for short-term pain control by inserting a catheter.

5. _____ When reporting 62290 at the same session as 62291, a –59 modifier is necessary to prevent bundling.

6. _____ Skull base surgery always requires the services of two or three surgeons.

7. _____ Never report codes from the musculoskeletal and nervous systems together.

8. _____ The meninges consist of the dura mater, the subarachnoid, and the pia mater.

9. _____ Nerve grafts, nerve wrapping, and suture repair are all part of the nerve repair services.

10. _____ Discectomy is always included in the laminectomy procedures.

Multiple Choice

Select the letter that best completes the statement or answers the question.

1. A patient is status post–inguinal hernia repair and is having chronic pain into the groin. The surgeon suspects nerve entrapment. The patient is referred for an ilioinguinal nerve block. Which code(s) should be reported?
   A. 64421
   B. 49505, 64425
   C. 64450
   D. 64425

2. Which of the following is *not* true about lumbar puncture?
   A. Contrast material is used during the fluoroscopy.
   B. It is used as a diagnostic test.
   C. Fluid is removed from between two vertebrae.
   D. It may have side effects.

3. A patient presented with nerve compression of the left hand secondary to entrapment of the nerve in scar tissue from previous hand surgery. Decompressive neuroplasty was performed with external neurolysis. Which code should be reported?
   A. 64722–LT
   B. 64704–LT
   C. 64702–LT
   D. 64834–LT

4. A patient is seen for total removal of implanted spinal neurostimulator pulse generator. Which code should be reported?
   A. 63661
   B. 63746
   C. 63685
   D. 63688

5. A patient suffers from pseudotumor cerebri and undergoes a lumbar puncture to reduce the CSF pressure. Which code should be reported?
   A. 62287
   B. 62272
   C. 62270
   D. 62273

6. A patient suffers from muscle spasms of the face. Chemodenervation is provided via injection of Botox type A, 1 unit. Provide the CPT code for the injection and the HCPCS code for the drug.
   A. 64612, J0585
   B. 64616, J0587
   C. 20552, J0585
   D. 64612, J0587

7. A patient is being treated for cervical radiculopathy. The physician performs a left greater occipital nerve root block. Which code should be reported?
   A. 64415
   B. 64405
   C. 64450
   D. 64418

8. Vertebral corpectomy was performed via a thoracolumbar approach to levels T12, L1, and L2 with discectomy. Which code(s) should be reported?
   A. 63087 x 2
   B. 63087, 63088 x 2
   C. 63081, 63082
   D. 63081, 63077–51

9. A patient has a malignant neoplasm of the brain stem. An otolaryngologist performs the approach via a transtemporal posterior cranial fossa and decompression of the sigmoid sinus. The neurosurgeon then excises the neoplastic lesion, extradural, from the brain stem. The neurosurgeon closes the operative field. Which codes should be reported?

	Otolaryngologist	Neurosurgeon
A.	61590, 61605	61605–62
B.	61590	61605
C.	61595	61615
D.	61595, 61615	61615–62

10. A patient is suffering from an intracranial hemorrhage resulting from an intracranial aneurysm in the right carotid artery. Emergent microdissection of the aneurysm is performed via an intracranial approach. Which code(s) should be reported?
    A. 61700, 69990
    B. 61700
    C. 61697
    D. 61697, 69990

11. The regions of the spine are
    A. Sacral, lumbar, brachial, pia
    B. Sacral, cervical, lumbar, thoracic
    C. Pia, arachnoid, vertebral, lumbar
    D. Lumbar, cervical, pia, thoracic

12. A patient is diagnosed with spondylolisthesis, lumbosacral, without myelopathy. The surgeon performs a bilateral laminotomy via a posterior approach. The nerve roots are decompressed, and a partial facetectomy is performed for interspace L4–L5. Which code should be reported?
    A. 63040
    B. 63040–50
    C. 63030–50
    D. 63030

CPT: Eye and Ear

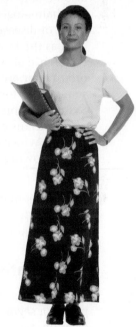

CHAPTER OUTLINE

Eye and Ocular Adnexa

Eye Anatomy

Diseases and Injuries of the Eye and Associated Procedures

Oculoplastic Surgery

Auditory System

Ear Anatomy

Common Problems of the Ear and Associated Procedures

LEARNING OUTCOMES

After studying this chapter, you should be able to:

1. Distinguish when codes from the Eye and Ocular Adnexa and the Auditory System sections of CPT are used versus those in the Integumentary System and Musculoskeletal System sections for removing lesions of the eyelid.
2. Differentiate between extracapsular and intracapsular cataract extraction and complex cataract extractions.
3. Distinguish between phototherapeutic keratectomy and photorefractive keratectomy procedures.
4. Explain how to determine when blepharoptosis repair is performed for cosmetic purposes versus a medical condition.
5. Explain the difference between an ectropion and an entropion repair.
6. Differentiate between tympanostomy and myringotomy for insertion of ventilation tubes.
7. Describe the purpose and components of a tympanoplasty.

This chapter presents the anatomical structures, common conditions surgically treated, and surgical techniques covered by the Eye and Ocular Adnexa and the Auditory System sections of the CPT. These body systems are grouped in the 65091–69990 code range and are related because they both process sensory information. Together, these systems allow us to sense and react to our environment through vision and hearing. This chapter discusses surgical services of low surgical complexity to high complexity of the eye, ocular adnexa, and ear.

EYE AND OCULAR ADNEXA

Codes in the Eye and Ocular Adnexa section include procedures on the eyeball, anterior and posterior segment, ocular adnexa, and conjunctiva. The codes are arranged by anatomical part and then by procedure on that part. The outline of this section mostly follows the template used in other surgical sections, grouping procedures by introduction, incision, excision, repair, and other procedures. Codes for eye examinations and vision screenings are captured in the Medicine section and not in the surgical Eye and Ocular Adnexa section of CPT. Nonsurgical and diagnostic ophthalmology services are reported from the Medicine section of CPT by reporting codes 92002–92499.

Procedures and services in this section are performed by an ophthalmologist and rarely by an optometrist. An optometrist is a doctor of optometry (OD) who specializes in improving vision and in diagnosing and providing nonsurgical treatment of various eye diseases and injuries. ODs are trained to prescribe and fit lenses for vision correction, treat conditions of the eye and ocular structures with oral and topical medications, and, depending on the state where licensed, may also be able to perform limited laser procedures to improve vision. An ophthalmologist is a surgeon who specializes in the diagnosis and treatment of diseases and injuries to the eye and areas surrounding the eye such as the lacrimal system and eyelids. Surgical codes related to the eye region are also located in other sections of CPT. For example, codes for orbit repair are located in the Musculoskeletal System section. Likewise, some codes for treating eyelid lesions are located in the Integumentary System section.

> When coding procedures for eyes and eyelids, remember to use modifiers. HCPCS Level II modifiers are required for use when billing eyelid procedures (E1, E2, etc.). Remember to use the –50 modifier when coding procedures on both eyes.

Physicians commonly use abbreviations to depict which eye is being treated, which can lead to errors in code assignment or modifier usage. The following abbreviations are used to describe which eye is being treated:

- OU: both eyes
- OS: left eye
- OD: right eye

Organization

Codes in this section are arranged by the compartments of the eye—eyeball, anterior segment, posterior segment, ocular adnexa, and conjunctiva—and then by procedure: introduction, incision, excision, removal, repair, destruction, and other.

Before assigning codes, read the documentation carefully. Some procedure code descriptors in this section are specific to whether a patient has had prior surgery on the affected eye. Be sure to read the section notes under each subheading for bundling rules and the parenthetical notes following codes for directions and instructions for going to other sections of CPT if necessary to capture all services provided and selecting the most appropriate anatomical code.

Modifiers

HCPCS includes alphanumeric modifiers specific to reporting procedures and services on the eye and eyelid. Table 26.1 includes some of the more common modifiers that may be reported with eye procedures.

Table 26.1 Modifiers for Eye Procedures

MODIFIER	DEFINITION
E1	Upper left eyelid
E2	Lower left eyelid
E3	Upper right eyelid
E4	Lower right eyelid
LT	Left side
RT	Right side
VP	Aphakic patient
LS	FDA-monitored intraocular lens implant
PL	Progressive addition lenses
AP	No determination of refractive state during diagnostic ophthalmologic examination
50	Bilateral procedure
76	Repeat procedure or service by same physician
77	Repeat procedure or service by another physician
78	Unplanned return to the operating room by the same physician following initial procedure for a related procedure during the postoperative period
79	Unrelated procedure or service by the same physician during the postoperative period

Bilateral ophthalmic procedures should be reported with modifier –50 and one unit of service on a single claim line. Procedures performed on eyelids should be reported with modifiers E1–E4. The maximum units per day or medically unlikely edit (MUE) values for eyelid procedures are one based on the use of –E modifiers when the same procedure is performed on more than one eyelid.

EYE ANATOMY

The eye is located inside the bony orbit of the skull (Fig. 26.1). The eyeball is referred to as the *globe*. The colored portion of the eye is the iris. The pupil is the dark circular opening in the center of the iris. The white portion of the eye is the sclera. The thin clear membrane that covers the eye is the conjunctiva. The cornea cannot be seen with the naked eye. It is clear and curved to help focus what we see. Light passes through the cornea into the anterior chamber through the pupil and into the posterior chamber where the lens brings the light into focus. The light then passes through the vitreous chamber to the back of the eye. The retina receives the light and converts this into nerve impulses that are sent to the brain via the optic nerve.

The anterior and posterior chambers are collectively referred to as the *anterior segment* of the eye. The aqueous flows from the posterior chamber to the anterior chamber and then drains from the anterior chamber through trabecular meshwork into the canal of Schlemm. The lens is encased in a capsule. The outer portion of the lens is called the *cortex* and the interior portion is called the *nucleus*.

The eyelids and lashes serve to protect the anterior surface of the eyeball or globe. They also serve other purposes including regulation of light reaching the eye, distribution of the tear film over the cornea during blinking, and circulation of tear flow by pumping the conjunctival and lacrimal sacs during blinking. The upper eyelid is called the *superior palpebra* and the lower eyelid is called the *inferior palpebra*. The eyelid is constructed of skin, orbicularis muscle, tarsus cartilage, and levator muscle. The eyelashes are attached to the eyelid on the outer edge of the lid margin. The eyelid margin is the 1-mm-wide edge of an eyelid where the front (anterior) and back (posterior) of the eyelid meet. The outer corner of the eye is referred to as the *lateral canthus* and the inner corner as the *medial canthus*. The insides of the eyelids are lined with conjunctiva.

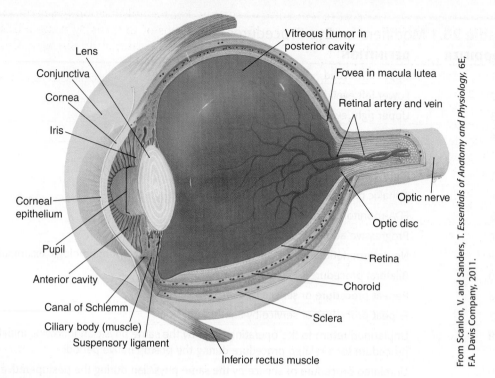

Figure 26.1 Eye anatomy.

Eye movement and alignment are controlled by the following six muscles:

1. Superior rectus
2. Inferior rectus
3. Lateral rectus
4. Medial rectus
5. Inferior oblique
6. Superior oblique

Further anatomy of the eyelid and its musculature is discussed in the Oculoplastic Surgery section of this chapter.

DISEASES AND INJURIES OF THE EYE AND ASSOCIATED PROCEDURES

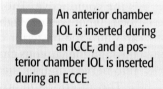

An anterior chamber IOL is inserted during an ICCE, and a posterior chamber IOL is inserted during an ECCE.

Typical procedures performed on the eye are cataract removal, glaucoma surgery, laser surgery for vision correction, strabismus surgery on the muscles of the eye, foreign body removal, and retinal procedures.

Cataract

A cataract is the clouding or opacification of the lens of the eye that impairs vision. Cataracts are caused by aging, diseases such as diabetes, excessive exposure to the sun, scar tissue from previous ocular surgery, or trauma to the eye. The degree of impairment depends on the size, location, and density of the cataract. When coding cataract extractions, the following must be determined: which technique was used, which type of cataract was removed, and whether an intraocular lens (IOL) was placed. Routine cataract surgery does not involve work on the cornea. Intracapsular cataract extraction (ICCE) (66983) includes removing the entire lens and its capsule in one piece. An anterior chamber IOL is simultaneously inserted. Extracapsular cataract extraction (ECCE) (66984) involves removing the front portion and nucleus of the lens, leaving the posterior capsule in place. An incision is made where the cornea and sclera meet (limbus). The front portion and nucleus of the lens are removed, leaving the capsule in place. A posterior chamber IOL is simultaneously inserted. ECCE is the most common cataract procedure performed because it requires no stitches. Phacoemulsification (*phaco* means "lens") is used to dissolve the hard nucleus of the lens by using ultrasound to break it up into tiny pieces (emulsification) and then aspirating or suctioning it away.

The following procedures are included in the cataract extraction and are not coded separately:

- Lateral canthotomy
- Iridectomy
- Iridotomy
- Anterior capsulotomy
- Anterior capsulorrhexis
- Posterior capsulotomy
- Use of viscoelastic agents
- Enzymatic zonulysis
- Pharmacological agents
- Subconjunctival injections
- Subtenon injections
- IOL insertion
- Partial vitrectomy (removal of the vitreous)

Anterior vitrectomy is most often associated with cataract extraction. Vitreous that moves into the wound during the cataract removal may cause complications. The surgeon must remove the vitreous in order to properly close the wound. The amount of vitreous that leaks through the wound determines whether the vitrectomy will be partial or subtotal.

Complex cataracts are reported with 66982. They are not to be confused with the common or conventional cataract. Cataracts such as a dense white cataract or those occurring in the pediatric age group would qualify. Look for the following indications in the record to assist in identifying complex cataracts before assigning 66982:

- Patient with small/miotic pupils that require multiple incisions
- Patient with a subluxed lens
- Eye trauma requiring the insertion of a capsular support ring for the new lens
- Patient with glaucoma whose surgery requires the use of iris retractors
- Pediatric patient with posterior cataract extraction
- Documentation of use of an iris expansion device, use of sutures to support the IOL, insertion of endocapsular rings, or a primary posterior capsulorrhexis
- Patient with dense cataracts removed in conjunction with application of indocyanine green (ICG) or trypan blue
- Patient with floppy iris syndrome

Read the medical record documentation carefully for whether an IOL was placed at the time of the cataract extraction and, if so, which kind of lens was implanted. The insertion of the lens and the supply thereof are included in the reimbursement of the cataract extraction procedure; however, according to Medicare, the supply code for the lens can be billed separately with HCPCS code Q1004 or Q1005 if it qualifies as a new technology intraocular lens. The list of special technology lenses that can be billed is located in the *Federal Register* at www.cms.gov.

On occasion, the intraocular lens may not be inserted at the same time as the cataract extraction, requiring the patient to return for lens placement at a different operative session than the cataract extraction. If the cataract is removed and the IOL is not immediately inserted during the operative session, report a code from 66840−66940. Code 66985 is assigned when the IOL is inserted at a different surgical episode.

Assign the CPT code(s) to the following procedure.

1. The physician performed an extracapsular cataract removal by phacoemulsification, with insertion of an IOL prosthesis. This was a complex procedure due to the density of the cataract. The patient had undergone prior intraocular surgery 6 months ago. _____

Secondary Cataract

Many patients develop what is called a *secondary membranous cataract* after initial cataract extraction and lens implant. The posterior portion of the lens capsule is left in place and tends to become "cloudy." This cataract can easily be treated by yttrium-aluminum-garnet (YAG) laser surgery to correct the "cloudiness" or "after-cataract" and destroy the opacification by incising the posterior capsule, allowing light to reach the retina to improve vision. Report CPT code 66821.

 The physician can report only one YAG performed on the same eye within the 90-day global period. The 66821 code description states "one or more stages," meaning that the code includes any number of subsequent YAG sessions within the 90-day global period.

IOL Procedures

At times, a patient may come in to have an IOL inserted because it was not done at the time of initial cataract extraction. In this circumstance, assign code 66985, not 66984, because the cataract extraction was already performed at the previous surgery. Situations may also necessitate the exchange of an IOL. Report the IOL exchange with 66986 with an ICD-10 diagnosis code describing failure of the implant. If the IOL becomes dislodged and requires repositioning, report 66825. Parenthetical instruction under code 66985 alerts the coder not to assign it with 66982, 66983, or 66984.

REIMBURSEMENT REVIEW

The *Medicare Carriers Manual* is very clear about coverage of IOL insertion at the same time as a cataract extraction. Medicare does not make separate payment for the supply of the actual IOL implant to the hospital or ambulatory surgical center (ASC) when inserted subsequent to extraction of a cataract. Payment for the IOL is packaged into the payment for the cataract extraction procedure. Medicare can legally penalize with civil money penalties parties who submit a bill for an IOL inserted during or subsequent to cataract surgery. For physician professional claims, a physician may not bill Medicare for an IOL inserted during a cataract procedure performed in a hospital or ASC setting because the payment for the lens is included in the payment made to the facility for the surgical procedure. However, the physician can bill Medicare for the lens if the cataract extraction is done in the ASC or hospital and the lens is subsequently inserted in the office with place of service (POS) 11.

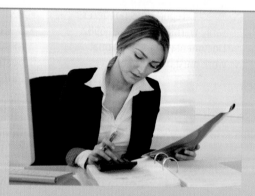

Ophthalmic Endoscope

An endoscope offers a more extended view of the eye anatomy that is currently not accessible through an operating microscope. In this procedure, an endoscopic probe tip is inserted into the eye via sclerotomy. By using the endoscope, the doctor can visualize the internal eye in patients with poor papillary dilation or pathological changes. CPT code 66990, *Use of ophthalmic endoscope*, is an add-on code and may be appended to the following series of surgical codes: 65820, 65875, 65920, 66985, 66986, 67036, 67039, 67040, 67041, 67042, 67043, and 67113.

CHECKPOINT 26.2

Assign CPT code(s) to the following procedures. Some scenarios also require HCPCS code assignment.

1. A Medicare patient is status post–cataract extraction 5 years ago. He is seen today for insertion of a replacement Alcon SN60WS intraocular lens, right eye, with ophthalmic endoscope. _____

2. A patient is seen in the office with decreased vision in the right eye 3 months after a cataract extraction. The eye is examined and it is determined that the patient has secondary opacification. The physician makes an incision at the limbus to remove the posterior lens membranous capsule. _____

3. A patient is seen in the office for his annual eye examination. He states he has decreased vision in his left eye where he had a cataract removed the previous year. The doctor examines the eye and discovers that the lens has become dislodged. The patient is taken to the operating room the next day and the IOL is repositioned. _____

If a surgeon electively performs a corneal re-laxing incision to correct astigmatism, this is a noncovered service and should be reported with 66999–GY to Medicare. If the astigmatism is not surgically induced, the procedure is generally a noncovered elective refractive surgery.

CPT codes 65420 and 65426 describe excision of pterygium without and with graft, respectively. Graft codes and the ocular surface reconstruction CPT codes 65780 –65782 should not be reported separately with either of these codes for the same eye.

Surgically Induced Astigmatism

Surgically induced astigmatism occurs during eye surgery, such as IOL placement, glaucoma surgery, and corneal transplants. Eye surgeons strive to eliminate or reduce the amount of corneal astigmatism created, particularly with patients receiving IOL implants. During the surgery, a small incision is made in the patient's cornea, through which instruments can be inserted into the eye to remove the natural lens and introduce an IOL. The incision is very small and heals without a need for sutures. However, the incision can induce postoperative corneal astigmatism or modify preexisting corneal astigmatism. Surgically induced astigmatism can vary from one patient to another. The corneal astigmatic aberrations or curvature of the cornea can lead to different magnifications, resulting in blurred vision. This astigmatism is not the same as a congenital astigmatism. To correct this, the surgeon incises the cornea to allow it to relax and lay flat, correcting the vision. Report codes 65772 or 65775.

Pterygium

Pterygium is an abnormal growth of the conjunctiva of the inner corner of the eye that obstructs vision by growing over the cornea. Most surgeries are done cosmetically, but they may also be needed when the condition involves the cornea to relieve the distortion of the cornea. The surgeon uses a blade and scleral scissors to remove the growth. Sutures are placed in the sclera and conjunctiva if needed. Report 65420 if the pterygium is removed with no graft and 65426 if a conjunctival graft or flap is placed. If the defect is repaired by using an amniotic membrane transplant, assign code 65780 instead of 65426. The facility should also report HCPCS code V2790 (*Amniotic membrane for surgical reconstruction, per procedure*) for the supply of the donor tissue.

Trichiasis

Trichiasis is a condition in which the eyelashes are ingrown or growing in the wrong direction. It is caused by infection, inflammation, and trauma such as burns or eyelid injury. Standard treatment involves destruction of the affected eyelashes with electrology, a specialized laser, or surgery. The method of treatment must be determined before the code can be assigned (laser, graft required). Codes from 67820–67835 are reported once per session, not per eye, regardless of the number of epilations performed. In 67825, either cryotherapy or electrosurgery is performed to destroy the hair follicles. Report 67830–67835 if the physician incises the eyelid to remove the area where abnormal eyelash growth is located. A split-thickness graft may be taken from the patient's mouth and placed to cover the defect if necessary.

Glaucoma

Glaucoma or *primary open-angle glaucoma (POAG)* is a condition in which the aqueous cannot drain from the anterior segment of the eye, causing pressure on the optic nerve. Glaucoma is the leading cause of blindness but can be treated with daily medication and/or surgery. Two techniques are used in glaucoma surgery: laser or incision. Trabeculoplasty, iridotomy, and iridoplasty are laser treatments. Trabeculoplasty is performed by using a laser to alter the trabecular meshwork, which is heated so that it shrinks, and pulling open the areas not treated to allow aqueous to drain. During iridotomy, the laser creates a hole in the iris, allowing the aqueous to reach the trabecular meshwork and canal of Schlemm through the iris instead of flowing around it. Iridoplasty requires the use of a laser to burn the edges of the iris, causing it to contract and pull away from the trabecular meshwork. Trabeculectomy is an incisional procedure that creates a drain for the aqueous. This procedure is usually performed ab externo, from the outside of the eye. Trabeculectomy procedures include the following:

- Incision through the limbus
- Conjunctival flap
- Removal of trabecular tissue
- Closure of the incision
- Restoring ocular pressure by injecting Healon or saline
- Injection/application of antibiotics

At times, when a trabeculectomy is not indicated, an aqueous shunt may be placed. This tube is placed into the anterior chamber between the cornea and the iris.

> **EXAMPLE**
>
> The physician performed a nonpenetrating deep sclerectomy with insertion of glaucoma drainage shunt of left eye. Assign code 66180–LT, *Aqueous shunt to extraocular reservoir.* The sclerectomy is part of the procedure for the aqueous shunt implant and not reported separately. Facilities may also report HCPCS code L8612, *Aqueous shunt,* for the implant.

> Do not confuse PTK with PRK. They are essentially the same procedure; however, they are used for different clinical indications. PTK is used to correct particular corneal diseases, and PRK involves the use of the excimer laser for correction of refraction errors (e.g., myopia, hyperopia, astigmatism, and presbyopia) in persons with otherwise nondiseased corneas.

Vision Correction Surgery

Many people are taking advantage of technological advances to eliminate the need for glasses. Three procedures are frequently done to correct vision by altering the surface of the cornea. Laser-assisted in-situ keratomileusis (LASIK) uses a laser to reduce curvature and correct nearsightedness. Because the corneal tissue has natural bonding qualities, the eye heals without stitches. LASIK is used to treat a broad range of vision problems. During this procedure, a thin layer of the surface of the cornea is lifted as a flap and the laser is used to reshape the underlying cornea. The flap is then laid back down over the resurfaced area. This procedure can also be performed by using a thermal probe to heat the edges of the cornea without making any incisions. At this time,

> Keratomileusis involves removing a portion of the cornea, reshaping it, and then suturing it back in place. Do not report HCPCS S codes when filing claims to Medicare.

there is no CPT code for this procedure; however, there is an HCPCS code: S0800. Photorefractive keratectomy (PRK) is a technique used to correct near- and farsightedness and mild astigmatisms. A laser is used to reshape the surface of the cornea. There is no CPT code for this procedure; however, there is an HCPCS code: S0810. Phototherapeutic keratectomy (PTK) is a corneal laser treatment that removes layers of corneal clouding and clears patients' vision when successful. There is no CPT code for this procedure; however, there is an HCPCS code: S0812.

Eyelid Lesions

Skin on the eyelid is susceptible to the elements and the same diseases as the rest of the body. Many eyelid infections and ailments are treated with medication and conservative measures. However, some lesions or growths may require surgical intervention or excision, including carcinoma, chalazion, and stye. If the excision involves only skin of the eyelid, use a code from the Integumentary System section. If it involves lid margin, tarsus, or otherwise, use codes 67840–67850 and 67961–67966. Code 67810, despite its description, involves removing (excising) tissue from a specific area of the eyelid and possibly eyelid margin, for biopsy purposes. The entire area is not excised. Notice the description says "tissue" and not "skin." The parenthetical note following this code says to use codes from the Integumentary section of CPT for biopsy of skin of the eyelid.

A chalazion is a raised lesion or cyst that appears on the edge of the upper eyelid. A chalazion may need to be drained or excised if it does not resolve on its own. Surgical excision is usually done from underneath the eyelid to avoid a scar on the skin by placing a clamp to expose the undersurface of the eyelid. The chalazion is incised and the wound is cauterized. Code assignment is dependent on how many chalazions are removed and if they are on the same eyelid. Code 67808 is assigned if general anesthesia is used regardless of the number of chalazions removed.

■ CASE SCENARIO

A patient complains of a nevus on the lower eyelid that over the years has grown in size and now partially obstructs her vision. The physician removes the 0.7-cm nevus by making a full-thickness incision into the dermis and excising the nevus in one piece. The wound is closed with 6-0 superficial nonabsorbable sutures. Assign code 11441.

Foreign Body

For foreign body (FB) removal from the eye, codes are differentiated by compartments of the eye and whether a corneal slit lamp is used. Numerous notes related to this are located prior to code 65205 and provide instructions on code assignment.

Any material such as dust, sand, sawdust, paint, metal shavings, or bugs that gets into the eye is considered a foreign body. Foreign bodies fall into two categories.

- Superficial foreign bodies: These stick to the front of the eye or get trapped underneath one of the eyelids and sit on the surface of the conjunctiva but do not enter the eyeball. They may be referred to as loose FBs or floating FBs.
- Penetrating foreign bodies: These penetrate the outer layer of the eye (cornea or sclera) and enter the eye. These objects are usually traveling at high speed and are commonly made of metal, glass, or wood. Penetrating eye injuries occur during car and recreational vehicle accidents and when people are hammering, sawing, or grinding.

The chapter has two sets of FB removal codes from which to choose, depending on whether the FB is in the conjunctiva or cornea. For conjunctival FB removal (65205–65210), the coder must be able to determine where it is embedded. An embedded conjunctival FB sits in the conjunctiva but has not penetrated the anterior chamber. A conjunctival FB is typically removed with a sterile cotton swab and, if embedded, by using a needle to act like a beveled edge to pry the object out. Similarly, for corneal FB removal (65220–65222), the coder should look for slit-lamp use before assigning a code. For intraocular FB removal, assign codes from 65235–65265.

On initial examination, the physician will perform a fluorescein stain and slit-lamp examination to identify the extent of injury, exact location, and whether there is any corneal abrasion caused by the foreign body. Superficial FBs can become trapped under the eyelid and, during blinking, cause scratches on the cornea called *corneal abrasion*.

> ### ■ CASE SCENARIO
> A house painter with a swollen right eye sees his ophthalmologist. The doctor examines the eye and finds a paint chip sitting atop the patient's conjunctival sac. Using a moistened cotton swab, the doctor removes the FB. Assign code 65205–RT.

Retinal Detachment

Retinal detachment occurs when the retina pulls away from the choroid. The detachment can be partial or total and/or may have many defects. Detachment usually begins as a tear in the retina subsequent to a traumatic blow to the head (e.g., as in boxing). Vitreous then seeps under the retina behind the tear. The retina becomes detached, is separated from the blood supply, and falls into the posterior segment of the eye, causing vision loss. Surgery is required to repair the retina by cryotherapy (67101), laser photocoagulation (67105), scleral buckle (67107), or injection of air or gas (67110). Cryotherapy uses a cold probe to freeze the tissue. Diathermy uses heat to burn through the back of the eye to destroy abnormal tissue and force the retina to seal back to the eye. When a vitrectomy is performed in a retinal detachment surgery, use 67108 because the code description includes both the vitrectomy and retinal detachment procedure. Photocoagulation uses a laser that emits green waves to coagulate tissue by sealing off blood vessels with the absorption of the laser wave. Scleral buckling is a technique used to treat retinal detachment by placing silicone material around the eye to indent the sclera to close the hole or reduce the vitreous traction after diathermy is performed. The buckle is like a belt around the eye to hold the silicone. This application compresses the eye so that the hole or tear in the retina is pushed against the outer scleral wall of the eye, which has been indented by the buckle.

> ### ■ CASE SCENARIO
> The surgeon treated a tractional retinal detachment with pan retinal endolaser photocoagulation, peripheral cryopexy, and air-fluid exchange. He relieved the area of tractional retinal detachment with a high-speed vitreous cutter. He also applied peripheral panendolaser photocoagulation to previously untreated areas of the retina and treated a small retinal tear with cryopexy. Assign code 67108.

CHECKPOINT 26.3

Assign the CPT code(s) to the following procedure.

1. A surgeon performed a repair of a retinal detachment by scleral buckling of the right eye. The patient previously underwent scleral buckling on the left eye approximately 4 months ago.

_____

Vitrectomy is also performed to provide access to the retina for treatment of other retinal disorders or infection. See codes 67015 and 67036–67040. The vitreous is removed mechanically with a probe or vitreous infusion suction cutter (VISC) accompanied by endolaser coagulation. Look for key words such as *microvit, ocutome,* or *daisy wheel probe* to indicate that a mechanical vitrectomy was performed. If a vitreous substitute is injected after the vitrectomy, assign code 67025, *Injection of vitreous substitute, pars plana or limbal approach, with or without aspiration.* Focal endolaser coagulation treats one or two small areas of the retina. Pan retinal photocoagulation treats all four quadrants of the retina.

> ● Some retinal detachment repair procedures include vitreous procedures that are not separately reportable. For example, the procedure described by CPT code 67108 includes the procedures described by CPT codes 67015, 67025, 67028, 67031, 67036, 67039, and 67040.

CHECKPOINT 26.4

Assign the CPT code(s) to the following procedure.

1. An ophthalmologist performs a pars plana vitrectomy with focal endolaser photocoagulation immediately following an ophthalmic endoscopy that revealed severe proliferative diabetic retinopathy with hemorrhage in the left eye. The patient is 26 years old. _____

Corneal Disease

Disease of the cornea can result in visual impairment. Common corneal problems include the following:

- Corneal edema: swelling of the cornea
- Corneal opacity: clouding of the cornea
- Keratoconus: abnormal cone-shaped cornea
- Trauma: penetration, abrasion, or burning

> ● Procedures of the cornea should not be reported with anterior chamber "separate procedures" such as CPT codes 65800, 65815, and 66020. The Centers for Medicare and Medicaid Services (CMS) payment policy does not allow separate payment for procedures, including the "separate procedure" designation in its code descriptor, when the "separate procedure" is performed with another procedure in an anatomically related area.

> ● Facilities should report HCPCS code V2785, *Processing, preserving, and transporting corneal tissue,* in addition to the corneal transplant procedure code.

> ● Read the operative report closely when assigning codes for keratoplasty. Some of the code descriptions are specific to a diagnosis, and the correct diagnosis must be linked to this procedure. For example, 65750, *Keratoplasty; penetrating (in aphakia)*.

Corneal grafts are performed on patients with damaged or scarred corneas due to disease or trauma that inhibits clear vision. Keratoplasty or corneal transplant is also known as a corneal graft or penetrating keratoplasty, which involves removing the central portion (called a *button*) of the diseased cornea and replacing it with a matched cadaver donor cornea. A lamellar keratoplasty uses a partial-thickness graft and includes removing the anterior layer of the cornea and cutting the donor cornea to the same size as the defect. A penetrating keratoplasty uses a full-thickness graft.

Keratoplasty codes are chosen based on whether the graft was partial thickness or full thickness and whether the eye is in aphakia or pseudophakia status. Aphakia describes an eye that had the lens removed surgically or by trauma. This would include patients who have had cataract surgery without an IOL replacement. Pseudophakia describes an eye that had the natural lens removed and replaced with a synthetic one.

Pneumatic retinopexy is performed on an outpatient basis under local anesthesia. Laser or cryotherapy is used to seal the hole or tear. The surgeon then injects a gas bubble directly inside the vitreous cavity of the eye to push the detached retina against the back outer wall of the eye (sclera). The gas bubble initially expands and then disappears over 2 to 6 weeks.

Ocular Trauma

Trauma to the eye often occurs from burns, chemical splashes, blunt force to the eye from assault or accidental injury from foreign objects, or dog bites. Eyelid lacerations may involve the lid margin, requiring a meticulous suturing technique; be extramarginal; or cause tissue loss. Codes for repair of the linear skin of the eyelid are located in the Integumentary System section. Codes for procedures of the eyelid margin, tarsus, or palpebral conjunctiva are located in the Eye and Ocular Adnexa section, as are codes for full-thickness eyelid reconstruction.

EXAMPLE
Partial-thickness suture repair of a 2-cm wound of the eyelid margin tarsus. The wound was sustained 1 day ago. Assign code 67930.

If skin grafting is also required to repair the wound or defect, the appropriate skin graft code is determined by whether greater than or less than one-fourth of the lid margin is involved. Code 67961 is assigned for preparation for skin graft or pedicle flap with adjacent tissue transfer or rearrangement of up to one-fourth of the lid margin. Code 67966 is assigned for transfer or rearrangement of greater than one-fourth of the lid margin.

Cancer

Neoplasms, or skin cancers of the eyelid, require treatment that involves surgical intervention to some degree, whether it be chemical cauterization or laser or scalpel excision. Basal cell carcinoma (BCC), the most common eyelid malignancy, usually appears in the lower lid and medial canthal region as a firm nodule. BCC typically does not metastasize but may be locally invasive. Squamous cell carcinoma (SCC), on the other hand, behaves more aggressively and occurs frequently on the upper lid as erythematous, raised, scaly, and centrally ulcerated lesions. Sebaceous carcinoma occurs in middle-age to elderly patients. It invades locally and spreads to regional preauricular or submandibular lymph nodes. Because of the aggressive nature of these tumors, surgical removal of the orbital contents may be required.

If the excision involves only the skin of the eyelid, use a code from the Integumentary System section. If it involves the lid margin, tarsus, or otherwise, use codes 67840–67850 and 67961–67966.

At times, the cancer or neoplasm is of the actual eyeball, or globe, which requires surgical removal of the eyeball and may also require removal of surrounding tissues, depending on the extent of the disease. Enucleation is the surgical removal of the eyeball that leaves the eye muscles and remaining orbital contents intact. Enucleation is performed because of large-size eye tumors when the eye cannot be spared or as a result of traumatic injury when the eye cannot be preserved. According to the U.S. National Center for Health Statistics, trauma is considered the most common cause of enucleation in children over 3 years of age. Sometimes in the case of tumors, the amount of radiation required to treat the tumor is too intense and consequently destroys the eye and causes vision loss, glaucoma, and tissue damage, requiring enucleation.

The eyeball is removed by resecting the conjunctiva with blunt scissors. The four rectus muscles are removed from their attachments to the globe. The optic nerve is severed, and the eyeball is removed.

Three codes exist for enucleation procedures and differ by whether an implant was placed at the time of the eyeball removal or whether the muscles were attached to the implant (65101–65105).

> Conjunctivoplasty done after enucleation is coded separately using code range 68320–68328.

> Remember to also report the HCPCS code for the prosthetic implant. Codes 65093–65105, 65130–65175, and 67550 describe the procedures for inserting the implant, not the implant itself. The facility or the physician supplying the implant should also report HCPCS codes V2623–V2629.

Implants

Two types of implants are associated with the eye. An *ocular implant* is placed inside the muscular cone of the eye socket. Implantation of ocular implants is reported using codes 65093, 65103–65105, and 65130–65175. *Orbital implants* are placed outside the muscular cone of the eye socket and reported using code 67550.

Two to six weeks after enucleation surgery, patients are sent for a fitting and creation of a synthetic ocular prosthesis. A subsequent surgery is performed to insert the implant and is reported using 65135 or 65140. A synthetic globe or ocular implant replaces the eyeball in the socket, and the rectus muscles are sutured around it.

If the surgeon immediately places the prosthetic implant at the same session as the enucleation, 65103 is reported if the implant is inserted but the muscles are not attached to the implant. Code 65105 includes muscle attachment to the implant.

Strabismus

Strabismus is a condition in which the eye is misaligned (this is commonly referred to as cross-eyed). This condition is typically diagnosed during childhood and may occur in one or both eyes. Strabismus can develop in adulthood as well. Strabismus results when the extraocular muscles do not work together to align the eye and focus on a single object. If the six muscles do not move the eye together, they focus on separate objects and send different images to the brain. If a muscle is too strong, it may cause the eye to turn in, turn out, or rotate too high or too low. Likewise, if a muscle is too weak, misalignment will also occur. *Esotropia* is when one of the eyes is turned inward. In *exotropia,* the eye is turned outward. The documentation may state that the condition is "monocular" or "alternating." Monocular means that only one eye is involved. Alternating means that both eyes are involved but not necessarily at the same time.

Table 26.2 Eye Muscles

MUSCLE NAME	MUSCLE GROUP
Superior rectus	Vertical
Inferior rectus	Vertical
Lateral rectus	Horizontal
Medial rectus	Horizontal
Inferior oblique	Vertical
Superior oblique	Vertical

Strabismus Correction

Repair is accomplished by resecting or recessing the appropriate ocular muscles in the affected eye (Table 26.2). Recession weakens a specific ocular muscle by altering where the targeted muscle is attached to the eyeball. A suture is placed through the muscle at the attachment site, and the surgeon detaches the outside (extraocular) muscle from the eye and reattaches it farther back on the eyeball to weaken the relative strength of the muscle if it is too strong, pulling the eye out of alignment. In contrast, if a muscle is too weak, the surgeon may use a recession procedure to reduce the strength of an *opposing* muscle (antagonist) to achieve more balanced function of the eye muscles.

A resection procedure is commonly used to strengthen the lateral rectus eye muscle as in esotropia. Resection involves removing a piece or portion of an affected muscle and reattaching it at the same or adjacent site, shortening or tightening the muscle, so to speak. The lateral rectus muscle is located on the side of each eye, toward the ear. Shortening the lateral rectus muscles strengthens them so that they can pull the eyes farther outward. This results in better eye alignment.

Codes are divided based on the muscles detached and reattached. It is very important to know which muscles are horizontal and which are vertical. The vertical muscles—superior and inferior rectus and superior and inferior oblique—move the eye up and down. The horizontal muscles—lateral rectus and medial rectus—move the eye side to side (see Table 26.2). These muscles are illustrated in the Strabismus Surgery section of CPT. Recession makes the muscles weaker, whereas resection makes the muscles stronger. Extraocular muscles are transposed to bring the eye into proper alignment (67320). The code description for transposition includes the term *specify*, alerting the coder that documentation is required to indicate which muscle was treated, along with the claim for payment of services.

For reporting strabismus surgery, several add-on codes may also be reported to capture all work and paint the most accurate clinical picture. To capture all applicable surgery codes, it is necessary to know if the patient has had prior eye surgery. If the patient has had prior strabismus surgery, the add-on code 67332 is listed in addition to the procedure performed. Also, if posterior fixation sutures are placed, 67334 is listed separately. In posterior fixation suturing, the extraocular muscle is sutured to the eye posterior or behind where it is inserted. Adjustable sutures may be placed to allow for further adjusting of the musculature after the anesthetic wears off. Add-on codes for adjustable suture insertion (67335), posterior fixation suture technique (67334), previous strabismus surgery status (67332), and transposition of extraocular muscles (67320) are used in addition to the base code for strabismus surgery.

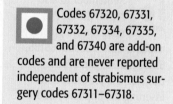

Codes 67320, 67331, 67332, 67334, 67335, and 67340 are add-on codes and are never reported independent of strabismus surgery codes 67311–67318.

OCULOPLASTIC SURGERY

This section specifically discusses diseases and oculoplastic procedures of the eyeball, adnexa, eyelid, and eyebrow. Oculoplasty, or oculoplastic surgery, is a subspecialty of ophthalmology that specializes in the plastic and reconstructive surgery of the eye and surrounding structures. This subspecialty concentrates on the medical and surgical management of deformities and abnormalities of the eyelids, lacrimal (tear) system, orbit, and the adjacent face (eyebrow). These specialists focus on procedures involving the skin, subcutaneous tissue, muscle, and fat of the eye involved in reconstructions and cosmetic repairs from trauma or extensive disease.

To accurately assign codes for these complex procedures, the coder must master the intricate anatomy of the eyelid and surrounding skin and musculature. Use illustrations located online or an anatomy text of the skin, musculature, and the accessory structures surrounding the eye as guides to find landmarks when reading descriptions of the procedures discussed next.

Eyelid and Muscle Anatomy

The upper eyelid extends superiorly to the eyebrow, which separates it from the forehead. The lower lid extends below the inferior orbital rim to join the cheek, forming folds where the loose connective tissue of the eyelid is side to side with the denser tissue of the cheek. The upper eyelid skin crease (superior palpebral sulcus) is approximately 8 to 11 mm superior to the eyelid margin and is formed by the attachment of the superficial insertion of levator aponeurotic fibers.

The nasojugal fold runs inferiorly and laterally from the inner canthal region along the depression of separation of the orbicularis oculi and the levator labii superioris, forming the tear channel. The malar fold runs inferiorly and medially from the outer canthus toward the inferior aspect of the nasojugal fold.

The open eye presents the palpebral fissure or crease between the lid margins. The palpebral fissure presents the lateral canthus; the medial; and the lacrimal papillae, which rest on the free lid margin, with the punctum lacrimale serving as an opening to the canaliculus.

Overview of Structure

Structures that must be considered in a description of lid anatomy are skin and subcutaneous tissue, orbicularis oculi muscle, submuscular areolar tissue, the fibrous layer consisting of the tarsi and orbital septum, lid retractors of the upper and lower eyelids, retroseptal fat pads, and conjunctiva.

The anatomy of the lid consists of many layers of tissue. The orbital septum represents the anatomical boundary between the lid tissue and the orbital tissue. Anatomically complex, the eyelids consist of an anterior layer of skin and orbicularis oculi muscle, and a posterior layer of tarsus and conjunctiva. In eyelid reconstruction these areas are referred to as *lamellae*, with the anterior lamella being the skin and orbicularis and the posterior lamella being the tarsus and conjunctiva.

Orbicularis Oculi Muscle. The orbicularis oculi muscle is one of the superficial muscles of facial expression. The muscle is divided into the orbital and palpebral parts, with the latter being further divided into the preseptal and pretarsal portions. The palpebral portion is used in blinking and voluntary winking, while the orbital portion is used in forced closure. The orbital portion extends in a wide circular fashion around the orbit, intertwining with other muscles of the face.

The preseptal orbicularis muscles overlie the orbital septum and take origin medially from a superficial and deep head associated with the medial palpebral ligament. The fibers from the upper and lower lid join laterally to form the lateral palpebral raphe, which is attached to the overlying skin. The pretarsal portion lies anterior to the tarsus, with a superficial and deep head of origin intimately associated with the medial palpebral ligament.

Submuscular Areolar Tissue. Submuscular areolar tissue consists of variable loose connective tissue below the orbicularis oculi muscle. The lid may be split into anterior and posterior portions through this potential plane, which is reached by division at the gray line of the lid margin. In the upper lid, this plane is traversed by fibers of the levator aponeurosis, some of which pass through the orbicularis to attach to the skin to form the lid crease. In the lower eyelid, this plane is traversed by fibers of the orbitomalar ligament.

Superior continuance in this submuscular plane arrives at the retro-orbicularis oculi fat (ROOF), which is best developed in the eyebrow region. In addition, the suborbicularis oculi fat (SOOF) is found in the lower lid in a continuance of this plane.

Tarsal Plates. The tarsal plates are composed of dense fibrous tissue and are responsible for the structural formation of the lids. The lower border of the superior tarsus forms the posterior lid margin. The rectangular inferior tarsus is located in the center of the eyelid. The posterior surfaces of the tarsi adhere to conjunctivae.

The medial palpebral ligament (medial canthal tendon [MCT]) is a fibrous band stabilizing the medial tarsi and is intricately related with the orbicularis oculi muscle and the lacrimal system.

The lateral palpebral ligament (lateral canthal tendon [LCT]) is formed by dense fibrous tissue arising from the tarsi. It passes laterally deep to the septum orbitale to insert into the lateral orbital tubercle posterior to the lateral orbital rim.

The lateral tarsal strap is described as a broad and strong structure connecting the lower lid tarsal plate to the inferolateral orbital rim.

> **INTERNET RESOURCE:** For additional information about human eye anatomy, visit
> **www.drmeronk.com/anatomy.html**

Eyelid Ptosis

Blepharoptosis is considered severe drooping (ptosis) of the eyelids or brow. This is frequently caused by aging and dehiscence of the levator muscle, myasthenia gravis, Horner's syndrome, stroke, and trauma. *Blepharochalasis* is an inflammation of the eyelid that occurs intermittently whereby the eyelid swells considerably, stretching the skin and causing atrophy of the eyelid tissue.

In blepharochalasis, the eyelid skin becomes lax and falls in redundant folds over the lid margins. It typically affects only the upper eyelids and may be unilateral or bilateral.

Repair

Blepharoplasty, or blepharoptosis repair, is correction of a drooping eyelid by repairing the levator muscle and removing excess skin that may weigh down the lid. This procedure may be performed by an ophthalmologist or plastic surgeon. An extensive blepharoplasty involves excision of the tarsal wedge and possibly fat from the lower orbit of the eyelid. The tarsus consists of dense connective tissue that contributes to the form and support of the eyelid. CPT codes 67900–67904 include the services of CPT codes 15820–15823 as part of the total service performed and should not be billed separately. If the procedure involves only skin, fat, and muscle (without the tarsus), use codes 15820–15823. These are considered cosmetic blepharoplasties. You must determine which approach was performed and which muscle was affected (tarsus, levator) before assigning a code. Most are done "externally," where the incision is made on the outside of the eyelid.

Lower Lid Ptosis

Canthoplasty is performed to reinforce lower eyelid support by detaching the lateral canthal tendon from the orbital bone and constructing a replacement (67950). Canthopexy is a less-invasive procedure designed to stabilize the existing tendon (as well as surrounding structures) without removing it from its normal attachment. Canthopexy is more of a cosmetic procedure commonly performed with transconjunctival fat trimming and chemical peel as part of a lower eyelid rejuvenation (21282, 21280). If no skin is to be removed, the external incision is much smaller.

> ● Blepharoplasty is often considered a cosmetic or plastic surgery. Insurance carriers routinely require preauthorization for this procedure, with photos taken of the patient's eyes and visual field examinations to determine the extent of vision loss due to the skin impairing the eyelid's ability to open fully. Because visual field examination (CPT codes 92081–92083) would be performed prior to scheduling a patient for a blepharoplasty (CPT codes 15820–15823) or blepharoptosis (CPT codes 67901–67908) procedure, the visual field examination CPT codes should not be reported separately with the blepharoplasty or blepharoptosis procedure codes for the same date of service.

Entropion Repair

Entropion is the turning inward of the lower or upper eyelid, causing it to rub against the eyeball. Entropion can be divided into the following classes: congenital, acute spastic, involutional, and cicatricial. It primarily occurs in the lower eyelid and is often caused by scarring from trauma or inflammation from certain diseases that involve the eyelids.

When the eyelid turns inward, the lashes rub against the eye, resulting in irritation, scratchiness, tearing, and redness. Entropion can be repaired either by using a suture technique or by a more complex technique involving removal of muscle and tarsus and skin grafting. Code 67921 is strictly suturing of the lid; no incision is made. Sutures are threaded through the inferior fornix or inferior cul-de-sac externally to the lash line. The sutures are placed mattress style in the medial, middle, and lateral third of the eyelid and tied on the skin side. Code 67923 is a triangular tarsal wedge excised along with exposed orbicularis muscle and then repaired with sutures. Repair with extensive blepharoplasty (67924) is carried out by making an incision about 80% the length of the eyelid. A triangular section of tarsus may be excised. Deep sutures are used to sever the eyelid margin, forcing the lid outward. Again, technique is key to assigning the proper code. If a skin graft is needed as in the case of a cicatricial entropion, use codes 67961–67975 instead.

> ● CMS policy does not allow separate payment for blepharoptosis (CPT codes 67901–67908) and blepharoplasty procedures (CPT codes 15822 and 15823) on the same (ipsilateral) upper eyelid. If these procedures are performed during the same operative session but on different lids, report the HCPCS –E anatomical lid modifiers to differentiate.

Ectropion Repair

Ectropion is the turning outward of the edge of the lower or upper eyelid, causing the margin to pull away. The turning outward of the lower or upper eyelid causes corneal exposure and drying of the eye because the eyelid cannot close completely to protect the eye or blink properly to lubricate it. Repair can be carried out in several ways, which differ based on the type of excision and

You must read the operative report to determine the ectropian repair technique. Look for key words like *tarsal wedge* (67916) or *tarsal strip* (67917). The coder must know the extent of tarsus involvement before assigning a code.

blepharoplasty performed. These techniques range from simple to extensive. In 67914, absorbable sutures are used to foreshorten the posterior tissues of the eyelid. No incision is made in this type of repair because the suture causes the eyelid to rotate posteriorly. In 67915, cautery is used to shrink the tissues of the eyelid margin to rotate them posteriorly toward the eyeball or globe. Code 67916 describes repair with blepharoplasty and excision of a tarsal wedge. A piece of the tarsus and conjunctiva is removed in the shape of a diamond or rhomboid from the back surface of the lower eyelid. The margin of the eyelid is then rotated posteriorly toward the eyeball with absorbable sutures. Code 67917 is considered an extensive blepharoplasty and is also referred to as a Kuhnt-Szymanowski operation. An incision is made in the lower lid to create a tongue or tarsal strip. This strip is then set apart in the lateral one-third of the lower lid by incising the tarsus or shortening the tarsus by incising it, not excising it. Sutures are placed into the tarsal strip through the periosteum of the lateral orbit where the sutures are then tightened to achieve the proper contour.

AUDITORY SYSTEM

Additional codes for otologic services are located in the Medicine section.

Codes for the Auditory System section include procedures on the external ear, middle ear, inner ear, and temporal bone. This section is the smallest surgical section in the CPT manual. Procedures and services in this section are performed by an otolaryngologist, otherwise referred to as an ear, nose, and throat (ENT) specialist. An otolaryngologist is a surgeon who specializes in the diagnosis and treatment of diseases and injuries to the ears, nose, and throat, including the sinuses. Codes in this section describe diagnostic and therapeutic procedures on the inner, middle, and outer ear. The codes are arranged by anatomical part and then by procedure on that part. The following abbreviations are used to describe which ear is being treated:

- AU: both ears
- AS: left ear
- AD: right ear

The ear is a paired body part and requires the use of the –LT or –RT modifiers with code assignment.

Organization

At times, Medicare coding and reporting policies differ from CPT guidelines or instructions. CMS guidelines for payment of CPT code 69990 differ from the CPT manual instructions following CPT code 69990. The Internet-only manuals (IOMs), *Medicare Claims Processing Manual* (Publication 100–04), Chapter 12, Section 20.4.5, limits the reporting of an operating microscope (CPT code 69990) to procedure codes 61304–61546, 61550–61711, 62010–62100, 63081–63308, 63704–63710, 64831, 64834–64836, 64840–64858, 64861–64870, 64885, 64891, and 64905–64907. CPT code 69990 should not be reported with other procedures, even if an operating microscope is utilized. The National Correct Coding Initiative (NCCI) bundles CPT code 69990 into all surgical procedures other than those listed in the *Medicare Claims Processing Manual*. Most edits do not allow use of NCCI-associated modifiers.

The Auditory System section is organized into the following sections and then by the standard subsections of Introduction, Incision, Excision, Removal, and Repair:

- External Ear
- Middle Ear
- Inner Ear
- Temporal Bone, Middle Fossa Approach

Included at the end of the Auditory System section is the Operating Microscope section. Instructional notes state that the surgical microscope is used when the microsurgery technique is employed. The microscope code 69990 represents the work of setting up, calibrating, positioning, and adjusting the operating microscope when brought into position to view the surgical area. Code 69990 may be assigned in addition to surgical procedure codes in specific circumstances. Many CPT procedures already include the work of 69990, and payer reimbursement for these procedures is valued accordingly. CPT provides a list of codes in the operating microscope introductory guidelines of codes that consider the use of an operating microscope to be an integral component, according to the American Medical Association. Based on the CPT manual, from a coding standpoint it is incorrect to assign 69990 in addition to the codes listed within these guidelines. Magnifying loupe glasses do not constitute microsurgery technique. The code 69990 cannot be reported alone or with a −51 modifier.

Commercial plans are not bound to the NCCI, so if the patient has commercial insurance adhere to CPT guidelines for reporting the operating microscope.

> **●** Read the guidelines for use of microscope BEFORE assigning the code. Do not assign 69990 unless the operative report specifies the use of a microscope. Loupes or magnifying lenses are not the same as a microscope.

Modifiers

Read the documentation carefully to determine which ear is treated. Physicians commonly use abbreviations to depict which ear is being treated; this can lead to errors in code assignment or modifier usage.

Table 26.3 includes some of the more common modifiers that may be reported with ear procedures. This by no means is an exhaustive list.

Table 26.3 Modifiers for Ear Procedures

MODIFIER	DEFINITION
LT	Left (ear)
RT	Right (ear)
50	Bilateral (ears)
76	Repeat procedure or service by the same physician
77	Repeat procedure or service by another physician
78	Unplanned return to the operating room by the same physician following initial procedure for a related procedure during the postoperative period
79	Unrelated procedure or service by the same physician during the postoperative period

EAR ANATOMY

The ear is essentially divided into three areas: external, middle, and inner ear (Fig. 26.2). The external ear consists of the auricle or pinna, external acoustic membrane, and tympanic membrane or eardrum. The external ear conducts sound to the middle ear. The middle ear comprises the tympanic cavity and eustachian tube. The tympanic cavity consists of the auditory ossicles: malleus, incus, and stapes. The attic is a cavity of the middle ear that lies above the tympanic cavity and contains the malleus and incus. The bones of the middle ear are responsible for amplifying sound and transmitting it to the inner ear via the oval window. The stapes has a footplate that fits into the oval window. The inner ear is located within the temporal bone, which consists of a complex system of bony chambers and tubes called an *osseous labyrinth*. Within this labyrinth lies a membranous labyrinth of fluid-filled spaces and tubes. The bony labyrinth is sectioned into the vestibule, semicircular canals, and cochlea. The cochlea serves a function in hearing, and the three semicircular canals and vestibule assist in providing a sense of equilibrium.

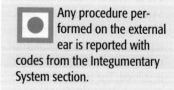

> **●** Any procedure performed on the external ear is reported with codes from the Integumentary System section.

COMMON PROBLEMS OF THE EAR AND ASSOCIATED PROCEDURES

Foreign Body in the Ear

It is very common for children to place objects into their ears (peas, crayons, beads, etc.), which then become lodged. More often than not, this requires surgical removal under anesthesia (69200–69205). Do not report these codes for ventilation tube removal. A specific code is available for this service (69424). Codes are assigned based on whether general anesthesia was required.

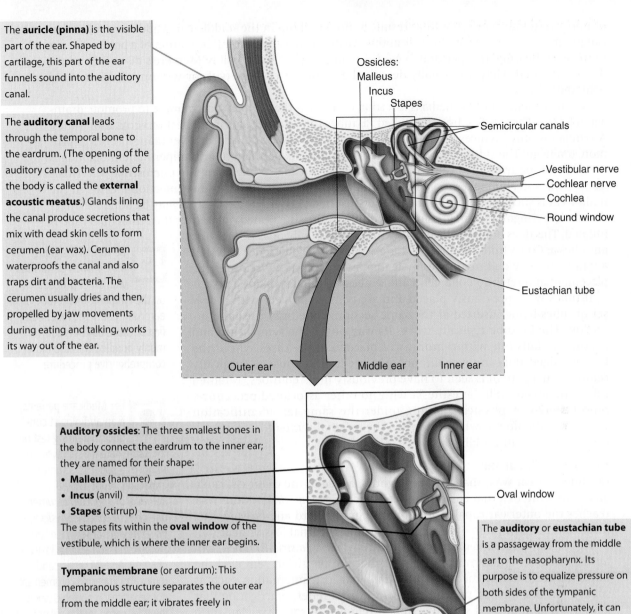

The **auricle (pinna)** is the visible part of the ear. Shaped by cartilage, this part of the ear funnels sound into the auditory canal.

The **auditory canal** leads through the temporal bone to the eardrum. (The opening of the auditory canal to the outside of the body is called the **external acoustic meatus**.) Glands lining the canal produce secretions that mix with dead skin cells to form cerumen (ear wax). Cerumen waterproofs the canal and also traps dirt and bacteria. The cerumen usually dries and then, propelled by jaw movements during eating and talking, works its way out of the ear.

Ossicles:
Malleus
Incus
Stapes
Semicircular canals
Vestibular nerve
Cochlear nerve
Cochlea
Round window
Eustachian tube

Outer ear   Middle ear   Inner ear

Auditory ossicles: The three smallest bones in the body connect the eardrum to the inner ear; they are named for their shape:
- **Malleus** (hammer)
- **Incus** (anvil)
- **Stapes** (stirrup)

The stapes fits within the **oval window** of the vestibule, which is where the inner ear begins.

Tympanic membrane (or eardrum): This membranous structure separates the outer ear from the middle ear; it vibrates freely in response to sound waves.

Oval window

The **auditory** or **eustachian tube** is a passageway from the middle ear to the nasopharynx. Its purpose is to equalize pressure on both sides of the tympanic membrane. Unfortunately, it can also allow infection to spread from the throat to the middle ear.

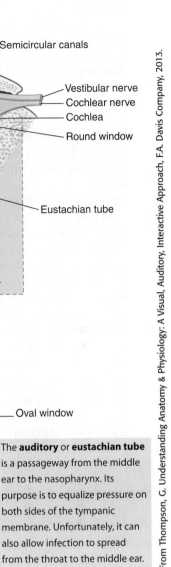

From Thompson, G. Understanding Anatomy & Physiology: A Visual, Auditory, Interactive Approach, F.A. Davis Company, 2013.

Figure 26.2 Ear anatomy.

Code 69200, *Removal foreign body from external auditory canal; without general anesthesia,* would be assigned in the physician office for foreign bodies that are easily accessible and for patients who do not require sedation. Children often require anesthesia due to lack of cooperation.

Otitis Media

Even though a surgeon uses the microscope to place the PE tube, the microscope code (69990) cannot be reported separately for Medicare recipients or those payers following the NCCI.

Otitis media (also known as middle ear infection) is the most common diagnosis for infants and toddlers. "Otitis" means inflammation of the ear and "media" means middle. Children are most affected by this because of their anatomy and young age. The middle ear is connected to the upper respiratory tract via the eustachian tube, and in children, the eustachian tubes are not fully developed, so they may not allow fluid to drain into the throat. Also, young children, particularly infants and toddlers, cannot blow their noses, causing fluid to collect in the middle ear. An ear infection or inflammation of the middle ear is typically caused by a cold or upper respiratory infection that results in fluid buildup in the middle ear. Middle ear infections can progress to more serious complications, including mastoiditis (inflammation of a bone adjacent to the ear), hearing loss, perforated eardrum, meningitis, and possibly Meniere's disease in adults if left untreated. They are usually described as acute or chronic with or without effusion (fluid behind eardrum).

One treatment for otitis media is insertion of tubes in the tympanic membrane to promote drainage (69436). These tubes are often called PE tubes (pressure-equalizing tubes) or ventilation tubes. A tympanostomy involves incising the tympanic membrane and inserting ventilation tubes to promote drainage. The suffix -ostomy implies that an artificial permanent or semipermanent opening is created to drain from the inside of the body to the outside. While using the microscope for visualization, the surgeon makes an incision in the tympanum, and any fluid or infection located in the middle ear is suctioned out. The tube is then inserted. A myringotomy alone may be done for infection. In a myringotomy, an incision is made and fluid is suctioned out and/or the eustachian tube is inflated. This does not involve inserting tubes and usually does not require anesthesia. Codes from 69420–69421 are assigned. The difference between a tympanostomy and myringotomy is that a tympanostomy requires the placement and retention of a ventilation tube and the use of anesthesia.

If tubes were previously placed and are being removed, with a new set of tubes being inserted at the same session, code only the tube insertion. The PE tube typically works its way out of the tympanum and eventually falls out within months of placement. In cases where the tube is lodged and cannot spontaneously free itself, it must be surgically removed. If a patient is seen to have previously inserted tubes (retained tubes) removed under anesthesia with no other associated procedure, report 69424. A physician billing under the same tax identification number as the doctor who performed the original tympanostomy with tube insertion cannot bill 69424.

Impacted Cerumen

Cerumen, or ear wax, that becomes tightly packed in the outer ear canal and blocks the external ear canal is referred to as *impacted*. As the wax reaches the outer ear canal it dries out, becoming hard and crusted. The most common symptom of cerumen impaction is partial loss of hearing.

To assign 69210, *Removal impacted cerumen requiring instrumentation, unilateral*, documentation must be present that the physician removed the impacted cerumen by mechanical means with instrumentation such as suction, probes, forceps, right angle hooks, wax curettes, or irrigation that goes above and beyond simple cerumen removal. If the physician (or a nonphysician practitioner) removes the cerumen with lavages or other solutions, 69210 cannot be reported; instead, report the evaluation and management (E/M) code for the service. Do not report 69210 with a –50 modifier because the code description already includes both ears.

Cholesteatoma

When eustachian tubes do not function correctly to regulate pressure in the middle ear, negative pressure builds. This pressure pulls the tympanic membrane into the middle ear, creating a pocket that fills with material called a *cholesteatoma*, a complication from chronic ear infections that may involve the middle ear and mastoid bone. This cyst can become infected and grow, breaking down some of the middle ear bones or other structures of the ear, affecting hearing, balance, and possibly function of the facial muscles. It actively erodes bone because it contains enzymes that are activated by moisture. A cholesteatoma must be removed promptly and many times requires mastoidectomy. Some cholesteatomas are very small and can be removed from the ear canal. Use of a microscope is required to properly remove all tissue (69990).

Mastoidectomy is commonly performed to treat infection and cholesteatomas. Mastoidectomy is the removal of disease from the bone behind

Be careful assigning 69424 when performed with other procedures on the tympanic membrane or eardrum. Check the NCCI edits first because 69424 is commonly bundled with the more comprehensive procedure.

For Medicare patients, if an audiologist conducts a hearing test on the same date that a physician removes a patient's cerumen impaction, report G0268, *Removal of impacted cerumen, one or both ears, by physician on same date of service as audiologic function testing*, instead of 69210. An E/M service and removal of impacted cerumen are not separately reportable when the sole reason for the patient encounter is for the removal of impacted cerumen. Reporting cerumen impaction removal separate from an E/M visit requires a separate diagnosis code. When reporting 69210 on its own, the corresponding diagnosis code is H61.23 (impacted cerumen). However, if the physician uses H61.23 for both the removal of the wax and the E/M code, the E/M service will be denied.

Search the following website to see if your state-specific Medicare carrier has a Local Coverage Determination on this topic: www.cms.gov/medicare -coverage-database/indexes/ national-and-local-indexes.aspx.

the ear. Ear canals and mastoid cavities (ear canals that have been surgically widened to treat chronic ear infections) produce wax and skin. The wax normally carries debris and bacteria out of the ear canal. Some ear canals and mastoid cavities do not readily clear this wax and skin, resulting in problems with recurrent drainage (infection). During the procedure, the surgeon drills into the mastoid cortex until the attic and antrum open. In a simple mastoidectomy, the incision is made behind the ear or from the ear canal. An incision is made into the antrum and the infected mastoid bone air cells are removed. During modified radical mastoidectomy (69505), the mastoid air cells and the posterior wall of the external auditory canal are removed. The surgeon removes the superior and posterior canal walls to create an open mastoidectomy cavity. The tympanic membrane is preserved or grafted and an attempt is made to preserve the middle ear ossicles. With a radical mastoidectomy (69511), no attempt is made to preserve any structure. The tympanic membrane, the malleus and the incus, and all of the mastoid cells are removed as well as the posterior wall of the external auditory canal. All of the ossicular structures, all of the middle ear mucosa, and the tensor tympani muscle are removed.

To assign codes for mastoidectomy, the coder should determine whether the surgery involved a mastoidectomy or a tympanoplasty with mastoidectomy. For a mastoidectomy alone, codes 69501–69511 from the first initial mastoidectomy section should be reported. If a tympanoplasty and mastoidectomy are performed, report a code from 69641–69646.

Perforation of Tympanic Membrane

Perforation of a tympanic membrane (TM) can occur from foreign objects being pushed too far into the ear canal, trauma, infection, and previous PE tube placement. It is not uncommon for a tympanic membrane repair to be required to patch the "hole" left from the PE tubes when they are removed. These codes are differentiated by whether the tympanic membrane was simply repaired or whether the eardrum was repaired or reconstructed. TM repair can be done via tympanoplasty, myringoplasty, or grafting. A patch commonly referred to as a cigarette patch or a paper patch is used to cover the "hole" left from the tubes. Code 69610 describes repair of the membrane that may or may not involve preparing the edges of the perforation to receive the patch. Myringoplasty is a procedure used to close a hole in the eardrum and is carried out in the operating room. There are a few ways to conduct the operation, but the most common is to take a piece of thin tissue from under the skin covering one of the muscles (temporalis fascia) and put this underneath the eardrum. The ear is approached from either an incision behind the ear or a small incision that comes from inside the ear canal out to the front of the ear. Code 69620 describes a myringoplasty of the drumhead and donor area. The edges of the perforation are freshened, then a fat plug graft or temporalis fascia graft is placed.

EXAMPLE

A physician performs bilateral middle ear exploration, with placement of bilateral PE tubes, foreign body removal (right), with fat graft myringoplasty. On evaluation of the left TM, it had a thick scar and effusion. The middle was widely opened and evacuated. The middle ear was fine, not requiring mastoidectomy. A PE tube was placed. On the right, an old tympanostomy tube was located and removed. A fat graft myringoplasty was performed. A wide anterior incision was made and thick effusion was suctioned. A PE tube was placed. Assign codes 69620–RT, 69436–59–RT, 69436–LT.

Tympanoplasty is performed to repair the perforated eardrum and sometimes the middle ear bones. Horst Wullstein created a classification scheme for tympanoplasty procedures involving five basic types:

- Type I tympanoplasty is actually a myringoplasty and involves only the restoration of the perforated eardrum by grafting. This is the simplest tympanic repair and may be performed in the physician office (depending on the age of the patient) under local anesthesia. It is often performed by using a paper patch and reported using 69610, *Tympanic membrane repair, with or without site preparation or perforation for closure, with or without patch.*

- Type II tympanoplasty is used for tympanic membrane perforations with erosion of the malleus. It involves grafting onto the incus or the remains of the malleus. A code to consider is 69631. This code describes an initial or revision tympanoplasty that does not require a mastoidectomy. The eardrum is reflected forward and the middle ear is explored. Fascia from the temporalis muscle or other tissue is used as a graft to repair the perforation.
- Type III tympanoplasty is indicated for destruction of two ossicles, with the stapes still intact and mobile. It involves placing a graft onto the stapes and providing protection for the assembly. The tympanic membrane/graft or a partial ossicular chain reconstruction prosthesis is placed.
- Type IV tympanoplasty is used for ossicular destruction, which includes all or part of the stapes arch. It involves placing a graft onto or around a mobile stapes footplate. Ossicular reconstruction may be indicated to repair the three small bones in the ear: malleus, incus, and stapes. These bones may be sculpted and repositioned using the patient's own ossicles or replaced with prosthetic bone (cadaver bone), referred to as a partial ossicular replacement prosthesis (PORP). Codes to consider include 69632 and 69633.
- Type V tympanoplasty is used when the footplate of the stapes is fixed.

The tympanoplasty CPT codes do not mimic this clinical classification system. There are 13 CPT codes and only five types of tympanoplasty, so there is not a direct correlation from type to code. One key difference between the classification and the code descriptors is that none of the classifications includes a mastoidectomy. Depending on its type, tympanoplasty can be performed under local or general anesthesia. It includes repairing or reconstructing the eardrum and may involve one or more of the following procedures:

- Canalplasty
- Atticotomy
- Mastoidectomy
- Antrotomy
- Ossicular chain reconstruction
- Ossicular chain reconstruction with prosthesis

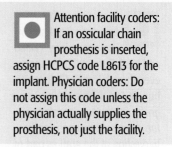

Attention facility coders: If an ossicular chain prosthesis is inserted, assign HCPCS code L8613 for the implant. Physician coders: Do not assign this code unless the physician actually supplies the prosthesis, not just the facility.

Myringoplasty is performed via the ear canal and confined to the eardrum head and perforation graft. The donor site for the graft must be known. Tympanoplasty is a more complex procedure, often uses a postauricular incision or canal wall incision, and usually includes an examination of the ossicular chain inside the middle ear. Because there are more than a dozen tympanoplasty codes, the coder must carefully review the operative report to select the correct code. A myringotomy (e.g., CPT codes 69420 and 69421) is included in a tympanoplasty or tympanostomy procedure and is not separately reportable.

If a cartilage graft is harvested from the outer ear (21235) or a temporalis fascia graft (20920, 20922, 20926) is utilized, bill it separately in addition to the tympanoplasty code. Assign 20926 when the graft is performed and no flap is done. Code 20920 is assigned when the graft is performed by a stripper tool. Code 20922 is used when the graft is performed by incision.

The surgeon uses an operating microscope to enlarge the view of the ear structures. If the perforation is very large or the hole is far forward and away from the surgeon's view, it may be necessary to perform an incision behind the ear (transauricular). This elevates the entire outer ear forward, providing access to the perforation. Tissue is then taken either from the back of the ear or the tragus. An absorbable gelatin sponge is placed under the eardrum to support the graft. The graft is inserted underneath the remaining eardrum remnant, which is folded back onto the perforation to provide closure.

Steps to Assign Tympanoplasty Codes

Answer these questions and review Pinpoint the Code 26.1 to correctly code for a tympanoplasty:

1. Is surgery performed in the office or the operating room?
2. Is surgery confined to drumhead or donor area?
3. Did the mastoid involved require mastoidectomy?
4. Was ossicular chain reconstruction done? Was it with the patient's own ossicular contents or was a prosthesis inserted?
5. Was this a revision?
6. Was a graft harvested and applied?

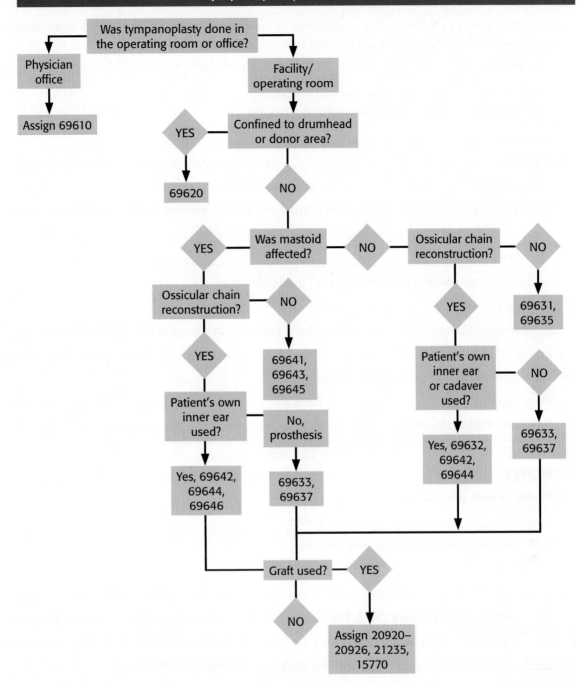

Oval or Round Window Fistula

The oval and round windows are special openings in the middle ear. The oval window and the round window assist in sound transmission and vibration. The space between the membranous and bony labyrinths is filled with perilymph, which is very much like normal cerebrospinal fluid. These openings between the air-filled middle ear and the fluid-filled inner ear can spontaneously develop fistulas where perilymph fluid becomes trapped, which causes hearing loss. Symptoms of perilymph fistula include hearing loss, dizziness, vertigo, imbalance, motion sickness, and nausea. Treatment consists of surgery to repair the fistula by placing a soft-tissue graft over the fistula defect in the oval and/or round window (69666, 69667).

Assign CPT code(s) to the following procedures. Some scenarios also require HCPCS code assignment. Assign codes for the physician and the surgical center (facility).

1. Myringotomy with removal of retained PE tubes, bilaterally, with replacement of new tubes

   Physician: _____ Facility: _____

2. Tympanoplasty and mastoidectomy, radical, both ears

   Physician: _____ Facility: _____

3. A patient has otosclerosis of the left ear. The patient is admitted for stapedectomy. The middle ear is entered and the ossicles are palpated. The stapes footplate is visualized and found to be thickened. Small and large Buckingham mirrors are used to drill out the stapes footplate. Once completed, a Schuknecht piston prosthesis is placed into position.

   Physician: _____ Facility: _____

4. Insertion of cochlear implant, left ear, with mastoidectomy

   Physician: _____ Facility: _____

5. A 3-year-old child with adhesive otitis media is placed under general anesthesia. The right ear is examined and debris and fluid are encountered. A PE tube is placed. The left ear is thoroughly examined and the previous tube is still intact.

   Physician: _____ Facility: _____

6. Tympanic membrane repair on right with operating microscope. Payer follows CPT guidelines and does not have separate policy for microscope use.

   Physician: _____ Facility: _____

7. Biopsy of both external ears

   Physician: _____ Facility: _____

8. Impacted cerumen is removed from both ears

   Physician: _____ Facility: _____

9. A mentally-handicapped patient in a nursing home placed a bead in her ear that is now lodged in the right external auditory canal. The patient's combativeness when she is examined requires that general anesthesia be used to extract the bead. Once the patient has been anesthetized, the physician is able to visualize the bead and extract it with forceps and suction.

   Physician: _____ Facility: _____

Hearing Loss

Hearing loss can be treated with cochlear implantation. Not all patients with hearing loss will qualify for the implant, but those with profound sensorineural hearing loss do. The implant is surgically placed under the skin behind the ear. First, a small area of the scalp directly behind the ear is shaved and cleaned. Then a small incision is made in the skin just behind the ear. The surgeon drills into the mastoid bone and the inner ear, where the electrode array is inserted into the cochlea (69930). The basic parts of the device include the following:

- External microphone that picks up sound from the environment
- Speech processor that filters sound

CPT © 2017 American Medical Association, All Rights Reserved.

- Transmitter that sends processed sound signals to the internal device by electromagnetic induction
- Internal receiver/stimulator that is secured in bone beneath the skin; it converts the signals into electric impulses and sends them through an internal cable to electrodes
- Array of up to 22 electrodes that is wound through the cochlea, which send the impulses to the nerves and the brain through the auditory nerve system

When a patient receives a cochlear implant, the audiologist must initially program the speech-generating device and then periodically adjust it. Initial analysis and programming of a cochlear implant are not included in 69930 and should be reported using 92601 or 92603. Code 69930, *Cochlear device implantation, with or without mastoidectomy,* carries a 90-day global period; however, diagnostic and aural rehabilitation are not included in the follow-up care allowance and should be reported using codes from the Medicine section 92507–92508, 92626–92627, 92630, and 92633.

Chapter Summary

1. Codes from the Integumentary System and/or Musculoskeletal System sections are necessary to capture services performed on the skin and deeper tissues in conjunction with procedures from the Eye and Ocular Adnexa and the Auditory System sections. Procedures on the eyelid may be reported from the Integumentary System section when only the skin and subcutaneous tissue are involved.

2. Extracapsular cataract extraction involves removing the front portion and nucleus of the lens, leaving the posterior capsule in place. A posterior chamber IOL is placed. Complex cataract surgery involves the same basic procedure components but may require the use of capsular support rings to hold the new lens or iris hooks to retract the pupil to obtain better access to the IOL. Complex cataracts are more difficult to remove for several reasons: small/miotic pupils that require multiple incisions, a subluxed lens, eye trauma requiring the insertion of capsular support rings for the new lens, glaucoma surgery that requires use of iris retractors, or surgery in a child who already had posterior cataract extraction. Documentation of use of an iris expansion device, sutures used to support the IOL, insertion of endocapsular rings, or a primary posterior capsulorrhexis are all indications of a complex cataract procedure. Intracapsular cataract extraction includes removing the entire lens and its capsule in one piece. An anterior chamber IOL is simultaneously inserted.

3. Phototherapeutic keratoplasty and photorefractive keratoplasty are often confused. They are essentially the same procedure; however, they are used for different clinical indications. PTK is used to correct particular corneal diseases and PRK involves the use of the excimer laser for correction of refraction errors (e.g., myopia, hyperopia, astigmatism, and presbyopia) in persons with otherwise nondiseased corneas.

4. A blepharoptosis procedure involving only skin, fat, and muscle (without the tarsus), is considered a cosmetic blepharoplasty and reported with codes 15820–15823. Correction of a drooping eyelid by repairing the levator muscle or removing a portion of the tarsus and removing excess skin weighing the lid down is considered a therapeutic procedure to treat a medical condition.

5. Entropion is the turning inward of the lower or upper eyelid, causing it to rub against the eyeball. Entropion can be repaired either by using a suture technique or by a more complex technique involving removal of muscle and tarsus and skin grafting. Ectropion is the turning outward of the edge of the lower or upper eyelid, causing the margin to pull away. Repair can be carried out in several ways, which differ based on the type of excision and blepharoplasty performed. These techniques range from simple incision to extensive by removing a tarsal wedge and a portion of the conjunctiva.

6. Both tympanostomy and myringotomy involve incising the tympanic membrane. The difference between tympanostomy and myringotomy is the placement and retention of a ventilation tube during tympanostomy.

7. The purpose of a tympanoplasty is to preserve hearing and prevent middle ear infections. The procedure includes repairing or reconstructing the eardrum and may involve one or more of the following procedures:

- Canalplasty
- Atticotomy
- Mastoidectomy
- Antrotomy
- Ossicular chain reconstruction
- Ossicular chain reconstruction with prosthesis

Review Questions

Matching

Match the key terms with their definitions.

A. tympanostomy
B. keratoplasty
C. pneumatic retinopexy
D. trabeculectomy
E. myringotomy

F. phototherapeutic keratectomy
G. photocoagulation
H. pseudophakia
I. photorefractive keratectomy
J. aphakia

1. _____ Procedure in which a gas bubble is injected directly inside the vitreous cavity of the eye to push the detached retina against the back outer wall of the eye

2. _____ Laser treatment that removes layers of corneal clouding and clears patients' vision

3. _____ Involves incising the tympanic membrane and inserting ventilation tubes

4. _____ Removal of the central portion of a diseased cornea and replacement with a matched donor

5. _____ Incisional procedure that creates a drain for the aqueous

6. _____ Status of eye that had a lens removed surgically or by trauma

7. _____ Incision of the tympanic membrane

8. _____ Use of a laser to reshape the surface of the cornea to correct vision

9. _____ A laser that emits green waves to coagulate tissue by sealing off blood vessels

10. _____ Eye that had the natural lens removed and replaced with a synthetic one

True or False

Decide whether each statement is true or false.

1. _____ A vitrectomy is separately reported when performed during a cataract extraction.

2. _____ Report 65130 for the insertion of an IOL after cataract removal surgery.

3. _____ All codes necessary for reporting procedures on the eye or ear are located in the Eye and Ocular Adnexa and Auditory System sections of CPT.

4. _____ A chalazion is an abnormal growth of the conjunctiva.

5. _____ All codes located within the Eye and Ocular Adnexa and Auditory System sections can be appended with modifier –50 because the eye and ear are paired body organs.

6. _____ Incision and drainage of a conjunctival cyst is assigned code 68020.

7. _____ Removal of a rock from a patient's ear, under anesthesia, with a microscope is assigned to 69205.

8. _____ An intracapsular cataract is considered a complex cataract.

9. _____ Removal of existing PE tubes is coded separately from the insertion of new tubes because the doctor has to make a new incision in the tympanic membrane.

Multiple Choice

Select the letter that best completes the statement or answers the question.

1. A patient undergoes extracapsular cataract extraction OD with phacoemulsification and IOL insertion. Which code should be reported?
   A. 66982–RT
   B. 66940–LT
   C. 66850–RT
   D. 66984–RT

2. A patient had a cataract removed 70 days ago on the right eye. The ophthalmologist finds opacification and incises the posterior capsule with a YAG laser. Which code should be reported?
   A. 66850–RT
   B. 66821–RT
   C. 66830–RT
   D. 66821–78–RT

3. An anterior capsulorrhexis was performed. The lens nucleus was hydrodissected and then removed by phacoemulsification. Cortical material was removed with irrigation. What procedure(s) was performed?
   A. Phacoemulsification of cataract
   B. Extracapsular cataract extraction
   C. Intracapsular cataract extraction
   D. Both A and C

4. A patient complains of pain and swelling in the right eye. He says he was tearing out drywall without safety glasses. The physician removed the conjunctival foreign body. Which code should be reported?
   A. 65220–RT
   B. 65235–RT
   C. 65210–RT
   D. 65205–RT

5. A 9-year-old Down syndrome patient with previous tympanostomies is seen for examination under anesthesia and debridement. The canal was debrided and an extruded tube was noted on the right and removed. On the left, a perforation is noted and there was granulation tissue and the tympanic membrane was debrided. Which codes should be reported?
   A. 69424–RT, 69799–LT
   B. 69220–LT, 69222–RT
   C. 69222–LT, 69799–RT
   D. 69424–RT, 69222–LT

6. Removal of FB from right cornea using slit lamp. The physician also repairs the corneal laceration. Which code(s) should be reported?
   A. 65222–RT, 65270–RT
   B. 65220–RT, 65285–RT
   C. 65275–RT
   D. 65280–RT

7. A patient is diagnosed with otitis media of the right ear with ossicular damage and erosion. The TM was totally perforated. Right tympanoplasty and canal split-thickness skin graft are performed. A posterior ear canal skin flap was made and then a postauricular incision. A temporalis fascia graft was harvested. Which code should be reported?
   A. 15770
   B. 20926
   C. 69631
   D. 69620

8. A patient has cataract surgery that involves using iris hooks and an endocapsular ring. Which code should be reported?
   A. 66984–22
   B. 66850–22
   C. 66984
   D. 66982

9. A patient is taken to the operating room for removal of retained foreign bodies of the left ear with chronic infection. The operating microscope was used and the canal was cleaned of infected debris. The ventilation tube was removed and a new one placed. The edges of the myringotomy were freshened and a paper patch applied. The patient has Cigna insurance, which utilizes the NCCI. Which code(s) should be reported?
   A. 69610–LT
   B. 69424–LT, 69436–LT
   C. 69436–LT
   D. 69631–LT

10. A patient has three chalazions removed under general anesthesia. Two were removed from the upper right eyelid and the third from the upper left eyelid. Which code should be reported?
    A. 67808
    B. 67805
    C. 67808–50
    D. 67801

CHAPTER 27

CPT: Radiology Codes

CHAPTER OUTLINE

Ancillary Services

Radiology

Radiology Section Guidelines

Diagnostic Radiology

Common Procedures

Assigning Radiology Codes

Radiological Supervision and Interpretation

Interventional Radiology

Radiation Oncology

Nuclear Medicine

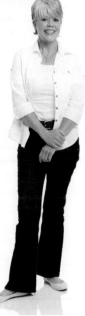

michaeljung/iStock/Thinkstock

LEARNING OUTCOMES

After studying this chapter, you should be able to:

1. Discuss the organization of and key guidelines for the Radiology section of CPT.
2. Discuss the importance of the modality and the number of views taken for code selection.
3. Discuss code selection for radiology procedures with, without, and without followed by with contrast material.
4. Explain the difference between the professional and technical components of radiology services and how to designate this by using modifiers.
5. Discuss the correct assignment of radiological supervision and interpretation services.
6. Discuss the difference between diagnostic imaging and interventional radiology procedures.

This chapter introduces CPT codes for the ancillary services that support the diagnosis and treatment of disease or injury. Ancillary services include work such as laboratory tests, radiological studies, pathology studies, physical therapy, and speech therapy. These services are provided for patients at the request of a physician to supplement or enhance medical treatment. They represent various important steps in the process of diagnosing and treating a patient from the onset of symptoms to recovery and maintenance.

Some ancillary services are typically provided by hospital departments. Others are done in physician practices, outpatient clinics, or separate facilities. Documentation in the form of physician orders, test requisitions, and ancillary reports is used to assign codes. Ancillary services documentation contains many acronyms and abbreviations; coders become familiar with their meanings as they work with these code sections of CPT.

This chapter reinforces basic radiology, and introduces uncomplicated interventional radiology, radiation oncology, and nuclear medicine coding concepts.

> Invest in an abbreviation resource or use websites such as www.AcronymFinder.com to determine the meaning of unfamiliar acronyms and abbreviations.

ANCILLARY SERVICES

Some of the professional ancillary services performed by hospital-based radiologists and pathologists are coded by technicians in the clinical areas of a hospital. More commonly, pathologists and radiologists contract with third-party billing companies that offer this highly technical specialty-specific service for coding and billing physician professional services. Diagnostic or therapeutic procedures performed in the laboratory and radiology departments are provided at the *order* of a physician and supplement or enhance medical treatment. According to Medicare, an order is a form of communication between the treating physician and another provider (physician or facility) requesting that a diagnostic test be performed. The requesting or ordering provider is required to authenticate all orders for hospital tests under Medicare's conditions of participation for hospitals.

Some ancillary services, however, may be provided and billed by physicians from varying specialties whose medical offices are equipped with x-ray or basic laboratory instruments. (Note that this definition of ancillary services relates to radiology and pathology/laboratory services, not extra services the physician may offer such as a weight-loss center or retail eyewear center.) When x-rays, urine and blood samples, and the like are obtained in an office setting, it is the coder's or biller's responsibility to capture the charges and accurately report codes for these services.

Coders must take heed of Medicare rules regarding ancillary testing in the *Federal Register* and in select *Program Memorandums*. Section 4317(b) of the Balanced Budget Act states that referring physicians are required to provide diagnostic information to the testing entity, whether it is a hospital, clinic, or lab, at the time the test is ordered. There is no specific requirement as to how this must be ordered. Physician offices supply this order in one of three ways: by faxing it directly to the lab or x-ray department, by calling the clinic and providing a verbal order or request for the testing, or by giving a copy to the patient to carry by hand to the facility where services are performed.

This diagnostic information may be referred to as a *diagnosis, clinical history*, or *clinical data*. This diagnostic statement must be "codable," meaning it must meet the criteria for assigning an ICD-10 code. If the test or service is performed on an outpatient basis, diagnoses cannot be assigned from "rule out, suspected, consistent with, etc." If this information is not provided, the coder is unable to assign a code even if the radiologist or pathologist has read and interpreted the findings and provided a *final* diagnosis.

RADIOLOGY

The codes in the Radiology section of CPT represent a subspecialty of medicine that concentrates on medical imaging to prevent, diagnose, and treat diseases and injuries. Radiologists diagnose diseases by obtaining and interpreting medical images rather than through laboratory testing or conventionally examining a patient. They correlate medical image findings with other examinations and recommend further studies or treatments to the ordering physician. Radiologists not only diagnose conditions, they also treat a number of diseases by means of radiation (radiation oncology) or minimally invasive, image-guided surgery (interventional radiology).

Many radiology terms end with the suffix *-graphy,* which means "a recording of or picture of"; for example, mammography. Radiology services, like surgical services, are divided into two categories: diagnostic and therapeutic. Diagnostic services identify or "magnify" locations of injury or determine the extent of a disease. Therapeutic services treat or repair an injury, disease, or defect in the body.

Radiologists frequently perform studies on the vasculature of the body that are reported with codes located outside of the Radiology section of CPT. Some of these studies are considered noninvasive vascular diagnostic studies (93880–93998) and are located in the Medicine section of CPT, while others involve invasive studies or interventional services located in the Surgery section, such as vascular injections (36200–36299).

Radiology coding can be especially complicated because the components are often "split" or "shared" between two physicians or between a physician and a facility. Further, there are numerous combination codes for various views, panels, and testing techniques. It is very important for the coder to read the documentation to choose the most comprehensive code that describes the services performed rather than billing multiple codes to describe the same service.

Codes in the Radiology section can be used by physicians of any medical specialty to report radiological services performed by the physician or under the physician's supervision. For example, a radiologist supervises a radiology technician (an RT or rad tech), who performs a service such as taking an x-ray and providing the images to the radiologist to interpret. Because of the expense of radiology equipment featuring advanced technology, such as positron emission tomography (PET) scans, many diagnostic services are offered only by hospital radiology departments. However, many physicians, particularly orthopedic physicians, have lower-cost x-ray equipment in their offices, and facilities also have portable x-ray equipment so that x-rays can be taken at the bedside.

The Radiology section of CPT is divided into seven main subsections according to method or "type" of radiology (i.e., diagnostic or therapeutic) that depicts the purpose of the service. These subsections and their code ranges are listed in Table 27.1.

Table 27.1 Radiology Subsections

SUBSECTION	CODE RANGE
Diagnostic Radiology (Diagnostic Imaging)	70010–76499
Diagnostic Ultrasound	76506–76999
Radiologic Guidance	77001–77022
Breast, Mammography	77053–77067
Bone/Joint Studies	77071–77086
Radiation Oncology	77261–77799
Nuclear Medicine	78012–79999

Each subsection is further subdivided by anatomical site and type of service or modality. A modality is a method, technique, or protocol used to treat or diagnose a disease or injury. As in other sections of CPT, notes, definitions, and special instructions are extremely important and must be read before assigning a code.

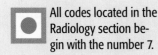 All codes located in the Radiology section begin with the number 7.

The subsections begin at the head and move down to the feet. Soft tissue body areas and vascular procedures follow. Each code designates the number of views and whether or not contrast was used. As in other sections of CPT, notes, definitions, and special instructions are located throughout this section.

Coders cannot assign codes directly from this section solely by looking up the anatomical area examined. Anatomical areas are listed separately in each of the four subsections. Codes are assigned based on "type" of radiology service.

RADIOLOGY SECTION GUIDELINES

The section guidelines explain unique terminology and review pertinent common terms such as *separate and unlisted procedures* as they apply to radiology codes. Important guidelines are located in usual CPT fashion throughout this section, and the section has many notes and instructions. Unlisted procedure codes are located at the end of the appropriate subsections. A unique annotation used in the *Professional Edition* of CPT is specific to this section. Similar to the use of the ⮌ symbol for *CPT Assistant* or *CPT Changes: An Insider's View* cross-references, the ⮌ symbol refers to the *Clinical Examples in Radiology* quarterly newsletter. Radiology coders refer to this newsletter for additional information regarding the procedure.

EXAMPLE
73525 *Radiologic examination, hip, arthrography, radiological supervision and interpretation.*

⮌ *CPT Assistant* Feb 07:11, Jun 12:14
⮌ *Clinical Examples in Radiology* Spring 05:6

> Read the documentation carefully. For skull or facial bone fractures, many radiology codes may actually be assigned due to the number of bones associated with the face, jaw, and skull. Determine the specific site being evaluated.

Required Order and Radiology Report

Diagnostic radiology services are ordered by a patient's treating physician (primary care, consultant, emergency department physician, etc.) to aid in diagnosing a patient's condition or assessing the extent of injury or disease. The order contains specific instructions on the type of study to be performed, the number of views, and why the study is requested (reason for examination). The order describes the patient's signs or symptoms and provides the radiologist with a working diagnosis.

> Under federal law, the ordering physician or practitioner (physician's assistant or nurse practitioner) must sign the radiology order. Most states allow either the physician or a practitioner to authenticate the order; some states require the physician to cosign orders from practitioners.

The radiology report is a written report signed by the radiologist or interpreting physician that accompanies all diagnostic or therapeutic radiological services. In response to the ordering physician's request for examination, the radiologist documents the results of the imaging exam in this report and sends a copy to the requesting physician for review. It is considered an integral part of a radiological professional service, so the work of providing this report should not be coded separately. Final reports, which are dictated and signed by a radiologist after viewing the images, include an impression or diagnosis and at times recommended follow-up care, as noted in Box 27.1 and Box 27.2. This report is a very important source document for a radiology coder to read, because it contains the clinical impression/diagnosis needed to assign the ICD-10 diagnosis code as well as vital information needed to assign the CPT code such as the specific imaging test performed, the number of views (i.e., individual radiological images) taken, and contrast type given for reporting the radiologist's professional service.

BOX 27.1 Elements of a Radiology Report

Patient name	Contrast used (if any)
Age or date of birth (DOB)	Limitations of the exam (if any)
Sex	Patient reactions (if any)
Date of exam	Description of findings
Requesting physician name	Impression or definitive diagnosis
Indications for exam	Suggestions for follow-up (if any)
Name of the examination	Name and signature of radiologist
Views taken	

Facility coders also read radiology reports to obtain the same information. However, in a hospital setting, inpatient coders are not permitted to code directly from this document. The attending or ordering physician must also document these results in progress notes and "confirm" the findings of the radiologist. If documentation is not present in the patient's medical record, the coder must query the attending or ordering physician to use the information present on a radiology report. Outpatient coders are allowed to assign codes based on ancillary reports if they are signed by the radiologist.

BOX 27.2 Sample Radiology Report

Radiology Report
Middletown Memorial Hospital
MR# 123-45-6789

Patient: Smith, Jacqueline

Date of Birth: 07/24/1946

Clinical History/Indications: Left lumpectomy 5 years ago. This woman is status post–left breast lumpectomy done April, 2000.

Exam: Diagnostic bilateral mammogram

Exam Date: 06/19/--

Requesting Physician: Ted Miller, MD

Report: There is a fibroglandular pattern. No mass, calcification, or architectural distortion suspicious for malignancy is seen. Magnification views with spot compression demonstrate architectural distortion consistent with postsurgical change. A few calcifications with benign characteristics are scattered in both breasts. Except for postsurgical changes in the left breast, there has been no other change since 5/22/01.

Impression: No evidence of malignancy or focal area of radiographic concern. Postlumpectomy and radiation therapy change in the left breast are visible with no apparent active disease. Recommend annual bilateral mammogram to compare films.

Attending Radiologist: Rosemary Tucker, MD

Diagnostic tests ordered in the absence of signs and/or symptoms or indications of illness or injury (e.g., screening tests) are reported by the physician interpreting the diagnostic test by using the *reason* for the test as the primary ICD-10-CM diagnosis code. The test results, if reported, may be recorded as additional diagnoses. On occasion the interpreting physician will not have clinical data or diagnostic information as to why the test was ordered, which is required by Medicare and must be obtained before the test is conducted. It can be gathered by calling the referring/ordering physician's office, from the patient's medical record, or by interviewing the patient. The last two sources are problematic for third-party billing companies, however, because they do not (in most cases) have access to patients or their medical records.

Administration of Contrast Materials

The ordering physician or the radiologist may decide that contrast is indicated to enhance a particular view or tissue of interest. The contrast material (media)—a substance that helps provide a clearer image—can be administered, or introduced, with an infusion or an injection, rectally or orally. The phrase *with contrast* in the code descriptor refers to contrast material administered either intravascularly, directly into a joint (intra-articularly), or into the space under the arachnoid membrane of the brain or spinal cord (intrathecally). Rectal or oral contrast administration alone does not qualify as a study with contrast.

It is common for imaging work to be done in a series—some images with contrast and some without. However, when this is the approach, two codes, one with contrast and the other without contrast, are not both coded for a service. Instead, a coder must use a code that describes *without contrast followed by contrast*. In other words, when a service is done first without contrast material, followed by contrast material and additional images, the coder should report a single code specifying both without and with contrast material. For example, for a CT scan of the head or brain, the coder has three codes to consider:

70450   *Computed tomography, head or brain; without contrast material*
70460   *with contrast materials*
70470   *without contrast material, followed by contrast material(s) and further sections*

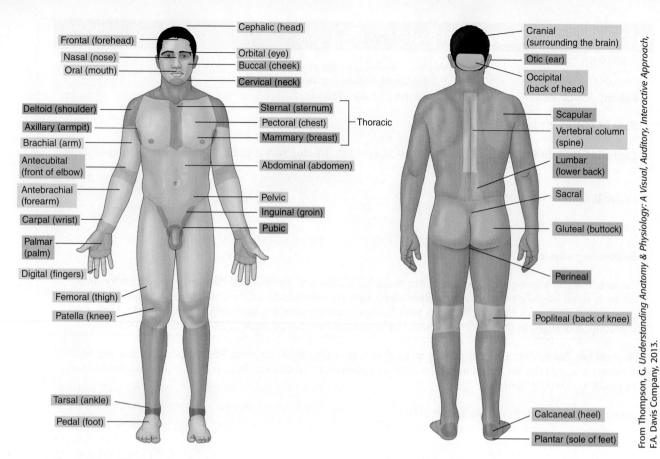

Figure 27.1 Anatomical regions.

From Thompson, G. *Understanding Anatomy & Physiology: A Visual, Auditory, Interactive Approach,* F.A. Davis Company, 2013.

Radiographic Positions

Usually, two images (from different angles) are taken; at times, three images are needed if the problem is around a joint (knee, elbow, or wrist). Anatomical references are common in the Radiology section, especially to refer to planes and positions of the body (Fig. 27.1). Code descriptions often differ just on the number of views obtained. To properly choose a code, the coder must be able to determine how many views were obtained based on the positions described or the abbreviations in the documentation. For reference, CPT provides illustrations of the planes of the body in the front of the CPT manual in the Illustrated Anatomical and Procedural Review section.

Patients are asked to lie or stand in various positions in order to capture the best image of the area being evaluated. The way a patient is positioned on the examination table directly correlates to the projection of the beam, providing varying angles of images obtained. Table 27.2 provides a summary of the positions and views. For example, for an x-ray of the hand, the patient may be asked to position a hand in several ways to view the bones from various angles. If the patient places a hand on an x-ray plate palm down, the x-ray projection is posteroanterior, meaning that the x-ray beam passes through the body from back to front. If the patient places the right hand on its side perpendicular to the x-ray plate, this is considered an oblique view, either anterior or posterior, depending on the angle of the machine.

> Due to the increased use of diagnostic imaging scans, particularly CT scans and MRIs, many payers require preauthorization in order to reduce the number of unnecessary scans ordered. Payers hire radiology management companies that quickly respond to requests for approval.

Table 27.2 Radiology Positions and Views

POSITIONS	VIEWS
Anteroposterior (AP)—front to back	Right anterior oblique (ROA)
Lateral side view (LAT)	Left anterior oblique (LOA)
Decubitus (DEC)—lying on side	Left posterior oblique (LPO)
Oblique (OBL)—angled view	Right posterior oblique (RPO)
Posteroanterior (PA)—back to front	Odontoid view (open mouth)
Prone (ventral)—lying on stomach	Swimmer's view (arm raised above head)
Supine (dorsal)—lying on back	Stereo view (images blended appear 3-D)
	Tangential (beam skims profile of body)
	Apical view (relating to the apex of a pyramidal or pointed structure)
	Frontal (head on, facing forward)
	Axial (beam is angled to pass through body lengthwise)

DIAGNOSTIC RADIOLOGY

Diagnostic radiology, also known as *diagnostic imaging*, refers to radiology methods that produce images or pictures of the body. Images may be in the form of shadows or very intricate color images with three-dimensional views. These studies include plain film examinations, gastrointestinal studies, genitourinary studies, arthrograms, hysterograms, and so forth. This first radiology subsection is arranged by anatomical site and then further by the *modality*, meaning the method used to obtain imaging. Codes are located in the Index under these terms:

- X-ray
- Computed tomography (CT) scan
- Magnetic resonance imaging (MRI)
- Magnetic resonance angiography (MRA)
- Mammography
- Fluoroscopy
- Dual-energy x-ray absorptiometry (DEXA)

INTERNET RESOURCE: MedlinePlus, a service of the U.S. National Library of Medicine and the National Institutes of Health, provides an overview of diagnostic imaging and links to additional resources. www.nlm.nih.gov/medlineplus/diagnosticimaging.html

Plain film radiography (x-ray) and fluoroscopy are the basis of diagnostic radiology. They are the least expensive methods of diagnostic radiology and most often the first radiological exams performed on a patient.

COMMON PROCEDURES

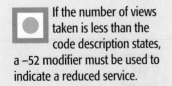
If the number of views taken is less than the code description states, a –52 modifier must be used to indicate a reduced service.

Radiography is the medical term for x-rays. An x-ray is the most commonly used radiology modality for diagnosing injuries. It uses a beam of ionizing radiation that travels through the body's soft tissue to create an image on film placed under the patient's body. X-rays are commonly used to evaluate the chest, spine, extremities, and abdomen. Coders thoroughly review the code descriptions before making a code selection. Codes specify *minimum number of views, with or without contrast, complete,* or *radiological supervision and interpretation.* When a specific number of views is listed, the coder must verify that the patient was positioned and images were taken for this number of views.

EXAMPLE

73650 *Radiologic examination; calcaneus, minimum of two views.* If only one view was taken, 73650–52 would be reported. If three or more views were obtained, 73650 is still appropriate to report.

Code descriptions that state *radiologic examination* refer to standard or conventional plain film x-rays of a particular site. Codes for other modalities are located in the same section but the code descriptions will vary depending on the method used.

EXAMPLES

70250 *Radiologic examination, skull; less than four views.*

70450 *Computed tomography, head or brain; without contrast material.*

70544 *Magnetic resonance angiography, head; without contrast material(s).*

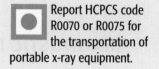

> If a minimum number of views is stated, no additional code or modifier is used if more than that number was obtained.

> Codes for x-rays in this section refer to "infant." According to coding guidelines, an infant is younger than 1 year old (365 days). A newborn is less than 30 days old. A toddler is a child over 1 year and under 5 years.

> Report HCPCS code R0070 or R0075 for the transportation of portable x-ray equipment.

Computerized Axial Tomography

A computerized axial tomography scan is more commonly recognized by its abbreviated name, CT or CAT scan. This x-ray procedure combines many x-ray images with the aid of computer enhancement. A CT scan can produce cross-sectional views and three-dimensional images of soft tissues, such as the internal organs, and other parts of the body. The scanners also can be used effectively to evaluate the spine and hip for osteoporosis. CT scans are also used to help guide the placement of instruments. CT scans often utilize contrast materials.

The scanner takes x-ray images at many different angles around the body. These images are processed by a computer to produce cross-sectional pictures. In each picture the body is seen as an x-ray "slice" recorded on film. The recorded image is called a *tomogram. Computerized axial tomography* refers to the processing of recorded slices at different levels of the body to create a three-dimensional picture of a body structure.

Codes for CT scans of the body are located by body area in the Diagnostic Imaging section. The terms *CT scan* and *CAT scan* are used to locate these codes in the CPT index.

EXAMPLE

72125 *Computed tomography, cervical spine; without contrast material.*

A contrast agent is sometimes used to block the x-rays from passing through the selected body areas in order to obtain clearer, more detailed images. Contrast may be introduced through an IV or catheter to more clearly see the urinary system, bowel, or other internal structures. X-rays are sometimes ordered prior to or for comparison with other imaging procedures.

Magnetic Resonance Imaging

A magnetic resonance image (MRI) uses radio-frequency waves and a strong magnetic field rather than x-rays to provide detailed pictures of internal organs and tissues. MRI images produce clear pictures of soft tissue structures near and around bones and an MRI is therefore the preferred examination for spine and joint problems and sports-related injuries. In the case of joint injury, an MRI may be useful in identifying ligament tears, joint effusions, or other problems. It is also a tool for diagnosing coronary artery disease and heart problems. Physicians can examine the size and thickness of the chambers of the heart and determine the extent of damage caused by a heart attack or observe the flow of blood through vessels. CPT codes 75557–75565 are used for

> Other imaging modalities, such as PET, bone scanning, or CT, may be more successful in diagnosing cancer metastases (spread) to bone or primary bone tumors.

cardiac magnetic resonance imaging and are differentiated by whether or not contrast material was used and if the procedure was performed with stress imaging.

MRIs can also be done with or without contrast. Gadolinium is a routinely used contrast agent. Codes for MRIs are located by body area in the Diagnostic Imaging section. They are found in the CPT Index under the entries *magnetic resonance imaging* and *MRI*.

○ According to the American College of Radiology (ACR), if a screening study results in a definitive diagnosis, report a screening ICD-10-CM Z code as primary and the diagnosis code as secondary.

EXAMPLE

73718 *Magnetic resonance imaging, lower extremity other than joint; without contrast material(s)* (an MRI of the foot).

Bone/Joint Studies

Although x-ray images are among the clearest, most detailed views of bone, they are not useful in evaluating the *density* of bone or adjacent soft tissues such as tendons and ligaments. Dual-energy x-ray absorptiometry (DEXA or DXA) is an accepted means of measuring bone mineral density (BMD).

There are two types of DXA equipment: the central device and the peripheral device. Central DXA devices measure bone density in the hip and spine, whereas peripheral devices measure it in the wrist, heel, or finger. The central DXA device is used in hospitals and medical offices; the smaller peripheral device is available in drugstores and on mobile health vans in the community. The DXA machine sends a thin, invisible beam of low-dose x-rays with two distinct energy peaks through the bones. One peak is absorbed mainly by soft tissue and the other by bone. The soft tissue amount can be subtracted from the total, and what remains is a patient's bone mineral density.

○ If a breast mass that was identified preoperatively by needle localization is sent back to radiology after the mass is removed for confirmation of removal, 76098 would also be assigned by the radiologist. The ACR and the Radiological Society of North America website "RadiologyInfo" provides information about diagnostic radiology exams: www.radiologyinfo.org/en/sitemap/

EXAMPLE

77080 *Dual-energy x-ray absorptiometry (DXA), bone density study, 1 or more sites; axial skeleton (e.g., hips, pelvis, spine).*

Magnetic Resonance Angiography

Magnetic resonance angiography (MRA) is an MRI study of the blood vessels. It utilizes MRI technology to detect, diagnose, and aid the treatment of heart disorders, stroke, and blood vessel diseases. MRA provides detailed images of blood vessels without using any contrast material, although contrast may also be used to make the pictures even sharper. Angiography focuses on the size and condition of vessels and is commonly used for diagnosing aneurysms; cardiovascular disease; venous malformations; and vessel disease of the head, lungs, kidneys, and legs.

BOX 27.3 Contrast Agents

Barium	Gastrografin
Iohexol	Iopamidol
Ioxaglate	Hypaque
Renografin	Gadolinium

Administration of Contrast Materials

If contrast medium is ordered, the radiology report indicates the substance that was used for the procedure. Common contrast materials are listed in Box 27.3. Some tests or procedures commonly performed using contrast are barium enema, angiography, cystogram, intravenous pyelogram (IVP), fistulogram, cholangiography and/or pancreatography, and retrograde pyelogram. Retrograde is a technique used to administer contrast in urologic procedures. The flow of contrast (up from the bladder to the kidney) is opposite the usual flow of urine. Antegrade is a technique used to administer contrast to visualize forward movement or the flow of blood or urine, or forward extension of an organ.

When a scan is done without contrast material, followed by contrast materials and additional scan sections, the coder should report a code specifying both without and with contrast material.

EXAMPLE

MRI of the right foot without contrast, followed by contrast and additional MRI sections. From the code range 73721–73723, the coder should assign code 73723.

IV injection of contrast for MRI and CT is not coded separately. The coder selects the proper code that states *with contrast* for the MRI or CT scan. The exception to this is if intrathecal injection of contrast into the subarachnoid space of the spine is performed. For the intrathecal injection, either 61055 or 62284 is reported in addition to the code for the imaging (72125). Read the note that appears at the beginning of code 72125 for instructions.

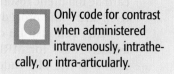

Only code for contrast when administered intravenously, intrathecally, or intra-articularly.

Spine Studies

X-rays may not be effective in diagnosing central nervous system conditions. A better radiology study is myelography, which involves injecting contrast into the subarachnoid space of the spine to visualize the spinal column and intervertebral discs. The radiologist will position the patient in various ways in addition to tilting the table to get pictures of the spinal column contents. Tilting the table allows the dye to move up and down the spinal column, allowing the nerves to also be visualized. CPT lists four codes to describe myelography:

> 72240 *Myelography, cervical, radiological supervision and interpretation*
> 72255 *thoracic . . .*
> 72265 *lumbosacral . . .*
> 72270 *two or more regions . . .*

Specific x-ray codes are used for patients with scoliosis (72081, 72082, 72083, 72084). Do not assign 72070–72080 in addition to these codes.

If two or more levels of the spine are examined, 72270 should be assigned.

With respect to x-rays, most of the codes referring to spine examination are dependent on the level of the spine (i.e., cervical, thoracic, lumbar) and the number of views taken. Because of the spine's intricate anatomy, several views may be obtained.

Epidurography is a radiographic technique whereby contrast is injected to visualize the epidural space. It is a diagnostic procedure commonly performed prior to injecting steroids into the spine. Visualizing this space is important to accurately determine the source of pain and inject medications in this location. An epidurogram is done under fluoroscopic guidance at a specific location (also known as "level") in the spine. Once a needle has been carefully inserted into this location, dye is injected. The x-ray allows the physician to document how the contrast dye disperses, assess a diagnosis, and confirm the exact location of pain.

If procedures must be repeated because of poor picture quality or if the radiologist requests additional views to render an opinion, the most comprehensive CPT code that describes the total service is reported even if the patient leaves the department and has to return later.

Fluoroscopy is an imaging technique that uses a continuous low-level x-ray beam to view the body in motion.

Discography, or discogram, is an x-ray procedure that attempts to recreate or "provoke" the patient's back pain in order to identify the source in the intervertebral discs. This procedure is a diagnostic tool used to pinpoint exact locations of pain in anticipation for spinal fusion. Codes 72285 and 72295 are used to report this service. This procedure code is coupled with pain management injection codes from the Nervous System section (62290–62291).

Diagnostic Ultrasound

Ultrasound refers to the inaudible ultra–high-frequency sound waves used for diagnostic scanning. Ultrasound technology is similar to the sonar that submarines use to navigate; the sound waves bounce off the body tissue and produce an echo. Ultrasound waves are emitted by a transducer (the part of the machine that is pressed against the body or placed inside an orifice such as the vagina or esophagus), and a picture of the underlying tissues is built up from the pattern of echo wave feedback that bounces back. Hard surfaces such as bone return a stronger echo than soft tissue and fluids, giving the bony skeleton a white appearance on the screen. There are four different ultrasound approaches

If an epidurography was performed in an office, the physician would report a code for the S&I with no modifier along with an injection code. However, if this service was provided in a facility such as an ambulatory surgery center, the physician would report the S&I with the –26 modifier in addition to the procedure code.

in terms of placement: transesophageal, transvaginal, transrectal, and external (placing the transducer on the outer body).

There are four types of ultrasound:

- *A-mode*—a one-dimensional ultrasonic measurement procedure
- *M-mode*—a one-dimensional ultrasonic measurement procedure with movement of the trace to record amplitude and velocity of moving echo-producing structures
- *B-scan*—a two-dimensional ultrasonic scanning procedure with a two-dimensional display
- *Real-time scan*—a two-dimensional ultrasonic scanning procedure with display of both two-dimensional structure and motion with time

Ultrasounds are routinely performed on the abdomen (liver, gallbladder, kidney, uterus, ovaries) to look for abnormalities or to measure the size of a fetus. They are also performed on the heart and extremities to observe blood flow (Doppler study).

EXAMPLE
76870 *Ultrasound, scrotum and contents.*

Ultrasound is also often used to guide needle placement and to perform percutaneous procedures and central venous catheter placement. Ultrasound ensures precision in positioning a needle or catheter placed percutaneously so as to avoid nerves, the spinal cord, a fetus, or other structures. The imaging confirms the needle placement before injecting material, aspirating fluid, ablating tissue, inserting radioelements, or biopsying a site. Palpation or standard x-ray was the approach traditionally used to guide needle placement.

Ultrasound guidance codes 76930–76965, 76998 must be reported in addition to codes from the Surgery section that describe the surgical procedure.

EXAMPLE
For example, when a physician performs a needle biopsy of the thyroid using ultrasound guidance, the following codes are reported:

76942 *Ultrasonic guidance for needle placement, imaging supervision and interpretation.*
60100 *Biopsy thyroid, percutaneous core needle.*

Parenthetical instructions are available following code 76942 listing the numerous codes that are not allowed to be reported in combination with 76942.

The Ultrasound section is arranged by anatomical site. Codes can be found in the Index under the words *ultrasound* and *echography*.

The Medicine section also contains codes for ultrasound imaging on certain areas:

93303–93355: Ultrasounds of the heart
93880–93895: Cerebrovascular arterial studies
93922–93931: Arterial studies of the extremities
93965–93971: Venous studies of the extremities
93975–93981: Visceral and penile vascular studies
93990: Duplex scan of hemodialysis access

Obstetrical Ultrasound

According to the American College of Obstetricians and Gynecologists, 60% to 70% of pregnant women undergo an ultrasound between weeks 18 and 20 of their pregnancies. Ultrasound is most commonly used during pregnancy to determine the due date of the baby. This is very important when mothers with irregular periods or who are perimenopausal do not know when they conceived. Ultrasound is also performed to measure and monitor the developing fetus, locate the placenta, diagnose ectopic pregnancy, and determine the number of gestational sacs (twins, triplets, etc.). Occasionally, these routine exams can unexpectedly discover intrauterine abnormalities or fetal emergencies. Some conditions such as hydrocephalus or heart valve defects can be identified and may be treated "in utero" now thanks to this technology.

The pelvic ultrasound section is divided into two subsections: obstetrical (76801–76828) and nonobstetrical (76830–76857). All ultrasounds conducted on pregnant women must be coded from the "obstetrical" codes. Code descriptions are specific to single or multiple gestations, trimester, and ultrasound technique. Most ultrasounds are performed transabdominally. Ultrasound codes are reported for each gestation or fetus. Add-on codes 76802, 76810, 76812, and 76814 are coded in addition to the base ultrasound for each additional gestation in the case of a multiple-gestation pregnancy.

Transvaginal ultrasound (TVU) imaging is coded separately in addition to the basic obstetrical ultrasound. At times, this may be necessary if the images are inadequate using the abdominal transducer. The transvaginal ultrasound is often required for ultrasounds prior to 8 weeks' gestation. When reporting TVU in addition to another OB ultrasound at the same visit, be sure to append modifier –59.

Radiology Modifiers

The common radiology modifiers are listed in Table 27.3. For facility reporting, two modifiers often apply—one to distinguish the facility (technical) charges from the physician's (professional) charges, and a second to describe the body part being examined.

EXAMPLE

73020–RT–TC *X-ray of the right shoulder, 1 view* reported by the facility.

Table 27.3 Radiology Modifiers

MODIFIER	DESCRIPTION
–22	Increased procedural service
–26	Professional component
–32	Mandated service
–51	Multiple procedure
–52	Reduced service
–53	Discontinued service
–59	Distinct procedural service
–76	Repeat procedure by same physician
–77	Repeat procedure by another physician
GG	Performance and payment of a screening and diagnostic mammogram on the same patient, same day
GH	Diagnostic mammogram converted from screening mammogram on the same day
ANATOMICAL MODIFIER(S)	
–FA to –F4	Left hand
–F5 to –F9	Right hand
–LT	Left side
–RC	Right coronary artery
–RT	Right side
–TA to –T4	Left foot
–T5 to –T9	Right foot

Read the ultrasound code descriptions carefully. Pregnancy ultrasound code descriptions indicate weeks of gestation or trimester of pregnancy and technique (e.g., transvaginal).

A common coding error occurs when the coder reports the abdominal ultrasound codes (76700–76705) for pregnancy ultrasound. The correct obstetrical ultrasound codes are located in the pelvis subsection, which refers to a pregnant uterus.

Payers have guidelines limiting the number of obstetric ultrasounds that are payable during a normal pregnancy. Many carriers only pay for one ultrasound in the second trimester; others pay for one in the second and one in the third trimester.

Avoid using the –50 modifier with radiology codes. Instead, check with the payer; most require reporting the code twice using the –RT or –LT modifiers.

Do not report both a diagnostic and a guidance ultrasound code during the same procedure or session.

Fluoroscopy

Fluoroscopy uses a continuous, low-level x-ray beam to view the body in motion. Fluoroscopy is used in orthopedic, podiatry, pain management, and gastrointestinal procedures and exams. It is used to follow barium through the intestinal tract to look for ulcers. It can also be used to verify placement of needles and catheters during joint injections, breast biopsies, insertion of venous access devices, and pain management procedures. The time descriptors in the codes apply to the time the technologist or physician is actually using the equipment to assist in a case, not the time the fluoroscopic unit is turned on.

Radiological Guidance

Guidance is used with a variety of codes, and all except ultrasound were previously scattered in multiple sections. Radiological guidance can be provided by fluoroscopy (77001–77003), computed tomography (77011–77014), and magnetic resonance (77021–77022).

The fluoroscopic guidance codes (77001–77003) pertain to guidance for central venous devices, needle placement, and localization of needles or placement of catheters. Numerous instructional notes beneath these codes direct the coder not to assign these codes in addition to specific radiological S&I procedures. Fluoroscopic guidance codes are not reported with codes that include *arthrography* in the code description. For example, 77002, *Fluoroscopic guidance for needle placement*, cannot be reported with code 73615, *Radiologic examination, ankle, arthrography, radiologic supervision and interpretation*. Instructional notes also instruct the coder to assign additional codes for the surgical procedure performed.

There are additional instructional notes under the computed tomography, magnetic resonance, and other radiological guidance codes as well.

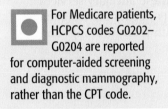

Pay close attention to the code descriptions for the words *bilateral* and *unilateral*. If only one breast is examined and the description states *bilateral*, a –52 modifier is appended.

For Medicare patients, HCPCS codes G0202–G0204 are reported for computer-aided screening and diagnostic mammography, rather than the CPT code.

Breast, Mammography

Mammography, or mammogram, uses a low-dose x-ray system for the examination of breasts. There are two different kinds of mammography, diagnostic and screening, based on the documented reason for the examination. This distinction is important for payers, because some cover the service to assess a suspected condition but not the screening service.

The referring physician's diagnosis on the mammography order determines whether it is a diagnostic or a screening service. A screening procedure is performed to detect a disease or condition in the absence of signs and symptoms. A diagnostic procedure is performed to assess the extent of an already-diagnosed disease or condition. However, a radiologist (but not a radiological technologist) who finds an abnormality in a screening can proceed with a diagnostic mammogram even though it was not ordered.

Screening Mammography

A screening mammography is usually limited to two images, craniocaudal and mediolateral oblique views. It is performed to detect unsuspected cancer in an early stage in an asymptomatic woman. CPT code 77067 is inherently bilateral, so the –50 modifier is not required when examining both breasts.

Diagnostic Mammography

A diagnostic mammography (CPT code range 77065–77066) is reported when a suspected mass or abnormality has been found during a physical examination, when the patient has previously had breast surgery, or for follow-up after a related surgery. Diagnostic mammography requires additional work, supervision, and interpretative skills.

Codes 77065–77067 are used to report computer-aided detection with further review for interpretation to provide a more in-depth study of a diagnostic or screening mammogram.

Bone/Joint Studies

The Bone/Joint Studies subsection is unique because varying methods of study are grouped into one subsection. For example, 77084, *Magnetic resonance imaging, bone marrow blood supply*, is not separately listed under a heading or subheading for magnetic resonance imaging and is grouped with codes for traditional x-ray and CT scan.

CHECKPOINT 27.1

Assign the correct modifiers to the following, based on whether the code is for the facility or the physician. Do not assign the radiology code.

1. Venography S&I of the right leg, facility _____

2. Physician use of fluoroscopic guidance for left wrist injection _____

3. MRI of the heart, without contrast followed by with contrast material for morphology and function _____

4. Upper GI imaging with KUB _____

5. Ultrasound of the gallbladder _____

6. Ultrasound-guided needle placement for thoracentesis _____

7. CT scan of chest, without contrast _____

8. MRI of the brain with contrast _____

9. Mammography of the right breast, facility _____

ASSIGNING RADIOLOGY CODES

Most coders do not assign radiology imaging and ultrasound codes. When these ancillary services are provided in hospital departments—whether for inpatients or outpatients—codes are assigned automatically during the coding and billing process. However, familiarity with their meanings and selection, and their modifiers, is required knowledge for coders.

Modifier Guidelines

As in all sections of CPT, modifiers are important for radiology coding.

Professional/Technical Components

For facility code reporting, two modifiers often are used to distinguish the facility charges from the physician's charges along with the laterality of the body part being examined. The –TC modifier is only for use for charges submitted by a facility. It is never applied to the codes reflecting the physician's professional charge.

> **EXAMPLE**
> 73020–RT–TC *X-ray of the right shoulder, 1 view.*

If a code description states *radiological supervision and interpretation (S&I)*, it may seem to indicate that it is a professional component only code; however, S&I codes have both a professional and a technical component. Radiology equipment is being used and supervision and interpretation of that test are being provided. Unless the physician who is doing the test also owns the equipment, modifier –26 is reported with the radiology code.

> **Do not use the –50 modifier for radiology codes. Use –RT and –LT and list the codes separately. Radiology codes are paid at 100% of the allowed amount and are not subject to the surgery rules where bilateral procedures reported with the –50 modifier are paid at 150%.**

EXAMPLE
A physician is injecting dye into the cervical spine (62291) and is viewing its progress and interpreting the findings (72285). If performed in a hospital or outpatient center, the physician does not own the equipment being used for the discography and would report 62291, 72285–26. The facility would report 72285–TC.

If a radiologist employed by the hospital or outpatient center provides the discography S&I, he or she would report 72285 without a modifier. The physician who provided the injection procedure would report 62291.

EXAMPLE
A physician uses fluoroscopy to verify placement of an epidural needle in the epidural space for a pain management procedure. The procedure is performed in the outpatient department of a hospital. The physician will report code 77003–26 and the facility will report 77003–TC.

Bilateral Procedures
The preferred way to report x-rays obtained on bilateral parts is by listing the code twice with the –RT and –LT modifiers.

EXAMPLE
A patient falls while ice skating. The physician obtains x-rays, two views, both elbows. Report codes 73070–LT, 73070–RT.

Reduced or Unusual Services
If a patient is an amputee and x-rays are obtained of the remaining limb, the –52 modifier should be appended to the radiology code to indicate this service was partially reduced because the full body is not examined.

EXAMPLE
73090 *Radiologic examination; forearm, 2 views.* If the patient had his hand removed above the wrist, the complete forearm is no longer present and the –52 modifier should be appended.

> **Modifier –52 can be appended to CT scan codes for limited study or for follow-up studies.**

> **When limited comparative studies are performed where films are obtained preprocedure and postprocedure, a code for the total radiological series should be billed with a –52 modifier. This demonstrates that the level of interpretation is reduced.**

Use the –22 modifier with CT scan codes when additional slices are needed for a more detailed exam than is usually conducted.

Let's Code It

The following example gives coders an idea of the questions they should ask to correctly assign radiology codes.

> A patient is seen in the emergency department (ED) after tripping on a curb and fracturing her right wrist. X-rays were ordered, and two views of the wrist were obtained. The radiologist reviewed the films, dictated a written report, and made a verbal report to the ED physician.
>
> | | |
> |---|---|
> | What service would you look up in the Index? | X-ray |
> | What is the body site? | Wrist |
> | Based on the documentation, was fluoroscopy used? | No |
> | How many views were obtained? | Two |
> | Based on the documentation, was any contrast used? | No |
> | Is a modifier applicable based on the body part examined? | Yes, –RT |
> | Does the physician own the equipment? | No |
> | Did the physician dictate a formal report? | Yes |
> | What is the correct code? | 73100–RT |

Steps in Assigning Radiology Codes

The following steps will result in correct radiology code assignment (Pinpoint the Code 27.1):

1. Review the complete medical documentation (x-ray report, imaging study, etc.) and identify the type of service performed.
2. Locate the body site being viewed.
3. Look in the CPT Index for the type of service performed or body part imaged. Common words to look for include *x-ray, CAT scan, magnetic resonance imaging (MRI), magnetic resonance angiography (MRA), ultrasound, echography, mammography, radiology, nuclear medicine, nuclear imaging,* or the actual body site (e.g., chest).
4. Reference the documentation and determine if fluoroscopy was used along with the exact positional views, the number of views, and any special views that might have been performed.
5. Determine if intravenous contrast was used. If so, this can be coded.
6. Watch for indented CPT codes and pay attention to the semicolon (;) placement.
7. Pay attention to the code descriptions for complete versus limited, obstetrical versus nonobstetrical, bilateral, with or without contrast, finger versus fingers (meaning more than one), minimum number of views, radiological S&I, and so forth.
8. Was this an interventional procedure? If so, make sure that each portion of the procedure is captured from injection to the definitive procedure. Do not code for the access to a vessel and code only the highest-order vessel treated or examined.
9. Pay attention to modifiers! Consider whether the assignment of modifiers will clarify the code being reported. If the code description does not say *bilateral*, use –LT or –RT. Make note of whether the physician prepares a written report. If the physician reads the x-ray (interprets) but does not provide a written report, a –26 modifier is required.

RADIOLOGICAL SUPERVISION AND INTERPRETATION

Many codes in the Radiology section include the phrase *radiological supervision and interpretation.* These codes are used to describe the radiological portion of a procedure that two physicians often perform in tandem. Typically, a surgeon will perform the "surgical" portion of a procedure, and the radiologist will conduct the "radiological" portion. At times, though, the radiologist will perform both. The codes in this section are used to describe *only* the radiological portion of a procedure. S&I codes do not include the procedure; they are for the "supervision and interpretation of the results" only. The radiological S&I codes are thus used in conjunction with the code for the surgery that required guidance or enhancement from the Surgery section.

Essentially, for every S&I code there should be a corresponding procedure code submitted either by the radiologist or the surgeon. In situations where one physician provides the S&I and performs the procedure, two codes are reported by that same physician: a radiological code and a code from another section of CPT, such as surgery. This is referred to as a *complete procedure.* A complete diagnostic radiology procedure involving injection of contrast media provided by one physician includes the following:

- Services provided prior to and immediately following the injection
- Injection of a local anesthetic
- Placement of the needle or catheter
- Injection of the contrast media
- Supervision of the study and interpretation of results

EXAMPLE
A physician who performed a transcatheter placement of an intravascular stent and also provided the catheter introduction into the vessel and the S&I in the hospital would report code 37238. The code description says that S&I is included in this code; therefore, no separate radiology code is reported.

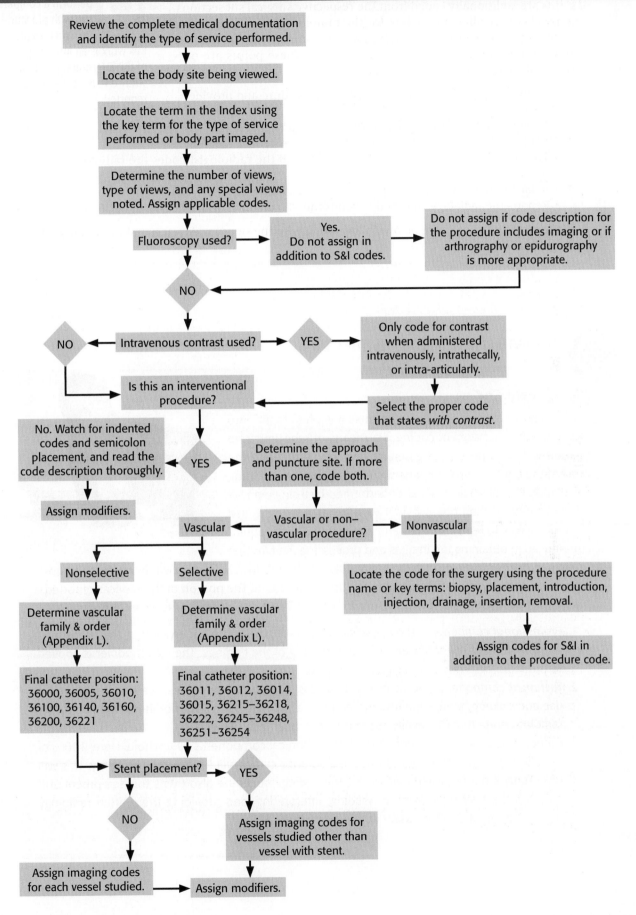

Review the complete medical documentation and identify the type of service performed.

Locate the body site being viewed.

Locate the term in the Index using the key term for the type of service performed or body part imaged.

Determine the number of views, type of views, and any special views noted. Assign applicable codes.

Fluoroscopy used? → Yes. Do not assign in addition to S&I codes. → Do not assign if code description for the procedure includes imaging or if arthrography or epidurography is more appropriate.

NO

Intravenous contrast used? → YES → Only code for contrast when administered intravenously, intrathecally, or intra-articularly.

NO

Select the proper code that states *with contrast*.

Is this an interventional procedure?

No. Watch for indented codes and semicolon placement, and read the code description thoroughly.

YES → Determine the approach and puncture site. If more than one, code both.

Assign modifiers.

Vascular ← Vascular or non–vascular procedure? → Nonvascular

Locate the code for the surgery using the procedure name or key terms: biopsy, placement, introduction, injection, drainage, insertion, removal.

Nonselective | Selective

Determine vascular family & order (Appendix L).

Determine vascular family & order (Appendix L).

Assign codes for S&I in addition to the procedure code.

Final catheter position: 36000, 36005, 36010, 36100, 36140, 36160, 36200, 36221

Final catheter position: 36011, 36012, 36014, 36015, 36215–36218, 36222, 36245–36248, 36251–36254

Stent placement? → YES

NO

Assign imaging codes for vessels studied other than vessel with stent.

Assign imaging codes for each vessel studied. → Assign modifiers.

Codes from the Radiology section only describe the radiology component of a procedure. Any injections, catheterizations, or placement of stents are additionally coded from the respective surgical subsections. Coders who are coding and billing for the radiologist would report the S&I codes and/or a procedure code. Facility coders would assign the code for the procedure itself with no S&I code. These points are outlined as follows:

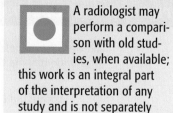

A radiologist may perform a comparison with old studies, when available; this work is an integral part of the interpretation of any study and is not separately reported.

1. The physician performs both the invasive procedure and provides the supervision and interpretation:
   • Assign radiology procedure and the surgical procedure.
2. The physician and the radiologist perform the procedure together:
   • The surgeon codes the surgical procedure and the radiologist codes the radiology procedure (S&I).
3. The facility that owns the equipment reports as follows:
   • Reports the radiology code and appends the –TC modifier and codes the surgical procedure.

While reading the example below, follow along with the steps for decision making as shown in Pinpoint the Code 27.2.

 REIMBURSEMENT REVIEW

Component Coding

Radiology coding can be difficult because it is often "split" into components. Component coding is a means of reporting who performed what portion of a service and who is bearing the cost of the equipment. Component coding allows the reporting of all radiological services whether performed by a single physician or by more than one provider working as a team. It also includes a way to report services and associated fees for equipment used in obtaining the images and processing the film that is owned by the physician or by a facility. This also allows the facility to cover its costs for equipment use and employee time spent in the procedure room. The portion of the services reported will depict payment made by the insurance carrier. There are basically three components: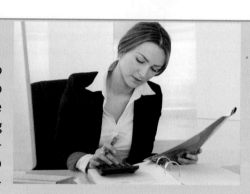

1. *Professional component:* The physician portion describes the supervision of the procedure, interpretation of the study, and official reporting of the findings. The –26 modifier is applied to the radiology code to indicate this portion.
2. *Technical component:* The facility or business portion encompasses overhead, equipment use and upkeep, time, supplies, and employee expenses. The –TC modifier is applied to the radiology code that the facility submits to the insurance carrier.
3. *Global:* This captures the professional and technical components as a whole. Here, 100% of the allowed payment amount from the insurance carrier will be paid to one entity. This will only apply if the physician performing the testing/procedure also owns the equipment and employs the staff in addition to reading, interpreting, and providing the written radiology report. No modifier is necessary in this circumstance.

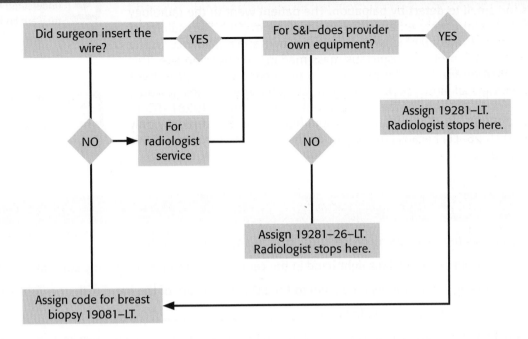

Did surgeon insert the wire? — YES — For S&I—does provider own equipment? — YES

NO → For radiologist service

Assign 19281–LT. Radiologist stops here.

NO

Assign 19281–26–LT. Radiologist stops here.

Assign code for breast biopsy 19081–LT.

Payment for each component is "shared" among all. The professional component typically allows for 40% of the "global" payment amount, and the technical component is allocated 60% of the global payment amount, so together they total 100% of what insurance carriers will allow (or pay) for the service.

EXAMPLE

A patient goes to the ED to have her hand x-rayed. The radiology technician takes two pictures of the right hand. The radiologist, who is not employed by the hospital, reads the films and dictates a written report of his findings. The radiologist would report code 73120–26, and the facility would report 73120–TC.

This example would be coded and billed differently, however, if the radiologist were an employee of the hospital. In that case, the hospital would report 73120 with no modifier, allowing them 100% of the reimbursable rate.

The same holds true for physician practices that own x-ray or ultrasound equipment. If the same woman went to her physician office and had a two-view x-ray performed for which the physician read the x-rays and completed a report, the office would report 73120. The practice is permitted to do this, because it owns the equipment and also provided the film interpretation.

A code that indicates "supervision and interpretation" can never be used to report services for a facility or the technical component.

What would happen if this office obtained the x-rays but then had to send the films to an outside radiologist for examination and interpretation? The office would report 73120–TC and the radiologist interpreting/reading the films would report 73120–26.

EXAMPLE

A surgeon needs to perform a left breast biopsy; however, the mass is too small to detect by palpation. The patient went to the radiology department prior to entering the operating room (OR). The radiologist inserted a radiographic wire using mammographic guidance in the exact location of the suspicious mass marking the excision site. This is called localization. The patient then proceeded to the OR to have the incisional biopsy performed by the surgeon. The radiologist would bill for 19281–26–LT. The facility would report codes 19281–TC–LT and 19081–TC–LT. The surgeon would bill for the breast biopsy only (19081–26–LT) because he did not do the radiological portion of this service.

CHECKPOINT 27.2

Assign codes to the following procedures. Include any necessary modifiers.

1. A 5-year-old boy closed his right hand in the car door. His thumb was clearly stuck in the door. After freeing it, the parents drove him to the ED where x-rays of the hand with one view and thumb (three views) were obtained. _____

2. A patient has been experiencing right hip and lower back pain for several weeks. Lumbar spine and hip x-rays were inconclusive. Myelography S&I was performed at the lumbosacral region by injecting Iopamidol at the L5–S1 interspace to rule out disc herniation or nerve impingement. Code for the injection and the S&I. _____

Use Box 27.2 to answer the following questions.

3. What type of radiological service was performed? Was it a diagnostic, screening, or therapeutic service? _____

4. Was clinical data or a preliminary diagnosis provided by the referring doctor? If so, is it adequate to allow you to assign the findings by Dr. Tucker? _____

5. Provided that the clinical data are adequate, what CPT code is assigned by the radiologist? What code is assigned by the facility? _____

INTERVENTIONAL RADIOLOGY

Interventional radiology (IR) is a subspecialty of radiology in which a radiologist uses image-guided minimally invasive or percutaneous techniques to diagnose and treat conditions as an alternative to traditional surgery. Endoscopic surgery is nicknamed "keyhole surgery," but interventional radiology takes it one step further to perform "pinhole surgery."

Interventional radiology focuses on evaluating and treating the vasculature of the body and providing a safe way to biopsy and destroy tumors or emboli within the organs themselves. IR utilizes needles or catheters guided by radiological imaging such as CT, fluoroscopy, and MRI to complete the procedures. IR procedures do not require incisions greater than a few millimeters, which allows for a shorter recovery time than open surgery.

IR is one of the most difficult specialties for which to code. Because of its complexity, IR is an advanced coding specialty; the goal of this introduction is to provide basic background information so that the coder can build skills through further study. Because this is a very multifaceted subspecialty for which to code and bill, there are not many trained professional coders working in this subspecialty. There is great opportunity for career growth in this area if one can master this content.

IR Procedures

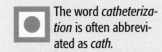
The word *catheterization* is often abbreviated as *cath.*

As shown in Table 27.4, interventional radiology has two types: vascular and nonvascular. Vascular IR involves accessing a vessel via catheterization as a means to reach the desired site. Nonvascular IR does not involve catheterization of a vessel to gain access to the desired site.

Table 27.4 Types of Interventional Radiology Procedures

VASCULAR IR	NONVASCULAR IR
Angiography	Percutaneous biopsies
Angioplasty	Cryoablation
Thrombolysis	Percutaneous vertebroplasty
Dialysis access	Nephrostomy tube insertion
Embolization	Percutaneous biliary drainage
	Insertion of drains

Unbundling occurs when a comprehensive procedure is broken into smaller component parts, each of which is coded. A comprehensive procedure by definition includes everything that was performed, so only one procedure code is reported to fully describe the service.

Typically, when coding an IR procedure, a code for the injection of dye or catheterization or imaging is assigned for each definitive or surgical procedure—*but not always.* Interventional radiology cases are complex. These cases can include anywhere from 1 to 20 or more procedure codes. Some codes include both the procedure and the injection, so only one code is reported; to code each separately would be wrong and considered unbundling.

EXAMPLE

42660 *Dilation and catheterization of salivary duct, with or without injection.* No additional code is reported for the catheterization or injection because this code description includes all services.

Vascular Interventional Radiology

Vascular IR procedures, commonly performed in a cardiac cath lab, imaging center, or peripheral vascular setting, are carried out on veins and arteries. Procedures commonly performed on the arteries are arteriograms, angioplasty, stent insertion, embolization, and thrombolytic infusion. Venous procedures include diagnostic studies, insertion of Greenfield filters, and insertion of vascular access devices.

Five vascular systems may be accessed during IR procedures. If procedures are carried out on more than one system during the same operative session, each should be coded separately. With that being said, coders must have a thorough knowledge of vascular anatomy and be able to differentiate among these five systems:

1. Systemic venous
2. Systemic arterial
3. Portal
4. Lymphatic
5. Pulmonary

The *Professional Edition* of CPT contains illustrations at the beginning of each CPT section, such as the arterial and venous systems, which are located at the beginning of the cardiovascular system; the anatomical illustration of the respiratory system is at the beginning of the respiratory section. The book does not, however, illustrate the portal system. The portal system drains the GI tract and forwards the blood to the liver for absorption. It is made up of the hepatic portal vein, mesenteric veins (inferior and superior), and splenic vein.

Vascular catheterizations are classified as either selective or nonselective. In the arterial vascular system, nonselective catheter placement involves placing the catheter into a small incision in the femoral artery and directing the catheter into the aorta, which is the main conduit of the arterial system, or placing the catheter directly into an artery. CPT code 36200 is for the nonselective code for the arterial system. CPT code 36010 is for the nonselective catheter placement into the venous system, specifically the superior or inferior vena cava. The superior and inferior venae cavae are the main conduits for the venous vascular system. Materials and supplies (drugs, contrast, catheters, stents) are not included in the code for catheterization and should be coded separately using HCPCS codes.

EXAMPLE

Abdominal aortogram: Catheter is inserted directly into the aorta. This is considered a nonselective catheterization because it is placed directly into the artery being studied. Report code 36200 for inserting the catheter into the aorta. The S&I code would be 75625–26.

Selective catheter placement means that the catheter is manipulated or guided through or to a specific arterial system other than the aorta or the vessel punctured to gain access. It includes placement and administration of contrast and repositioning of the catheter, which is done under fluoroscopic guidance and usually involves the use of a guidewire. This type of catheterization is more complex and requires more skill than nonselective catheterizations.

IR Vascular Order

Visualizing the arterial system aids in reading and interpreting catheterization reports. The arterial system can be thought of as a river, as illustrated in Figure 27.2. The aorta is the river and gives rise to many primary streams. When a primary stream diverts and branches off, tributaries or secondary streams or "brooks" are formed. These secondary brooks can then divide off and branch into tertiary creeks. Catheter placement in a primary branch is considered a first-order catheterization. First-order vessels are those that are primary branches off of the aorta or vena cava (the main conduits). Selective catheterization of a secondary stream or "branch" is considered a second-order catheterization. Second-order vessels branch from first-order vessels. Similarly, the selective catheterization of the creeks or tributary vessels is considered third-order catheterization.

A primary stream or "branch" plus all of its brooks and creeks is considered a vascular family. Appendix L in CPT demonstrates the concept of vascular family. A vascular family is a group of vessels that branch off from the aorta (primary branch of the arterial system) or a primary branch of the vessel punctured. Coders must be familiar with the arterial anatomy and understand to which vascular family each artery belongs. The specific selective catheterization code assigned is determined by the number of branches within a specific vascular family that are passed to reach the desired site. Always select a code that describes the most selective (or farthest destination reached within a vessel) catheter placement performed. This concept also applies to the venous system. First-order veins are primary branches of the vena cava or vessel punctured. Second-order vessels are branches of the primary vein.

> The physician performs three steps: (1) placement of the catheter, (2) injection of the contrast agent, and (3) interventional procedures.

> Notice that there is no mention of the cardiac vasculature in these five systems. Cardiac catheterizations are located in the Medicine section.

> Before attempting to assign codes for selective catheter placement, read the CPT guidelines carefully. The more extensive guidelines are in the Cardiovascular section preceding codes 36000 and 36200.

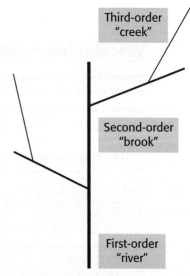

Figure 27.2 Vascular order.

Only the most selective catheterization is coded when both selective and nonselective placements are performed except in cases with more than one access site. A nonselective catheterization is not coded in addition to a selective catheterization when a single access puncture is used. Even if a nonselective catheter placement is conducted first, the highest selective placement is coded. The following example provides a case and code-assignment rationale. The coder needs to determine the vascular order and assign the correct code.

- Only the most selective catheterization is coded when both selective and nonselective placements are performed except in cases where more than one access is used.
- The most selective or highest-order vessel is coded for each vascular family. Do not code the primary and secondary vessel passed along the way to the IR procedure site.

Coders must have an anatomy book and access to Appendix L in the CPT when coding catheterizations to determine which artery belongs to which vascular family.

Some code descriptions include both the injection and the definitive procedure in one code. Read the code descriptions carefully.

EXAMPLE

A patient is experiencing portal hypertension and cirrhosis of the liver. On CT exam, a lesion of the splenic artery is also found. At angiography, the catheter is inserted into the common femoral artery and manipulated into the aorta. From the aorta, it is advanced to the celiac trunk and into the splenic artery. Marked focal dilation of the splenic artery was found.

Rationale: The puncture to the femoral artery does not count. We know this is a selective catheterization because the catheter is manipulated out of the abdominal aorta and into the celiac trunk and ultimately in the splenic artery. Use Appendix L of CPT to locate the first-order vessel, which is the celiac trunk. The second-order vessel is the splenic artery. From here, look up the term *catheterization* in the Index. Do you find celiac trunk or splenic artery? No. The logical next best entry is *Abdomen* or *Pelvic Artery* in the code range 36245–36248. We have already said that we are coding for a second-order vessel, so code 36246 is the correct choice. We still have to code for the angiography. Review codes 75600–75774. Because the angiography was performed in the splenic artery, 75726 is the correct code. Report codes 36426, 75726–26.

Review the cardiovascular chapter for more details on the nonselective and selective catheterization codes.

If more than one second- or third-order vessel in the arterial vascular family is catheterized, the additional branch catheterization is assigned add-on code 36218, 36227, 36228, or 36248 in the arterial system. Each vascular access is coded separately. If two separate punctures are performed, each is assigned a code.

INTERNET RESOURCES: Suggested Professional References
Dr. Z's Medical Coding Series Interventional Radiology Coding Reference
www.zhealthpublishing.com

Journal of Vascular and Interventional Radiology
http://www.jvir.org

Nonvascular Interventional Radiology

Nonvascular procedures are routinely performed on the genitourinary, gastrointestinal, spinal canal, liver, and biliary systems. Nonvascular IR does not involve catheterization of a vessel to gain access to a specific site. Typical procedures include biopsies, aspirations, insertion of drains, joint aspirations/injections, and diagnostic injections (myelography, sialography, arthrography, etc.).

EXAMPLES

- Nonvascular procedures: A patient has lumbar spondylosis. The pain specialist performs a bilateral L4, L5, and S1 medial branch block under fluoroscopy. The physician will report codes 64493–50, 64494–50, 64495–50. The fluoroscopy services are included in these codes.

- A patient was involved in a motor vehicle accident and suffered severe whiplash. An MRI of the C1–C3 cervical discs is performed with contrast. The radiologist injects dye into the base of the skull and reads and interprets the MRI. The radiologist would bill for the S&I, the MRI, and the injection of dye. Report codes 70542–26, 61055.

IR Coding Guidelines

Specific instructions pertaining to IR procedures are located under the subheadings: Aorta and Arteries, Veins and Lymphatics, and Transcatheter Procedures. These guidelines must be read carefully for correct code assignment. Here are the major points:

- Diagnostic procedures performed before therapeutic IR services (at a separate setting) such as stents, angioplasty, or thrombolysis are *not* included in the therapeutic service and may be coded separately even if they are performed at the same time *if* the purpose is arriving at a diagnosis.
- Diagnostic angiography/venography performed at the same time as an IR procedure is *not* separately reportable if it is included in the IR code description.
- With respect to vascular catheterizations, S&Is are reported for *each visualization technique* performed. This is dissimilar to the rules for catheterization where only the highest-order vessel in a family is reported. The exception is the code series 36221–36228. These codes include the S&I.
- If a catheter is reinserted into a distinct and separate site, this procedure is coded separately.
- Selective catheterizations include nonselective catheterizations.
- Code each vascular family to the highest order selected.
- Each vascular access is coded separately.
- Each vascular family catheterized is coded separately.
- Modifiers: Do *not* use –50 or –RT/–LT with catheterization codes. Instead use modifier –59 to indicate separate vascular families. For S&I codes, use –RT/–LT or –59 when applicable.

EXAMPLE

A patient is experiencing significant cold sensitivity and complains of both hands blanching white. Upper extremity catheterization is recommended. The catheter is inserted at the right common femoral artery. The catheter is advanced to both the right and left subclavians, which are selectively catheterized with injection and imaging.

Because the right and left subclavians are in separate families, you must report each of those catheterizations separately. The left subclavian is a first-order cath, the right subclavian is a second-order cath. Note that 75716 is a bilateral S&I. Report 36216 for the right subclavian cath, 36215–59 for the left subclavian cath, and 75716–26 for the S&I, bilateral.

IR Abdominal Aortic Aneurysm Repair

Radiologists may participate in an abdominal aortic aneurysm (AAA) treatment either prior to diagnosing the condition or while providing therapeutic intervention. Endovascular graft placement is a less invasive technique relying heavily on IR. During this procedure, a catheter is introduced, usually through the groin, and fed through the vessels to the aneurysm site. The stent or prosthesis is placed. When selecting codes for this procedure, the coder must determine the location of the repair, the approach, and what device (prosthesis) is used or inserted, because the CPT code will vary between the Cardiovascular and Radiology chapters. The IR radiologist usually teams with a cardiologist to carry out this procedure. There are codes for the endovascular repair and open repair. The S&I codes 75956 and 75957 can be assigned in addition to the surgical code. Notes in the Radiology and Surgery sections direct the coder to assign codes for both the surgical and radiology components.

Component Coding and Billing

The component coding and billing concept must be applied for IR procedures because codes from the Radiology section in addition to codes from the Surgery section of CPT are reported. The procedural aspect of the service is coded outside of the Radiology section and the S&I is coded from the 70000 code series. Interventional radiology services are different from other services using contrast in that there is a direct correlation of the "timing" of the study to the injections. Single services are described by one procedure code and one supervision and interpretation code. Refer to Pinpoint the Code 27.3.

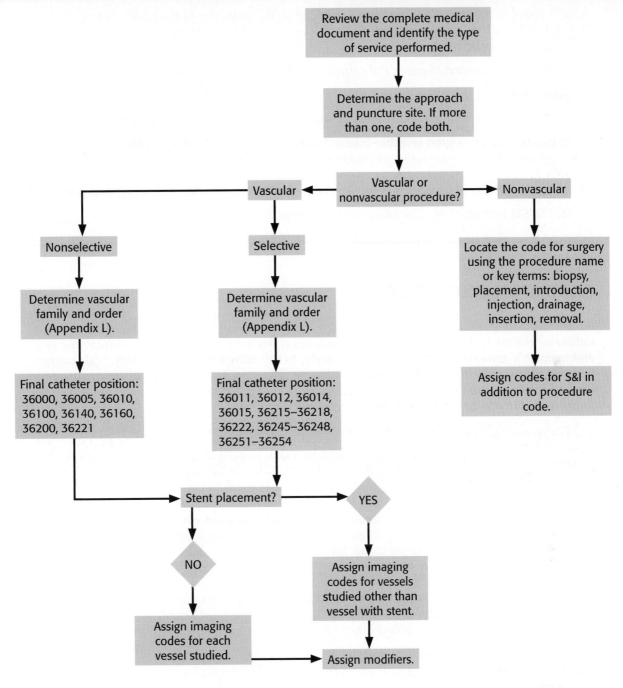

Review the complete medical document and identify the type of service performed.

Determine the approach and puncture site. If more than one, code both.

Vascular or nonvascular procedure?

Vascular

Nonvascular

Nonselective

Selective

Locate the code for surgery using the procedure name or key terms: biopsy, placement, introduction, injection, drainage, insertion, removal.

Determine vascular family and order (Appendix L).

Determine vascular family and order (Appendix L).

Assign codes for S&I in addition to procedure code.

Final catheter position: 36000, 36005, 36010, 36100, 36140, 36160, 36200, 36221

Final catheter position: 36011, 36012, 36014, 36015, 36215–36218, 36222, 36245–36248, 36251–36254

Stent placement?

YES

NO

Assign imaging codes for vessels studied other than vessel with stent.

Assign imaging codes for each vessel studied.

Assign modifiers.

To be successful in coding IR, you must disconnect the surgical procedure aspect from the radiological aspect of the service and assign a separate CPT code for each of these.

EXAMPLES

- Injection for elbow arthrography. The physician performs the invasive procedure and provides the supervision and interpretation. The physician bills the radiology and surgical procedure. Report codes 24220, 73085–26.

- CT-guided renal biopsy in the hospital radiology department. The physician and the radiologist perform the procedure together. The surgeon codes the surgical procedure and the radiologist codes the radiology procedure. The radiologist would report 77012–26 and the surgeon would report 50200.

Assign codes to the following procedures provided by the physician in the facility setting. Assign the S&I code. Include any necessary modifiers. Remember, S&I codes are assigned for each vessel accessed—diagnostic and therapeutic.

1. Access: right common femoral. The catheter is advanced into the aorta and contrast is injected for aortography. _____

2. A 73-year-old patient with a history of pulmonary embolism complains of acute shortness of breath. She undergoes selective bilateral main (R) and (L) pulmonary arteriograms.

   _____

3. Selective catheter placement was provided into the left common carotid. Will the physician code for the S&I portion of the procedure, and if so what modifier will be used? _____

RADIATION ONCOLOGY

Radiation oncology is a therapeutic radiology service. Fifty percent of patients with cancer undergo radiation treatment. This subsection of CPT includes codes for radiation therapy to treat diseases and neoplastic tumors of various areas of the body. In this subspecialty of radiology, high-energy ionizing radiation is used in the treatment of malignant neoplasms and certain nonmalignant conditions. Radiation oncology codes are organized around distinct therapeutic modalities such as radiation treatment, brachytherapy, teletherapy, and dosimetry.

Radiation therapy, or radiotherapy, may be administered externally or internally. Teletherapy is external radiation therapy that uses a beam of radiation (x-ray or gamma ray) directed from the outside of the body through the patient's skin toward a designated area. This is also referred to as external beam radiation therapy (EBRT). Internal radiation therapy, better known as brachytherapy, involves inserting a radioactive substance into the patient via tubes, wires, seeds, needles, or other small containers. Dosimetry determines the amount of radiation needed during the treatment. Essentially, it measures how much radiation exposure you get from substances or machines that produce radiation. The technical component of radiation oncology codes includes simulation, dose planning, dosimetry, radiation and proton treatment delivery, treatment devices, and special services.

Weekly treatment management (77427) includes the evaluation and management (E/M) services while the patient is being treated for her or his current diagnosis.

The first paragraph of guidelines under the Radiation Oncology header provides important information for the coder. It stipulates the five basic services associated with this specialty:

1. Initial consultation with the radiologist
2. Clinical treatment planning
3. Simulation
4. Medical radiation physics, dosimetry (calculating the radiation dose), treatment devices, and special services
5. Clinical treatment management procedures

Normal follow-up care during the patient's treatment and for 3 months after completion of treatment are also included in the radiation oncology codes. The following sections provide more specific descriptions of the basic services.

The Radiation Management and Treatment Table located within this section of the CPT manual is very useful in helping coders with determining the codes for radiation treatment management, radiation delivery, when guidance for localization of target volume for radiation treatment delivery is separately reported, and which codes have a professional component.

Initial Consultation

Initial consultations with the radiation oncologist are reported with E/M codes 99201–99215 or 99241–99255. When radiation therapy is incorporated as part of a cancer treatment plan, a consultation with a radiation oncologist, a physician specially trained in using radiation therapy for treating cancer, is required. The radiation oncologist meets with the patient prior to treatment to discuss the therapy and examine the patient. A detailed history is taken and a physical examination is performed. This visit is coded with an E/M or medicine code as appropriate. Following this visit, the physician discusses the findings with the primary oncologist and/or surgeon so that all chemotherapy treatments and surgeries are coordinated. The radiation oncologist at this time recommends what kind of radiation therapy is necessary.

Clinical Treatment Planning

Clinical treatment planning (77261–77263) is a complex service including interpretation of special testing, tumor localization, treatment volume determination, treatment time and dosage determination, choice of treatment modality, allocation of the number and size of treatment ports, and selection of appropriate treatment devices. A *port* or *portal* refers to the site on the skin where the radiation beam enters the body. *Field* is often used as a synonym for port. *Treatment volume* or *area of interest* refers to that volume within the body to which the radiation therapy is directed.

Three levels of clinical treatment planning are defined in CPT and structure this code range as simple, intermediate, or complex. Simple treatment planning requires no interpretation of special tests and only involves one area. The area easily encompasses the tumor while not involving normal tissue. With intermediate planning, a moderate amount of planning difficulty is involved. Interpretation of tests, localizing tumor volume, and up to three ports or structures are involved. Complex planning includes interpreting complex tests, localization of the tumor, and no more than two critical structures.

> Remember to assign modifier –26 for the simulation codes 77306–77307, because the facility will be filing these codes for the technical component.

> If block check simulation is used after the regular simulation, assign 77280 even if it is complex blocking. Not all radiation treatments require block check simulation.

> The treatment plan should be documented separately from the history and physical (H&P) examination. This treatment plan is for a course of radiation treatment. A different or new condition requiring a new course of treatment justifies filing another treatment plan and service code.

Simulation

Simulation (77280–77293) is included in the treatment planning process. It is a "run through" before treatment to confirm that the treatment machine will treat the exact site on the body. A map of the area on the body where the radiation is to be delivered, referred to as the *treatment field(s)*, is created. A machine called a *simulator*, which is designed to mimic the movements and settings on the actual treatment machine, is used.

In some situations, a special CT scanner will be used along with simulation to help plan some radiation therapy treatments. In these instances, the CT scanning process will be performed in the radiation oncology department several days prior to the simulation. Information from the CT scan is used to precisely locate the treatment fields.

At the end of the simulation visit, tattoos are created on the body to outline the treatment field(s). When the simulation is complete, data are sent to medical radiation dosimetrists and medical physicists who perform calculations that will be used to set the treatment machine (linear accelerator). The dose of radiation is determined by the size, extent, type, and grade of tumor, along with its response to radiation therapy. Complex calculations are done to determine the dose and timing of radiation in treatment planning. Often, the treatment is given over several different angles in order to deliver the maximum amount of radiation to the tumor and the minimum amount to normal tissues.

Large alloy blocks may be custom made and placed inside the treatment machine to limit, or "block," the amount of radiation delivered to normal tissue in and around the treatment field. If three-dimensional simulations are used, assign 77295.

Radiation Treatment Delivery

Codes from the range 77385–77387, 77401–77417, 77424–77425 capture the actual treatment provided and the technical component associated with providing treatment and equipment use. Radiation energy is measured in megaelectron-volts (MeV). The amount of radiation actually absorbed or deposited into a patient's body is measured in rads (radiation-absorbed dose). Radiation treatment code descriptions are specific to the number of treatment areas, block and ports used, and total megaelectron volts administered. Codes 77402–77406 are used when a single treatment area is involved and single or parallel opposed ports and/or simple or no blocks are used. Codes 77407–77412 involve two separate treatment areas with three or more ports on one of these areas and use of multiple blocks.

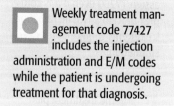 Radiation treatment delivery codes are only reported by the facility providing the treatment. There is no need to append the –TC modifier because there is no professional component allocated to these codes.

Radiation Treatment Management

Radiation treatment management is represented by codes 77427–77470, but special attention should be given to codes 77427–77431. These two codes have specific criteria associated with them in conjunction with the radiation treatment codes. Refer to the Radiation Management and Treatment Table that follows these codes in the CPT manual.

- Code 77427 represents five units of treatment, also referred to as fractions.
- Report 77427 when five units of treatment have been provided regardless of the time period in which they were furnished. They do not need to have been furnished on consecutive days. For example, two treatments were provided in week 1, one treatment during week 2, and two treatments in week 3. For this scenario, code 77427 would be reported once those five treatments were provided.
- If at the end of the complete treatment course there are three or four treatments remaining, code 77427 may be reported again. If, however, only one or two treatments remain, they are included in the final reporting of the last five treatments.
- If two or more treatments are provided on the same day, each treatment may be counted as a separate treatment as long as there has been a distinct break in the treatment sessions, and the treatments are of the same character as those provided on separate days.
- The actual services associated with code 77427 require a minimum of one examination of the patient by the physician for medical E/M such as assessment of the patient's response to treatment, coordination of care and treatment, and review of imaging and/or lab test results for each reporting of code 77427.
- Code 77431 is reported only when the complete course of treatment for the patient is one or two treatments. Do not report this code in addition to 77427.

EXAMPLES

- A patient received a total of 17 treatments over a period of 4 weeks. Report code 77427 three times (once after each set of five treatments). Do not report code 77431 in addition.

- A patient received a total of 18 treatments over a period of 4 weeks. Report code 77427 four times to cover the three treatments remaining after the 15th treatment.

- If a patient receives treatments twice a day for 5 days, two radiation treatment management services will be reimbursed for the calendar week.

Weekly treatment management code 77427 includes the injection administration and E/M codes while the patient is undergoing treatment for that diagnosis.

Proton Beam Treatment Delivery

Proton beam therapy (77520–77525) is a radiation treatment that delivers high-dose radiation to a localized site. Protons, which are particles not x-rays, slow down faster than photons and deposit more energy as they slow down. This allows the majority of radiation to be delivered to the target site with less scattering of radiation to the adjacent tissues, resulting in less damage and fewer side effects. It is an optional method of delivering radiation instead of the traditional x-ray or Gamma ray (*photon* beam).

Hyperthermia (77600–77615) is another mechanism for destroying cancer cells. Heat is used to raise the temperature of a site to speed up cell metabolism and increase the destruction of cancer cells. Hyperthermia codes are used in addition to radiation therapy codes. Hyperthermia can be induced by using microwave, ultrasound, or low-energy radio-frequency conduction, or by probe. The listed treatments include physician management during the course of the therapy and for 3 months after the therapy is complete. Preliminary consultations are not coded in this section but from the E/M section.

To assign these codes, the following details must be documented:

- Number of areas treated
- Number of ports utilized
- Number of shielding blocks utilized
- Total megaelectron-volts administered

Clinical Brachytherapy

Brachytherapy (77750–77790) requires the assistance of a surgeon to place the radioactive source (e.g., seed, capsule, ribbon) inside the body while the radiation oncologist provides supervision of the radioelements and dose interpretation. Given this dual effort, the use of modifiers is crucial to obtaining proper reimbursement for both physicians.

Radioactive seed placement is a low-dose brachytherapy method that utilizes either loose or stranded seeds. Loose seeds are individually placed into or nearby a tumor by using a needle. With stranded seeds, the radioactive seeds are linked together and embedded in a polymer strand of glycolide, lactide, and polydioxanone spaced from 5 mm to over 50 mm apart. The strand is then placed inside an 18-gauge needle and transferred to the patient. An example trade name for this product is Vari-Strand. The stranded product reduces the number of needles required to place the seeds.

There are three types of brachytherapy administration. *Interstitial* therapy places the substance (source) directly into the tissues. *Intracavity* therapy involves implanting sources into the body cavities. *Surface application* brachytherapy (strontium plaque therapy) uses plaques that contain radioactive material that is applied directly to the surface of the patient. Common radioactive materials used in brachytherapy treatment are radium-226, iodine-125, cobalt-60, and cesium-137.

There are two brachytherapy methods: low-dose rate and high-dose rate. With low-dose rate (LDR) brachytherapy, a radioactive source is placed inside or adjacent to the tumor for a minimum of several days but can be left in the tissue permanently. LDR brachytherapy is most commonly used to treat prostate cancer and brain tumors. LDR requires an overnight stay in the hospital.

When billing for stranded sources, you should report the number of units on the claim form based on the number of brachytherapy sources in the strand and not as one unit per strand. If both stranded and nonstranded sources are applied to a patient in a single treatment, bill the stranded and nonstranded sources separately.

For Medicare patients, facilities report brachytherapy sources using HCPCS C codes. Remember, HCPCS C codes are reported only for facility (technical) services and not for physician offices or ASCs.

■ **CASE SCENARIO**

A patient receives brachytherapy for brain metastases requiring five radioactive seeds placed at the time of craniotomy for tumor removal. The neurosurgeon and radiation oncologist work together to place the seeds using the intracavitary method. Report code 77799–66. Two physicians worked as a team to accomplish proper placement. The radiation oncologist is not a surgeon so modifier –62, the cosurgery modifier, would not be appropriate.

With high-dose rate (HDR) brachytherapy, a radioactive source is placed in the tumor temporarily, for just a few minutes at a time, and is then removed. The source is guided to the correct position using plastic catheters and a special machine called a remote afterloader. Because the source position can be precisely adjusted, this allows for customized dose distributions to meet each patient's needs. HDR brachytherapy is most commonly used to treat prostate, cervical, and head and neck cancer and is performed on an outpatient basis.

To correctly report brachytherapy, the coder must account for five basic elements. Each step or component of the therapy is assigned its own code. It is not uncommon to submit a claim with five or more codes for patients treated with brachytherapy. When assigning codes, locate the pertinent information by using this checklist:

1. *Consultation.* Was the consultation performed by the radiation oncologist to determine treatment options? If so, report E/M codes 99201–99215 or 99241–99255.

2. *Clinical treatment planning* (77261–77263). This visit includes interpreting special testing, localizing the site where the source or catheter will be placed, and so forth. These codes reflect the skill of the physician and are used to report the physician professional services. No –26 modifier is necessary. Treatment planning is only reported once for a course of therapy.

3. *Simulation* (77280–77299). The radiation oncologist may conduct a simulation to ensure that radiation therapy is delivered only to the diseased tissue. For the physician component reporting, append a –26 modifier.

4. *Dosimetry and isodose planning* (77295, 77300–77331). To determine the proper amount of radiation delivered by the source, technicians will perform calculations based on the radiation oncologist's orders.

5. *Treatment.* Codes are assigned based on the type of radioactive source and the delivery method. Radiation oncologists can also separately assign codes for surgical procedures that require implanting devices such as virginal cones, oral catheters, or tubes.
   a. What was the delivery method: interstitial, intracavity, or surface? Select a code.
   b. Was liquid radiation utilized? If so, report liquid radioactive sources with 77750, *Infusion or instillation of radioelement solution (includes three months follow-up care).*
   c. Report interstitial radiation source application with one of these:
      77778 *Interstitial radiation source application, complex, includes supervision, handling, loading of radiation source, when performed (10 or more)*
      77799 *Unlisted procedure, clinical brachytherapy*
   d. If ultrasound was used to guide placement of sources/ribbons, also assign 76965, *Ultrasonic guidance for interstitial radioelement application.*
   e. Assign code 77295 if three-dimensional simulation is carried out.
   f. If assigning codes for the facility, coders may assign HCPCS code(s) when they supply the agents.

6. *Postoperative services/follow-up.* A second brachytherapy plan (77316–77318) or simulation (77280–77299) may be performed after the original source is placed, about 1 month after the procedure. This is done to measure the actual dose of radiation delivered, as opposed to the projected dose.

CHECKPOINT 27.4

Assign codes to the following procedures. Include any necessary modifiers.

1. A radiation oncologist reviews the port films, dosimetry, dose delivery, and treatment parameters, and also does a medical evaluation each week for a patient who receives eight treatments in a period of 2 weeks. Code for the radiation oncologist's services related to the eight treatments. _____

2. Prior to the patient's course of radiation treatment, the radiation oncologist sets up intermediate simulation procedures. _____

3. A patient diagnosed with a primary endometrial carcinoma receives intracavitary brachytherapy using 10 sources with applicators left in place for 2 days. _____

NUCLEAR MEDICINE

Nuclear medicine, another subspecialty of radiology, provides doctors with another way to look inside the human body. This modality combines the use of computers, detectors, and administration of radioactive substances (thallium-201, technetium-99m) for diagnostic imaging or for therapy. It consists of diagnostic examinations of the body that produce images and measure organ function.

Nuclear medicine imaging tests differ from most other imaging modalities in that the tests primarily show the physiological function of the system being investigated as opposed to the anatomy. The images are developed based on the detection of energy emitted from a radioactive substance given to the patient, either intravenously or by mouth. Nuclear medicine imaging is useful for detecting:

- Tumors
- Aneurysms (weak spots in blood vessel walls)
- Irregular or inadequate blood flow to organs
- Blood cell disorders and inadequate functioning of organs, such as thyroid and pulmonary function deficiencies
- Metastasis
- Myocardial infarction
- Fractures

Codes are arranged by the nature of the procedure, meaning whether it was diagnostic or therapeutic, and further subdivided by body system. Codes are also differentiated by the extent of the area examined (i.e., limited area versus multiple areas versus whole body). Nearly 100 different nuclear medicine procedures are available. Common scans performed are bone scans to determine cancer metastasis and osteomyelitis and cardiac scans to evaluate cardiac output and myocardial infarction. Thyroid scans for nodules and renal scans for kidney function are also commonly performed. In therapy, radionuclides are administered to treat disease or provide palliative pain relief. Radioactive iodine (I-131) may also be used to treat Graves' disease.

Positron Emission Tomography

When billing Medicare for PET scans, use HCPCS codes (currently G0219, G0235, G0252) instead of a code from the Radiology section.

Positron emission tomography (PET) codes are found within the Nuclear Medicine subsection of the Radiology section and represent exams that produce high-energy, three-dimensional, computer-reconstructed images of the function of an organ. Specific organ studies such as thyroid, liver and spleen, bone, cardiovascular, kidney, and single-proton emission computerized tomography imaging are performed using PET. PET can show images of glucose metabolism in the brain or rapid changes in activity in various areas of the body. PET scans can also detect biochemical and pharmacological changes in body tissues before structural damage is caused by disease. The United States has only a few PET centers because they must be located near a particle accelerator device that produces the short-lived radioisotopes used in the technique. Box 27.4 shows a PET scan report.

BOX 27.4 Sample PET Scan Report

A 62-year-old woman with a history of invasive ductal carcinoma and ductal carcinoma in situ had undergone bilateral mastectomy and chemotherapy. She had one positive right axillary lymph node at dissection. She now presents for staging evaluation.

Radiopharmaceutical:
4.3 mCi F-18 Fluorodeoxyglucose IV

Findings:
PET images demonstrate areas of decreased uptake in the anterior chest corresponding to breast implants. Mild increased uptake is seen in the right axilla, probably representing postsurgical inflammation. There is no abnormal uptake to suggest recurrent or metastatic disease. There are several foci of markedly increased uptake conforming to the bowel in the region of the ileum, cecum, and right lower abdomen.

Single-Proton Emission Computerized Tomography

Single-proton emission computerized tomography (SPECT) codes are also found within the Nuclear Medicine subsection. SPECT services provide three-dimensional, computer-reconstructed images of an organ. They are documented as shown in Box 27.5. SPECT studies use radioactive materials to study blood flow and organ activity and function. Radioactive materials are inhaled or injected and then move through the blood to the organ being tested. Codes for lung scans (ventilation/perfusion [V/Q] scans), HIDA (hepatobiliary) scans, renal scans, thyroid scans, and cardiac stress tests are also located here.

SPECT is a technique similar to PET; however, some of the radioactive substances used in SPECT (xenon-133, technetium-99m, iodine-123) have longer decay times than those used in PET, and emit single instead of double gamma rays. SPECT can provide information about blood flow and the distribution of radioactive substances in the body. Its images are less sensitive and less detailed than PET images, but the SPECT technique is less expensive than PET. Also, SPECT centers are more accessible than PET centers, because they do not have to be located near a particle accelerator.

Radioimmunoassay tests are located in the Pathology section of CPT. These codes can be reported by any specialist performing these tests in a laboratory. Some nuclear studies are assigned codes from the Medicine section of CPT. For example, nuclear tests that are performed during exercise, or pharmacologically induced stress tests, are located in the 93015–93018 range. These codes should be reported in addition to the actual code from the Nuclear Medicine subsection.

The provision of radium or another radiation source may or may not be included in the nuclear medicine service. If not packaged, these are coded separately using the appropriate HCPCS supply codes. Best practice is to report each radiopharmaceutical on claims, whether or not it is paid.

The supply of radio-pharmaceuticals used in nuclear medicine is not included in the nuclear medicine services and should be reported separately with HCPCS codes A9500–A9699.

The injection of a radionuclide is included in the scope of the procedure itself and not reported separately.

■ CASE SCENARIO

A patient with a long-standing history of coronary artery disease and arrhythmia is required to have a cardiac stress test every year. Due to recent back surgery, the patient cannot walk on the treadmill, so he has a pharmacological stress test along with a technetium-99m ventriculogram scan, multiple studies. Report codes 93015, 78452.

BOX 27.5 Sample SPECT Report

A 57-year old with dizziness and black, tarry stools requires a transfusion. Physician is suspicious of a GI bleed.
Radiopharmaceutical:
Tc99m tagged RBC
Findings:
Sequential images demonstrate tracer activity accumulation in a small bowel pattern in the midline/left upper quadrant beginning at 5 to 10 minutes.
Diagnosis:
Crohn's disease

Assign codes to the following procedures. Include any necessary modifiers.

1. PET tumor imaging, whole body _____

2. SPECT myocardial imaging _____

3. Diagnostic nuclear medicine procedure, gastrointestinal, unlisted _____

4. Multiple determinations of thyroid uptake _____

5. High-dose rate brachytherapy, remote afterloading, 11 channels _____

6. A radiation oncologist provides clinical treatment planning services to patients who are receiving radiation therapy for cancer. Code for the clinical treatment planning that encompasses a single treatment area in a single port with no blocking. _____

7. How would you report the CPT code for the study in Box 27.5? _____

8. Patient is status postchemotherapy and radiation treatment for lung cancer 1 month ago. He is here today for PET scan follow-up to evaluate response to therapy and any distant metastatic lesions. A whole-body PET scan was performed. Radiopharmaceutical: 15.0 mCi F-18 FDG i.v. Findings: Images of the body show a photopenic focus with a rim of minimal FDG uptake in the left lower lobe. _____

9. A 79-year-old male was brought to the imaging center by his daughter who states that he is becoming very lethargic, forgetful, and less able to care for himself. He got lost driving home from the grocery store. PET scan shows hypometabolism in the temporoparietal and reduced glucose uptake in the cranial portion of both frontal lobes. Radiologist confirms Alzheimer's disease.

_____

10. A 53-year-old man with a history of end-stage renal disease underwent kidney transplant 2 years ago. His post-transplant creatinine has remained elevated and has increased to 2.8. A nuclear medicine diagnostic study was provided for kidney function imaging with vascular flow.

_____

Chapter Summary

1. The Radiology section has seven subsections organized according to method or type of radiology and its purpose. Codes in this section begin with the number 7. Coders must read key guidelines and notes at the beginning of the section as well as those in the subsections and in parentheses.

2. A *modality* is a method used to obtain images. Understanding the difference between modalities such as radiological examination (x-ray), CT scan, MRI scan, and MRA scan is essential to determining the correct code for radiology services. Also, coders

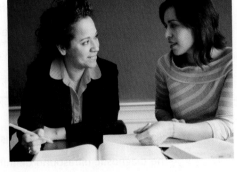

must identify the number of radiological views taken in order to properly assign the correct code. To assign a code identified as complete, all views of that specific area must be taken.

3. Many radiology codes are selected on the basis of whether contrast was introduced. Oral or rectal contrast administration alone does not qualify as a study with contrast because the phrase "with contrast" represents contrast material administered intravascularly or directly into a joint. CT and MRI scans break down into specific contrast methods. The coder must be aware of the distinction between "without contrast," "with contrast," and "without contrast followed by with contrast." To report two codes to represent the scenario of without contrast followed by with contrast is incorrect. A code is already available for that type of CT or MRI.

4. A complete code in the Radiology section has component parts. The technical component is the allocation of staff or the technologist, use of equipment, supplies, and related services. The professional component encompasses the physician's time and skill in reading and interpreting the test and providing a written report rendering an opinion, advice, or assessment of findings.

5. The radiological S&I services represent the professional component of viewing the contrast as it flows through the anatomical area being examined and interpreting the findings. If contrast is injected into an extremity and cannot pass through an artery, the physician can determine that some type of occlusion is present and the patient will need a therapeutic intervention to correct the problem.

6. Diagnostic imaging is the radiology method used to produce images of the body to diagnose a problem. X-rays are the most common diagnostic technique followed by CT scans, MRI scans, and MRA scans. In interventional radiology, the radiologist can provide both diagnostic and/or therapeutic services via minimally invasive or percutaneous methods as an alternative to traditional surgery. Abdominal aortic aneurysms, artery occlusions, and embolizations are just a few examples of therapeutic services.

Review Questions

Matching

Match the key terms with their definitions.

A. fluoroscopy
B. nuclear medicine
C. vascular family
D. ultrasound
E. selective catheter placement
F. magnetic resonance angiography
G. charge description master
H. technical component
I. portal
J. retrograde

1. _____ Uses ultra–high-frequency sound waves for diagnostic scanning

2. _____ Encompasses the allocation of staff or use of equipment

3. _____ Uses a continuous low-level x-ray beam to view the body in motion

4. _____ Against the normal flow pattern

5. _____ Placement of a catheter into a branch off the main conduit of a vascular system

6. _____ A computerized master list of hospital services with associated fees and codes

7. _____ All arteries or veins branching off of the main conduit of a vascular system

8. _____ An MRI study of the blood vessels

9. _____ Entry point for a radiation beam

10. _____ The use of computers, detectors, and radioactive substances for diagnosis or therapy

True or False

Decide whether each statement is true or false.

1. _____ The diagnostic ultrasound definition of an A-mode implies a one-dimensional ultrasonic measurement procedure.

2. _____ The time descriptors for fluoroscopic exam codes apply to the actual time the fluoroscopic unit is turned on.

3. _____ When the physician owns the equipment and provides the S&I, the global x-ray service has been provided.

4. _____ Nuclear medicine involves imaging that uses injection or infusion of radioelements to allow visualization of a specific area.

5. _____ The abbreviation PC stands for professional charge.

6. _____ For situations in which contrast is provided orally, codes with contrast are chosen.

7. _____ There is a separate unlisted procedure code for diagnostic ultrasounds.

8. _____ The −26 modifier reports the professional and technical component of a procedure.

9. _____ In radiation oncology, the consultation with a radiation oncologist is part of the clinical management of the patient during treatment.

10. _____ Selective catheter placement includes nonselective catheter placement.

Multiple Choice

Select the letter that best completes the statement or answers the question.

1. What does the abbreviation S&I mean?
   A. Search and intervention
   B. Supervision of iodine
   C. Supervision and interpretation
   D. Supervision of injection

2. Two views of the thumb and two views of the second digit on each hand are coded as
   A. 73140–RT, 73140-LT
   B. 73120–FA, 73120–F5, 73140–F1, 73140–F6
   C. 73120–50, 73140–50
   D. 73120–LT–RT, 71340–LT–RT

3. When a diagnostic mammogram is performed on the same day as a screening mammogram, which modifier is used on the diagnostic mammogram?
   A. −76
   B. −GA
   C. −22
   D. −GH

4. Diagnostic ophthalmic ultrasound of the eye with quantitative A scan only is coded as
   A. 76511
   B. 76513
   C. 76516
   D. 76519

5. A physician not employed by the hospital provides a shoulder arthrography S&I to an inpatient. What is the code?
   A. 73020–26
   B. 73050–TC
   C. 73040–26
   D. 73040–TC

6. A complete cervical x-ray with flexion and oblique views is coded as
   A. 72082
   B. 72052
   C. 72050
   D. 72040

7. An x-ray of the paranasal sinuses, two views is coded as
   A. 70160
   B. 70250
   C. 70210
   D. None of the above

8. A CT scan of the lumbar spine without contrast and with contrast is coded as
   A. 72131, 72132
   B. 72120
   C. 72100
   D. 72133

9. A hysterosalpingography, S&I is coded as
   A. 74740
   B. 58340
   C. 58345
   D. 74742

10. A barium enema with KUB is coded as
    A. 74246
    B. 74270
    C. 74280
    D. 74241

CHAPTER 28

CPT: Pathology and Laboratory Codes

CHAPTER OUTLINE

Pathology and Laboratory Overview

Modifiers

Major Pathology/Laboratory Procedures

LEARNING OUTCOMES

After studying this chapter, you should be able to:

1. Explain the difference between the professional and technical components of the pathology and laboratory medicine services and determine whether a pathology/laboratory service requires modifier –26 or modifier –TC.
2. Explain the specific coding rules associated with reporting panel codes.
3. Distinguish between qualitative and quantitative drug testing.
4. Describe the basis for code selection in molecular pathology.
5. Determine if one or more pathology codes are needed based on the specimens received by the surgical pathology department.
6. Understand the different types of pathology consultation services.

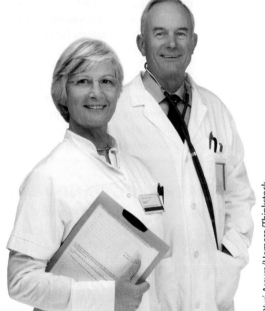

Yuri Arcurs/Hemera/Thinkstock

The information contained within the pathology and laboratory section of the CPT is very technical. Some of the tests described in this chapter can be performed in a physician office, while others require the use of sophisticated equipment and review by a pathologist and, hence, are only performed in a hospital or by an independent laboratory. Coders can review documentation in the form of physician orders, test requisitions, laboratory reports, and pathology reports to build a complete clinical picture of a patient's workup and may capture applicable procedure codes. This type of documentation, however, is never used to assign diagnosis codes (pathology reports are the only exception to this rule).

The Pathology and Laboratory section of CPT contains numerous combination codes for various panels and testing techniques. It is very important for the coder to read the documentation to choose the most comprehensive code that describes the services performed rather than billing multiple codes to describe the same service.

The laboratory section of CPT is the most difficult to master because of the various testing methods used and the chemistry terminology. It is also a section subjected to layers of regulation and Medicare coverage determinations. Inpatient coders in particular must become familiar with common tests performed on the many body systems and why the tests are being performed. This enables them to assign diagnosis codes to the highest specificity. It also provides a mechanism for coders to query physicians when documentation is not detailed enough or if lab results are indicative of a condition that is not documented by the physician. Inpatient coders seldom code for pathological or laboratory services, but they must be able to read and understand the results of these examinations. Outpatient coders, on the other hand, are charged with assigning codes for pathology and laboratory services. To expedite the coding process, coders should become acclimated to the various abbreviations used throughout this highly technical section of CPT. The CPT manual contains a table of definitions and abbreviations located within the Drug Assay section.

> Documentation pertaining to physician orders for laboratory tests and their results are predominantly based on abbreviations. Invest in an abbreviation resource or use websites to determine the meaning of unfamiliar laboratory or pathology definitions.

This chapter discusses basic pathology/laboratory coding concepts, new terminology, and laboratory testing methods.

INTERNET RESOURCES: Acronyms specific to pathology can be found at the following two websites, and a Web search will produce many others. Just specify in the search box pathology or laboratory medicine.
www.allacronyms.com
www.acronymfinder.com

The College of American Pathologists (CAP) is the best source to use for coding laboratory and pathology procedures. Their website has a References Resources and Publications menu with links to guidelines and various resources for this specialty.
www.cap.org

ARUP Laboratories: A National Reference Laboratory provides an extensive searchable test directory, specialty-specific resources, Medicare coverage, and educational opportunities.
https://www.aruplab.com/#

PATHOLOGY AND LABORATORY OVERVIEW

The Pathology and Laboratory section of CPT contains the codes relating to a broad range of services—from routine diagnostic testing that may be performed in a physician office lab, hospital lab, or independent laboratory to very complex tests that require sophisticated equipment at a specialized laboratory.

Pathology and laboratory (or "path/lab") services are performed to diagnose or monitor diseases by examining specimens obtained from the body in the form of body fluid (sputum, blood, urine, mucus) or tissue. Common procedures include urinalysis, culturing bacteria, organ or disease panels, microscopic examination of tissue or blood, and dissection of surgical specimens.

The lab tech identifies and designates codes for the lab tests performed onsite. If you are working for a billing service, you must be familiar with this type of coding and billing for professional fees. It is an important part of a coder's general knowledge to be able to verify path/lab codes against documentation.

Services provided in this chapter are performed by a physician or by technologists (such as medical laboratory technicians, or MLTs) under a physician's supervision. A few tests may actually be performed by a medical assistant, nurse, or patients themselves.

Some services combine the *professional component* (the physician's supervision and interpretation), but most of the path/lab codes are for the technical component only. The *technical component* represents the use of equipment for the handling and actual testing of the material submitted and is not commonly done by a physician. (See Chapter 27.) The techniques for testing are very complex and involve methods and terminology that must be carefully studied to assign codes. Good references to use that explain the test performed include the *Coder's Desk Reference for Procedures*, the *Laboratory Cross Coder*, and the *Coding and Payment Guide for Laboratory Services*.

Pathology plays a particularly important role in preventive medicine by ruling out diseases or detecting them early. The medical laboratory is one of the first stops in preventive medicine. Because it is predicted that preventive medicine will continue to become even more important in the next decade, laboratory and medical testing will be in greater demand to rule out incorrect diagnoses and to detect diseases early. There are many specific fields of pathology outside of surgical pathology, including the following:

- Blood banking
- Clinical chemistry
- Cytopathology
- Dermatopathology
- Forensic pathology
- Hematopathology
- Immunopathology
- Neuropathology
- Pediatric pathology

Pathology and Laboratory General Guidelines

As in all other sections of CPT, guidelines are located before the codes themselves. Notes are also located at the beginning of code ranges or as parenthetical notes. The chapter also has several tables with abbreviations, definitions, and crosswalks to codes for reference. It is appropriate to list as many CPT codes from this section as necessary to capture all of the services performed, regardless of whether they have been performed on the same date of service. Unlisted procedures are also available for use for most subsections but should be assigned only after checking for a Category III or HCPCS Level II code. In this section, codes do not include specimen collection unless otherwise stated in the parenthetical notes or in the instructions prior to or below the code for the test.

Physician laboratory and pathology services are limited to the following:

- Surgical pathology services
- Specific cytopathology, hematology, and blood-banking services that require performance by a physician, including clinical consultation services and clinical laboratory interpretation services

NOTE: HCPCS Level II codes are covered in Chapter 30 of this text.

Location of Testing

Labs can be performed in physician offices, clinics, reference labs, or hospital-based labs. Where the test is performed is of great interest to the carrier to assess proper payment and compliance with CLIA practices.

Table 28.1 Examples of CLIA-waived Tests

CPT CODE/MODIFIER	DESCRIPTION
81025–QW	Urine pregnancy test (various manufacturers)
86318–QW	Acon® *H. pylori* test device
85018–QW	HemoCue Hemoglobin 201
83001–QW	Synova Healthcare Menocheck Pro

All lab work is regulated by Clinical Laboratory Improvement Amendments (CLIA) rules. Most offices do easy-to-administer, low-risk tests (ovulation, blood glucose, dipstick or tablet reagent urinalyses, and rapid strep test), which are "waived" under CLIA and are subject to minimal requirements (Table 28.1). Providers who want to perform these tests file an application and pay a small fee. Offices that handle more complex testing (such as complete blood cell counts, prostate-specific antigen tests, routine chemistry panels, and antibiotic susceptibility tests) must apply and be certified and inspected for accreditation.

INTERNET RESOURCE: View a list of CLIA-waived tests at www.cms.gov. Search for "CLIA waved tests."

Organization of the Path/Lab Section

All codes in this section begin with the number 8. This section has 20 subsections, with guidelines located at the beginning of the section. The section includes services that are performed behind the scenes in a laboratory setting such as urinalysis, culturing bacteria, organ or disease panels, microscopic examination of tissue or blood, and dissection of surgical specimens. Take a few moments now to peruse this section. Make note of the miscellaneous codes located under the "Other Procedures" subsection. This subsection contains codes for sweat collection, nasal smears, and gastric aspiration, to name a few. Table 28.2 is a list of the subsections in the Path/Lab section. (*Note:* These code ranges are organized by the type of service, not by anatomy.)

Table 28.2 Path/Lab Subsections

SUBSECTIONS	CPT CODES
Organ or Disease-Oriented Panels	(80047–80081)
Drug Assay	(80305–80377)
Therapeutic Drug Assay	(80150–80299)
Evocative/Suppression Testing	(80400–80439)
Consultations (Clinical Pathology)	(80500–80502)
Urinalysis	(81000–81099)
Molecular Pathology	(81105–81479)
Genomic Sequencing Procedures and Other Molecular Multianalyte Assays	(81410–81471)
Multianalyte Assays with Algorithmic Analyses	(81490–81599)
Chemistry	(82009–84999)
Hematology and Coagulation	(85002–85999)
Immunology	(86000–86849)
Transfusion Medicine	(86850–86999)
Microbiology	(87003–87999)
Anatomic Pathology	(88000–88099)
Cytopathology	(88104–88199)
Cytogenetic Studies	(88230–88299)
Surgical Pathology	(88300–88399)
In Vivo (e.g., Transcutaneous) Laboratory Procedures	(88720–88749)
Other Procedures	(89049–89240)
Reproductive Medicine Procedures	(89250–89398)
Proprietary Laboratory Analyses	(0001U–0017U)

To bill Medicare for waived tests performed onsite, the office must have a CLIA certificate of waiver, must follow the manufacturers' test instructions, include the CLIA number on the claims, and add modifier –QW (for a CLIA-waived test) to the codes. (Note that this modifier does not apply to private payers.) Offices billing waived tests stay current on new additions to the list with the CMS Medicare Laboratory National Coverage Determination edit module.

With respect to hospital lab billing under Medicare Part B, neither the deductible nor the coinsurance applies to labs paid under the lab fee schedule.

- Path/lab test codes do not usually include the specimen collection, so this service can be separately coded. Venipuncture (code range 36400–36425; usually 36415) can be coded if lab personnel actually draws the blood.
- When specimens are obtained in a physician's office or other setting and sent offsite for testing, the office should assign code 99000 or 99001 (from the Medicine section) for the handling and transferring of the specimen.

Physician Orders and Test Requisitions

Every laboratory test must be ordered by a physician (MD), physician assistant (PA), or registered nurse practitioner (RNP). When a specimen is obtained in the office (urine, blood, sputum, saliva, tissue, etc.), a lab requisition is completed and sent along with the specimen to an outside lab for analysis or processing. Alternatively, patients are instructed to go to an independent lab or a hospital-based lab to provide their sample. For every laboratory test ordered, a test requisition (Fig. 28.1) must be sent that specifies which tests to perform on the specimen and supplies a diagnosis or reason for the test, even if it is a sign or symptom, to justify its medical necessity.

IMMUNOSCIENCES LAB., INC.

822 S. Robertson Blvd., Ste. 312, Los Angeles, CA 90035   Tel (310) 657-1077 · Fax (310) 657-1053
E-mail: immunsci@ix.netcom.com   Website: www.immunoscienceslab.com

TEST REQUEST FORM

IF THE INFORMATION BELOW IS INCOMPLETE OR INCORRECTLY FILLED OUT, THERE MAY BE A DELAY IN THE PROCESSING OF YOUR SAMPLE.

PATIENT'S NAME (LAST)	(FIRST)
BIRTH DATE SEX DATE & TIME COLLECTED SAMPLE COLLECTOR'S INITIALS	
ADDRESS	
CITY STATE ZIP CODE	
PHONE (INCLUDE AREA CODE) PATIENT ID	

DOCTOR'S NAME (LAST)	(FIRST)	UPIN#
ADDRESS		
CITY STATE ZIP CODE		
PHONE NO. FAX NO.		
DIAGNOSIS:		
DOCTOR'S SIGNATURE If signature is not available, please attach doctor's prescription.		

BILLING INFORMATION

BILL TO
❏ DOCTOR ❏ LAB
by permission or request

PREPAID
❏ CASH ❏ CHECK ❏ MC ❏ VISA

CARDHOLDER'S NAME _____

CREDIT CARD NO. _____

EXPIRATION DATE _____

CARDHOLDER'S SIGNATURE

SPECIMENS RECEIVED: **FOR ISL USE ONLY**
❏ RED/SST
❏ SERUM
COMMENTS _____

DATE RECEIVED: _____   TIME RECEIVED: _____

Immunosciences Lab., Inc. (ISL) is a fee-for-service provider.
ISL does not bill any insurance provider, including Medicare.

I agree to pay the costs for the analysis requested. I understand the testing will be performed upon receipt of full payment. I understand I will receive a statement for the testing performed by ISL, and if I choose, I can submit this invoice to my insurance carrier.

Responsible Party's Name _____   Relation to Patient _____

Responsible Party's Signature _____   Date _____

❏ **2010 - Autoimmune Profile-Basic**
(ANA, RF, C1Q)

❏ **2011 - Autoimmune Panel-Comprehensive**
(ANA, ENA, DNA, RF, C1Q, Actin IgG, Mitochondrial IgG)

❏ **2013 - Autoimmune Liver Disease**
(Actin IgG, Mitochondrial IgG)

❏ **2015 - B. burgdorferi IgG, IgM by ELISA**
(IgG, IgM against B. burgdorferi by ELISA)

❏ **2016 - B. burgdorferi IgG, IgM by Western Blot**
(IgG, IgM against B. burgdorferi by Western Blot)

❏ **2017 - Immunoserology of Lyme Panel A**
(IgG, IgM against tickborne antigens by Multi-Peptide ELISA)

❏ **2018 - Immunoserology of Lyme Panel B**
(IgG, IgM against tickborne antigens by Multi-Peptide ELISA & Western Blot)

❏ **2019 - Epstein-Barr Virus (EBV) Panel**
(VCA IgG, IgM; EA IgG; EBNA IgG, IgM)

❏ **2020 - Viral Screen**
(EBV-VCA IgG, IgM; CMV IgG, IgM; Herpes 1+2 IgG, IgM)

❏ **2022 - Viral Panel Premier**
(EBV-VCA IgG, IgM; EA IgG; EBNA IgG, IgM; CMV IgG, IgM; Herpes 1+2 IgG, IgM; HHV-6 IgG, IgM; VZV IgG)

❏ **2023 - Viral Panel Comprehensive**
(EBV-VCA IgG, IgM; EA IgG; EBNA IgG, IgM; CMV IgG, IgM; Herpes 1+2 IgG, IgM; HHV-6 IgG, IgM; VZV IgG; Measles IgG, IgM)

v.120914

Figure 28.1 Sample test requisition form. (© 2015 Immunosciences Lab., Inc. Used with permission.)

Complete Lab Codes

To properly code and bill for a *physician,* the coder must determine the following:

- Whether the physician performed the complete procedure or only a component of the procedure
- Whether the procedure was performed onsite or offsite

A complete lab test includes ordering the procedure/test, obtaining the sample/specimen, handling the specimen, performing the actual procedure/test, and analyzing and interpreting the results. Blood can be collected via a vein (venipuncture), capillary (fingerstick), or port-a-cath. Some offices have sophisticated in-house equipment and can perform a wider variety of laboratory procedures. However, if the physician sends the sample/specimen to a freestanding lab or a hospital-based lab for testing and analysis, only the collection and handling fee for preparation of the specimen is coded.

CHECKPOINT 28.1

Read the following scenario and answer the question.

1. An internal medicine physician did a venipuncture to obtain blood for lab analysis and then sent the blood specimen to an outside lab for testing. The lab will bill the patient for the testing. How will the internal medicine physician's services be reported? _____

Physicians may also send a patient for lab testing to a local hospital or freestanding laboratory, which obtains the sample/specimen, performs the test/procedure, and analyzes and interprets the results. Or, in the case of a surgical procedure performed at a facility, the physician will remove a surgical specimen and send it to pathology for examination. In the latter situation, three sets of services are coded and billed:

1. The surgeon bills for the surgical procedure using a surgical code.
2. The pathologist bills for the professional interpretation of the specimen using a path/lab code with the professional component modifier.
3. The facility bills both the surgery and path/lab codes with the technical component modifiers to be paid for the associated facility fees.

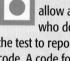 Medicare does not allow any provider who does not perform the test to report the path/lab code. A code for the venipuncture only should be reported (only once, even if more than one specimen is drawn). Other payers do allow physicians to report the lab code with a –90 modifier when specimens are sent offsite for analysis.

EXAMPLE

A bone marrow biopsy performed by a surgeon with the specimen sent to a pathologist for review and interpretation. The surgeon reports 38221 for the actual biopsy of the bone marrow. The pathologist reports 88305–26 for the review and interpretation of the specimen. The facility reports both 38221 and 88305–TC for the surgery and the technical component of the specimen processing.

If a physician is requested to review a test result due to abnormalities or is asked to interpret the test or specimen, the –26 modifier is appended to show the professional component. In the example above, the pathologist renders opinions after examining tissue or cultures, so the –26 modifier is used to capture this professional service.

MODIFIERS

As with every chapter of CPT, modifiers may be used to further describe a service or circumstance surrounding a procedure:

 Medicare has very specific requirements for reporting modifier –90. Medicare will not pay for more than one clinical lab test with matching patient name, date of service, and CPT code with the –90 modifier per day.

- –22 Increased procedural services
- –26 Professional component
- –32 Mandated services
- –52 Reduced services
- –53 Discontinued procedure
- –59 Distinct procedural service

−90 Reference (outside) laboratory
−91 Repeat clinical diagnostic laboratory test
−92 Alternative laboratory platform testing
−GA Waiver of liability
−QW CLIA-waived test

EXAMPLE

A blood sample was obtained by Dr. Simmons' office and sent to an outside laboratory for testing, analysis, and interpretation. Dr. Simmons has an arrangement with the lab to bill for the lab test even though it is not performed in his office. He reported the venipuncture code 36415 and 80061–90 to describe the lab test with interpretation and analysis being performed at an offsite laboratory.

The Centers for Medicare and Medicaid Services (CMS) limits payments for diagnostic testing to tests that are "medically necessary." This is problematic for physicians and labs alike. The diagnosis codes submitted are very important in establishing this foundation. CMS contends that physicians should only order individual tests or less-inclusive profiles when all of the tests in a profile are not performed. They also state that customized panels may include tests on which they will deny payment. If physicians submit charges for a noncovered lab, they must have an Advance Beneficiary Notice (ABN) signed by the patient to protect them and the lab from penalty from Medicare.

■ CASE SCENARIO

A patient feels run down and lethargic but has otherwise been healthy to date. A physician orders a CBC to get a baseline study. The physician should report CPT code 85027–GA on the Medicare claim.

Modifier −91 is used to alert the carrier that a test is performed or repeated more than once in a given day. This is not used when there is a problem with a specimen or when the equipment necessitates the need to do the test again. This also cannot be appended to codes to confirm initial results.

■ CASE SCENARIO

A 49-year-old male experiences chest pain while playing basketball at the local gym. He goes to the emergency department (ED) and the physician orders a troponin test. Qualitative study shows the presence of troponin and the physician orders a level. The patient is kept in a holding room and the test is repeated 6 hours later. Assign codes 84512, 84484, 84484–91.

CHECKPOINT 28.2

Read the following scenario and answer the question.

1. Evocative/suppression testing was done to determine adrenal insufficiency and cortisol was administered twice in the course of testing. The lab reported 82533, 82533–91. Is the lab correct? _____

The date of service for a lab test is the date the *specimen was collected*, not the date the test was actually performed.

Modifier −51 (multiple procedures) is not used with laboratory/pathology codes. Fees are not reduced for multiple procedures.

Modifier −59 can be used in this section but with caution. The coder must know if a test is performed multiple times at the same time but on separate or different specimens. The documentation must clearly state which test is performed and on which specimens.

EXAMPLE

A physician obtains cultures from two nonhealing pressure ulcers: one on the heel and the second on the right hip. The physician orders a bacterial culture for both specimens. Assign codes 87070, 87070–59.

INTERNET RESOURCE: Visit Medicare's website for questions related to coding and billing clinical lab tests. www.cms.gov/. Search for "Medicare Claims Processing Manual Chapter 16 Laboratory Services."

MAJOR PATHOLOGY/LABORATORY PROCEDURES

Organ or Disease-Oriented Panels

Common laboratory tests (Table 28.3) that are performed in a group are referred to as a *panel*. Table 28.3 lists the CPT panels. Remember, this is not an all-inclusive list of panels. CPT maintains these organ- or disease-oriented laboratory panels as a convenient way for physicians to order tests and subsequently bill. The CPT panels contain a limited number of lab test options. Physicians and labs create panels that test organ-specific functions or diseases not provided by CPT; some of these tests are listed in Table 28.4. There are other tests that commonly appear on lab requisition forms under a test title that indicates a group of related procedures to the lab; therefore, each lab's policy may differ. These panels are referred to as customized panels. For example, a rheumatologist orders what his office calls an "arthritis panel"; CPT does not have a panel for "arthritis," even though this is a routine battery of tests he regularly orders.

Table 28.3 Common Laboratory Tests

TEST	ORGAN SYSTEMS OR DISEASES
Albumin	Renal disease with proteinuria
Alkaline phosphatase	Liver and bone disorders
Alpha-fetoprotein test (AFP)	Prenatal birth defect marker, liver, testes, ovary
Bilirubin direct	Liver and biliary disorder
Bilirubin indirect	Liver and biliary disorder
Bilirubin total	Liver and biliary disorder
Bleeding time	Vascular diseases, bleeding disorders
Blood culture	Blood infections, bacteremia, sepsis
Blood urea nitrogen (BUN)	Renal diseases
Complete blood count (CBC)	General health, cellular components of blood
Creatinine	Renal failure
Electrolytes (chloride, sodium, potassium, CO_2)	Hypertension, water metabolism, electrolyte balance, endocrine system
Eosinophils	Allergies, parasitic and collagen diseases
Erythrocyte sedimentation rate (ESR)	Infections, inflammatory processes, autoimmune diseases
Ferritin (iron)	Investigation of anemia
Full blood count (FBC)	Hematologic disorders, infections, bleeding, malignancies
Gamma-glutamyl transferase (GGT)	Hepatic and biliary disorders
Globulins	Immune status and antibodies
Glucose, glucose tolerance test (GTT)	Diabetes, hypoglycemia, hyperglycemia
Hematocrit	Anemia and hematologic disorders
Hemoglobin	Anemia and hematologic disorders
High-density lipoprotein (HDL)	Cholesterol, risk of heart disease, arteriosclerosis
Iron saturation	Iron metabolism disorders
LDL/HDL ratio	Heart risk prognosis
Lipase	Digestion, pancreas
Liver function test (LFT)	Hepatic disorders, hepatitis, cirrhosis
Low-density lipoprotein (LDL)	Cholesterol, heart risk prognosis
Occult blood (feces) (FOBT)	GI bleeding, intestinal cancer

Table 28.3 *Continued*

TEST	ORGAN SYSTEMS OR DISEASES
Partial prothrombin time (PTT)	Blood test for measuring blood clotting
Platelet count	Bleeding disorders, thrombosis
Prothrombin time (PT)	Blood test for unusual bleeding or bruising, vitamin K deficiency
Red cell distribution width (RDW)	Anemia, Hb
Rh typing	Red blood cell, transfusion medicine, pregnancy
Serum glutamic oxaloacetic transaminase (AST)	Liver and heart disorders
Serum glutamic pyruvic transaminase (ALT)	Liver function test
Sodium	Acid–base balance, water balance, dehydration
TORCH	Pregnancy screening for harmful viruses, toxoplasmosis, rubella, cytomegalovirus, and herpes
Total iron binding capacity (TIBC)	Anemia, sideropenia
Triglycerides	Lipid metabolism disorders, heart risk prognosis
Urea	Kidney function test
Uric acid	Gout, nonrheumatic arthritis
White blood cell count (WBC)	Number and type of WBC, infection, immune system

Table 28.4 Lab Panels

PANEL	COMPONENTS (INDIVIDUAL TESTS INCLUDED)
Acute hepatitis	Hepatitis A antibody (HAAb), IgM antibody, hepatitis B core antibody (HBcAb), IgM antibody, HBsAg, hepatitis C antibody
Basic metabolic	Calcium–ionized, carbon dioxide, chloride, creatinine, glucose, potassium, sodium, blood urea nitrogen (BUN)
Basic metabolic	Total calcium, carbon dioxide, chloride, creatinine, glucose, potassium, sodium, BUN
Comprehensive metabolic	Albumin, total bilirubin, calcium, carbon dioxide, chloride, creatinine, glucose, phosphatase, alkaline, potassium, total protein, sodium, alanine amino transferase (ALT), serum glutamic-pyruvic transaminase (SGPT) aspartate amino transferase (AST), serum glutamic-oxaloacetic transaminase (SGOT), BUN
Electrolyte	Carbon dioxide, chloride, potassium, sodium
General health	Comprehensive metabolic panel, automated complete blood count (CBC) with manual differential white blood cell count (WBC), or automated CBC and platelet count with automated differential WBC count; thyroid-stimulating hormone (TSH)
Hepatic function	Albumin, bilirubin total, bilirubin direct, alkaline phosphatase, total protein, ALT, SGPT, AST, SGOT
Lipid	Total serum cholesterol, high-density lipoprotein (HDL), low-density lipoprotein (LPL) triglycerides
Obstetrical	Automated CBC with manual differential WBC or automated CBC and platelet count with automated differential WBC count, hepatitis B surface antigen (HBsAg), antibody screen, RBC, blood typing ABO, blood typing Rh (D)
Renal function	Albumin, calcium, carbon dioxide, chloride, creatinine, glucose, phosphorus, potassium, sodium, BUN
NOT LISTED AS PANELS IN CPT BUT COMMONLY PERFORMED	
Arthritis	Uric acid, sedimentation rate, fluorescent antinuclear antibody (FANA), Rh factor (qualitative)

Continued

Table 28.4 Continued

PANEL	COMPONENTS (INDIVIDUAL TESTS INCLUDED)
Complete blood count	WBC, RBC, hemoglobin, hematocrit, mean corpuscular volume (MCV), mean corpuscular hemoglobin (MCH), mean corpuscular hemoglobin concentrations (MCHC) red cell distribution width (RDW), platelet count, absolute neutrophils, absolute lymphocytes, absolute monocytes, absolute eosinophils, absolute basophils, neutrophils, lymphocytes, monocytes, eosinophils, basophils
Hepatic function panel A (with bilirubin total and direct)	Albumin, bilirubin, alkaline phosphatase, AST, SGOT, ALT, SGPT
TORCH antibody	Cytomegalovirus (CMV) antibody, herpes simplex antibody, rubella antibody, toxoplasma antibody

To bill a panel code, *all* of the listed tests must be performed. No substitutions are permitted. If fewer tests are performed, individual CPT codes for each test should be reported, not the panel code. In CPT, the individual test codes can be located quickly because each test listed under the panel has its associated CPT code next to it for quick reference. Typically, a single diagnosis code is sufficient to justify the necessity of using a panel code. Tests ordered in addition to a panel, however, must be justified separately with a diagnosis.

EXAMPLE

A physician orders a comprehensive metabolic panel. CPT code 80053 is assigned. If, however, one of the tests included in this panel is not performed, the panel code would not be assigned and the tests that were performed would be listed individually.

Customized labs are problematic for Medicare recipients. Laboratories are required by the inspector general's office to have ordering physicians sign annual notices and acknowledgments that Medicare will not pay for unnecessary medical tests. The notices describe what Medicare will reimburse for each component of this customized profile and explain that Medicare may not cover these tests. An ABN may be necessary when billing Medicare for customized profiles. CPT maintains organ- or disease-oriented laboratory panels as a convenient way for physicians to order tests and subsequently bill. However, this doesn't mean that the tests in a given panel are the only tests that will be ordered. If all of the stated tests in a predefined panel as listed in CPT are not performed, each test must be reported separately.

EXAMPLE

80048, *Basic Metabolic Panel* includes the following tests: calcium, carbon dioxide, chloride, creatinine, glucose, potassium, sodium, and urea nitrogen. If the sodium level was not tested, it would be inappropriate to report this code. Each test must be reported individually in this case.

It is the coder's responsibility to recognize and bill a panel code, even if the physician orders each test individually. This is extremely challenging and can be somewhat time consuming to compare each panel and its associated tests to determine the correct one. As mentioned, physicians may create their own "custom panels" outside of what is designated in CPT; however, the tests should be billed with the existing CPT panel codes and any additional codes to account for all of the tests ordered without overlapping or double billing for labs that are part of other panels. All labs ordered must include documentation to support medical necessity.

EXAMPLE

A primary care physician orders a comprehensive health panel on a 40-year-old male. He considers this panel to include albumin, BUN, electrolytes, LDL, HDL, iron, LFT, SGPT, SGOT, glucose, calcium, protein total, creatinine, bilirubin total, CBC, TSH, and uric acid. How would this be coded? According to CPT, there is no single code that lists all of these tests as a panel. The general health panel lists some of these, as well as the basic metabolic panel, electrolyte, and comprehensive metabolic panels. To bill this battery of tests properly, the coder must look at the available panels in CPT and assign any that do not overlap tests. Any tests that remain would be assigned separate codes. Assign codes 80050, *General Health Panel*, and 83718, 83721, 83540, 84550.

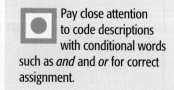

Pay close attention to code descriptions with conditional words such as *and* and *or* for correct assignment.

Read the following scenario and answer the questions.

The lab performs the following tests: total calcium, carbon dioxide, chloride, creatinine, glucose, potassium sodium, and blood urea nitrogen (BUN).

1. Can a panel code be used? If so, which one? _____

2. Is an additional code required? _____

When reading medical documentation, coders should be able to associate lab tests ordered with signs and symptoms and determine for which disease or condition the physician is testing.

Drug Testing

Drug testing or toxicology screening can be performed by sampling urine, blood, hair, saliva, or sweat. CPT lists 18 common drug classes assayed in this section. Some of these classes include alcohol, barbiturates, and amphetamines. Once a drug is detected, the screening test is followed by a confirmation test with a second method. However, drugs tested in this section can be prescription medications or illicit drugs. The most common sample used to perform drug testing is urine. There are four types of testing methods: immunoassay, high-performance liquid chromatography, gas chromatography, and gas chromatography/mass spectrometry.

Qualitative testing refers to tests that detect the presence of a particular analyte, constituent, or condition. (Is it there or not?) A positive result indicates that a drug or metabolite is present. An analyte is a chemical or substance being measured or analyzed. Because this is a screening test, there is a chance that it will detect substances other than the drug for which the urine is being screened, called *interfering substances*.

Quantitative testing provides specific results of numerical amounts of an analyte in a specimen/sample. (How much of the drug is in the patient's system?) Typically, quantitative tests are performed after a qualitative study to identify the specific amount of a particular substance in the sample. Once a drug is detected through the qualitative screening process, confirmation is commonly performed to test for the presence of the specific drug without the interfering substances for a more accurate level. Definitive drug testing may be qualitative, quantitative, or a combination of both for a patient on a given day. Drug confirmation is a repeat of the definitive test to reduce the risk of a false-positive or false-negative result. Confirmation tests can be performed on qualitative and/or quantitative testing.

> If an analyte is measured in more than one specimen from different sources or in specimens that are obtained at different times, assign a code for each source and for each specimen and append the –59 modifier.

> Medicare requires HCPCS codes instead of the 80000 series codes for qualitative presumptive drug testing (G0431 and G0434). Note that the Medicare codes specify "per patient encounter," rather than per procedure or per analyte.

■ CASE SCENARIO

A patient comes to the ED in a coma; the patient reeks of alcohol. The ED physician ordered a drug screen (80306) (multiple class A, one procedure). The presence of barbiturates, opiates, and alcohol was noted. Confirmatory tests for each of these drug classes were run. In this case, there were three drug classes to confirm: 80345, 80361, 80320.

Drug Assay

Drug assay procedures are divided into subsections: Therapeutic Drug Assay, Drug Assay, and Chemistry. Codes are selected based on why the test was ordered and what kinds of test results were obtained. *Assay* means testing drug purity or absorption level of prescribed drugs in the body.

Drugs are routinely assayed first by a presumptive screening method that can be visually interpreted (i.e., dipstick), immediately followed by definitive drug identification. Codes are assigned by the drug class list—single (A *or* B) or multiple (A *and* B)—with or without chromatography. Read the code descriptions carefully because some are reported *per day*, while others are reported *per procedure*. Report codes 80305–80307 for presumptive screening.

Definitive testing identification identifies individual drugs and distinguishes between structural isomers. CPT provides a Definitive Drug Class listing within the Drug Assay section to assist in assigning codes based on the drug being tested and drug class. This listing provides the respective code or code range from which to select the correct code.

Therapeutic Drug Assay

Codes in the Therapeutic Drug Assay section describe the quantitative determination of blood levels of various therapeutic compounds. These tests are performed to help the clinician monitor the best level of medication for the patient or to monitor compliance with a given medication regimen, such as Coumadin (blood thinner) levels. Testing is also performed to evaluate the drug's effect on kidney and liver functioning. Common medications tested for are as follows:

- Antidepressants
- Anticonvulsants
- Antipsychotic medication
- Antiarrhythmic medication for blood thinning

Drugs in this section are referred to by their generic name, not their brand name. For example, if a patient is being treated with Digitek, code 80162 is assigned because this is a brand name for digoxin. Many drugs are separately identified, but this is not an exhaustive list of therapeutic drugs. If a code is not available for the drug being monitored, the unlisted code 80299 is assigned.

Codes for these tests are located in the Index under the main term *drug assay* or by looking up the drug names.

EXAMPLE

A patient is diagnosed with bipolar disorder. Every month, the patient must have his blood drawn to measure his lithium level. Assign code 80178.

CHECKPOINT 28.4

Read the following scenario and answer the question.

1. An elderly patient has been taking digoxin for many years but now appears sleepy all the time. The physician is concerned that the patient is not able to excrete the digoxin and has increased levels in her blood. The patient's blood is drawn and sent to the lab for testing. Report the lab's CPT code for the test. _____

Evocative/Suppression Testing

Tests in the evocative/suppression code range measure how endocrine glands are working, evaluating a patient's endocrine status and the response to certain agents that are intended to stimulate or suppress a particular hormone. The physician will administer agents to evoke or provoke a response or production of analytes or to suppress them. The analyte being measured is something that a person must take as a supplement because his or her body does not produce it. Sometimes, it may be a product that is given to suppress production of a different substance. Each code depicts a panel listing the specific analyte and number of times it must be tested.

EXAMPLE

80430 *Growth hormone suppression panel (glucose administration).* This panel must include the following:

Glucose (82947 x 3).

Human growth hormone (HGH) (83003 x 4).

This code description means that the glucose must be tested three times on blood samples and the HGH four times. The administration of the agent is reported with codes from the Medicine section (96365–96376) and the supply of the agent is reported with a supply code from HCPCS.

Urinalysis

This CPT section is dedicated to tests performed on urine. Urinalysis is commonly performed in physician offices as part of a preventive examination. It is a quick, easy, and inexpensive means of detecting glucose, protein, nitrates, and ketones that are indicative of urinary tract infections, diabetes, and nephritic disease. In the process used to analyze patients' urine, the technician observes the sample and normally notes its specific gravity, opacity, color, and appearance. The code descriptions in this area will identify the method of testing, color of the urine, and volume of urine. Urinalysis can be performed either manually or automatically and with or without microscopy. Automated testing utilizes a machine to analyze the specimen, speeding up the process. Manual testing does not use a machine to conduct the test. Manual urinalysis can be performed by dipstick. The color change occurring on each segment of a dipstick is compared to a color chart. Dipsticks are used to determine the urine's pH (acidity); specific gravity (density); and protein, ketone, nitrite, and glucose content; and the number of WBCs in the urine. Instructional notes at the beginning of this section direct the coder to refer to another section when testing for a specific analyte; for example, 83069, *Hemoglobin; urine.*

Some diseases such as renal disease require monitoring of the volume of urine expelled during a specified time period. This is called a *timed volume measurement.* The time period may only be 2 hours or as much as 24 hours, during which all urine is collected in a special container and a log is kept of each time urination occurred.

Steps for Assigning Urinalysis Codes

1. Determine if the method used for visual color comparison was automated or manual.
2. Determine if microscopic study was performed. Some labs routinely do this as their standard protocol for all urinalysis.
3. If a timed urine collection urinalysis was performed, assign code 81050 for each timed sample.

■ CASE SCENARIO

A 30-year-old female presents for her annual gynecology examination. A medical assistant performs a urinalysis using a dipstick. She compares the colors on the strip to the control colors on the box. The physician also viewed the sample under a microscope. Assign code 81000.

The examples in this section give you the code that depicts the testing done. When you must read and code from a report, however, it is a more difficult task. The key is to know that you are looking for a molecular pathology code. When you look in the CPT Index under *molecular pathology*, it guides you to check "gene testing." You will then look up *gene testing* in the Index, and at that point you will need the test name, such as HTT or ASPA.

Molecular Pathology

The Molecular Pathology (often called *MoPath*) section of CPT contains over 100 codes representing the rapidly evolving field of molecular pathology. This rapid evolution reflects medicine's efforts to understand the molecular basis of disease and the need for knowledge of the basic elements of medical afflictions. Definitions of terms encountered in this field of laboratory testing are given at the beginning of the section. As a result, molecular pathology coding is a two-tier structure categorizing the most commonly performed tests into Tier 1 codes and the lower-volume tests into Tier 2 codes. Molecular pathology procedures are medical laboratory procedures involving the analyses of nucleic acid to detect variants in genes that may be indicative of germline or somatic conditions, or to test for histocompatibility antigens. Code selection is based on the specific gene being analyzed.

When the gene name is represented by an abbreviation such as F5, the full gene name is then italicized in parentheses (*coagulation Factor V*) with some exceptions. The molecular pathology codes include all analytical services performed in the test process; however, any procedures required prior to cell lysis should be reported separately. An example would be microdissection codes 88380 and 88381. If a physician provides only the interpretation and report of the test results, modifier –26 would be added to the molecular pathology code.

The Molecular Pathology Gene Table is located at the beginning of the Pathology and Laboratory chapter of the CPT manual and should be referenced to assist in assigning codes from this subsection. Coders can locate the gene abbreviation or full name within the table and select an appropriate CPT code provided. The Tier 1 section contains 110 codes (81105–81162, 81170–81383) and describes specific gene and genomic procedures. The Tier 2 section contains nine codes (81400–81408) and is used to report molecular pathology procedures that are not specifically described in the Tier 1 section. Tier 2 categorizes services based on the complexity of the methodologies required to perform the tests and the resources. If the specific molecular pathology procedure is not specified in the Tier 1 codes, then coders should refer to the Tier 2 codes. If the specific procedure is not found in either Tier 1 or Tier 2, use the unlisted code 81479.

For Tier 2 codes, CPT guidelines indicate that the codes are arranged by the level of technical resources and interpretive work required. The parenthetical examples given in each code description provide general guidelines used to group procedures for a given level and are not all inclusive.

Any updates to these codes are located at www.ama-assn.org/ama/pub/physician-resources/solutions-managing-your-practice/coding-billing-insurance/cpt/about-cpt

Use of *ie* and *eg* in molecular pathology is very important. Use of *ie* indicates that the term that follows clarifies the intent of the preceding word or phrase. Use of *eg* means that the term that follows represents an example or examples of the preceding word or phrase.

These analysis codes are qualitative unless otherwise noted.

■ CASE SCENARIOS

• A patient of Jewish ancestry is being seen for prenatal care and has not been tested to determine if she carries the mutation for Canavan disease. Her blood sample is submitted to the lab for testing of the two variants in the ASPA gene. The lab would report code 81200 (Tier 1).

• An asymptomatic male patient has a family history of Huntington disease and requests genetic testing. The blood test is submitted for HTT mutation testing. The lab would report 81401 (Tier 2).

CHECKPOINT 28.5

Read the following scenario and answer the question.

A patient presents with fatigue, dyspnea on exertion, and easy bruising. The patient's hemogram shows leukocytosis anomalies. Bone marrow is submitted for NPM1 exon 12 mutation testing.

1. Assign the CPT code and any applicable modifier reported by the lab. _____

Multianalyte Assays With Algorithmic Analyses

Multianalyte assays with algorithmic analyses (MAAAs) are also known as in vitro diagnostic multivariate index assays (IVDMIAs). These tests use the results derived from multiple tests/assays using an algorithmic analysis method to provide a single result in a numeric score, index, or as a probability. For example, code 81500, *Oncology (ovarian), biochemical assays of two proteins (CA-125 and HE4), utilizing serum, with menopausal status, algorithm reported as a risk score,* is used for a qualitative serum test to combine the results of two analytes and the patient's menopausal status to provide a numeric score using an algorithm. The patient presented with symptoms and pain, and a mass was found in the left adnexal area. An ultrasound was done and the physician requested a risk of ovarian malignancy algorithm (ROMA) test to determine how best to proceed with the patient's treatment.

Chemistry

The chemistry code range reports individual chemistry tests that are not performed as part of the automated organ or disease-oriented panels. They can be performed on any body source. Some of the code descriptions, however, do state a specific source. For example, 82040, *Albumin; serum, plasma or whole blood,* states that serum is the source, so this could only be

If the exact test is performed on two different specimens on the same day, use modifier –91.

performed on blood. In contrast, code 82127, *Amino acids; single, qualitative, each specimen,* can be used for any specimen. Calculations in reporting the results are included in the code description. The majority of the tests in this section are considered to be quantitative. Code descriptions in this section state that the amount of an analyte is being measured. When an analyte is measured in multiple specimens from different sources, a –59 modifier is necessary. The analyte is reported separately for each source and for each specimen. This would also apply to specimens obtained at different times.

When reviewing codes from this section, look for a code that describes the specific analyte being analyzed. If a code specific to the analyte is not located, search for a code that describes the methodology used to test such as chromatography.

EXAMPLE

A PA performs a glucose screening by Dextrostix method (reagent strip) using capillary blood. Assign codes 82948, 36416.

Hematology and Coagulation

Tests performed in this section are done on blood and blood components. High-tech equipment is used to count, type, and size blood cells. Hematology—the study of blood—involves counting the cells in blood. Coagulation measures how fast the blood clots. Coagulation testing involves semiautomated and automated techniques. Tests commonly performed in this section are bleeding times, hemograms, blood count, clotting factor analysis, prothrombin time, coagulation time, viscosity, and thromboplastin time. Serology testing is also performed in this section. In serology testing, blood serum is used to test for pregnancy, infectious mononucleosis, and mycoplasma screening. A hemogram includes CBC, differentials, and platelets. A CBC includes white blood cell (WBC), red blood cell (RBC), hemoglobin (Hgb), hematocrit (HCT), mean corpuscular hemoglobin (MCH), mean corpuscular hemoglobin concentrations (MCHC), mean corpuscular volume (MCV), and red cell distribution width (RDW) levels.

A CBC is typically performed with automated equipment. It is routinely ordered to diagnose anemia, polycythemia, and hemolytic disease; monitor the side effects from high-risk drug therapy; and evaluate bone marrow function. It is extremely important that the coder know and understand the parameters of a CBC and be able to verify the validity of a code assigned by the lab. Physician documentation must support the need for laboratory tests.

EXAMPLE

Automated CBC with *automated* differential. The WBC is abnormal and a manual differential is performed to confirm this value. Assign codes 85027, 85007.

The code for a blood marrow smear is located in this section (85097); collection of the bone marrow is reported with a Musculoskeletal section bone-biopsy code.

Immunology

Immunology is the study of the immune system. The immune system is a complex network involving multiple organ systems, such as the blood and lymph systems, whereby bone marrow, white blood cells, lymph nodes, and the skin contribute to the immunity of people. Because the immune system is so broad, encompassing everything from blood cells to skin, immunology is an extensive field of study. Autoimmune disorders are those in which an individual's immune system attacks its own tissues. Rheumatoid arthritis is an example of an autoimmune disease. Immunology codes represent tests performed to measure immunity to specific diseases and the presence of antigens. Antigens are substances that stimulate a reactive response from the body. The response creates antibodies. Antibodies, also called *immunoglobulins,* are actually proteins that are triggered by antigens to neutralize or "flag" foreign bodies such as bacteria and viruses in the body to be destroyed.

Methods for routine immunology testing include the following:

- Particle agglutination
- Complement fixation tests
- Fluorescent antibody tests
- Immunodiffusion

Steps for Assigning Immunology Codes

1. Identify the specific organism or disease related to the test.
2. Determine if the procedure performed was to detect antigens or antibodies.
3. If performed on antibodies, which type and number of antibodies were being tested?
4. Did the test measure multiple antibody subclasses or species?
5. Determine the method used to perform the test.
6. When performing allergen testing, code for each allergen during IgE testing.

■ **CASE SCENARIO**
A patient is experiencing joint pain and a nodule on her right middle finger. The physician orders an antinuclear antibody (ANA) test to rule out rheumatoid arthritis or lupus. Assign code 86038.

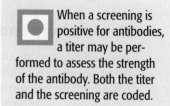 When a screening is positive for antibodies, a titer may be performed to assess the strength of the antibody. Both the titer and the screening are coded.

INTERNET RESOURCE: Visit the Amarillo Medical Specialists webpage to learn how to read laboratory test results. www.amarillomed.com/howto.htm

Transfusion Medicine

Many code descriptions in the transfusion medicine code range are reported per "each technique," "each elution," or "each panel." CPT specifies that each procedure performed in the blood bank must be separately identified. Separate procedures exist for typing blood, screening antibodies, identifying antibodies, and processing blood and blood products. Category III codes may also be used for harvesting, preparing, and injecting platelet rich plasma and white blood cells.

Microbiology

Microbiology covers bacteriology, virology, parasitology, and mycology. Blood, urine, and cerebrospinal fluid (CSF) cultures are performed to determine the type of infection present. Code descriptions include the terms *presumptive* and *definitive identification*. Presumptive identification is identifying or recognizing a microorganism based on the characteristics of growth, colony morphology, and Gram stains; for example, consider code 87081, *Culture, presumptive, pathogenic organisms, screening only*. Definitive identification narrows the classification down to the specific genus or species level by performing additional tests; for example, consider code 87106, *Culture, fungi, definitive identification, each organism; yeast*.

The coder must know several important factors about the specimen, including source, method of handling, identification techniques, and stains performed. Three types of staining techniques are commonly used in microbiology: Gram stains, methylene blue stain, and acid-fast stain. Gram stains are used to stain microorganisms from a culture. Gram-positive organisms, such as *Staphylococcus aureus*, stain purple-black. Gram-negative organisms, such as *Escherichia coli*, stain pink-red. Methylene blue is used when a Gram stain shows increased WBCs but no bacteria. Bacteria will turn blue. Acid-fast stain confirms the presence of mycobacteria, such as tuberculosis. If a specific

■ **CASE SCENARIO**
A patient sustains a superficial wound while hunting. Five days later, the wound appears to be infected and is oozing exudate. The physician orders a C&S of the exudate for anaerobic and aerobic organisms. The sensitivity was conducted by disk method. The lab results showed *Clostridia* with resistance to penicillin G. Assign codes 87070, 87076, 87184.

Some codes indicate screening for the presence of any organism, some are screenings for specific organisms, and others indicate a sensitivity study.

agent is not specified, a general methodology code should be used (87299, 87449, 87450, 87797, 87799, 87899). Once an organism is identified, further testing may be carried out to look for susceptibility to antibiotics to guide the physician in choosing a medicinal treatment. This is called *culture and sensitivity* (C&S) and is ordered by the physician as such.

Steps for Assigning Microbiology Codes

1. Determine if smears were performed on the specimen. If so, assign code for smear (87205–87207).
2. Determine culture source or type. Sources can be blood, urine, stool, sputum, and pus. Culture types include pathogen screening, fungal, bacterium, or viral.
3. Assess whether the culture report was a final diagnosis or a presumptive identification. The lab report will indicate this. If presumptive, assign a code that states presumptive identification.
4. For final or definitive identification, determine if the isolate type was anaerobic or aerobic.
5. Assign codes for any additional studies, including antimicrobial sensitivity studies.

> ◼ If additional tests, such as chromatography or molecular probes, are carried out after the definitive identification is made, code these separately.

> ◼ Medicare requires submission of HCPCS codes for papanicolaou (Pap) screening. Code Q0091 is submitted for obtaining and preparing a smear and conveyance to the laboratory. Laboratories would also assign HCPCS codes P3000–P3001 and G0123–G0124, G0141–G0148.

> ◼ Medicare will pay for a Pap smear every 2 years. If a patient is at high risk for cervical or vaginal cancer or is of childbearing age and has had an abnormal Pap in the last 36 months, Medicare will then pay for one smear every 12 months.

Cytopathology

Cytology is the study of individual cells to detect abnormal cells. This method of examination is used extensively to diagnose cancer. Cytology is also used in screening for fetal abnormalities and in diagnosing infectious organisms. Cytopathology services include the examination of cells from fluids, washings, brushings, fine-needle aspiration, needle biopsy, or smears under a microscope but generally exclude hematology. Code assignment depends on the method of screening and examining the slide. Examination of cervical and vaginal smears is the most common service in cytopathology. Cervical and vaginal smears do not require interpretation by a physician unless the results are or appear to be abnormal. In such cases, a physician personally conducts a separate microscopic evaluation to determine the nature of an abnormality. This code range has both professional and technical component services. Code 88141 reports the physician interpretation of a smear and is coded in addition to the technical component. Codes for vaginal or cervical screening are selected based on whether the slides were prepared by the Bethesda or non-Bethesda reporting system. The 2001 Bethesda System is used for reporting results of gynecological specimens. The pathological interpretation is shown between asterisks on the final report. This reporting system has three general categories:

1. Unsatisfactory for evaluation: The smear does not yield diagnostic information. Additional statement(s) will indicate why the specimen is unsatisfactory.
2. Negative for intraepithelial lesion or malignancy: This indicates that the findings are normal.
3. Epithelial cell abnormality: This category is used to indicate that abnormal cells are present.

A report may have comments to describe the severity and type of the abnormality, and at times these may include a recommendation for further action.

Consultations (Clinical Pathology)

> ◼ Codes 88321–88325 are not assigned if a pathologist is providing a second opinion on slides or tissue reviewed by his or her own physician group.

Two types of clinical pathology consultation codes are available in the Clinical Pathology section. As with all consults in CPT, this service must be requested by an attending physician and requires the interpretive judgment of a specialist, in this case, the pathologist. There are times when a physician wants this expertise in reviewing abnormal or complex test results. Test(s) reviewed must be outside the clinically significant normal range before this service is requested. A written report must be prepared by the pathologist and sent to the requesting physician with findings and included in the patient's record. Codes 88321–88325 are used when slides or tissue are obtained and prepared at a different location and sent to a pathologist for a second opinion.

Surgical Pathology

Surgical pathology codes report tests conducted on specimens—biopsies, abnormal tissue, growths, fluids, or organs—submitted from the operating room. Physician pathologists examine the tissue specimens to help diagnose a disease and determine a treatment plan. Surgical pathology codes do not include autopsies, which are not covered by Medicare. Specimens are placed in containers and sent to the pathology department for examination and analysis.

Surgical pathology services include accession, macroscopic (gross) and microscopic examination, and reporting. Accession is the recording or pathology registry tracking system where a number is assigned to each specimen that is received and examined. Macroscopic or gross examination is viewing the specimen with the naked eye and making note of color, appearance, size, weight, texture, and so on. Some specimens can be diagnosed adequately with the naked eye. Microscopic examination involves slicing the specimen, preparing slides, and viewing the specimen under a microscope. Tissue blocks refer to the specimens for making slides.

Of the six levels of surgical pathology, Level I identifies gross examination of tissue only, and Levels II through VI refer to gross and microscopic examination of tissue. Each level represents a degree of difficulty and interpretation for the physician as well as the type of specimen examination that falls into each level. Level I is the least difficult examination in regard to viewing the external tissue, with Level VI being the most difficult and requiring the greatest physician effort and skill.

Rules for Billing Surgical Pathology Codes

Correct coding follows these rules:

- If several specimens were received in the same container without separate identification, bill only one surgical pathology code.
- If several specimens were received in the same container and were identified separately, bill each specimen separately.
- If several specimen bottles were received, one with, for example, the uterus, one with the right tube and ovary, and another with the left tube and ovary, bill per specimen using applicable codes for each, based on anatomical part.

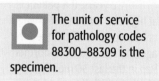

The unit of service for pathology codes 88300–88309 is the specimen.

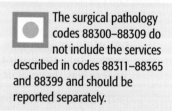

The surgical pathology codes 88300–88309 do not include the services described in codes 88311–88365 and 88399 and should be reported separately.

EXAMPLE

A patient undergoes a septoplasty for chronic nasal obstruction and severe septal deformity. The tissue removed was nasal cartilage. Gross description: specimen is labeled with the patient's name and "nasal cartilage" and consists of multiple fragments of tan tissue. Fragments of bone are also noted. Gross diagnosis: nasal septum. Microscopic diagnosis: nasal cartilage and bone.

How is this coded? First, the coder looks up pathology in the CPT Index. The coder knows there was a gross and a microscopic examination, but not at which level. Because of this, the coder skips Level I and begins at 88302 (Level II). Which kind of specimen was it? It was nasal cartilage. The coder keeps reading through the levels until the tissue type is found.

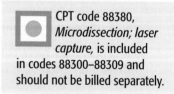

CPT code 88380, *Microdissection; laser capture,* is included in codes 88300–88309 and should not be billed separately.

Code 88304 is assigned because it lists bone fragments and cartilage. The pathologist would report 88304–26 for the service and the facility would report 88304–TC.

EXAMPLE

A physician removes two ulcerated skin lesions: one from the right ear and the other from the back of the neck. Each lesion was labeled and separately contained and sent to pathology. Code 88305 is coded

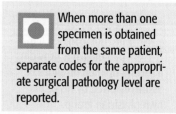

When more than one specimen is obtained from the same patient, separate codes for the appropriate surgical pathology level are reported.

twice with a −59 modifier on the second code because each sample required separate examination and was labeled individually. Assign codes 88305, 88305−59.

If gross and microscopic examinations are performed on *separate* specimens, report the second pathology code with a −59 modifier.

CHECKPOINT 28.6

Read the following scenario and answer the question.

A specimen of a portion of the lung from a left lower segmental resection is sent for gross and microscopic examination.

1. Assign the CPT code and any applicable modifier reported by the lab. _____

Pathology Report

Every specimen sent to the pathology department for examination requires a written pathology report (Box 28.1). This report is used to determine the level of pathological examination performed. The pathological diagnosis is most important to surgeons and patients. The diagnosis provided by the pathologist from a surgical biopsy or removal of tissue can change the course of a patient's treatment.

BOX 28.1 Sample Pathology Report

Department of Pathology
Surgical Pathology Report

Patient Name: Nobody, Sue   **DOB**: 11/15/59   **Sex**: Female
Collection Date: 10/25/--   **Location**: ASU/A228-A   **Hospital Number**: 007811234
Surgeon: Cutter, Barry   **ACC#**: 268-9682

Clinical Information: Enlarged fibroid uterus, pelvic pain, menometrorrhagia

Gross Description: The specimen is received in formalin, labeled with the patient's name and designated "uterus." The specimen consists of an aggregate of tan tissue with foci of white nodules weighing 124 gm and measuring 15 x 15 x 4 cm, consistent with uterine fundus and leiomyomata. The serosa is smooth and glistening. The endometrium is tan and has average thickness of less than 1 mm.

Microscopic Description: Sections of the myometrium demonstrate no additional abnormalities. Representative sections of the specimen are submitted.

Summary of Sections:
1. Endometrium
2. White whorled nodule
3. Five myometrium and serosa

Pathological Diagnosis:
1. Proliferative endometrium with no specific histopathology
2. Leiomyomata

Sophie C. Miler, MD
Sophie C. Miler

Electronically signed Oct 27, 20-- 4:45 p.m.

SCM/jw
10/25/--

Frozen Section

Frozen section evaluation is available to surgeons intraoperatively. At times, surgeons must know if surgical margins are clear after removing a tumor before ending the procedure, or they may discover something unexpected and need biopsy results to determine the course of the surgical procedure. The surgeon removes a sample of tissue and sends it to the pathology department. The pathologist freezes the tissue in a cryostat machine, cuts it with a microtome, and then stains it with various dyes so that it can be examined under the microscope. The reason for requesting a frozen section is that it can be processed very quickly, which is necessary because the patient is in the operating room (OR) under anesthesia. Results are obtained in approximately 10 minutes. Obtaining results while the patient is still in the OR can prevent the need for a second surgery. Frozen sections and permanent sections are coded separately.

For coding purposes, CPT provides codes 88329–88332 for the intraoperative pathology consultations. Code 88329 is gross examination, eyes only, no frozen sections are performed. Codes 88331 and +88332 represent the services of freezing the tissue and examining it and are based on the number of blocks that are examined from each individual specimen. To correctly code these services, it is important to understand the terms *block* and *section*. Once the specimen is received by the surgical pathologist, it is frozen and blocks of tissues are taken from the specimen. A section is a thin slice of tissue taken from the block for examination.

When the first block of tissue from a specimen is examined, report code 88331. When more blocks are taken from the same specimen, report add-on code 88332 for each additional block. If an additional specimen is sent from the OR and frozen sections are done on the second specimen, the same coding process is followed, but modifier –59 must be added to show that the second set of services is separate and distinct from the original or first specimen sent from the operating room.

EXAMPLE

A portion of lung tissue is removed from a patient intraoperatively and a pathology consultation is requested with frozen sections to be performed. The pathologist examines three blocks of tissue from the original specimen. Report 88331, +88332 x 2. Because the pathology findings indicate that there may be additional metastasis in other areas, a second specimen is sent from the operating room and the pathologist examines two blocks from the second specimen. Report 88331–59, +88332–59 for the work done on the second specimen.

Proprietary Laboratory Analyses

New for 2018 are alpha-numeric CPT codes assigned to Proprietary Laboratory Analyses (PLA) tests that are developed and branded by laboratories and manufacturers. These tests consist of advanced diagnostic lab tests (ADLTs) and clinical diagnostic laboratory tests (CDLTs) such as multianalyte assays with algorithmic analyses (MAAA) and genomic sequencing procedures (GSP). The tests are given a special code within CPT that includes a designated label to identify the particular laboratory or manufacturer.

EXAMPLE

0001U Red blood cell antigen typing, DNA, human erythrocyte antigen gene analysis of 35 antigens from 11 blood groups, utilizing whole blood, common RBC alleles reported.

The tests located within this section are defined by the Protecting Access to Medicare Act (PAMA) of 2014. Laboratories must apply with the AMA to obtain a PLA code. PAMA, in part, changes the way Medicare pays for clinical laboratory tests to more closely align the reimbursements with market rates. The act requires the reporting of private sector payment rates for advanced diagnostic laboratory tests to establish Medicare payment rates. This act also invokes special rules for payment for new tests. Specifically, it requires the Department of Health and Human Services to consult with an outside expert advisory panel of molecular pathologists, researchers, and experts on health economics to provide input on establishing payment rates.

AMA publishes on their website additional information about these tests, the application process, and long descriptions of these tests with the corresponding laboratory that submitted the test: www.ama-assn.org/practice-management/cpt-pla-codes.

Assigning Pathology and Laboratory Codes

For laboratory coding, follow the steps in Pinpoint the Code 28.1 to assign procedure codes.

■ CASE SCENARIO

A company required an employee to have a random drug test (screening) performed as part of his drug rehabilitation program. He is a recovering crack cocaine addict. When he arrived at the lab, he submitted a urine sample. A qualitative drug test was performed. Which code would the lab report?

1. What test was performed? Drug screening

2. Which specimen or substance was being tested for? Cocaine in a urine sample

3. Which method of testing was conducted? Qualitative drug test

4. Which words can be located in the Index? "Drug" or "screening" or "cocaine"

5. Was testing done offsite from where the sample was obtained? No

6. What code should be assigned? 80305

PINPOINT THE CODE 28.1: Laboratory

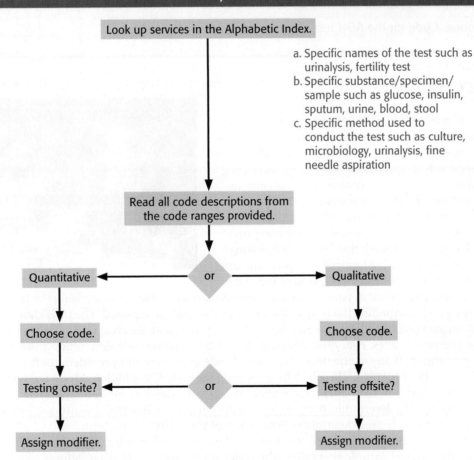

Look up services in the Alphabetic Index.

a. Specific names of the test such as urinalysis, fertility test
b. Specific substance/specimen/ sample such as glucose, insulin, sputum, urine, blood, stool
c. Specific method used to conduct the test such as culture, microbiology, urinalysis, fine needle aspiration

Read all code descriptions from the code ranges provided.

Quantitative — or — Qualitative

Choose code. — Choose code.

Testing onsite? — or — Testing offsite?

Assign modifier. — Assign modifier.

Assign codes to the following procedures. Include any necessary modifiers.

1. hCG, quantitative _____

2. Cholesterol, HDL, triglycerides, LDL _____

3. Rubella screen (antibody testing) _____

4. Cryopreservation of five cell lines _____

5. HGH antibody _____

6. Comprehensive clinical pathology consultation with history and record review _____

7. Mandated alcohol screen (single drug class) _____

8. A cardiologist suspects a blockage in the coronary arteries and needs to do a cardiac catheterization. One test that the hospital will need both before and after surgery is the test that shows how long it takes for the blood to clot (bleeding time). Code for this test. _____

9. After his most recent chemotherapy treatment, a patient was quite weakened. His oncologist ordered a complete CBC, automated. _____

10. A patient with chronic edema, despite years of treatment with diuretics, is considered to have a pituitary gland problem that may be secreting excessive amounts of vasopressin, an antidiuretic hormone. Code for the ADH test. _____

Chapter Summary

1. Codes in the Pathology and Laboratory section are broken into component parts. The technical component encompasses the allocation of staff and/or technologists, use of equipment, processing/developing the film, injection of the contrast material, and related pre- and postinjection services. The professional component encompasses the physician's time and skill in reading and interpreting the test and providing a written report rendering his or her opinion, advice, or assessment of findings. The predominant issue is modifier –26 versus –TC. Most of the codes 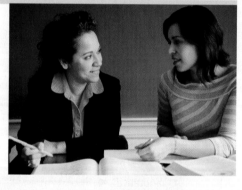 are considered technical in nature, but if a physician is responsible for supervising the test and reviewing and interpreting the results, then two services will be reported. The physician will report the code with modifier –26 and the lab facility will report the code with modifier –TC.

2. To use the panel codes, every test designated within the panel code description must have been performed. If any of the designated panel code tests were not provided, then the panel code cannot be reported and each individual test is reported. If additional tests were done other than what is in the panel code, each of those tests may be reported separately.

3. Qualitative testing determines the presence or absence of an analyte, constituent, or condition. Quantitative testing determines how much of the analyte is present.

4. In molecular pathology, codes are selected based on the particular gene being analyzed.

5. To code for surgical pathology services, the coder must understand what defines a specimen. Based on that description, the coder will know if one, two, or more codes are needed to complete the surgical pathology service. A specimen is defined as tissue or tissues that are specifically designated for individual attention. It may be that they are placed into separate containers or that the tissue itself requires a different level of surgical pathology service from any other specimen submitted at the same time.

6. There are two types of pathology consultation codes: clinical pathology and surgical pathology. The clinical consultation reflects an opinion requested by another physician or healthcare professional on a test that requires additional medical judgment. It is not a physical specimen submitted to a pathologist but a test result that needs more interpretation. The surgical pathology consultation also reflects an opinion requested by another physician (surgeon) regarding a physical specimen obtained by a surgical procedure.

Review Questions

Matching

Match the key terms with their definitions.

A. analyte
B. antibody
C. antigen
D. assay
E. block

F. coagulation
G. gross examination
H. panel code
I. qualitative
J. quantitative

1. _____ Portion of frozen tissue from a specimen

2. _____ Substance that causes a reaction in the body

3. _____ Measurement of how much of a substance is present in the body

4. _____ A substance that is being measured or analyzed

5. _____ One code that represents a group of tests

6. _____ Measurement of whether a substance is present in the body

7. _____ Pathology examination with eyes only

8. _____ A measurement of how fast the blood will clot

9. _____ Analysis of a substance in the body

10. _____ The body's response to an antigen

True or False

Decide whether each statement is true or false.

1. _____ Unlisted procedure codes are listed under their specific subsections.

2. _____ The –26 modifier reports the professional and technical component of a procedure.

3. _____ Multiple procedures that are rendered on the same date should be reported as separate entries.

4. _____ When a panel code is reported and an additional test not listed in the panel code is performed, the test should be reported separately in addition to the panel code.

5. _____ Pathology and laboratory services are provided by a physician only.

6. _____ The codes in the Surgical Pathology subsection represent levels of difficulty of the particular specimen examined.

7. _____ A physician office with an in-house lab draws blood and performs a TSH. The physician would report code 84443 and no other code.

8. _____ The organ and disease panels located in CPT are clinical parameters for such.

9. _____ Confirmation of a drug assay is only coded once per drug class per procedure.

10. _____ Surgical pathologists do not ever examine people but rather specimens obtained from people.

Multiple Choice

Select the letter that best completes the statement or answers the question.

1. Your lab offers a hepatic function panel with the following components: albumin, bilirubin (total and direct), alkaline phosphatase, total protein, SGOT, SGPT, and GGT. Which code(s) should be reported?
   A. 80076
   B. 80076, 82977
   C. Code each test separately
   D. 80076–52

2. Code a nonautomated microscopic examination of urine by dipstick performed in a doctor's office. A CLIA waiver is on file.
   A. 81000
   B. 81000–26
   C. 81002
   D. 81025

3. The source of the specimen for a chemistry test coded to 82000 through 84999 is
   A. Urine
   B. Blood
   C. Sputum
   D. Any source

4. Code for a glucose tolerance test, four specimens taken.
   A. +82952
   B. 82951
   C. 82950
   D. 82951, +82952

5. A patient is being tested for the presence of cocaine in his system. The lab used the single drug class procedure and also confirmed its findings. What code(s) would the lab report?
   A. 80305
   B. 80305, 80353
   C. 80353
   D. 82542

6. A urine pregnancy test was performed in the office using Hybritech ICON (visual color comparison). Which code(s) should be reported?
   A. 84703
   B. 81025, 36415
   C. 84702
   D. 81025

7. Which code should be reported for a stool culture for salmonella?
   A. 87102
   B. 87046
   C. 87045
   D. 86768

8. Which code should be reported for a Pap smear, screening by automated system with manual rescreening under physician supervision?
   A. 88166
   B. 88153
   C. 88175
   D. 88148

9. Which code should be reported for a pathological gross and microscopic examination of the entire left testicle?
   A. 88302
   B. 88304
   C. 88305
   D. 88307

10. Which code should be reported for a pathology consultation in which the physician reviews complete medical records and provides a written report?
    A. 88355
    B. 80500
    C. 88321
    D. 80502

CHAPTER 29

CPT: Medicine Codes

CHAPTER OUTLINE

Immune Globulin Administration and Products

Immunization Administration for Vaccines/Toxoids

Psychiatry

Dialysis

Gastroenterology

Ophthalmology

Special Otorhinolaryngologic Services

Cardiovascular

Pulmonary

Allergy and Clinical Immunology

Neurology and Neuromuscular Procedures

Medical Genetics and Genetic Counseling Services

Health and Behavior Assessment/Intervention

Hydration, Therapeutic, Prophylactic, Diagnostic Injections and Infusions, and Chemotherapy and Other Highly Complex Drug or Highly Complex Biologic Agent Administration

Chemotherapy Administration

Physical Medicine and Rehabilitation

Non–Face-to-Face Services

Special Services, Procedures, and Reports

Moderate (Conscious) Sedation

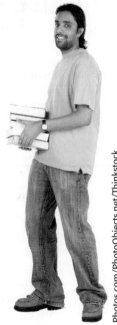
Photos.com/PhotoObjects.net/Thinkstock

LEARNING OUTCOMES

After studying this chapter, you should be able to:
1. Apply conventions specific to administering immunizations and immune globulins.
2. Apply rules for therapeutic or diagnostic infusion and injection codes.

3. Differentiate between infusion and injection, and properly report these services.
4. Assign ESRD codes based on time factor and physician assessments.
5. Describe cardiography tests and their purposes.
6. Describe the components of cardiac catheterization procedures, and assign codes for them, including appending HCPCS Level II modifiers as appropriate.
7. Describe allergy and clinical immunology services.
8. Differentiate between the electrodiagnostic studies of EEG and EMG.
9. Discuss the chemotherapy administration codes and circumstances in which additional codes are appropriate to reflect services provided.
10. Describe the rules for coding and reporting assessment and management services on the telephone and Internet by nonphysician staff members.

The Medicine section of CPT includes codes for noninvasive or minimally invasive (primarily percutaneous access) services that are not considered surgical, evaluation and management (E/M), pathology, laboratory, or radiology services. These codes are reported for a variety of specialty procedures and services.

This CPT section is unique in that it includes codes for services that are primarily evaluative and diagnostic in nature, but therapeutic procedures are also located here. Many of the Medicine CPT codes are specialty specific such as psychiatry, neurology, oncology, cardiovascular and ophthalmology codes, Many are associated with primary care practices that provide services and treatments to patients with a variety of medical problems. Family practice physicians, internists, pediatricians, and general practitioners are primary care providers. In some cases, services listed in this section are performed in conjunction with or adjunct to services or procedures listed in other sections of CPT.

The Medicine section is divided into 34 subsections, as shown in Table 29.1. Many include specific guidelines. These special instructions precede the procedural listings and refer specifically to the subsection. Unlisted procedure code numbers for the individual subsections are shown.

IMMUNE GLOBULIN ADMINISTRATION AND PRODUCTS

Immune globulin is medication provided to a patient who has been exposed to a disease to which he or she is known to have no immunity. Also referred to as *gamma globulin* or *immune sera*, its purpose is to provide immediate, short-term protection or to prevent the patient from becoming ill. Immune globulins consist of antibodies that have been manufactured by another person in response to the disease. It is obtained from the infected person's blood and injected into the patient. Immune globulin can provide immediate protection if given within 3 to 4 days of exposure to an illness.

The codes in this subsection represent broad-spectrum and anti-infective immune globulins, antitoxins, and various isoantibodies. They represent the immune globulin products only and must be reported in addition to administration codes 96365–96368, 96372, 96374, and 96375, as well as E/M codes to account for evaluation of patients and decisions to perform injections. The codes in this subsection are modifier –51 exempt.

> ■ CASE SCENARIO
> An established patient is seen in the office for an exam, and the physician sees that the patient needs an updated injection of the hepatitis B immune globulin. The patient is injected with the hepatitis B immune globulin intramuscularly. Report code 90731 for the immune globulin and code 96372 for the injection.

Table 29.1 CPT Medicine Subsections

SUBSECTION	CODE RANGE
Immune Globulins, Serum, or Recombinant Products	90281–90399
Immunization Administration for Vaccines/Toxoids	90460–90474
Vaccines, Toxoids	90476–90749
Psychiatry	90785-90899
Biofeedback	90901–90911
Dialysis	90935-90999
Gastroenterology	91010–91299
Ophthalmology	92002–92499
Special Otorhinolaryngologic Services	92502–92700
Cardiovascular	92920–93799
Noninvasive Vascular Diagnostic Studies	93880–93998
Pulmonary	94002–94799
Allergy and Clinical Immunology	95004–95199
Endocrinology	95249–95251
Neurology and Neuromuscular Procedures	95782–96020
Medical Genetics and Genetic Counseling Services	96040
Central Nervous System Assessments/Tests	96101–96127
Health and Behavior Assessment/Intervention	96150–96161
Hydration, Therapeutic, Prophylactic, Diagnostic Injections and Infusions, and Chemotherapy and Other Highly Complex Drug or Highly Complex Biologic Agent Administration	96360–96549
Photodynamic Therapy	96567–96574
Special Dermatological Procedures	96900–96999
Physical Medicine and Rehabilitation	97010–97799
Medical Nutrition Therapy	97802–97804
Acupuncture	97810–97814
Osteopathic Manipulative Treatment	98925–98929
Chiropractic Manipulative Treatment	98940–98943
Education and Training for Patient Self-Management	98960–98962
Non–Face-to-Face Nonphysician Services	98966–98969
Special Services, Procedures, and Reports	99000–99091
Qualifying Circumstances for Anesthesia	99100–99140
Moderate (Conscious) Sedation	99151–99157
Other Services and Procedures	99170–99199
Home Health Procedures/Services	99500–99602
Medication Therapy Management Services	99605–99607

IMMUNIZATION ADMINISTRATION FOR VACCINES/TOXOIDS

Immunization, or vaccination, helps the body develop protection against certain diseases. It involves administering a small amount of antigen prior to the patient's exposure to the disease so that antibodies will be produced. An antigen is a substance considered foreign to the body, and as a result of its presence, the body forms antibodies to protect the body from that substance.

Immunization codes include administrative staff services such as scheduling and registration as well as clinical services, including taking vital signs, giving the vaccine, and completing the record. Two codes are reported: one for the substance injected and the other for the actual administration of the injection (Table 29.2). Vaccines can be administered orally, intranasally, or by injection. The administration codes are further broken down by whether counseling has been provided along with the administration. For example, many parents have expressed concern over the side effects of vaccination, particularly in regard to autism. Physicians have found themselves in the position of discussing the pros and cons of vaccination with the parents and/or patient to allay these fears. When counseling is provided, specific codes should be reported for the administration service—90460 and +90461—and they are applicable through 18 years of age and represent any route of administration.

> Vaccines for hepatitis B and *Haemophilus influenzae* type b (Hib) can be purchased separately or combined. When combined, the vaccine is coded as 90748. When purchased separately, the hepatitis B vaccine is coded as 90740, 90743, 90744, 90746, or 90747 (depending on the patient's age and circumstances), and the Hib vaccine is coded as 90647 or 90648. The vaccine code is reported in addition to codes 90471 and +90472 to capture the administration of the injection.

Table 29.2 Examples of Vaccine and Administration Codes (Same patient, same session)

VACCINE	ROUTE	VACCINE CODE	ADMINISTRATION CODE
PCV13 w/counseling	IM	90670	90460
Rotavirus, two-dose	Oral	90681	+90474
DTaP	IM	90700	+90461

Additionally, the counseling administration codes represent the components of each vaccine/toxoid administered. Many vaccine/toxoid codes combine several different components. One example is the DTaP code 90700. DTaP represents diphtheria (D), tetanus (T), and acellular pertussis (aP)—three components. If a physician or other qualified health-care professional (QHP) counsels the patient/family on all three components, then the service would be coded as 90700, 90460, and +90461 ×2 to capture the vaccine/toxoid product and the administration and counseling for the three components of DTaP.

If the administration method is not associated with counseling, then coders will report code range 90471–90474 based on the method of administration and the number of vaccines, whether single or in combination. The vaccine administration code selected must correlate with the mode of administration in the vaccine toxoid code descriptor. For example, 90473, *Immunization administration by intranasal or oral route,* is only reported with vaccine substances that can be administered orally or intranasally. Using the example of DTaP administered by one intramuscular injection, the service would be reported by codes 90700, 90471, because one injection incorporated all three vaccines. If the patient had received one injection of DTaP and another injection of the mumps vaccine, the codes would be 90700, 90704, 90471, +90472. Nurse visits are common in situations where the patient is only being seen for an injection and not seeing a physician. In this case, the immunization administration code (injection codes 90471–90474) along with the vaccine (substance injected) is reported.

Medicare has different requirements from commercial carriers for reporting certain immunizations. HCPCS G codes are reported for the vaccine administration instead of the Medicine section administration codes when the hepatitis B, influenza, and pneumococcal vaccines are administered to Medicare recipients. A second code is reported for the vaccine product. Information regarding how to code and report vaccines and immunizations to Medicare are available on the Centers for Medicare and Medicaid Services (CMS) website (www.cms.gov).

INTERNET RESOURCE: Visit the CMS website and download a copy of "Quick Reference Information: Medicare Immunization Billing." Go to www.cms.gov and type "immunization billing" into the search box.

> Read the code descriptions carefully. Some immunization codes are assigned based on the age of the patient and the route of administration. For example, the following two codes describe vaccines but for different age groups:
>
> 90732, *Pneumococcal polysaccharide vaccine, 23-valent, adult or immunosuppressed patient dosage, when administered to individuals 2 years or older, for subcutaneous or intramuscular (IM) use*
>
> 90644, *Meningococcal conjugate, vaccine, 4 dose schedule, when administered to children 6 weeks-18 months of age, for intramuscular use*

■ CASE SCENARIO

A 5-year-old child is seen by a pediatrician for a preventive medicine visit. During that visit, the child receives DTaP, measles-mumps-rubella (MMR), polio (IPV), and varicella immunizations. The administration methods are intramuscular and subcutaneous. The Medicine codes are reported for the immunizations, and an E/M code is reported for the office visit, resulting in codes 99393 for the preventive medicine visit, 90471, +90472 × 3, 90700, 90707, 90713, 90716.

When reporting multiple vaccines administered at a given episode of care, only one initial administration code is reported, followed by the appropriate add-on codes for each additional vaccine. It is an error to report more than one single/first/initial immunization administration per encounter.

■ CASE SCENARIO

A 2-month-old infant is seen by the doctor, and the mother is counseled regarding side effects and immunization schedule. The baby receives the DTaP intramuscular, the rotavirus (two-dose series) oral, and pneumococcal conjugate (PCV13) vaccines intramuscular. Report 90640, +90641, +90474.

> If a provider administers a vaccine that is supplied by the state at no cost to the provider and the patient is uninsured or underinsured, the –SL HCPCS modifier (state-supplied vaccine) is appended to the vaccine code (Medicine section 90000 or HCPCS code) with no charge for the vaccine supply. Each state's immunization program is available online with a list of vaccines that are supplied by the state.

Symbols

The Medicine section utilizes the lightning bolt symbol, which is not often seen throughout the CPT manual. The coder should take special note before assigning codes.

The lightning bolt symbol (⚡) represents vaccine products that have not yet received approval by the U.S. Food and Drug Administration (FDA). Codes designated with this symbol will be tracked by the American Medical Association (AMA) to monitor FDA approval status. When the FDA approval is obtained, the symbol will be removed. The most up-to-date information on codes with this symbol can be obtained on the AMA website as indicated in CPT guidelines for vaccines and toxoids.

Multiple Procedures

Multiple procedures that are rendered on the same day are listed in separate entries on the claim form and are represented by modifier –51; however, do not use modifier –51 when a patient sees a physician and also receives a vaccination during a single visit. In such cases, the coder assigns an E/M code for the office visit if the E/M service is significant and separately identifiable from the vaccination, and modifier –25 would be appended to the E/M code. A separate code from the Medicine section would be reported for the vaccination without modifier –51.

PSYCHIATRY

Coders should give specific attention to four main coding areas in the psychiatry section: diagnostic services, interactive complexity, psychotherapy, and psychotherapy for crisis. CPT has emphasized the importance of correct coding in these specific areas, which is addressed here.

Psychiatry coding represents diagnostic services, psychotherapy, and other services provided to a patient, family, or group. Some patients will require a specific type of diagnostic or psychotherapy treatment referred to as *interactive* and some will require crisis treatment. The psychiatry codes are relevant to all settings of care; no distinction is made for place of service (office versus hospital, for example). Some psychiatry codes should be reported with E/M codes based on the services provided during that episode of care; at other times, the provider should report only an E/M code. For example, if a consultation is provided by a psychiatrist or other QHP, that provider will report the E/M consultation codes 99241–99255. These codes are based on office/outpatient versus inpatient place of service. At times, the psychiatrist or other QHP will report initial or subsequent hospital care codes 99221–99233. Documentation must be carefully reviewed to determine if the service provided should be E/M or psychiatry coding.

Psychiatric Diagnostic Procedures

The diagnostic services are the patient assessments including history, mental status, and recommendations. The assessment includes communication with the patient's family or other sources and review and ordering of diagnostic studies. There are two CPT codes for this area of psychiatry coding: 90791 and 90792. These two codes differentiate between diagnostic services provided *without* medical services (90791) and *with* medical services (90792). Code 90791 does not include E/M services, but it does include history, mental status, review and/or ordering of studies, and recommendations, and it is typically reported by mental health professionals not licensed to perform E/M services. Code 90792 includes all components of 90791 *in addition to* a physical exam (psychiatric specialty exam), prescription of medications, and ordering lab tests as needed. Medical services may consist of any medical activities such as performing elements of a physical exam or considering writing a prescription or modifying psychiatric treatment based on medical comorbidities.

> CPT guidelines say it is an error to report psychotherapy services on the same date of service as 90791 or 90792.

Interactive Complexity

Under specified circumstances, the add-on code 90785 will be reported in addition to the psychiatric diagnostic codes and the psychotherapy

An adult with comorbid medical conditions is anxious, irritable, and cannot sleep. The patient takes antidepressant medication but continues to be depressed and cannot work. The psychiatrist obtains a psychiatric history, a history of present illness, past medical history, and past family and social history. After examining the patient the psychiatrist modifies the patient's psychiatric treatment based on his medical comorbidities. The psychiatrist arranges for other tests and evaluations, and a treatment plan is developed. Report code 90792.

codes to reflect any communication difficulties the patient may have that complicate the delivery of care. CPT guidelines state that this code cannot be reported alone and must be reported with an E/M code and a psychotherapy code (90833, 90836, 90838, 90853). Some patients are too young to communicate their symptoms or situation, or some patients have lost that ability. The difficulties may also be due to others involved with the patient's care such as emotional family members or caregivers, or there is a language barrier between the provider and the patient. There may also have been a sentinel event that has caused the patient to be unable to communicate.

EXAMPLES

- The patient's parents are present and constantly challenge the provider's interaction with the patient and each other's observations regarding their child. The provider would report 90791 and +90785.

- The provider uses play equipment, other physical devices, and an interpreter or translator to communicate with the patient to overcome barriers to psychotherapy. The interaction between the provider and the patient lasts 45 minutes. The provider would report 90834 and +90785.

Psychotherapy

Psychotherapy is the use of definitive therapeutic communication to alleviate the patient's emotional disturbances, to reverse or change maladaptive patterns of behavior, and to encourage personality growth and development. This process may also include the involvement of family members or others. These are face-to-face services with the patient and may include informant(s), and the patient must be present for all or most of the services. There is a specific code for family psychotherapy without the patient present (90846).

The psychotherapy codes are broken down into those performed without an E/M service and those performed with an E/M service. Codes 90832–90838 offer options to the provider when choosing a psychotherapy code based on two factors: (1) time spent with the patient performing psychotherapy only and (2) psychotherapy performed in conjunction with an E/M service. The add-on codes 90833, 90836, and 90838 represent psychotherapy services based on psychotherapy time when performed with an E/M service. These codes are reported <u>in addition to the applicable E/M code.</u> The E/M codes are based on the three key components of an E/M visit, and the E/M service must be significant and separately identifiable from the psychotherapy service.

To report psychotherapy with E/M services, keep the following in mind:

- First, determine the level of E/M code based on the key components.
- The psychotherapy must be at least 16 minutes or more.
- Time may not be used as the basis of the E/M service.
- The same diagnosis is allowed for both the E/M and psychotherapy services.

The add-on codes in this section are meant to be reported by psychiatrists and should not be reported by providers who are not licensed or not permitted by their scope of practice to report E/M services.

Note that the psychotherapy codes are timed codes and CPT provides a time range for each code. For example, 90832 is a 30-minute code but the time range is from 16–37 minutes. Do not report psychotherapy of less than 16 minutes. Carefully review the time criteria for this range of codes and the parenthetical coding notes associated with each code.

When psychotherapy extends beyond 68 minutes, CPT instructs the coder to report prolonged service codes (99354–99357).

When reporting the interactive complexity services (+90785) with psychotherapy, the additional time spent due to the interactive complexity should be included in the timed psychotherapy code. For example, the provider spent 10 minutes working with the patient and then realized the communication difficulty would require an interactive component, so an additional 35 minutes were spent for the interactive complexity of the visit. Report codes 90834 and +90785 reflecting 45 minutes of psychotherapy including interactive complexity.

> The time associated with the add-on codes for psychotherapy should not be added to the time associated with the E/M service. They are two separate services.

Psychotherapy for Crisis

The psychotherapy in crisis codes (90839, +90840) are used when a patient in a crisis state requires an urgent assessment. The assessment includes a history of the crisis state, a mental status exam, and a disposition. The presenting problem is usually life threatening or complex and requires immediate, urgent attention. The provider will perform psychotherapy, mobilizing resources to defuse the crisis and to restore safety. If time spent for crisis psychotherapy is less than 30 minutes, codes 90832 or 90833 should be reported instead of 90839, +90840.

The time associated with the crisis state codes is face to face with the patient and/or family even if the time spent on that date is not continuous. The time reported must represent the provider's full attention, and there should be no services provided to other patients during that time. Code 90839 is a 60-minute code representing the first 30 to 74 minutes on a given date. Do not report this code if less than 30 minutes were spent. If less than 30 minutes were spent, report the psychotherapy code 90832. Report +90833 if an E/M service was also provided.

> **■ CASE SCENARIO**
> A 45-year-old woman who has been in therapy for 7 years due to depression indicates she has an imminent plan for committing suicide. The provider assesses the patient's depression and the level of risk and contacts a family member. The provider discusses what has happened to bring on this situation, and a safety and protection plan is discussed with the patient and family member. The provider would report code 90839.

> Do not report these codes with the diagnostic evaluation codes 90791, 90792, or the psychotherapy codes 90832–90838, 90785–90899.

DIALYSIS

Dialysis is used to manage end-stage renal disease (ESRD), chronic renal failure (CRF), and acute renal failure (ARF). It is used in patients whose kidneys fail to work or fail to adequately remove waste from the blood. In acute renal failure, the patient's kidneys temporarily fail, requiring inpatient dialysis. The kidneys of patients with ESRD and CRF cannot function because of disease and progressive deterioration.

Hemodialysis

The hemodialysis codes (90935, 90937) include the hemodialysis procedure for cleansing the blood (Fig. 29.1) and any associated E/M services. Code 90935 includes one E/M service per day; code 90937 includes any repeated E/M services that are required in one day. CPT will allow the separate reporting of an E/M code if a significant and separately identifiable E/M service is provided on the same day as the dialysis procedure if it is <u>unrelated</u> to the dialysis procedure or to the patient's renal failure *and* it cannot be rendered during the dialysis session. Modifier –25 would be appended to the E/M service under those circumstances.

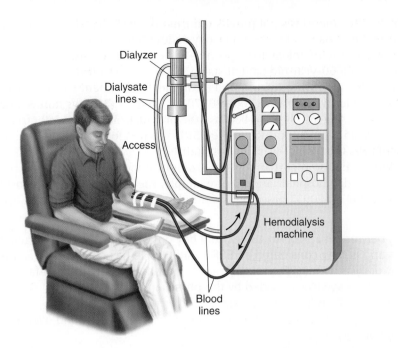

Figure 29.1 Hemodialysis.

Miscellaneous Dialysis Procedures

The miscellaneous dialysis codes (90945, 90947) are for dialysis other than hemodialysis and have the same guidelines as the hemodialysis codes. Other types of dialysis are peritoneal, hemofiltration, or other continuous renal replacement therapies.

End-Stage Renal Disease Services

For patients classified as having ESRD, coding requirements were set up to report the related services provided by physicians. The premise for use of codes 90951–90970 is that a patient is designated as having ESRD and is receiving outpatient dialysis treatment. The physician or other QHP provides management of the dialysis visits, telephone calls, and patient management during a full month or less of dialysis.

Several parameters must be considered when coding for ESRD:

- These are outpatient services.
- The services are divided into per-month codes, per-month codes for home dialysis, and less than a full month of services.
- For coding purposes, every month is considered 30 days.
- The per-month codes are further divided by the patient's age and how many face-to-face visits were provided during that month.
    - First, the coder must find the code that correlates to the patient's age—younger than 2 years through 20 years of age or older (90951–90962).
    - Within the age category, find the number of face-to-face visits that were provided during the month.
    - For patients younger than 2 years through 19 years of age, the code requirements include "monitoring for the adequacy of nutrition, assessment of growth and development, and counseling of parents" per CPT. This requirement is not part of the code range for patients 20 years of age and older.
    - If the patient receives ESRD-related services for home dialysis, then age is the only consideration in the selection of codes (90963–90966).
- In addition, when per-month services are interrupted by hospitalization, travel, recovery, death, or a kidney transplant was provided, the coding is affected by whether or not a complete assessment was performed by the provider during the interrupted month.
    - If a complete assessment was provided during the less-than-full-month period, coders will still use the per-month codes.

- If a complete assessment was not provided during the less-than-full-month period, coders will report the less-than-full-month, per-day codes 90967–90970.
- There is a specific methodology for reporting these per-day codes:
  - For example, if a 60-year-old patient starts ESRD services on August 1, but is then hospitalized for 5 days during August, and a complete assessment was not provided during August, the coder would report code 90970 for 25 days (30 days minus 5 days).
  - It may be confusing at this point because the provider did not actually treat the patient each of those 25 days, but provided the ESRD services for outpatient care during the balance of days the patient was not hospitalized.
  - The provider will also report any hospitalization services provided to the patient during the patient's 5-day hospitalization. For example, the provider would report the hemodialysis codes 90935, 90937 based on the number of evaluations provided each day.

EXAMPLES

- *Code 90958, per-month ESRD:* An 18-year-old boy has suffered from glomerulosclerosis for several years and is now considered an ESRD patient. He has completed his fourth month of outpatient dialysis. During the fourth month, he has had two face-to-face visits by his physician. The ESRD services provided by the physician are as follows:
  - Evaluation of the patient's dialysis access
  - Changing the dialysis prescription based on growth, weight, and fluid overload
  - Review of laboratory results
  - Modifying long- and short-term care plans in relation to social services, school personnel, and overall care coordination
  - Determining dietary supplements needed
  - Counseling parents

(This list is not exhaustive but does represent typical services.)

- *Code 90970 × 18, less-than-full-month, per-day ESRD:* A 60-year-old woman had one kidney removed due to renal cancer 9 years ago. She developed an infection that compromised her remaining kidney and has been on dialysis for 6 months and is considered an ESRD patient. Due to a flare-up of her infection, she was hospitalized for 12 days.

CHECKPOINT 29.2

Assign codes to the following procedures for the physician. Include any necessary modifiers.

1. A nurse sees a patient in the outpatient dialysis clinic for dialysis training. The nurse educates the patient on how to keep the catheter site clean, how to connect and disconnect the dialysis tubing, and what to do in an emergency. The patient completes the course. _____

2. A patient receives hemodialysis in the hospital and is evaluated by her physician for her renal disease, respiratory issues, and chronic leg pain. Can the physician report an E/M service? Explain your answer. _____

GASTROENTEROLOGY

Gastroenterology (GE) codes are assigned when studies are performed to assess the functionality of the stomach or esophagus. Many of these tests require the patient to swallow a capsule or probe to measure movement of these parts or the level of acid in the stomach. For example, tests are performed for the presence of *H. pylori* and for lactase deficiency. Specimens may be taken and sent to the laboratory.

OPHTHALMOLOGY

Ophthalmology services in the Medicine section are broken down into two sections: general and special. The general services are the E/M ophthalmoscopy codes, while the special services are evaluations of parts of the visual system beyond the services included in the general ophthalmological services. In effect, special treatment is given. These special services are reported in addition to the general services.

General Ophthalmology Services

The general ophthalmological services codes 92002–92014 have "new" and "established" designations. They differ from the E/M codes, because they are defined as intermediate and comprehensive and do not require the three key components of history, examination, and medical decision making and do not use the CMS documentation guidelines to determine the proper code selection. Physicians do have a choice of using the E/M codes or the ophthalmology general services codes. In determining which codes are appropriate, consider the E/M codes as an evaluation of the body's systems and the ophthalmology codes as an evaluation of eye function. To further clarify, the general ophthalmological codes are for services provided to new or established patients for medical examinations when those examinations include routine ophthalmic examination techniques such as slit-lamp exam, keratometry, routine ophthalmoscopy, or retinoscopy. Intermediate and comprehensive ophthalmological services constitute integrated services in which medical decision making cannot be separated from the examination techniques. The slit-lamp examination, keratometry, routine ophthalmoscopy, retinoscopy, tonometry, and motor evaluation are not reported separately; they are part of the general services codes 92002–92014.

> ◉ Codes from the E/M section are assigned when the patient is being seen for an ocular injury or as part of a medical examination to monitor a disease with ocular involvement such as diabetes and glaucoma.

EXAMPLE
An established patient is seen and the ophthalmologist does a review of the patient's history, an external examination, ophthalmoscopy, and biomicroscopy for acute iritis. The provider would report code 92012, intermediate general ophthalmological service.

SPECIAL OTORHINOLARYNGOLOGIC SERVICES

> ◉ Pay close attention to the code descriptions in otorhinolaryngology, because many of these codes are inherently bilateral. If the examination was performed on one ear, a –52 modifier is appended.

Much like the Ophthalmology section, the Special Otorhinolaryngologic Services section includes specialized examinations of the ears, nose, and throat (ENT) that are performed in the office or procedure room. Services range from audiology exams, hearing aid checks, and speech-language communication to swallowing studies. A code from 92601–92604 is assigned and may be used many times during the training period after cochlear implantation. Implants must be programmed after they are placed, and the patient must be taught about the sounds generated.

EXAMPLE
Assessment of tinnitus (includes pitch, loudness matching, and masking). Report code 92625.

CARDIOVASCULAR

Cardiovascular services include both diagnostic and therapeutic procedures. Codes 92920–93799 are considered cardiac-related nonsurgical services. Procedures in this section may be performed by a cardiologist or an interventional radiologist. A *cardiologist* is an internal medicine physician who specializes in the diagnosis and treatment of diseases and disorders of the heart and vasculature. Cardiologists are not surgeons; unlike cardiovascular surgeons, they do not perform open procedures on the heart or vessels. *Interventional radiologists* subspecialize in diagnosing and treating diseases of the vasculature using image guidance.

NOTE: Anatomy of the cardiovascular system is presented in Chapter 20 of this text.

Therapeutic Services

Cardioversion

Physicians may elect to perform **cardioversion** after reviewing event monitor recordings in patients who have arrhythmia, particularly atrial fibrillation or flutter, and where medication cannot regulate the heartbeat. Also referred to as *cardiogenic shock*, cardioversion utilizes external defibrillators or paddles to deliver an electrical shock through the chest wall to the heart. This is performed in a controlled hospital setting, and the patient is given a sedative. Electrodes are placed on the patient's chest and back to receive the electricity, and one or more synchronized electric shocks are administered to force the patient's heart back into a normal sinus rhythm. Assign code 92960 for external cardioversion and code 92961 for internal cardioversion. Note that 92961 is a designated separate procedure and would be included in any other major cardiovascular procedure performed during the same session.

> It is not appropriate to report the cardioversion codes for reviewing the telemetry monitor strips taken from a monitoring system.

For example, if the surgeon is doing aortic valve repair (the chest is open, and the heart is exposed) and sees that cardioversion is needed, the only code to be reported is the aortic valve repair code. The cardioversion would be included and not separately reported.

Percutaneous Transluminal Coronary Thrombectomy

Percutaneous transluminal coronary thrombectomy (PTCT) involves excision of a thrombus (blood clot) by inserting a balloon catheter into the vein. The thrombus is either pressed against the walls to restore most of the patency of the artery, or the balloon is passed by the thrombus, inflated, and then carefully backed out of the vein. Thrombectomy is typically performed prior to angioplasty (Fig. 29.2) or stent placement (Fig. 29.3) to remove the blood clot, allowing the angioplasty procedure to be safer and more effective.

> Percutaneous transluminal angioplasty and atherectomy in the same artery as the stenting are not coded separately. However, percutaneous thrombectomy (add-on code 92973), coronary brachytherapy (add-on code 92974), and intravascular ultrasound (add-on codes 92978–92979) are separately reportable. Note the parenthetical instructions listed under these codes indicating which codes to report with the add-on codes.

Percutaneous Coronary Interventions

A percutaneous coronary intervention (PCI) is the placement of a catheter through the skin to treat a blockage within the coronary arteries and/or their branches. The coding for interventions in the coronary arteries to correct blockages has become more and more precise over the years. The CPT guidelines for PCIs are extensive and require careful review. Coders need to understand how CPT categorizes the coronary arteries into "main" and "branch" designations and the coding hierarchy that indicates which services are included in others. Also emphasized in the guidelines are the diagnostic angiography coding rules related to when you can report these services with PCIs and when you cannot. What follows is a review of the PCI guidelines to assist coders with this complex area of coding.

Codes 92920–92944. Coders must know how CPT designates the main coronary arteries: left main (LM), left anterior descending (LD), left circumflex (LC), right coronary artery (RC), and ramus intermedius artery (RI).

You can report PCI in each of these vessels and in up to two branches of the following:

- LD, the branches referred to as the *diagonals*
- LC, the branches referred to as the *marginals*
- RC, the branches referred to as the *posterior descendings* and the *posterolaterals*

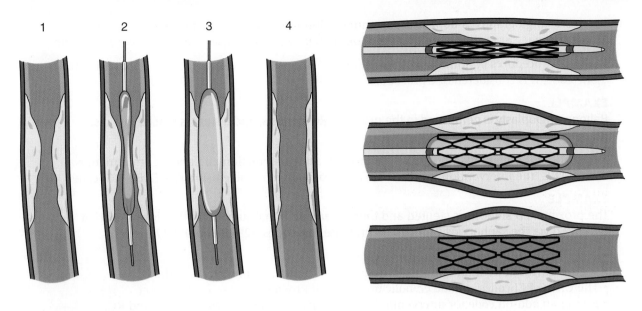

Figure 29.2 Angioplasty.

Figure 29.3 Coronary artery stent.

Percutaneous Revascularization Services

Percutaneous revascularization services may be provided in the following:

- The major coronary arteries
- The coronary artery branches
- Any coronary artery bypass grafts (CABGs), which are considered major coronary arteries for these coding purposes

The less intensive services are included in the more intensive services:

- Stent placement includes atherectomy and balloon angioplasty.
- Atherectomy includes balloon angioplasty.
- The balloon angioplasty intervention can be reported if that is the only intervention being provided.
- Review each code description carefully to determine which type of intervention(s) is being provided.

PCI codes include the following:

- Accessing and selectively catheterizing the vessel
- Traversing the lesion
- Radiological supervision and interpretation (RSI) directly related to the intervention
- Closure of the arteriotomy site
- Imaging done to document the completion of a procedure

Codes 93454–93461 (diagnostic angiography) and injection codes (93563–93564) are not reported with 92920–92944 for the following services: injecting and viewing contrast, road mapping, fluoroscopic guidance; measuring the vessel for the intervention procedure; and doing any intervention angiography after the intervention is completed.

Diagnostic angiography is separately reportable if the following conditions are met:

- There is no prior base angiography study.
- A full study is done at the time of the intervention.
- The decision to do the intervention is based on concurrent angiography, *or*
- A prior study is available but:
  - The patient's condition changed, or
  - There is inadequate visualization, or
  - A clinical change occurs during the intervention that requires a new evaluation outside of the target area.

If diagnostic angiography is done at a separate session it is separately reportable.

Major coronary artery issues include the following:

- All PCI procedures performed within one major coronary artery or branch are reported with one code; it is considered one procedure.

EXAMPLE

Balloon angioplasty is performed in the proximal RC stenosis, and a stent is placed in a distal RC stenosis. Report only 92928.

- Exception: If one intervention is via the normal artery circulation and another treatment is via CABG, the intervention via the CABG is separately reportable using the CABG PCI code.

EXAMPLE

The proximal LD stenosis is stented and there is an additional stenosis in the distal LD but it is stented via the saphenous vein bypass graft. Report codes 92928 and 92937.

- Each CABG is considered a coronary vessel.
- A CABG with more than one anastomosis (rejoining) is still one bypass graft.
- The CABG PCI codes include embolic protection if provided.
- Report an add-on code for interventions in up to two branches of the LD, LC, and RC.

EXAMPLE

A stent is placed in the LC, and angioplasty is performed in two of its branches (the obtuse marginal 1 and 2). Report codes 92928, +92921 × 2.

- Report two interventions when the lesion is at a bifurcation of two vessels.

EXAMPLE

There is a bifurcation lesion at the left anterior descending and the first diagonal. Report codes 92928, +92929.

- If a single lesion extends from one main coronary artery, one of its branches or a CABG into another main coronary artery, one of its branches or a CABG, *and* it is treated with one intervention, report with one code. This is referred to as *bridging*.

EXAMPLE

A left main coronary lesion extends into the left circumflex and a single stent is used to treat the entire lesion. Report code 92928.

- Use 92941 for PCI during an acute myocardial infarction.

EXAMPLES

- A patient presents with a 90% stenosis in the left anterior descending artery, and coronary balloon angioplasty is performed. Report code 92920.

- A patient presents with a 90% stenosis in the left anterior descending artery and 80% stenosis in the first diagonal artery (a branch of the LD). Report both 92920 and +92921.

- A patient presents with 80% stenosis in the right coronary artery. PCI atherectomy and coronary balloon angioplasty are performed. Report code 92924.

- A patient presents with 80% stenosis in the right coronary artery and also has 80% stenosis in the posterior descending artery (a branch of the RC). Atherectomy and balloon angioplasty are performed. Report 92924 and +92925.

- A patient presents with 80% stenosis in the circumflex coronary artery, and after coronary balloon angioplasty a stent is placed. Report code 92928.

- The patient in the previous example also has stenosis in the first obtuse marginal (a branch of the LC). Report 92928 and +92929.

- A patient presents with stenosis in both the left and right coronary arteries and an additional stenosis in the left circumflex artery. Both atherectomy and a stent are provided. Report only code 92933.

Cardiography

The cardiography subsection includes diagnostic tests such as routine electrocardiograms, cardiovascular stress tests, rhythm electrocardiograms, and event monitors worn by patients.

Electrocardiography is a diagnostic procedure that measures and records the heart's electrical activity. An electrocardiogram (ECG or EKG) records the electrical activity of the heart over a period of time and is used to measure and diagnose abnormal heart rhythms and myocardial infarctions (MIs), or heart attacks.

With each heartbeat, an electrical impulse (or wave) moves through the heart, causing the muscle to contract and pump blood through the heart. By performing an ECG and interpreting the results, a doctor can determine how long the electrical wave takes to pass through the heart. The amount of time it takes a wave to move from one part of the heart is indicative of the condition of the heart. For example, if the wave takes too long to travel through the heart, bradycardia may be involved. Measuring the amount of electrical activity can also indicate whether the heart is overworked or if portions are enlarged. This test can identify damaged heart muscle, but it cannot measure the heart's ability to pump blood.

ECGs are commonly performed in the physician office but are also performed in facilities and in ambulances. The choice of a CPT code is based on whether the ECG is routine or has been triggered by an event. Code range 93000–93010 represents the routine ECG services, and the codes break down into the components of the global service. *Global service* in this coding scenario refers to the professional and technical components of an ECG. CPT code 93000 is the global code representing both the professional and technical components of the ECG. This means the physician owns the ECG equipment and interprets and reports the results. Code 93005 is the technical component; it represents the tracing only, without interpretation and report. Code 93010 represents the professional component only. If the provider only interprets and provides the report, code 93010 is assigned.

An ECG is part of the Welcome to Medicare Exam and is reported with a HCPCS G code. If the physician performs the ECG in the office using his or her own equipment and interprets the test, report code G0366 (*Electrocardiogram, routine ECG with at least 12 leads; with interpretation and report, performed as a component of the initial preventive physical examination*) instead of a Medicine code. Code G0367 is reported if the physician provides tracing and no interpretation. The provision of interpretation and report only is reported as code G0368.

■ **CASE SCENARIO**
A patient is seen in the office for a 6-month follow-up visit with his cardiologist. An ECG is performed with interpretation and report. Report code 93000.

Rhythm ECGs are different from routine ECGs in that the patient is currently experiencing symptoms or recently had some type of event, warranting the necessity of an ECG. Instructional notes at the beginning of the cardiography subsection explain that codes 93040–93042 are appropriate to report when an order for the test is present along with documentation of the trigger of the event or reason for the exam. A separate written and signed report by the physician reading and interpreting the ECG or rhythm strips is required. Codes 93040–93042 also break down into the global code 93000, the technical code 93041, and the professional code 93042.

■ **CASE SCENARIO**
A patient went to his primary care doctor's office complaining of intermittent chest pain. The physician performed a rhythm ECG to rule out potential heart attack. He did not read the ECG or produce a report. Code 93041 was reported.

CPT and Medicare require physicians to properly document ECG testing and results in the patient's medical record. Documentation of watching the telemetry screen or stating that the ECG was performed and interpreted is not adequate. According to Medicare, notation in the medical record stating "ECG is normal" is not enough to qualify as a separately payable interpretation service but is instead considered a review of findings that is part of the E/M service. A separate dictated or handwritten entry should address the ECG findings, relevant clinical issues (the need for the ECG or rhythm strip), and comparative data from previous studies. The computer interpretation generated by the ECG machine is also not considered a suitable interpretation and report. All computer-interpreted ECGs must be verified and corrected by the interpreting physician, if necessary, and the physician should sign and date the report to indicate that it was verified. A separate entry should be made in the patient's record indicating that the physician reviewed and agreed with the computer interpretation.

Cardiovascular Monitoring Services

The cardiovascular monitoring services (93224–93278) are also diagnostic and use both in-person and remote technology to assess patients' ECG data. Cardiologists use the data to detect heart arrhythmias. Some cardiac monitors are small, portable ECG machines worn around the clock by patients for a specified period of time. A physician typically prescribes a monitor upon a patient's discharge from the hospital after a myocardial infarction, for a patient with arrhythmia after changing antiarrhythmic medications, or for a patient with intermittent chest pain or syncope that is difficult to diagnose. Such patients wear the monitor and go about their normal daily activities.

Several devices are used for monitoring: Holter monitors (93224–93227), mobile cardiac telemetry (MCT) monitors (93228, 93229), and event monitors (93268–93272). Some monitors require the patient to push a button on the machine when he or she experiences symptoms, while others record continuously. Data are transmitted over the telephone to a central processing unit, which produces a printout of the data for physician interpretation. In general, a patient wears a Holter monitor for only 24 to 48 hours, and the monitor records the entire time the patient is wearing it. Event monitors are worn for extended periods of time to record ECG activity, with the results stored in the devices. Codes 93268–93272 are used to report this service per 30-day period.

Event recorders may also be placed internally and are part of the implantable and wearable cardiac device evaluation services covered later in this chapter. To report the implantation, use code 33282; to report the programming of this device, use code 93285; and to report the interrogation of the device, use code 93291 or 93298.

Implantable and Wearable Cardiac Device Evaluations

The various cardiovascular devices covered previously and in the cardiovascular chapter need programming, reprogramming, and interrogation to assess the device and determine physiological data. Pacemakers, implantable defibrillators, MCT devices, implantable cardiovascular monitors (ICMs), and implantable loop recorders (ILRs) all require these services, which are coded with codes 93279–93299. Programming and interrogations can be done in person or over the telephone.

Echocardiography

Echocardiography (ECHO) is a noninvasive study that uses ultrasound to visualize all four chambers of the heart, all four valves, the great vessels, and the pericardium. It is widely used to study the heart's function, blood flow, and valve movement to diagnose cardiovascular diseases. It can provide information about the heart's size, shape, and pumping capacity; the location and extent of tissue damage; valve function; blood flow patterns; and back flow (regurgitation). The biggest advantage of echocardiography is that it is noninvasive and can be done in the office or facility. ECHO utilizes two-dimensional or Doppler ultrasound.

ECHO is performed transthoracically or transesophageally. In transthoracic echocardiography (TTE), transducers are placed directly on the skin of the chest. Two-dimensional (2-D) echocardiography is performed using multiple transducers or a rotating transducer. The images are recorded either digitally or via videotape. M-mode provides additional detail of the specific

When "attended surveillance" is part of a code description, it refers to the fact that the immediate availability of a remote technician is required when responding to a monitoring device's alert.

The Medicine section, as with many sections of CPT, has many parenthetical notes. Most of the notes instruct the coder not to report a specific code with another code or set of codes. For example, under code 93282 for single-lead transvenous implantable defibrillator programming, the note instructs that the code not be reported with codes 93287, 93289, 93745.

portions of the heart. With M-mode, a stationary ultrasound beam is directed at the area of the heart being studied.

The primary codes for TTE are 93303–93308. Coders should be aware of code 93306, which includes spectral Doppler echocardiography and color-flow Doppler echocardiography. Because of these inclusions, 93306 would not be reported with the add-on codes 93320, 99321, and 99325, which are the codes for spectral and color Dopplers. If neither spectral nor color Dopplers are provided during the TTE, use code 93307. The spectral and color Dopplers provide information on intracardiac blood flow and hemodynamics. CPT further emphasizes in the parenthetical note below 93307 that this code is not to be reported with the add-on codes 93320, 99321, and 99325. If all the services are provided, use code 93306. Also note that code 93303 is specific to patients with congenital cardiac anomalies, and while that may seem to indicate that it is used for children only, that is not the case. Many patients do not discover their congenital anomalies until they are adults.

Carefully review how CPT delineates what a complete transthoracic ultrasound encompasses.

NOTE: At times, identification and measurement of some of these structures may not be possible. When that happens, the provider is to document the reason an element could not be visualized.

A follow-up or limited echocardiographic study (93308) is one that does not evaluate or document the attempt to evaluate all the structures required for the complete transthoracic echocardiogram.

Transthoracic Stress Echocardiography

Transthoracic stress echocardiography (TSE) imaging is recorded using codes 93350, 93351. TSE images are recorded before, after, and sometimes during a cardiac stress test. When a stress echocardiogram is performed with a *complete* cardiovascular stress test, report code 93351 for the stress echocardiogram. A complete cardiovascular stress test includes continuous ECG monitoring with physician supervision, interpretation, and report.

If only the professional components of the stress test are provided by the physician because the test is performed in a facility that provides the technical component, and the same physician provides the professional component of the echocardiogram, report 93351–26 to indicate that only the professional component was provided.

If, in the facility setting, all professional components are not provided by the same physician (e.g., one provides the stress test, the other provides the echocardiogram), use code 93350 with the appropriate stress test codes 93016–93018. Do not report 93350 with the complete stress test code 93015.

Transesophageal echocardiography (TEE) is performed by placing a transducer on the end of an endoscope and inserting it into the patient's esophagus to record 2-D images of the heart and the great arteries. Codes are selected by anatomical site, purpose of the test, and whether the ECHO is complete or limited. There are seven codes for TEE: 93312, 93313, 93314, 93315, 93316, 93317, 93318. Carefully review their descriptions.

Doppler and mapping studies are not separately reportable for screening purposes and must meet medical necessity requirements when reported in addition to the ECHO.

Congenital Anomalies

Again, a caution about considering congenital anomalies as being for children only. Consider the following example: A 57-year-old male with a history of cardiac and respiratory issues undergoes a TEE using pulse wave, continuous wave, and color Doppler. The physician documented a patent foramen ovale (PFO), prolapse of the anterior leaflet of the mitral valve, and mild mitral regurgitation.

A PFO is a small hole located in the atrial septum that is used during fetal circulation. Normally, it closes at birth; however, if it does not close properly, it is called the *patent foramen ovale*. This patient would be considered as having a congenital cardiac anomaly that was not discovered until 57 years of age. The physician will report 93315, +93320, and +93325. The pulsed wave and Doppler color-flow mapping are add-on codes, so coders should report them in addition to the TEE code. The add-on codes are 93320, 93321, 93325.

Diagnoses reported with codes 93307 and 93320 may not meet medical necessity for the color flow. Check Local Coverage Determinations before reporting this procedure in addition to the ECHO.

Cardiac Catheterization

Cardiac catheterization is an invasive diagnostic and therapeutic medical procedure that includes several components. It involves passing a catheter into the heart through a vein or artery, withdrawing samples of blood, measuring pressures within the heart's chambers or great vessels, and injecting contrast media. A cardiac catheterization most often begins as a diagnostic procedure and evolves into a therapeutic one once the cause of the patient's problem has been identified.

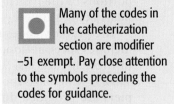 Many of the codes in the catheterization section are modifier –51 exempt. Pay close attention to the symbols preceding the codes for guidance.

Codes are differentiated by whether a professional fee or a technical fee is being submitted. The professional component is reported with a –26 modifier unless the physician owns the catheterization equipment.

Catheter Procedure

The most common catheter entry site is the femoral artery. It is used for left heart catheterizations, aortography, coronary angiography, internal mammary artery injection, vein bypass graft injection, and other left heart procedures and coronary artery interventions. One or more catheters are inserted into the femoral artery in the groin. (The catheter can be inserted into the basilic vein in lieu of the femoral artery if necessary.) From there, the catheter is advanced under x-ray guidance (fluoroscopy) through the aorta with the help of a guidewire to a branch vessel. It reaches the aortic valve, which separates the left ventricle from the arterial system.

Once the catheter crosses this valve, the procedure is officially considered a left heart catheterization. Confirmation that the aortic valve has been crossed includes documentation of left ventriculography performed or mention of intracardiac pressure measurements. If the catheter does not cross this valve, the left heart catheterization codes cannot be reported. When the catheter does not cross the aortic valve, the procedure is considered a limited left heart catheterization because there are no ventriculogram or intracardiac pressure measurements, and a right heart catheterization code is reported instead.

When the catheter is inserted into the heart, a contrast medium is injected into the coronary arteries, which branch off the aorta, to highlight the course of these vessels, and an angiogram is performed. This is done to assess vessel patency (i.e., to assess how open the vessels are). Any coronary blockage or narrowing can be detected. During the catheterization procedure, recordings are made of intracardiac and intravascular pressures; blood samples are obtained for measurement of oxygen saturation or blood gases; and cardiac output measurements are made.

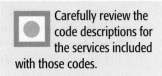 Carefully review the code descriptions for the services included with those codes.

Depending on the findings on the angiogram, an angioplasty, atherectomy, or stent placement may be performed. At the conclusion of the catheterization procedure, the physician removes the catheters that were inserted and stops the bleeding from the catheterization site. Later, a final evaluation of hemodynamic and other data is completed, and a report of the procedure is made.

Coding for Cardiac Catheterizations

CPT does provide a Table of Catheterization Codes to assist with the coding for these services. The codes are either for congenital heart disease or noncongenital heart disease. The two types are never reported together.

EXAMPLES
- A left heart catheterization is performed percutaneously with dye injection and visualization of venous bypass grafts, the left ventricle, and coronary angiography. Radiological supervision and interpretation are also provided. You cannot report 93452 with the coronary angiography code 93454. Go to the indented codes under 93454 to find the code that has coronary angiography, RSI, left ventriculography, bypass graft angiography, and the LHC. Report code 93459. All services are captured by that one code.

- A left and right heart catheterization is performed percutaneously with dye injection and visualization of right and left ventricles, pulmonary angiography, and selective coronary angiography. Radiological supervision and interpretation are also provided. There is no one code that incorporates all these services. The primary code is 93460, which represents the coronary angiography, RSI, right and left heart catheterizations, and left ventriculography. The services not represented within this code are the right ventriculography and the pulmonary angiography. Those are add-on codes 93566 and 93568.

Cardiac Catheterization Report

Cardiac catheterization procedure reports are generated for every procedure performed in a cath lab. For the coder to assign codes for all components of the diagnostic or therapeutic procedures, the following essential information should be included:

- Indications for procedure; history
- Indication of whether the patient has a congenital anomaly
- Preoperative and postoperative diagnoses
- Procedure(s) performed
- Anesthesia provided
- Techniques:
  - Catheter access site(s)
  - Each vessel entered
  - Each vessel subjected to angiography
  - Hemodynamics
  - Stent insertion
  - Angioplasty
  - Thrombectomy
  - Atherectomy
- Additional procedures:
  - Intravascular ultrasound
  - Doppler velocity
  - Coronary and fractional flow measurements

Certain medical supplies used during catheterization procedures can be reported separately by the facility for reimbursement under the Ambulatory Payment Classification or Diagnosis-Related Group payment system. Facilities report these supplies with HCPCS C codes:

- Drug-eluting stent:
  - Coated stent (codes C1874, C1875): Coated stents are bonded with drugs to prevent future blockage by inhibiting the ability of plaque to adhere to them.
  - Covered stent (codes C1784, C1785): Covered stents are layered with silicone.
  - Stent delivery system (C1874, C1876): Certain stents are prepackaged as a complete delivery system, with a stent mounted on a balloon angioplasty catheter, introducer, and sheath.
- Vascular closure device (C1760): At the end of the procedure after the catheter is removed, this device is used to stop bleeding at the catheter puncture site. Two codes are required to report the complete service: C1760 for the device and G0269 for the placement.
- Transluminal angioplasty catheter (C1725, C1885): This catheter is made to dilate vessels that are stenotic.
- Guiding catheter (C1887): This catheter assists in introducing diagnostic devices into vessels. It can be used to inject contrast, pass instruments through, and measure arterial pressure.

Angiography

Angiography involves injecting contrast medium and imaging the contrast in the vessel (angiogram) to determine the vessel obstruction or abnormality. To assess the coronary arteries, each of the two main arteries off from the aorta are injected with contrast. Imaging may be done from several different angles by repositioning the catheter to perform the injection of contrast. Injection of dye is usually done manually, but when angiography of a ventricular or atrial chamber is performed, a power injector may be used to deliver contrast in a short time to achieve an image with good resolution.

Deciphering the Catheterization Report

Box 29.1 is a sample catheterization report with key elements highlighted. Items highlighted in green are reported by the catheterization lab (facility). Notes are provided in parentheses and highlighted in yellow to indicate the physician services.

Based on the documentation in Box 29.1, a left heart catheterization was performed with coronary angiography, left ventriculography, and RSI. One code captures the physician's professional component of this procedure: 93458–26. While there may not be any specific wording in the report that states "radiological supervision and interpretation," it is the physician's statement regarding his or her findings that indicates the RSI was provided. For example, "The left anterior descending coronary artery had 100% ostial occlusion" indicates that the physician followed the dye through the coronary arteries and determined the occlusion. That is RSI.

BOX 29.1 Catheterization Report

Cardiac Catheterization Report
History: Patient has been feeling very sluggish and fatigues easily. Patient has had intermittent chest pain.

Pre-op Diagnosis: Abnormal stress test. Valvular disease.

Post-op Diagnosis: 100% occlusion of the left anterior descending coronary artery. Mitral valve prolapse.

Procedure Performed: Left heart catheterization. Left ventriculogram. Coronary angiogram.

The patient was prepped and draped in the usual sterile fashion for percutaneous coronary procedures. Local lidocaine anesthesia was injected in the right groin. IV sedation of Versed was accomplished. A 6-French sheath (C1894) was placed in the right femoral artery. An Outlook 5-French angiographic catheter (C1887) was passed over the guidewire (C1769) and into the left ventricle. A hemodynamic study measured the left ventricular end diastolic pressure to be 12. Using this same catheter, the right coronary artery was visualized. It had minor plaquing present.

Another Outlook 5-French catheter (C1887) was passed over the guidewire and into the ostia of the left coronary artery. The left main was normal. The left anterior descending coronary artery had 100% ostial occlusion. A ramus intermedius branch had less than 50% ostial stenosis. The circumflex had mild plaquing (this is coronary angiography).

A 5-French pigtail catheter (C1887) was passed retrograde across the aortic valve into the left ventricle (this is the left heart catheterization procedure). Left ventriculogram was performed (this is left ventriculography). The left ventricular ejection fraction was 50%. There was mild anterior wall hypokinesis and mild mitral valve regurgitation.

The procedure was completed, and the catheter was removed. The incision site in the right femoral artery was closed with 6-French (G0269) Angio-Seal device (C1760).

Cardiac Catheterization for Congenital Cardiac Anomalies

Codes 93530–93533 are reported for cardiac catheterizations for congenital cardiac anomalies. There is no age requirement or limit for these services. The coding guidelines for these services differ from the cardiac catheterizations previously covered. Codes 93530–93533 do not include the injection of contrast, which is reported separately with codes 93563–93568.

These codes also include RSI. For example, a patient recently diagnosed with a congenital cardiac anomaly undergoes right heart and retrograde left heart cardiac catheterization (93531). Contrast injection is performed for selective coronary angiography including imaging supervision, interpretation, and report (+93563).

> Most of the cardiovascular National Correct Coding Initiative (NCCI) edits have the modifier indicator of 1, so the use of an appropriate modifier (usually –59) can override them.

Catheterization Modifiers

HCPCS modifiers specific to vessels of the heart are located in the HCPCS manual. They should be appended to catheterization procedures to indicate which procedure was performed on which vessel. They are required by Medicare but may not be recognized by all carriers. When a carrier does not recognize the HCPCS Level II modifiers, the –59 modifier with either –RT or –LT is used to describe the vessels instead. Coding can be very confusing when between 5 and 20 codes describe the services. Examples of the more common modifiers for the heart vessels are RCA for the right coronary artery, LAD for the left anterior descending, and LC for the left circumflex.

Intracardiac Electrophysiological Procedures/Studies

Intracardiac electrophysiological procedures (EPS) are invasive medical procedures used to diagnose and treat heart rhythm disorders. These diagnostic and/or therapeutic procedures involve insertion and repositioning of electrode catheters, recording of electrograms before and during pacing, programmed stimulation of multiple locations in the heart, analysis of recorded information, and report of the procedure.

Carefully review the parenthetical note listed below EPS study codes 93619, 93620, 93653, and 93654 indicating the codes that are not to be reported in conjunction with these study codes.

If the patient is evaluated and treated at the same encounter, the procedure will involve the electrophysiological study, induced tachycardia, mapping of the tachycardia and ablation of the tissue causing the tachycardia.

The study codes specific to right atrial and right ventricular pacing are as follows:

93619: "*without* induction or attempted induction of arrhythmia"
93620: "*with* induction or attempted induction of arrhythmia"
93653: includes the treatment of supraventricular tachycardia by ablation
93654: includes the treatment of ventricular tachycardia

The left-sided pacing and recording codes are as follows:

+93621, add-on code:
- For left *atrial* pacing and recording from coronary sinus or left atrium
- Use with 93620

+93622, add-on code:
- For left *ventricular* pacing and recording
- Use with 93620, 93653, 93654, 93656

The mapping codes are as follows:

+93609, add-on code:
- To identify origin of tachycardia
- Use with 93620, 93653

+93613, add-on code:
- Three-dimensional mapping
- Use with 93620, 93651, 93652

The ablation codes are as follows:

93650, modifier –51 exempt:
- Ablation of atrioventricular node function
- Creation of complete heart block
- With or without temporary pacemaker placement

93651, modifier –51 exempt:
- Ablation of supraventricular tachycardia

93652, modifier –51 exempt:
- Ablation of ventricular tachycardia

EPS study codes include the following:

- Inserting and repositioning of electrode catheters
- Recording of electrograms before and during pacing or programmed stimulation of the heart
- Analysis of recorded information
- The report
- Can be both diagnostic and therapeutic
  - Evaluation and treatment provided during same encounter
- Two or more electrodes placed within the heart to evaluate the heart's electrical system
  - May also provide pacing services
  - May also provide ablation services

Inducing arrhythmia:

- Is accomplished via catheters placed in one or more chambers of the heart
- Provides recording and pacing
- Involves stimulating chambers of the heart until clinical arrhythmia is induced or the protocol required is achieved
- Involves terminating the arrhythmia by pacing methods or by countershock and is included in the EPS services

The process is as follows:

- The sinoatrial node initiates the cardiac cycle.
- The electrical impulse travels to both atria causing each to contract.
- As the atria contract, blood is forced into each ventricle.
- Concurrently, the AV node depolarizes and the impulse follows the bundle of His.
- Electrical impulses are then sent from the bundle of His to the right and left bundle branches.
- The impulse is then distributed over the medial surface, which stimulates the Purkinje fibers located at the apex of the heart.
- When these are stimulated, the ventricles contract and blood is forced to the lungs and the body.
- Induction of arrhythmia is an important element.
- Cardiac catheterization is included in EPS.

Indications include the following:

- Palpitations
- Near syncope
- Syncope (fainting or blacking out)
- Cardiac arrest

Home and Outpatient International Normalized Ratio (INR) Monitoring Services

The codes in this section of CPT represent services provided for anticoagulation therapy, including management of the warfarin drug that keeps the patient's blood at a therapeutic level. The services include the training required for the patient to schedule and perform the INR test, and review and interpret the new international normalized ratio (INR) results Also included are communication of the findings to the patient and adjustment of the warfarin dosage. Most commonly, these services are provided when a patient has had a heart valve replaced or open-heart surgery or when a patient has vascular disease. Anticoagulation therapy is required so that the patient's blood does not clot too easily or get too thin (in which case the patient bleeds too easily).

93792: Training for initiation of home INR monitoring under direction of physician or QHP. This is a face-to-face that includes use and care of the INR monitor, obtaining the blood sample, instructions for reporting the results and documentation of the patient's or caregiver's ability to perform testing, and report results.

93793: This code represents the anticoagulant management of a patient taking warfarin. It includes the review and interpretation of a new home, office, or lab INR test result (wherever the patient performs the INR test). It also includes patient instructions, dosage adjustments, and scheduling of additional tests. This code is reported only once per day and cannot be reported with an E/M service.

The INR levels can vary over time, so the levels must be monitored and the patient's dosage carefully adjusted. If an E/M service is provided on the same day as code 93792 the E/M services may be reported with modifier –25 if it is significantly and separately identifiable from the INR service. Code 93793 is not reportable with an E/M service. Do not report these codes in addition to codes 98966–98969, 99441–99444, 99487, 99489, 98490, 99495, 99496.

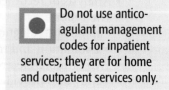 Do not use anticoagulant management codes for inpatient services; they are for home and outpatient services only.

Noninvasive Vascular Diagnostic Studies

The noninvasive vascular diagnostic studies subsection (codes 93880–93998) is organized by the following subheadings:

- Cerebrovascular Arterial Studies
- Extremity Arterial Studies
- Extremity Venous Studies
- Visceral and Penile Vascular Studies
- Extremity Arterial-Venous Studies
- Other Noninvasive Vascular Diagnostic Studies

These studies require no incisions to assess blood flow and stenosis of the arteries. The services in this section are further identified by the terms *duplex scan* and *physiological studies*:

- The duplex scan is an ultrasound scanning procedure that shows the pattern and direction of blood flow in arteries or veins. It produces real-time images and integrates B-mode, two-dimensional vascular structure, Doppler spectral analysis, and color-flow Doppler imaging. The use of a simple handheld or other Doppler device that does not produce a hard copy or that produces a record that does not permit analysis of bidirectional vascular flow is not part of this code range. Those services are considered to be part of the physical examination of the patient's vascular system.
- Physiological studies use equipment that is separate and distinct from the duplex ultrasound. These studies describe the evaluation of nonimaging physiological recordings of pressures with Doppler analysis of bidirectional blood flow, plethysmography, and/or oxygen tension measurements appropriate for the area studied.

The noninvasive physiological peripheral arterial examinations (93922–93990) are performed when there are significant signs and/or symptoms of either upper or lower limb ischemia. This allows the provider to determine whether to perform an invasive therapeutic procedure.

Noninvasive vascular studies codes 93922, 93923, and 93924 include the performance and supervision of studies using technology capable of producing a hardcopy output record (not imaging) of study results that permits physician analysis and written interpretation. Review of the complete CPT code descriptions is essential for each of these services.

Codes 93922, 93923, and 93924 may involve functional measurement procedures, including ankle/brachial index (ABI), blood pressure (BP), and physiological waveform measurements, segmental pressure measurement, plethysmography, and stress testing. These studies do not involve imaging because they are performed using equipment that is separate and distinct from the duplex scanner. For example, the ABI test uses a Doppler stethoscope to measure sound within the vessels at the ankle or the elbow's antecubital fossa. Doppler velocity signals, called *waveforms*, can be measured to localize vascular disease at a single level (93922) or at various limb levels (93923). Exercise testing can be used to analyze the functional significance of vascular disease by reassessing the blood pressure with the Doppler stethoscope, after completion of an appropriate amount of stress testing (93924).

Another example is plethysmography, a measurement of the volume of a limb section or flow rate, in response to the inflation and deflation of a specially calibrated blood pressure cuff. A transcutaneous oxygen tension measurement, which is typically performed on the foot or calf, measures the influx of blood providing oxygen for diffusion to the skin in the area of study.

In terms of the use of modifiers with these services, it is not appropriate to append modifier –50, the bilateral modifier, because codes 93922, 93923, and 93924 are inherently bilateral. Modifier –52 for reduced services may be used to indicate when a unilateral procedure was performed and the code represents bilateral services.

Modifier –59 would be used when a single-level upper extremities study was performed (93922) and a multiple-level study of the lower extremities (93923) was also performed. In this circumstance, modifier –59 may be appended to code 93922 to indicate that a separately distinct study was performed.

Assign codes to the following procedures for the physician. Include any necessary modifiers.

1. A patient was seen in the office, and the cardiologist performed an ECG with interpretation and report, with an office visit. Due to an abnormal ECG finding, the cardiologist also does a limited transthoracic echocardiogram that same day. What codes should be reported? Are any modifiers needed? _____

2. A patient was seen in the outpatient cardiology clinic for a real-time maximal stress ECHO. The patient walked for a total of 10 minutes and achieved 91% of age-predicted maximal heart rate. The test was stopped early because of fatigue. A baseline ECG showed normal sinus rhythm. An exercise ECG showed the same. The preexercise heart wall motion was normal. The postexercise wall motion showed an increase in the ejection fraction. _____

3. A patient was admitted for 23-hour observation for elective cardioversion. Oral medications had not been successful in maintaining his rhythm. The patient's A-fib was putting him at risk for stroke. The patient was sedated, and 300 synchronized joules were conducted through the electrodes by placing the paddles on the chest. A normal sinus rhythm was achieved, and cardioversion was successful. _____

4. A combined left heart catheterization and retrograde right heart catheterization were performed with right ventricular angiography and selective coronary angiography, including imaging supervision and interpretation. _____

PULMONARY

Physicians and respiratory therapists use codes from the Pulmonary section. Pulmonary function tests (PFTs) or studies are performed for many reasons: to obtain preoperative surgical clearance for individuals who are smokers or have histories of breathing problems, to diagnose lung disease, to assess the extent of a patient's pulmonary disability, and to manage or monitor a patient's treatment regimen. Codes 94010–94799 include laboratory procedure(s) and interpretation of the test results. Reporting E/M services with pulmonary services must clearly document a separately identifiable E/M service from the pulmonary service. Use modifier –25 with the E/M codes.

The most common pulmonary test is spirometry (94010), which measures the volume of air in the lungs by measuring how much air is expelled from the lungs and how quickly it is expelled. Patients are asked to take a deep breath and blow into a machine. Patients with asthma or other problems that obstruct airflow to the lungs require nebulizer treatments, which are commonly performed in the physician office or at home. When a nebulizer treatment is performed in the office, a HCPCS supply code for the medication is also reported. When spirometry is performed before and after administration of a bronchodilator, report code 94060.

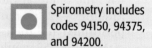
Spirometry includes codes 94150, 94375, and 94200.

Pulmonary function test codes 94011–94013 are specific to infants and young children through 2 years of age. CPT codes 94014–94016 are for patient-initiated spirometric recording for a 30-day period. Code 94014 is the global code representing both the professional and technical components. Code 94015 is technical only, and code 94016 is professional only. Do not report either modifiers –26 or –TC with these codes. Code 94070 represents a bronchodilation provocation evaluation after exposing the patient to an agent, antigen, cold air, or methacholine. A spirometer is used to measure the lung function after the exposure.

Carefully review the parenthetical notes for coding instructions related to the pulmonary codes.

ALLERGY AND CLINICAL IMMUNOLOGY

The Allergy and Clinical Immunology subsection of the Medicine chapter consists of codes for allergy testing and immunotherapy. A patient with chronic allergic symptoms or with acute allergic reactions to substances is often referred to one of two specialists for evaluation and treatment: an *allergist* (a physician who specializes in diagnosing and treating allergies) or an *immunologist* (a physician who specializes in diagnosing and treating malfunctions of the immune system pertaining to autoimmune diseases, hypersensitivities, and immune deficiencies). Both kinds of specialists are certified through the American Board of Allergy and Immunology.

Allergy Testing

Allergy testing is performed to determine which substance is triggering an allergic response. Typical allergy symptoms are itchy eyes, runny nose, congestion, hives, and sneezing. Some people are severely allergic and may experience a serious allergic response such as anaphylaxis, cramping, or diarrhea after eating certain foods or being stung by an insect. Allergy tests provide tangible results about specific substances to which patients may or may not be allergic.

There are many allergy testing techniques, including percutaneous tests (skin-prick tests or intradermal), skin endpoint titrations (SETs), patch or application tests, ophthalmic mucous membrane tests, blood tests, and direct nasal mucous tests. The percutaneous skin-prick tests and the blood tests are used most commonly. A small puncture is made in the skin during the skin-prick technique, and a drop of the allergen is placed into the puncture site. Intradermal testing involves injecting a small amount of allergen under the skin with a syringe and watching for swelling at the injection site. This form of testing is more sensitive than the skin-prick method and may be performed secondarily if the skin-prick test is negative. Skin endpoint titration, or serial endpoint titration, consists of administering increasing concentrations of an allergen known to cause a reaction. The first dilution that initiates a wheal that is 2 mm larger than that produced by the preceding dilution is called the *endpoint*. This endpoint is intended to determine the optimal dose, with immunotherapy beginning with 0.5 mL of the endpoint dilution. It is used in conjunction with immunotherapy to determine the starting point for a patient's sensitivity to the allergen and immunoglobulin E (IgE).

> Pay close attention to the code description for the type of testing performed and the number of tests performed.

Allergy Testing Code Assignment

Before codes for allergy testing can be assigned, the coder must identify the type of test that was performed and the substances that were administered. Code descriptions indicate "specify number of tests," prompting the coder to count the number of allergens tested. Allergy testing is reported in units. For CPT codes 95004–95028, there is a one-to-one correlation between units reported and antigens tested. Histamine and saline control skin tests may be billed as two antigens. These substances are injected into the skin to get a baseline or benchmark for the skin reaction and size of the local swelling.

EXAMPLE
Ten prick tests are reported with 10 in the units column on the claim form instead of being listed 10 times on 10 different lines of the claim form.

Code 95076 is assigned for the ingestion challenge test and should be reported for a time period of the initial 120 minutes. Add-on code 95079 represents each additional 60 minutes of testing.

Documentation is important in reporting allergy testing services and appealing denials. Allergy tests require direct or personal physician supervision because of the risk of the patient having a severe reaction and possibly requiring emergency treatment. Direct supervision requires the physician to be in the office and readily accessible if needed by the nursing staff; the physician does not have to be present in the examining room in which the procedure is performed. Personal supervision requires the physician to be in personal attendance in the examining room in which the procedure is performed. Codes 95004, 95017, 95018, 95024, 95027, 95028, 95044, 95052, and 95056 require direct supervision, whereas codes 95060, 95070, and 95071 require personal supervision.

Immunotherapy

Once allergy testing has confirmed to which substance the patient is allergic, the physician proceeds with remedying the patient's symptoms with immunotherapy, or allergy shots. The purpose of immunotherapy is to increase the patient's tolerance to the substances (allergens) that provoke allergy symptoms by giving the allergens in increasingly large doses to gradually develop immunity. Allergy shots alter the way in which the immune system reacts to allergens.

Coders must pay close attention to code descriptions. Some code descriptions include such statements as "specify number of vials" and "specify number of doses." Codes in this section sound similar yet are distinctly different. The language in the code descriptors differentiates professional services by the prescribing physician, professional services for the supervision of the preparation and provision of antigens in multiple-dose vials, professional services for the supervision of preparation and provision of antigens when the physician provides the antigen to be injected somewhere else in a single-dose vial, and professional services for the immunotherapy injection without the provision of the extract. There are also codes specific to immunotherapy for stinging insect venoms.

E/M office visit codes can be reported on the same day as an allergy injection in limited circumstances. The CPT note states: "Do not report Evaluation and Management (E/M) services for test interpretation and report. If a significant, separately identifiable E/M service is performed, the appropriate E/M service code should be reported using modifier –25."

 CPT states that a single-dose vial contains a single dose of antigen administered in one injection. CPT describes the allergen dose as the amount of antigen administered in a single injection from a multiple-dose vial.

Medicare does not reimburse for CPT codes 95120–95134. Medicare requires the use of multidose vials. Medicare does recognize codes 95115–95117 and 95144–95170.

> ### ■ CASE SCENARIO
> A physician sees a patient who has acid indigestion, after which the patient receives a scheduled bimonthly series of two allergy injections for allergic rhinitis due to dust mites. The preparation for the allergen dose was provided elsewhere. The physician performs and documents a level 2 E/M service. Codes 99212–25, 95117 are reported.

Immunotherapy Code Assignment

Before assigning immunotherapy codes, coders should determine whether the physician provided the allergenic extracts, simply administered the injection, or did both. There are sets of codes for each circumstance. If the allergist provided the injection and provided or prepared the antigen, two codes must be submitted: one for the injection (codes 95115–95117) and a second for the antigen. Use Pinpoint the Code 29.1 to assist in assigning codes for immunotherapy.

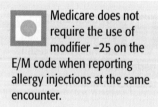 Medicare does not require the use of modifier –25 on the E/M code when reporting allergy injections at the same encounter.

Injection Service

Two codes exist for reporting the injection service alone: code 95115 (*Professional services for allergen immunotherapy not including provision of allergenic extracts; single injection*) and code 95117 (*. . . two or more injections*). These codes are reported if the office administering the injection does not prepare or provide the extract being injected. The codes are reported based on the number of injections given. Code 95117 is reported only once regardless of how many injections over two are reported.

Antigen Provision

An antigen is a foreign substance that reacts with antibodies in the body in a way that may evoke an immune response. In immunotherapy, the antigen is slowly introduced so that the

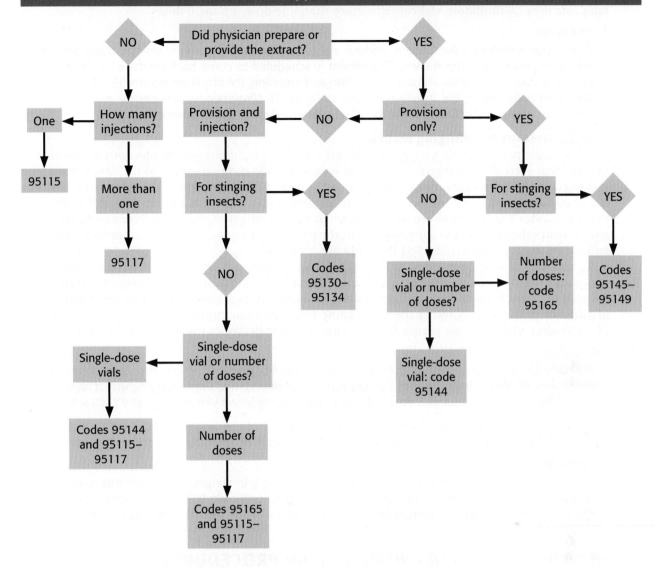

body will produce antibodies to the antigen and eventually the antigen will no longer be effective. When reporting codes for the antigen, physicians must specify the number of doses provided in the multidose vial. Code 95144 (*Professional services for the supervision of preparation and provision of antigens for allergen immunotherapy; single-dose vial[s] [specify number of vials]*) is submitted by an allergist who prepared and provided an antigen extract to another provider to be injected. This code is not used frequently because most extracts are packaged in multidose vials. Code 95165 (*Professional services for the supervision of preparation and provision of antigens for allergen immunotherapy; single-dose vial(s) [specify number of vials]*) represents the supervision and provision of the antigens. Code 95165 is for preparation and provision of antigen(s) in a multidose vial. The actual injection of the antigen from the multidose vial is billed using CPT code 95115 for one injection. The number of units billed is the number of doses in the vial. Code 95165 is billed once for each dose prepared.

> If the physician prepares more than one vial with separate antigens and the patient is injected with antigens from both vials on the same day, append the –59 modifier to indicate that the preparation of the second vial is for a different antigen and is not duplicate billing. Code 95117 is submitted instead of code 95115 in this case.

Codes 95120–95134 (*Professional services for allergen immunotherapy in the office or institution of the prescribing physician or other qualified health-care professional, including provision of allergenic extract*) are used to describe complete services, meaning they include both the injection and the preparation of the antigen. If the physician prepares the antigen and administers one injection, code 95115 is reported along with code 95165. Staff members must pay particular attention to the number of doses available in a vial. CPT translates a dose as equivalent to the amount of serum drawn up in the injection. A single-dose vial contains one dose. A multidose vial contains more than one dose, up to 10 doses.

> **EXAMPLE**
>
> A physician prepares a five-dose multidose vial for a patient and administers one injection containing one dose from the vial. The patient is scheduled to come back for the other four one-dose injections. For the antigen preparation and provision, the physician reports 95165 × 5. A second code reports the injection service: code 95115 (*Professional services for allergen immunotherapy not including provision of allergenic extracts; single injection*).

Immunotherapy for Stinging Insects

Physicians see patients with a variety of allergic reactions, including severe reactions to insect venom from such stinging insects as bees and wasps. Specific code sets apply to the preparation and injection of extract containing stinging insect venom. Code submission is based on whether the physician provided and injected this extract or simply prepared it for another provider to administer. Codes 95130–95134 are submitted when the allergist prescribing the immunotherapy also provides the antigen and administers it to the patient. When the physician just prepares the antigen for another office, codes 95145–95149 are submitted.

To correctly report these codes, the physician must document the number of stinging insect venoms in the vial. The number of insect venoms and the number of doses are important. This is vastly different from allergen antigen coding, in which codes are not selected by the number of antigens in the vial. Whether the doses come from the same multiple-dose vial or a series of single-dose vials does not matter here because the code describes the dose, not the bottle.

> **EXAMPLE**
>
> For code 95146, *Professional services for the supervision of preparation and provision of antigens for allergen immunotherapy (specify number of doses); two single stinging insect venoms.* If the physician prepares 5 doses of two single stinging insect venoms, report 95146 × 5.

Codes 95145–95149 do not include the administration of the antigen. If the office is also administering the injection, a code from 95130–95134 must be selected.

> **EXAMPLE**
>
> If an allergist prepares two doses of an antigen containing four stinging insect venoms, code 95148 × 2 is reported. The office injecting the antigen reports code 95117. If the same allergist prepared, provided, and administered the injection, he or she reports code 95133 instead.

NEUROLOGY AND NEUROMUSCULAR PROCEDURES

Neurological services in this chapter of CPT are mostly diagnostic and consultative in nature. They include sleep studies, electroencephalography (EEG), nerve conduction studies, and neurostimulator programming and testing.

Sleep Studies

According to the National Institute of Neurological Disorders and Stroke, more than 40 million Americans a year suffer from some sort of sleep disorder. While insomnia and narcolepsy are the best known sleep disorders, more than 100 types actually exist. To obtain proper diagnoses, sleep studies are conducted. Sleep medicine procedures (95782–95811) evaluate both adult and pediatric patients. A sleep study is a 7- to 8-hour recording of the body's electrical and physiological activity. Append modifier –52 to the sleep study codes for the following scenarios:

- Fewer than 6 hours of recording time was done for codes 95800, 95801, 95806, 95807, 95810, 95811.
- Fewer than 7 hours of recording time was done for codes 95782, 95783.
- Fewer than four nap opportunities were recorded for code 95805.

Polysomnography is the recording of brain activity, heart rate, muscle movements, oxygen levels, and breathing while the patient sleeps (Fig. 29.4) Unlike sleep studies, it includes sleep

CPT © 2017 American Medical Association, All Rights Reserved.

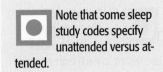
staging, which involves an electroencephalogram, electrooculogram, and electromyography, and both sleep and staging are recorded. In an electroencephalogram (EEG), electrodes are placed on the scalp to record electrical activity produced by the brain. An electrooculogram (EOG) is produced by placing electrodes strategically around the eyes to measure their activity, which aids in determining when sleep occurs and when REM sleep occurs. Electromyography (EMG) is defined as the study and recording of the electrical properties of muscles and the action generated by the muscle cells. It uses electrodes to measure muscle tension in the body and monitor for excessive muscle movement.

Codes are assigned based on how many parameters of sleep are measured and monitored. Additional parameters are indicated within CPT.

Codes 95808–95783 are assigned for polysomnography. The coder must know what stages of sleep are monitored and whether the patient is tested during a full night's rest or during daytime naps. Coders should also review the code description for the patient's age. If the test is conducted during daytime naps, code 95805 is assigned. This test is commonly done for excessive daytime sleepiness.

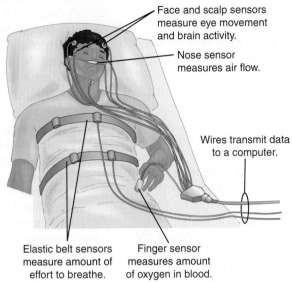

Face and scalp sensors measure eye movement and brain activity.

Nose sensor measures air flow.

Wires transmit data to a computer.

Elastic belt sensors measure amount of effort to breathe.

Finger sensor measures amount of oxygen in blood.

Figure 29.4 Polysomnography.

Routine Electroencephalography

Routine EEGs (95812–95830) are used for many purposes other than recording brain activity during sleep studies. They are used primarily for the investigation of epilepsy and other disorders of consciousness. They are also used in diagnosing encephalitis, coma, and dementia due to neurodegenerative disease. If a patient exhibits symptoms of altered mental status, severe migraines, or convulsions, an EEG may be ordered to assist in diagnosing the underlying problem.

Coders must rely on a thorough EEG report in order to assign the most specific codes for this service. According to the American Clinical Neurophysiology Society (ACNS), the EEG report should consist of three principal parts: an introduction, a description of the actual EEG and the patient's behavior during the test, and an interpretation of the test. The interpretation consists of an impression regarding the test's normality or degree of abnormality and correlation of the EEG findings with the clinical picture. The report should include the following items:

The ACNS states that coding for any testing or monitoring that lasts for more than 12 hours—which is half the prescribed 24-hour monitoring period for special EEGs—is adequate to justify reporting special EEG codes. The AMA states, "For recording more than 12 hours do not use modifier –52. For recording 12 hours or less, use modifier –52."

- State of the patient's consciousness when the test was performed. Codes are differentiated by whether the patient is awake and drowsy, awake, or asleep.
- How long the study was performed. An EEG must be performed for at least 20 minutes to report the service. For example, was the EEG recorded all night?
- Whether video was recorded during the procedure.

The Special EEG Tests subsection (95950–95967) includes the codes for long-term brain function monitoring. They are used to report long-term monitoring for seizure activity and are reported for each 24 hours monitored.

EXAMPLE
A pediatric patient was monitored for a total of 9 hours. The patient was experiencing mild seizure activity. The patient was in and out of a sleep state. Video was recorded. CPT code 95951–52 was assigned.

Electromyography

Needle electromyography codes 95860–95864 cover all muscles tested in the extremity, so only one unit of service is reported for the study. According to CMS, a minimum of five muscles in each limb must be studied to report EMG codes 95860–95864. Code 95870 is considered a limited study and reported with one unit per extremity when fewer than five muscles are examined.

> **EXAMPLE**
>
> A physician uses EMG to test five muscles in the right arm for ulnar neuropathy. He tests three muscles in the left arm. Codes 95860 and 95870–59 are reported.

EMG studies on bilateral extremities where five muscles are tested in each extremity are reported with code 95861. Code 95860–50 will not work because the code description is not specific to any one extremity. Code 95861 can hypothetically be used to report EMG studies on one leg and one arm.

Nerve Conduction Studies

Nerve conduction studies (95907–95913) are performed to detect and diagnose nerve damage, dysfunction, and demyelination such as carpal tunnel syndrome, metabolic and immune peripheral neuropathies, ulnar neuropathy, radiculopathy, and tarsal tunnel syndrome. They assess the capacity of electrical conduction of the motor and sensory nerves. Nerve conduction tests are performed with individually placed stimulating, recording, and ground electrodes, and their placement and test design are individualized to the patient's unique anatomy. The amount of time it takes a peripheral nerve to receive the stimulation is measured and recorded. Results determine the efficacy of the connection between the nerve and the muscle and the integrity of the muscle itself. An electromyogram is the actual recording of the study, showing the M-wave (the compound motor action potential [CMAP] that is recorded when the motor nerve is stimulated) and the F-wave (a late response used to assess the proximal segments of the motor nerve function). The EMG is also performed to monitor nerve localization and viability during surgical procedures to prevent accidental injury to the nerve. Code +95920 is assigned in addition to the surgical procedure code.

Nerve conduction studies and EMGs can also be performed by physical therapists who are certified by the American Board of Physical Therapy Specialties, because these codes are assigned supervision levels by CMS.

Neurostimulators, Analysis–Programming

Codes in this subsection are assigned for the testing and programming of a neurostimulator. They are reported when testing a previously placed generator system for battery status, pulse amplitude, duration, rate, and so on. These codes do not include the actual insertion of the device.

Neurostimulator analysis and programming are described as simple or complex. CPT says that a simple neurostimulator analysis is one capable of affecting three or fewer of the following:

- Pulse amplitude
- Pulse duration
- Pulse frequency
- Eight or more electrode contacts
- Cycling
- Stimulation train duration
- Train spacing
- Number of programs
- Number of channels
- Phase angle
- Alternating electrode polarities
- Configuration of waveform
- More than one clinical feature (such as rigidity, dyskinesia, tremor)

Component billing must be used if the interpreting physician does not own the equipment. The physician would report the code with modifier –26. Modifier –TC is appended to the code for the facility.

A complex neurostimulator analysis is capable of affecting more than three of the above.

Six codes are available in this section for neurostimulator analysis and reprogramming. Two of them, +95973 and +95975, are add-on codes assigned with codes 95972 and 95974, respectively, only after the first hour of programming. These add-on codes can be reported if the documented time extends at least 16 minutes beyond the previously billed hour or 30-minute unit of time.

Assign codes to the following procedures for the physician.

1. A patient complaining of pain in the thumbs and numbness of both hands is seen in the neurologist's office. The physician performs needle myography of bilateral forearms. _____

2. A patient reports to her doctor that for the past three summers she has caught a cold that turns into a sinus infection. She says that she does not have this problem year-round. The physician decides that allergy testing is warranted. The patient is tested for mold, ragweed, and grass pollen. Intradermal testing immediate-type reaction is performed with allergenic extracts. _____

3. The above patient's allergy tests show she is allergic to ragweed. She has agreed to immunotherapy. She returns to the allergist's office and receives an injection of the antigen. The serum to determine tolerance is prepared and provided by the allergist in a single-dose vial. _____

4. A patient was status post–insertion of deep-brain neurostimulator to combat tremors from Parkinson's disease. The system generator was tested, the battery was tested, and the parameters were also adjusted because the patient was still experiencing some tremor. Electronic analysis and programming of the single-array generator were performed. The overall session lasted 2 hours. _____

EXAMPLE
Eighty minutes of programming are reported with codes 95972 (first hour) and +95973 (additional 20 minutes).

The codes in the 95970 series are selected for the professional service to program and test the device. Code 95970 is assigned if the provider tests the neurostimulator pulse generator system without reprogramming anything.

MEDICAL GENETICS AND GENETIC COUNSELING SERVICES

Genetic testing identifies the likelihood of parents' passing of specific genetic diseases or disorders to offspring. Genetic counseling involves interviewing pregnant couples or those considering conceiving about the likelihood of passing genetic disorders, such as Down syndrome, cystic fibrosis, and Tay-Sachs disease, to their offspring. In genetic counseling, the family history and family tree are evaluated, medical records are reviewed, genetic tests are ordered, the results are analyzed, and the couple's risk is assessed. Counseling is reported in 30-minute increments. Only nonphysician genetics counselors may report the codes in this section. If a physician conducts genetic counseling, E/M codes are submitted from the Preventive Medicine section. Report code 96040 for each 30 minutes face to face with the patient/family.

HEALTH AND BEHAVIOR ASSESSMENT/INTERVENTION

Codes 96150–96155, 96160, and 96161 are reported by nonphysician health-care professionals such as psychologists, advanced practice nurses, and clinical social workers. These are professionals who have specialty or subspecialty training in health and behavior assessment/intervention procedures. Physicians do not use these codes. If these services are provided by a physician, they would use the E/M codes or preventive medicine codes. These services are face-to-face services;

therefore, questionnaires given to the patient without face-to-face contact are not reported with these codes. Health and behavior assessments and/or interventions are not psychiatric services; they identify situations in which a patient's physical health problems have led to psychological and/or emotional complications for the patient. The codes are time based and break down into assessment codes and intervention codes.

> ■ **CASE SCENARIO**
> A 40-year-old female patient has had chronic illnesses for more than 20 years: diabetes, asthma, and hypertension. She recently fell and broke her elbow and is now experiencing anxiety and almost daily panic attacks and refuses any type of treatment. She is combative with family and health professionals. Her physician has referred her for a health and behavior assessment. There was an extensive interview to evaluate how the patient reacts to the hospitalizations and treatments associated with her illnesses and injury. A pain questionnaire was used as well as a coping strategy inventory. Family members and medical staff involved in her care were also interviewed. The patient agreed to see her physician, and behavioral observations were made during the encounter. Report 96150 for each 15 minutes spent face to face with the patient.

● Do not use the preventive medicine codes for counseling and risk factor reduction for these services. Health and behavior services are associated with patients who have physical health problems.

HYDRATION, THERAPEUTIC, PROPHYLACTIC, DIAGNOSTIC INJECTIONS AND INFUSIONS, AND CHEMOTHERAPY AND OTHER HIGHLY COMPLEX DRUG OR HIGHLY COMPLEX BIOLOGIC AGENT ADMINISTRATION

CPT has divided this section into guidelines for administering hydration, nonchemotherapy injections and infusions, and chemotherapy in addition to other highly complex drugs or biological agents, injections, and infusions. The guidelines clarify the role of physicians and other QHPs in these services as well as the training required for ancillary personnel involved in the administration services (Table 29.3).

Table 29.3 Physician and QHP Roles in Complex Injections and Infusions

	PHYSICIAN OR QHP	ANCILLARY PERSONNEL
Hydration	Predominantly involves affirmation of the treatment plan and direct supervision of staff	Does not require advanced practice training
	Not reported by the physician or QHP in the facility setting	
Nonchemotherapy	Direct supervision for patient assessment, provision of consent, safety oversight, and intraservice supervision of staff	Requires practice training and competency for staff who administer the infusions and requires periodic patient assessment for vital sign monitoring during the infusion
	Not reported by the physician or QHP in the facility setting (i.e., hospital)	
Chemotherapy, etc.	Direct supervision for patient assessment, provision of consent, safety oversight, and intraservice supervision of staff	Requires advanced practice training and competency for staff who administer the infusions and requires periodic patient assessment for vital sign monitoring during the infusion
	Not reported by the physician or QHP in the facility setting	

Infusion is intravenous (IV) therapy in which medication from a bag or bottle is infused (dripped) into a patient's vein over a course of time. Infusion can also be performed subcutaneously. Subcutaneous (SC) infusion differs from IV infusion in that a needle is placed in the upper arm, abdomen, or flank to administer fluids or medication directly into subcutaneous tissue. The primary purpose of SC infusion is to provide hydration with saline water or electrolytes, such as lactated Ringer's solution. It is also used to deliver opioid medications to terminally ill patients in hospice care rather than trying to do so via IV access, which is much more difficult to achieve.

Table 29.4 Infusion Categories

THERAPEUTIC/ PROPHYLACTIC/DIAGNOSTIC	CHEMOTHERAPY/OTHERS	HYDRATION
96365: IV infusion for therapy, prophylaxis, or diagnostic, 16 minutes up to 1 hour. Report HCPCS code for the drug.	96413: Chemotherapy administration, IV infusion, 16 minutes up to 1 hour. Report HCPCS code for the drug.	96360: IV infusion, hydration only, no drug to report. 31 minutes up to 1 hour. Minimum is 31 minutes.
+96366: Each additional 31 minutes to 1 hour, considered a sequential infusion of same drug.	+96415: Each additional 31 minutes to an hour up to 8 hours.	+96361: Each additional 31 minutes to an hour.

Infusions can be performed in the physician office, home, or facility. The drugs are classified into three categories: therapeutic/prophylactic/diagnostic, chemotherapy/others, and hydration (Table 29.4). They all require different administration codes.

Coding IV Infusion

In order for IV infusion to be coded and billed, the coder must have an order from the physician naming the specific type of IV solution and flow rate. Nurses must also document infusion start and stop times. They may use a term such as *piggyback, mini-infuser, IV drip,* or *infusion* to indicate that IV infusion was performed. According to CMS Transmittal 566, a first-hour infusion code cannot be billed until the infusion has run for more than 15 minutes and up to 90 minutes. An infusion that lasts 15 minutes or less should be coded and billed as an intravenous or intra-arterial push (code 96374, +96375).

The AMA defines an intravenous push (IVP) as (1) an infusion in which the health-care professional who administers the substance is continuously present to administer the injection and observe the patient or (2) an infusion of 15 minutes or less.

A code for IVP should also be reported if the patient is premedicated with a drug such as diphenhydramine (Benadryl) or acetaminophen (Tylenol). There are different codes for an additional IVP of the same substance (+96376) as opposed to an additional IVP of a different substance (+96375).

EXAMPLES
• In the facility setting code an IVP of Demerol at 1:00 and a second IVP of Demerol at 1:45 as 96374, +96376. Note that more than 30 minutes have passed since the first IVP.

• Code an IVP of Demerol at 1:00 and a second IV push of Zofran at 1:10 as 96374, +96375.

Infusion codes should be reported to describe prolonged intravenous infusion requiring the presence or direct supervision of the physician. These codes are based on time. An example is code 96365, *Intravenous infusion for therapy, prophylaxis, or diagnosis; initial up to 1 hour.* Time must be sequential with no break in treatment, and start and stop times must be documented as lasting 16 minutes or more. Code 96366 is assigned for each additional hour for intervals of *more than* 30 minutes after the first hour of therapy for the same drug/substance.

When determining infusion time, use only the actual time of the drug administration service.

Additional codes from the E/M and HCPCS code sets may also apply in infusion coding. Hospitals report HCPCS C codes for infusion services instead of CPT Medicine section codes, along with J codes for the substances infused.

Situations in Which Infusion Is Not Coded

An infusion performed during a procedure is not coded if the infusion is part of the standard of care or routine practice. For example, the infusion of IV sedation for a colonoscopy procedure is not coded. This infusion is inherent in the code for the colonoscopy, which would not be performed without it.

EXAMPLE

A patient comes to the emergency department for chest pain, and a thrombolytic agent is infused. The facility bills for the infusion (a HCPCS C code) and the thrombolytic agent (a HCPCS J code). It also reports HCPCS codes for other supplies—such as the sterile needle (A4215) and infusion supplies (A4222). These codes are hard-coded in the facility's charge master.

According to CPT, the following services are included in the infusion service and are not reported separately:

- Use of local anesthesia
- IV start
- Access to indwelling IV, subcutaneous catheter, or port
- Flush at conclusion of infusion
- Standard tubing, syringes, and supplies

Medicare includes the preparation of agents in this list.

What Is the Initial Infusion?

The initial infusion is an important coding issue for infusion services. For multiple infusions, injections, or combinations, only one initial service code is reported unless protocol requires the use of two separate IV sites. The code that best describes the key or primary reason for the encounter is reported as the initial service. Once the primary service has been established, second or subsequent services are coded separately. At times, more than one initial or primary service code can be reported on the same day.

■ CASE SCENARIO

A patient was seen in the morning for chemotherapy. That afternoon the patient received IV steroids through a second IV site. In this case, two different primary services can be reported because two different IV access sites were involved at different encounters. The second infusion service would be reported with a −59 modifier. If, however, these two drugs were infused through the same IV access sites at the same time the code would reflect concurrent infusion for the second drug.

Concurrent and Other Infusion Situations

Concurrent infusion codes are reported when multiple infusions are provided simultaneously through the same IV. A smaller IV bag is hung piggyback style onto the main bag.

EXAMPLE

Infused with IV Rocephin and with a second antibiotic, doxycycline. Code 96365 is reported for the first antibiotic, code 96368 for the concurrent infusion of antibiotic. Code 96368 is reportable only once per date of service.

Code descriptions differ in the distribution of the increments of infusion time. Pay close attention to how the increments of time are broken out. For example, code 96360 states 31 minutes to 1 hour, whereas code 96365 states up to 1 hour.

Code 96368, *Concurrent infusion (list separately in addition to code for primary procedure)*, is reported only once per date of service.

The coding guidelines at the beginning of the hydration, therapeutic, prophylactic, and diagnostic injections and infusions subsections describe a hierarchy for facility reporting of infusions and injections. If chemotherapy or prophylactic, therapeutic, or diagnostic infusion and hydration all occur on the same day, chemotherapy is primary, the drug infusion is secondary, and the hydration is tertiary. Infusions are primary to IV pushes, which are primary to injections. (This hierarchy does not apply to physician reporting.) Regardless of the order in which the internist administers the infusions, the facility coder should report the initial code for the service that falls highest on the hierarchy list.

Subcutaneous infusion codes 96369–96371 are used to describe the physician work and practice expense when administering subcutaneous immune globulin in the office. Codes include placement of multiple subcutaneous accesses and infusion pumps. Code +96370 is reported for 30-minute increments of time beyond the initial 60 minutes. Code +96371 is reported when a new subcutaneous site is accessed, because the original site is full and is unable to absorb more fluid; it is reported in addition to code 96369. Report only once per encounter.

Table 29.5 can be used to help the coder report code combinations for infusion services from the 96365–96379 code range. Using the table will help the coder ensure proper code pair reporting of base codes, add-on services, and codes that should be reported in conjunction with one another.

<table>
<tr><td colspan="2">**Table 29.5** Code Pair Reporting</td></tr>
<tr><td>**CODE THAT CANNOT STAND ALONE**</td><td>**PAIRED CODES**</td></tr>
<tr><td>+96366</td><td>96365, 96367</td></tr>
<tr><td>+96368</td><td>96365, 96413</td></tr>
<tr><td>+96367</td><td>96365, 96374, 96409, 96413 (Report when a new drug or substance is provided after the initial drug through the same IV site.)</td></tr>
<tr><td>+96375</td><td>96365, 96374, 96409, 96413</td></tr>
</table>

Use codes 96372–96379 to bill for each intramuscular or subcutaneous injection other than vaccine administration and allergen immunotherapy injections. Vaccines are reported with codes 90476–90749. Allergy immunization is also covered in this chapter.

When coding injections, keep the phrase "stick and substance" in mind. Two codes are required in most cases to report injections—one for the stick, and the other for the drug or substance.

Do not report code 96523, *Irrigation of implanted venous access device for drug delivery systems*, if an injection or infusion is provided on the same day.

Therapeutic, Prophylactic, and Diagnostic Injections

Unlike an infusion, which delivers a substance over time, an injection delivers the substance in a single shot. Injections can be therapeutic, prophylactic, or diagnostic, and they are provided to achieve an immediate effect—typically within 3 to 5 minutes. An injection provided directly through a saline lock is considered an IV injection.

Intramuscular and subcutaneous injections are reported using CPT code 96372 for each injection. This code is considered a component of infusion codes and requires modifier −59. The code descriptor requires that the specific substance injected be reported with an additional HCPCS code. When additional services are performed at the same time, they should be reported separately. Code 96372 is also used to report non-antineoplastic hormonal therapy injections. Injections administered without direct physician supervision are reported with code 99211 instead of code 96372.

■ CASE SCENARIO

A patient sees her gynecologist for her monthly Depo-Provera shot. The office bills for the injection (code 96372) and the Depo-Provera (HCPCS code J1050 times the number of milligrams injected). Whether an E/M service can also be reported will depend on the documentation representing a significant and separately identifiable E/M service.

Assign codes to the following procedures for the physician.

1. A patient receives an infusion of a noncancer drug (including hydrating solutions) for 3 hours 27 minutes. _____

2. A patient receives a 2-hour infusion of a hydrating solution to which a cancer drug has been added. Documentation does not have a specific order for the hydration. _____

3. A cancer patient receives an antiemetic given by infusion over 10 minutes prior to chemotherapy. Chemotherapy starts at 10:00 a.m. and ends at 12:30 p.m. _____

CHEMOTHERAPY ADMINISTRATION

Chemotherapy is the treatment of cancer with drugs that destroy cancer cells by impeding their growth and keeping them from spreading (metastasizing) to adjacent body parts. Facilities and oncologists report services from this section. An *oncologist* is a physician who specializes in the diagnosis, treatment, and prevention of cancer and tumors. Oncologists are responsible for ordering treatment therapy (chemotherapy, radiation, surgery) for cancer. They study cancer cells and tumor growth and are trained to determine which chemotherapy protocol—type of chemotherapy drug, dose, duration, radiation—to use with which cancer type and location.

Codes from this subsection are selected for the administration of chemotherapeutic agents using various administration techniques. The codes are subdivided to describe the method of administration and the technique: intravenous and injection, intra-arterial, and other. Coders must be able to distinguish between the various techniques in order to capture codes for all agents administered at a given encounter. Intravenous and injection methods include intramuscular, subcutane-

 If extensive time or extensive preparation of the drug is involved, append the –22 modifier, but carefully document the time and the reason for the extensive preparation and/or time.

REIMBURSEMENT REVIEW

Coverage of Codes for Telephone and Online Services

CPT codes are used to report these services rendered by physicians and various midlevel providers. Not all services are reimbursable by third-party payers simply because CPT codes exist for them. Medicare has classified all six codes for telephone and online medical evaluations as a status N, which means they are not payable by Medicare. However, some private payers cover these services. Nevertheless, CMS has assigned relative value units (RVUs) for these nonphysician codes based on the following minute-to-minute breakdowns:

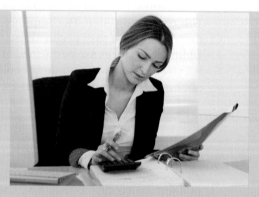

MINUTES	QUALIFIED STAFF CODE	RVU
5–10	98966	0.35
11–20	98967	0.66
21–30	98968	0.98

Report drug administration given sequentially with chemotherapy. If medications are administered before or after chemotherapy, they are reported separately using HCPCS Level II J codes and the appropriate administration code from +96366, +96367, or +96375. Remember the initial service rule.

ous, intralesional, push intravenous, and infusion intravenous. The intra-arterial method consists of push intra-arterial. Other chemotherapy includes various methods that are not as common, such as intrathecal or injection into the pleural cavity. The provision of the chemotherapy access or catheterization service is coded separately. Preparation of the drug is included in the administration code. A code is submitted for each method used to administer the antineoplastic agent.

Code 96409 (*Chemotherapy administration; IV push, single or initial substance/drug*) is submitted once for each drug administered. It can be reported only once per encounter regardless of the number of IV pushes of the same chemotherapy agent.

■ CASE SCENARIO

A patient receives one injection of antineoplastic drugs and an infusion for 2 hours of antineoplastic drugs in one encounter. Codes 96401, 96413, +96415, plus the J codes for the drugs are reported. Note that codes 96401–96406 do not specify the word "injection," but these codes do represent injection services.

Per CMS, CPT codes 96415 and 96423 are add-on codes used to report an additional infusion hour, up to a maximum of eight units per line billed. When infusions last longer than 9 hours, additional infusion hours are reported on a separate line of the claim form using the add-on code as appropriate.

IV hydration provided along with chemotherapy is reportable only if done before or after chemotherapy, not during the chemotherapy infusion. For IV hydration done during the chemotherapy infusion, it is appropriate to report the HCPCS code for the supply of the substance infused, even though the administration service will not be separately reimbursed. Certain chemotherapeutic agents, such as cisplatin, require hydration before or after infusion, whereas others, such as carboplatin (Paraplatin), do not require any hydration.

The CPT guidelines clarify when an E/M service code can be reported in addition to chemotherapy administration. If the E/M history, exam, and medical decision making are documented in addition to the description of chemotherapy services, both can be reported by appending a –25 modifier to the E/M service.

If physician practices are charging all patients across the board (non-Medicare and governmental carriers), without exception, for telephone or online E/M services, the Medicare patient may also be billed for the services. The office should notify the patient prior to providing the service that it is not a covered service and have the patient sign an Advance Beneficiary Notice (ABN) of noncoverage form.

A Medicare claim does not need to be filed for these services unless the patient requests it. If a claim is filed, the –GY modifier must be appended to the CPT code, signifying that the practice is not expecting Medicare to pay for the service. Before submitting these codes to insurance carriers, staff members should ask whether they reimburse for telephone or online assessments or management. The current policies of most major carriers are available on their websites.

Actinotherapy

Actinotherapy uses ultraviolet B (UVB) light to treat skin diseases, especially cancer. UVB is the ionizing ray of the sun's spectrum that causes sunburn and tanning. According to CMS policy, certain diagnoses are appropriate indications for actinotherapy, including but not limited to atopic dermatitis, psoriasis, and acne. Code 96900 is reported once per session. Therefore, if actinotherapy is performed on different anatomical areas, for example, the hand and forehead, code 96900 should be reported one time only.

Photochemotherapy

Photochemotherapy (PUVA) is a type of treatment used for severe skin diseases that uses a combination of medication application and ultraviolet A (UVA) light to destroy the skin lesion. Drugs such as methoxsalen (8-methoxypsoralen), 5-methoxypsoralen, and trisoralen are applied to the skin, making the skin photosensitive, and then the UVA light is applied.

Ultraviolet A is closer to visible light and less damaging than ultraviolet B, which is ionizing. According to CMS policy, several diagnoses are appropriate indications for 96910–96913, including, but not limited to psoriasis, atopic dermatitis, lichen planus, and vitiligo. Photochemotherapy should not be billed for more than 30 units in 45 days.

Active Wound Care Management Codes

The Medicine section also has debridement codes that may be provided by physicians and nonphysician practitioners. Codes in the Active Wound Care Management series provide a mechanism for reporting services performed by licensed nonphysician professionals, such as physician assistants (PAs), nurse practitioners (NPs), enterostomal therapy nurses, physical therapists (PTs), and occupational therapists (OTs). Only those individuals licensed by a particular state to perform the described services should use the codes to report services. State laws and requirements determine who may perform these specific types of services. Codes 97597–97606 involve wound care and removal of tissue that is nonexcisional, commonly performed by PTs and nurses, and the procedures do not require the use of anesthesia. Codes 97597–97598 are reported per session, as described in the code descriptor, using the total wound(s) surface area as the determinant of the appropriate code, not each wound treated.

Codes are chosen based on debridement type: selective or nonselective. Whirlpool therapy and maggot therapy are some examples of nonselective debridement. The Centers for Medicare and Medic-

Remember that all procedures on the MPFS are assigned a global period of 000, 010, 090, XXX, YYY, or ZZZ. The global concept does not apply to XXX procedures. The global period for YYY procedures is defined by the carrier. All procedures with a global period of ZZZ are related to another procedure, and the applicable global period for the ZZZ code is determined by the related procedure. During this time, the surgeon cannot bill for a follow-up visit that is related to that surgery, including E/M visits.

Debridement codes are reported for each site treated. The additional sites would be coded and appended with the –59 modifier.

Codes 97597–97606 cannot be reported in conjunction with 11040–11044. Codes 97597, 97598, 97602 include chemical cauterization code 17250.

■ **CASE SCENARIOS**

A 78-year-old male has developed a pressure ulcer on the sacrum from being bedridden due to total hip replacement. He reports pain from the ulcerated area. The wound is covered with black eschar and is surrounded by chronic inflammation with dark pigmentation. At this time, he is not a safe candidate for surgery, but it is felt that he would benefit from sharp debridement of the necrotic tissue.

The wound is measured and cleansed. The sacral wound measures 5.5 cm × 1.5 cm with a black wound bed. No active drainage is present. The surrounding tissue is palpated to identify the wound margin. Sharp debridement was carried out using scissors and forceps to remove the devitalized tissue and facilitate subsequent wound healing. An enzymatic agent, saline gauze, and a composite dressing are placed directly on the wound bed. Codes: 97597, A6203.

aid Services (CMS) has many wound care policies that are specific to the type of selective or nonselective debridement performed, the respective diagnosis, and what type of therapist is performing the service—an OT or PT. Wound care management services billed by therapists must be submitted with either the GO or GP modifier. GO is defined as "services delivered under an outpatient occupational therapy plan of care." GP is reported by PTs to depict "services delivered under an outpatient physical therapy plan of care." CPT codes 97597 and 97598 require the presence of devitalized tissue. If any secretions are present, these codes should not be reported.

The procedures associated with CPT codes 97597, 97598, 97605, and 97606 are not expected to be needed more frequently than once a week. If the debridement of chronic ulcers requires more than eight units of service to promote healing, the rationale and medical necessity for more frequent services must be clearly documented in the medical record.

PHYSICAL MEDICINE AND REHABILITATION

This area of coding encompasses physical therapy evaluations, occupational therapy evaluations, athletic training evaluations, modalities, therapeutic procedures, active wound care management, test and measurements and orthotic management and prosthetic management. All of these services are considered distinct procedures; therefore, modifier 51 would not be appended to codes 97010–97763

Physical Therapy Evaluations

To report physical therapy evaluations, the following components must be documented: history, examination, clinical decision making, and development of plan of care. Do not confuse these terms with similar terms in the evaluation and management codes. This section's terminology has different meanings.

The code levels require documentation of the clinical decision making and the severity of the patient's condition. Coders should know the body regions, and body systems, body structures and personal factors. As an example, code 97161 requires a physical therapy evaluation of low complexity and the following components: history without personal factors; examination with 1 to 2 elements from body structures, body functions, activity limitations and/or participation restrictions; a clinical presentation with stable and/or uncomplicated characteristics and low complexity clinical decision making. The time factor is 20 minutes face-to-face with patient and or family.

Occupational Therapy Evaluations

To report occupational therapy evaluations, the following components must be documented: occupational profile and the client's medical and therapy histories, assessments of occupational performance, and the development of plan of care.

The code levels require documentation of the performance deficits, physical skills, cognitive skills and psychosocial skills. As an example, code 97165 requires a brief history including the review of medical and/or therapy records that relate to the presenting problem, identification of 1 to 3 performance deficits that resulted in activity limitations and/or participation restrictions, and clinical decision making of low complexity. The time factor is 30 minutes spent with the patient and/or family.

Athletic Training Evaluations

To report athletic training evaluations, the following components must be documented: a history and physical activity profile, an examination, clinical decision making, and the development of a plan of care. As an example, code 97169 requires a history and a physical activity profile, no co-morbidities affecting physical activity, examination of affected body area and other symptomatic or related systems addressing 1 to 2 elements from any of the following: body structures, physical activity, and/or participation deficiencies, and clinical decision making of low complexity. The time factor is 15 minutes spent with patient and/or family.

NON–FACE-TO-FACE SERVICES

CPT has provisions for reporting E/M services that do not require the provider to be face to face with the patient, such as via the telephone and Internet. Online assessments and consultations are referred to as *e-visits, online E/M visits,* or *Web visits.* These are nonemergent or nonurgent communications between a qualified nonphysician practitioner and an established patient and must be initiated by the patient or the patient's caregiver.

Code set 98966–98969 is used to report telephone and Internet E/M services provided by qualified nonphysician health-care professionals. Included in this group are staff members to whom the physician delegates responsibility for performing telephone E/M services, typically registered nurses and nurse practitioners. Codes are based on time spent on the phone or online with the patient.

To report a non–face-to-face code, the service cannot be an integral part of the preservice work of a subsequent E/M visit or part of the postservice workup for previous service. Coders and providers must be aware of when the physician last saw the patient in order to submit these codes. This concept is similar to the surgical global period, where services are bundled into one comprehensive service for a period of time. Non–face-to-face services are subject to a 7-day preservice or visit global period.

EXAMPLE

A physician treats a patient in the office for a problem. Five days later, a qualified staff member discusses the problem with the patient on the phone. The telephone service cannot be reported.

If the qualified staff member provides an e-visit, code 98969 (*Online assessment and management service provided by a qualified nonphysician health-care professional to an established patient or guardian not originating from a related assessment and management service provided within the previous 7 days, using the Internet or similar electronic communications network*) is assigned. If the patient schedules an appointment with the provider to take place within 24 hours of the online or telephone service, or schedules the soonest available appointment, only the office visit can be billed.

Telephone service codes 98966–98968 can be reported only if the telephone call is unrelated to any service within the past week. To appropriately document this service, be sure that the provider develops separate documentation to show that the call is significant and independent of other recently provided services and was initiated by the patient or guardian of the patient.

For example, when a nurse provides a telephone service and the physician sees the patient for the same problem within 24 hours of the call, or sees the patient at the next available visit after the call, the office must forgo billing for the call. The provider reports only the E/M service for the office visit.

Non–face-to-face services such as telephone services and online medical evaluations must be carefully documented. Documentation must include information on the total time spent communicating with the patient by the health-care professional and when the previous E/M face-to-face visit occurred to establish a timeline. If a patient received E/M services during the period following the call or online contact, or 7 days prior to the non–face-to-face services, the services cannot be reported separately. If the Internet or telephone communication results in the patient subsequently being seen in the office within 24 hours or at the next available appointment, the services cannot be reported.

SPECIAL SERVICES, PROCEDURES, AND REPORTS

Codes 99000–99091 identify adjunct services that are reported in addition to basic services such as E/M services. Modifier –51 is not reported with codes 99050–99060. This coding area represents services such as the handling and/or conveyance of a specimen transferred from the physician's office to a laboratory for testing. If an E/M service was provided and blood was taken for analysis and then prepared for conveyance to the lab, the provider would report the E/M code, the code for venipuncture (36415, if that was the method of obtaining the blood), and 99000. For services that would normally be provided in the physician's office but were provided out of the office at the patient's request, the provider would report the E/M service and code 99056. Coders must carefully review this area to be sure they have captured all services provided.

MODERATE (CONSCIOUS) SEDATION

Moderate sedation is moderate anesthesia carried out by intravenously injecting a sedative and/or analgesic to relieve pain and anxiety during a medical procedure. Analgesics, unlike most anesthesia, relieve pain without the loss of consciousness. The patient remains awake and relaxed and may have amnesia after the procedure is completed. The patient breathes on his or her own, so no airway intervention is needed. Procedures performed under moderate sedation are typically performed in an office or clinic setting, not in the operating room.

> The moderate sedation codes are age based and timed. Carefully review the code descriptions for age and time.

Instead of involving an anesthesia provider, moderate sedation is done by the surgeon who is performing the surgery and also requires the presence of an independent, trained observer. The surgeon must supervise the assistant delegated to monitor and document the patient's condition throughout the procedure. The supervising physician must be able to recognize deep sedation, manage the consequences, and adjust the level of sedation to a moderate or lesser level. The nurse or assistant administering the medication must continually assess patient consciousness and cardiac and respiratory function.

When moderate sedation is provided by another physician or qualified individual, the services are reported with codes 99155–99157. Intraservice time and the age of the patient are additional requirements in the selection of the codes. CPT also provides extensive guidelines as to what is preservice and postservice work. Coders will need to be aware of these services, which are included in the intraservice work associated with moderate sedation, but for reporting purposes the time needed to provide pre- and postservice work is not used to determine the code time. For example, the patient may be under moderate sedation for 30 minutes but the preservice work took 15 minutes and postservice work took 20 minutes. The only time that is allowed for code selection is the 30 minutes of intraservice work.

EXAMPLES

- A urologist performs an ablation of renal tumor (code 50593) in the office on a 50-year-old male patient. The urologist contracts with a certified registered nurse anesthetist (CRNA) to come to the office to perform conscious sedation. The conscious sedation code can be reported separately by the CRNA, who is not employed by the practice and whose service is separate from the professional service of the physician. If the procedure requires 30 minutes of conscious sedation, the CRNA will report 99156 and 99157.

- A physician performs a dilation of the esophagus (code 43453) under conscious sedation in the practice-owned surgery center on a 35-year-old patient. The physician supervises the nurse administering Versed IV push for 45 minutes. The surgeon will report 43453, 99152, and 99153 x 2.

Assign codes to the following procedures for the physician.

1. A patient is seen in the OB/GYN oncology office for nonhormonal chemotherapy injection.

_____

2. An established patient with a history of rhinitis leading to sinusitis calls the physician to discuss new acute sinusitis symptoms. The nurse speaks to the patient for 15 minutes to obtain a history via telephone and assess the patient's condition, then talks to the doctor. The doctor decides to call in an order for an antibiotic rather than have the patient come to the office for examination.

_____

3. A 65-year-old patient needs to have a percutaneous gastrostomy tube inserted with fluoroscopic guidance in the outpatient surgery center. The physician does the procedure and provides moderate sedation, and a qualified trained nurse is present to monitor the patient during the procedure. The physician reports codes 49440, 99151, 99153 × 3 for the 45-minute procedure. The physician spent an additional 20 minutes in pre- and post-service work. Is the physician correct? Explain your answer.

_____

4. A patient is seen for the first chemotherapy session for recently diagnosed bone cancer. An infusion of 100 mcg of Kytril is provided. Kytril is infused at 1:15 p.m. and ends at 1:35 p.m. The RN administering the infusion is continuously present for the infusion. Code for the administration.

_____

Chapter Summary

1. Immunization services have their own administration codes (90460–90474), and the selection of the codes is based on whether or not counseling was provided to the patient or patient's family and on the method of administration. The immune globulin codes also have their own administration codes in the therapeutic, prophylactic, and diagnostic injections and infusions codes (96365–96379).

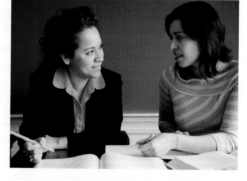

2. Infusion is performed primarily as a therapeutic service but can also be done for diagnostic purposes. Infusions are used for intravenous immune globulins, drugs and other substances, and hydration. All require different administration codes. For IV infusion to be coded and billed, an order from the physician with the specific type of IV solution and flow rate must be present. Total infusion time must be known and documented in the record. The first-hour infusion codes cannot be billed until the infusion has run for more than 15 minutes, and then they cover up to 90 minutes. Infusions of 15 minutes or less should be coded and billed as intravenous (or intra-arterial) pushes (codes 96374–96375). An IV push of the same substance more than once is coded differently from a second IV push of a different substance. Infusion of two substances simultaneously is considered concurrent, subsequent, or sequential administration. Facilities have a hierarchy for reporting infusions and injections. If chemotherapy, prophylactic, therapeutic, or diagnostic infusion occurs on

the same day as hydration, chemotherapy is primary, the drug infusion is secondary, and the hydration is tertiary. Infusions are primary to IV pushes, which are primary to injections. This hierarchy does not apply to physician reporting.

3. Infusion is IV therapy in which medication from a bag or bottle is infused (dripped) into a patient's vein over time. Subcutaneous infusion differs from IV infusion in that a needle is placed in the upper arm, abdomen, or flank to administer fluids or medication directly into subcutaneous tissues. Therapeutic, prophylactic, or diagnostic injection, unlike infusion, delivers a dosage of medication or other substance in one shot, rather than slowly over time. An injection is provided to achieve an immediate effect, typically within 3 to 5 minutes. Injections provided directly through a saline lock are considered IV injections. Code assignment is based on the purpose of the infusion or injection and the substance administered.

4. ESRD codes are assigned by whether or not the services were provided for a full month (30 days) or on a per-day basis. Further distinction is made based on the number of physician assessments provided during that time period. Location is another factor, because specific codes are used for patients receiving their dialysis at home. There are also codes for inpatient dialysis treatments (90935–90937) that are additionally based on the number of physician assessments.

5. The cardiography section contains several noninvasive tests to assess heart rate, rhythm, heart muscle damage, and the heart's ability to pump. Many of them measure the amount of electrical activity. An echocardiogram can provide information on the heart's size, shape, and pumping capacity; on the location and extent of any damage to its tissues and valve function; on blood flow patterns; and on back flow (regurgitation). Codes for routine ECGs allow the coder to choose the level of service based on whether the physician is billing globally or only provided components of the test. Routine ECGs are different from rhythm ECGs. Rhythm ECGs require an order prompted by some type of event, followed by a report. Stress test code assignment is based on whether the physician provided the global service.

6. Basic cardiac catheterization services are captured within one code that represents the placement of the catheter, the angiography services, and the imaging supervision and interpretation. An example is code 93458: The coronary angiography and imaging supervision and interpretation are captured within the parent code 93454. Code 93458 then adds the left heart catheterization and the left ventriculography. Add-on codes are reported for additional services such as right ventriculography and pulmonary angiography, which are also reported. The congenital cardiac anomaly codes for cardiac catheterization are coded differently. One code captures the catheterization, and a separate code is reported for the injection angiography and the imaging supervision and interpretation.

7. Allergy testing by such methods as blood tests, intracutaneous testing, and percutaneous testing is conducted to identify to what the patient is allergic (allergen). Documentation should state how many allergens are being tested for and how they are being tested. Before assigning immunotherapy codes, coders should determine whether the physician provided the allergenic extracts, simply administered the injection, or both. Sets of codes are provided for each circumstance. Codes are based on whether the preparation dose is from a single dose or based on a number of doses. Separate codes are provided for stinging venom insect immunotherapy.

8. EEG and EMG electrodiagnostic studies are similar in that each measures electrical activity, but of different anatomical areas and for different purposes. EMG is the study and recording of the electrical properties of muscles and the action generated by the muscle cells. It uses electrodes to measure muscle tension in the body and monitor for excessive muscle movement. EEG involves placing electrodes on the scalp to record electrical activity produced by the brain.

9. Chemotherapy can be administered in several ways; code descriptions are specific to mode of administration. Infusion time must be documented by nursing staff. The provision of the chemotherapy access or catheterization service is coded separately. Preparation of the drug is included in the administration code. A code is submitted for each method used to administer the antineoplastic agent. IV hydration provided along with chemotherapy is reportable only if done before or after, not during, chemotherapy. Code 96409 (chemotherapy administration, subcutaneous or intramuscular; intravenous, push technique, push, single or initial substance/drug) is submitted once for each drug administered, but can be reported only once per encounter regardless of the number of IV pushes of the same chemotherapy agent administered.

10. Online assessments and consultations are referred to as e-visits, online E/M visits, and Web visits. Codes 98966–98969 report telephone and Internet assessment and management services provided by qualified nonphysician health-care professionals. To report these codes, the service cannot be an integral part of preservice work prior to an E/M service or postservice work for a previous E/M service. If as a result of this service the patient is seen within 24 hours or at the soonest available appointment, the services cannot be reported. Non–face-to-face services are subject to a 7-day preservice or visit global period.

Review Questions

Matching

A. intravenous push
B. percutaneous transluminal coronary intervention, angioplasty
C. angiography
D. antigen
E. infusion
F. electroencephalogram
G. immunization
H. percutaneous transluminal coronary thrombectomy
I. electromyography
J. immune globulin

Match the key terms with their definitions.

1. _____ Injecting contrast medium and imaging the contrast in the vessel

2. _____ Helps the body develop protection against certain diseases by injecting a small amount of antigen

3. _____ A foreign substance in the body

4. _____ Therapy in which medication is dripped into a patient's vein over a course of time

5. _____ Physician threads a balloon-tipped catheter from the groin or the arm to the site of a narrow or blocked artery

6. _____ Inserting a balloon catheter into the vein to remove a clot

7. _____ Infusion of 15 minutes or less

8. _____ Produce antibodies prior to exposure to the disease

9. _____ Recording brain activity

10. _____ Recording of the electrical properties of muscles and the action generated by the muscle cells

True or False

Decide whether each statement is true or false.

1. _____ If the patient receives an infusion of a single drug that lasts 1 hour 45 minutes, the physician reports code 96365 for up to 1 hour and code +96366 for the additional 45 minutes.

2. _____ A pregnant mother is seen in the OB/GYN office for an injection of RhoGAM because she is a different blood type than the baby. CPT code 96372 should be submitted.

3. _____ Code 99026 from the Medicine section may be assigned to indicate a postoperative follow-up office visit.

4. _____ ESRD codes include monitoring of nutrition, assessment of growth and development, and parental counseling for patients under the age of 20 years.

5. _____ Moderate sedation is a form of anesthesia in which the patient is awake but still needs assistance in breathing.

6. _____ Separate cardiac catheterization codes exist for pulmonary artery angiography.

7. _____ Hierarchy rules for the complexity of percutaneous coronary therapeutic services and procedures state that if an angioplasty, atherectomy, and stent procedure are done on the same vessel, only the stent procedure is reported.

8. _____ Medicare considers CPT codes 95120–95134 to be invalid and does not recognize them.

9. _____ The lightning bolt (⚡) symbol located in CPT alerts the coder that this is a highly reimbursable product.

10. _____ CPT codes 90957 and 90959 can be reported together for the same month.

Multiple Choice

Select the letter that best completes the statement or answers the question.

1. A patient receives an antiemetic via IV infusion for 10 minutes, followed by 2 hours 30 minutes of chemo infusion. Report codes
   A. 96413, +96415, +96375
   B. 96413 × 2, 96365
   C. 96372, 96413, +96415
   D. 96413 × 2, +96372

2. A patient arrives in the ED with a 2-day history of gastroenteritis, nausea, and vomiting. IV hydration is begun at 100 mL/hour at 0300 hours. The patient receives one IV push Versed, and IV is continued until the patient is discharged at 0435. Report codes
   A. 96365, +96366, 96374
   B. 96360, +96361, +96375
   C. 96360, 96374
   D. 96365, 96360

3. A patient receives one antibiotic infusion for 45 minutes. The patient requires two different antibiotics, but the two drugs cannot be administered simultaneously. The second antibiotic is infused for an additional 25 minutes. What is the correct code assignment?
   A. 96365, +96376
   B. 96365 × 2
   C. 96365, +96367
   D. 96365

4. A young child's behavior has dramatically changed over a period of weeks. Her internist has recommended that she see a psychiatrist. The child is unable to speak, even though she is 8 years old and capable of speech. The first visit with the patient goes well, and the psychiatrist recommends psychotherapy. Code for the initial visit with the child.
   A. 90791
   B. 90791, +90785
   C. 90792
   D. 90792, +90785

5. A 45-year-old patient received outpatient ESRD-related services for 5 days and then was admitted to the hospital for inpatient dialysis and evaluation. The patient remained in the hospital for 4 days and returned to resume his outpatient dialysis for the rest of the month. Once back in outpatient dialysis, he had two face-to-face visits with the physician but no complete assessment was provided during that month. What code(s) will be reported for the outpatient services provided during that month?
   A. 90961
   B. 90961 × 26
   C. 90967
   D. 90970 × 26

6. Percutaneous transluminal coronary thrombectomy and percutaneous coronary atherectomy performed in the left circumflex artery are coded as
   A. 92924
   B. 92924, +92973
   C. 92924–22
   D. 92933, +92973

7. What is the correct code assignment for bilateral EMG of cranial nerves?
   A. 95867
   B. 95867–50
   C. 95868
   D. 95868–50

8. Moderate sedation codes are based on
   A. Age of patient and duration of service
   B. Duration of service, location
   C. Age of patient, duration of service, provider of service, location
   D. Age of patient, type of agent used, duration of service

9. A 2-year-old patient is seen for his measles, mumps, and rubella vaccine. The patient's parents are very concerned about the side effects of vaccination and ask to consult with the physician before the vaccination administration. The parents then agree to the vaccine, and it is administered subcutaneously. What is the correct code assignment?
   A. 90707, 90704, 90460
   B. 90707, 90471
   C. 90707, 90460, +90461
   D. 90707, 90460, 90461 × 2

10. For left heart catheterization with coronary angiography, left ventriculography, and pulmonary angiography, the physician reports code(s)
    A. 93452, 93454, +93568
    B. 93458, +93568
    C. 93458
    D. 93452

11. Coronary thrombolysis by IV infusion is coded as
    A. 92977
    B. 92975
    C. 92977, 92975
    D. 92977–22

12. What does ⊘ mean?
    A. The coder cannot append a –51 modifier.
    B. Conscious sedation is separately reportable.
    C. The code is likely to be audited.
    D. Conscious sedation is included in the surgical service and not separately reported.

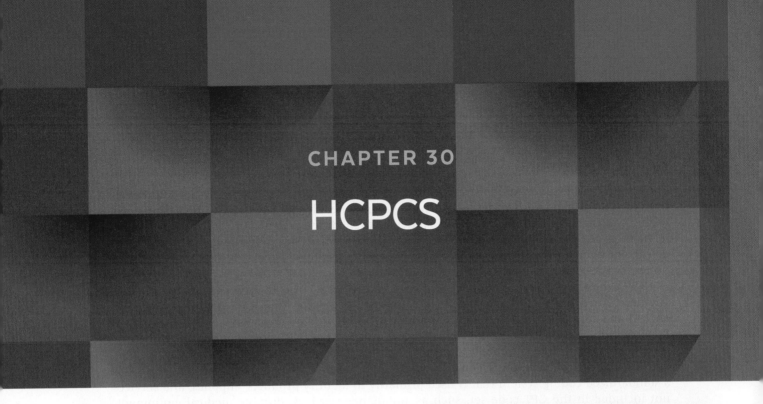

HCPCS

CHAPTER OUTLINE

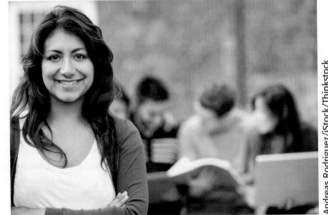

Andreas Rodriguez/iStock/Thinkstock

LEARNING OUTCOMES

After studying this chapter, you should be able to:

1. Explain the purpose of the HCPCS code set.
2. Differentiate between HCPCS Level I (CPT) and HCPCS Level II codes.
3. Identify circumstances under which codes from both HCPCS Level I and HCPCS Level II are required.
4. Compare permanent and temporary HCPCS codes.
5. Describe the content and organization of the Index, Table of Drugs, and main text in HCPCS.
6. Discuss the sources of information needed to keep current with HCPCS changes.
7. Understand the HCPCS A–V code sections.
8. Describe the purpose and correct usage of HCPCS modifiers, including ABN modifiers.
9. Choose the correct medication code based on the route of administration and the amount of medication administered.
10. Apply rules for choosing which level of HCPCS code to assign.

The national codes for products, supplies, and those services not included in CPT are located in the Healthcare Common Procedure Coding System (HCPCS). Establishing the medical necessity of these items for reimbursement is handled through the correct coding process for assigning HCPCS codes, as explained in this chapter.

HISTORY AND PURPOSE OF HCPCS

HCPCS Background

The Health Care Finance Administration (HCFA) Common Procedure Coding System was developed in 1983 to standardize codes for Medicare program health-care claims based on a three-level coding system for services and procedures provided to Medicare patients. In 2002, HCFA changed its name to the Centers for Medicare and Medicaid Services (CMS), and the code set was given its current name of the Healthcare Common Procedure Coding System (HCPCS), which is pronounced "Hic-Picks."

HCPCS has two main parts: HCPCS Level I and HCPCS Level II. Level I of HCPCS is CPT (Current Procedural Terminology), which is maintained by the American Medical Association (AMA) and contains codes that are used primarily to identify medical services and procedures furnished by physicians and other health-care professionals. CPT does not include the codes required to separately report medical supplies, drugs, or certain services that are regularly billed by health-care providers, physicians, or suppliers. Level II of HCPCS fills this need. Level II is a standardized coding system that is used primarily to identify products, supplies, and services not included in the CPT code set, such as ambulance services, durable medical equipment, prosthetics, orthotics, drugs, and supplies when provided outside of a physician office. Physician offices also use the codes for supplies provided to patients as well as certain services such as immunizations, examinations, and counseling rendered to government insurance program beneficiaries, such as Medicare and Medicaid patients. HCPCS codes are reported for supplies and drugs used for treating a patient or for supplies dispensed to a patient in any place of service regardless of the type of insurance a patient may possess. Medicare developed this coding system, but all insurance carriers use it to reimburse for these services and supplies (with the exception of the G, H, Q, S, and T codes discussed later in this chapter). Medicare and Medicaid require that certain procedural services be reported with HCPCS codes for proper reimbursement, whereas a corresponding CPT code would be reported for the same service for a patient with commercial insurance. For example, Medicare requires providers to submit code G0008, *Administration of influenza virus vaccine*, for reimbursement instead of CPT codes 90471, 90653–90658, 90661–90662, and 90666–90756.

> For Medicare and most Medicaid programs, if a Level II code exists for a service to be reported, select it rather than a CPT code (e.g., G and Q codes). HCPCS codes were developed even when there were existing identical CPT codes because of specific CMS reimbursement policies. If the patient is a member of a commercial plan, submit the appropriate Level I (CPT) code.

Purpose of HCPCS

HCPCS is a system for identifying medical services and supplies, not a payment methodology. The fact that a HCPCS code is available for assignment does not guarantee payment for the item. Decisions regarding coverage and allowed amounts are made by carriers and are independent of the decision for adding, deleting, or revising a HCPCS code. Physicians, facilities, and suppliers select HCPCS codes for items they are billing to the insurance carrier. Most often, the HCPCS code represents the physical supply of an item and not a professional service or procedure for actually applying or inserting the item, for which a code would be selected from HCPCS Level I (CPT). Refer to Table 30.1 for a comparison of these two levels.

There are well over 4,000 HCPCS codes for products and supplies. The code description represents the definition of the item or service provided. The descriptors do not refer to specific products by brand name or trade name. Items can be located only in the HCPCS codebook by type of product or supply or service.

Table 30.1 HCPCS Level Comparison

Level I	CPT	Level II	HCPCS (national codes)
Location	CPT book	Location	HCPCS book, CMS website
Publisher	AMA	Publisher	CMS
Code format	Five-digit numeric, except for Category II and Category III codes; codes begin with a number	Code format	Five-digit alphanumeric codes begin with A–V
Modifiers	Two-digit numeric	Modifiers	Two-digit alphanumeric or alphabetic
Use	Physician procedures and services; facility outpatient procedures and services	Use	Physician and nonphysician services; supplies, drugs, durable medical equipment, ambulance
Updated	Annually: the AMA CPT Editorial Panel meets quarterly and new codes may be released throughout the year but typically do not become effective until January 1 of each year; biannually for Category II and Category III	Updated	Quarterly for temporary codes, annually for permanent codes

Level II codes are used to report physician and nonphysician services (e.g., physician assistants, nurse practitioners, audiologists, speech pathologists, chiropractors), surgical supplies, medications dispensed or administered, ambulance transports, and durable medical equipment. Durable medical equipment (DME) is ordered by a physician, used at home, primarily and customarily used to serve a medical purpose, generally not useful to a person in the absence of illness or injury, and designed to withstand repeated use. Some examples of DME include hospital beds, walkers, wheelchairs, transfer benches with commode seats, and oxygen tents. An example of DME listings in the HCPCS book is shown in Box 30.1. Medical supplies of an expendable nature, such as bandages, rubber gloves, and irrigating kits, are not considered by Medicare to be DME.

BOX 30.1 Example of HCPCS Durable Medical Equipment Listings

L8000 Breast prosthesis, mastectomy bra
L8001 Breast prosthesis, mastectomy bra, with integrated breast prosthesis form, unilateral
L8002 Breast prosthesis, mastectomy bra, with integrated breast prosthesis form, bilateral
L8010 Breast prosthesis, mastectomy sleeve
L8015 External breast prosthesis garment, with mastectomy form, post mastectomy
L8020 Breast prosthesis, mastectomy form
L8030 Breast prosthesis, silicone or equal, without integral adhesive
L8031 Breast prosthesis, silicone or equal, with integral adhesive
L8032 Nipple prosthesis, reusable, any type, each
L8035 Custom breast prosthesis, post mastectomy, molded to patient model

Medicare contracts with four durable medical equipment regional carriers (DMERCs), also known as durable medical equipment Medicare administrative contractors (DME MACs). These carriers process Medicare claims for durable medical equipment, prosthetics, orthotics, and supplies (DMEPOS). Each DME MAC covers one of four geographic regions of the country, and is responsible for processing DMEPOS claims. Claims jurisdiction (i.e., the place to which the provider sends the claim) is determined by the state in which the beneficiary permanently resides. DMEPOS dealers or supply companies provide patients with DME and supplies. DMEPOS claims for items provided to patients by physicians or suppliers are sent to one of the regional DME MACs.

Providers and DME suppliers must comply with CMS quality standards in order to obtain a provider or supplier billing number or to furnish any DME, prosthetic device, or orthotic item or service for which Medicare Part B makes payment. If physicians intend to supply patients seen in their office with DME (e.g., wrist splint), they must obtain a DME provider number and report it on each DME claim submitted to the DME MAC. When providers treat patients in their office and provide DME, two claims must be generated and sent to two different locations to obtain payment for the service rendered and the supply of the item.

EXAMPLE

A patient is seen in the podiatrist's office for diabetic foot care. The physician issues the patient a special diabetic shoe that is direct formed, compression molded to the patient's foot. The claim for the evaluation and management (E/M) service will go to the local Medicare carrier claims processing center, and a separate claim with the provider's DME provider number for the shoe (HCPCS code A5510) will be sent to the regional MAC claims processing center for that area.

DME items are not payable under the Medicare Physician Fee Schedule (MPFS) because they are priced and reimbursed under the DMEPOS fee schedule. Codes are indicated as such with a specific symbol. Table 30.2 provides an excerpt of the fee schedule and an example of how applying modifiers to a code affects payment received. Modifiers are discussed later in this chapter.

For certain items or services billed by a supplier to a DMERC, the supplier must first receive a signed certificate of medical necessity (CMN) from the treating physician. Suppliers are required to have a faxed or copied original signed order or CMN in their records before they can submit a claim for payment to Medicare. CMNs communicate required medical necessity information and must be maintained by the supplier and made available to the DMERCs, who can ask for additional documentation to support the claim.

Table 30.2 DMEPOS Fee Schedule Example

HCPCS CODE	MODIFIER	JURISDICTION	ALABAMA
E0140	–NU	D	$333.94
E0140	–RR	D	$33.40
E0140	–UE	D	$250.47

INTERNET RESOURCE: To obtain timely and accurate payment for DME, the claim must be sent to the correct DME MAC. Determine the jurisdiction in which the provider resides by reviewing the jurisdiction map located on the CMS website. Additional information, such as the DMEPOS fee schedule, *Medicare Claims Processing Manual* chapter specific to DME, and links to the DMERC sites, can be obtained by visiting the DME specialty page on the CMS website. https://www.cms.gov/Center/Provider-Type/Durable-Medical-Equipment -DME-Center.html

HCPCS Today

In October 2003, the U.S. Department of Health and Human Services, acting under the Health Insurance Portability and Accountability Act (HIPAA), authorized CMS to maintain, update, and distribute HCPCS Level II codes. The CMS HCPCS Workgroup, made up of representatives from CMS and private insurance agencies as well as consultants from federal agencies, manages this process while also providing input as to what is necessary to meet each party's operational needs.

HCPCS codes are submitted to insurance carriers by physicians' offices, facilities, and other providers such as medical supply companies and home health agencies. HCPCS codes are required for reporting services, injections, materials, and supplies to federally funded programs (i.e., Medicare, Medicaid, TRICARE, and CHAMPVA) and private insurance

HCPCS is the mandated code set for reporting supplies, orthotic and prosthetic devices, and DME under the HIPAA Electronic Health Care Transactions and Code Sets standards.

carriers. Payer-specific reporting requirements for procedures, services, and supplies are located in the contracts between the providers and payers.

Who accepts HCPCS codes? All health plan entities are required to, per HIPAA as follows:

- HMO
- Medicare Part A and Part B and supplemental issuer
- Medicaid
- Long-term care (LTC) policy issuer
- Employee welfare benefit plan or other plan intended to provide benefits to employees of two or more employers
- Military and veteran personnel health-care programs
- CHAMPUS, FEHBP
- State child health plan
- High-risk pools
- Any other individual or group plan

Regularly used HCPCS codes should be on the office encounter form, superbill, or charge description master (CDM) and updated quarterly.

HCPCS codes can have a significant impact on the financial bottom line for practices and facilities. Revenue is lost each time a supply is used or an injection is given and the health-care claim does not reflect a HCPCS code. For example, if Medicare is billed for an injection using only a CPT code, the office will be paid for the injection but not for the actual drug administered. For physicians and facilities, the most commonly used HCPCS codes are for medical/surgical supplies and injections. Other providers, such as skilled nursing facilities (SNFs), use many of the HCPCS codes that describe equipment sold or rented as DMEs or medical appliances provided by supply companies.

HCPCS Code Format

HCPCS Level II codes are five alphanumeric characters in length. Each code begins with a letter from A through V followed by four numbers.

EXAMPLE
J1100 is the code for *Injection, dexamethasone acetate, 1 mg.*

Like CPT, HCPCS Level II has a unique set of modifiers. Discontinued (deleted) procedure codes and modifiers will appear in the HCPCS file located online at CMS for 4 years to facilitate claims processing. Unlike CPT, deleted HCPCS codes are also printed in the HCPCS codebook in their previous location with a line drawn through them for 1 year following the deletion. (This may vary depending on the publisher of the HCPCS code book.) Deleted codes are also listed either at the beginning of the code book or in an appendix.

EXAMPLE
E0192, *Low pressure and positioning equalization pad, for wheelchair,* was deleted but printed in the next year's edition of the HCPCS book as follows: ~~E0192 Low pressure and positioning equalization pad, for wheelchair.~~

CHECKPOINT 30.1

Determine whether the following codes are CPT HCPCS (Level I) or HCPCS (Level II) codes. Two are given as examples.

28285 CPT   A4649 HCPCS

1. 15002 _____   4. J0520 _____

2. A0430 _____   5. 69990 _____

3. 72040 _____   6. E0992 _____

HOW HCPCS CODES ARE CREATED

HCPCS national Level II codes are categorized based on the purpose of the codes and on whom is responsible for establishing and maintaining them. The CMS HCPCS Workgroup is a code advisory committee made up of representatives from CMS and other government agencies. Its role is to identify services for which new codes are needed.

To create a new HCPCS code, physicians, suppliers, or manufacturers start the process by submitting an application. The application outlines requirements that must be met to constitute a need for a new code. Application requirements include the following:

- U.S. Food and Drug Administration (FDA) approval if regulated by the FDA
- Not capital equipment or exclusively used in an inpatient setting
- Product must be primarily medical in nature
- There must be a national program operating need for Medicare, Medicaid, or private insurers
- Product must have significant sales volume

Permanent Codes

The CMS HCPCS Workgroup maintains the permanent codes that are available for use by all government and private payers. No code changes can be made unless all panel members agree. Advisers from private payers provide input to the workgroup. This workgroup is responsible for making decisions about changes to existing permanent codes, including additions, revisions, and deletions to alphanumeric codes. Because HCPCS codes are available to all payers, the workgroup and the Statistical Analysis Durable Medical Equipment Regional Carriers (SADMERC) group participate. SADMERC is responsible for providing suppliers and manufacturers of devices, drugs, and supplies with guidance and assistance in determining the appropriate HCPCS Level II code to be used for their product. Decisions on any permanent code change are discussed and voted on by the workgroup. Once a code is assigned to a product, the manufacturer of the drug or supply provides the respective HCPCS code to sale representatives, documents it in paperwork associated with the supply, and often publishes the code on the manufacturer's webpage.

Temporary Codes

Temporary codes can be added, changed, or deleted on a quarterly basis. They serve the purpose of meeting the immediate needs of a particular payer. Once established and approved, temporary codes are usually implemented within 90 days. Time is needed to prepare and issue implementation instructions to providers and to enter the new code into CMS and contractor computer systems. This also allows time for bulletins and newsletters to be sent out to suppliers to provide them with information and assistance regarding the implementation of temporary codes.

Temporary codes, which begin with C, G, H, K, Q, S, and T, are updated quarterly. The changes are posted to the CMS website under the *HCPCS Releases and Code Sets* menu. Coders who regularly use these codes must stay current with the new and deleted items. Temporary codes may later be given permanent status if they are widely used; otherwise, they will remain temporary indefinitely.

> **INTERNET RESOURCE: HCPCS quarterly updates are posted on the CMS website.**
> www.cms.gov/Medicare/Coding/HCPCSReleaseCodeSets/HCPCS_Quarterly_Update.html

FEATURES OF HCPCS CODEBOOKS AND OTHER CODING RESOURCES

Several publishers offer the HCPCS codes in book format. The codebooks have varying features such as color coding, general instructions for use, guidelines for each section, symbols to identify deleted codes, new codes, quantity alerts, age and gender edits, and appendixes. Each section begins with a short paragraph that describes the purpose of the section.

Introduction

The introduction to each publisher's HCPCS codebook is a valuable section that is often overlooked by coders. It provides instructions for using the book and how to decipher the color coding and symbols used throughout it. Read this section of your codebook before assigning any codes.

HCPCS Index and Code Sections

The HCPCS Index is arranged alphabetically, with the main term in bold print followed by the HCPCS Level II code. The listing of codes—the equivalent of the Tabular List section in the ICD and CPT sections—is organized alphabetically by the code range. Unlike CPT, very few anatomical terms are found in the Index. Pages are not tabbed in the books, but the edges are color typically coded to differentiate the various sections.

The books contain most, if not all, of the following additional material:

- Table of Drugs and Biologicals
- Modifiers (some books may print the modifiers on their inside covers)
- Common Abbreviations
- PUB 100 References
- New, Changed, Deleted, and Reinstated HCPCS Codes
- Place of Service and Type of Service
- National Average Payment Table for HCPCS
- Medically Unlikely Edits
- Deleted Code Crosswalk

The *Medicare Carriers Manual* (MCM) directs Medicare payers on coverage of services based on the two levels of coverage guidance (as explained in the Reimbursement Review on the following page).

Publishers of HCPCS codebooks, such as AMA, AAPC, and Optum, use their own system of symbols and color coding to indicate non-Medicare-covered codes, special coverage instructions, and carrier discretion. The legend for colors and symbols is located at the bottom of each page and in their manual's introduction. Many codes marked with special coverage instructions will provide reference to CMS *Medicare Claims Processing Manual* (MCPM), also known as Publication 100 (Pub 100)-04 or National Coverage Determination (NCD) (Pub 100-03). Pub 100 is the electronic version of the MCPM, which is located in the CMS *Internet-Only Manual* (IOM). The entries cited in the HCPCS Appendix Pub 100 References are taken straight from the manuals for easy reference. Many codes are followed by a number that references the specific manual where the respective policy or guideline is located.

> **INTERNET RESOURCE:** The IOM is located at
> https://www.cms.gov/Regulations-and-Guidance/Guidance/Manuals
> /Internet-Only-Manuals-IOMs.html Save this link to your favorites
> for future reference. This manual is a valuable source
> for coders and billers and applies to services performed
> in any place of service. Links to the official transmittals
> for changes in coverage decisions are located within the manual.

EXAMPLES

- E0782, *Infusion pump, implantable, non-programmable.* In some codebooks, the code is notated to indicate that a CMS policy applies to the item and to read and follow this guideline. For example, if 100-4, 4, 190 appears with the code, the 100-4 is PUB 100-4, 4 is the chapter reference, and 190 is the section number where this specific guideline can be read in its entirety.

- A4250, *Urine test or reagent strips or tablets (100 tablets or strips) 100-2,15,110.* Based on the notation, this supply is not covered by Medicare. However, when you read the reference, an explanation is provided that this may be covered if certain criteria are met.

Medicare Coverage Compliance

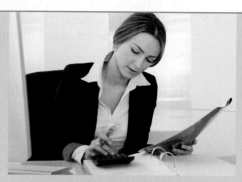

The CMS is responsible for promoting health-care services and delivery for its beneficiaries and maintaining payment processes that pay claims only for covered, medically necessary services at correct payment amounts and in a timely manner. Medicare coverage is regulated by federal laws that specify which procedures to treat conditions and illnesses are reimbursed, as well as which screening tests are paid.

For reimbursement, Medicare services must be covered and must meet Medicare's medical necessity criteria. To be considered medically necessary, a treatment must be:

- Appropriate for the symptoms or diagnoses of the illness or injury (i.e., in line with clinical practice standards)
- Not an elective procedure
- Not an experimental or investigational procedure
- An essential treatment; not performed for the patient's convenience
- Delivered at the most appropriate level that can safely and effectively be administered to the patient

Claims may be denied because the service provided is *excluded* by Medicare or because the service was *not reasonable and necessary* for the specific patient. Excluded services are not covered under any circumstances. The services that are excluded change from year to year. Other services that are not covered are classified as "not medically necessary" unless certain conditions are met, such as particular diagnoses. For example, a vitamin B_{12} injection is a covered service only for patients with certain diagnoses, such as pernicious anemia, but not for a diagnosis of fatigue. If the patient does not have one of the specified diagnoses, the B_{12} injection is categorized as not reasonable and necessary.

Determining Medicare Coverage

There are two coverage policies: National Coverage Determinations and Local Coverage Determinations. National Coverage Determinations (NCDs) describe whether specific medical items, services, treatment procedures, or technologies can be paid for under Medicare. The *NCD Manual* (Pub 100-03) is organized by categories, such as medical procedures, supplies, and diagnostic services. Local Coverage Determinations (LCDs) are developed to specify under which clinical circumstances a service is reasonable and necessary. It serves as an administrative and educational tool to assist providers in submitting claims correctly for payment. LCDs are also posted to an online Medicare manual.

NOTE: NCDs and LCDs are available online: https://www.cms.gov/medicare -coverage-database//search/advanced-search.aspx

Actions Required for Noncovered Services

Generally, providers may bill Medicare beneficiaries for services that are not covered by the Medicare program. Giving a patient written notification that Medicare will not pay for a service before providing it is a good policy, but it is not required. When patients are notified ahead of time, they understand their financial responsibility to pay for the service. CMS Form No. 20007, Notice of Exclusions from Medicare Benefits (NEMB), is available for this purpose. Providers use NEMBs on an entirely voluntary basis. Their purpose is to advise beneficiaries, before they receive services that are not Medicare benefits, that Medicare will not pay for them and to provide beneficiaries with an estimate of how much they may have to pay. Providers may also choose to design their own NEMBs based on the services they offer.

NEMB: Service not covered under Medicare. **ABN:** Medicare does not consider a service reasonable and necessary in this situation.

NOTE: Notice of Exclusions from Medicare Benefits form: www.cms.gov/Medicare/Medicare-General-Information/BNI

Providers also may not bill patients for services that Medicare declares as being not reasonable and necessary unless the patients were informed ahead of time in writing and agreed to pay for the services. If a provider thinks that a procedure will not be covered by Medicare because it is not reasonable and necessary, the patient is notified of this before the treatment by means of a standard Advance Beneficiary Notice (ABN) from CMS. A completed form is given to the patient for signature. The ABN is designed to:

- Identify the service or item that Medicare is unlikely to pay for
- State the reason Medicare is unlikely to pay
- Estimate how much the service or item will cost the beneficiary if Medicare does not pay

- Medicare prohibits the use of blanket ABNs given routinely to all patients just to ensure payment.
- Never have a patient sign a blank ABN for the physician to fill in later. The form must be completed before the patient signs it.

The ABN for general use is form CMS-R-131-G. Variations of the form for laboratory use (CMS-R-131-L) and home health care (CMS-R-296) are also available.

NOTE: Advance Beneficiary Notice form: www.cms.gov/Medicare/Medicare-General-Information/BNI/ABN.html

For inpatient services, a similar form is available called a *hospital-issued notice of noncoverage (HINN)*. This document has several formats instead of one mandated form.

Symbols

Symbols in HCPCS (Box 30.2) are similar to those used in CPT, although they can be located to the left of the code as well as to the right of the code description. HCPCS books have varying color coding and symbols; the legend at the bottom of each page depicts all of the symbols and color coding used and includes definitions to guide the coder in proper code selection. Coders must pay close attention to these. Remember, HCPCS is published by more than one publisher and color coding, symbols, and appendices may vary. The codes identified as revised, new, and reinstated change each year.

> CMS is not responsible for any errors in translation that might occur in private printings of HCPCS Level II codes or errors from the use of these publications.

BOX 30.2 Examples of Codebook Alerts and Notations Identified by Possible Symbols

◇ **Age Edit**
Example: G0101 Cervical or vaginal cancer screening; pelvic and clinical breast examination

■ **Maternity Only**
Example: E0602 Breast pump, manual, any type

▲ **Revised Code**

⊘ **SNF Excluded**
Example: L7170 Electronic elbow, Hosmer or equal, switch controlled

MED: Pub 100
Example: E0580 Nebulizer, durable, glass or autoclavable plastic, bottle type, for use with regulator or flowmeter

♂ **Male Only**
Example: E0325 Urinal; male, jug-type, any material

A2–Z3 ASC Payment
Example: J8501 Aprepitant, oral, 5 mg

♿ **DMEPOS Paid**
Example: E0618 Apnea monitor, without recording feature

☑ **Quantity Alert**
Example: L4205 Repair of orthotic device, labor component, per 15 minutes

● **New Code**

☐ **Reinstated Code**

A–Y APC Status Indicator or OPPS Status Indicator
Example: L5684 Addition to lower extremity, below knee, fork strap

♀ **Female Only**
Example: J7303 Contraceptive supply, hormone containing vaginal ring, each

---

HCPCS CODING RESOURCES

HCPCS Updates

Each January 1, HCPCS Level II codes are updated, the exception being the temporary codes that begin with C, G, H, K, Q, S, and T, which are updated quarterly. HCPCS codes are available from CMS or any local Medicare carrier in computer-generated list form. HCPCS codes are public-domain codes (unlike CPT codes, which are owned by the AMA) and can be accessed without purchasing a coding manual. The code list provided by CMS does not have any symbols, color coding, or references to assist the coder with code assignment.

> Stay current with this year's HCPCS codes by purchasing annual HCPCS codebooks and periodically checking the CMS website for updates.

HCPCS codes can be modified at the request of a provider. A document explaining the HCPCS revision process, as well as a format for submitting a request for revision or addition, is available on the HCPCS website. The HCPCS code review process is an ongoing effort. Requests may be submitted at any time throughout the year for inclusion in the next annual update.

INTERNET RESOURCE: HCPCS review process.
www.cms.gov/Medicare/Coding/MedHCPCSGenInfo/HCPCSCODINGPROCESS.html

As with HCPCS Level I, (CPT), errata (corrections of mistakes) are available online at the CMS website.

HCPCS Clearinghouse

The American Hospital Association (AHA) and CMS developed a clearinghouse to provide official interpretations of HCPCS codes. The AHA is a nonprofit association of health-care organizations that promotes uniformity of coding and classification standards and guidelines across health-care settings. The clearinghouse provides information on the proper use of Level I HCPCS (CPT) codes in the facility environment (hospital providers) and certain Level II HCPCS codes for hospitals, physicians, and other health-care professionals. The clearinghouse is available to anyone with questions regarding HCPCS coding. Questions and supporting documentation may be faxed or mailed to the AHA central office of HCPCS.

> **INTERNET RESOURCE: Form for submitting questions:**
> www.cms.gov/Medicare/Coding/MedHCPCSGenInfo/HCPCS_Coding_Questions.html

AHA Coding Clinic for HCPCS

The *AHA Coding Clinic for HCPCS* is published on a quarterly basis and provides information on the use of HCPCS codes related to the payment system for outpatient facility billing, called APCs. It is arranged much like the *AHA Coding Clinic for ICD-10-CM and ICD-10-PCS* used by hospitals. References to this publication are made beneath a code to alert the coder when there is guidance printed in a particular issue. For example, J0887 *Injection, epoetin beta, 1 microgram, (for ESRD on dialysis)* has an AHA: 1Q, `15,6 reference. The coder would then review that edition of *AHA Coding Clinic* for instructions on how to report that code.

CHECKPOINT 30.2

Using a current HCPCS codebook, write the notation(s) that appear for each code. Code J1960 is filled out for you with generic symbols and color coding as an example. Indicate the action taken by Medicare in the first column. Look at the color coding, symbols, and instructional notes to determine if information on coverage is supplied and list it in the second column. Alert/Action is the notification that Medicare has given or action taken since the last publication. Symbols and references may vary between book publishers.

	Alert/Action:	*Coverage:*
J9160	E APC Status Indicator for Outpatient PPS ☑ Quantity Alert ⊘ SNF Excluded	Yellow highlight means coverage at carrier discretion
1. J9390	_____	_____
2. L3217	_____	_____
3. A6206	_____	_____
4. G0105	_____	_____

HCPCS CODE SECTIONS

HCPCS Level II classifies medical products and supplies into categories for ease of coding and claims processing. The first character of each alphanumeric code identifies the category into which a product or supply is classified. Some are correlated, such as M for Medical Services, but most sections have no association with the first character, as in A for Medical and Surgical Supplies. Each code category is discussed in the following sections.

> **INTERNET RESOURCE: To stay current with changes to coding and reporting HCPCS codes, remember to check the CMS website for transmittals, updates to the *Claims Processing Manual*, or *MLN Matters* articles. CMS publishes quarterly updates for providers that can be accessed online.**
> www.cms.gov/Regulations-and-Guidance/Regulations-and-Policies/QuarterlyProviderUpdates/index.html

Section A: Transportation Services Including Ambulance, Medical/Surgical Supplies, and Administrative, Miscellaneous, and Investigational (A0000–A9999)

Codes for ambulance, chiropractic, and medical/surgical supplies are located in Section A. Ambulance services are billed by a third-party ambulance service company and considered to be a specialty area of coding. Codes are assigned primarily based on whether the transport was an emergency or nonemergency, by air or ground, and had wait time incurred. Ambulance transportation services include ground and air transportation and ancillary transportation-related fees.

EXAMPLE

A0429 *Ambulance service, basic life support, emergency transport (BLS, emergency).*

Ambulance transportation services require origin and destination modifiers, as listed at the beginning of Section A. These are single-digit modifiers. The first modifier indicates the origin (where the patient was transported from) and the second modifier indicates the destination (where the patient was transported to).

HCPCS code A4550 is commonly reported for surgical tray use when minor procedures are performed in a physician office. When a physician's office bills supplies, if the payer does not recognize a HCPCS code for a medical or surgical supply, CPT code 99070 is used. Facilities typically use A4649 for miscellaneous supplies and L8699 for implants surgically placed that do not have a specific HCPCS code assignment.

> ● At times, ambulance origin and destination modifier combinations may be confused with other existing HCPCS modifiers. For example, modifier –GH, *Diagnostic mammogram converted from screening mammogram on the same day,* can also be used as an ambulance modifier meaning the place of origin was a (G) *Hospital-based ESRD facility* and the destination was (H) *Hospital.*

INTERNET RESOURCE: Criteria for coding and reporting ambulance services is located in the *Medicare Claims Processing Manual* (Chapter 15: Ambulance): www.cms.gov/Regulations-and-Guidance/Guidance/Manuals/Downloads/clm104c15.pdf

Section B: Enteral and Parenteral Therapy (B4000–B9999)

Section B includes codes for supplies, formulas, nutritional solutions, and infusion pumps. Documentation in the patient's record may indicate a particular brand name that may not be listed in HCPCS. The physician should be queried for help in matching code descriptions for the formula provided.

Codes from this section are submitted when patients require tube feedings. Feedings can be administered in several ways: enterally through the intestine, parenterally into the body other than through the digestive tract (e.g., IV therapy, nasogastric tube), or via a percutaneous endoscopic gastrostomy (PEG) tube inserted into the patient's stomach. Some codes include the administration set and some only pertain to the formula given. The supplies and the administration set are not changed with each feeding. Modifier –BA is the only modifier specific to enteral feedings at the time of this writing and reported only with E0776, B4149, B4150, B4152, B4153, B4154, and B4155.

> 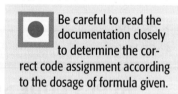 Be careful to read the documentation closely to determine the correct code assignment according to the dosage of formula given.

EXAMPLE

B4102 *Enteral formula, for adults, used to replace fluids and electrolytes 500 mL = 1 unit.*

If medication was given through a feeding tube or parenteral method, an additional J code for the medication should be assigned.

Section C: Outpatient Prospective Payment System (C1300–C9999)

Section C has temporary codes used in hospital-based surgery centers and hospital-based outpatient services. They cannot be used by freestanding ambulatory surgery centers (ASCs) or physician offices. C codes are used according to the Medicare Outpatient Prospective Payment System (OPPS) reimbursement methodology for hospital outpatient services and supplies. Most services are packaged into ambulatory payment classifications (APCs) with predetermined

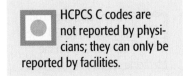
payment amounts. C codes identify transitional pass-through payments under OPPS, providing temporary additional payments (over and above the APC payment) made for certain medical devices, drugs, and biologicals provided exclusively to Medicare patients.

EXAMPLE

C2625 *Stent, non-coronary, temporary, with delivery system.*

Section E: Durable Medical Equipment (E0100–E9999)

The E codes are designated for DME such as canes, crutches, hospital beds, pacemakers, and dialysis kidney machines. The title of this section is somewhat misleading because codes located in other sections of HCPCS are also considered to be DME (e.g., A codes, B codes, L codes).

DME codes may be reported by all providers, regardless of specialty, that supply DME services to their patients, not just DME supply companies.

The primary non-DME specialties that routinely report DME codes are as follows:

• Orthopedic medicine
• Podiatry
• Family/general practice
• Home health
• Physical therapy

EXAMPLE

E0148 *Walker, heavy duty, without wheels, rigid or folding, any type, each.*

CPT services and HCPCS supply/services are subject to frequency and quantity limitations. This limitation is referred to as a *medically unlikely edit (MUE)*. An MUE for a HCPCS/CPT code is the maximum unit of service that a provider may report for an item or service, under routine circumstances, for a single patient on a single date of service. MUEs do not exist for all HCPCS/CPT codes. CMS publishes many of the MUE values for codes but not all. MUEs are developed based on HCPCS/CPT code descriptors, CPT coding instructions, anatomical considerations, established CMS policies, nature of service or procedure, nature of analyte, nature of equipment, prescribing information, and clinical judgment. The MUE is specific to Medicare as part of its payment integrity program, but most commercial plans adopt these same values. The MUE for E0148 is set to 1, meaning only one walker may be provided to a patient on a given day. MUEs, particularly for DME, are not all based on a per-day quota; some are based on per-month or per-year frequencies.

> INTERNET RESOURCE: The MUE table is located on the CMS website and is updated quarterly. Notice that the MUEs are broken out by physician, outpatient facility, and DME.
> https://www.cms.gov/Medicare/Coding/NationalCorrectCodInitEd/MUE.html

Section G: Procedures/Professional Services (G0000–G9999)

Section G contains temporary codes assigned to services being evaluated and reviewed for inclusion in the CPT codebook. The G codes may or may not be used by commercial insurance plans and are required and reported in lieu of CPT codes for Medicare patients. The section description for G codes indicates that the codes are for procedures and services that do not have a CPT code designation. This is not an entirely accurate statement. For example, for G0027, *Semen analysis; presence and/or motility of sperm excluding Huhner,* the CPT equivalent code would be 89321, *Semen analysis; sperm presence and motility of sperm, if performed.* The caveat to this is that the code is an exact match *if* presence and motility are performed. If only one or the other is performed, there is no exact CPT match. Consider the following examples of similar Level I and Level II codes where the G code is chosen over the CPT code.

EXAMPLES

• G0105 *Colorectal cancer screening; colonoscopy on individual at high risk* is preferred over CPT code 45378 in this case.

• G0289 *Arthroscopy, knee, surgical, for removal of loose body, foreign body, debridement/ shaving of articular cartilage (chondroplasty) at the time of other surgical knee arthroscopy in a different compartment of the same knee* is preferred over CPT code 29877.

Section H: Alcohol and Drug Abuse Treatment Services (H0001–H2037)

Codes in Section H are used by state Medicaid agencies, some of which are mandated by state law to establish separate codes for mental health services that include alcohol and drug treatment.

EXAMPLE
H0001 *Alcohol and/or drug assessment.*

Section J: Drugs Administered Other Than Oral Method, Chemotherapy Drugs (J0000–J9999)

This section is for reporting the supply of drugs administered subcutaneously, intramuscularly, or intravenously. These drugs cannot be self-administered.

EXAMPLE
J0585 *Injection, onabotulinumtoxin A, 1 unit.*

When reporting J codes in addition to CPT injection codes from the Medicine section, be careful to report the correct administration code that corresponds to the route by which the medication was given. For example, J0636, *Injection, Calcitriol, 0.1 mcg,* cannot be reported with administration code 96374, *Therapeutic, prophylactic, or diagnostic injection (specify substance or drug); intravenous push, single or initial substance/ drug,* because the drug is only administered intramuscularly.

When coding for injectables, the dose injected must be determined for proper billing in addition to maintaining inventory and tracking waste of unused drugs. Most drugs have a quantity limitation.

NOTE: J codes and the Table of Drugs are discussed later in this chapter.

INTERNET RESOURCE: Visit the *Medicare Claims Processing Manual*, Publication 100-04, Transmittal 1204, to read more about Medicare Part B drug pricing and reporting claims for J codes.
www.cms.hhs.gov/transmittals/downloads/R1204CP.pdf

REIMBURSEMENT REVIEW

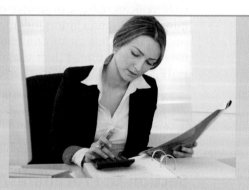

Section 303(d) of the Medicare Modernization Act requires the implementation of a Competitive Acquisition Program (CAP) for Medicare Part B drugs and biologicals not paid on a cost or prospective payment system basis. Effective January 1, 2005, the vast majority of drugs and biologicals are not paid on a cost or prospective payment basis will be paid based on the average sales price (ASP) methodology. HCPCS codes for drugs are not listed on the MPFS. A search must be done on the CMS website for the payment allowance limits for Medicare Part B drugs to determine reimbursement for drugs.

CAP is the newest alternative to the previous payment method and is comparable to "buy and bill" for certain Part B drugs that are administered. CAP geographic areas are established for contract award purposes for acquisition of and payment for categories of competitively biddable drugs and biologicals. If a physician elects to participate in this program, the claim for such drugs and biologicals is submitted by the contractor that supplied the drugs and biologicals, not the physician. The collection of amounts of any deductible and coinsurance applicable to such drugs and biologicals is the responsibility of the contractor and the payment is made to the contractor directly. CAP for Part B drugs and biologicals is only for injectable and infused drugs currently billed under Part B that are administered in a physician office, "incident to" a physician's service. To determine allowed amounts and reimbursement for drugs, the coder must access the CMS website and search for the Medicare Part B CAP. HCPCS J codes, along with the drug description and corresponding NDC codes and reimbursable amounts, are also located here.

Section K: Durable Medical Equipment for Medicare Administrative Contractors (Temporary Codes) (K0000–K9999)

These codes are used by MACs when there is no a permanent Level II code is available to implement a MAC coverage policy.

EXAMPLE
K0552 *Supplies for external drug infusion pump, syringe type cartridge, sterile, each.*

Section L: Orthotic and Prosthetic Procedures, Devices (L0000–L9999)

The L codes describe orthotic and prosthetic procedures and devices as well as orthopedic shoes and prosthetic implants. When a DME item is billed that can accommodate either side of the body, the anatomical modifiers (–LT/–RT) should be used to define which side (or both) is being supported (orthotic) or replaced (prosthetic). If a lower limb prosthetic is billed, a functional modifier (K0–K4) should also be billed to define the patient's functional state or potential ability to ambulate.

EXAMPLE
L0120 *Cervical, flexible, non-adjustable, prefabricated, off-the-shelf (foam collar).*

Section M: Medical Services (M0000–M0301)

The M codes include office services, cellular therapy, IV chelation therapy, and fabric wrapping of abdominal aneurysms. As of 2015, this section had only six codes.

EXAMPLE
M0300 *IV chelation therapy (chemical endarterectomy).*

Section P: Pathology and Laboratory Services (P0000–P9999)

P codes include chemistry, toxicology, microbiology tests, Papanicolaou tests, and travel allowance for clinical staff to drive to a patient's home to collect a specimen.

EXAMPLE
P2031 *Hair analysis (excluding arsenic).*

Section Q: Miscellaneous Services (Temporary Codes) (Q0000–Q9974)

The Q codes identify drugs, medical equipment, and services that have not been given CPT codes and are not identifiable in the permanent Level II codes but are needed to process a billing claim. These would be for items that typically would not receive a CPT code.

EXAMPLE
Q0114 *Fern Test.*

Section R: Diagnostic Radiology Services (R0000–R5999)

R codes are used for transportation of portable x-ray and/or electrocardiogram (EKG) equipment.

EXAMPLE
R0076 *Transportation of portable EKG to facility or location, per patient.*

Section S: Temporary National Codes (Non-Medicare) (S0000–S9999)

The codes in Section S were developed by Blue Cross/Blue Shield and other commercial payers to report codes for supplies and services. These codes are used by private payers to report drugs, services, and supplies for which there are no national codes but codes are needed to implement policies. These codes can also be used by Medicaid. Even though these codes are located within the HCPCS codebook, they are not reportable to Medicare. It is very important that a copy of the carrier contract be reviewed to determine which payers accept these codes.

EXAMPLE

Arthroscopic thermal capsulorrhaphy (capsular shrinkage). Code assignment can be S2300 if the payer accepts S codes. Otherwise, CPT code 29999 must be submitted depending on payer requirements.

Section T: National T Codes (T1000–T9999)

National T codes are used by state Medicaid agencies when no HCPCS Level II code is available but a code is needed to administer the Medicaid program. These are not used by Medicare but can be used by private insurers.

EXAMPLE

T1021 *Home health aide or certified nurse assistant, per visit.*

Section V: Vision, Hearing, and Speech–Language Pathology Services (V0000–V5999)

The V codes are for vision and hearing screenings and supplies including glasses, contacts, intra-ocular lenses, audiology services, and prostheses.

EXAMPLE

V2623 *Prosthetic eye, plastic, custom.*

Miscellaneous/Unclassified Codes

Under certain circumstances, a coder must assign an item or service to an unclassified HCPCS code. Health care is in a constant state of change. New drugs, devices, and equipment are developed and marketed at various times throughout the year. It is impossible and impractical to revise the HCPCS code sets each time a new item or service is introduced. An item or service may be newly approved by the FDA—the federal organization that protects against public health hazards by ensuring the safety and, in most cases, the quality and effectiveness of products and services—and not yet assigned a HCPCS code.

Services or items without a specific Level II code are assigned to an unclassified code in the interim until a new code can be implemented. Several unclassified codes exist in each section of HCPCS. Unclassified and unlisted codes allow providers a way to submit claims and carriers to process claims for items or services without a designated code. In CPT, any procedure that does not have a designated code is assigned to an "unlisted" procedure code within the appropriate body system. In HCPCS, as opposed to CPT, terminology is inconsistent throughout the book. The code description may include any of the following terms: *unlisted, not otherwise specified, unspecified, unclassified, other,* and *miscellaneous.*

> When coding an un-classified code, contact the local Medicare carrier in case the carrier prefers a specific Level II code.

EXAMPLE

A4649, *Surgical supply; miscellaneous,* may be used for an implanted device that does not have a permanent or temporary code that is more specific.

CHECKPOINT 30.3

In which sections are the following HCPCS services located?

1. Motorized wheelchair _____

2. Alcohol wipes, box _____

3. PET imaging, whole body _____

4. Ambulance waiting time _____

5. Contact lens, gas permeable _____

MODIFIERS

HCPCS Level II modifiers serve the same purpose as CPT professional modifiers. Level II modifiers do not change the definition of the procedure or service but give more explanation about where the procedure was performed, type of equipment used, or who provided the service. Level II modifiers may be used with Level I or Level II codes. In a situation where the coder has two modifiers, one a Level I and the other a Level II, the Level II modifier is sequenced first followed by the Level I modifier.

Frequently Used Modifers

There are nearly 300 HCPCS Level II modifiers. Level II modifiers are two characters: either alphanumeric or alphabetic only. They are located on the inside covers of the HCPCS codebook or in an appendix. A limited number of these commonly used modifiers are located on the front inside cover of the CPT codebook as well. Frequently used modifiers are discussed next.

Anesthesia Modifiers

Anesthesia modifiers are appended to CPT anesthesia codes reported by a certified anesthesia provider. These modifiers directly influence payment to the provider and represent who provided and supervised the provision of anesthesia. Anesthesia coding and modifier usage are discussed in Chapter 15 of this book.

> **EXAMPLE**
>
> –AA is a modifier appended to an anesthesia code to indicate that anesthesia services are performed personally by the anesthesiologist.

Anatomical Modifiers

HCPCS Level II modifiers include anatomical modifiers to show exact body location and help describe precisely which digit received treatment. These should be used with procedures on toes, eyes, and fingers instead of –LT or –RT.

- TA–T9 for procedures that are performed on the phalanges, or toes, rather than on the "foot." They are specific to individual toes on each foot and are the modifier of choice when doing multiple procedures on different toes.

> **EXAMPLE**
>
> A tarsal tunnel release is performed on the left foot and a hammertoe repair is reported on the fourth toe, right foot.
>
> 28035–LT.
>
> 28285–T8–51.
>
> In this example, the –T8 modifier specifically describes the fourth toe on the right foot and is preferred over modifier –RT.

- E1–E4 for procedures performed on the eyelids specifically, not the actual eye. These are specific to the upper and lower lids of each eye.

> **EXAMPLE**
>
> 67840–E1 *Excision of lesion of left upper eyelid without closure or with simple direct closure.*

- FA–F9 for procedures done on the phalanges, or fingers, rather than on the "hand." They are specific to individual fingers on each hand and are the modifier of choice when doing multiple procedures on different fingers.

> **EXAMPLE**
>
> 26110–F2 *Arthrotomy with biopsy; interphalangeal joint, each.*

Modifiers Relating to Medicare Coverage

Many of the HCPCS modifiers correspond to Medicare coverage of an item or service.

- GA is used when a waiver of liability or ABN is on file for a Medicare patient. This document must be signed for cases where the service will not be covered by Medicare. This modifier notifies Medicare that the patient is aware of the noncoverage and has a signed waiver on file. This way, the patient is liable for the cost of the services provided. Modifier –GA must be used when suppliers want to indicate that they expect that Medicare will deny an item or supply as not reasonable and necessary and that they have a signed ABN by the beneficiary on file. Modifier –GA can be used on either a specific or miscellaneous HCPCS code.
- GH is used when a diagnostic mammogram is converted from a screening mammogram on the same day.
- GG is used when a screening mammogram and diagnostic mammogram are performed on the same patient, same day.
- GY is used when an item or service is statutorily excluded or does not meet the definition of any Medicare benefit. A –GY modifier does not require a signed ABN to be on file. Some examples of this use would be cosmetic surgery, dentures, acupuncture, and hearing aids. It is very important that coders read the local and national coverage determinations to ascertain which services are deemed not reasonable and necessary. Use of the –GY modifier acknowledges that Medicare will deny the item or service as noncovered but allows any secondary insurer to consider coverage following Medicare's denial. This modifier is not used to file services *expected* to be denied for medical necessity; the –GZ modifier would apply in that circumstance. If the service or supply is statutorily excluded, thus resulting in an automatic denial, an ABN is not required.
- GZ is used when an item or service is expected to be denied as not reasonable and necessary (used when an ABN is not on file). Modifier –GZ is applied when physicians, practitioners, or suppliers want to indicate that they expect that Medicare will deny an item or service as not reasonable and necessary and no signed ABN is on file. In cases where there is no specific procedure code to describe services, a "not otherwise classified code" (NOC) is reported with the –GZ modifier. Even though the provider understands that Medicare will not allow payment, the code for the service is still submitted with this modifier for data collection purposes.

Lab Test Modifier

- QW is used for a CLIA-waived test. This modifier is appended to codes for laboratory tests performed in a physician office for tests that have been deemed "waived" and safe to perform outside a certified lab.

EXAMPLE

81025–QW *Urine pregnancy test, by visual color comparison methods.*

Technical Component Modifier

- TC refers to a technical component. Charges may be submitted by facilities for use of equipment. A –TC modifier is not used by physicians unless they are billing for the facility charge in their office and own the equipment. For every claim received that has the –TC modifier appended, there should be a corresponding claim for the same patient, date of service (DOS), and procedure code with a –26 modifier appended to balance out the charges between the facility and the provider.

EXAMPLE

76817–TC *Ultrasound, pregnant uterus, real time with image documentation, transvaginal.*

How does a coder know or confirm which codes may be reported with a –TC? The MPFS provides a listing of all CPT or HCPCS codes payable by CMS to providers for professional services rendered. The MPFS has a column labeled "PC/TC Indicator." The numerical indicator located in this column explains whether it is appropriate to append a –TC. Box 30.3 is an excerpt from the MPFS file explaining the meaning of the numerical values.

BOX 30.3 Explanations of MPFS PC/TC Indicators

0 = Physician Service Codes. Identifies codes that describe physician services. The concept of PC/TC does not apply because physician services cannot be split into professional and technical components. Modifiers –26 and –TC cannot be used with these codes.

1 = Diagnostic Tests for Radiology Services. Identifies codes that describe diagnostic tests. These codes have both a professional and technical component. Modifiers –26 and –TC can be used with these codes.

2 = Professional Component Only Codes. This indicator identifies stand-alone codes that describe the physician work portion of selected diagnostic tests for which there is an associated code that describes the technical component of the diagnostic test only and another associated code that describes the global test. Modifiers –26 and –TC cannot be used with these codes.

3 = Technical Component Only Codes. This indicator identifies stand-alone codes that describe the technical component (e.g., staff and equipment costs) of selected diagnostic tests for which there is an associated code that describes the professional component of the diagnostic test only. It also identifies codes that are covered only as diagnostic tests and therefore do not have a related professional code. Modifiers –26 and –TC cannot be used with these codes.

4 = Global Test Only Codes. This indicator identifies stand-alone codes that describe selected diagnostic tests for which there are associated codes that describe (a) the professional component of the test only, and (b) the technical component of the test only. Modifiers –26 and –TC cannot be used with these codes.

5 = "Incident To" Codes. This indicator identifies codes that describe services covered incident to a physician's service when they are provided by auxiliary personnel employed by the physician and working under his or her direct personal supervision. Payment may not be made by carriers for these services when they are provided to hospital inpatients or patients in a hospital outpatient department. Modifiers –26 and –TC cannot be used with these codes.

6 = Laboratory Physician Interpretation Codes. This indicator identifies clinical laboratory codes for which separate payment for interpretations by laboratory physicians may be made. Actual performance of the tests is paid for under the lab fee schedule. Modifier –TC cannot be used with these codes.

7 = Physical therapy service, for which payment may not be made. Payment may not be made if the service is provided to either a patient in a hospital outpatient department or to an inpatient of the hospital by an independently practicing physical or occupational therapist.

EXAMPLE

Physician performs a colorectal cancer screening using a barium enema in an outpatient facility. The MPFS indicates that this procedure code has a PC/TC indicator of 1, meaning it has a professional and a technical component associated with the examination. The facility would report G0106–TC and the physician would report G0106–26.

HCPCS	MODIFIER	DESCRIPTION	PC/TC INDICATOR
G0106		Colon cancer screen; barium enema	1
G0106	–TC	Colon cancer screen; barium enema	1
G0106	–26	Colon cancer screen; barium enema	1

ASC-Only Modifier

SG is used when filing surgical procedures rendered in an ASC. This modifier is to be used only by ASC providers. They must append the –SG modifier to the surgical procedure/CPT code(s). This modifier indicates that the charge is for the ASC facility service and is used to determine the appropriate reimbursement rate for the ASC. This modifier should be used in addition to any other applicable modifiers. It is also important to note that this modifier is applicable to surgical procedures only and should not be used on supply codes billed by the ASC, because the reimbursement for supplies is not affected by the ASC payment groups. Physicians performing services in the ASC setting should not use the –SG modifier when billing for their services.

Denial of Payment

In some situations, insurance carriers instruct suppliers and providers to use a modifier to provide information about the service or item. Payment may be denied or reduced due to lack of a modifier. Although both the alphabetic and alphanumeric modifiers are used across the country, some carriers may not recognize them. It is important for each carrier contract or coverage manual to be referenced and appropriate documentation submitted with a claim in times of question.

CMS no longer accepts modifier –59 for pricing claims due to problems with the incorrect usage of this modifier. To curb confusion and misuse of this modifier, CMS created four modifiers for use in reporting specific scenarios that meet the specification of a separate and distinct encounter.

- XE Separate encounter, *a service that is distinct because it occurred during a separate encounter*
- XS Separate structure, *a service that is distinct because it was performed on a separate organ/structure*
- XP Separate practitioner, *a service that is distinct because it was performed by a different practitioner*
- XU Unusual non-overlapping service, *the use of a service that is distinct because it does not overlap usual components of the main service*

> As of January 2008, ASCs are no longer required to report the –SG modifier with every surgical CPT code billed to Medicare. The facility instead can report the type of service "F" with specialty "49" and place of service "24." However, some commercial plans may still require the use of this modifier to link services to the correct carrier fee schedule if they are still reimbursing ASCs by ASC group method. Check with the carrier to obtain this information.

Therapy Modifiers

Therapy modifiers are available to providers who perform physical, occupational, rehabilitative, and habilitative services. Modifiers –GO (Services delivered under an outpatient occupational therapy plan of care), –GP (Services delivered under an outpatient physical therapy plan of care), and –GN (Services delivered under an outpatient speech language pathology plan of care) should accompany the CPT or HCPCS therapy codes submitted to insurance plans.

Effective January 1, 2017, federal regulations require individual and small group market plans to have separate therapy visit limits for habilitative and rehabilitative services. Habilitative services help a person keep, learn, or improve skills and functioning for daily living. Rehabilitative services help a person keep, restore, or improve skills and functioning for daily living that have been lost or impaired because a person was sick, hurt, or disabled (i.e., stroke, brain injury). To aide in tracking the separate visit limits, providers have to identify whether a provided service is habilitative or rehabilitative. Thus far, habilitative services have been flagged with the –SZ modifier (Habilitative Services). There isn't a HCPCS modifier to indicate rehabilitative services; however, there is a CPT modifier –97 (Rehabilitative Services). CPT modifier –96 (Habilitative Services) does not replace the –SZ modifier for Medicare patients.

Before appending a therapy modifier, coders can check online with CMS to see if a particular service is categorized as such at https://www.cms.gov/Medicare/Billing/TherapyServices/AnnualTherapyUpdate.html.

CHECKPOINT 30.4

Indicate which Level II modifier applies to the following scenarios.

1. Physician assistant, nurse practitioner, or clinical nurse specialist services for assistance at surgery

   _____

2. Outpatient occupational therapy service _____

3. Medicare beneficiary elected to purchase an item _____

4. Service is not reasonable and necessary _____

5. Office performed CLIA-waived test _____

ASSIGNING HCPCS CODES

Looking a code up in the HCPCS Index is similar to the process used in CPT or ICD-10. Keeping in mind that HCPCS codes are for services and supplies only, look up the medical or surgical supply, the service provided (such as *screening* or *implant*), the orthotic/prosthetic device, or generic/brand name of a drug. Some codes may be indexed by the condition or body part, but this is not the norm. The Index, however, only points to the general area of the code listings. Coders must locate the appropriate code in the appropriate section.

EXAMPLE

A podiatrist performs a complex bunionectomy with implant insertion. The code for the procedure is 28291 but the code for the supply of the implant itself must be located in HCPCS. If a HCPCS code is not assigned, the physician or facility will not be reimbursed for the device implanted. The HCPCS code L8642 is also reported to account for the supply component of the implant inserted.

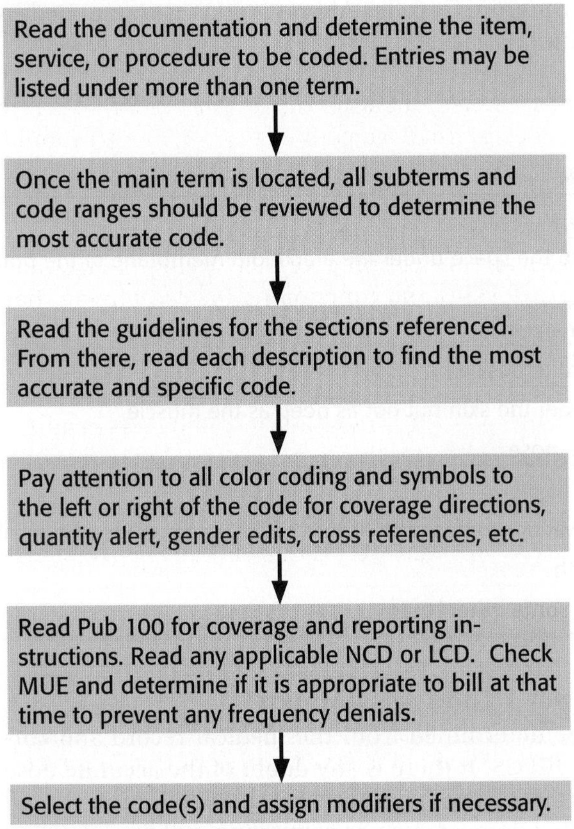

Coding Steps

As illustrated in Figure 30.1, coders follow a series of steps to assign HCPCS codes:

1. Read the documentation and determine the item, service, or procedure to be coded.
2. Find the terms in the Index. Entries may be listed under more than one term.
3. Once the main term is located, all subterms and code ranges should be reviewed to determine the most accurate code. Do not code straight from the Index.
4. Read the guidelines for the sections referenced.
5. Read each description to find the most accurate and specific code.
6. Pay attention to all color coding and symbols to the left or right of the code for coverage directions, quantity alert, gender edits, and cross references. An example of a cross reference is E0235, *Paraffin bath unit, portable* (see medical supply code A4265 for the paraffin).
7. Select the code(s) and assign modifiers if necessary.

Read the documentation and determine the item, service, or procedure to be coded. Entries may be listed under more than one term.

↓

Once the main term is located, all subterms and code ranges should be reviewed to determine the most accurate code.

↓

Read the guidelines for the sections referenced. From there, read each description to find the most accurate and specific code.

↓

Pay attention to all color coding and symbols to the left or right of the code for coverage directions, quantity alert, gender edits, cross references, etc.

↓

Read Pub 100 for coverage and reporting instructions. Read any applicable NCD or LCD. Check MUE and determine if it is appropriate to bill at that time to prevent any frequency denials.

↓

Select the code(s) and assign modifiers if necessary.

Figure 30.1 HCPCS coding process.

Practice by using your codebook to find the code for *Urinary indwelling catheter, Foley type, 2-way*.

Urinary is the main term and *catheter* is the subterm. You see the code ranges A4338–A4346 and A4351–A4353. Each code within these code ranges must be located and reviewed to determine the "best" code. You can also find this code by looking up *catheter* first and then *indwelling* and reviewing each code in the code range A4338–A4346. After examining the codes within this range, A4344 is the appropriate code to assign. The code is notated indicating that special coverage instructions apply and that a quantity alert is present. From here, the coder should research carrier-specific policies pertaining to urinary catheters and read any NCDs/LCDs before reporting the code.

Hierarchy of Assigning a HCPCS Level II Code Versus a HCPCS Level I CPT Code

Occasionally, a coder must decide from which level of HCPCS to choose a code. Use of a HCPCS code versus a CPT code depends greatly on the carrier. When dealing with Medicare, if there is no CPT code that describes the procedure or service, then use a HCPCS code before assigning an unlisted code. Medicare creates G codes for use in this situation, and this supersedes any other CPT code such as with screening colonoscopies (G0105, G0121, etc.) and arthroscopy with removal of loose body (G0289). Some commercial plans may accept HCPCS G codes. Check with the carrier to confirm. There are codes in CPT and HCPCS with the same code narrative. For non-Medicare patients, if the CPT code has the same description as a HCPCS code, use the CPT code.

Using the Table of Drugs

HCPCS Level II J codes describe drugs by using their generic names, amounts, and routes of administration. In most cases, the Table of Drugs is a more effective way to find a code than using the Index. The table is included as an appendix to the HCPCS codebook. This table lists trade names and generic names, along with the amount and mode of administration. Depending on the publisher, the brand name drugs are capitalized and generic drugs are in lowercase.

When injections are given and documented, the coder must determine the amount of drug given and the mode of administration before assigning a code. Abbreviations, summarized in Table 30.3, are used to indicate the mode of administration.

Table 30.3 Modes of Drug Administration

ROUTE	DESCRIPTION
IA (Intra-arterial)	Introduced via an artery
IT (Intrathecal)	Introduced into the space under the arachnoid membrane of the brain or spinal cord
IV (Intravenous)	Introduced via a vein
IM (Intramuscular)	Introduced into a muscle
SC (Subcutaneous)	Introduced under the skin but not as deep as the muscle
INH (Inhalant solution)	Inhaled via the nose
INJ (Injection, not otherwise specified)	Injected
VAR (Various routes)	Introduced by various routes, such as into a joint, cavity tissue, or topically
ORL (Oral)	Given by mouth
OTH (Other routes)	Introduced by some other route

Determining Units of Medication for Proper J Code Assignment

The dosage of medication administered must be determined from the medical record and correctly matched to the available dose amount in HCPCS. If there is any doubt of the accurate dose of a medication provided, the nurse or other provider who administered the medication should be queried. Coders should not be calculating actual dosages such as converting milliliters (mL) to cubic centimeters (cc) or milligrams (mg) to grams (gm). This is a clinical responsibility. Coders are responsible for choosing the correct units of the drug and the mode of administration based on the nurse or physician documentation.

EXAMPLE

A patient was injected with 40 mg of Elavil. The coder would look up the drug in the Table of Drugs. (See the excerpt from the Table of Drugs.)

DRUG NAME	UNIT	ROUTE	CODE
Elavil	20 mg	IM	J1320

The table indicates that the dose administered is 20 mg. To account for the 40-mg dose provided, the coder must bill J1320 with 2 units (J1320 × 2). The amount of medication given, or dose, has been provided. The coder calculates the units.

Be careful when reading the code descriptions. Some may say "up to" a specific amount of medication: Anything less than that should be coded by assigning the code one time.

EXAMPLE

A patient was given 80 mg of phenobarbital. The Table of Drugs indicates the following:

DRUG NAME	UNIT	ROUTE	CODE
phenobarbital sodium	120 mg	IM, IV	J2560

Do not code from the Table of Drugs. J codes must be verified in the J code section of the book for a complete description of the code.

The unit notes 120 mg and only 80 mg were given. Look at code J2560 in the code section of the book. The code description states: *Injection, phenobarbital sodium, up to 120 mg.* Thus, this code would be appropriate to assign.

CHECKPOINT 30.5

Assign the HCPCS Level I or II codes for the following scenarios. Append any HCPCS Level II modifiers as needed.

1. Blood glucose monitor with integrated lancing _____

2. Injection Depo-Estradiol Cypionate, 2.5 mg _____

3. Thoracic lumbar sacral orthosis back brace _____

4. LPN nursing care in the home, per diem _____

5. Blood glucose reagent strips for home blood glucose machine _____

6. Injection of Cordarone IV, 45 mg _____

7. Patient received 1 hour of outpatient speech therapy by a speech pathologist in the office

_____

8. Prostate screening in a 69-year-old patient _____

Chapter Summary

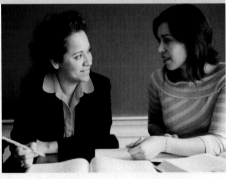

1. The HCPCS code set is the HIPAA-mandated coding system for products, supplies, and services not included in the AMA CPT code set.
2. HCPCS Level I (CPT) codes are five-digit numeric codes with the exception of Category II and Category III codes. HCPCS Level II codes are five-digit alphanumeric codes starting with the letters A–V.
3. HCPCS codes are assigned along with a CPT code for an encounter to identify supplies and drugs used or provided. These are required for claims for services, supplies, and drugs for all federal health insurance programs.
4. The HCPCS code set contains both permanent and temporary codes. Permanent codes change just once a year, based on the recommendations of the CMS HCPCS Workgroup. Temporary codes are updated quarterly.
5. Sources for keeping current include the HCPCS website, the AHA/CMS HCPCS Clearinghouse, and the AHA Coding Clinic for HCPCS.

6. The HCPCS Index is arranged alphabetically, as is the Table of Drugs included in HCPCS codebooks. The main text is made up of sections of codes arranged numerically according to their initial letter, from Section A through Section V. The category sections are as follows:

- Section A: Transportation Services Including Ambulance, Medical/Surgical Supplies, and Administrative, Miscellaneous, and Investigational
- Section B: Enteral and Parenteral Therapy
- Section C: Outpatient Prospective Payment System
- Section E: Durable Medical Equipment
- Section G: Procedures/Professional Services (temporary)
- Section H: Alcohol and Drug Abuse Treatment Services
- Section J: Drugs Administered Other Than Oral Method, Chemotherapy Drugs
- Section K: Durable Medical Equipment for Medicare Administrative Contractors (Temporary Codes)
- Section L: Orthotic and Prosthetic Procedures, Devices
- Section M: Medical Services
- Section P: Pathology and Laboratory Services
- Section Q: Miscellaneous Services (Temporary Codes)
- Section R: Diagnostic Radiology Services
- Section S: Temporary National Codes (Non-Medicare)
- Section T: National T Codes
- Section V: Vision, Hearing, and Speech–Language Pathology Services

7. HCPCS Level II modifiers, such as CPT professional and facility modifiers, are used for reporting that the circumstances of a service changed, but not enough so that another code should be selected. The –GA, –GZ, and –GY modifiers relate to the status of the ABN.

8. Paying close attention to the units and the route columns in the Table of Drugs is required to correctly assign the J code that accurately reflects the dose provided and method of administration.

9. There is a hierarchy for assigning HCPCS codes. Identifying the patient's insurance will assist in determining if a Level I or Level II HCPCS code is required.

Review Questions

Matching

Match the key terms with their definitions.

A. durable medical equipment (DME)
B. HCPCS
C. *Medicare Carriers Manual* (MCM)
D. permanent national codes
E. temporary national codes
F. Level II modifiers
G. Pub 100-03
H. CMS HCPCS Workgroup

1. _____ HCPCS Level II codes that are maintained for the use of all payers

2. _____ Reference containing guidelines established by Medicare related to covered services in HCPCS Level II

3. _____ HCPCS Level II codes that are used by individual payers for items not covered in permanent national codes

4. _____ Reference containing information whether specific medical items, services, treatment procedures, or technologies are payable under Medicare

5. _____ Code set providing national codes for supplies, services, and products

6. _____ Reusable medical equipment for use in the home

7. _____ Two-character codes that are assigned to clarify Level II codes

8. _____ Government committee that maintains and advises on HCPCS Level II codes

True or False

Decide whether each statement is true or false.

1. _____ HCPCS Level II codes have six digits.

2. _____ HCPCS Level II codes are used only by hospitals.

3. _____ HIPAA mandates the use of HCPCS codes.

4. _____ CPT modifiers and HCPCS Level II modifiers are the same.

5. _____ HCPCS permanent national codes can be altered or deleted by a single payer alone.

6. _____ HCPCS permanent national codes are issued on January 1 of each year and must be used as of their effective date.

7. _____ HCPCS codebooks use symbols to show new, revised, and deleted codes and descriptors.

8. _____ Coding drugs involves paying attention to both the method of administration and the quantity administered.

9. _____ DME supplies are located in the K section of the main listing.

10. _____ Private payers are not permitted to use HCPCS codes; use is restricted to government programs.

Multiple Choice

Select the letter that best completes the statement or answers the question.

1. Transportation services are HCPCS _____ codes.
   A. A
   B. B
   C. C
   D. D

2. Vision and hearing services are HCPCS _____ codes.
   A. D
   B. E
   C. H
   D. V

3. Temporary codes are HCPCS _____ codes.
   A. D
   B. Q
   C. T
   D. V

4. DME codes are HCPCS _____ codes.
   A. D
   B. E
   C. H
   D. V

5. Prosthetic procedures are HCPCS _____ codes.
   A. D
   B. E
   C. H
   D. L

6. Temporary national codes for private insurers to identify drugs, services, supplies, and procedures that are not reimbursable under Medicare are HCPCS _____ codes.
   A. D
   B. E
   C. S
   D. V

7. Diagnostic radiology services are HCPCS _____ codes.
   A. R
   B. E
   C. H
   D. V

8. Chemotherapy drugs are HCPCS _____ codes.
   A. D
   B. E
   C. H
   D. J

9. Laboratory and pathology are HCPCS _____ codes.
   A. D
   B. E
   C. P
   D. V

10. Modifiers –A1 through –A9 are
    A. Anatomical modifiers
    B. Reported with wound care services
    C. Anesthesia modifiers
    D. Accepted by all payers

Abbreviations and Acronyms

3-D	three-dimensional
AA	anesthesiologist assistant
AAA	abdominal aortic aneurysm
AAFPRC	American Academy of Facial Plastic and Reconstructive Surgery
AAOS	American Academy of Orthopaedic Surgeons
AAPC	American Academy of Professional Coders
AB	missed abortion
ABI	ankle/brachial index
ABN	Advance Beneficiary Notice
AC	acromioclavicular
ACA	Affordable Care Act
ACE	angiotensin-converting enzyme
ACL	anterior cruciate ligament
ACNS	American Clinical Neurophysiology Society
ACTH	adrenocorticotropic hormone
ADHD	attention deficit-hyperactivity disorder
AFP	alpha fetal protein
AHA	American Hospital Association
AHIMA	American Health Information Management Association
AHRQ	Agency for Healthcare Research and Quality
AIDS	acquired immunodeficiency syndrome
AK	actinic keratosis
AKA	above-knee amputation
ALS	amyotrophic lateral sclerosis
ALT	serum glutamic pyruvic transaminase
AMA	advanced maternal age
AMA	American Medical Association
AMI	acute myocardial infarction
A-mode	one-dimensional ultrasonic measurement procedure
ANA	antinuclear antibody
AP	anteroposterior
APC	ambulatory payment classifications
APE	anterior posterior ethmoidectomy
APMA	American Podiatric Medical Association
APR-DRG	All Patient Refined Diagnosis-Related Group
ARB	angiotensin II receptor blocker
ARC	AIDS-related complex
ARF	acute renal failure
AROM	artificial rupture of membranes
ART	assisted reproductive technology
ASA	American Society of Anesthesiologists
ASC	ambulatory surgery center
ASHD	arteriosclerotic heart disease
ASMBS	American Society for Metabolic and Bariatric Surgery
ASP	Active Server Pages
ASP	average sales price
AST	serum glutamic oxaloacetic transaminase
ATFP	arcus tendineus pelvic fascia
AV	artery to vein
AVF	arteriovenous fistulate
AVG	arteriovenous graft
AVM	arteriovenous malformation
BCBS	Blue Cross and Blue Shield

BCC	basal cell carcinoma
BGC	bacillus Calmette-Guerin
BiPAP	bilevel positive airway pressure
BKA	below-knee amputation
BLS	basic life support
BMD	bone mineral density
BMI	body mass index
BMT	bone marrow transplantation
BNO	bladder neck obstruction
BOO	bladder outlet obstruction
BP	blood pressure
BPH	benign prostatic hypertrophy
BRBPR	bright red blood per rectum
B-scan	two-dimensional ultrasonic scanning procedure with a two-dimensional view
BUN	blood urea nitrogen
C-section	cesarean section
CABG	coronary artery bypass graft
CACS	computer-assisted coding system
CAD	coronary artery disease
CANPC	Certified Anesthesia and Pain Management Coder
CAP	College of American Pathologists
CAP	competitive acquisition program
CAT scan	computerized axial tomography scan
Cath	catheter
CBC	complete blood count
CC	chief complaint
CCA	Certified Coding Associate
CCI	Correct Coding Initiative
CCS	Certified Coding Specialist
CCS-P	Certified Coding Specialist–Physician-based
CDC	Centers for Disease Control and Prevention
CDM	charge description master
CEU	continuing education unit
CHF	congestive heart failure
CHPS	Certified in Healthcare Privacy and Security
CIC	Certified Inpatient Coder
CIN	cervical intraepithelial neoplasia
CKC	cold knife colonization
CKD	chronic kidney disease
CKC	cold knife conization
CLIA	Clinical Laboratory Improvement Amendments
CMC	carpometacarpal (joint)
CMG	cystometrogram
CMN	certificate of medical necessity
CMS	Centers for Medicare and Medicaid Services
CMV	cytomegalovirus
CNS	central nervous system
COC	Certified Outpatient Coder
COMP	comprehensive
COPD	chronic obstructive pulmonary disease
CPAP	continuous positive airway pressure
CPC	Certified Professional Coder
CPC-A	Certified Professional Coder–Associate
CPCD	Certified Professional Coder in Dermatology
CPC-P	Certified Professional Coder–Payer
CPM	continuous passive motion
CPRC	Certified Plastic and Reconstructive Surgery Coder
CPT	Current Procedural Terminology

CR	change request
CRC	Certified Risk Adjustment Coder
CRF	chronic renal failure
CRM	cryptococcal meningitis
CRNA	Certified Registered Nurse Anesthetist
CS	cardiology specialist
CS	conscious sedation
CSF	cerebrospinal fluid
CT scan	computerized axial tomography scan
CTR	Certified Tumor Registrar
CTR	carpal tunnel release
CUG	cystourethrogram
CVA	cerebrovascular accident
CVAD	central venous access device
CVC	central venous catheter
D&C	dilation and curettage
D&E	dilation and evacuation
DDD	degenerative disc disease
DEC	decubitus
DES	diethylstilbestrol
DET	detailed
DG	documentation guidelines
DHHS	Department of Health and Human Services
DIP	distal interphalangeal joint
DJD	degenerative joint disease
DM	diabetes mellitus
DME	durable medical equipment
DME MAC	Durable Medical Equipment Medicare Administrative Contractors
DMEPOS	durable medical equipment, prosthetics, orthotics, and supplies
DMERC	durable medical equipment regional carrier
DOB	date of birth
DOL	Department of Labor
DPM	doctor of podiatric medicine
DRA	Deficit Reduction Act
DRE	digital rectal examination
DRG	diagnosis-related group
DRS	designated record set
DSM-V	*Diagnostic and Statistical Manual of Mental Disorders*
DTaP	diphtheria, tetanus, acellular pertussis
DUB	dysfunctional uterine bleeding
E&O	error and omission
EBRT	external beam radiation therapy
ECCE	extracapsular cataract extraction
ECG	electrocardiogram
ECHO	echocardiography
ECLS	extracorporeal life support services
ECMO	extracorporeal membrane oxygenation
ED	emergency department
EDC	estimated date of confinement
EDI	electronic data interchange
EEG	electroencephalogram
EEO	equal employment opportunity
EGD	esophagogastroduodenoscopy
EHR	electronic health record
EKG	electrocardiogram
E/M	evaluation and management
EMG	electromyography

EMR	electronic medical record
EMS	emergency medical systems
EMS	Evaluation and Management Specialist
EMT	emergency medical technician
ENT	ear, nose, and throat
EOG	electrooculogram
EP	established patient
EPF	expanded problem-focused
EPS	electrophysiological procedure
ER	emergency room
ERCP	endoscopic retrograde cholangiopancreatography
ESR	erythrocyte sedimentation rate
ESRD	end-stage renal disease
ESWL	extracorporeal shock-wave lithotripsy
FB	foreign body
FBC	full blood count
FCA	False Claims Act
FDA	Food and Drug Administration
FDS	flexor digitorum superficialis
FESS	functional endoscopic sinus surgery
FNA	fine-needle aspiration
FNG	free nipple graft procedure
FOBT	occult blood (feces)
FTG	full-thickness graft
Fx	fracture
GE	gastroenterology
GE	gastroesophageal
GEMs	General Equivalency Mappings
GERD	gastroesophageal reflux disease
GFR	glomerular filtration rate
GGT	gamma-glutamyl transferase
GI	gastrointestinal
GPO	Government Printing Office
GSS	General Surgery Specialist
GTT	glucose tolerance test
GU	genitourinary
GYN	gynecology
H&P	history and physical
HAAb	hepatitis A antibody
HBsAg	hepatitis B surface antigen
HBO₂	hyperbaric oxygen therapy
HCC	Hierarchical Condition Categories
HCFA	Health Care Financing Administration
HCPCS	Healthcare Common Procedure Coding System
HCT	hematocrit
HDL	high-density lipoprotein
HDR	high-dose rate
HEDIS	Healthcare Effectiveness Data and Information Set
HGH	human growth hormone
HHA	home health agency
Hib	*Haemophilus influenzae* type b
HIGH	high complexity
HIM	health information management
HINN	hospital-issued notice of noncoverage
HIPAA	Health Insurance Portability and Accountability Act of 1996
HIT	health information technology
HITECH	Health Information Technology for Economic and Clinical Health Act

HIV	human immunodeficiency virus
HMO	health management organization
HPI	history of present illness
HPV	human papillomavirus
HTA	Hydro ThermAblator
I&D	incision and drainage
IC	interstitial cystitis
ICCE	intracapsular cataract extraction
ICD-10-CM	International Classification of Diseases, Tenth Revision, Clinical Modification
ICD-9-CM	International Classification of Diseases, Ninth Revision, Clinical Modification
ICDA	International Classification of Diseases, Adapted for Indexing of Hospital Records and Operation Classification
ICF	intermediate care facility
ICM	implantable cardiovascular monitor
IDET	intradiscal electrothermal therapy
IFD	interspinous fusion device
IgE	immunoglobulin E
IGS	image-guided surgery
ILR	implantable loop recorder
IM	intramuscular
Index	Index to Diseases and Injuries
INR	international normalized ratio
IOL	intraocular lens
IOM	Internet-Only Manual
IOP	increased intraocular pressure
IP	inpatient
IPPS	Inpatient Prospective Payment System
IPV	polio
IR	interventional radiology
IUD	intrauterine device
IUI	intrauterine insemination
IV	intravenous
IVDMIA	in vitro diagnostic multivariate index assays
IVF	in vitro fertilization
IVP	intravenous push
IVP	intravenous pyelogram
LAC	laser ablation of the cervix
LAD	left anterior descending
LASGB	laparoscopic adjustable gastric silicone band
LASIK	laser-assisted in situ keratomileusis
LAT	lateral side view
LAVH	laparoscopically assisted vaginal hysterectomy
LC	left circumflex
LCD	Local Coverage Determination
LCL	lateral collateral ligament
LCT	lateral canthal tendon
LD	left anterior descending
LDL	low-density lipoprotein
LEC	left external carotid
LEEP	loop electrosurgical excision of the cervix
LES	lower esophageal sphincter
LFT	liver function test
LIC	left internal carotid
LIMA	left internal mammary artery
LLETZ	large-loop excision of the transformation zone
LM	left main
LOA	left anterior oblique

LOS	length of stay	
LOS	level of service	
LOW	low complexity	
LPO	left posterior oblique	
LTAC	long-term acute care	
LTC	long-term care	
LTCF	long-term care facility	
LUTS	lower urinary tract symptoms	
LVRS	lung volume reduction surgery	
MAAAA	multianalyte assays with algorithmic analyses	
MAC	monitored anesthesia care	
MAC	*Mycobacterium avium* complex disease	
MAGPI	meatal advancement and glanuloplasty	
MCC	major complications and comorbidities	
MCH	mean corpuscular hemoglobin	
MCHC	mean corpuscular hemoglobin concentrations	
MCL	medial collateral ligament	
MCM	*Medicare Carriers Manual*	
MCP	metacarpophalangeal (joint)	
MCPM	*Medical Claims Processing Manual*	
MCT	medial canthal tendon	
MCT	mobile cardiac telemetry	
MCV	mean corpuscular volume	
MD	medical doctor	
MDM	medical decision making	
MDS	minimum data set	
MEC	mutually exclusive code	
MeV	megaelectron volts	
MI	myocardial infarction	
MLT	medical laboratory technician	
MMR	measles, mumps, and rubella	
MOD	moderate complexity	
MPFS	Medicare Physician Fee Schedule	
MPFSDB	Medicare Physician Fee Schedule Database	
MPJ	metatarsal phalangeal joint	
MRA	magnetic resonance angiography	
MRI	magnetic resonance imaging	
MRSA	methicillin-resistant *Staphylococcus aureus*	
MS-DRG	Medicare Severity Diagnosis-Related Group	
MSSA	methicillin-susceptible *Staphylococcus aureus*	
MTP	metatarsophalangeal (joint)	
MUE	medically unlikely edit	
NAM	nasoalveolar moulding	
NCCAA	National Commission for Certification of Anesthesiologist Assistants	
NCCI	National Correct Coding Initiative	
NCD	national coverage determination	
NCHS	National Center for Health Statistics	
NCQA	National Committee for Quality Assurance	
NCRA	National Cancer Registrars Association	
NCS	nerve conduction study	
NEC	not elsewhere classified	
NEMB	Notice of Exclusions from Medicare Benefits	
NGT	nasogastric tube	
NLP	natural language processing	
NLP	no light perception	
NOS	not otherwise specified	
NP	new patient	

NP	nurse practitioner
NPI	National Provider Identifier
NPP	nonphysician provider
NPUAP	National Pressure Ulcer Advisory Panel
NSAID	nonsteroidal anti-inflammatory drug
NSTEMI	non-ST myocardial infarction
OA	osteoarthritis
OB	obstetrics
OBL	oblique
OCR	Office for Civil Rights
OD	doctor of optometry
OFR	Office of the Federal Register
OGS	Obstetrics and Gynecology Specialist
OIG	Office of the Inspector General
OLC	online learning center
OMC	osteomeatal complex
OP	outpatient
OPPS	Outpatient Prospective Payment System
OR	operating room
ORIF	open reduction with internal fixation
OS	Orthopedics Specialist
OSHA	Occupational Safety and Health Administration
OT	occupational therapist
P4P	pay-for-performance
PA	physician assistant
PA	postanterior
PACU	postanesthesia care unit
PAP	Papanicolaou
PBSCT	peripheral blood stem cell transplantation
PC	professional component
PCA	patient-controlled anesthesia
PCI	percutaneous coronary interventions
PCL	posterior cruciate ligament
PCP	*Pneumocystis carinii* pneumonia
PCP	primary care physician
PCS	Procedure Classification System
PCV13	pneumococcal conjugate
PDR	proliferative diabetic retinopathy
PEG	percutaneous endoscopic gastrostomy
PET	positron emission tomography
PF	problem-focused
PFO	Patient foramen ovale
PFS	physician fee schedule
PFSH	past, family, and/or social history
PFT	pulmonary function test
PHI	protected health information
PICC	peripherally inserted central catheter
PIN	prostatic intraepithelial neoplasia
PIPJ	proximal interphalangeal joint
PMP	practice management program
POA	present on admission
POAG	primary open-angle glaucoma
PORP	partial ossicular replacement prosthesis
POS	place of service
PPS	prospective payment system
PRK	photorefractive keratectomy
PSA	prostate-specific antigen

PSB	protected specimen brush
PT	physical therapist
PT	prothrombin time
PTCT	percutaneous transluminal coronary thrombectomy
PTK	phototherapeutic keratectomy
PTT	partial prothrombin time
PUVA	photochemotherapy
QHP	qualified health professional
RA	remittance advice
RA	rheumatoid arthritis
RAI	resident assessment instruments
RAP	resident assessment protocol
RBC	red blood cells
RBRVS	resource-based relative value scale
RC	right coronary artery
RCA	right coronary artery
RCC	right common carotid
RDS	respiratory distress syndrome
RDW	red cell distribution width
REC	right external carotid
RFA	radio-frequency ablation
RHIA	Registered Health Information Administrator
RHIT	Registered Health Information Technician
RI	ramus intermedius artery
RIC	right internal carotid
ROA	right anterior oblique
ROI	release of information
ROM	range of motion
ROMA	risk of ovarian malignancy algorithm
ROS	review of systems
RPO	right posterior oblique
RSI	radiological supervision and interpretation
RVF	relative value file
RVU	relative value unit
S&I	supervision and interpretation
SAB	spontaneous abortion
SADMERC	Statistical Analysis Durable Medical Equipment Regional Carriers
SCAN	stereotactic computer-assisted navigation
SCC	squamous cell carcinoma
SCM	sternocleidomastoid
SET	skin endpoint titrations
SF	straightforward
SIADH	syndrome of inappropriate secretion of antidiuretic hormone
SIRS	systemic inflammatory response syndrome
SLAP	superior labrum anterior and posterior
SMAS	superficial musculoaponeurotic system
SNF	skilled nursing facility
SOAP	subjective, objective, assessment, plan
SPECT	single proton emission computerized tomography
SRT	submucous resection of the turbinate
STD	sexually transmitted disease
STI	sexually transmitted infection
STEMI	ST elevation myocardial infarction
STG	split-thickness graft
Sx	surgery
T3	triiodothyronine
T4	thyroxine

TAA	thoracic aorta aneurysm
TAVI	transcatheter aortic valve implantations
TAVR	transcatheter aortic valve replacement
TB	tuberculosis
TBSA	total body surface area
TC	technical component
TCM	transitional care management
TCS	HIPAA Electronic Health Care Transactions and Code Sets
TEE	transesophageal echocardiography
TENS	transcutaneous electrical nerve stimulator
THA	total hip arthroplasty
TIA	transient ischemic attack
TIBC	total iron binding capacity
TIP	tubularized incised plate
TKR	total knee replacement
TM	tympanic membrane
TOT	transobturator
TPI	trigger point injection
TPN	total parenteral nutrition
TPO	treatment, payment, and health-care operations
TSH	thyroid-stimulating hormone
TTE	transthoracic echocardiography
TUMT	transurethral microwave therapy
TURBT	transurethral resection of the bladder
TURP	transurethral resection of prostate
TVT	transvaginal tape
UA	urinalysis
UCL	ulnar collateral ligament
UE	upper extremity
UHDDS	Uniform Hospital Discharge Data Set
UPJ	ureteropelvic junction
UPP	urethral pressure profile
US	ultrasound
USAN	United States Adopted Name
UTI	urinary tract infection
UUO	unilateral urethral obstruction
VA	ventriculoatrial
VAD	ventricular assist device
VAP	ventilator-associated pneumonia
VAPPL	venous, arterial, pulmonary, portal, and lymphatic
VATS	video-assisted thoracic surgery
VBAC	vaginal delivery after C-section
VBG	vertical banded gastroplasty
VC	virtual colonoscopy
VIN	vulvar intraepithelial neoplasia
VISC	vitreous infusion suction cutter
VLAP	visual laser ablation of prostate
VP	voiding pressure
VP	ventriculoperitoneal
WBC	white blood cell count
WC	workers' compensation
WHO	World Health Organization
WIT	water-induced thermotherapy
YAG	yttrium-aluminum-garnet

Professional Resources

GOVERNMENT SITES AND RESOURCES

CCI
The Medicare National Correct Coding Initiative automated edits:
www.cms.gov/Medicare/Coding/NationalCorrectCodInitEd

CDC
ICD-10-CM codes are used for statistical reporting (e.g., causes of death) by federal health agencies such as the Centers for Disease Control and Prevention (CDC):
www.cdc.gov/nchs/nvss/deaths.htm

CDC NCHS Injury Data and Resources
www.cdc.gov/nchs/injury.htm

CMS
Coverage of the Centers for Medicare and Medicaid Services: Medicare, Medicaid, SCHIP, HIPAA, CLIA topics:
www.cms.gov

Medicare Learning Network:
www.cms.gov/Outreach-and-Education/Medicare-Learning-Network-MLN/MLNGenInfo

Online Medicare manuals:
http://cms.hhs.gov/Regulations-and-Guidance/Guidance/Manuals/Internet-Only-Manuals -IOMs.html

Medicare Physician Fee Schedule:
www.cms.gov/Medicare/Medicare.html (scroll through the list to find the current direct link)

Conditions of Participation:
www.cms.gov/Regulations-and-Guidance/Legislation/CFCsAndCoPs/index.html

Present on Admission (POA):
www.cms.gov/Medicare/Medicare.html (scroll through the list to find the current direct link)

Hospital-acquired conditions that impact payment when POA code cannot be found:
www.cms.gov/Medicare/Medicare.html (scroll through the list to find the current direct link)

Hospital Outpatient Prospective Payment Systems:
www.cms.gov/Medicare/Medicare.html (scroll through the list to find the current direct link)

Medicare National and Local Coverage Determinations database:
www.cms.gov/medicare-coverage-database

Federal Register
ICD-10-CM and ICD-10-PCS code changes are published annually in the *Federal Register*:
www.federalregister.gov

HIPAA Administrative Simplification: Modification to Medical Data Code Set Standards to adopt ICD-10-CM and ICD-10-PCS: Proposed Rule, *Federal Register*, August 22, 2008 (Volume 73, Number 164 [Proposed Rule] [Pages 49795–49832]):
www.gpo.gov/fdsys/pkg/FR-2008-08-22/pdf/E8-19298.pdf

The final rule, published in the January 16, 2009, issue of the *Federal Register*:
www.gpo.gov/fdsys/pkg/FR-2009-01-16/pdf/E9-743.pdf

GEMs

General Equivalence Mappings (GEMs) have been created to assist in the data transition from ICD-9 to ICD-10:
http://cms.gov/Medicare/Coding/ICD10/downloads/GEMs-CrosswalksBasicFAQ.pdf

HCPCS

General information on Healthcare Common Procedure Coding System (HCPCS):
www.cms.gov/Medicare/Medicare.html (scroll through the list to find the current direct link)

Alphanumeric HCPCS System file:
www.cms.gov/Medicare/Medicare.html (scroll through the list to find the current direct link to HCPCS Release & Code Sets)

Durable Medical Equipment (DME) Center:
www.cms.gov/Center/Provider-Type/Durable-Medical-Equipment-DME-Center.html
Durable Medical Equipment (DME) Center:
www.dmepdac.com/dmecs/index.html

HIPAA

HIPAA for Professionals Home Page
www.hhs.gov/hipaa/for-professionals/index.html

Questions and Answers on HIPAA Privacy Policies:
www.hhs.gov/answers /hipaa

HIPAA Privacy Rule, "Standards for Privacy of Individually Identifiable Health Information; Final Rule," 45 CFR Parts 160 and 164m. *Federal Register* 65, no. 250 (2000).
www.hhs.gov/hipaa/for-professionals/privacy/index.html

ICD

NCHS ICD-10-CM full text, Conversion Table, and *Official Guidelines for Coding and Reporting*:
www.cdc.gov/nchs/icd/icd10cm.htm

NCHS (National Center for Health Statistics) ICD-9-CM addenda and guidelines:
www.cdc.gov/nchs/icd/icd9cm.htm

NCHS Coordination and Maintenance Committee:
www.cdc.gov/nchs/icd/icd9cm_maintenance.htm

WHO's International Statistical Classification of Diseases and Related Health Problems, tenth revision, is posted on the World Health Organization site:
www.who.int/whosis/icd10

NUBC

The National Uniform Billing Committee develops and maintains a standardized data set for use by institutional providers to transmit claim and encounter information. This group is in charge of the 837I and the CMS-1450 (UB 04) claim formats:
www.nubc.org

NUCC

The National Uniform Claim Committee develops and maintains a standardized data set for use by the noninstitutional health-care community to transmit claim and encounter information. This group is in charge of the 837P and the CMS-1500 claim formats:
www.nucc.org

OCR

The Office for Civil Rights of the U.S. Department of Health and Human Services (DHHS) enforces the HIPAA Privacy Rule. Privacy information is online:
www.hhs.gov/hipaa

OIG

The DHHS's Office of Inspector General home page links to fraud and abuse, advisory opinions, exclusion list, and other topics:
www.oig.hhs.gov

TRICARE and CHAMPVA

TRICARE is the health-care program for uniformed service members (active, Guard/Reserve, retired) and their families around the world:
www.tricare.mil

CHAMPVA Overview
The Civilian Health and Medical Program of the Department of Veterans Affairs (CHAMPVA) is a health benefits program in which the Department of Veterans Affairs shares the cost of certain health-care services and supplies with eligible beneficiaries:
www.military.com/benefits/veterans-health-care/champva-overview

WPC

Washington Publishing Company is the link for HIPAA Transaction and Code Set implementation guides. It also assists several organizations in the maintenance and distribution of HIPAA-related code lists that are external to the X12 family of standards:
Provider Taxonomy Codes
Claim Adjustment Reason Codes
Claim Status Codes
Claim Status Category Codes
Health Care Services Decision Reason Codes
Insurance Business Process Application Error Codes
Remittance Remark Codes
www.wpc-edi.com

DISEASE INFORMATION

Cancer
National Cancer Institute: Resource for tumor types:
www.cancer.gov

American Cancer Society
www.cancer.org

Diabetes
American Association of Diabetes Educators: Current information on disease management of diabetes mellitus:
www.diabeteseducator.org

General Disease Information
Medline: The Government source for information on diseases:
www.nlm.nih.gov/medlineplus

WEBMD
www.webmd.com

HIV-AIDS
Information on HIV-related conditions and AIDS:
www.nlm.nih.gov/medlineplus/aidsandinfections.html
www.aids.org
www.who.int/hiv/pub/en

Kidney Disease
www.kidney.org/kidneydisease

Pressure Ulcers
www.nlm.nih.gov/medlineplus/pressuresores.html
www.npuap.org

Sepsis
Background on sepsis and explanations of
clinical etiology, signs, and symptoms:
https://www.cdc.gov/sepsis/basic/index.html

ELECTRONIC MEDICAL RECORDS

AHIMA

The American Health Information Management Association has played a leadership role in the
effective management of health data and medical records needed to deliver quality health care
to the public:
www.ahima.org

HIMSS Electronic Health Records Association

EHRA is a partner of the Healthcare Information and Management Systems Society and operates
as an independent organizational unit within HIMSS for companies who are EHR software solution providers:
www.ehra.org

ASSOCIATIONS

AAFP American Academy of Family Physicians
www.aafp.org

AAHAM American Association of Healthcare Administrative Management
www.aaham.org

AAMA American Association of Medical Assistants
www.aama-ntl.org

AAPC American Academy of Professional Coders
www.aapc.com

ACA International Association of Credit and Collection Professionals
www.acainternational.org

ACHE American College of Healthcare Executives
www.ache.org

AHDI Association for Healthcare Documentation Integrity
www.aamt.org

AHIMA American Health Information Management Association
www.ahima.org

AHIP America's Health Insurance Plans
www.ahip.org

AHLA American Health Lawyers Association
www.healthlawyers.org

AHA American Hospital Association
www.aha.org

AHA Coding Clinic Advisor
www.codingclinicadvisor.com

AHA Coding Clinic Home Page
www.ahacentraloffice.org

AHA Coding Clinic® for ICD-10-CM
www.aha.org/aha/issues/Medicare/IPPS/coding.html

AMA American Medical Association
www.ama-assn.org

AMBA American Medical Billing Association
www.ambanet.net/AMBA.htm

AMT American Medical Technologists
http://www.americanmedtech.org

ANA American Nursing Association
www.ana.org

HBMA Healthcare Billing and Management Association
www.hbma.org

HFMA Healthcare Financial Management Association
www.hfma.org

MGMA Medical Group Management Association
www.mgma.com

PAHCOM Professional Association of Health Care Office Management
www.pahcom.com

SELECTED PROFESSIONAL CODING RESOURCES

AHA Coding Clinic for ICD-10-CM
AHA Order Services
PO Box 933283
Atlanta, GA 31193-3283
800-242-2626
www.ahaonlinestore.com
Official Coding Guidelines for ICD-10-CM

American Academy of Professional Coders (AAPC)
2480 South 3850 West, Suite B
Salt Lake City, UT 84120
800-626-CODE
www.aapc.com
Certification courses/examinations and coding-related publications

American Association of Health Information Management (AHIMA)
233 North Michigan Avenue, 21st floor
Chicago, IL 60601-5809
312-233-1100
www.ahima.org
Certification courses/examinations and coding-related publications

NCHS
National Center for Health Statistics
3311 Toledo Road
Hyattsville, MD
301-458-4000
www.cdc.gov/nchs/icd/index.htm
ICD-10-CM code set, addenda, and coding guidelines available for downloading

INDEX